The Difficult Case in
Head and Neck Cancer Surgery

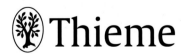

The Difficult Case in Head and Neck Cancer Surgery

Paul J. Donald, MD
Department of Otolaryngology
University of California Davis School of Medicine
Sacramento, California

Thieme
New York • Stuttgart

Thieme Medical Publishers, Inc.
333 Seventh Avenue
New York, NY 10001

Editorial Director: Michael Wachinger
Executive Editor: Timothy Hiscock
Managing Editor: J. Owen Zurhellen IV
Editorial Assistant: Jacquelyn DeSanti
Vice President, Production and Electronic Publishing: Anne T. Vinnicombe
Production Editors: Martha L. Wetherill, Donald Whitehead
Vice President, International Marketing and Sales: Cornelia Schulze
Chief Financial Officer: Peter Van Woerden
President: Brian D. Scanlan
Compositor: MPS Content Services Inc.
Printer: Everbest Printing Company

Library of Congress Cataloging-in-Publication Data

Donald, Paul J.
   The difficult case in head and neck cancer surgery / Paul J. Donald.
      p.; cm.
   Rev. ed. of: Head and neck cancer / Paul J. Donald. 1984.
   Includes bibliographical references and index.
   ISBN 978-0-86577-984-6
   1. Head—Cancer—Surgery.   2. Neck—Cancer—Surgery.   I. Donald, Paul J. Head and neck cancer.   II. Title.
   [DNLM: 1. Head and Neck Neoplasms—surgery.   2. Head—surgery.   3. Neck—surgery.   4. Postoperative Complications—prevention & control.
WE 707 D675d 2009]
   RC280.H4D66 2009
   616.99'491—dc22
                                                    2009008387

Important note: Medical knowledge is ever-changing. As new research and clinical experience broaden our knowledge, changes in treatment and drug therapy may be required. The authors and editors of the material herein have consulted sources believed to be reliable in their efforts to provide information that is complete and in accord with the standards accepted at the time of publication. However, in view of the possibility of human error by the authors, editors, or publisher of the work herein, or changes in medical knowledge, neither the authors, editors, or publisher, nor any other party who has been involved in the preparation of this work, warrants that the information contained herein is in every respect accurate or complete, and they are not responsible for any errors or omissions or for the results obtained from use of such information. Readers are encouraged to confirm the information contained herein with other sources. For example, readers are advised to check the product information sheet included in the package of each drug they plan to administer to be certain that the information contained in this publication is accurate and that changes have not been made in the recommended dose or in the contraindications for administration. This recommendation is of particular importance in connection with new or infrequently used drugs.

Some of the product names, patents, and registered designs referred to in this book are in fact registered trademarks or proprietary names even though specific reference to this fact is not always made in the text. Therefore, the appearance of a name without designation as proprietary is not to be construed as a representation by the publisher that it is in the public domain.

Printed in China

5 4 3 2 1

ISBN 978-0-86577-984-6

This book is dedicated to my family. My loving wife, Roz, has been a source of inspiration, patience, and support during the often tedious hours I've spent with this text. My love and thanks go out to her. It is also dedicated to my children, Scott, Alison, Heather, and Andy, and to their spouses, Leslie, Danny, Scott, and April. It is further dedicated to my dear grandchildren, Jack, Ben, Lizzy, Anna, William, and Piper.

Contents

Foreword

Paul J. Donald approached the writing of this book, *The Difficult Case in Head and Neck Cancer Surgery*, with the same degree of passion with which he approaches life. He is to be admired for undertaking the task of producing this fully updated volume more than a quarter of a century after his well-received standard, *Head and Neck Cancer: Management of the Difficult Case*. The "difficult case" is usually a patient with advanced cancer who has had inadequate or unsuccessful previous treatment, or both. Most of the patients with cancer of the head and neck referred to a center for head and neck surgery fall into this category, so that these are not uncommon problems. This book fills an important niche in addressing these issues, and the book is best suited for physicians in more advanced stages of their training or in the practice of head and neck surgery.

In reviewing Dr. Donald's older book again, I was impressed with the enormous advances that have been made in our field during the past 25 years. Although many of the extirpative procedures are still with us, many new approaches, particularly endoscopic procedures, have been introduced. Much of the credit for the development of these techniques goes to the companies that invented the computed tomographic scanner, enabling surgeons to make more precise diagnoses and visualize areas that were previously obscure, such as the parapharyngeal space, and to the companies that developed endoscopes and appropriate accompanying instrumentation to enable surgeons to operate safely in areas that previously required an external approach.

Almost the entire approach to reconstruction has changed. Most of the reconstructive procedures that were described, for example, the forehead flap for intraoral reconstruction, the Zovikian flap, the deltopectoral flap, and the intentional pharyngostoma, are now virtually obsolete.

The introduction of the pectoralis major myocutaneous flap and later the microvascular free tissue transfer completely changed what we could do for this group of patients with advanced cancer by carrying out definitive reconstruction at the time of the extirpative surgery. The two most im-

portant advances were in the immediate reconstruction of the mandible using osseocutaneous free flaps with compression plates and the reconstruction of the total laryngopharyngectomy wound with a menu of free flaps, including jejunum, radial forearm, and lateral thigh. The use of these flaps has allowed the patient to heal rapidly, regain the ability to swallow, and enter postoperative adjunctive therapy with radiation with or without chemotherapy in a timely way. Previously, the use of delayed or undependable forms of reconstruction prolonged the time interval to radiation that resulted in the cancer recurring before the patient healed or entered adjunctive therapy.

The improved quality of life for these patients as a result of improved reconstruction has been emphasized in the literature, but we should also recall that local and regional control has improved as well, and recent data from the Surveillance, Epidemiology and End Results (SEER) Program indicate that the overall cure rate has improved somewhat. In my view, this is due to the fact that the extirpative surgeon can now carry out the most radical surgery without the worry of not having sufficient or appropriate tissue to close the wound. The systematic use of intraoperative frozen sections has also helped to ensure local control. This results in a better opportunity to obtain clear margins of resection without which, according to the literature, there is little hope for either local control or survival. The use of the selective neck dissection in the N0 neck has replaced the "watch and wait" attitude of the past, and most series of patients reported in the literature indicate that local-regional disease-free survival is enhanced.

In an era where textbooks are almost universally multiauthored, Dr. Donald has undertaken the herculean task of writing all the chapters on site-specific surgery himself, with the exception of the chapter on cancer of the larynx, which he co-authored with Dr. Bruce Pearson. There is also a new chapter on the treatment of advanced skin cancer.

Dr. Donald emphasizes the all-important concept of the team approach to cancer of the head and neck, including the latest techniques for reconstruction. To that end he has recruited Dr. John Beumer, a pioneer and leader in the field of maxillofacial prosthodontics, for the chapter on the restoration of oral and facial defects secondary to tumor ablation, and Dr. Rachel H. Chou for the chapter on radiotherapy. Ann Sievers, RN, addresses nutrition and nursing aspects, and Rebecca J. Leonard, PhD, addresses speech and swallowing issues; both are seasoned veterans of Dr. Donald's earlier book who (along with the other contributors) round out the multidisciplinary team.

The specialty of head and neck surgery must now be thought of in the broader context of head and neck oncology. The enormous strides made by our colleagues in radiation and medical oncology, aided and abetted by industry, have changed the approach to many of these difficult-to-treat cancers. The concept of "organ preservation," which became popular after the results of the Veterans Administration Study in the early 1990s were revealed, made a huge impact on referral patterns and patient choice of treatment. In a recent article in the *New England Journal of Medicine*, Dr. Arlene Forastiere announced that "the standard of care"—a legal rather than a medical term—for advanced cancer of the larynx is treatment with chemoradiation. This type of "organ preservation program" was offered to patients in their prospective, randomized study without offering the option of organ preservation by conservation laryngeal surgery. Lest we as head and neck surgeons lay down our scalpels prematurely, we should note that many of these patients, though cured of their cancer by nonsurgical treatment, will not be able to swallow and breathe and will choose laryngectomy as an option for solving this problem. Salvage surgery for patients who have failed treatment made more difficult by radiation intensified by the radiation-sensitizing effect of chemotherapy will also need to be carried out.

Congratulations to you, Paul Donald, for the industry and courage that you have brought to this task. Surely those who read this textbook will be rewarded by the exposure to your philosophy of aggressive surgery and the details of surgical techniques such as those you have passed on to your residents and fellows over the years. The readers will also gain valuable insight into the imagination, tenacity, and humanism that make up the character of Paul J. Donald.

Eugene N. Myers, MD, FACS, FRCS (Hon)Edin

Preface

Today's surgeons have at their disposal a number of outstanding textbooks that cover the basic principles of head and neck cancer management, but since my 1984 book *Head and Neck Cancer: Management of the Difficult Case*, there has been no text devoted to the difficult and problematic cases. Most of the unfortunate patients who fall into this category suffer from tumors that are either massive in size or extend beyond the cervicofacial area to encroach upon adjacent anatomical regions (such as the brain or thorax). Patient management often requires a unique set of intricate surgical steps, both for ablation of the tumor and for the eventual reconstruction. Some of the tumors in this category exhibit unusual histological and biological behavior. Because of the debilitation resulting from the tumor and the extensiveness of the surgery, many of these patients are difficult to manage postoperatively. Later, they often require the assistance of both a maxillofacial prosthetist and a speech therapist in their rehabilitation. The surgeon faced with these enigmatic lesions must often conduct an exhaustive literature search for a solution to a particular problem.

This thoroughly revised and updated book provides a concise and comprehensive reference source for those cases in which complete excision is difficult or complex, and reconstruction to restore function and cosmesis is problematic. This book is not intended for the beginning resident or the practitioner who does occasional head and neck tumor surgery. It is directed at the senior resident level, specifically those surgeons regularly engaged in head and neck tumor exenterative surgery who from time to time are faced with difficult and problematic cases.

Each chapter of *The Difficult Case in Head and Neck Cancer Surgery* begins with a brief outline of the pertinent points of pathology, etiology, and presentation of the lesions in each major anatomical area of the head and neck. Concentration is directed toward the natural history of the disease, the peculiar anatomical details, the pathophysiology of the tumors, and most especially the surgical management of the area involved. There is some variation in emphasis among chapters. Those on malignant melanoma and pediatric tumors, for instance, are a little more general in nature because these diseases are very uncommon, exhaustive treatises on them are wanting, and their management is highly controversial. On the other hand, chapters such as the one on the oral cavity provide detailed discussions of conservation surgery, the management of lesions in specific areas of the region, and excision of massive tumors with the subsequent reconstruction. Procedures such as wedge resection of the tongue and composite resection are not covered because they are so well described in the standard textbooks on head and neck surgery.

Overlap of some material is unavoidable, such as the application of mediastinal resection both in thyroid cancer and in malignancy of the cervical esophagus. The details of mediastinal resection are carefully outlined in the chapter on surgery of the hypopharynx and cervical esophagus, and only the modifications peculiar to thyroid cancer with mediastinal involvement are described in the chapter on the thyroid. The thyroid chapter also presents a guide to attempt the differentiation of benign from malignant tumors, as well as details on how to avoid injury to the recurrent laryngeal nerve.

The management of tumors in some areas (such as the base of the tongue, the posterior pharyngeal wall, and the cervical esophagus) remains somewhat controversial, with solid statistical information on the best choice of procedure as yet unavailable. The author's usual methods of handling these difficult lesions are outlined as well as the appropriate techniques to reconstruct the gullet.

The chapter on the nose and paranasal sinuses concentrates on the management of two major problem areas: lesions of the nasal dorsum and vestibule, and those large paranasal sinus tumors that require craniofacial resection. The combined procedures are detailed, and anesthesia and postoperative management are thoroughly discussed. Particular attention is paid to the physiological considerations of altered intracranial homeostasis and its necessary restoration during and after these operations. This problem is dealt with in even greater detail in the chapter on the skull base. This latter chapter presents a number of avant-garde procedures with which to successfully exenterate neoplasms that invade the base of the skull from a host of cervicofacial areas, such as the deep lobe of the parotid gland, the nasopharynx, and neurovascular structures under the temporal and sphenoid bones.

The chapter on the ear and temporal bone presents a detailed account of the author's approach to the excision of lesions at the various levels in the temporal bone. A meticulous recounting of each step in temporal bone resection combines the best features of contributions by many of the giants in the field of head and neck surgery.

The chapter on the salivary glands attempts to clarify the classification of salivary gland tumors. The surgical approach concentrates on the more unusual problems: dealing with recurrent pleomorphic adenoma; the excision of large, extensive malignancies that invade the infratemporal fossa or temporal bone; and the management of adenoid cystic cancers. The management of tumors of the minor salivary glands is detailed as well.

The chapter on the larynx deals mainly with conservation surgery, transoral laser microsurgery, and voice-preserving techniques. The excellent contribution of Dr. Bruce Pearson of the Mayo Clinic is an outstanding embellishment to this book. His description of the voice-conserving procedure he developed is easy to follow and, with some practice, easy to duplicate.

The final chapters concern those specialized fields that are integral to the management of these difficult cases. In many anatomical areas, the ultimate resection has been achieved and become established. Irradiation and antitumor drug therapy are often vital adjuncts to the surgical management and represent the only hope to improve both local control and patient survival. There is increasing evidence that tumor eradication and reasonable patient survival can be hoped for only when these three modalities are judiciously combined.

The main focus of the chapter on irradiation is its utilization in combination with surgery. The basic principles of antitumor activity are clearly and briefly outlined in the beginning of the chapter. The utility of modalities in each site is reviewed, but the main thrust is the discussion of various formats of combined therapy and their success rates.

A smooth postoperative course and the ultimate recovery of the patient are often heavily dependent upon the quality of the nursing care. The prevention of complications and their diligent management by the bedside nurse are of paramount importance. The chapter on nursing aspects provides a detailed account of the treatments involved in the "control of the wound," as aptly coined by Conley, and the management of the often difficult and complex psychosocial problems of these patients. Organization of the flow of nursing care, both pre- and posttreatment, as well as in the home following discharge, is also included. Good nutritional care is essential to the healing of the wound and rapid recovery of the patient. Risk factors that impact nutrition status are identified and means of mitigating the adverse impact on the nutrition state and healing are discussed. The majority of patients have their nutrition met by gastric / enteral tube feeding or oral route. Intervention options are discussed in detail along with strategies for dealing with complications. Choices of methods of enteral feeding are outlined.

Maxillofacial prosthodontics is one of the most rapidly advancing fields in dentistry. Over the past decades it has become an integral part of the rehabilitation of the problem of head and neck cancer patients. The chapter on maxillofacial prosthetics concentrates more on the application of prosthetic rehabilitation in the difficult case than on the basic principles of the specialty, with considerable attention given to the surgical details that will facilitate the fitting and retention of the prosthesis.

Saving "the best for last" is aptly applied to the final chapter of this book. The chapter on speech rehabilitation is one of the best, most orderly approaches to an understanding of the effects of head and neck surgery on speech production and its possible remediation that I have encountered. Dr. Leonard has done an exceptional job in reviewing the pertinent literature, then clearly and succinctly coalescing the facts in a lucid and meaningful way. The effects of the various surgical procedures in the oral cavity on speech are discussed in great detail, and rehabilitative measures for the pharyngectomized as well as the laryngectomized patient are beautifully described.

An important caveat is essential at this juncture. The nature and extent of these lesions dictate that the surgery, in order to be successful, must be radical. Problem surgery is not for the faint of heart. Armed with the knowledge that with extensive exenteration of the tumor the patient has a good chance of being rid of the malignancy, and that most can be surgically and prosthetically rehabilitated, the surgeon is able to approach these lesions with considerable optimism.

Lastly, the patients themselves must not be forgotten. Often during the deliberations of the complexities of the preoperative workup, the intricacies of the surgery, and the coordination of the specialists involved in the patient's care, there is a tendency to concentrate on the tumor rather than on the unfortunate person who possesses it. The patient is in pain and suffers not only the compromises of disturbed function but also the agony of an often grossly altered physiognomy and its devastating social consequences. Eclipsing these adversities is the pervasive fear of possible impending death and the helplessness of being the victim of a complex surgical procedure, the comprehension of the nature and consequences of which defy the surgeon's detailed explanation. Compassion, empathy, and patience are vital tools in the management of these severely afflicted individuals.

It is hoped that *The Difficult Case in Head and Neck Cancer Surgery* will fill a need relevant to the practice of the head and neck surgeon engaged in the treatment of these challenging patients.

◆ Acknowledgments

I would first like to acknowledge my administrative assistant Ms. Mary McCarthy for the tireless effort she put forward in the preparation of this book. She spent many extra hours and weekends toiling over this difficult project, and for this I extend my heartfelt gratitude. I would also like to thank Ms. Nelva Richardson for coming out of semiretirement to do the excellent artwork. I would further like to thank J. Owen Zurhellen, Jacquelyn DeSanti, and their colleagues at Thieme Publishers for their patience and forbearance in awaiting the completion of this work. Many deadlines passed, but they thankfully persisted in encouraging me, and they pleasantly extended my time for completion.

Contributors

John Beumer III, DDS
Department of Maxillofacial Prosthetics
UCLA
Los Angeles, California

Rachel H. Chou, MD
South Sacramento Radiation Oncology Center
South Sacramento, California

Paul J. Donald, MD
Department of Otolaryngology
University of California Davis School of Medicine
Sacramento, California

Rebecca J. Leonard, PhD
Department of Otolaryngology
University of California Davis School of Medicine
Sacramento, California

Beverly Lorens, RD, MS
Clinical Dietitian
Food & Nutrition Department
University of California Davis Health System
Sacramento, California

Bruce W. Pearson, MD
Department of Otolaryngology–Head and Neck Surgery
Mayo Clinic
Jacksonville, Florida

Eleni D. Roumanas, DDS
Professor, Division of Advanced Prosthodontics,
    Biomaterials and Hospital Dentistry
Director, Advanced Prosthodontics
Department of Dentistry
UCLA
Los Angeles, California

Ann E. F. Sievers, RN, MA, CORLN
Department of Otolaryngology
University of California Davis School of Medicine
Sacramento, California

Bhavani Venkatachalam
Assistant Clinical Professor
Division of Advanced Prosthodontics
School of Dentistry
UCLA
Los Angeles, California

Richard B. Wilder, MD
Assistant Professor
Division of Radiation Oncology
University of Texas MD Anderson Cancer Center
Houston, Texas

1

Cancer of the Oral Cavity

Paul J. Donald

In 1999, carcinoma of the oral cavity accounted for approximately 5% of all human malignancies in the United States, representing an estimated 21,500 cases.[1] The lesion is histologically squamous cell carcinoma in 95% of cases.[2,3] The worldwide variation of incidence of oral cancer is striking; the oral cavity is the site of 1% of all cancers in Germany, strongly contrasting with a 45% incidence in Bombay, India. Male predominance is characteristic in the United States; however, some notable exceptions are seen elsewhere in the world. In the state of Andra Pradesh in India, on the island of Singapore, and in the city of Durban, South Africa, there is a considerably higher incidence in females than in males.[2] This is also true in Scandinavia, where the Plummer-Vinson syndrome is common.

◆ Pathology

Etiology

Oral lesions commonly occur in the so-called salivary puddle,[4] a horseshoe-shaped area that encompasses the lateral regions of the tongue, the floor of the mouth, the retromolar trigone, and the anterior tonsillar pillar. **Figure 1.1** shows the distribution of a series of oral cavity carcinomas seen at the Memorial Hospital in New York.[5] It is interesting to note that the distribution of oral carcinomas has not changed in more than 30 years. Eighty percent of the lesions are confined to only 20% of the oral cavity surface. Thus Lederman's[4] conception of the etiologic implication of these mucosal areas being continuously bathed in saliva in which carcinogens are suspended has considerable relevance.

The precise etiology of these neoplasms remains obscure, but several factors have been elucidated. A common association has been noted between the interstitial glossitis of tertiary syphilis and lingual cancer. The predilection of syphilis-induced malignancy for the dorsum of the tongue (**Fig. 1.2**), in contrast to the usual site of origin of these cancers, is distinctive. Trieger et al[6] reported an 18% incidence

of serologically positive syphilis in their series of patients. Gorlin and Vickers[7] state that carcinoma of the tongue is four times more common in patients afflicted with syphilis. Trauma, sepsis, alcohol, tobacco, and dietary deficiencies have all been implicated. The presence of broken and carious teeth and infected gingiva has long been thought to be etiologically significant, and although no consistent statistical proof of a link with cancer has been forthcoming, the association appears to be common. The importance of chronic irritation in the genesis of cancer at any site is frequently noted. The fact that half of all patients with oral cancer are edentulous and are therefore usually denture wearers, lends some credence to this opinion. In fact, oftentimes, the "denture sore" produced by the irritation of a denture is indistinguishable on gross examination from a carcinoma (**Fig. 1.3**).

Heavy tobacco use and alcohol consumption are undoubtedly implicated in the genesis of oral cancer. Whether these substances act directly on the mucosa or as a trigger mechanism on a predisposed cellular situation is not yet clear. There is substantial evidence showing that the cellular immunocompetence of an individual is markedly diminished with heavy cigarette smoking[8] and high alcohol intake.[9,10] The role of marijuana smoking as a possible etiologic agent in oral cavity cancer has been suggested.[11] The concentration of known carcinogens in tobacco smoke are in higher concentration in marijuana; in addition other known carcinogens not in tobacco as well as several primary irritants unique to cannabis are present as well. The role of delta-9 tetrahydrocannabinol, the active euphoria-producing agent in marijuana, as an immunosuppressant has been investigated by Nehas[12] and others. In a small cohort of cases Molin et al[13] have found a series of alterations in the altered p53 genome that appear to be unique to this group of patients. The author has had in his experience a series of 70 cases of patients under the age of 40 (range 19 to 39 years) with an average age of 32.6 years who contracted a squamous cell carcinoma of the head and neck. Most of these tumors were in the oral cavity or oropharynx. Of the 70, 60 (85.7%)

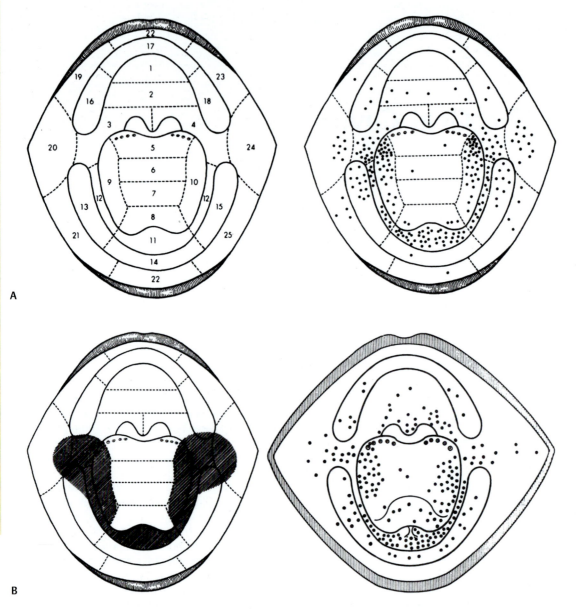

A

B

Fig. 1.1 (**A**) *Left,* Segmental distribution of the incidence of oral cavity cancer in 252 cases. Each segment occupies an approximate equivalent area of mucosa. *Right,* A scattergram indicating the distribution of 256 cases of oral carcinoma. (**B**) *Left,* Preferred site of predilection for squamous cell carcinoma of the oral cavity. *Right,* Scattergram of 209 consecutive cases of oral cavity cancer. (From Moore C, Catlin D. Anatomical origins and locations of oral cancer. Am J Surg 1967;114:511.)

had been or were at the time of diagnosis marijuana smokers. Only eight patients were either nonsmokers or had only tried the drug once or a few times.

Several lesions that are thought to be the precursors of malignancy have been identified in the mouth. The importance of leukoplakia (**Fig. 1.4**) as a progenitor of carcinoma has been debated. The fact that carcinomas are commonly found in leukoplakic areas, including some previously proved histologically benign, lends some support to their importance. A study by Waldron and Shafer[14] showed that between 14 and 18% of leukoplakias are dysplastic or malignant on the first biopsy. Subsequent sampling of the benign ones showed that a further 5% eventually became carcinomatous. Queyrat erythro-

plasia is seen most commonly in the region of the soft palate and the anterior tonsillar pillar, but it has also been observed on the buccal mucosa. Its premalignant potential is well established. The condition of so-called erythroplakia, an ostensible hybrid of leukoplakia and erythroplasia, is considered to be more malignant still.[15] In most instances of erythroplakia, there is histological evidence of at least severe dysplasia and often carcinoma in situ or microinvasive carcinoma.

Lichen planus oris is a not uncommon mucosal diathesis sometimes associated with the cutaneous lesion of the same name. It appears as a white, lacy-patterned, flat leukoplakia. There are occasionally erosive areas that look suspicious for carcinoma. The lesions are often painful, especially the ero-

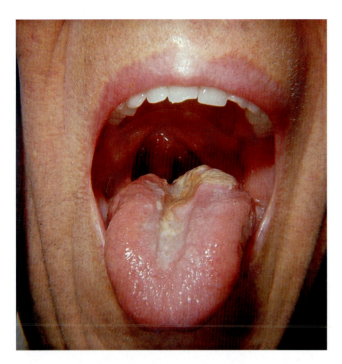

Fig. 1.2 Carcinoma on the dorsum of the tongue.

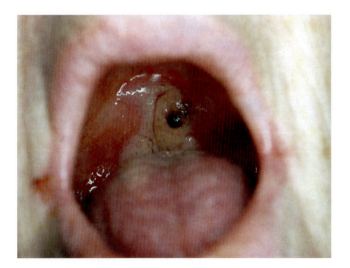

Fig. 1.3 Denture sore on hard palate, closely resembling an exophytic carcinoma.

sive type. The disease commonly waxes and wanes in severity. Carcinoma is said to be associated with this lesion rarely.[16,17] In my experience, carcinoma occurs in about 10% of patients with lichen planus and is more common in the erosive type.

A further complexity in the management of patients with oral cavity cancer is the problem of multicentric carcinoma. There is a tendency in some individuals to develop multiple foci of squamous cell carcinoma. These may be either in situ or frankly invasive. These patients have a mucosa often predisposed to cancer formation by chronic heavy tobacco abuse and alcohol consumption. This so-called field cancerization[4] renders the definitive treatment of these lesions most difficult.

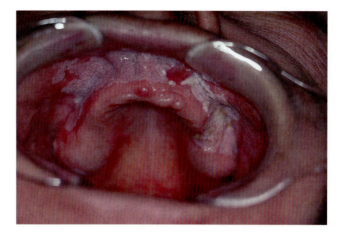

Fig. 1.4 Extensive leukoplakia on upper alveolar ridge. Arrow denotes verrucous carcinoma.

Metastasis

The local aggressiveness, the regional metastatic potential, and even the distant metastatic rate increase as distal progression of tumor location is made from the tongue tip to the oropharynx. Lesions of the tongue base generally have a dismal prognosis compared with those of the oral tongue. Unilateral cervical metastases are usually present, and bilateral disease is common. Throughout the tongue, but especially in the posterior one third, the intrinsic musculature acts like a "muscular pump," disseminating tumor cells in the interstices between muscle fibers that are a considerable distance from the primary tumor.

The incidence of regional metastases varies among series. Strong[18] reported on 314 patients with carcinoma of the anterior two thirds of the tongue gathered in a 5-year period between 1957 and 1963. The number of patients with palpable lymph node metastasis on presentation was 98, an incidence of 31.2%. Only four patients had contralateral or bilateral nodal involvement. **Table 1.1** illustrates the incidence of regional lymph node metastases in a large composite group of 4841 patients with oral cavity carcinoma from different sources.[19] In this group, a total of 59.1% had either manifest or occult metastases. In approximately one third of each anatomical group, the metastasis was occult in nature. However, the incidence of occult metastases is highly variable among series.

Table 1.1 Regional Lymph Node Involvement by Site

	Tongue (2751)	Floor of Mouth (1013)	Gingiva (423)	Buccal Mucosa (654)
Nodes present at admission	36%	38%	33%	32%
Nodes involved later (occult)	29%	18%	17%	13%
Total lymph node involvement	65%	56%	50%	45%

Source: From DiTroia JF. Nodal metastasis and prognosis in carcinoma of the oral cavity. Otolaryngol Clin North Am 1972;5:335, Table 1.

The employment of computed tomographic (CT) scanning and magnetic resonance imaging (MRI) to enhance the accuracy of metastatic lymph node diagnosis in the neck is somewhat controversial. It is most helpful in the previously irradiated neck or in the necks of individuals who are obese. In the author's experience, these modalities are of moderate value in the detection of metastatic nodes. Batsakis[20] depicts this variability with a table reproduced here as **Table 1.2**.[21–25]

Table 1.2 Incidence of Clinically Occult Cervical Metastases

Authors	Incidence
Lyall and Shetlin[21]	60%
Kreinen[22]	50%
Southwick et al[23]	40%
Sako et al[24]	27.6%
Ward et al[25]	25%

Nodal metastasis varies with both size and site of the tumor. T3 and T4 lesions are much more commonly seen with metastases than are smaller lesions. Cancers on the tongue tip have a much lower metastatic rate than those in the middle third, and these in turn have a lower rate than those of the posterior third of the oral tongue.[26] This also holds true for the bilaterality of the nodal metastases. Fries et al,[27] in a combined study of oral cavity tumors from Germany, Switzerland, and Austria, found that cancer of the buccal mucosa had the highest metastatic rate: 75%. The mandibular alveolar ridge was next highest at 61.2%, followed by the floor of the mouth at 59.9%. The tongue itself had metastases in 40% of cases. In the smaller series of buccal mucosal carcinomas quoted by Batsakis, the metastatic rate was lower, varying

from 37 to 50%.[20] There was, however, some concurrence in the rates cited for the alveolar ridge, which ranged from 30 to 80% in both his and the European group.

Sites of Predilection

The oral cavity is generally divided into the lips, buccal mucosa, tongue, floor of the mouth, hard palate, and alveolar ridges. However, the area of the distal oral cavity—the retromolar trigone, adjacent floor of the mouth, anterior tonsillar pillar, and soft palate—is a unit (**Fig. 1.5**) that anatomically and biologically forms a kind of transition zone between the oral cavity and the oropharynx.[28] Tumors in this region are managed in a similar fashion to those involving the oropharynx and often extend into it. Malignancies remain asymptomatic in this region for a considerable time before becoming manifest as localized pain, trismus, or cervical adenopathy. Lesions of the distal floor of the mouth adjacent to the retromolar trigone of the mandible are particularly pernicious. This area has been dubbed the "coffin corner" because of the ability of tumors therein to remain occult until they obtain substantial size. The examining physician must move the tongue well to the side and illuminate this area adequately to pick up these lesions while they are still small.

The buccal mucosa is not nearly as common a site for primary carcinoma as the other regions in the oral cavity. Batsakis[20] classifies these lesions according to their presentation on gross examination as ulcer infiltrative, exophytic, or verrucous. The verrucous variety is the most benign in its natural course, almost never metastasizes, and can most easily be adequately encompassed by a local resection. The ulcer-infiltrative type is the most locally aggressive, has the highest metastatic rate, and requires the most radical excision. The anatomical composition of the area predisposes it

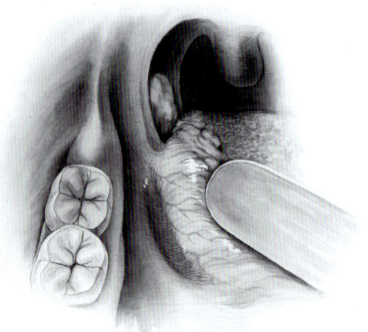

Fig. 1.5 The distal oral cavity. Note the retromolar trigone area behind the third molar tooth and the posterior extreme of the floor of the mouth, the co-called coffin corner.

to rapid through-and-through penetration by aggressive tumors. The buccal mucosa lies against the buccinator muscle, which is sheathed in the buccopharyngeal fascia. Superficial to this lie the buccal fat pad, the subcutaneous fat, and skin.

The alveolar ridge is an area in which the diagnosis of cancer may be mistaken for some time. In the upper jaw and palate, the appearance of an exophytic mass must raise the suspicion of the maxillary sinus as the site of origin. It is important to note in this regard that expansion of the maxillary sinus into the alveolar process occurs in 50% of persons.[29] Carcinoma is two to three times more common in the lower jaw than in the upper.[30] The exophytic and ulcerative character of the neoplasm in its early stages is grossly indistinguishable from the infected granulation tissue accompanying pyorrhea. A high index of suspicion in susceptible individuals is mandatory. Following extraction of a carious tooth, a failure of the site to heal—the so-called dry socket—must be equally suspiciously viewed in the same population. However, according to Thoma[31] most alveolar ridge lesions occur in the edentulous patient. Sharp and Wood[32] stated that 50% of the tumors in their series arose in previously leukoplakic areas.

Method of Spread

Lip carcinomas are the least aggressive of the oral cavity malignancies. They are usually the squamous cell type in the lower lip and basal cell carcinoma in the upper. They are slow growing and local infiltrative. The regional metastatic rate is less than 10% and the nodes most commonly involved are the submental and submandibular. Manifest neck nodal involvement carries a poor prognosis. The survival rate of lip cancer without metastasis is ~90%. With nodal metastasis, the rate drops to as low as 30%.[33,34]

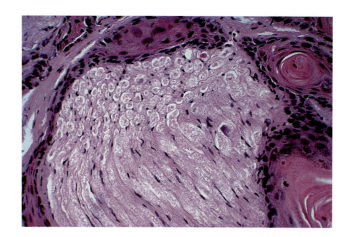

Fig. 1.6 Photomicrograph of perineural spread of squamous cell carcinoma. (From Donald PJ. Surgery of the Skull Base. New York: Lippincott-Raven; 1995:57, Fig. 12.)

The tumors tend to retain their relatively innocuous behavior until they begin to invade periosteum or the nerve fibers leading to the mental nerve (**Fig. 1.6**). The neoplasm then assumes a vicious behavior with wide soft tissue infiltration, cortical and cancellous bone invasion, and spread of the tumor along the inferior alveolar nerve (**Fig. 1.7**).

Tongue carcinomas spread to the floor of the mouth and encroach upon the loose gingiva in the same way.[35] These malignancies can also penetrate the lingual plate of cortical bone of the mandible. In this bone, local spread is usually quite limited. Once the cortex is breached to the level of the marrow space, then the tumor spread is much easier within the cancellous bone. It spreads throughout this space and

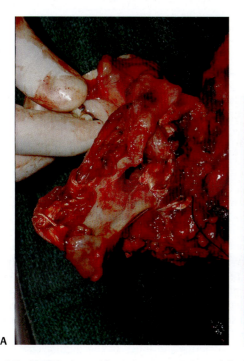

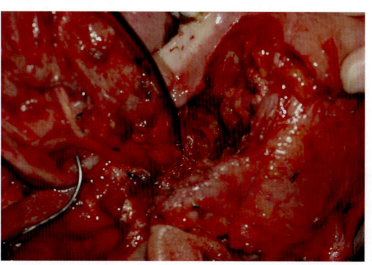

A   B

Fig. 1.7 (**A,B**) Patient with a primary carcinoma of the lip with extensive spread along the alveolar nerve to the region of the foramen ovale. (Harold Mathews)

often invades the inferior alveolar nerve. In the tongue itself, the only limiting factor is the midline septum. Tumor may even spread to the adjacent laryngeal framework or the hypoglossal nerve.

Buccal mucosal carcinoma tends to spread through the buccinator muscle and may invade the overlying cheek subcutaneous fat. In more aggressive lesions, the facial skin may be penetrated (**Fig. 1.8**). Many of the buccal mucosal lesions are verrucous in type and are contained by the subcutaneous fascia (**Fig. 1.9**). Soft tissue lesions may occur within the cheek substance and extend to the mucosa and the overlying skin.

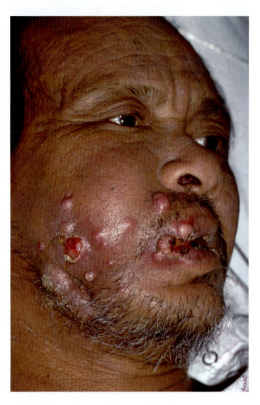

Fig. 1.8 Buccal carcinoma with penetration of the skin.

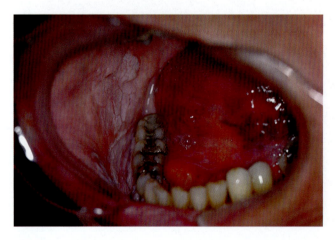

Fig. 1.9 Verrucous carcinoma of the buccal mucosa; tumor is usually contained by the subcutaneous fascia or buccinator muscle.

Tumors of the hard palate are usually benign (**Fig. 1.10**). The pleomorphic adenoma is commonest. Unlike the tongue and floor of the mouth, malignancies of the minor salivary glands are the most usual, especially adenoid cystic carcinomas. Cancers of the palate tend to erode the thin palatal bone and extend into the floor of the nose. They may be ulcerative or mucosally covered. Malignancies of the maxillary sinus commonly present as tumors of the palate or upper alveolar ridge. Recurrent pleomorphic adenoma must be treated as malignant tumors with an aggressive resection.

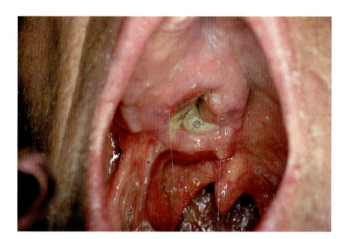

Fig. 1.10 Pleomorphic adenoma of the hard palate. Note ulceration that resembles the appearance of a malignancy. (Iowa)

◆ Management Principles

In keeping with the philosophy of this monograph, the basic principles of management of oral cavity lesions will be merely overviewed, with detailed discussion reserved for specialized areas. Generally speaking, T1 lesions (less than 2 cm in size) may be treated equally well with irradiation or surgery. This decision depends on several factors. For example, the proximity of the tumor to bone tends to favor the choice of surgery because of concern that irradiation therapy may lead to the development of osteoradionecrosis of the mandible (**Fig. 1.11**). The presence of mandibular tori (**Fig. 1.12**) is similarly a deterrent. Often the final decision as to modality of therapy is primarily the patient's.

The treatment of T2 lesions (between 2 and 4 cm) is a little more controversial. Lesions that are 2.0 to 2.5 cm, or occasionally even 3 cm, in size, are superficial in type, and are not accompanied by cervical lymphadenopathy generally do fairly well with irradiation therapy alone. All T2 lesions that are larger or deeply infiltrative, especially when accompanied by cervical lymph node metastasis, are resected en bloc. The so-called suprahyoid neck dissection should not be done except to establish an adequate soft tissue margin around the tumor. The fact that metastatic tumor may bypass the submandibular nodes and lodge in the jugular chain militates against use of this procedure as a definitive attempt at nodal clearance.[36]

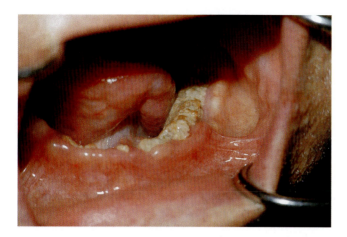

Fig. 1.11 Extensive osteoradionecrosis of the mandible.

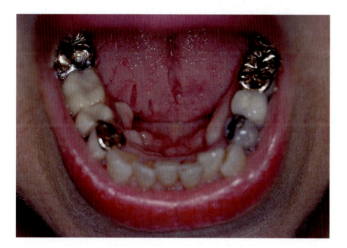

Fig. 1.12 Torus mandibularis.

The management of cervical nodal metastasis has evolved considerably over the past 15 years. The most notable has been the treatment of the N0 neck. The emergence of the selective neck dissection initially introduced by Suarez[37] and then popularized by Medina and Byers[38] and Gavilan et al[39] has significantly altered the approach to neck disease. The selective neck dissection of levels I, II, and III in patients with an N0 neck has obviated the need for postoperative prophylactic radiation therapy to the neck in most patients with small T1 and T2 lesions. If the neck is negative clinically but positive on histological sectioning, then a completion modified neck dissection is done saving the spinal accessory nerve if uninvolved by tumor. In the vast majority of patients, the remaining nodes are clear. More recently Meyers has recommended postoperative radiation therapy rather than completion neck dissection to treat those necks whose occult nodes unsuspectedly are histologically positive on permanent section.[40] The use of the selective neck has markedly diminished the incidence of regional recurrence in the neck and has enhanced survival.[41]

The radical neck dissection is the gold standard by which its modifications must be judged. In manifest neck disease at the time of initial diagnosis of an oral cavity tumor, a radical neck dissection is done and the spinal accessory nerve preserved. If the nerve is close to tumor, then the nerve is resected. If bilateral nodes are present, a bilateral radical neck dissection is done, with an attempt made to save the internal jugular vein in the least affected side.

Gilbert et al[42] reported a local control rate of 77% in T1N0, but only 21% in T2N0 lesions of the anterior floor of the mouth treated with radiotherapy. The incidence of osteoradionecrosis in their patients was 22%. This study is reflective of the fact that it was published in 1975 and reviewed the experience of 15 years. Many patients would have been treated with Cobalt 60 or even 250 kilo voltage irradiation. The more modern experience with patients treated by the linear accelerator has resulted in a much lower incidence of osteoradionecrosis. Berthelsen et al[43] found a 79% control rate with T1 lesions and a 76% rate in T2 carcinomas similarly treated by radiation. These patients were all N0 at the time of first examination. Pierquin et al[44] noted an astoundingly high local control rate of 95% in 153 patients with lesions 4 cm and less in diameter treated with interstitial irradiation. The telling statistic, however, is that at 4 years the actual survival rate was only 40%. Those who succumbed did so to metastatic disease. Fu et al[45] recorded optimistic results with irradiation therapy for neoplasms less than 4 cm in size. In 50 patients, a 76% control rate was experienced. Similarly, Delclos et al[46] reported an 82% local control rate in 34 patients with tumors less than 4 cm.

Table 1.3 illustrates the collective experience of several surgeons in their management of small lesions by conservation-type surgery.[47] It is important to note that many of the patients had cervical metastases. In a further series of 26 patients published by Schramm et al,[48] a 100% control rate was observed with surgical resection of this type. This was a series of anterior oral cavity tumors, 5 cm or less in diameter, and only 15% of the entire group eventually developed metastases to the neck. With one exception, all the patients were followed for longer than 2 years, and all patients who had cervical metastases developed them within 18 months.

Table 1.3 Five-Year Control and Survival Rate with Conservation Therapy for Oral Cavity Carcinoma

THERAPY FOR ORAL CAVITY CARCINOMA.*				
	5-Year Survival		Local Control	
Author	(No.)	(Per Cent)	(No.)	(Per Cent)
King	38/65	59%	53/65	82%
DeSanto	32/46	70%	36/46	73%
Keim and Lowenberg	27/34	79%	27/34	79%
Flynn and Moore	Not stated		19/23	82.6%
Marchetta	14/23	61%	17/23	76%
Som and Nussbaum	8/18†	44%	Not stated	
TOTALS	119/186	64%	182/229	80%

*From Donald PJ: Conservation therapy for oral cavity carcinoma. Trans Pacific Coast Oto-Ophthalmological Soc 58:111, 1977.

†Two years or more.

Large lesions are frequently accompanied by cervical metastases, either manifest or occult. Surgical excision combined with irradiation has provided the best survival rates. This was dramatically illustrated by the review of Krause et al[49] on the University of Iowa study of 472 patients. The determinant 5-year survival after surgical excision alone was 45%, and that following primary irradiation therapy alone was 35%. A regimen combining 4500 rads of irradiation to the lesion and both necks followed 4 weeks later by excision improved the determinant 5-year survival to 76%. A similar combined therapy program utilized by La Ferriere et al[50] produced comparable results. Postoperative combined therapy, popularized by the M.D. Anderson group, allows the surgeon the luxury of operating in an unirradiated field, thus lowering the postoperative complication rate while at the same time making it possible to use a higher total irradiation dose.[51]

We adopted the postoperative radiotherapy strategy in the late 1970s and found it to be far superior to the preoperative regimen. There are fewer postoperative complications, and they are of a much less serious degree than when preoperative irradiation is used or when surgery is done for failure of primary irradiation therapy. The most devastating complications are seen in those patients who fail combined surgery and chemotherapy.

Postoperative radiotherapy is now utilized in those individuals with multiple nodal metastases, lymph nodes with extracapsular spread, and tumors with vascular or perineural spread. Postoperative irradiation is not used for patients with positive margins. They are reoperated upon.

An ambitious cooperative study directed by Snow et al[52] has produced some revealing statistics regarding combined therapy. The patient population is composed of those with stage III and stage IV lesions, with the patients randomly assigned to one of three treatment groups: a preoperative combined therapy group, a postoperative combined therapy group, and a radical radiation group. Although the Snow paper is a preliminary report, it showed no statistically significant difference in 18-month survival rates between the preoperative and postoperative combined therapy group. Interestingly, the radical radiation group, which had a comparable patient mix with regard to lesion site and size, had a respectable 18-month survival compared with the combined group. Sixteen of the original group of 38 who received radiation only are alive and free of disease, but at 18 months, two in the surviving group had required surgery for local recurrence. Surgical salvage was attempted in nine failures of the original 38, but only one third of those survived free of disease—two for 18 months and one for a shorter follow-up period. The problems of high complications rates and poor survival of patients in their surgical salvage group is a common finding in our own experience.

Composite resection of the tongue, floor of the mouth, and mandible is a standard procedure found in several surgical atlases.[53–56] Some modifications of this time-honored method that produce superior functional and cosmetic results without compromising survival have been recently described by La Ferriere et al.[50] Instead of using a lip-splitting incision, they use a horizontal curvilinear neck incision that extends from the mastoid tip to the level of the midbody of the opposing side of the mandible, remaining 4 cm below the mandible through its course (**Fig. 1.13**). Although a McFee incision can be constructed using a parallel incision 2 cm above the clavicle, we do not recommend it in cases that have been irradiated (**Fig. 1.14**). The watershed area of cutaneous blood supply, the area that is nourished by opposing vertically disposed blood vessels responsible for the nutrition of the skin of the head and neck, is isolated by this incision. Rather, a curvilinear or lazy S-shaped vertical incision should be dropped from the submandibular cut. The intersection should be at right angles and located posteriorly to the carotid artery (**Fig. 1.13**). La Ferriere makes intraoral incisions in the gingival–labial and gingival–buccal sulci that communicate with the neck incision so that the soft tissue of the lip and chin can be retracted superiorly like a knight's visor (**Fig. 1.15**). Care must be taken

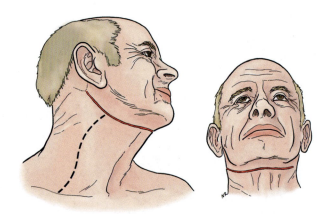

Fig. 1.13 Incision for a visor flap. The dotted line represents extension if radical neck dissection is necessary.

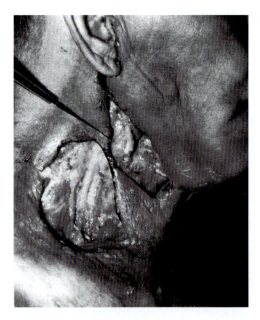

Fig. 1.14 Patient treated with preoperative irradiation. The McFee incision was employed, and a large area of cervical skin flap necrosis resulted.

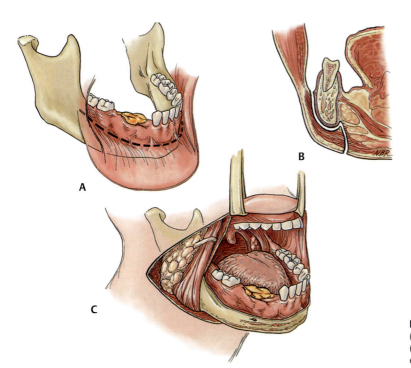

Fig. 1.15 (**A**) Vestibular incision in the oral cavity. (**B**) Connection between the intra- and extraoral incisions. (**C**) Lip retraction with soft rubber Penrose drains gives excellent tumor exposure.

to avoid damage to the mental nerve on the side of the mandible opposite the lesion. A totally insensible lower lip will not register the presence of saliva or food and is a serious social incapacity. Gentle retraction of the flap using Penrose drains produces little flap damage and permits excellent visualization for performing the definitive resection. The damage to the mental nerves is difficult to avoid and this procedure is most useful in the more anteriorly located lesions. In more distal lesions we still use the lip-splitting incision. This can be constructed in such a way as to minimize any cosmetic or functional impairment. A V-shaped incision is begun in the apex of the vermilion of the lip that is oriented horizontally (**Fig. 1.16**). This is carried through the muscle so a wedge of muscle will later fit into a triangular notch during reconstruction and thus avoid a whistle deformity from scar contracture. The vermilion cutaneous white roll is marked with a methylene blue tattoo to facilitate precise approximation at the time of closure. A vertical limb is extended to the chin button and then circumvents the chin button and sweeps under the chin in the upper neck to facilitate the submental dissection. This connects to the aforementioned modified Schobinger incision in the neck.

In tumors that are located more distally in the mouth, it is often necessary to dissect the cheek flap well beyond the initial midline incision through the lip. It is important to leave some soft tissue, especially over the bone, to maintain the integrity of the underlying periosteum. This will reduce the chances of devascularizing the mandibular bone that may lead to later complications such as osteomyelitis of the jaw.

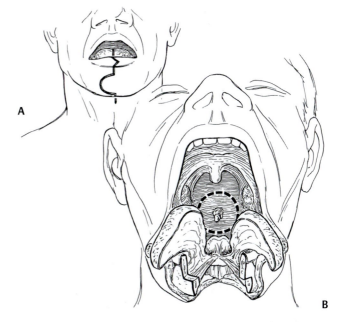

Fig. 1.16 Incision in the lower lip constructed in such a fashion as to avoid contracture. (**A**) Note the tattoo mark at the white roll for pinpoint approximation at the end of the procedure and that the apex of the "V" on the vermilion surface is halfway between the white roll and the wet lip. (**B**) The "V" extends through the entire lip thickness.

More soft tissue needs to be removed than bone when resecting the primary. This is especially true when only the cortex has been invaded. Local recurrences are most commonly seen in the soft tissue rather than the bone. Once the cancellous bone of the marrow cavity has been reached by the tumor, then a wide-field resection of bone is essential to clear the malignancy. In tumors greater than 3 cm in diameter and especially when deeply infiltrative, a minimum of a 2 cm margin of tongue is needed.

Once the tumor extirpation has been done, postoperative lingual mobility is made possible by skin grafting the defect or by reconstruction with a radial forearm free flap. A split-thickness skin graft is sutured medially to the lingual edge and, if the oropharynx is involved, the pharyngeal and palatal resection edges, and laterally to the buccal and labial mucosa (**Fig. 1.17**). The authors stresses that a substantial pouch of skin must be created that actually descends a short distance into the upper neck. The graft will shrink to ~50% of its original size. The pouch is then packed firmly with antibiotic-soaked cotton balls. This bolster is firmly anchored with tie-over sutures. The bolster is removed at 10 days, and lingual mobility is encouraged.

Free flap reconstruction has come a long way in providing a lining to the oral cavity that consists of thin pliable tissue that easily conforms to the defect and can even be rendered sensate. The most utilitarian flap in this regard is the radial forearm free flap pedicled on the radial artery and vein and in some instances carrying the antebrachial cutaneous nerve of the forearm. The artery is usually anastomosed to the lingual, facial, its common trunk (if present), or the external carotid artery. An attempt is made to suture the flap's vein end to side to the internal jugular vein. In desperate situations when both internal jugular veins need to be resected for oncological reasons, a jump graft of the saphenous vein may be required to reach the jugular stump low in the neck.

If an attempt to establish sensation is made, then the lingual nerve is sewn to the antebrachial cutaneous nerve. Although touch and two-point discrimination sensation is established in a significant percentage of cases, the utility of this function has yet to be proven in terms of improved swallowing.

The forehead flap, which was popular in the 1960s and early 1970s, has been entirely supplanted by the radial forearm free flap. The cosmetic defect left by the forehead flap at the donor site and the necessity of a second stage to return the flap has relegated the flap to be largely of historical interest.

The musculocutaneous flaps have provided several successful one-stage procedures for the restoration of resected oral cavity soft tissues. The advantage over free flap reconstruction is the lesser amount of time it takes to raise and insert the musculocutaneous flaps. Islands of skin from the neck and upper trunk receiving their blood supply through blood vessels perforating underlying attached muscle are pedicled on axial vessels and swung into the defect. The skin provides the lining while the muscle provides bulk (**Fig. 1.18**). For most resections, the trapezius and sternomastoid flaps would seem to be ideally suited. Unfortunately, although the blood supply to the muscles in these flaps is generally quite good, that to the overlying skin is less vigorous and cutaneous viability is unpredictable. The workhorse musculocutaneous flap in the oral cavity continues to be the pectoralis major musculocutaneous flap, either with or without the skin. The trapezius flap was developed by Demergasse in Argentina and is eloquently described by Bertotti.[57] He notes that it works best when it is pedicled on the transverse cervical artery, or as a second choice the posterior scapular artery, and then swung into the defect. However, if these vessels have been compromised by the resection, a trapezius flap can be constructed that will depend on the descending branches of the occipital artery and perforators from the ver-

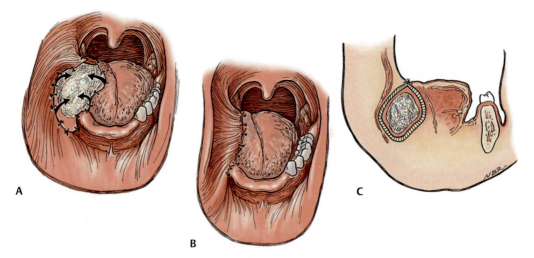

Fig. 1.17 (**A**) Split-thickness skin graft used to line defect. This is inserted like a pouch and held in place by a pad of medicated gauze or cotton balls. (**B**) Cheek to tongue approximated to oversew the bolster on the skin graft. (**C**) Coronal view showing the bolster in place.

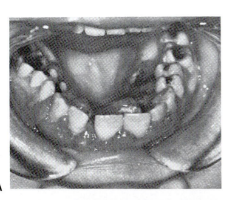

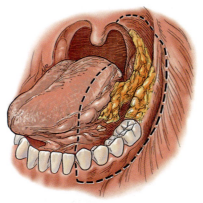

A

B

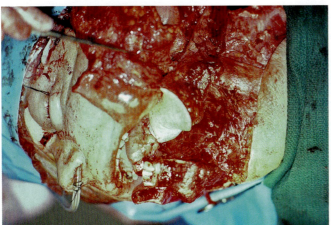

C

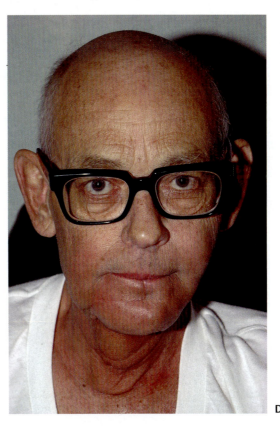

D

Fig. 1.18 (**A**) Large oral cavity tumor extending into the oropharynx. Tumor begins just above the canine tooth and extends onto the soft palate of the same side. (**B**) Resection margin outlined. (**C**) Following composite resection of the jaw, tongue, lateral pharyngeal wall, and soft palate, and radical neck dissection, the defect is replaced with a trapezius musculocutaneous flap. (**D**) Postoperative result.

tebral and paraspinal arteries for its viability (**Fig. 1.19**). The sternomastoid flap, despite its supply from three sources at three levels,[58] is probably the least dependable of the musculocutaneous flaps. In this flap even more than the others, the principle of loosely suturing the subcutis to the underlying muscle is absolutely essential because the skin is so loosely attached to the underlying muscle. The shearing action of skin over muscle during this flap's dissection has great potential for damaging the perforating vessels. It is a common experience to witness some degree of epithelial necrosis in this flap. Fortunately, reepithelialization is the rule and fistulization is rare.[58,59] In both the sternocleidomastoid and trapezius flaps, the donor site can often be closed primarily. Occasionally, especially with the trapezius flap taken from

the back, a split-thickness skin graft is needed to complete the closure of the donor site.

The pectoralis flap and the radial forearm free flap and more laterally the anterolateral free flap have mostly supplemented the trapezius and the sternomastoid flaps for oral cavity reconstruction. However, it is wise for the surgeon to have these two latter flaps in their reconstructive armamentarium when the fact of prior use or other conditions preclude their use.

The details of the pectoralis major musculocutaneous flap reconstruction are well known to most head and neck reconstructive surgeons; therefore, only key points in the raising and employment of this flap will be touched on here. Although Ariyan's[60] original description of the flap outlined its

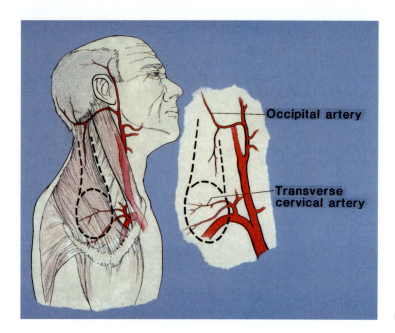

Fig. 1.19 Superiorly based trapezius musculocutaneous flap.

employment as a flap whose pedicle would be returned at a second stage, most surgeons use it as an island flap and obviate this second stage. It is prudent, however, to remember that, under certain circumstances, the flap's pedicle should be left outside the skin of the neck flaps. This is particularly important in the patient who has had prior irradiation therapy and has suffered radiation damage with thick, nonpliable skin or in the case of prior neck dissection with resultant scarring of the cervical tissues. At particular risk is the patient who is having a bilateral neck dissection wherein an acute angulation of the flap at the level of the clavicle will produce strangulation of the flap pedicle. This is especially the case when the patient has been given a large fluid volume during the operation. Part of the problem of flap compression at the base of neck can be alleviated by resecting the medial one third of the clavicle and inserting the flap pedicle into the gap.

In most instances the flap pedicle can be buried under the neck flaps raised for the neck dissection. In approaching the flap, I have abandoned the idea of creating a skin bridge over the pectoralis muscle pedicle on the chest previously advised to potentially preserve a deltopectoral flap for possible future use. This creates more difficulty in identifying the pectoral branch of the thoracoacromial artery as it emerges at the medial border of the pectoralis minor muscle. As the flap is elevated, it is important to secure the skin to the underlying deep muscular fascia to avoid shearing forces on the perforating vessels. Leaving a small cuff of pectoralis muscle around the artery and vein will help to protect it from later compression.

In oral cavity reconstruction oftentimes the cutaneous paddle and the subcutaneous tissues are too bulky and fill the oral cavity, impeding speech and deglutition. Using the bare pectoralis muscle covered with a skin graft, or as the exposed muscle, will cover the defect and fill in for missing soft tissue but not impede lingual mobility. At times there is insufficient fixed gingiva or it is too friable to hold a suture.

In such cases the flap can be anchored into position by encircling the teeth adjacent to the defect with the sutures in the flap's edge.

The use of the levator scapulae flap and nasolabial flaps for reconstruction will be described in the section on conservation surgery.

◆ Conservation Surgery

Conservation surgery for carcinoma of the larynx has become highly developed over the past 3 decades. The increased awareness of medical and dental practitioners with regard to oral cavity carcinoma has made its early diagnosis more commonplace. Although irradiation and surgery result in roughly equivalent survival rates in patients with these small neoplasms, often the complications, expense, and time lost from gainful employment favor the latter over the former modality. This is especially true when the principles of conservation surgery are applied. Transoral microscopic laser resection of the tongue, floor of the mouth, and buccal mucosa is the most recent innovation in conservation surgery of the oral cavity. The prior notion of needing a 1 to 2 cm margin of healthy tissue around the tumor to establish tumor-free margins is obviated by the laser technique. Narrow margins of tumor resection are enabled by the high magnification provided by the dissecting microscope. This combined with the relatively easy discernment between the laser cutting of normal tissue compared with that of tumor tissue permits the essential discrimination between tumor and nontumor. High magnification allows the surgeon to detect balls of tumor as small as 750 μm at the edge of the neoplasm thereby guiding the surgeon to a tumor-free zone. Because a small spot size of laser energy is used, in the range of 0.2 mm in diameter, the power density of a 10 W laser beam has excellent cutting potential while leaving a negligible amount of char.

The setup is relatively simple. The head is dropped into the Rose position. After draping the patient with wet towels in the vicinity of the oral cavity, applying wet sponges and a reflective barrier over the eyes, and assuring that the oxygen tension of the anesthetic mixture is near room air, the mouth is propped open with a side gag. The cheek is retracted with a Pierce cheek retractor. In tongue resections the tongue is grasped with a towel clip (**Fig. 1.20**).

The tumor is outlined with a narrow margin of 1 to 3 mm using short pulses of the laser (**Fig. 1.21**). To determine the depth of invasion but in total violation of traditional surgical oncological principles, the tumor is completely transected (**Fig. 1.22**). The tumor is cut through from side to side until normal tissue is reached at its depth. The microscope is turned up to high power and with the cutting beam the tumor periphery is skirted by a margin of ~2 mm from its visual and palpable limits. As the peripheral cut deepens, if tumor is encountered, then a narrow cuff of healthy tissue is taken around it. Once the depth of tumor is reached at its edges then by retracting the tumor with a grasping forceps

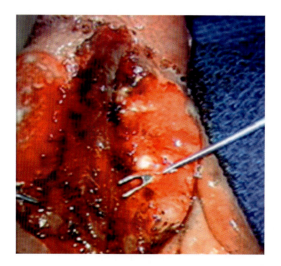

Fig. 1.22 The tumor is completely transected.

the vertical dissection can now become horizontal and the resection proceeds to the point of initial transsection (**Fig. 1.23**). Hemostasis is ensured by use of the fine-tipped bipolar cautery and vascular clips. The first piece of tumor is carefully removed from the field to maintain its anatomical orientation. It is mounted on wax affixed to a square of cork board by colored pins (**Fig. 1.24A**). The surgeon constructs a labeled drawing using the pin colors for orientation (**Fig. 1.24B**). The specimen is covered by a saline-soaked gauze sponge to prevent dessication.

In a similar fashion the laser is used to excise the remaining tumor. The second specimen is mounted on the same wax and cork platform, and the drawing is completed. Numerous frozen sections are taken, especially in areas where there is some doubt as to the integrity of the resection. Often the margins in the tumor bed are best left for permanent sections, and any revision resection can be delayed until the time of the neck dissection, which is done 7 to 10 days later.

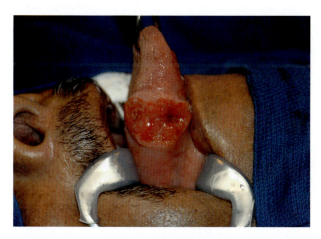

Fig. 1.20 The tongue is stabilized with a tongue clip.

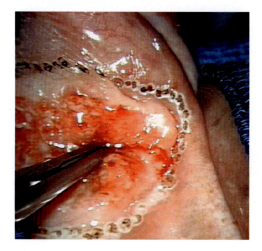

Fig. 1.21 The tumor is outlined using short-duration pulses with the CO_2 laser.

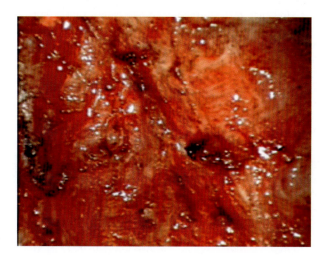

Fig. 1.23 The initial laser cut to determine depth has now become a horizontal dissection.

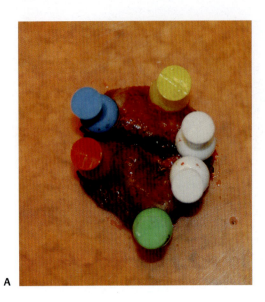

A

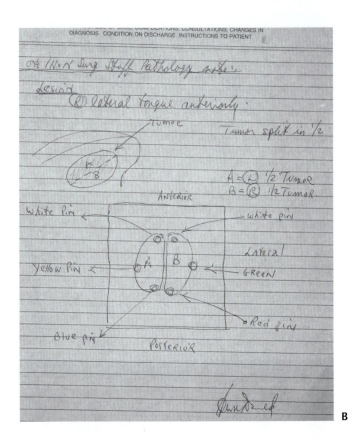

B

Fig. 1.24 (**A**) The specimen is mounted on a square of wax on cork board with colored pins for orientation. (**B**) A drawing accompanies the specimen to further aid the pathologist in orientation.

The wound is closed with interrupted catgut sutures in the same fashion as a wedge resection. It is essential that the surgeon takes the specimen and drawing to enhance the pathologist's understanding of the resection and surgical margins.

The margins of resection are not infrequently reported as positive by the pathologist. This is in part because of the shrinkage artifact secondary to the fixative and the proximity of the resection to the tumor enabled by high-power microscopic resection with the laser. The surgeon is obligated to do a revision resection even though the presence of tumor in the revision specimen will be seen in only ~20 to 30% of cases. However, if the surgeon can be assured that a biopsy of the margin taken at the initial resection was at the precise site that the pathologist judged the margin on the main specimen to be positive then further resection is unnecessary.

Local recurrence rates and survival rates are the same as classical wide field resection. With close follow-up any local recurrences can be managed by revision excision with the laser. Transoral microsurgical laser excision is especially valuable in patients with so-called field cancerization. The tissue sparing with this technique enables much better functional results than standard resection.

Although function-preserving procedures for the larynx are found in most standard texts, similar procedures for the oral cavity are more difficult to find. A corollary between the narrow tissue margin of resection necessary to ensure adequate tumor extirpation relative to the true vocal cord is also found in the mandibular periosteum. The work of Marchetta et al[61,62] indicates that the lymphatics that drain the floor of the mouth and tongue do not circle the mandible but pass directly into the upper cervical lymph nodes. In general, the sparse lymphatics that drain the meager lymph from the osseous tissue encircle the bone they drain between the two layers of investing periosteum. Contrary to the earlier notions of Polya and Narratel,[63] there is presently no evidence to indicate that continuity exists between those sparse lymphatics of the mandible and those in the floor of the mouth or in the tongue. In a review of 80 cases of oral cavity carcinoma, Marchetta and his associates found no evidence of tumor in bone, periosteal lymphatic, or periosteum when a tumor of the floor of the mouth was up to 1 mm away from the mandibular periosteum.[61,62] In the 15 patients in whom the periosteum was involved, the incidence of lymph node metastasis was 27%. In the remaining 65 patients without periosteal involvement, the metastatic rate was 65%, implying an extraperiosteal route of metastatic spread.

The work of Marchetta and coworkers prompted the development of procedures that split the mandible in a horizontal or vertical plane, permitting adequate tumor excision and the preservation of mandibular continuity. Such "face-saving" operations[64] eliminate the need for extensive reconstructive efforts in areas that are particularly difficult to rebuild. This is especially true of the anterior regions of the oral cavity. Fortunately, mandibular bone invasion by squamous cell cancer is a slow process. Byars[65] has shown that this remains true until the medullary cavity or the major neurovascular foramina have been invaded, at which time tumor spread becomes more rapid.

Although these procedures have withstood the test of time, the work of Ossoff and colleagues[66,67] has cast some

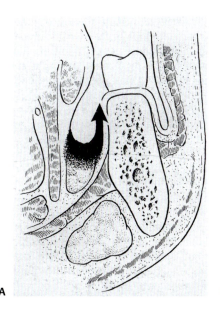

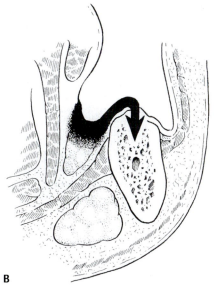

Fig. 1.25 Patterns of tumor spread in the (**A**) dentulous and (**B**) edentulous mandible. (From McGregor IA, McGregor JM. Floor of mouth. In: McGregor IA, McGregor FM, eds. Cancer of the Mouth and Face. Edinburgh: Churchill Livingstone; 1986:443–444.)

doubt as to their safety. By injecting lymph vessels in the floor of the mouth of dogs, they found that some of the efferent lymphatics were tightly adherent to the mandibular periosteum. As yet, no studies have been done to establish a human corollary.

Floor of mouth carcinomas have only a thin layer of loose areolar tissue between the mucosal surface and the diaphragm of the floor of the mouth, the mylohyoid muscle. Tumor can extend from this site medially to the adjacent tongue musculature or laterally to the loose and then fixed gingival tissues. The route of spread of tumor to the bone and thence to the medullary cavity has been clearly elucidated and described by McGregor and McGregor (**Fig. 1.25**).[35] The presence of teeth influences the route and rapidity of the spread of cancer through the bone. The edentulous mandible is much more susceptible to the penetration of cancer of the floor of the mouth because of the proximity of the mucosa to the mylohyoid line coupled with thinness of the bone at the occlusal surface of the mandible once the teeth are lost. In the intact mandible, the mylohyoid muscle inserts on the mylohyoid line on the basal bone, and the alveolar bone adds significant height and distance for tumor to travel over the fixed gingiva until it reaches the occlusal surface of the mandible. Tumor penetration of the cortical bone is slow and pushing in character. It is not until the medullary cavity is reached that more extensive local extension occurs. Perineural spread along the alveolar nerve is not uncommon and can extend all the way to the foramen ovale. Such perineural spread can very occasionally occur in extensive lip carcinoma along the mental nerve. Once the foramen ovale is reached and tumor has been positively identified in the mandibular branch of the trigeminal nerve, then skull base surgery must be done to achieve a negative margin, initially either through the transmandibular approach if the intracranial invasion is minimal or through the infratemporal fossa-middle fossa approach if the degree of extension goes into the Meckel cave.

Marginal Mandibulectomy

This procedure is indicated for the excision of tumors of the attached gingiva (**Fig. 1.26**) that extend no more than 2 to 3 mm into the gingival, labial, buccal, or lingual mucosa. There must be no evidence of bone erosion radiographically or on radionuclide scanning. The tumors are generally of the superficially invasive and exophytic varieties and will seldom be larger than 4 cm. Tumors that are more extensive require either a full-thickness excision of mandibular bone or a combination of marginal mandibulectomy and a lingual or buccal split.

The excision is done entirely intraorally. The area of resection, allowing a 2 cm margin of healthy tissue around the tumor, is outlined with methylene blue, using a non-siliconized needle. The cutting cautery is used to make the incision down to the bone and into the adjacent soft tissues to the estimated depth of the bony resection. Care must be taken to keep the soft tissue cuts vertical, avoiding the natural tendency to slant the incisions toward the tumor

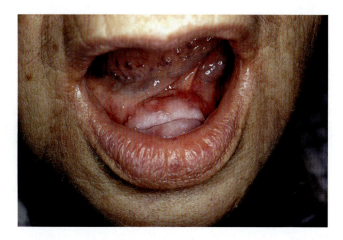

Fig. 1.26 Alveolar ridge carcinoma.

(**Fig. 1.27**). A bone saw or cutting bone needle, such as the Midas Rex drill system (Medtronic, Inc., Minneapolis, MN), is used to make vertical cuts through the mandible to a depth of 1.5 to 2.0 cm. Shallower cuts are made in the edentulous mandible in which alveolar bone is lost and only basal bone remains. In the atrophic mandible, the marginal resection must often be abandoned and full-thickness bone excised.

Horizontal incisions in the soft tissue now extend from the vertical incisions on the labial-buccal and lingual aspects of the resection. Once these deep incisions abut the mandible, a sagittal saw or bone-cutting needle is used to complete the bony cuts, and the bloc is removed. Alternatively, the bone incision can be done by making multiple penetrating bur holes and then connecting them with an osteotome. The danger imposed by the osteotome is the risk of fracturing the mandibular remnant. Larger areas can be nicely covered with one or both nasolabial flaps.[68] These are created as island flaps with the flap passed through a puncture through the orbicularis muscle into the defect.

During the resection it is important to remember that the invasion of alveolar bone is more often minimal, whereas the spread to the soft tissues is more extensive. Therefore it is wise to take a much narrower margin of bone than adjacent soft tissue. If radiographic evidence of minimal cortical bone invasion is visualized on the preoperative CT scan or occlusal view of the mandible then a wider margin of bone is taken. Assessment of the residual bone stock after resection is vi-

tally important, especially in the edentulous mandible. If the patient has osteoporosis the potential for future mandibular fracture is even more acute. The placement of a low-profile titanium reconstruction plate will protect the patient from a later fracture. The plate should be bent and the drill holes registered prior to the actual resection because fracture during the ostectomy may occur.

Smaller raw areas are readily covered by a dermis graft or split-thickness skin graft. It is best to stent these grafts in position. Numerous quilting sutures may be inserted as suggested by McGregor,[69] but the surest means of anchoring the graft in place is with some form of bolster or stent. A preformed acrylic stent (**Fig. 1.28**) can be fixed to the dentition by prosthetic clips or anchored to the lower jaw by circum-mandibular wires. Any necessary reshaping of the splint to accommodate the graft is done at the operating table prior to fixing it in place. If sufficient acrylic is present to adequately obdurate the graft, additional cold cure acrylic may be added. The splint is left in place for 10 to 14 days. Some means of continuous splinting is essential until a permanent denture is fashioned. This splinting will reduce the graft shrinkage that invariably ensues during the subsequent weeks of healing. If a prosthetist is not available to provide a splint, bolstering of the graft can be accomplished with cotton dental rolls. However, keeping the bolster in place is often difficult because of the considerable movement of the tongue.

A radial forearm free flap can be used in much larger defects when the soft tissue resection is considerable. In most

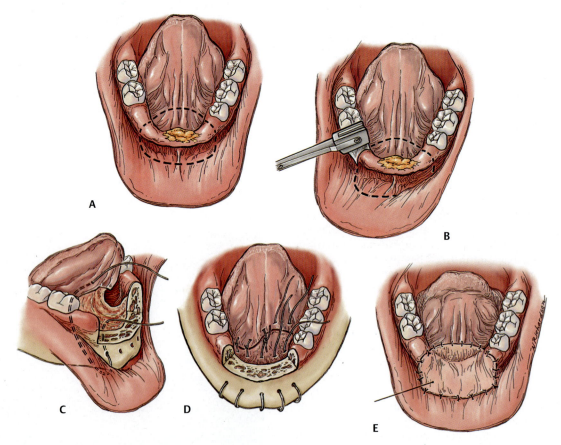

Fig. 1.27 Marginal mandibulectomy. (**A**) Tumor of fixed gingiva outlined with a 2 cm margin. (**B**) Stryker saw used to make bony cuts. (**C**) Chronic sutures through drill holes in mandible used to close dead space. (**D**) Dead space effaced. (**E**) Skin graft placed to cover remaining defect.

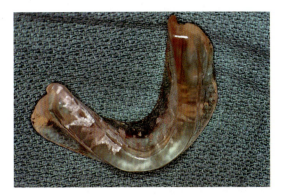

Fig. 1.28 Preformed acrylic stent.

marginal mandibulectomy defects, the free flap is overkill; easier and quicker methods should be employed. In our hands, the most utilitarian method for such reconstructions is the combination of a levator scapulae flap and a nasolabial island flap. A relative contraindication to this combination of flaps is in a male with a heavy beard. The hair growing in the floor of the mouth is unpleasant and aesthetically repugnant. The levator muscle may be quite large, especially in muscular persons, but even in slender individuals it is usually large enough to cover the defect. In midline lesions bilateral flaps can be used. The levator muscle takes its origin from the transverse processes of C1 to C4 and inserts on the medial border of the scapula. It sometimes exists as several slips that may seem somewhat distinct from one another but are indeed one single muscle. The blood supply is segmental, and during the flap elevation the arteries and veins for each

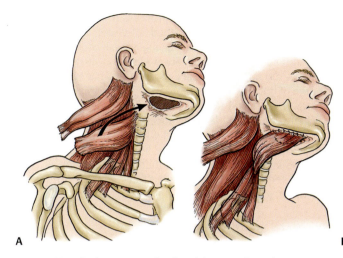

Fig. 1.29 The levator scapulae flap. (**A**) Arrow shows levator scapulae flap being sewn into place. (**B**) Flap used to reconstruct floor of mouth.

segment are ligated, with care to preserve those branches at the C1 and C2 levels. The muscle is dissected from the underlying deep muscles in the neck down to the level of the scapula. A right-angled clamp is placed around the muscle at its insertion, and the muscle transected then rotated into the defect (**Fig. 1.29**). The muscle is then sutured to the soft tissues on the lingual and labial or buccal side of the mandibular defect and draped over the raw bony surface. The surface epithelium is supplied by the nasolabial island flap. A triangular or elliptical flap is designed in the melolabial fold. It is completely circumscribed by the incision (**Fig. 1.30**). The flap

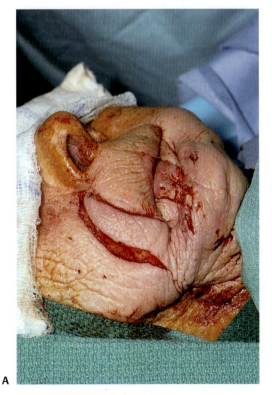

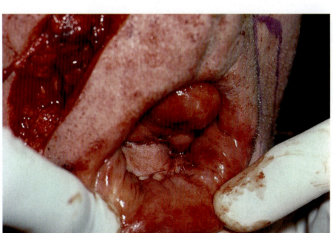

Fig. 1.30 Nasolabial flap. (**A**) Flap elevated. (**B**) Flap placed into floor of mouth.

elevation begins superiorly and proceeds to the base. As the inferior third of the flap is reached, all vessels are carefully preserved and circumvented, leaving a small protective cuff of fat and connective tissue. Scant elevation of the inferior aspect of the flap is necessary to the limit that will permit rotation of the flap into the oral cavity and permit cutaneous closure of the facial skin. A puncture is made through the buccinator muscle wide enough to allow passage of the flap into the region of the defect and without compromising its pedicle. The flap is sewn over the levator muscle, approximating the flap skin to the oral mucosa. The region of the vascular pedicle must be carefully protected from compression and stricture at the site of closure.

Lingual and Buccal Plate Excisions

Vertical excisions of mandibular bone are indicated in oral cavity tumors that extend to the proximity of the buccolabial or lingual portions of the mandible (**Fig. 1.31**). An adequate margin of resection necessitates the excision of partial-thickness bone in the vertical plane. Primary tumors of the lip or buccal mucosa uncommonly extend to the depths of their reflection on to the mandibular gingiva. On the other hand, lingual and floor of mouth tumors often extend onto the gingiva or close to it. According to Marchetta's[61] studies, a slim margin of 1 mm of uninvolved tissue between the mandibular periosteum and the tumor ensures the safety of a conservation procedure.

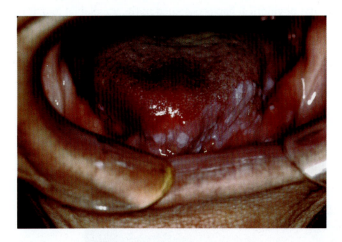

Fig. 1.31 Carcinoma of the anterior floor of the mouth and associated leukoplakia. Malignancy approximates the lingual plate of the mandible on the left.

Unlike to the marginal mandibulectomy, vertical plane excisions can only occasionally be done entirely intraorally. Usually the lesions are more extensive, and the excision must extend through the mylohyoid muscle. In these instances, a cervical incision should be added. It is placed horizontally about two fingerbreadths below the body of the mandible (**Fig. 1.32**). Flaps are elevated over an area that enables sufficient exposure of the submandibular and submental triangles. In the absence of cervical lymph node involvement, a selective neck dissection including levels I, II, and III is per-

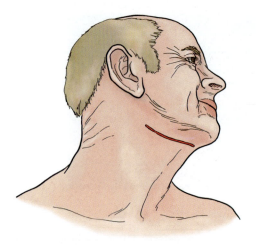

Fig. 1.32 Cervical excision for inferior exposure in lingual or buccal plate excision.

formed. The excision often entails the removal of one submandibular salivary gland and occasionally both. Although care should be exercised to preserve the ramus mandibularis, no compromise of the tumor resections should be made to achieve this. A simple rapid means of preserving the nerve is to incise the fascia overlying the submandibular salivary gland at the inferior pole. As the fascia is dissected from the gland in a superior dissection, the nerve is carried with it. The dissection is carried to the body of the mandible, and the nerve's safety is ensured. An alternative method of nerve protection is to isolate the posterior facial vein, transect it, and dissect the fascia of the gland and the vein superiorly. Because the ramus marginalis always runs superficial to the posterior facial vein the nerve is protected. If palpable adenopathy is detected, a radical neck dissection is done in continuity. The incision is outlined in **Fig. 1.13**.

The intraoral part of the excision is marked out using multiple punctures with a nonsiliconized needle dipped in methylene blue. A lip split is seldom, if ever, necessary for adequate exposure. The soft tissue excision usually extends through the mylohyoid muscle. The adequacy of the excision width is best controlled from below. The necessity of making the soft tissue cuts precisely vertical must be reemphasized, and the natural tendency to slant the incision toward the tumor as the deeper planes are reached must be firmly resisted.

Any teeth in the line of excision are now extracted. Care must be taken to leave an adequate shell of alveolar bone surrounding the teeth adjacent to the resection margin. An exposed tooth root may lead to infection, poor healing, and eventual tooth loss. The vertical incision through the bone is made with a sagittal cutting saw (**Fig. 1.33**). A quick, easy, and precise excision can be done using a bone cutting needle such as the Midas Rex S4–218 cutting tool (Medtronic, Inc.). The incisions from the cortex to the marrow cavity of the bone running in the anterior-posterior direction can be made with a precision that facilitates preservation of the lamina dura of the teeth adjacent to the line of the incision. The curve of the incision along the occlusal surface of the mandible can be accomplished more smoothly with bone

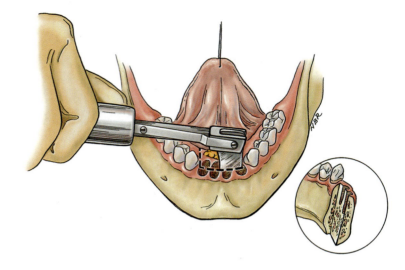

Fig. 1.33 Bony cuts for lingual plate excision. Notice how the plane of the incision is at right angles to the mandible.

needle than with the saw. This is especially important in excisions done in the symphyseal area and even more vital in the edentulous mandible when inadvertent cuts with the saw tip weaken the residual bone predisposing it to fracture. It is important to remember that the buccal plate of the mandible is much thicker than the lingual, and the inferior aspect of the mandible is much broader than the alveolar portion. The vertical bone cut is directed as nearly perpendicular to the inferior plane of the mandible as possible. It can also be accomplished with multiple closely spaced bur holes that are then connected with an osteotome. This cut in the sagittal plane of the mandible is now connected by vertical cuts at right angles to, and at the extremities of, the sagittal cut.

Once the specimen is free, all soft tissue attachments are severed and it can be "pulled through" the floor of the mouth.

Reconstruction is similar to that of the marginal mandibulectomy. However, especially in buccal plate excisions, care is taken to reconstruct a sulcus. An effaced gingival-buccal sulcus may thwart even the best attempts at prosthetic rehabilitation.

Combined Excisions

Probably the most commonly performed conservation procedure is the combination of the vertical and horizontal mandibulectomy (**Fig. 1.34A,B,C**). This is used for tumors that

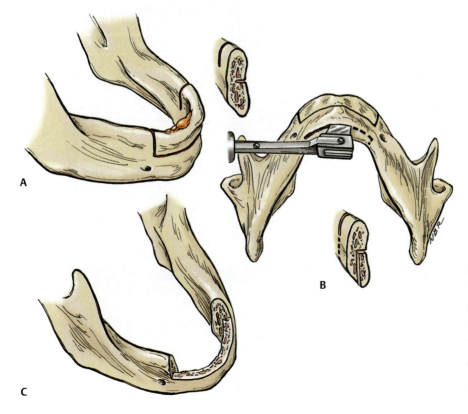

Fig. 1.34 Combined marginal mandibulectomy and lingual split. (**A**) Marginal incisions made through the alveolar ridge. A horizontal cut is made on the buccal but not the lingual surface. (**B**) A lingual plate incision made with a sagittal saw connects with the horizontal cut of the marginal mandibulectomy. (**C**) Resection is completed with residual buccal-inferior bone strut remaining to connect both mandibular bodies, thus retaining mandibular arch configuration.

originate in the tongue or floor of the mouth on the lingual side, or for those on the lip or buccal mucosa on the buccolabial side that encroach on the alveolar gingiva (**Fig. 1.31**).

Once the mucosal cuts are completed, the marginal mandibulectomy incisions are made in the usual way, with the exception of the horizontal portion. This cut is carried through only half the thickness of the mandible, from the plate on the side opposite the tumor to the midportion of the medullary cavity. For example, in a floor of mouth tumor encroaching on the gingiva, the horizontal bony incision would be from the buccal plate to the midportion of the medullary cavity. The sagittal cut is begun at the inferior aspect of the jaw and carried superiorly to meet the horizontal cut of the marginal portion of the operation (**Fig. 1.34B**). The residual bar of bone is often thin and fragile, especially if the buccal plate is excised. Because this procedure is most applicable in the anterior aspect of the mandible, this bony strut is usually sufficiently strong, except in the markedly atrophic mandible.

Reconstruction of the area is the same as in the previously mentioned conservation procedures. If an accidental fracture occurs through the residual bone in the operative defect or if the strength of the residual bony bar appears precarious, then the bone should be reinforced with a titanium reconstruction plate (**Fig. 1.35**). This form of fixation has resulted in bone healing in all of our patients despite postoperative irradiation, which has been done in the majority of cases. Several authorities feel that these tumors merit a full-thickness bony excision. Som and Nussbaum[68] state strongly that periosteal involvement mandates a full-thickness resection. On the other hand, Keim and Lowenberg[70] showed no bone invasion in 22 consecutive cases of oral cavity tumors that invaded the gingiva. King[71] had excellent local control in 65 patients of whom many had periosteal involvement; however, none of the tumors were greater than 4 cm in size and all were superficial in type. Whereas the arch area in the anterior region is notoriously difficult to reconstruct, in the lateral aspect of the mandible, a segmental resection and replacement with a plate is probably technically easier than the conservation procedure. For large segmental defects, a fibular free flap can be done.

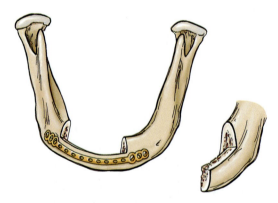

Fig. 1.35 Titanium reconstruction plate reinforcing the residual mandible following combined marginal mandibulectomy and lingual splitting.

◆ Rehabilitation following Anterior Resections

Most standard texts of head and neck surgery adequately describe the procedure of composite resection of the anterior aspects of the oral cavity. Little attention is paid to either the details of the incapacity this surgery inflicts on these patients or the rectification of these disabilities. Unfortunately, surgical resections, especially of extensive lesions, often leave patients severely orally handicapped by incompetence with drooling, problems with alimentation, and severe articulation defects, in addition to an often hideous appearance, frequently making them an anathema to family and friends (**Fig. 1.36**). These problems are so grave that several head and neck surgeons elect irradiation therapy for these tumors, accepting a reduced survival, and reserve surgery for salvage of those who fail this modality, despite the increased morbidity and the poor survival that result from salvage surgery.

Surgical reconstruction and rehabilitation of patients who have had extensive resections of the anterior aspects of the oral cavity provides one of the greatest challenges in head and neck surgery. A detailed consideration of each anatomical area reveals a unique group of specific functional contributions to each facet of normal oral physiology. In managing the defects as a consequence of extirpative surgery, a clear

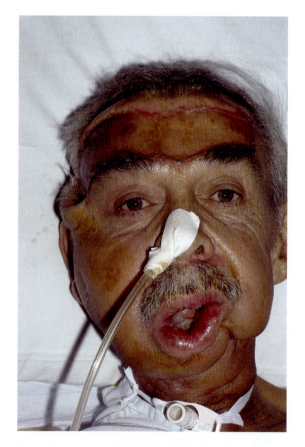

Fig. 1.36 A flaccid, inactive lower lip secondary to denervation resulting from tumor excision.

plan of action must be formulated based upon the restoration of function of these structures and utilizing a host of surgical, prosthetic, and physiotherapeutic measures.

Although each anatomical area of involvement will be dealt with individually in a sequential manner, reconstruction of several contiguous areas is usually demanded in many commonly encountered resections.

Lips

The lips are the guardians of the oral cavity. Their ability to approximate prevents drooling during rest or speech, and during mastication they are responsible for maintaining the food in the mouth. Although the orbicularis oris is often thought to be solely responsible for these functions, important contributions are made by several other facial muscles. The deepest muscular layer lying adjacent to the labial mucosa is made up principally of the buccinator and the deepest fibers of the orbicularis oris. At this level, the middle portions of the buccinator muscle decussate at the angle of the mouth, with the lower fibers seeking and then traversing the upper lip, and the upper fibers, the lower lip. The buccinator fibers that lie superior and inferior to the decussating ones course straight across the upper and lower lips, respectively. These fibers blend with those of the orbicularis oris muscle, which are similarly disposed, and the two muscles together are responsible for drawing the lips together and against the adjacent surface of the teeth and alveolar gingivae (**Fig. 1.37**).

The most superficial layer of the lip musculature is made up principally of the depressor and levator anguli oris muscles and their interdigitation with the orbicularis oris, whose fibers are now oriented in an oblique direction. This enables the lips to be pursed and pouted. The levator anguli oris alaeque nasi, the zygomaticus major and minor, and the mentalis muscles are all integrated at this level. They insert into the decussating fibers of the levator and depressors, the oblique fibers of the orbicularis oris, and the skin of the lips.[72]

The lower lip is functionally more important than the upper, in part owing to the action of the lower jaw. Even though the upper lip may hang like a curtain, the active lower lip will perform all of the activities essential to normal functioning.[73] On the other hand, even if the upper lip is fully innervated and operative, oral continence will be lost if the lower lip is flaccid and inactive (**Fig. 1.36**). In reconstructing the lip, whenever possible, replacement of lost labial tissue is done with adjacent labial tissue; hence the success of the Abbe and Estlander flaps as well as the Karapandzic technique.[74] Reconstruction of the lower lip from adjacent nonlabial tissue is far less successful than that of the upper.

Following anterior resection of the oral cavity for large tumors, the lower lip is often partially or completely denervated. Despite heroic attempts to restore the integrity of the mandible and mobility of the tongue, rehabilitation will be thwarted if oral continence is not ensured. Often the lower lip is quite large, usually the result of edema secondary to the effects of the surgery alone or in combination with irradiation. This is especially frequent in cases of bilateral neck dissection. A reduction in bulk by wedge resection of the lip will usually restore continence, especially if some semblance of muscle activity remains.

The more severe condition of the prolapsed, totally denervated lip can be rehabilitated by a wedge resection followed by the use of a fascial sling.[75] In constructing the sling, a small incision is made just above the zygomatic arch, and about 6 mm of arch is divested of soft tissue covering. The fascial strip is fed around the arch with an aneurysm needle. This sling of fascia lata is then tied around one zygomatic arch, knitted through one half of the lower lip, and brought out in the midline. A second fascial strip is similarly placed on the opposite side, the lip is cinched into position (**Fig. 1.38**), and the two strips are sutured together. Once the lower lip approximates the upper lip, oral continence is greatly improved (**Fig. 1.39**). When motor function is lost to the lip secondary to trauma or surgical excision for tumor, sensation is also often lost. This precludes the patient's appreciation of the presence of saliva or oral contents on the lip. Occasionally some return of tactile sense will occur by regrowth of the sensory nerves from the least involved side; however, it is often incomplete and continues to be a vexing problem.

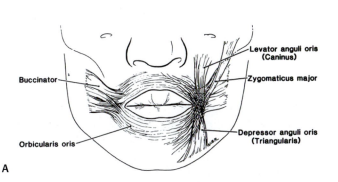
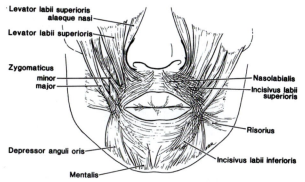

Fig. 1.37 Muscle layers of the lip. (**A**) Deep layer, composed principally of the buccinator and orbicularis oris muscles. Note how the central slips of the buccinator decussate at the corners of the mouth (right), then interdigitate with the orbicularis oris. (**B**) Superficial layer, composed of more obliquely oriented orbicularis fibers, showing their interdigitation with the muscles of facial expression that act on the mouth.

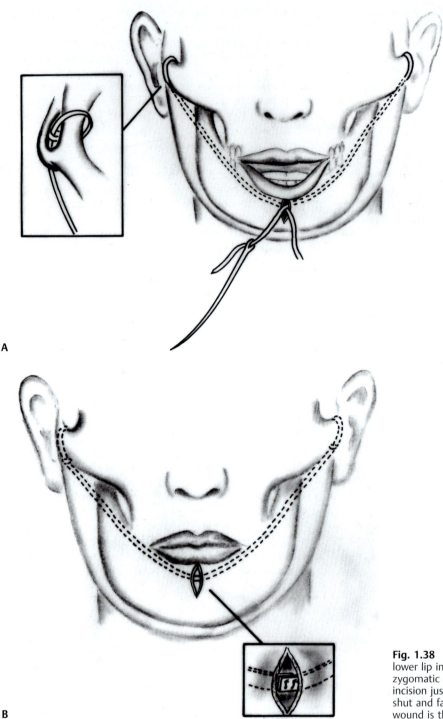

A

B

Fig. 1.38 Fascial sling used to cinch inactive functionless lower lip into position. (**A**) Fascia lata loop is slung over the zygomatic arch and brought out through a central midline incision just below the lower lip. (**B**) The lip is cinched shut and fascia strips are approximated in the midline. The wound is then closed.

Mandible

The key to retention of both oral functioning and aesthetics is the preservation or the adequate reconstruction of the mandibular arch. The arch has a unique configuration that is extremely difficult to reproduce. Moreover, it forms an anchor for one of the major tongue muscles, the genioglossus; serves as a point of stabilization for the hyoid bone through the gen-

iohyoid and the anterior belly of the digastric; and is the origin of the diaphragm of the floor of the mouth, the mylohyoid. Loss of this arch results in collapse of the anterior aspect of the oral cavity, resulting in total oral incompetence, dysphagia, severely distorted speech, and aesthetic deformity.

Numerous methods have been described to reconstruct this keystone of the oral cavity. Immediate free bone grafting in a tumor patient who is often elderly, chronic alcoholic,

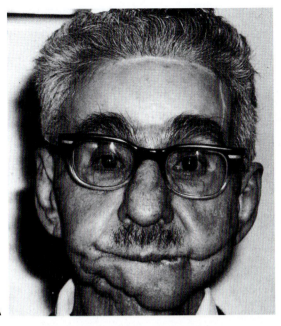
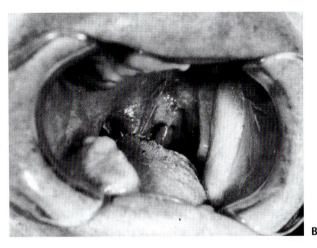

Fig. 1.39 Patient who had a large carcinoma of the anterior tongue done many years ago reconstructed with an old-fashioned forehead flap. (**A**) Patient prior with severe oral incompetence. (**B**) Continence restored ~90% with a fascial sling.

protein-depleted, and with grossly carious dentition, is usually doomed to failure. If the patient has had prior irradiation, an even higher extrusion rate can be anticipated. The same holds true for reconstruction of the arch with a titanium plate; ~80% will spontaneously extrude.

In the past, several methods have been attempted to reconstruct the mandible, especially the anterior arch. Various trays to carry cancellous bone to the reconstruction site have been used. The most promising among them have been those made of stainless steel, Vitalium, titanium, Tantalum, or Dacron mesh. Although a few successes have been reported, many have met with failure, especially if they are implanted at the time of the exenterative surgery. However, even if the reconstruction has been done in a delayed fashion, the extrusion rate is significant and the regenerated bone is of poor quality. An exception to this may be the use of an absorbable tray with cancellous bone. As the tray is absorbed, the bone is in the process of regenerating and remodeling. With the weakening of the tray the bone is enabled to respond according to Wolff's law and ultimately be stronger than that usually experienced with the permanent trays. Preliminary work in dogs by Strong and Rubinstein has been very encouraging.[76]

Cadaver mandible that has been freeze-dried then implanted with cancellous bone as described by DeFries et al[77] saw an initial flush of success when implanted into young, healthy combatants during the Vietnam War but did not withstand the test of time when used in the civilian population, especially in the head and neck cancer patient, and was subsequently abandoned. The experiences of Cantrell and Boyne[78] and the author have established this fact.

Cummings[79] has attempted removing the mandibular arch, excising the attached cancer, freezing the bone twice in liquid nitrogen, and then reimplanting it. He expresses guarded optimism regarding the efficacy of this procedure because he found local persistence of tumor in adjacent soft tissue. Popescu and Spirescu[80] described four cases done in the same way: two patients with squamous cell tumors and two others with benign lesions invading the mandible. Although they had no instances of local recurrence, they had a high rate of serious local complications. Panje[81] attempted this procedure three times without success, reporting that the bone became septic and extruded. Haymaker[82] has had short-term success with gross excision of tumor from the resected jaw, after which the bone is exposed to 10,000 rads of gamma irradiation and then reinserted as a free graft. However, subsequent irradiation of the patient as part of a combined therapy program often results in transformation of the graft to fibrous tissue.[83]

The greatest innovation in the reconstruction of the mandible is the introduction of osseous free flaps. Free flaps containing either the radius, scapula, iliac crest, or fibula have all been employed but the most utilitarian has been the fibula. The scapular bone is thin, and it is difficult or impossible to install titanium intraosseous implants to later employ a bone-anchored dental prosthesis. On the other hand the iliac crest free flap, which brings with it a large piece of bone, is particularly difficult to harvest and carries with it a large unwieldy block of muscle that is often difficult to work into the intraoral reconstruction. The split radius often provides less than adequate bone for reconstruction in both length and thickness and is also fraught with a significant incidence of spontaneous fracture of the residual bone in the arm.

The fibular free flap, initially described by Taylor et al,[84] is the most useful flap for the reconstruction of the mandible. It can provide up to 22 to 25 cm of bone, and its thickness enables the implantation of titanium dental implants. An additional advantage is that the harvest of the bone can be done at the same time as the cancer resection. Preoperatively it is important to establish the patency of the peroneal artery, which is the nutrient artery to the flap. Some controversy exists regarding the routine use of arteriography in assessing the health of this vessel. Some feel that the presence of a strong pulse at the ankle ensures a sufficiently patent peroneal artery. Care is taken to preserve the distal one third of the bone so as not to destabilize the ankle joint. A skin paddle is usually included to serve as a flap monitor and may be included in the reconstruction. The flap is inserted in such a way that the vascular pedicle lies on the lingual surface of the mandible. The curve of the mandible can be achieved by making a series of wedge-shaped ostectomies on the lingual side of the bone preserving the periosteum on that facing the labial side of the bone to maintain the integrity of the blood supply. The osteotomies can be stabilized with mini-plates and the fibular graft fixed to the residual mandible with thicker mandibular plates. A detailed description of the surgical technique in harvesting and implantation of the fibular free flap is beyond the scope of this text. The reader is advised to consult such sources as the text by Urken et al[85] for an excellent dissertation on the details of this technique.

The skin paddle on the flap not only acts as a monitor but can also be employed in the resurfacing of the surgical defect. Unfortunately the color and texture of this skin are a poor match to that of the neck and face. In addition, its hair-bearing quality as well as thickness and texture make it less than ideal for intraoral reconstruction. At times its bulk may displace the residual tongue posteriorly into the oropharynx interfering with speech and deglutition. This will require revision at a second sitting some months later once the flap has healed.

Chin

One of the most disfiguring consequences of anterior resection is the markedly receding chin or Andy Gump deformity. This is often brought about by a deficiency in the bony component, but in its severest forms it results from the loss of both bone and overlying soft tissue.

Before a bone graft can be inserted to establish the continuity of the mandible, it must have adequate soft tissue coverage. When the malignancy is so extensive that a through-and-through excision is necessary, reconstruction requires a flap often of substantial size. Musculocutaneous and free flaps often of considerable size are necessary to cover these defects. However, in instances where previous surgery and irradiation have failed, it is often wise to suture the skin to the oral mucosa, delaying the reconstruction to a time when healing is complete, the danger of local recurrence has passed, and the patient's nutritional and metabolic status has sufficiently recovered (**Fig. 1.40**). In these patients another impediment to immediate reconstruction other than their poor general health is a history of previous radical neck dissection and radiation therapy. This renders the cervical tissues woody, hard, difficult to dissect, and nonresilient. In these cases, a free flap is risky in that no cervical veins of sufficient caliber are present to which to anastomose the donor vein. This then would necessitate installing a jump graft from the flap vein to the subclavian vein, increasing the vulnerability of the vessel to coagulation with consequent flap

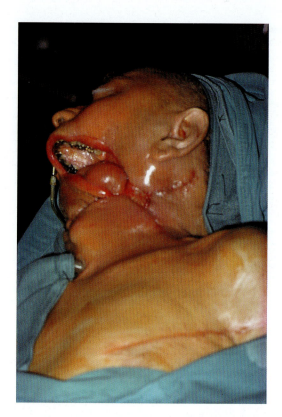

Fig. 1.40 Skin-to-mucosa closure is performed and reconstruction is delayed because of extensive tumor resection done on a previously irradiated patient who is markedly malnourished. Tumor had eroded through the skin, causing fistulization, and a pathological fracture eventuated because of extensive tumor involvement and osteoradionecrosis of the mandible.

loss. Placing a musculocutaneous flap such as the pectoralis or latissimus dorsi flaps would have to be done extracutaneously, similarly jeopardizing flap viability.

Conley[86–88] used several osteocutaneous composite flaps to reconstruct these defects in a few patients with some success. He used both attached rib and clavicle as the osseous components, but frequent bone extrusion and absorption were encountered and the results were little better than with immediate bone grafting. The reason for this is the nature of the blood supply to the bones in these flaps. In their usual anatomical site, they are supplied from two sources: the small periosteal arteries and the nutrient artery. The nutrient artery piercing the head of the bone is responsible for the supply of the medullary and most of the compact bone of the diaphysis.[89,90] The periosteal supply, which is preserved in chest flaps that include either rib or the shaft portion of the clavicle, nourishes the outer portion of the compact bone. The principal periosteal artery in the rib is the anterior intercostal branch of the internal mammary artery, and, unfortunately, this is sacrificed in most composite flap transfers. Therefore, the only blood supply to the bone in these flaps is through collaterals from overlying muscle.

Using the goat as an experimental model, Medgyesi[91] showed an extensive and rich capillary blood supply from the overlying muscle and soft tissue to the periosteum of bone in several osteomyocutaneous flaps. Snyder et al[92] found some evidence of actively growing bone in several tubed flaps in humans. The cases of Conley and associates, with the exception of one temporal flap, all showed either necrosis or creeping substitution on microscopic examination.[88] However, Cuono and Ariyan[93] showed evidence of viable medullary bone in a rib graft taken with a pectoralis major myocutaneous flap. Ostrup and Fredrickson[94] state that an intact medullary blood supply is required for bone transfer, to avoid the creeping substitution seen in free bone grafts and commonly experienced in composite flaps.

Panje and Cutting[95] have used a trapezius musculocutaneous flap with attached scapular spine with excellent functional and cosmetic results in four patients. They fracture the bony fragment in the middle to achieve a semblance of the arch configuration. Fluorescein studies at the operating table and bone scans done later in the postoperative period reveal the maintenance of an excellent blood supply. The main disadvantages of this procedure are the difficulty in maintaining an intact blood supply to the flap from the transverse cervical artery during the neck dissection, the uncomfortable position of the patient's shoulder during the early postoperative weeks, and the difficulty in creating a satisfactory arch configuration from the graft. McCraw and Arnold[96] have commented quite aptly that the trapezius osteomyocutaneous flap may qualify as a "gee whiz" flap, and that one is quite enough for anyone's collection. From my own experience I am in agreement with this statement. Ariyan[97] found that composite free flaps of skin muscle and rib grafted to the mandible by microvascular anastomoses survived and were adequately maintained on the anterior intercostal artery. This is fortunate because primary medullary circulation can be established only by an anastomosis between the recipient artery and the nutrient artery piercing the head of the rib. The dissection necessary to preserve this nutrient vessel is exceedingly difficult. The artery of Adamkiewicz, an important artery to the lumbar spine, is in jeopardy during the maneuvers necessary to free up this vessel. Obtaining sufficient vessel length to provide an adequate cuff for anastomosis to the recipient artery is also very difficult.

If the anterior intercostal artery is chosen as the main nutrient vessel to the rib in the graft, serial wedge cuts in the posterior rib surface and a series of greenstick fractures on the anterior surface further endanger the periosteal supply. The survival of the microvascular anastomosis in a previously irradiated bed was dramatically illustrated by Ostrup and Fredrickson in dogs.[94] These anastomoses appear to be able to withstand a full course of irradiation.

The most difficult problem in the various techniques of reconstruction in the oral cavity is the reproduction of a smoothly contoured but sufficiently strong mandibular arch. An arch that produces an aesthetically pleasing chin is a challenge of significant magnitude. Although the smooth curve required to reproduce the form of the chin can be established with a rib graft with multiple osteotomies, the bone is thin and weak. In latter years the costal free flap has been pretty much abandoned by most surgeons.

The difficulty in arch reproduction and the problem of obtaining a medullary blood supply may have been answered by the work of Ostrup and Fredrickson,[98] and Taylor[99] They utilized the inner surface of the iliac crest with attached muscle and accompanying deep circumflex vessels. An outline of the required mandibular arch graft is inscribed on the inner cortex, and it and the underlying medullary bone are taken. A generous cuff of overlying muscle must be included to protect the nutrient vessels that branch from the deep circumflex artery. Although the reported clinical experience of Ostrup and Fredrickson[98] is with only one patient, the procedure shows much promise. Most of Taylor's[99] cases were either in patients with nonmalignant disease or in young patients. None were reported in patients following failed prior radiation therapy or prior neck dissection. As previously mentioned, the major drawbacks to this flap are the difficulty in flap harvest and the bulk of the overlying muscle.

Once the epithelial coverings of the lower third of the face have been restored, the mandibular graft inserted, and the continuity of the jaw reestablished, the chin prominence is occasionally deficient. The insertion of an irradiated cartilage graft in a small pocket over the mentum restores a more normal appearing profile (**Fig. 1.41**).

Tongue

The fine, precise movements of the tongue result from the delicate coordination of its intrinsic muscles, which are oriented in longitudinal, vertical, and transverse planes. The verticalis linguae fibers are located only in the margins of the anterior tongue and are responsible for some of the delicate movements of the tongue tip. This may explain why, in cases in which tumor resection in the anterior oral cavity in-

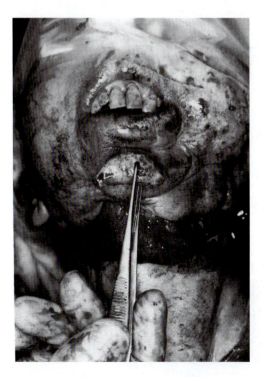

Fig. 1.41 Instillation of irradiated cartilage graft to improve projection of the chin in a patient whose mandibular replacement graft rib was inadequate to produce sufficient mental projection.

volved the removal of only relatively small portions of anterior tongue, the residual impairment of function is markedly out of proportion to the amount of resected tissue.

Clearly enunciated speech requires not only precise muscular coordination but adequate tongue length to contact the other oral articulatory structures, as well as intact sensation to maintain the necessary kinesthetic sense. Often following extensive resections of large tumors, a longitudinal hemisection of the oral tongue is performed. Excellent function is commonly retained because of sufficient residual length and sensation, despite the fact that half of the bulk has been removed.

Marked improvement in speech can be achieved by reconstruction of the anterior tongue with a flap, but the loss of normal lingual sensation and fine movement markedly diminish the potential for perfectly articulated discourse. The success of this reconstruction also depends on the degree of fibrosis incurred during subsequent healing. The forehead flap in the past has been excellent for reconstructing both the anterior tongue and the floor of the mouth. However, the residual cosmetic deformity of the donor site has largely precluded its use.

The pectoralis musculocutaneous flap may be used and is good for restoration of large defects. The flap is usually too large for most hemiglossectomy defects but may be used without the cutaneous component. If a hemimandibular defect is replaced with a reconstruction plate without a bone graft, then the plate may be covered by the muscular flap.

The raw surface of the tongue may be covered with a split-thickness skin graft, but this usually undergoes shrinkage of up to one fourth of its original size. The radial forearm free flap is the best cover for the lingual defect; it provides an excellent lining without shrinkage and can even be made to supply sensation. By anastomosis of the antebrachial cutaneous nerve of the flap to the lingual nerve Urken et al[101] have shown the restoration of touch and two-point discrimination. Whether or not this aids at all in the improvement of deglutition is unproven at this time.

Often the principal limitation to good oral functioning is tethering of the anterior tongue in the floor of the mouth. Lingual release by sharp dissection, followed by lining of the defect with split-skin or dermis is a simple procedure with excellent results. The graft must be initially splinted with either dental rolls or some kind of dental stent for immobilization or fixed into place by multiple "quilting" sutures. When the restriction is more in the form of a band, a simple Z-plasty is all that is required as long as sufficient mobile tissue is present in the lateral oral gutters (**Fig. 1.42**).

Despite vigorous surgical efforts, the ultimate goal of acceptable speech is often not realized. Concentrated speech therapy usually improves the quality of articulation immensely. The surgeon's encouragement of both patient and therapist in their strenuous participation is often rewarded with a surprising degree of success.

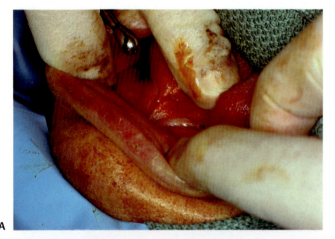

A

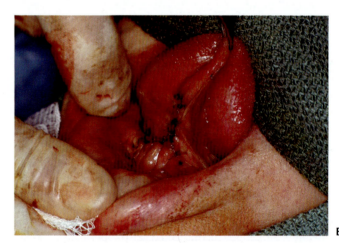

B

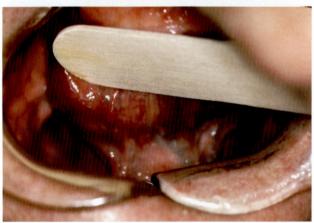

C

Fig. 1.42 (**A**) The tongue is bound to the floor of the mouth by scarring following lingual plate excision of the mandible and partial glossectomy. (**B**) Z-plasty is complete. (**C**) Result 18 months later.

◆ Prosthetic Rehabilitation

In prior years adequate dental rehabilitation was dependant on an alveolar ridge of sufficient height covered in a durable epithelial cover and gingival-buccal and gingival-labial sulci of sufficient depth to retain a dental prosthesis. The innovation of the intraosseous titanium implants by Branemark has revolutionized the oral rehabilitation of these patients. The procedure will be described in more detail in the chapter on prosthetic rehabilitation. The problems related to implantation are those of mandibular bone thickness, bone density, the nature of the epithelium over the alveolar ridge, and whether the patient had been irradiated. Irradiated patients need to have the implants in place for up to 1 year before they can be loaded with the second-stage abutments. The tendency to lose the implanted fixtures because of inadequate bony integration is much more common in irradiated bone. In most cases, an over denture is used rather than a fixed appliance because it is better tolerated, especially when irradiation is employed as part of the therapy.

◆ Management of Massive Lesions

The massive T4 lesion that invades bone, erupts through skin (**Fig. 1.43**), and extends beyond the confines of the oral cavity may present with a distant metastasis or a metabolism that is too fragile to permit a potentially curable resection. Lesions of this magnitude often present with bilateral cervical adenopathy as well, and as a group their prognosis is generally poor. However, a defeatist philosophy in the face of such horrendous tumors should be tempered with the knowledge that a significant number of patients can be cured if an appropriately radical approach is adopted.

The surgeon who is courageous and skilled enough to undertake these heroic procedures must have a thorough knowledge of head and neck anatomy and physiology, as well as an understanding of the biology of these aggressive lesions. The techniques of radical tumor ablation must also be accompanied by considerable skills in reconstructive surgery to achieve a satisfactory result.

Adequate excision in these cases often requires removal of most of the mandible. Many of the patients represent failures of previous resections or irradiation therapy, and winning in these cases can be equated to "playing catch-up football." An extra-wide resection margin is essential to get ahead of a rapidly advancing tumor that has already eluded at least one previous therapist. Postoperative irradiation is of great help in the management of these patients, but it can never be considered a method of shrinking the surgical margins. In general, surgical salvage of radiation failure is a poor concept as a therapeutic plan and should be heartily discouraged because of low survival and high complication rates.

Possibly the best way to illustrate the basic principles involved in the ablation of these large neoplasms, and especially the reconstruction of the extensive residual defects, is with several case examples.

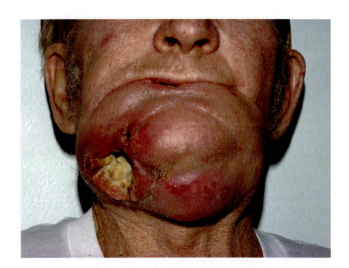

Fig. 1.43 Massive oral cavity carcinoma that began as a primary tumor in the lip and then extended through bone and fistulized through the skin.

Case 1 (Fig. 1.44–Fig. 1.48, pp. 32–34)

The patient depicted in the radiograph (**Fig. 1.44A**) had a metastasis from an unknown primary tumor. This massive tumor, measuring ~15 cm in diameter, deeply invaded the bone and penetrated the skin. A generous excision of mandible and overlying skin with a bilateral neck dissection was required for adequate excision (**Fig. 1.44B**).

Resections in these cases usually require a full-thickness excision from skin to mucosa, including intervening bone. Cutaneous excision in penetrating lesions should include a 3 to 4 cm margin of uninvolved skin. This is because of the frequent tendency of rapid tumor spread in the subepithelial plane once skin involvement occurs.

As previously mentioned, tumor spread through cortical bone is slow but progresses rapidly once the medullary cavity of the mandible is reached. In this patient, the tumor had extensive medullary involvement, and resection from one condyle to the opposing ramus was necessary. The tongue and floor of the mouth could be spared because of their lack of involvement. The resected tissue was reconstructed with a deltopectoral flap (**Fig. 1.44C**).

This patient was lost to follow-up for 2 years. When he was finally located, his hideous countenance, oral incompetence (**Fig. 1.45**), and unintelligible speech had made him a socially unacceptable recluse. His own self-image was so severely affected that he tucked his head into his chest and hid the lower third of his face from view by a Styrofoam coffee cup fastened in place by an attached elastic band that was slung around his head. This posture, combined with soft tissue contractures of his neck, resulted in a permanent cervical flexion deformity.

His rehabilitation began with correction of the flexion contracture in his neck. This was accomplished by effacing the cervical webs, using multiple Z-plasties, and then manipulating his cervical spine under general anesthesia once bone ankylosis had been ruled out. He was immobilized in the upright position with a halo brace (**Fig. 1.46**). The next stage was to supply a large flap of soft tissue to provide a bed for the installation of a bone graft. A pectoralis major musculocutaneous flap was selected because it would supply more than adequate skin coverage and would also provide the necessary muscle bulk to augment the deficient chin and anterior neck (**Figs. 1.47A,B,C**).

An incision was made at the junction of the previously transposed deltopectoral flap and the residual chin skin. Skin flaps were developed so that a raw area of sufficient dimension was created to accept the flap. An important principle in reconstructing these cases, and one absolutely vital to their success, is to provide an excess of tissue in the flap. Touch-up trimming of a superfluous flap can always be done once all the reconstructive steps have been completed. The disaster of being caught short of tissue in the middle of reconstruction thwarts any hope of a successful functional or cosmetic result. In this particular instance, concern regarding pressure on the flap pedicle precluded its subcutaneous placement. The hollowed supraclavicular aspect of the previously dissected neck posed such an acute angulation with the clavicle that the nutrient arteries and the pectoral branch of the thoracoacromial artery would likely be severely compromised. The flap was rotated into position extracutaneously and the pedicle tubed. The pedicle was returned 3 weeks later.

Mandibular reconstruction posed several serious problems. The amount of graft material necessary eliminated the possibility of an osseous or osteocutaneous free flap. There were no available recipient veins in the neck for a free flap, and interposition vein grafts in our hands have had a limited degree of success. Resections that stretch from one mandibular condyle to the opposite angle leave little hope for functional restoration; however, bone grafting can give some projection to the chin and, by supporting the tongue and floor of the mouth, assist in oral continence. It was elected to use two ribs, notch their posterior cortical surfaces to make them malleable, and skewer them with Kirschner wires. The Kirschner wires, in addition to skewering the two grafts together, lent them some stability and helped to anchor one bend into the mandibular ramus. They were bent into a horseshoe shape to reproduce the arch configuration of the mandible. Although the temporomandibular joint, mandibular ramus, and body of the mandible have been adequately restored by Obwegeser[102] in congenital anomalies, such attempts in cancer patients are generally futile. Reconstruction of a temporomandibular joint in this patient was not attempted. The distal end of the graft was inserted into a fibrous tissue pocket, which was tunneled into the area roughly corresponding to the site of the opposing mandibular angle.

The patient was tumor free for almost 6 years, had oral continence, was free of his nasogastric and tracheotomy tubes, and had understandable speech (**Fig. 1.48**). He unfortunately succumbed to a lymphoma 6 years postoperatively.

Case 2 (Fig. 1.49–Fig. 1.51, pp. 34–36)

Primary tumors of the buccal mucosa (**Fig. 1.49**) often require through-and-through excision. When internal and external linings are required for closure, the use of a musculocutaneous flap with a deepithelialized bridge can be employed. The young woman in **Fig. 1.50** had a resection for an adenocarcinoma of the buccal mucosa that was fixed to skin and close to the anterior maxillary periosteum. The excision included the anterior wall of the maxillary sinus with preservation of the sinus mucoperiosteum. In addition, the oral commissure and lateral upper lip were removed to achieve a satisfactory margin. The upper lip was reconstructed with an Estlander flap (**Fig. 1.50A**).[103] A sternocleidomastoid musculocutaneous flap was constructed with its skin paddle bifurcated by a narrow, transverse, deepithelialized bridge (**Fig. 1.50B**). A wider margin of muscle than skin is included in the flap to compensate for the soft tissue resection extending under the facial skin.

The Difficult Case in Head and Neck Cancer Surgery

The flap is tunneled under the skin and the donor defect closed primarily (**Fig. 1.50C**). The distal end of the flap is folded into the mouth to replace the excised mucosa. Muscle is sutured under the skin to the soft tissue, and cutaneous closure is done. **Figure 1.51** illustrates the final result after scar revision. She was tumor free, able to speak and swallow normally, but suffered from depression. She was followed for 5 years and then lost to follow-up.

Case 3 (Fig. 1.52–Fig. 1.63, pp. 36–40)

This patient was a 22-year-old Haitian female who had a history of a slow-growing mass in the left mandible for 9 years. She complained of malocclusion and an obvious deformity. On examination, she had a massive tumor that had invaded the left hemimandible and crossed over the symphysis to the right parasymphyseal area (**Fig. 1.52A,B**). The tumor bulged the buccal mucosa on the left (**Fig. 1.52C**) and could be palpated up along the lateral wall of the maxilla. Her teeth were in remarkably good shape as a result of chewing raw sugarcane, a common practice in her homeland. CT scanning revealed replacement of two thirds of the mandible by an invasive tumor (**Fig. 1.53A**) that produced a thin honeycombed appearance (**Fig. 1.53B**) on three-dimensional reconstruction. A fine needle aspiration cytology revealed a diagnosis of ameloblastoma. Prior to resection, a tracheotomy was done and a nasogastric tube was inserted. The surgical approach was through an extended Risdon incision combined with splitting the lower lip (**Fig. 1.54**). Skin and soft tissue were attenuated but not invaded by tumor. The periosteum, although greatly expanded, had no neoplasm that penetrated through to the overlying soft tissue (**Fig. 1.55A**). The gingival incision intraorally encompassed the teeth of the affected mandible. The tumor attenuated the overlying masseter and superiorly the buccinator but, as mentioned, was limited by the periosteum. The buccal mucosa was not invaded (**Fig. 1.55B**). The tumor was seen to extend alongside and indented the lateral maxillary sinus wall but did not invade it (**Fig. 1.56**). The mandible was disarticulated at the left temporomandibular joint (**Fig. 1.57**) and transected at the level of the left midbody (**Fig. 1.58**). The diagnosis was ameloblastoma (**Fig. 1.59**).

A fibular free flap was harvested from the leg (**Fig. 1.60**). The curve of the mandible was duplicated with a reconstruction plate, and a series of osteotomies were performed to produce a mandibular arch (**Fig. 1.61**). The anterior peroneal artery and vein were anastomosed to the lingual artery and external jugular vein. The graft was fixed to the right mandibular body with three locking screws through the reconstruction plate (**Fig. 1.62A**), and the wound was closed (**Fig. 1.62B**).

The patient suffered some facial swelling for about 6 weeks but otherwise had an uneventful recovery. On 2-year follow-up, she was tumor free and had an excellent contour to her jaw and good function (**Fig. 1.63**).

Case 4 (Fig. 1.64–Fig. 1.67, pp. 41–42)

A 65-year-old male had a history for almost 2 years of a painful ulcer in the mouth that became erosive through his lower lip and chin over the past 1 month. He had lost 10 pounds of weight and was a heavy smoker and drinker. On examination, he had an extensive endophytic, ulcerative lesion in the anterior floor of the mouth and extensive invasion of his anterior tongue (**Fig. 1.64**). The tumor eroded through the mandible, and there was widespread involvement of the chin (**Fig. 1.64A,B**). Palpation of the neck revealed a 3 cm diameter lymph node in the right submandibular area and a 1 cm diameter node in the posterior triangle of the left neck.

His chest x-ray was clear, and liver function studies were within the normal range. A biopsy of the intraoral lesion revealed squamous cell carcinoma. Panendoscopic examination revealed no other primary tumors.

Surgical resection involved taking a 4 cm margin of healthy skin surrounding palpable tumor. This has been found to be necessary to encompass the widespread microscopic disease, sometimes even in the dermal lymphatics, that is common when skin is penetrated by underlying upper aerodigestive tract squamous cell carcinoma. The inferior aspect of the skin incision extended into the upper neck and became the horizontal limb connecting the two lateral lazy-S incisions made to do the bilateral neck dissection (**Fig. 1.65A,B**).

Following the bilateral neck dissections, the lower third of the face was resected (**Fig. 1.65D**). This included a considerable portion of the anterior tongue and the mandible from angle to angle (**Fig. 1.66A,B**).

The wound was closed with a large pectoralis major musculocutaneous flap (**Fig. 1.67**). The mandibular reconstruction was delayed because of his poor general condition. He underwent a full course of irradiation therapy and remained tumor free up to his death 1 year later from a myocardial infarction. Although his residual deformity was considerable, he declined further surgery to have his mandible reconstructed. He maintained a cheery and positive demeanor up to the time of his death from cardiac disease. It is notable that his girlfriend drove him to his follow-up appointments.

Case 5 (Fig. 1.68, p. 42)

It is wise to remember that not all reconstructive efforts are successful. The patient in **Fig. 1.68** required a bilateral radical neck dissection, an angle-to-angle mandibular resection, and a skin excision that involved the removal of a third of the upper lip, the entire lower lip, the skin of the lower third of the face, the inferior third of the tongue, and the larynx. The defect was covered with a pectoralis major musculocutaneous flap containing an area of ~400 cm^2 of skin. The flap was inserted through a wide subcutaneous tunnel. It remained healthy for ~26 hours and then became dusky in color. By the time the neck skin bridging the pedicle was incised, most of the flap's circulation was lost, and ~70% of the skin and muscle sloughed (**Fig. 1.68**). The marked edema of the face and neck skin resulted from ligation of both jugular veins as well as the extensive dissection and had squeezed off the circulation in the flap's nutritional supply. The flap may have been saved by extracutaneous positioning of the pedicle at the time of surgery or by vigilance in the early morning hours of the second postoperative day. The patient subsequently underwent debridement and had a skin graft performed. He underwent postoperative irradiation but died, tumor free, 6 months later of a myocardial infarction.

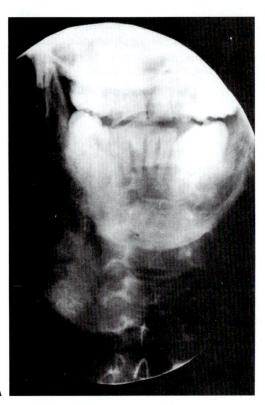

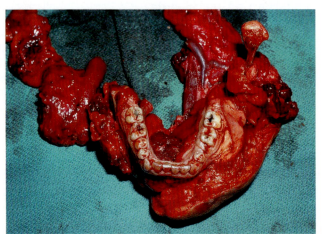

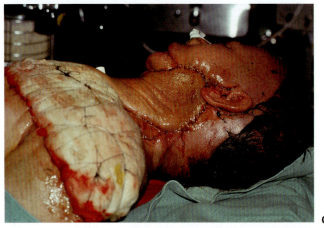

Fig. 1.44 *Case 1* (**A**) X-ray of a middle-aged patient with massive metastatic carcinoma from an unknown primary tumor that involved the skin of the chin and lateral neck in a mass that was approximately half the diameter of the patient's head. Soft tissue detail reveals the size of the mass, and the radiograph shows extensive mandibular erosion. (**B**) Resection included bilateral radical neck dissection and mandibular excision from the left condyle to the right angle. The tongue was spared, but the skin of the left chin and neck was included in the specimen. (**C**) Deltopectoral flap used to cover the defect.

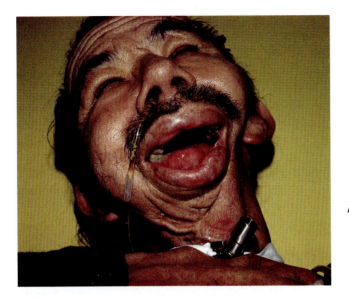

Fig. 1.45 *Case 1* Grotesque visage results from inadequate soft tissue replacement and lack of bony support.

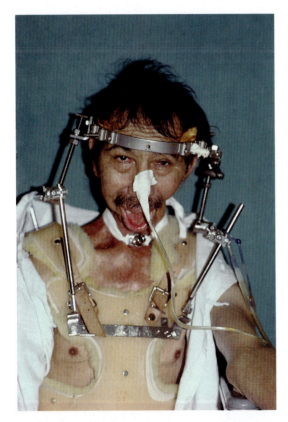

Fig. 1.46 *Case 1* Initial step in rehabilitation is the straightening of the patient's spine following multiple Z-plasties in the neck to alleviate soft tissue contracture. A halo brace maintains head position.

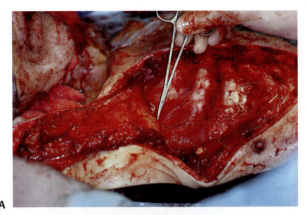

A

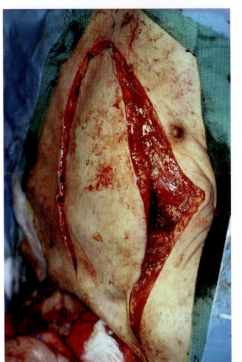

B

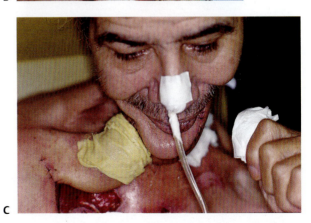

C

Fig. 1.47 *Case 1* Reconstruction of the chin and anterior neck is begun by the use of a pectoralis major myocutaneous flap. (**A**) Flap incised. (**B**) Flap raised; hemostat points to vascular pedicle. (**C**) Flap is rotated into position and placed outside the usual skin bridge to avoid compromising the pedicle of this massive flap by its compression between the lower cervical skin and the underlying clavicle.

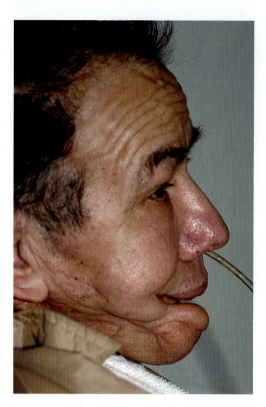

Fig. 1.48 *Case 1* Patient shown 6 months after the instillation of two tandem rib grafts extending from right to left mandibular angles. Nasogastric and tracheotomy tubes were eventually discontinued.

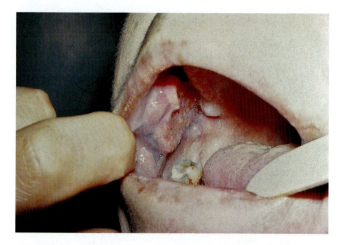

Fig. 1.49 *Case 2* Extensive carcinoma of the buccal mucosa.

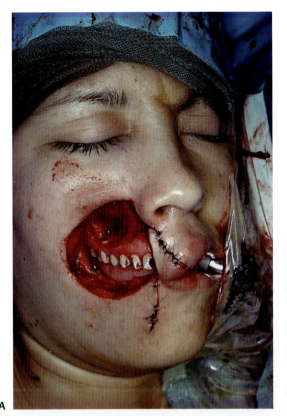

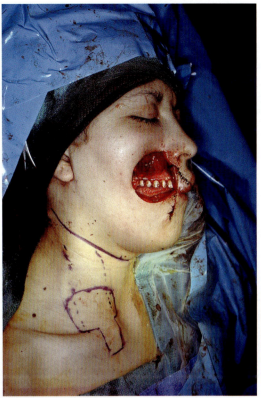

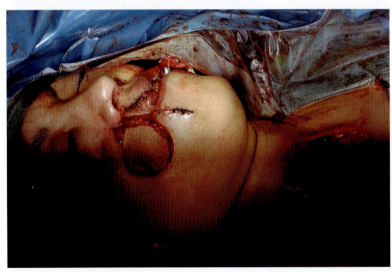

Fig. 1.50 *Case 2* Young woman with adenocarcinoma of the buccal mucosa requiring through-and-through excision. (**A**) Surgical defect following Estlander reconstruction of the right lateral mouth and commissure. (**B**) Sternocleidomastoid island flap marked out on the skin. Note the inferior paddle extending over the clavicle. A thin strip of epithelium is excised between the paddle and the flap proper. (**C**) The flap is tunneled under a skin bridge and inserted into the defect. The paddle is turned into the oral cavity to provide lining.

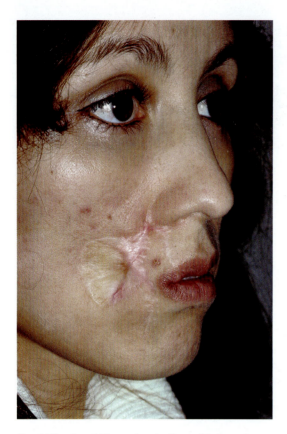

Fig. 1.51 *Case 2* The patient in Figure 50, 2 years postoperatively, following scar revision.

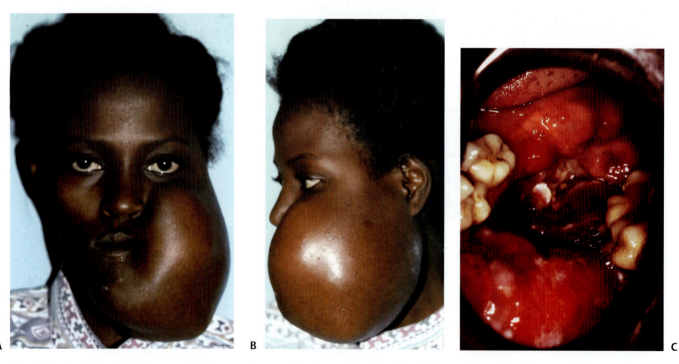

A   B   C

Fig. 1.52 *Case 3* Young Haitian woman with a massive ameloblastoma of the mandible. (**A**) Frontal view. (**B**) Lateral view. (**C**) Intraoral view showing submucosal tumor. Note excellent status of dentition, although in severe malocclusion.

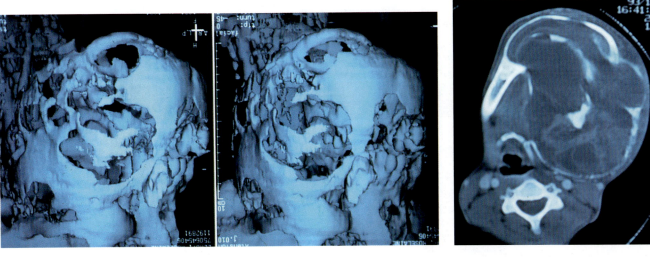

Fig. 1.53 *Case 3* (**A**) Computed tomographic (CT) scan illustrating marked bone erosion caused by ameloblastoma. (**B**) Three-dimensional reconstruction of CT scan showing honeycomb pattern of bone erosion.

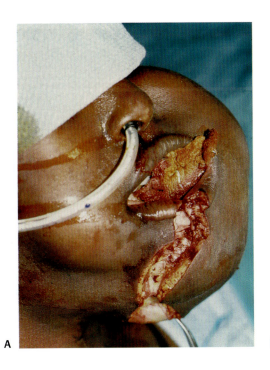

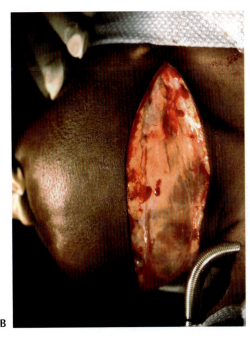

Fig. 1.54 *Case 3* Surgical incision. (**A**) Lip and chin incision. (**B**) Cervical incision.

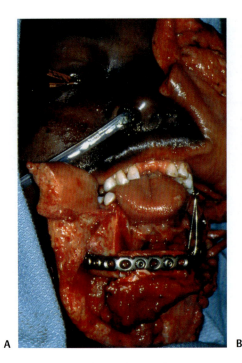

A

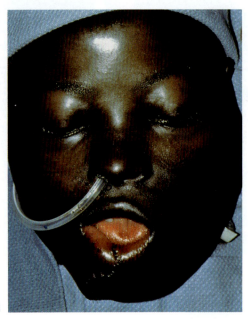

B

Fig. 1.62 *Case 3* (**A**) Free flap placed and (**B**) wound closed.

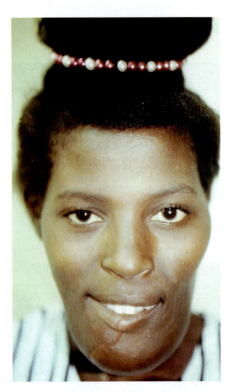

Fig. 1.63 *Case 3* Patient 2 years postoperative, tumor free, and with excellent function.

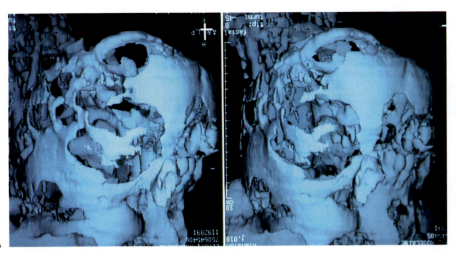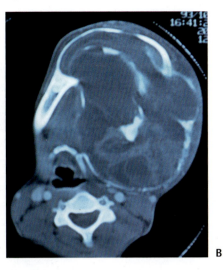

Fig. 1.53 *Case 3* (**A**) Computed tomographic (CT) scan illustrating marked bone erosion caused by ameloblastoma. (**B**) Three-dimensional reconstruction of CT scan showing honeycomb pattern of bone erosion.

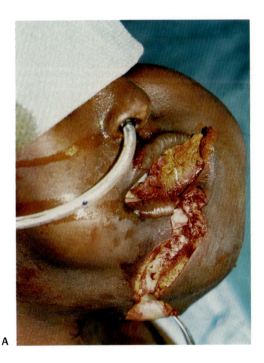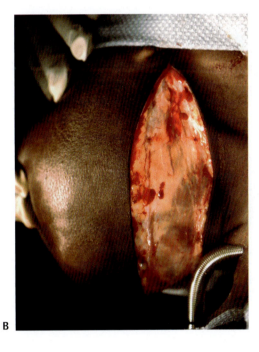

Fig. 1.54 *Case 3* Surgical incision. (**A**) Lip and chin incision. (**B**) Cervical incision.

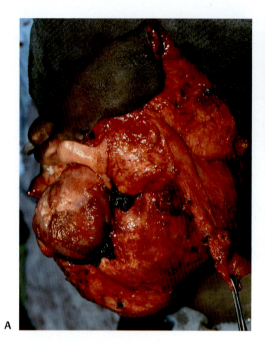

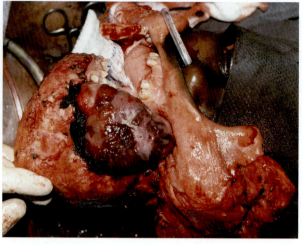

Fig. 1.55 *Case 3* (**A**) Tumor exposed. (**B**) Intraoral extent of tumor. No invasion of buccal mucosa seen.

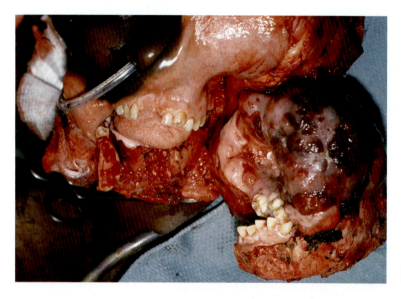

Fig. 1.56 *Case 3* Tumor indenting but not invading the lateral wall of the maxillary sinus.

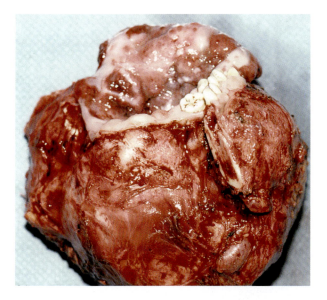

Fig. 1.57 *Case 3* Mandibular resection.

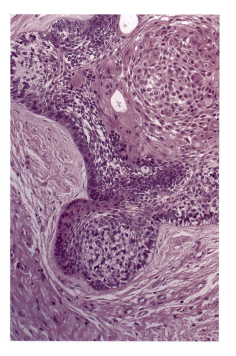

Fig. 1.59 *Case 3* Histological appearance of ameloblastoma (H&E ×200). (Photo courtesy of Regina Gandour-Edwards, M.D., Department of Pathology, University of California, Davis.)

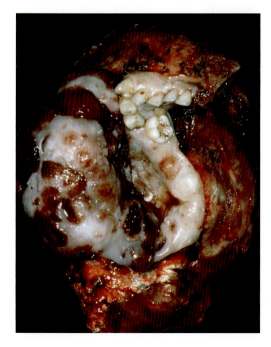

Fig. 1.58 *Case 3* Resected specimen from the mandibular condyle to the anterior body of the mandible on the opposite side.

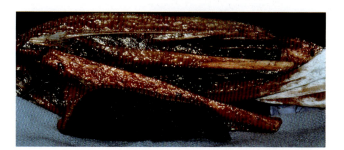

Fig. 1.60 *Case 3* Fibular free flap being harvested. (Photo courtesy of Thomas Stevenson, M.D., Division of Plastic Surgery, University of California, Davis.)

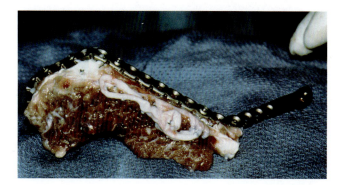

Fig. 1.61 *Case 3* Osteotomies created to reproduce the arch of the mandible and fixed to a contoured reconstruction plate.

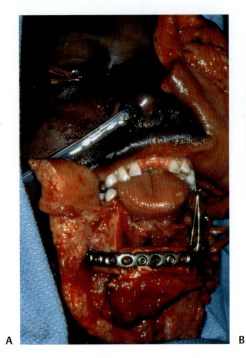

A

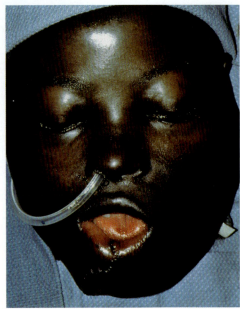

B

Fig. 1.62 *Case 3* (**A**) Free flap placed and (**B**) wound closed.

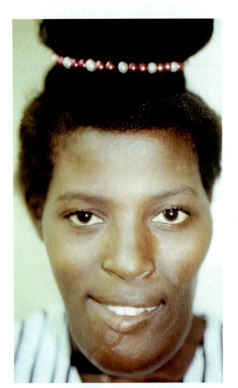

Fig. 1.63 *Case 3* Patient 2 years postoperative, tumor free, and with excellent function.

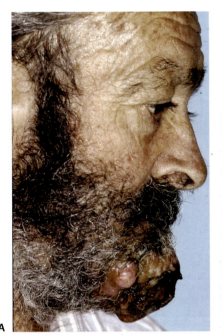

Fig. 1.64 *Case 4* Middle-aged man with extensive floor of mouth carcinoma. (**A**) Tumor penetrating through the chin. (**B**) Intraoral view.

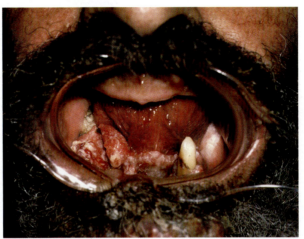

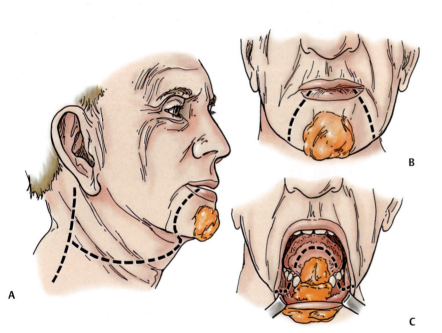

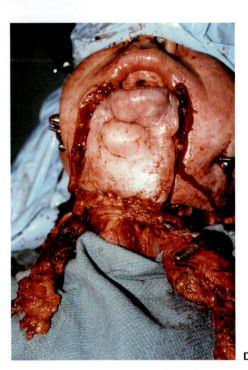

Fig. 1.65 *Case 4* Extent of incisions outlining resection. (**A**) Lateral view. (**B**) Frontal view. (**C**) Resection of lower third of the face including the lip, chin, anterior tongue, and mandibular arch. (**D**) Cut patient.

Fig. 1.66 *Case 4* Resection completed. (**A**) Surgical specimen. (**B**) Defect.

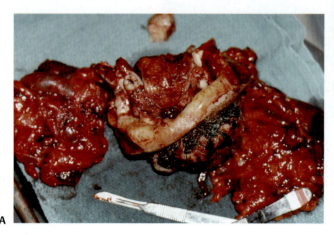

A

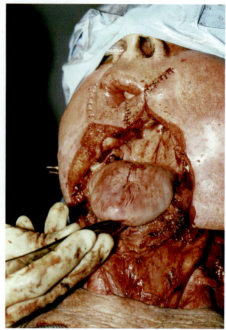

B

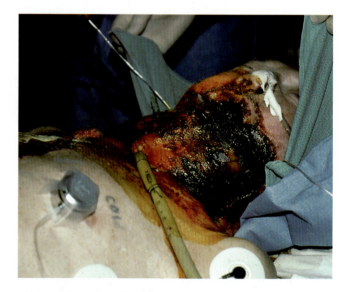

Fig. 1.68 *Case 5* Slough of the major portion of a large (400 cm²) pectoralis major myocutaneous flap used to cover defect from the oral commissures to the skin of the clavicles. Patient subsequently healed and had postoperative radiation therapy but died in his home of a myocardial infarction 6 months later.

Fig. 1.67 *Case 4* Wound closed with large pectoralis major musculocutaneous flap with a biphase appliance maintaining the mandibular fragments in good position for later reconstruction.

References

1. Landis SH, Murray T, Bolden S, Wingo PA. Cancer statistics. CA Cancer J Clin 1999;49:8–31

2. Sellars SL. Epidemiology of oral cancer. Otolaryngol Clin North Am 1979;12:45–55

3. Conley J, ed. Concepts in Head and Neck Surgery. New York: Grune & Stratton; 1970:99

4. Lederman M. The anatomy of cancer. J Laryngol Otol 1964;78:181–208

5. Moore C, Catlin D. Anatomic origins and locations of oral cancer. Am J Surg 1967;114:510–513

6. Trieger N, Shipp II, Taylor GW, et al. Cirrhosis and other predisposing factors in carcinoma of the tongue. Cancer 1958;11:357–362

7. Gorlin RJ, Vickers RA. In: Anderson WAD, ed. Pathology. 6th ed. St. Louis: CV Mosby; 1971:1084

8. Chretien PB. The effects of smoking on immunocompetence. Laryngoscope 1978;88(1 Pt 2, Suppl 8):11–13

9. Palmer DL. Alcohol consumption and cellular immunocompetence. Laryngoscope 1978;88(1 Pt 2, Suppl 8):13–176

10. Lundy J, Raaf JH, Deakins S, et al. The acute and chronic effects of alcohol in the human immune system. Surg Gynecol Obstet 1975;141:212–218

11. Donald PJ. Marijuana smoking: possible cause of head and neck carcinoma in young patients. Otolaryngol Head Neck Surg 1986;94:517–521

12. Nehas GG. Psychoactive drugs and immune response. Presented at Drugs of Abuse and Immune Response Symposium, Clearwater, FL, December 13–15, 1990

13. Molin LJ, Deng D, Shi SB, Gandour-Edwards R, Donald PJ, Gumerlock PH. The identification of marijuana-induced p53 mutations in head and neck carcinomas. In preparation.

14. Waldron CA, Shafer WG. Leukoplakia revisited. Cancer 1975;36:1386–1392

15. Shafer WG, Waldron CA. Erythroplakia of the oral cavity. Cancer 1975;36:1021–1028

16. Moschella SL, Hurley HJ. Dermatology. Vol 2. 2nd ed. Philadelphia: WB Saunders; 1985:1860

17. Pindborg JJ. Atlas of Diseases of the Oral Mucosa. 4th ed. Philadelphia: WB Saunders; 1985:254–256

18. Strong EW. Carcinoma of the tongue. Otolaryngol Clin North Am 1979;12:107–114

19. DiTroia JF. Nodal metastases in carcinoma of the oral cavity. Otolaryngol Clin North Am 1972;5:333–342

20. Batsakis JG. Tumors of the Head and Neck: Clinical and Pathological Considerations. Baltimore: Williams & Wilkins; 1974:86–111

21. Lyall D, Schetlin CF. Cancer of the tongue. Ann Surg 1952;135:489–496

22. Kreinen AJ. The case for elective (prophylactic) neck dissection. In: Conley J, ed. Cancer of the Head and Neck. Washington DC: Butterworths; 1967:183–185

23. Southwick HW, Slaughter DP, Trevino ET. Elective neck dissection for intraoral cancer. Arch Surg 1960;80:905–909

24. Sako K, Pradier RN, Marchetta FC, et al. Fallibility of palpation in the diagnosis of metastases to cervical nodes. Surg Gynecol Obstet 1964;118:989–990

25. Ward GE, Edgerton MT, Chambers RG, et al. Cancer of the oral cavity and pharynx and results of treatment by means of the composite operation (in continuity with radical neck dissection). Ann Surg 1959;150:202

26. Skolnik EM, Saberman MN. Cancer of the tongue. Otolaryngol Clin North Am 1969;2:603–615

27. Fries R, Platz H, Wagner RR, et al. Carcinoma of the oral cavity: on the prognostic significance of the primary tumor site (by organs) in the oral cavity. J Maxillofac Surg 1980;8:25–37

28. Litton WB, Krause CJ. Surgical management of carcinoma of the oral cavity. Otolaryngol Clin North Am 1972;5:303–320

29. Vidic B, Melloni BJ. Applied anatomy of the oral cavity and related structures. Otolaryngol Clin North Am 1979;12:3–14

30. Cady B, Catlin D. Epidermoid carcinoma of the gum. Cancer 1969;23:551–569

31. Waldron CA. Oral epithelial tumors. In: Gorlin RI, Goldman HM, eds. Thoma's Oral Pathology. 6th ed. Vol 2. St. Louis: CV Mosby; 1970:834

32. Sharp GS, Wood RC. Treatment of cancer of the gums. J Oral Surg 1950;8:185–203

33. Renner GJ, Zitsch RP. Cancer of the lip. In: Myers EN, Suen JY, eds. Cancer of the Head and Neck. 3rd ed. Philadelphia: WB Saunders; 1999:294–360

34. Baker SR, Krause CJ. Carcinoma of the lip. Laryngoscope 1980;90:19–277356766

35. McGregor IA, McGregor JM. Floor of mouth. In: McGregor IA, McGregor JM, eds. Cancer of the Mouth and Face. Edinburgh: Churchill Livingstone; 1986:442–446

36. Schuller DE. Cancer of the oral cavity. SIPac. American Academy of Otolaryngology; 1980

37. Suarez O. El problema de las metastasis linfaticas y alejadas del cancer de laringe e hipofaringe. Rev Otorrinolaringol 1963;23:83–99

38. Medina JR, Byers RM. Suprahyoid neck dissection: rationale, indications, and surgical technique. Head Neck 1989;11:111–122

39. Gavilan J, Gavilan C, Herranz J. Functional neck dissection: three decades of controversy. Ann Otol Rhinol Laryngol 1992;101:339–341

40. Meyers EN. Management of Neck Metastasis. The Wullstein Lecture. Guest of Honor Address, Combined American Academy of Otolaryngology and German Society of Otolaryngology, Mannheim, Germany, May 2006

41. Diaz FL, Kligerman J, Matos de Sa G, et al. Elective neck dissection versus observation policy. In: Annual Meeting of the American Academy of Otolaryngology–Head and Neck Surgery; September 24–27, 1999, New Orleans, LA

42. Gilbert EH, Goffinet DR, Bagshaw MA. Carcinoma of the oral tongue and floor of the mouth: 15 years experience with linear accelerator treatment. Cancer 1974;35:1517–1524

43. Berthelsen A, Hansen HS, Rygard J. Radiation therapy of squamous carcinoma of the floor of the mouth and the lower alveolar ridge. J Laryngol Otol 1977;91:489–499

44. Pierquin B, Chassagne D, Cox JD. Toward consistent local control of certain malignant tumors. Radiology 1971;99:661–667

45. Fu KK, Chan EK, Phillips TL, et al. Time, dose, and volume factors in carcinoma of the oral tongue. Radiology 1976;119:209–213

46. Delclos L, Lindburg R, Fletcher GH. Squamous cell carcinoma of the oral tongue and floor of the mouth. AJR Am J Roentgenol 1976;126:223

47. Donald PJ. Conservation therapy for oral cavity carcinoma. Trans Pac Coast Otoophthalmol Soc Annu Meet 1977;58:111–124

48. Schramm VL, Myers EN, Sigler BA. Surgical management of early epidermoid carcinoma of the anterior floor of the mouth. Laryngoscope 1980;90:207–215

49. Krause CJ, Lee JG, McCabe BF. Carcinoma of the oral cavity: a comparison of therapeutic modalities. Arch Otolaryngol 1973;97:354–358

50. LaFerriere KA, Sessions DG, Thawley SE, et al. Composite resection for oral cavity and oropharyngeal cancer. Arch Otolaryngol 1980;106:103–110

51. Donald PJ. Complications of combined therapy in head and neck carcinoma. Arch Otolaryngol 1978;104:329–332

52. Snow JB, Gelber RD, Kramer S. Randomized preoperative and postoperative radiation therapy for patients with carcinoma of the head and neck: preliminary report. Laryngoscope 1980;90:930–945

53. Lore JM. An Atlas of Head and Neck Surgery. 2nd ed. Vol 2. Philadelphia: WB Saunders; 1973:506–509

54. Spiessl B, Tschopp HM. Surgery of the jaws in head and neck surgery, face, and facial skull. In: Naumann HH, ed. Head and Neck Surgery. Vol 2. Philadelphia: WB Saunders; 1980:149–154

55. Barbosa JF. Surgical Treatment of Head and Neck Tumors. San Francisco: Grune & Stratton; 1974:93–104

56. Freund HR. Principles of Head and Neck Surgery. 2nd ed. New York: Appleton-Century-Crofts; 1979:152–175

57. Bertotti JA. Trapezius-musculocutaneous island flap in the repair of major head and neck cancer. Plast Reconstr Surg 1980;65:16–21

58. Ariyan S. One-stage reconstruction for defects of the mouth using a sternomastoid myocutaneous flap. Plast Reconstr Surg 1979;63:618

59. Sasaki CT. The sternocleidomastoid myocutaneous flap. Arch Otolaryngol 1980;106:74–76

60. Ariyan S. The pectoralis major musculocutaneous flap. Plast Reconstr Surg 1979;63:73–81

61. Marchetta FC, Sako K, Babillo J. Periosteal lymphatics of the mandible and intraoral carcinoma. Am J Surg 1964;108:505–507

62. Marchetta FC, Sako K, Murphy JB. The periosteum of the mandible and intraoral carcinoma. Am J Surg 1971;122:711–713

63. Polya SJ, Narratel D. Experiments on lymph ducts of the buccal mucous membranes. Orvostud ertek gyujt magy orz. Arch Budapest v.f. III:4885, 1902.

64. Cunningham MP, Slaughter DP. A face-saving procedure: marginal resection of the mandible for anterior oral cavity cancer. Ill Med J 1968;133:166–169

65. Byars LT. Extent of mandibular resection required for treatment of oral cancer. Arch Surg 1955;70:914–922

66. Ossoff RH, Bytell DE, Hast MH, et al. Lymphatics of the floor of the mouth and periosteum. Presented at Research Forum, American Academy of Otolaryngology, 1978

67. Ossoff RH, Sisson GA. Lymphatics of the floor of the mouth and periosteum. Otolaryngol Head Neck Surg 1980;88:652

68. Som ML, Nussbaum M. Marginal resection of the mandible with reconstruction by tongue flap for carcinoma of the floor of the mouth. Am J Surg 1971;121:679–683

69. McGregor IA. "Quilted" skin grafting in the mouth. Br J Plast Surg 1975;28:100–102

70. Keim WF, Lowenberg S. Marginal mandibulectomy in the treatment of carcinoma of the floor of the mouth. Laryngoscope 1970;80:1566–1579

71. King GD. Transoral resections for carcinoma of the oral cavity. Otolaryngol Clin North Am 1972;5:321–325

72. Goss CM, ed. Gray's Anatomy of the Human Body. 29th ed. Philadelphia: Lea & Febiger; 1976:383–386

73. Bratcher GO. Personal communication, 1979

74. Karapandzic M. Innervated myocutaneous arterial flap in lip reconstruction. Transactions of the Third International Symposium on Plastic and Reconstructive Surgery, New Orleans, 1980

75. Norante JD, McCabe BF. Fascial sling suspension of the chin following resection of the anterior mandible. Laryngoscope 1973;83:336–346

76. Strong EB, Rubinstein B. Mandible reconstruction with a resorbable alloplastic bone tray. Otolaryngology Head and Neck Surgery Journal 2003;129:417–426

77. DeFries HO, Marble HB, Sell KW. Reconstruction of the mandible: use of a homograft combined with autogenous bone and marrow. Arch Otolaryngol 1971;93:426–432

78. Cantrell RW. Personal communication, 1976

79. Cummings CW, Leipzig B. Replacement of tumor-involved mandible by cryosurgically devitalized autograft. Arch Otolaryngol 1980;106:252–254

80. Popescu V, Spirescu IE. Bone resection, extracorporeal cryotherapy and immediate reimplantation in the treatment of mandibular tumors. J Maxillofac Surg 1980;8:8–16

81. Panje WJ. Personal communication, 1980

82. Haymaker R. Symposium on Head and Neck Cancer: Principles of Reconstruction. Cincinnati, June 17–19, 1982

83. Haymaker R. Personal communication, 1982

84. Taylor GI, Miller DH, Ham FJ. The free vascularized bone graft: a clinical extension of microvascular techniques. Plast Reconstr Surg 1975;55:533–544

85. Urken ML, Cheny ML, Sullivan ML, Biller HF. Atlas of Regional and Free Flaps for Head and Neck Reconstruction. New York: Raven Press; 1995

86. Conley J. Regional Flaps of the Head and Neck. Stuttgart: Thieme; 1976, pp 247–266

87. Conley J. Use of composite flaps containing bone for major repairs in the head and neck. Plast Reconstr Surg 1972;49:522–526

88. Conley J, Cinelli PB, Johnson PM, et al. Investigation of bone changes in composite flaps after transfer to the head and neck region. Plast Reconstr Surg 1973;51:658–661

89. Brookes M, Elkin AC, Harrison RG, et al. A new concept of capillary circulation in bone cortex: some clinical applications. Lancet 1961;1:1078–1082

90. Brookes M, Harrison RG. The vascularization of the rabbit femur and tibiofibula. J Anat 1957;19:61–72

91. Medgyesi S. Observations on pedicle grafts in goats. Scand J Plast Reconstr Surg 1972;7:110–115

92. Snyder CC, Bateman JM, Davis CW, et al. Mandibulofacial restoration with live osteocutaneous flaps. Plast Reconstr Surg 1970;45:14

93. Cuono CB, Ariyan S. Immediate reconstruction of a composite mandibular defect with a regional osteomusculocutaneous flap. Plast Reconstr Surg 1980;65:477–484

94. Ostrup LT, Fredrickson JM. Reconstruction of mandibular defects after radiation using a free living bone graft transferred by microvascular anastomosis. Plast Reconstr Surg 1975;55:563–572

95. Panje W, Cutting C. Trapezius osteomyocutaneous island flap for reconstruction of the anterior floor of the mouth and mandible. Head Neck Surg 1980;3:66–71

96. McCraw JB, Arnold PG, eds. McCraw and Arnold's Atlas of Muscle and Musculocutaneous Flaps. Norfolk: Hampton Press; 1986:60

97. Ariyan S. The viability of rib grafts transplanted with the periosteal blood supply. Plast Reconstr Surg 1980;65:140–151

98. Ostrup LT, Fredrickson JM. Reconstruction of mandibular defects after irradiation using a free living bone graft transferred by microvascular anastomoses. Plast Reconstr Surg, 1975;55:563

99. Taylor GI, Miller GDH, Ham FJ. The Free Vascularized Bone Graft. A Clinical Extension of Microvascular Techniques. Plast Reconstr Surg, 1974;54:274.

100. Fredrickson JM. Free flap reconstruction of the head and neck. Submitted to Otolaryngol Head Neck Surg, September 1999

101. Urken ML, Weinberg H, Vickery C, et al. The combined sensate forearm free and iliac crest free flaps for reconstruction of significant glossectomy-mandibulectomy defects. Laryngoscope 1992;102:543–558

102. Obwegeser HL. Advances in reconstructive maxillofacial surgery. Presented at the Third International Symposium of Facial Plastic Surgeons, New Orleans, 1979

103. Estlander JA. Méthode d'autoplastie de la joue ou d'une lèvre par un lambeau emprunté à l' autre lèvre. Rev Mens Med Chir 1877;1:344–356

2

Cancer of the Oropharynx and Tongue Base

Paul J. Donald

In the decades prior to modern surgical and radiotherapeutic techniques, tumors of the oropharynx and tongue base had a dismal prognosis, the only exceptions being small tonsillar or tongue lesions that were usually picked up incidentally on examination. The patient was usually doomed to early recurrence. Today, however, newer, more radical surgical procedures, especially when combined with radiation therapy, have vastly improved the situation, making many of these patients surgically salvageable. There is currently a great deal of interest in "organ sparing" protocols utilizing various combinations of chemotherapy and irradiation in an attempt to avoid radical surgery in the responders. The early results have produced mixed reviews, and only the test of time will prove their efficacy. My own experience with poor survival results and frequent complications when attempting surgical salvage on patients who have failed such treatment at other institutions has encouraged me to continue with my philosophy of radical surgery followed by full-course radiation therapy until more definitive data emerge proving the efficacy of such strategies.

◆ Anatomy

The inferior anatomical boundary of the oropharynx is somewhat obscure. *Gray's Anatomy*[1] describes this limit to be the hyoid bone, which is about level with the depths of the valleculae. Some clinical textbooks[2-4] agree with this definition, whereas others[5,6] place the inferior border at the tip of the epiglottis. This leaves uncertain the locale of the base of the tongue. By one definition, only that area adjacent to the circumvallate papillae would be included, whereas by the other, the entire tongue base would be oropharyngeal in location. This problem frequently makes unclear survival statistics quoted for patients with tumors in this region. Discussions of oropharyngeal tumors often refer only to tumors of the tonsil, soft palate, and pharyngeal walls. The base of the tongue is frequently an orphan.

In this chapter, the areas of surgical management will include not only the aforementioned areas and the tongue base but also the retromolar trigone area. The *retromolar trigone* (see chapter 1, Fig. 1.5), in a strict anatomical sense, resides in the oral cavity. However, because of its proximity to the mandibular ramus and anterior tonsillar pillar, as well as the biological similarity of its tumors to those of the tonsillar region, it is included in the discussion of the management of oropharyngeal cancer. Retromolar tumors (**Fig. 2.1**) are particularly

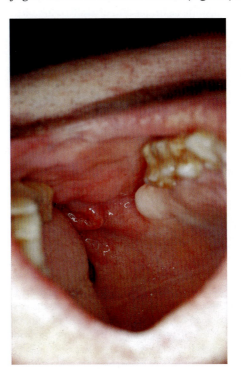

Fig. 2.1 Squamous cell carcinoma of the retromolar trigone. Despite combined therapy with preoperative irradiation, this man died of local recurrence in the pterygoid muscles and distant metastatic disease.

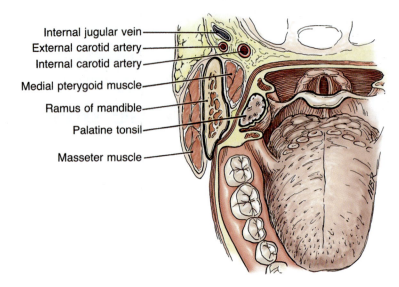

Internal jugular vein
External carotid artery
Internal carotid artery
Medial pterygoid muscle
Ramus of mandible
Palatine tonsil
Masseter muscle

Fig. 2.2 Proximity of the tonsil to the inner surface of the mandibular ramus.

aggressive locally and have high metastatic rates similar to those of the anterior tonsillar pillar and soft palate.

The *pharynx* is a muscular tube suspended from the skull base. It opens anteriorly to the nose in its superior or nasopharyngeal portion and to the oral cavity in its middle or oropharyngeal part. The inferior border of the nasopharynx—thus the superior limit of the oropharynx—is clearly established at the level of the soft palate.

The *tonsillar fossa* is separated from the medial surface of the mandibular ramus by a thin sheet of superior constrictor muscle and some scant fat and areolar tissue of the lateral pharyngeal space (**Fig. 2.2**). Tumors of the fossa are frequently endophytic. Invasion and attachment to bone can occur early in the course of the disease. Early detection of this phenomenon radiographically is difficult. Computed tomographic (CT) scanning and magnetic resonance imaging (MRI) show evidence of bone invasion only when the lesions are advanced. The MRI is especially sensitive to showing invasion of the marrow space, but in lesions this deeply erosive, the detection can usually be made clinically. CT scans show proximity to bone but not early cortical invasion.

As progression is made posteriorly around the lateral aspect of the oropharynx, the *posterior pharyngeal wall* appears to be a simple structure composed of mucosa, submucosa, pharyngobasilar fascia, superior constrictor muscle, and overlying buccopharyngeal fascia.[7] Loose areolar tissue is contained in a potential space between the buccopharyngeal fascia and the thick prevertebral fascia. This loose connective tissue permits the easy gliding movement of the pharynx and cervical viscera over the cervical spine required by normal activity. It is a common experience to see extensive mucosal, submucosal, and muscular involvement of the posterior oropharyngeal wall with cancer, but no penetration of the buccopharyngeal fascia. The hardiness of this layer in resisting the penetration of malignant cells allows for an exception to the 2 cm resection rule. Although a minimum margin of 2 cm of healthy tissue is required for adequate resection of mucosal disease in the pharynx, a free dissection plane between the prevertebral and buccopharyngeal fascial

layers almost always ensures a tumor-free plane. This is seen even in tumors with deep muscular penetration. However, once the tumor has transgressed the prevertebral space, it penetrates the paraspinous muscles and becomes fixed to the vertebral bodies of the cervical spine.

◆ Clinical Pathological Behavior and Survival

By far the most common malignancy in the oropharyngeal region is squamous cell carcinoma.[8] These tumors may be exophytic and bulky (**Fig. 2.3**) or deeply infiltrating and ulcerating (**Fig. 2.4**). Occasionally, we see a tumor described as "superficially invasive" (**Fig. 2.5**). The grossly innocuous appearance of these sinister lesions must not tempt the surgeon to tailor a more conservative approach. The frequent finding of deeply extending chords of tumor cells in these cases dooms conservative measures to certain failure.

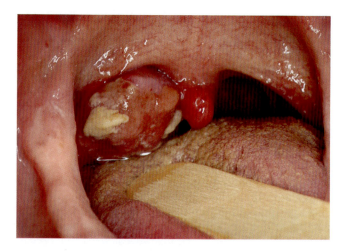

Fig. 2.3 Large, bulky, squamous cell carcinoma of the tonsil.

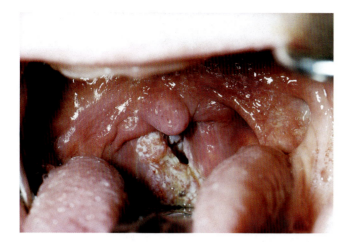

Fig. 2.4 Endophytic ulcerative cancer of the posterior pharyngeal wall eroding into the cervical spine.

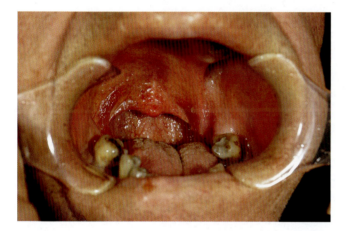

Fig. 2.5 Carcinoma of the left tonsillar fossa of the "superficially invasive" variety.

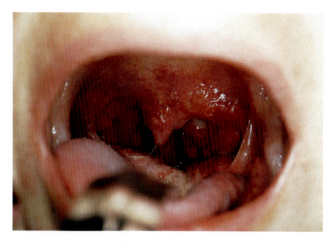

Fig. 2.6 Epidermoid cancer of the tonsillar fossa and anterior pillar extending onto the soft palate and maxillary tuberosity. Lesion is surrounded by a brilliant scarlet-colored arc of Queyrat erythroplasia.

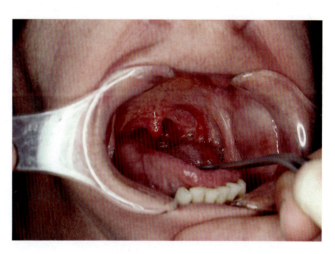

Fig. 2.7 Lymphoma of the left lateral pharyngeal wall.

Many of these lesions in the faucial-palatine arch are surrounded by an area of Queyrat erythroplasia (**Fig. 2.6**). As mentioned in the preceding chapter, these regions harbor numerous foci of carcinoma in situ and microinvasive cancer. Multifocal cancer and "field cancerization" seen in the oral cavity continue to be problems in the oropharynx.

The lymphocytic aggregations of the ring of Waldeyer may become a source of lymphoma (**Fig. 2.7**). In a compendium of several series reported by Parkhill,[8] analysis of 416 malignancies of the palatine tonsil revealed 47, or 11.3%, to be malignant lymphoma. If the unusual Mayo Clinic experience is extracted from these data (27 out of 64 of their cases being lymphoma), the incidence of lymphoma in the remaining 352 is 5.7%. In general, the male incidence slightly exceeded that of the female, and the average age at diagnosis was 59 years. Following the palatine tonsil, the nasopharynx is the next most common site, with the lingual tonsil and the pharyngeal lymphoid aggregations being the least frequently involved. Accompanying cervical lymph nodal disease is common. In a large series of lymphomas involving the Waldeyer

ring, Banfi et al[9] reported 62.3% with cervical lymph node involvement. Only 22.5% of the entire group of patients had lymphoma limited exclusively to the pharyngeal arch. In 74 of the 225 patients, lower limb angiography was done, and 44.6% were found to have lymph node involvement outside the cervical area. Lymphoid malignancy in the head and neck is usually a manifestation of a systemic disease. This is especially true in Hodgkin disease.[10] Surgery is rarely the method of choice for control in these disorders. The pathologist occasionally experiences considerable difficulty in differentiating between a so-called anaplastic carcinoma and lymphoma. A high index of suspicion must be maintained in such patients, and further studies, such as the identification of cell surface markers and cytogenetics, may be required to establish the diagnosis (**Fig. 2.8**).

The incidence of cervical lymph node metastases is high in oropharyngeal cancer. Toomey[11] quotes an overall figure of 50 to 75%, and Lindberg[12] cites 60 to 80% for cervical metastases from oropharyngeal carcinoma. Truluck and Putney[13]

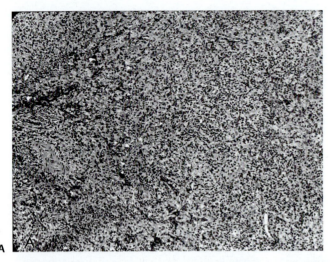

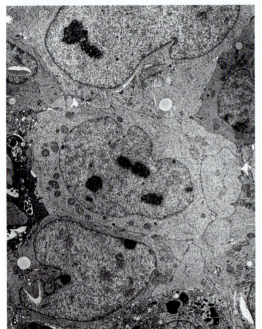

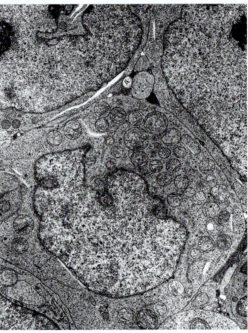

Fig. 2.8 (**A**) Photomicrograph of lymphoma of the tonsil that was initially diagnosed as anaplastic carcinoma (H&E ×110). (**B**) Electron micrograph showing three adjacent lymphocytic cells. There is a very primitive, diffusely distributed chromatin pattern with prominent nucleoli. The cytoplasm contains only scattered endoplasmic reticulum (×8250). (**C**) Higher-power magnification electron micrograph showing a single cell possessing very primitive cytoplasm and nucleus. Some nuclear pores are seen adjacent to the nucleus. There are no modifications of the cytoplasmic membranes such as desmosomes that would characterize squamous cells (×13,800). (**Figs. 2.8B** and **C** are used courtesy of Dr. R. D. Cardiff, Department of Pathology, University of California, Davis.)

in 1971 reported on 168 cases of tumors in the tonsil, tongue base, and hypopharynx. Of the patients with tongue base lesions, 66% had cervical metastases, whereas 56.3% of those with tonsillar lesions had cervical spread. Civantos and Goodwin[14] reported a 66 to 76% incidence of neck nodal metastases in their review of tonsillar carcinoma with a 22% incidence of contralateral involvement. They found a 60% incidence of clinically positive nodes in carcinoma affecting the tongue base, with 20% of patients presenting with bilateral involvement. The majority of their cases that were either T3 or T4 by staging had either manifest or occult metastases in the neck. Wang[15] quotes a 33 incidence of secondary tumors in 124 patients with anterior tonsillar pillar and retromolar trigone lesions. In T3 lesions of the area, the metastatic rate rose to 43% in his series. Quenelle et al[16] reported a 55% metastatic rate in tonsillar fossa carcinoma in a series of 58 patients, whereas Edström et al[17] found cervical metastases

in 27 of 37 patients (73%) with tonsil tumors. When the tumor crosses the palatine arch or invades the tongue, contralateral metastases are seen in 10 to 20% of cases.[12,18] Aijax, in his series from the University of Pittsburgh,[19] saw a 39% incidence of nodal involvement in retromolar trigone lesions with occult disease in another 10 to 20%.

Cancers involving the base of the tongue are frequently poorly differentiated, extend rapidly among the muscle bundles of the structure, and often remain occult until a substantial size is reached. Cervical metastases are common. In an article by Ogura et al[20] discussing the utility of elective neck dissection, it was reported that of 42 patients with cancer of the base of the tongue, 25 (59%) had lymph node metastases. Bilateral disease was present in eight of 42 patients, or 19.1%. Out of a group of 102 patients with base-of-tongue carcinoma described by Whicker et al[21] 56 patients had metastatic disease in the neck, and seven patients (6.8%)

had bilateral disease. Strong[22] reported a 76.5% incidence of unilateral cervical involvement and a 22.8% incidence of bilateral disease in his series of 136. Skolnik et al[23] report that cervical metastases to the ipsilateral lymph nodes occur in 40 to 60% of cases, and to the contralateral nodes in 5% of cases. Wang[15] lumps together retromolar trigone lesions and anterior faucial pillar lesions. He found an overall cervical metastatic rate of 33% and emphasized the locally aggressive nature of these lesions. Infiltration into the adjacent tongue is common with these lesions and caused a precipitous drop in survival rate in his series when radiation was used as the principal therapeutic modality.

◆ Oropharyngeal and Tongue Base Cancers

Tonsillar Carcinoma

In a more recent review of the Sloan Kettering experience Kraus et al[24] noted that 62% of 100 patients with tongue base carcinoma had clinically positive lymph nodes in the neck, of which 55 cases were histologically positive. In 27 cases that had elective neck dissections there were 13 whose histological examination showed the presence of metastatic cancer, for an overall true incidence of metastatic modal disease of 50%. Survival rates in carcinoma of the tonsil are, as expected, relative to the size of the tumor and the extent of metastatic disease. Treatment of larger lesions needs to be tailored according to the site of lesion and tumor extent and to the needs and requirements of the individual. Until the 1960s, the primary modality of therapy for oropharyngeal lesions was irradiation therapy. Surgery alone was popular for awhile, and then combined surgery and irradiation especially for advanced lesions was invoked. Currently, clinical trials are being conducted utilizing organ-sparing protocols that involve various combinations of chemotherapy and irradiation therapy. In the author's experience, radiation therapy for small primary lesions in the T1 size range is very close in efficacy to surgery. Lesions from 2 to 4 cm have a modest cure rate with irradiation but have better results with surgery. Currently, the gold standard for T3 and T4 lesions is combined therapy using radical surgery followed by postoperative irradiation.

Because the theme of the book is management of the difficult case, the focus will be on the management of the T3 and, especially, the T4 lesions. The most difficult cases of all are those who have failed irradiation or combined irradiation/chemotherapy protocol. Survival results in the latter group are poor and the complication rate is high. Not only is the complication rate high but these complications are often devastating in extent and slow to heal. For limited lesions of the tonsillar fossa that have not approximated the inner surface of the mandible, transoral laser excision with microscopic control is simple and highly efficacious. The margin of healthy tissue can be seen to be normal under the microscope, and this is reaffirmed by frozen section control. Mounting and labeling the specimen for the pathologist in a clearly understood, nonambiguous manner is essential for successful establishment of tumor-free margins.

One of the larger series of tonsillar tumors treated by radiotherapy has been published by Wang.[15] He followed 124 patients with lesions of the anterior pillar and retromolar trigone, one third of whom had metastases to cervical lymph nodes. His 3-year disease-free survival rate was 36%. In those patients who had T3 lesions, the survival rate dropped to 20%. Furthermore, in any tumor that encroached on the tongue, the survival was only 28%. There were no survivors among the patients who had bilateral lymph node metastases or in those whose nodes were fixed. Of the 79 failures, 30 were eligible for surgical salvage, and 21 (70%) of these survived disease free for 3 years. It is important to note that, because only 38% of the patients were eligible for surgical salvage, the *overall* surgical salvage rate was only 27%.

There is little doubt that the T1 lesion of the tonsil itself responds well to radiotherapy. In an analysis of 201 tonsillar fossa lesions by the same author, 85% of patients with T1 lesions had a disease-free 3-year survival. A series of 125 tonsillar lesions at the University of Iowa reviewed by Krause[25] demonstrated a 5-year determinant survival rate of 75% for T1N0 lesions when radiotherapy was the modality employed. These figures have been unimproved upon in more recent reports as exemplified in the report by Jackson et al.[26] However, in Krause's series, the survival rate fell to 25% when the lesion became T1N1. In the Iowa group, 94 patients with all varieties of T and N lesions had primary radiotherapy; 49% were alive without disease at 3 years, and 39% at 5 years.

There is a general agreement that some form of combination therapy is best for management of lesions that extend beyond the confines of the tonsillar fossa, involve the base of the tongue, or present with cervical adenopathy. Wang[15] recommends this modality in all large oropharyngeal lesions, although he presents no results. In the Iowa series,[27] there was a 67% 2-year survival rate among 36 patients. The data of Snow and coworkers,[28] who compared the efficacy of preoperative and postoperative irradiation, are inconclusive and show survival rates for both at 18 months to be around 65%. Our own experience using postoperative combined therapy shows about the same results. Hinerman and his colleagues at the University of Florida[29] report a series of 134 patients treated by either external beam irradiation therapy alone or in combination with neck dissection. The local control rates were 90% for T1, 73% for T3, and 35% for T4 tumors. At 5 years the probability of survival in all groups was 44%. One must remember that this survival rate is based on an *estimated value* calculated from a statistical prediction and not the actual counting of real patients who were alive after the prescribed period of 5 years. Our local control rates are in the range of 85 to 90%, and the attrition rate is mainly due to intercurrent disease, distant metastasis, and second primary tumors.

Although Wang speaks optimistically about the surgical salvage of patients who fail to be cured with irradiation, others report grim statistics in their attempts at salvage surgery. In one study, of 21 patients who had failed to be cured by irradiation, 12 had tumors in the tonsillar fossa, four had disease of the anterior pillar, and five had tumors primarily in the base of the tongue. Following an attempt at salvage surgery, 48% died of their disease and 43% died of complications. More than 50% of the original group died of locally recurrent disease. A similarly dismal experience is cited by Schleuning and Summers,[30] in the management of tongue base carcinoma. Radiotherapy was employed in 79 such tumors, with only 10 cures. Surgical salvage was successful in only 13 (18.8%) of the 69 patients with locally recurrent disease. In more recent years there has arisen an interest in combined neoadjuvant chemotherapy in combination with radiation therapy for primary treatment of advanced tumors of the oropharynx. In a meta-analysis of this form of primary treatment by the working group of the Federation Nationale des Centres de Lutte Contre le Cancer in France,[31] they found no evidence of efficacy of this therapeutic approach compared with the standard approaches using surgery and postoperative radiation therapy.

Del Campo et al from Barcelona[32] conducted a phase 2 trial in which they used simultaneous chemotherapy and radiation therapy as a preoperative regimen in patients with oral cavity and oropharyngeal cancer that were deemed inoperable. The irradiation was given as a split course; half preoperatively and half postoperatively. In this cohort of 40 patients, 30 were located in the oral cavity and 10 in the oropharynx. Of the oral cavity tumors, five were in the retromolar trigone area and two were located in the soft palate. The criteria for inoperability were unclear, but statements defining inoperability, such as, the tumor was "fixed to a bone structure in the region" and "was fixed to a lymph node," describe tumors that would clearly not be inoperable in many institutions. Thirty-two of the 40 patients subsequently underwent surgery; four patients refused surgery, and four others were still considered inoperable. A complete response (CR) to preoperative treatment was 52%, and partial response (PR) was 37%. At surgery no pathological evidence of tumor was seen in 12 of the 14 CR patients. Survival with an average follow-up of 21 months yields a 71% rate for those with a CR and 55% for those with a PR. This very interesting study raises some key issues. Did the resection margins include the original tumor volume plus a projected margin of healthy tissue? How many patients recurred locally and/or in the neck? What was the time from resection to the first detection of local recurrence? The follow-up on these patients is far too short to say anything definitive about treatment efficacy. This is unfortunately one of the major problems involving giving adequate informed consent to our patients, who are currently being given a choice between a chemotherapy–radiation therapy protocol based on preliminary data and standard surgical excision followed by full-course radiation, which has an established efficacy over many years. The veiled promise that surgical salvage of those individuals who fail chemoradiation will produce similar results as those who undergo standard therapy is irresponsible.

An article by Pfister et al[33] outlines in detail the management of 33 patients with advanced oropharyngeal cancer who underwent an attempt at organ salvage by various combinations of chemotherapy and irradiation therapy. Of the original 33, 26 were able to complete the course, two patients died secondary to the chemotherapy regimen, and another died no evidence of disease (NED) 1 month following treatment. Of the seven who did not complete the initial course of chemotherapy nothing is mentioned of their even-

tual survival. Of the 26 who completed treatment, 20 eventually died over an 8.5-year period, and many within months of the completion of therapy. One died of a second primary in the lung and two of a disease likely related to the chemotherapy. It is presumed that the 20 were out of the 26 and not out of the original 33. It appears that in the final analysis four patients died secondary to the effects of chemotherapy and 15 died of local disease. The overall determinant survival was 6/20 or 30%. Presuming that the seven that did not complete treatment also died (which may not be a fair assumption) the determinant survival then would be 6/40 or 18%.

It is important to keep in mind that 50 to 60% of patients with appropriately radical surgery, which may require total laryngectomy and partial, but rarely total, glossectomy, plus timely postoperative radiation therapy will survive disease free for at least 5 years. Moreover, they will have an almost nonexistent intraoperative and extremely low postoperative mortality rate. The price in mortality against the hope of organ and life preservation must be carefully weighed.

Carcinoma of the Base of the Tongue

Patients with tumors of the tongue base have a notoriously poor survival rate. Occult spread beyond the palpable limits of the tumor; frequent neck metastasis occurring, often bilaterally; and a relatively high incidence of distant metastases combine to yield a poor prognosis. A large series of oral cavity lesions reported by Trible included 58 patients with tongue base cancer.[34] Several different treatment modalities were used, and the overall 5-year survival was 27.6%. Of the 16 survivors, seven were treated with radiotherapy, seven by surgery alone, and two with planned combined therapy. Unfortunately, no specific data were given representing how many total patients were treated by each specific modality.

Truluck and Putney[13] analyzed 36 patients with tongue base carcinoma. Combined therapy using preoperative irradiation was employed in 18 patients, with six (33%) surviving 5 years. Strong[22] presented the results of treating 136 patients with carcinoma of the tongue base. The overall cure rate was 30%, with stage II disease having a 63.6% and stage IV a 21.7% cure rate. Cure was not analyzed according to therapeutic regimen; the recommendation for therapy is either combined irradiation and surgery or triple therapy using cisplatin and bleomycin in combination with the other two modalities. In a review of previously untreated cases with tongue base carcinoma from 1986 to 1996 that were treated at our institution by surgery followed by postoperative radiation therapy 60% were alive and disease free at 2 years. When the surgical salvage cases were included that had been treated by prior radiation or surgery or both and failed, the combined 2-year survival dropped to 47%.[35]

Carcinoma of the Soft Palate

Carcinomas that involve primarily the soft palate produce cervical metastases in an average of one third of cases, with statistics varying from a high of 48.1% reported by Ash[36] to a low of 27% in the series of Russ et al,[37] with other studies yielding rates of 29.2 and 33%.[38,39] Small lesions less than

2 cm in size may be managed equally well by local resection or radiotherapy. Laser resection for smaller lesions of the soft palate, especially the uvula, can be easily done with the handheld CO_2 laser pencil (**Fig. 2.9**). Selected, more com-

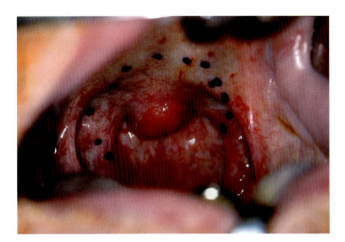

Fig. 2.9 Small soft palate lesion amenable to excision with the pencil laser.

plex lesions are amenable to the laser but are best done with microscopic control. The limitations are bony involvement of the maxilla, mandible, and pterygoid plates, or extension up the eustachian tubes. Larger lesions are probably best managed by combined therapy.[38] In the series of 80 patients studied by Konrad et al,[39] it was curious to note that the survival results of irradiation, surgery, and combined therapy were almost the same (36, 50, and 44%, respectively). The 38 patients followed by Russ and coworkers[37] were treated primarily by radiation, with 33% having a 5-year survival rate. It is astonishing that this should be their recommended modality of treatment when most of their patients succumbed to local recurrences.

Carcinoma of the Pharyngeal Wall

Little statistically significant information is available on the survival rate relative to management techniques in lateral and posterior pharyngeal wall malignancy. Rider in 1962 reported a 9% success rate in controlling lesions of the oropharyngeal walls and 0% when the disease was bilateral.[40] Fletcher et al[41] had a series of 145 patients treated by surgery, radiation, and combinations of the two. The overall 5-year actual survival rate was 41.3%. In the Iowa series of 108 patients,[27] the 5-year determinant survival rate for those treated with irradiation therapy was 35%; with surgery alone, 40%; and with combined therapy using 4500 rads of preoperative irradiation, 67%. The often-encountered pessimistic attitude regarding the prognosis for these patients is probably based on the early experience of individuals such as Rider.

Some controversy exists regarding metastasis to retropharyngeal lymph nodes. The dissections of Lucas de Clercq and Chole,[42] who were investigating the pathophysiology of retropharyngeal abscesses, revealed no definitive lymph node

material in this space in adults. *Gray's Anatomy*[43] describes one to three lymph nodes in the retropharyngeal space, within the buccopharyngeal fascia anterior to the arch of the atlas and draining the mucosa of the nasal area, the nasopharynx, and the eustachian tubes. Gray discusses the passage of lymphatic radicals to the retropharyngeal nodes but does not elaborate on precise number or location. Rouviere[44] found a few small lymph nodes in only one out of every five dissections. The paucity of lymph nodes in the retropharyngeal space and the relative infrequency of metastases to this site from cancers of the oropharynx coupled with the resistance of the fascial envelopes of the pharyngeal musculature to tumor penetration render these lesions eminently resectable. Very few reviews of the results of treatment at this site have been published since the first printing of this book (1984). Thawley et al,[45] in their review of the management of hypopharyngeal tumors printed in 1999, devoted a single paragraph to lesions of the posterior pharyngeal wall. The most recent review they quoted was published in 1988. For those lesions treated by radiotherapy there was a very high incidence of failure in the neck and at the local site. In another report, tumor-free survival rates of 3 to 11% are quoted with radiation therapy alone and 32 to 50% with combined surgery and postoperative radiation therapy.[14] In Spiro et al's series of 78 patients with posterior pharyngeal wall carcinoma the overall disease-free 5-year actuarial survival rate was 32%. Most of the patients in the series had surgery alone, surgery combined with postoperative irradiation, or surgery for irradiation failure. Although the exact percentage was not stated the control rate with radiation therapy was very poor, and they advised surgery and postoperative radiation as their treatment of choice.[46]

Our treatment of choice is wide resection either transorally with the laser under high-power microscopic control for smaller lesions or open resection for the larger ones and reconstruction with a radial forearm or anterolateral thigh free flap.

◆ Surgical Procedures

Transpharyngeal Tongue Base Resection

Occasionally, a tumor that would be amenable to laser therapy cannot be resected by virtue of inadequate exposure with the laryngoscope. Moreover, the extent and depth of penetration make laser resection very difficult to achieve. A common means of resection is via a midline lip splitting incision followed by a midline mandibular split and exposure gained by incising along the gingival lingual sulcus back to the level of the tonsillar base. I have abandoned this approach because of the limited exposure of bulky tumors and the addition of the morbidity of the mandibular and labial split.

The approach I use is well established and nicely described by Moore and Calcaterra.[47] This is by the way of a lateral pharyngotomy. Once the neck dissection is completed, attention is given to the lateral area of the pharynx. The common tendon of the digastric muscle is divided if not already done so as part of the removal of metastatic disease in the neck.

The hypoglossal nerve is dissected throughout its length from its tethering point over the external carotid artery to its early insertion into the tongue musculature deep to the mylohyoid muscle. The occipital artery, which creates this tethering point over the carotid, is clamped and tied. The stylohyoid and stylopharyngeus muscles are transected. Care is taken to avoid cutting the stylopharyngeus, mainly to protect cranial nerve IX that runs on its inferior surface. Inferiorly, the separation of the pharynx from the common carotid is done to the level of the external laryngeal nerve and vessels. This separation creates a complete exposure of the lateral pharynx from the external laryngeal nerve to the stylopharyngeus. Dissection is carried around the lateral curve of the pharynx, separating it from the prevertebral muscles in the prevertebral space. This medial dissection is only carried as far as it is necessary to encompass the tumor.

Entry into the inferior oropharynx is made with cutting cautery between the external laryngeal neurovascular bundle inferiorly and the stylopharyngeus superiorly. A determination is made from the information gleaned at endoscopy to know how far medially into the pharynx this entry is made to have a sufficient resection margin around this lateral aspect of the tumor. Once the opening in the pharynx is made the tongue base neoplasm can be rolled by finger pressure above the hyoid and the tumor extent determined by both direct visualization and palpation. With one blade of the scissors inside the pharyngeal lumen and the other outside the suprahyoid muscles, the inferior tongue base cut is made, often at the level of the vallecula. If tumor is penetrating the hypoepiglottic ligament but is not close to the epiglottis, the preepiglottic space can be resected. Usually, extent beyond this, such as into the thyrohyoid ligament or epiglottis, should have been visible on the preoperative CT scan and a modification such as a supraglottic laryngectomy anticipated. However, if this surprise occurs, the inferior resection can be extended into a supraglottic laryngectomy.

In the usual scenario, the inferior margin of resection can be very easily visualized and the horizontal cut in the vallecula continued medially. If tumor is clearly not penetrating the mylohyoid muscle, this muscle can often be spared to some extent. Once the

medial extent of tumor is reached, the cancer is grasped with a large tenaculum, and the medial vertical and finally the superior horizontal transection completes the encirclement of the tumor.

The exposure in this approach is so good that superior involvement of the tonsil, lateral pharyngeal wall, and even a portion of soft palate can be clearly seen and excised. Frozen section margins are taken. If the initial entry into the pharynx miscalculated tumor extent and a dangerous proximity to the cancer was made at entry, then an additional strip of pharyngeal mucosa and muscle is done.

In most instances, closure is made by advancing the residual tongue muscle into the defect, and primary closure is achieved. This is the best-case scenario for achieving optimal function. A double layer of the residual pharyngeal muscle to the remaining supraglottic musculature provides a second layer.

Total Glossectomy

Total glossectomy is a formidable procedure, but it is the best chance of survival for several patients severely stricken with extensive malignancies of the tongue. The denial of this chance to patients desperate for life, by surgeons who fear the mutilation of such a procedure and then attempt to assuage their conscience by directing such unfortunate patients to other therapeutic modalities that give vain hope for survival, is to be condemned. The curious dichotomy in the minds of some surgeons, who do not hesitate to perform a radical maxillectomy with orbital exenteration and extensive facial skin, but balk at total glossectomy, defies reason.

Recent advances in reconstructive surgery, prosthetics, and speech therapy have greatly improved the rehabilitative potential for these patients. The patient in **Fig. 2.10** had a total glossectomy for a massive lingual malignancy. The larynx was preserved, and protection to the airway was afforded by the replacement of the excised tissue with a deltopectoral flap. Although oral alimentation is impossible without aspiration, the patient does not aspirate her saliva. She takes her meals by the periodic insertion of a nasogastric tube. Her speech is sufficiently articulate, especially with the use of an artificial tongue, to permit her to retain her employment as

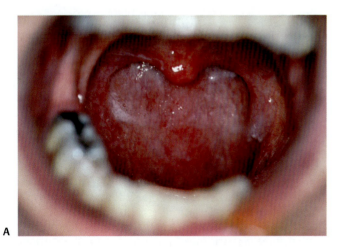
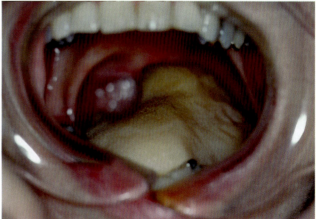

A   B

Fig. 2.10 (**A**) Patient with total glossectomy. (**B**) Prosthetic tongue in place.

an office supervisor, which includes regular communication over the telephone. She was lost to follow-up 10 years postoperatively. The patient in case number 2 had a total glossectomy with laryngeal preservation and was able to swallow some liquids and had understandable speech.

Because of the frequency of cervical metastasis on presentation, the operation is done in continuity with a radical or modified neck dissection. If bilateral nodal disease is present, a simultaneous bilateral neck dissection should be done. A staged neck dissection may be considered, but two factors militate against it. First, cutting the primary specimen from a region of known metastatic disease violates the principle of en bloc dissection and runs the risk of tumor spillage. Second, the delay required between the first and second operations, in addition to the necessary time for healing of the staged neck, may take the patient beyond the "golden period" for postoperative irradiation. The morbidity of simultaneous bilateral neck dissection is considerable, and a good deal of judgment is essential in this situation. In the performance of over 150 simultaneous neck dissections we have had no deaths, but one case of bilateral blindness probably secondary to fluid overload (24 units of crystalloid and blood) and consequent increased intraocular pressure. Transient facial edema and headache are common in most patients.

A modified H incision or an apron flap is used in the skin. We prefer the former. On completion of the neck dissection the primary lesion is approached, with care taken to preserve a connection to the lymphatic drainage route to the neck. Unless at least a 2 cm margin of healthy tissue can be achieved by an incision in the vallecula, the larynx should be taken. A supraglottic laryngectomy has no place in a total glossectomy because continuous aspiration is inevitable.

When the larynx can be spared, the lingual excision begins through an entrance in the vallecula or upper piriform sinus on the side with the least tumor involvement (**Fig. 2.11**). Care must be taken on entering the pharynx to avoid the superior laryngeal nerve and its sensory branch, the internal laryngeal nerve, which after piercing the thyrohyoid membrane courses submucosally through the anterior apex of the piriform sinus. Its sensory innervation to the upper laryngeal mucosa is essential to airway protection. If a laryngectomy is indicated because of direct invasion of this structure or the spread of tumor to the preepiglottic space, a pharyngotomy through the piriform sinus on the side of least involvement is done. The larynx is excised, separating it as high as possible from the remainder of the hypopharynx and preserving a maximal amount of pharyngeal mucosa. As the resection proceeds into the contralateral side of the pharynx, the entire tongue base is displayed, and resection can proceed superiorly (**Fig. 2.12**). In the laryngeal preservation procedure, the tongue musculature is cut from its origins on the hyoid bone and resection proceeds along the lateral pharyngeal gutters (**Fig. 2.13**). In both resections, the line of incision continues from the pharyngeal gutters to the base of the tonsillar fossae. If either tonsillar area is involved with tumor, a tonsillectomy with a margin of 2 cm of healthy mucosa and adjacent muscle is taken in continuity. When the mandibular periosteum is uninvolved it is not necessary to remove any bone. When the periosteum is positive on frozen section a mandib-

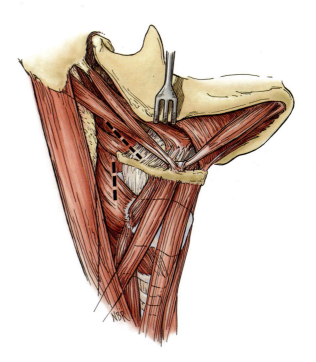

Fig. 2.11 An excision of the tongue base and either total or subtotal glossectomy is approached through an entrance in the vallecula (small upper set of dashed lines) or upper pyriform sinus (long lower set of dashed lines) of least tumor involvement. If a larynx-sparing procedure is to be done, care is taken to avoid injury to the superior laryngeal nerve.

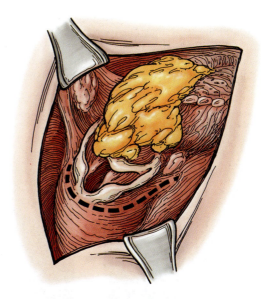

Fig. 2.12 When the resection cannot spare the larynx, the hypopharyngeal mucosa (see dashed lines) is maximally preserved. The trachea is excised at the first ring and the procedure proceeds superiorly.

ular splitting procedure may be done. If there is any evidence of cortical invasion then a partial mandibulectomy is performed on that side. Similarly, when tumor extends into the oral tongue and involves adjacent mandible, the bone must be sacrificed. If the malignancy spares the mucosa of the

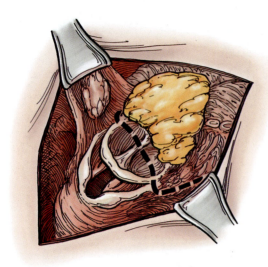

Fig. 2.13 In the larynx-sparing procedure, an incision is made in the depths of the vallecula (see dashed lines) and along the superior border of the hyoid bone. The lesion is cleared by a 2 to 3 cm margin of healthy tissue.

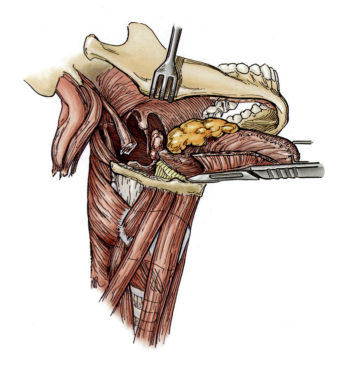

Fig. 2.14 Outline of oral and tonsillar portion of resection of subtotal glossectomy when the tumor spares some anterior tongue.

floor of the mouth, resection proceeds along the reflection of the mucosa onto the lingual aspect of the mandible (**Fig. 2.14**). Whenever possible, a small cuff of oral floor mucosa is preserved to aid in closure. A cuff of lingual gingiva may be raised to improve the approximation of tissues. In instances when only a narrow margin of fixed gingiva remains and the patient's dentition is intact, sutures that pass through this tissue and around the teeth may anchor the reconstructive flap into position. As the oral incisions are made, great care must be taken to incise through the entire thickness of the mylohyoid, taking the underlying anterior bellies of the di-

gastrics so that the superficial margin of excision here is the platysma (**Fig. 2.14**).

Once the tumor is removed, the defect is assessed and the method of reconstruction chosen. Even in patients with a subtotal resection, some form of flap reconstruction is necessary. With total glossectomy a large bulky flap that will substitute for a tongue will best serve the patient (**Fig. 2.15**).

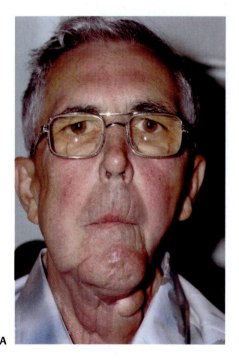

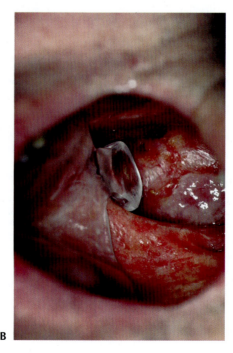

Fig. 2.15 Patient 4.5 years after subtotal glossectomy and partial pharyngectomy. Tongue is replaced with a deltopectoral flap. (**A**) Facial symmetry is aided by flap. (**B**) With the help of an oropharyngeal obturator the patient's speech and swallowing are vastly improved.

A

B

The forehead flap, once the workhorse of oral cavity and oropharyngeal reconstruction, has entirely been supplanted by the myocutaneous and free flaps. A common objection to the use of the myocutaneous flaps in the oral cavity—that of redundant tissue—is a tremendous asset in reconstruction following total glossectomy. One of the major problems in completing the oral phase of swallowing and in articulation during speech is the approximation of the tongue to the palate. If a bulky flap is used to replace lost lingual tissue, approximation of the jaws will permit this important palate-to-flap contact. The pectoralis major flap is most useful here, and inclusion of fat and muscle wide of the skin paddle will add to the flap's bulk. The deltopectoral flap is also suitable (**Fig. 2.16**). This latter, however, carries the major disadvantage of requiring a second procedure to return the pedicle and has been replaced by the radial forearm or anterolateral thigh free flap. The rectus abdominis and even latissimus dorsi free flaps can also be used. However, the pectoralis musculocutaneous flap is quicker and easier to do. Pharyngeal approximation is done in the usual way, with the carotid arteries protected by dermis grafts and the neck wounds closed and drained. Oral closure is done with interrupted absorbable sutures supported by a second running suture of the same material.

Irradiation with a full dose of 6000 to 7010 rads to the primary area and 4500 rads to both necks is given 4 to 6 weeks following surgery. Care is taken to keep the fields high enough on the side of the face, preferably to the zygomatic arches, to include the highest lateral pharyngeal lymph nodes. Bitter experience has taught us that these massive tumors with their proclivity for aggressive cervical metastasis do so even in a retrograde manner. We have seen several cases in which the uppermost part of the neck, containing the parotid gland, was spared from the radiation field for the sake of the patient's comfort, only to have the patient succumb to recurrent tumor in that high nodal region.

Rehabilitation of deglutition following surgery involves careful instruction by the surgeon and the clinical nurse specialist. It is hard to improve upon the excellent review by Myers[48] describing the physiology of normal swallowing and the alterations incurred and adjustments required in the glossectomized patient. In the immediate postoperative period, all patients have a nasogastric or gastrostomy tube and a tracheostomy in place. Once the wounds are healed, attempts at oral alimentation commence. The performance of a generous cricopharyngeal myotomy at the time of surgery often prevents many of the difficulties encountered with pharyngeal pooling. As Meyers so aptly points out, the principal problem in the glossectomized patient is the absence of the "oral hold" phase of swallowing. Ingested material is immediately delivered to the oropharynx and proceeds directly over the insensate flap to the hypopharynx. The material tends to pool in the piriform recesses and spill into the larynx. A myotomy will prevent this "pharyngeal hold" phase of the swallowing sequence. Because effective delivery of ingested material to the pharynx has been precluded by the excision, gravity is the principal force that initiates the movement of the material to the digestive tract. The patient is instructed to "toss the material back" by extending the head back on the neck, which allows the upper digestive conduit to become a straight pipe with the funnel at the top. The patient uses small 10 to 15 mL boluses at first and works from liquids up to semisolids.

The cricopharyngeal myotomy is relatively easy to perform (**Fig. 2.17**). A dull tracheostomy hook is placed around the posterolateral border of the thyroid cartilage and the pharyngeal musculature exposed by retracting the larynx anteromedially. A strip of muscle 3 to 4 mm wide is removed from the posterolateral aspect of the cricopharyngeus and the inferior constrictor. Cutting against an index finger placed through the pharyngotomy will allow the surgeon to incise down to the submucosa without violating the mucosa. Care

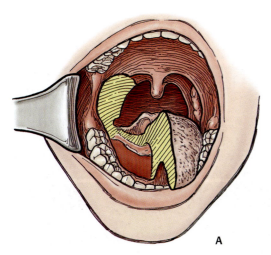

A

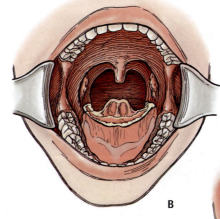

B

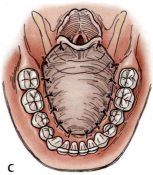

C

Fig. 2.16 (**A**) Resection completed. The deep margin is the platysma of the skin flap. All muscles deep to the tumor are resected. (**B**) Total glossectomy completed in tumors with extensive posterior and anterior lingual involvement. (**C**) Reconstruction with pectoralis major musculocutaneous flap.

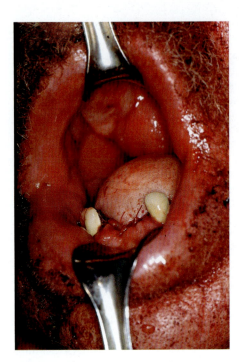

Fig. 2.17 Large pectoralis major musculocutaneous flap reconstruction following total glossectomy.

is taken to excise the muscular strip far enough posteriorly to avoid damage to the recurrent laryngeal nerve on that side.

The laryngectomized patient, of course, need not be concerned about aspiration during swallowing, but is similarly hampered by the loss of whatever lip anesthesia eventuates from the mandibulectomy if it is done. The problem of the immobile and insensate flap in propelling the bolus into the pharynx needs compensation by the artificial tongue prosthesis and the head tilt.

The early introduction of vigorous speech therapy is essential (see chapter 17). It is surprising how good the speech of a totally glossectomized patient can be. If the larynx is taken, however, speech using a trachea-esophageal puncture and speech valve is difficult at best. When total glossectomy is done then total laryngectomy is most often done usually due to the compromised respiratory status of these patients, who have usually been heavy smokers. Even young otherwise healthy patients are in danger of chronic aspiration with total glossectomy and laryngeal preservation. Close supervision in the first postoperative months is mandatory, and recurrent respiratory infections are an absolute indication for laryngectomy. Pharyngeal mucosal sparing, as already mentioned, would aid in subsequent swallowing.

Surgery for Tongue Base and Vallecular Invasion

Carcinoma of the tongue base may invade the vallecula. Past wisdom mandated tongue base resection as well as supraglottic laryngectomy as the necessary steps to effect complete tumor removal. The author has shown that the hyoepiglottic ligament provides a temporary but resistant barrier to the penetration of tumor.[49] Even large tumors of the tongue base at this site (**Fig. 2.18**) can be held out of the preepiglottic space by this structure. Preoperative assessment with MRI will often suggest whether the membrane has been broached and the space entered. This combined with the clinical examination and the findings at direct laryngoscopy will give a firm idea of whether a resection of the preepiglottic space without supraglottic laryngectomy will safely encompass the tumor.

All patients in our series had cervical adenopathy. Our policy in tongue base carcinomas with unilateral metastasis is to perform a radical or modified radical neck dissection on the side of nodal involvement and a selective neck dissection on the opposing side. The tongue base tumor is approached

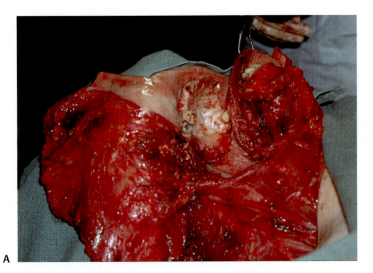

A

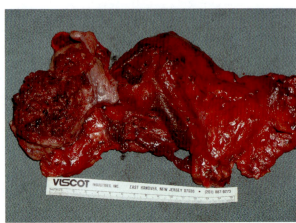

B

Fig. 2.18 (**A**) Large tongue base tumor completely removed with tongue base and preepiglottic space resection. (**B**) Tumor specimen with radical neck dissection.

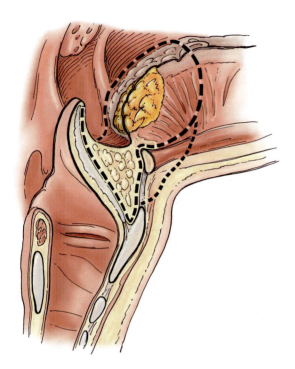

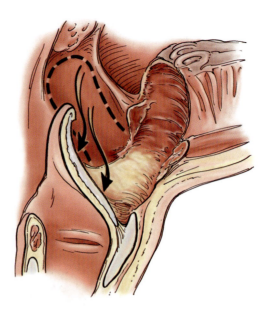

Fig. 2.20 A flap of lateral oropharyngeal wall is transposed over the epiglottic defect.

Fig. 2.19 Resection of tumor is cleared by a margin of at least 2 cm around the neoplasm. The entire preepiglottic space is included, but the epiglottis is left intact. The hyoid bone may be preserved (*long dashed lines*) in more superficially invasive tumors, but is more usually resected (*short dashed lines*).

through a lateral pharyngotomy on the side of least involvement staying away from the tumor by a margin of 2 cm. The incision is carried around from this entrance in the pharynx to along the aryepiglottic fold and over the rim of the epiglottis to the opposite aryepiglottic fold. The epiglottic mucosa is dissected with perichondrium to the base of the preepiglottic space. Gross tumor invasion of the space, especially invasion of the epiglottis, mandates either supraglottic or total laryngectomy, and this more conservative procedure is abandoned. With no gross invasion or minimal penetration of the hyoepiglottic ligament the resection of the fat of

the preepiglottic space proceeds to its inferior apex and then is carried superiorly along the deep surface of the thyrohyoid membrane up to the inner surface of the hyoid bone (**Fig. 2.19**). If the tumor is close or invades the hyoid bone, it is included in the resection. The tongue base tumor along with its minimum of 2 cm of uninvolved tissue is resected in continuity. Once the margins are established by frozen section then the reconstruction can begin.

The denuded epiglottis is covered by a flap of mucosa from the lateral pharyngeal wall pedicled at the level of the aryepiglottic fold incision on the side of greatest tumor involvement. The donor site is closed on itself primarily. The flap is rotated 90 degrees and slightly twisted to the epiglottic rim and the aryepiglottic folds of each side (**Fig. 2.20**). The tongue base is approximated either to the hyoid bone, if present, or the epiglottic base (**Fig. 2.21**).

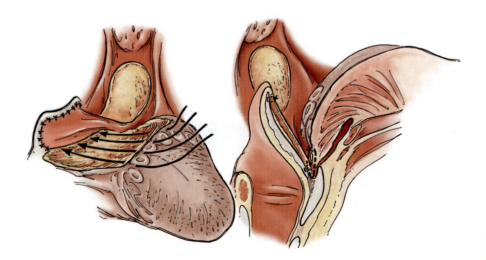

Fig. 2.21 The tongue-base is sutured to the base of the epiglottis to achieve final closure.

Seven patients have undergone this procedure with follow-up from 2 to 13 years. All patients had a full course of post-operative radiation therapy. Most were T4 and all had cervical adenopathy. One patient developed a glottic carcinoma 14 months after his tongue base and preepiglottic space resection, required laryngectomy, and is over 5 years free of disease. All patients are tumor free and alive at this time.

Resection of Tumors of the Lateral and Posterior Pharyngeal Walls

Tumors originating in the region of the lateral and posterior pharyngeal walls have a remarkable inability to penetrate the fascial envelope that encircles the constituent musculature. This factor permits successful resection of tumors in which a 2 cm deep margin cannot be obtained. On the other hand, because of the tendency of these tumors to spread submucosally, a mucosal margin of 2.5 to 3.0 cm is advised when encircling the neoplasm. Small lesions less than 2 cm in diameter are curable by radiotherapy or local excision. Transoral endoscopic laser excision under high power microscopy provides excellent control of margins and resection depth.[50] Closure in these T1 tumors is obtained either by primary approximation or by swinging in a flap of sternocleidomastoid muscle and skin grafting. The defect may even be allowed to granulate in, with epithelialization usually being complete in 3 weeks. This open method, which is also used in the pharyngeal flap operation for velopharyngeal incompetence, is usually less painful than primary approximation.

The excision can be done with the patient's head in the Rose position, the tongue being retracted with a Dingman or other variety of self-retaining mouth gag if the lesion is relatively small, and cautery rather than the laser is to be used to excise the lesion. If laser is to be used the Steiner oropharyngoscope and suspension provides excellent exposure, and the high power setting on the microscope permits safe excision of the tumor.[48] Margins will necessarily be wider than those will be when this technique is used in the larynx. In my experience this technique is suitable for smaller lesions of T1 and T2 size; however, those with wider experience feel comfortable in resecting malignancies of larger size (**Fig. 2.22**). Alternatively, exposure can be achieved through a median labial-mandibuloglossotomy (**Fig. 2.23**). The latter approach is discussed in chapter 9.

There is usually extension of the larger tongue base tumors to the lateral pharyngeal wall and the tonsillar fossa. Once the fossa is reached, a hemimandibulectomy is usually necessary. Spread to the soft palate in these cases is common, as is involvement of the nasopharyngeal wall mucosa. Involvement of the eustachian tube torus used to be an absolute contraindication to surgery. At our present stage of knowledge and technical development, however, it is now possible to excise the pharyngeal end of the eustachian tube, drilling away the bone at the apex of the petrous temporal bone and a portion of the clivus to get a satisfactory resection margin. It is important to note that the internal carotid artery is at risk because of its exit at the petrous apex and its subsequent course through the superior half of the foramen lacerum. Therefore, as the surgeon approaches this artery, careful control from below and above is essential.

In most instances, however, control of the tumor margins can be achieved at a level below the eustachian tube. The first step in the procedure must be an exploration of the retropharyngeal space to verify lack of tumor fixation to the anterior longitudinal ligament. The neck dissection is performed and the primary approached through a lateral pharyngotomy incision. This provides excellent access to the tumor, and the resection proceeds, with maintenance of a wide margin of healthy tissue around the neoplasm. Excision is relatively bloodless provided that careful control of the ascending pharyngeal arteries is maintained. Because of the

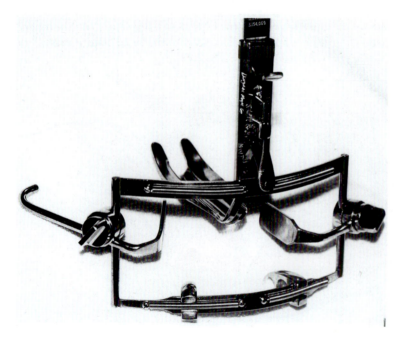

Fig. 2.22 Dingman mouth gag.

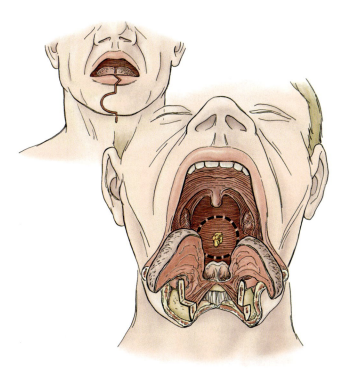

Fig. 2.23 Labiomandibuloglossotomy.

proximity of the carotids, vigilance is necessary throughout the excision as each successive cut is made.

Reconstruction of the pharyngeal defect has undergone a significant evolution during the past 15 years. The trapezius musculocutaneous flap, especially that which is superiorly based, has supplanted the forehead flap in most cases. A one-stage reconstruction can be done that will leave a minimal cosmetic defect (**Fig. 2.24**). In addition, if the tumor extends into the oral cavity and the mandibulectomy extends beyond the angle of the jaw, the muscle bulk now helps to restore the esthetics of the area. Although still a viable alternative, the trapezius flap has largely been abandoned. The jejunal free flap has been good for circumferential defects and can be split along the antimesenteric border to be used when a strip of residual pharyngeal mucosa has been left. The disadvantage of the jejunum is its overproduction of mucous, the friability of the mucosa following postoperative irradiation, and the problem of curvature and redundancy necessitated in the preservation of the segmental mesenteric arcade essential for the flap's survival. The curvature is particularly problematic if the stenosis of the distal anastomoses occurs because dilatation even under general anesthesia is very difficult. An easier reconstructive solution is the use of the radial forearm free flap. The harvest time is considerably less than the jejunal flap, and a laparotomy with its problems of ileus and postoperative pain can be avoided. The flap usually has vessels of adequate caliber and adapts well to its new pharyngeal location. It can be used as a gusset type of reconstruction or for circumferential defects. For noncircumferential defects a patch type of flap utilizing the gastro-omental free flap provides an excellent mucosal lining.[51,52]

With loss of the posterior and lateral walls of the oropharynx, there is no stripping action of this part of the tube to propel a bolus of food into the hypopharynx. In these patients, this early stage of swallowing is a passive phenomenon, but passage of ingesta can be aided by a cricopharyngeal myotomy. When the soft palate is also excised, the problem of initiating deglutition is further compounded by the lack of

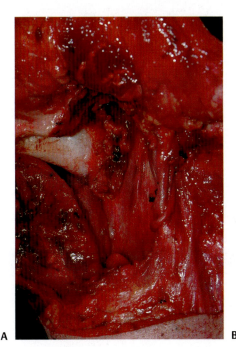
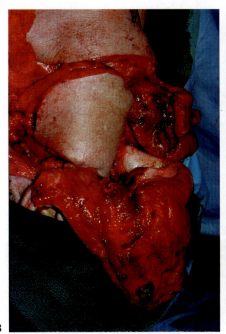
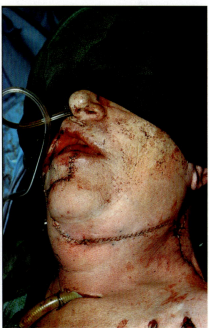

A   B   C

Fig. 2.24 (**A**) Defect following wide-field resection of tonsillar fossa, lateral pharyngeal wall, and soft palate to the level of the torus tubarious. (**B**) Reconstruction with a trapezius musculocutaneous flap. (**C**) Wound closed.

closure of the velopharyngeal port, and nasal regurgitation becomes an annoying problem. Much of this can be avoided by the use of a nasopharyngeal obturator, which is most effective when used intraoperatively. A more complete discussion of this is found in chapter 14.

Surgery for Extensive Malignancies

Each extensive neoplasm in the oropharynx presents with its own unique set of problems. The basic principle of the composite resection for large pharyngeal neoplasms is similar to that for distal oral cavity resections. With few exceptions, a radical neck dissection is done in continuity. The mandible is resected from the coronoid notch to just beyond the angle, depending on the oral extent of the tumor. All mucosal disease is skirted by a 2 cm margin of healthy tissue, but as the hypopharynx is approached, this margin is widened to 2.5 to 3 cm. All or part of the soft palate often needs to be resected, and it must be kept in mind that areas of Queyrat erythroplasia should be included in the specimen. When the maxillary tuberosity or the hard palate is involved, a partial maxillectomy must be done.

The deep aspect of resection in tonsillar fossa and lateral pharyngeal wall neoplasms includes the medial pterygoid muscle. A generous margin of muscle should be resected, even though bleeding from this area—usually from the pterygoid venous plexus—is often profuse. Once the specimen has been removed, hemostasis is initially attempted with pressure. This must be augmented with stick ties and even pledgets of hemostatic gauze or cotton. Reconstruction is done either with simple approximation of pharyngeal wall mucosa to buccal mucosa or the interposition of a flap and a palatal obturator.

Bimaxillary Resection

This type of resection has been dubbed the bimaxillary resection because both a maxillary and a mandibular resection are required given the tumor extent and the fact that the mandible used to be called the inferior maxilla. This is the best method of encompassing those oropharyngeal tumors that have invaded the pterygoid muscles or the posterior maxilla. These patients usually present with trismus from invasion of these muscles of mastication, but in some instances there will be only minor invasion of the muscles,

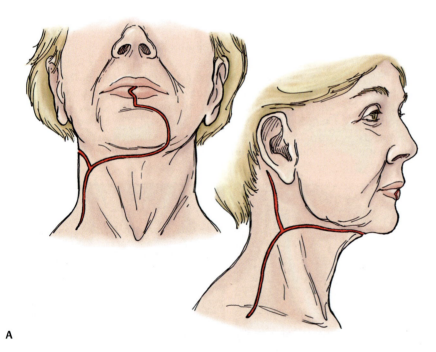

A

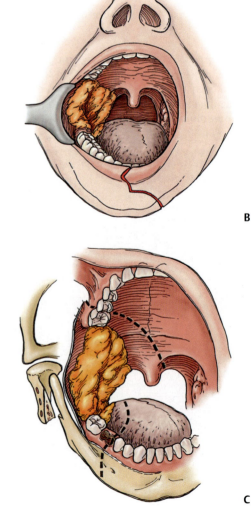

B

C

Fig. 2.25 Bimaxillary resection. (**A**) Skin incision similar to the Conley modification of the modified Schobinger incision. (**B**) Lip-splitting component of facial incision. (**C**) Intraoral component necessary to encompass a large retromolar trigone lesion invading the mandible and inferior maxilla.

and little restriction will be seen. Another symptom that will often require this type of resection for both complete removal of tumor and the necessary exposure of the skull base is that of numbness over the distribution of the third division of the trigeminal nerve. Deeply invasive tumors with an endophytic growth pattern may invade the inferior alveolar nerve as it enters the mandibular canal and then spread retrograde up the mandibular branch of cranial nerve V. The initial symptom is usually numbness over the mental nerve distribution, then numbness in the mandibular dentition of the affected side. When auriculotemporal nerve distribution anesthesia or paresthesia occurs then the mandibular division and even the Gasserian ganglion may be involved. The most effective way of removing tumor in the pterygoid muscle is removing the bones of origin and insertion.

The incision for the bimaxillary resection is depicted in **Fig. 2.25**. An upper lip split is not required. The lower lip split and the cervical portions of the incision are depicted in the illustration. The incision in the anterior tongue is carried from the most distal point of visualization nearer the tongue base in an anterior direction to the limits of the tumor anteriorly then across the lateral tongue and floor of the mouth through the extraction site of the tooth at the anterior extent of the mandibulotomy then into the buccal mucosa. The incision usually needs to stop short of the anterior tonsillar pillar and the pterygomandibular raphe to obtain a good margin and then proceeds into the gingivobuccal sulcus over the maxilla. The maxillary incision passes through the socket of either the second or the third molar tooth and onto the hard palate. Any tumor on the palate is skirted by the usual margin. Usually, a partial removal of the hard palate and total removal of the soft palate will be done. At least a 2 cm margin of healthy tissue is maintained around the tumor.

If the tumor extends into the tongue base and down the oropharyngeal wall toward the larynx the most posterior extremity of the lesion cannot be outlined until the mandibulotomy and the initial part of the resection are done. The mandibulotomy is done in the body of the mandible sparing as much bone as possible. The inferior incision through the tongue can now be carried into the tongue base, extended laterally into the lateral or posterior pharyngeal walls, and brought superiorly into the nasopharynx. The gingival-buccal sulcus incision is carried anteriorly enough so that the soft tissue can be dissected over the posterior wall of the maxilla to expose the pterygoid plates.

Once the initial incisions are made in the soft tissues then the bony work may proceed. After the mandibulotomy the pterygomaxillary sling is incised under the angle and distal body of the mandible. The masseter muscle is dissected from the lateral aspect of the mandibular ramus and carried up to the temporal-mandibular joint. The masseter will be the lateral margin of the resection (**Fig. 2.26**). Occasionally, the condyle and the mandibular neck can be preserved, but in most instances they need to be included in the resection. The temporomandibular joint is separated and the internal maxillary artery ligated and cut. The mandible is now mobilized from the glenoid fossa. Attention is now directed toward the upper jaw. A bone saw is used to cut through the maxillary alveolus along the posterolateral wall of the maxillary sinus

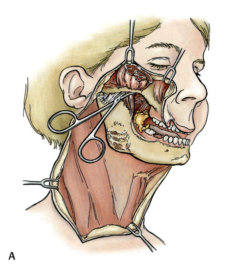

A

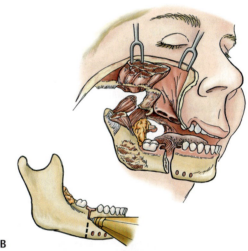

B

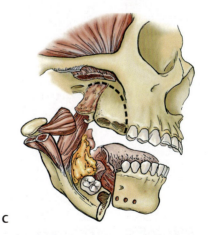

C

Fig. 2.26 (**A**) Cheek flap elevated exposing mandibular and maxillary extent of tumor. Scissors on the temporalis muscle at its insertion into the coronoid process of the mandible. (**B**) Mucosal incisions made including those on the tongue. Mandibulotomy done. Note the condyle is to be removed to remove the insertion of the lateral pterygoid muscle. (**C**) The incision on the posteroinferior maxilla is marked out.

and then directed superiorly just anterior to the pterygoid plates until the undersurface of the basisphenoid is reached (**Fig. 2.27**). The last step in the resection will be the separation of the pterygoid plates from their origin from the base of the sphenoid bone. This final cut of the operation is delayed until all the soft tissue incisions have been made, the tumor is totally mobilized, and the specimen is pedicled at the pterygoids. This is because of the profuse bleeding from the pterygoid plexus of veins and branches of the internal maxillary artery during this last step.

The resection of the involved tongue and the pharynx will then be done, carried into the nasopharynx, and the palatal portion is incised completely up to the maxillary tuberosity. The pterygoid plates are severed from their base (**Fig. 2.28A,B**), the medial maxillary wall incised to the hard palatal incision previously made, the last soft tissue attachments separated, and the specimen removed. In this way the entire tumor can be exenterated en bloc with the involved pterygoid muscles being removed from their origin to insertion.

Closure is often done by simple approximation of the oral and pharyngeal tissues and the use of a previously fabricated palatal appliance (**Fig. 2.29**). A flap will be needed in those cases in which a large circumference of pharyngeal mucosa is resected. The radial forearm free flap is probably the most useful in these instances because of its thinness, suppleness, and reliability. As an alternative a pectoralis musculocutaneous flap can be employed. Reconstruction of the mandible can be done with a fibular free flap but is usually not done when the mandibular resection is at or just beyond the mandibular angle. The reconstruction of the mandibular condyle is problematic. A condyle fashioned from rib or from the metatarsal head from the foot is usually not worth the trouble in terms of restoration of function. Reconstruction of the distal mandibular body and

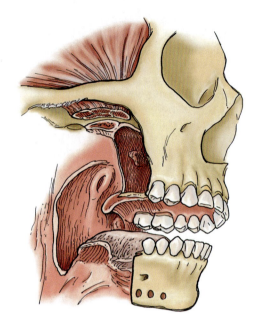

Fig. 2.27 The bone saw, or in this case the cutting bone needle, of the Midas Rex drill (Medtronic, Inc., Minneapolis, MN) is used to cut through the lateral maxillary wall up to the base of the pterygoid plates.

ramus can be done with a titanium reconstruction plate and covered by a flap, usually a pectoralis flap, but only one plate is currently available in the United States as an attached condyle. The big disadvantage of this prosthesis is that it is not adjustable and cannot accommodate the variances in each individual glenoid fossa. Postoperative full dose of irradiation is administered in all previously unirradiated cases.

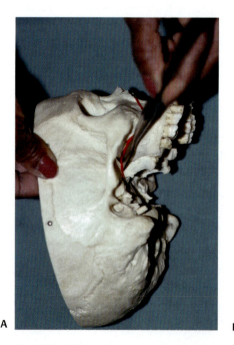
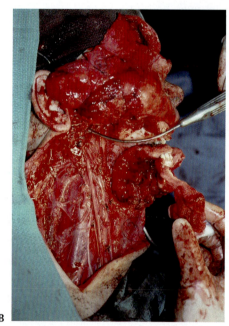
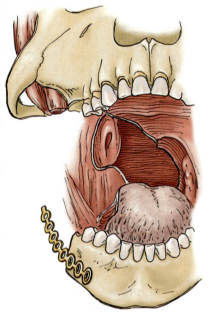

A

B

C

Fig. 2.28 (**A**) An osteotome is used to separate the pterygoid plates from the basisphenoid. *Case 1* Osteotome placed against the base of the pterygoid plates to ensure complete excision of the pterygoid muscles. (**B**) Defect after tumor resection. *Case 1* Resection completed. Suction tip is at the skull base. (**C**) Defect after tumor resection with reconstruction plate in place.

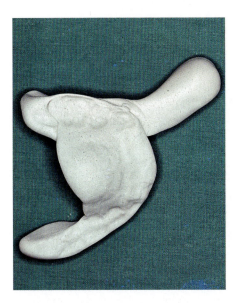

Fig. 2.29 Palatal appliance for speech and oral rehabilitation following bimaxillary resection.

Resection of Nasopharyngeal Extension

In the not-too-distant past, the extension of oropharyngeal carcinoma into the nasopharynx was considered to be a sign of inoperability. The problem of obtaining a margin of healthy tissue around this extension was the key issue that established this notion. The core of the problem centers around the fact that the superior constrictor origin from the pharyngeal tubercles of the clivus renders the muscle tightly bound to bone and devoid of the easy resection plane that exists between the rest of the pharynx located inferiorly and the underlying cervical spine. This in fact is an easy problem to overcome. The major theoretical impediment to the consideration of tumor removal in this area is the traditional notion that all oncological resections need to be en bloc. Although a laudable goal in those resections in which this type of resection is feasible it cannot always be accomplished. The violation of the en bloc principal is more usual than not in skull base surgery. Furthermore, it is the commonplace method of removing parotid salivary gland tumors and in detaching the radical neck dissection specimen from a supraglottic laryngectomy. Resections of tumors in the nasopharynx are not piecemeal but are a modification of the en bloc principal. In this technique the main specimen is removed with most of the margins intact but with the exception that the tumor is cut away from initially inaccessible areas such as the deep surface of the nasopharyngeal muscles, leaving remaining residual tumor attached to the clivus (**Fig. 2.30**). This initial specimen containing the bulk of the tumor is the first layer. The second layer is outlined with a healthy tissue margin laterally, and the clival bone is removed with a bur (**Fig. 2.31**).

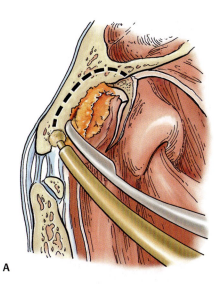

A

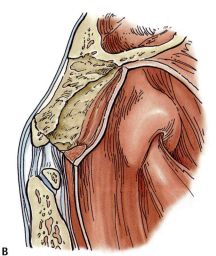

B

Fig. 2.30 Main composite resection specimen removed carrying with it most of the tumor. Residual tumor of the "second layer" is left for the next step in resection. Dotted line outlines the projected resection.

Fig. 2.31 (**A**) Tumor with a margin of uninvolved tissue is dissected up to the area of clival involvement, which is removed with the cutting bur (see dashed lines). (**B**) Tumor removed.

This method of a modified en bloc resection relies heavily on frozen sections control. Frozen sections of the lateral soft tissues establish integrity of the more superficial margins, and curetting of clival cancellous bone and marrow can establish negative margins in the deep aspects of the resection.

Tumor may extend laterally into the fossa of Rosenmüller or into the cartilage of the eustachian tube (**Fig. 2.32**). The palatal muscles and even their origins on the undersurface of the temporal and sphenoid bones may be involved with the malignancy. The limitation of resection at these lateral extensions is usually at the level of the bony portion of the eustachian tube. If this area is involved it is best addressed by the infratemporal fossa approach, which is fully described in chapter 9. After the first layer of resection has been removed, tumor involvement of the palatal muscles, the cartilaginous portion of the tumor and adjacent deep sphenoid bone, temporal bone, and anterior portions of the occipital contribution to the clivus are resected. The soft tissue is removed first with a periosteal elevator dissecting it from the underlying bone, and the bone itself is removed with the cutting bur. The TAC attachment of the Midas Rex drill (Medtronic, Inc., Minneapolis, MN) is ideal for this resection (**Fig. 2.33**). The posterior limitation of the resection is the pontine dura, and the lateral limit is the foramen lacerum. Involvement of the foramen lacerum or the petrous carotid artery will need the infratemporal fossa/middle fossa approach for possible control. Superiorly, the roof of the nasopharynx is made up mainly by the floor of the sphenoid sinus. This is easily removed with the drill. The raw area is left to granulate in. If the pontine dura has been penetrated and a cerebrospinal fluid (CSF) leak occurs, an attempt to suture it is made. This is possible if a wide enough hole in the bone has been made, or if this is not feasible, then a fascial graft is welded in place

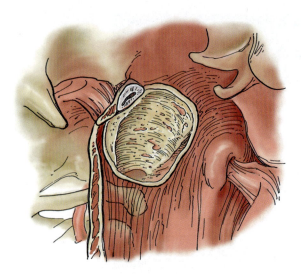

Fig. 2.33 Defect after cartilaginous eustachian tube as well as palatal muscles are incised and retracted. TAC attachment of the Midas Rex drill (Medtronic, Inc., Minneapolis, MN) used to remove parts of the involved clivus, bony eustachian tube, and petrous tip and roof of the nasopharynx, which is the floor of the sphenoid sinus.

with fibrin glue and covered over with a superiorly pedicled septal flap (**Fig. 2.34**).

The posterior oropharyngeal wall can be replaced with a pectoralis myocutaneous flap, but even better is the radial forearm musculocutaneous free flap. The clival area granulates in quickly unless the patient has been previously irradiated.

Surgery for Cervical Spine Extension

Traditionally, when squamous carcinoma invades paraspinous muscles and especially the cervical vertebrae themselves, patients have been deemed unresectable. Clearly, spread of malignancy to multiple levels of the spine with extensive invasion of the adjacent intervertebral forearm and plastered against the adjacent paraspinous muscles presents a limited to zero chance of surgical rescue. However, in certain carefully selected cases the interdisciplinary effort of the head and neck surgeon, the orthopedic surgeon, and the neurological surgeon can conjointly achieve complete resection of the tumor and stabilization of the cervical spine. Some of the more obvious contraindications include involvement of both common or internal carotid arteries, involvement of both vertebral arteries, and invasion of the spinal cord, in addition to those previously cited. Relative contraindications are a past history of radiation therapy or the presence of a pharyngocutaneous fistula.

The modified en bloc resection is done with the final layer being that on the cervical spine (**Fig. 2.35**). A 1 to 2 cm margin of healthy muscle, fascia, and periosteum is incised down to the spinal bone and dissected toward the region of the invaded vertebra. The involvement may be only at the level of the transverse process. After dissecting out the vertebral artery, the transverse process is removed with a rongeur or

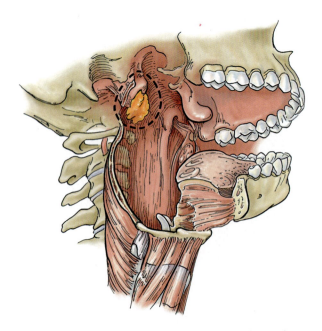

Fig. 2.32 Tumor invading the eustachian tube and extending into the fossa of Rosenmüller.

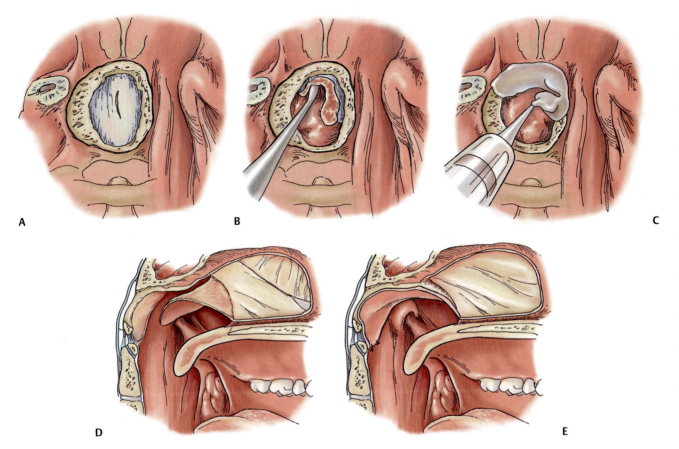

Fig. 2.34 (**A**) Rent or small resection of pontine dura. (**B**) Replaced with fascia graft. (**C**) Sealed with fibrin blue. (**D**) Septal flap elevated. (**E**) Septal flap turned into position.

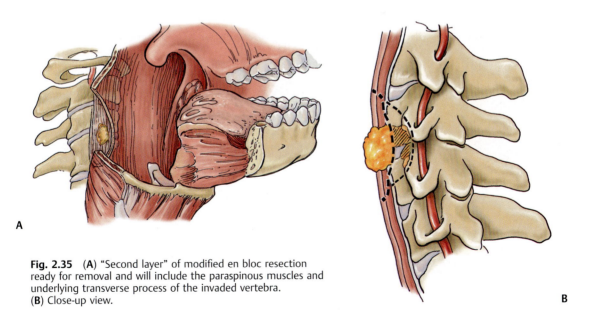

Fig. 2.35 (**A**) "Second layer" of modified en bloc resection ready for removal and will include the paraspinous muscles and underlying transverse process of the invaded vertebra. (**B**) Close-up view.

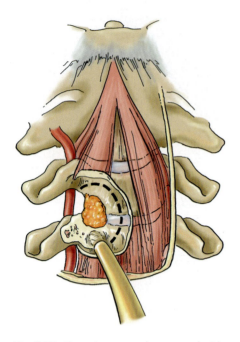

Fig. 2.36 Paraspinous muscles resected with an adequate margin and bur used to resect transverse process avoiding injury to the underlying vertebral artery.

a cutting bur (**Fig. 2.36**). If the vertebral artery is invaded it can usually be sacrificed without any untoward neurological event as long as the contralateral vertebral artery is intact and patent and both common and internal carotids are patent. The safest way to minimize postoperative stroke is to perform a preoperative balloon test occlusion and Single Proton Emission Computerized Tomography (SPECT) scan to estimate the effect on flow through the circle of Willis of vertebral artery occlusion. Involvement of the vertebral body is removed with a bur or a rongeur (**Fig. 2.37A,B**). Invasion of spinal nerves can be resected down to the dentate ligament by the neurological surgeon.

The resected spine, if deemed unstable, is fused with cancellous bone from the hip and stabilized with a plate (**Fig. 2.37B**). Invasion of the transverse process with or without sacrifice of the vertebral artery has not adversely affected the postoperative courses or overall prognosis for survival. Resection of potions of one or two adjacent vertebrae has been done on a limited number of patients with good local control, but some of the patients succumbed to distant disease.

Various problems arise that are peculiar to each case. The following case histories illustrate the basic principles as well as offer some possible solutions to several troublesome problems.

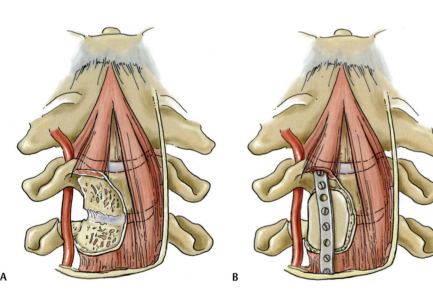

A   B

Fig. 2.37 (**A**) Tumor resected from bodies of two adjacent cervical vertebrae and intervening disk. (**B**) Resected area fused with a bone graft and reconstruction plate.

Case 1 (Fig. 2.38–Fig. 2.40, pp. 68–69)

A 37-year-old woman was first seen with a T2N1M0 lesion of the right tonsillar fossa and anterior pillar. She elected not to have conventional therapy and after a year of attempting quack cures re-presented herself for definitive therapy. The lesion was as depicted in **Fig. 2.38**. A photo could not be obtained because of the severity of her trismus. She had a 1.5 cm hard mass in the right posterior triangle of the neck.

A bimaxillary resection of the right side was done that included lateral tongue, lateral pharyngeal wall, tonsillar fossa, soft palate, hemimandible, maxilla, some buccal mucosa, and a right radical neck dissection (**Fig. 2.39**). The mandibulectomy and massive oropharyngeal resection gave excellent access to the skull base. The osteotome could then be placed against the basisphenoid and the pterygoid plates excised at their origin (**Fig. 2.28B**). The excision of the posterior and posteroinferior maxilla along with the distal upper alveolus encompassed the palatal extent of the tumor and that invading the posteroinferior maxillary sinus, and completed the excision of the pterygoid muscles in their entirety (**Fig. 2.28A**). No flaps were turned, and reconstruction was by primary approximation of the wound edges. A course of postoperative irradiation completed the therapy.

Discussion

At the time the patient presented with trismus, the generally accepted dictum was that this symptom indicated a hopeless prognosis. Pterygoid plate erosion and involvement of the pterygoid muscles with tumor had been considered an unresectable situation. Because of the patient's youth and her willingness to try anything for a potential cure, the pterygoid resection was advised.

Speech was remarkably enhanced by a nasopharyngeal obturator. Swallowing was greatly improved by a cricopharyngeal myotomy done some months later. The patient survived disease free for 17 years (**Fig. 2.40**), until she succumbed to ovarian carcinoma.

Case 2 (Fig. 2.41–Fig. 2.43, pp. 69–70)

Mr. G.C. was a 46-year-old man who presented with a 2.5-week history of pain in the tongue, often biting it, but noted no masses in the neck. On physical examination he had a 4 cm diameter mass in the anterior lateral tongue extending to the tongue base. No masses were palpable in the neck. He underwent a partial pull-through glossectomy and a right radical neck dissection. Six months later he presented with the sudden appearance of a massive local recurrence. The recurrent tumor had invaded most of the residual tongue base and was fixed to the fight mandibular ramus and body. He underwent a total glossectomy, partial mandibulectomy, and antralateral modified radical neck dissection (**Fig. 2.41**) sparing the larynx. Reconstruction was done with a pectoralis major myocutaneous flap and a titanium hollow locking screw plate (**Fig. 2.42**). The pectoralis flap substituted for the tongue and, also, portions were wrapped around the plate to prevent subsequent erosion through the skin (**Fig. 2.43**). He had a full course of postoperative irradiation and chemotherapy. The patient was able to take some liquid by mouth and had understandable speech. Although he remained tumor free at the resection site, he died of pulmonary metastasis 6 months later.

The decision to preserve the larynx was based upon his age, his other wise good state of health, and his motivation. In the older patient or one that has had prior irradiation it is much safer to take the larynx. Despite a 10% breakage rate and a 20% exposure rate of the titanium plates over prolonged periods of plate retention, especially after postoperative irradiation, they remain the mainstays of mandibular reconstruction in these cases.

Discussion

This case demonstrates the most common mode of reconstruction we employ in cases of mandibular involvement and our most usual approach to the problem of massive invasion of the tongue.

Case 3 (Fig. 2.44, p. 71)

Mrs. H.M. was a 65-year-old woman who complained of a sore throat and a "plugged-up" ear for 12 months. On examination she had a massive oropharyngeal neoplasm that extended from the nasopharynx to the region just above the aryepiglottic fold. The geographic center of the tumor was in the left tonsil extending almost to the opposite posterior tonsillar pillar. The extension in the nasopharynx was within 2 cm of the choanae and invaded the left eustachian tube (**Fig. 2.44**). Multiple large metastatic lymph nodes were palpable in both necks.

A resection that included the walls of the oropharynx and the nasopharynx, as well as the soft palate, the left tonsillar fossa, and mandibular ramus, a portion of the tongue base and bilateral radical neck dissections were done. The nasopharyngeal portion of the operation included the entire cartilaginous eustachian tube, all the nasopharyngeal mucosa to the top of the vomer and sphenoid rostrum, and the origins of the palatal muscles. The bony resection included the beginnings of the bony part of the eustachian tube and approximately one half of the thickness of the clivus (**Fig. 2.32 and Fig. 2.33**). Reconstruction was with a pectoralis major musculocutaneous flap.

Postoperatively, the pectoralis flap pulled away from the nasopharynx and prolapsed into the oropharyngeal isthmus, interfering with swallowing. Debulking of the flap with the CO_2 laser was required to enable swallowing, which is still limited. A full course of irradiation followed.

She has now been decannulated but still takes most of her nutrition through a gastrostomy. At 8 years postoperatively, she has no evidence of recurrent disease.

Discussion

Traditionally the nasopharynx was thought to be an area where cancer resection was impossible. The problem of determining margins is inherent in the inability to do a classic mono bloc excision. The clival bone was thought to be an inviolable barrier. Using the techniques acquired from skull base surgery these types of resection are feasible and yield favorable survival results. Diligent attention to the tumor margins is essential for complete removal of the neoplasm. The interdigitation of the cartilaginous eustachian tube into its bony counterpart is the limit of the excision through this approach. Further tumor spread must be addressed through an approach to the infratemporal fossa.

Case 4 (Fig. 2.45, p. 72)

Mr. G.G. was a 62-year-old man who presented with a sore throat for 6 months. On examination, he had a 3 by 5 cm exophytic ulcerating tumor of the right third molar tooth socket extending onto the tonsillar area, both the hard and soft palate, and the lateral pharyngeal wall. There were no palpable lymph nodes in the right neck. He had a serous otitis media in the right ear. CT scanning revealed erosion of the posterior maxillary wall and opacification of the right maxillary sinus.

At endoscopy a biopsy of the pharyngeal lesion revealed squamous cell carcinoma. Metastatic screening revealed no evidence of distant tumor spread.

Resection of the primary lesion employed the classical steps of the bimaxillary excision (**Figs. 2.25, 2.26, 2.27,** and **2.28**). A right radical neck dissection was done as the initial step in the resection. An en bloc removal of the mandibular ramus including the condyle; the posterior maxilla, including the pterygoid plates; the lateral pharynx; and a portion of the tongue base was done. Reconstruction was with a pectoralis musculocutaneous flap. Weeks later he underwent a full course of irradiation to the primary site and both necks. He was fitted with a surgical obturator and has excellent speech and swallowing. He is now 13 years postoperative and free of disease (**Fig. 2.45**).

Discussion

The bimaxillary excision was developed precisely to address this type of tumor. Complete excision of the pterygoid muscles by including both their origins and insertions eliminates the problem of local recurrence in these muscles by a more limited resection. The skull base can be clearly visualized such that perineural invasion of the inferior alveolar nerve or the main trunk of the mandibular nerve can be addressed. Excellent functioning can be anticipated in most cases with a well-fitting palatal obturator.

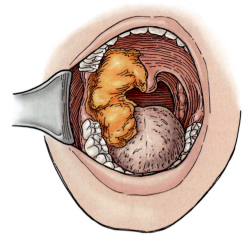

Fig. 2.38 *Case 1* Large oropharyngeal carcinoma originating in the tonsillar fossa.

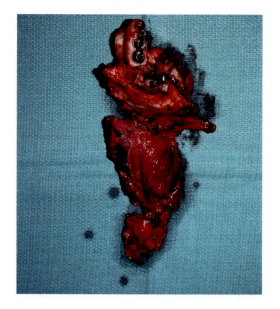

Fig. 2.39 *Case 1* Composite resection includes posterior maxilla.

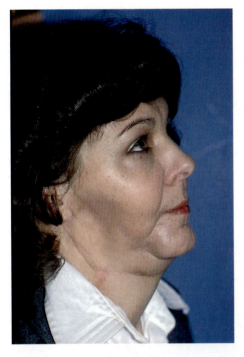

Fig. 2.40 *Case 1* Patient alive and well at 5 years after resection, with acceptable cosmetic appearance.

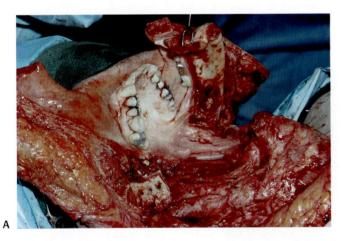

A

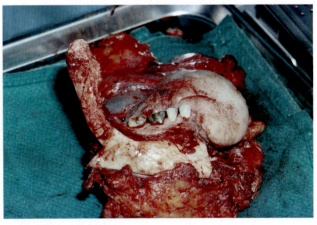

B

Fig. 2.41 *Case 2* Patient with massive tongue base carcinoma. (**A**) Defect after total glossectomy. (**B**) Surgical specimen including tongue and hemimandible.

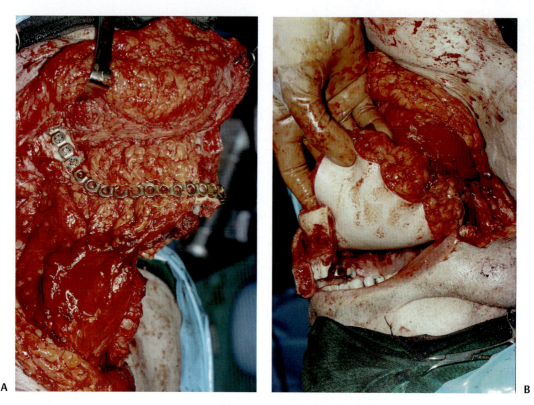

A   B

Fig. 2.42 *Case 2* Reconstruction with a large pectoralis major musculocutaneous flap and a locking screw plate. (**A**) Locking screw plate in place. (**B**) Pectoralis flap placed over plate. Anterior flap replaces resected tongue.

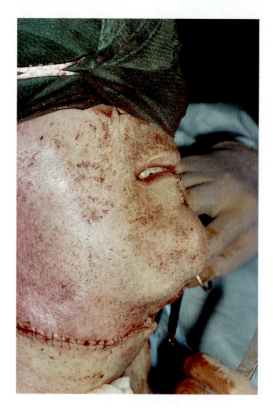

Fig. 2.43 *Case 2* Patient's appearance after closure.

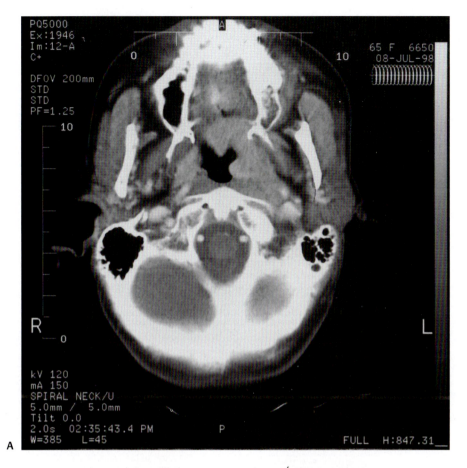

A

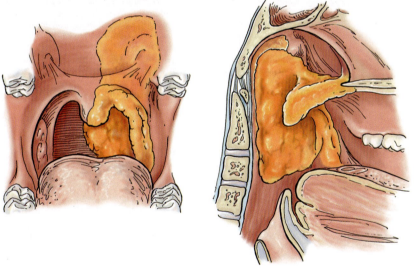

B

Fig. 2.44 *Case 3* (**A**) Magnetic resonance imaging scan showing tumor extent. (**B**) Drawing showing tumor extent.

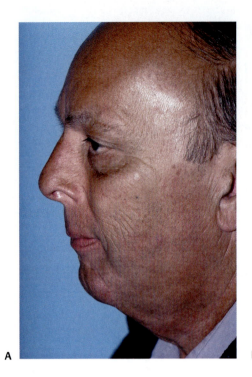

A

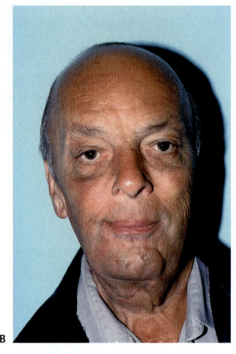

B

Fig. 2.45 Patient 2 years postoperatively. (**A**) Side view. (**B**) *Case 4* Frontal view (patient is still alive 13 years postoperatively).

References

1. Goss CM, ed. Gray's Anatomy. 29th ed. Philadelphia: Lea & Febiger; 1973:1197

2. Fletcher GH, Jesse RH, Healey JE, et al. Oropharynx. In: MacComb WS, Fletcher GH, eds. Cancer of the Head and Neck. Baltimore: Williams & Wilkins; 1968:180

3. Ballenger JJ. Diseases of the Nose, Throat, and Ear. 12th ed. Philadelphia: Lea & Febiger; 1977:237

4. DeWeese DD, Saunders WH. Textbook of Otolaryngology. 2nd ed. St. Louis: CV Mosby; 1964:69

5. Davies J. Embryology and anatomy of the head and neck, face, palate, nose and paranasal sinuses. In: Paparella MM, Shumrick DA, eds. Otolaryngology. Vol 1. 2nd ed. Philadelphia: WB Saunders; 1980:116

6. English GM. Otolaryngology. Hagerstown, MD: Harper & Row; 1976: 414

7. Romanes GJ. Cunningham's Manual of Practical Anatomy. Vol 3. 13th ed. New York: Oxford University Press; 1968:147

8. Parkhill EM. Tumors of the palatine tonsil. In: Dockerty MB, Parkhill EM, Dahlin DC, eds. Tumors of the Oral Cavity and Pharynx. Washington, DC: Armed Forces Institute of Pathology; 1964:243

9. Banfi A, Bonadonna G, Carnevali G, et al. Lymphoreticular sarcoma with primary involvement in Waldeyer's ring. Cancer 1970;26:341–351

10. McNelis FL, Pai VT. Malignant lymphoma of the head and neck. Trans Am Soc Laryngol Rhinol Otol June:79(6)10:76–86

11. Toomey JM. Cysts and tumors of the pharynx. In: Paparella MM, Shumrick DA, eds. Otolaryngology. Vol 3. 2nd ed. Philadelphia: WB Saunders; 1980:2323

12. Lindberg R. Distribution of cervical lymph node metastases from squamous cell carcinoma of the upper respiratory and digestive tracts. Cancer 1972;29:1446–1449

13. Truluck CH Jr, Putney FR. Survival rates in cancer of the tongue, tonsil, and hypopharynx. Arch Otolaryngol 1971;93:271–274

14. Civantos FJ, Goodwin JW. Cancer of the oropharynx. In: Myers EN, Suen JY, eds. Cancer of the Head and Neck. 3rd ed. Philadelphia: WB Saunders; 1989:361–380

15. Wang CC. Radiation therapy in the management of oral malignant disease. Otolaryngol Clin North Am 1979;12:73–80

16. Quenelle DJ, Crissman JD, Shumrick DA. Tonsillar carcinoma: treatment results. Laryngoscope 1979;89:1842–1846

17. Edström S, Jeppsson PH, Lindstrom J. Carcinoma of the tonsillar region: aspects on treatment modalities with reference to a study on patients treated by radiation. Laryngoscope 1978;88:1019–1023

18. Healy GB, Strong MS, Uchmakli A, et al. Carcinoma of the palatine arch: the rationale of treatment selection. Am J Surg 1976;132:498–503

19. Aijax A, Meyers EM, Johnson JT. Cancer of the oral cavity. In: Myers EN, Suen JY, eds. Cancer of the Head and Neck. 3rd ed. Philadelphia: WB Saunders; 1989;18, 19:321–360

20. Ogura JH, Biller HG, Wette R. Elective neck dissection for pharyngeal and laryngeal cancers: an evaluation. Ann Otol Rhinol Laryngol 1971;80:646–650

21. Whicker JH, DeSanto LW, Devine KD. Surgical treatment of squamous cell carcinoma of the base of the tongue. Laryngoscope 1972;82:1853–1860

22. Strong EW. Carcinoma of the tongue. Otolaryngol Clin North Am 1979;12:107–110

23. Skolnik EM, Campbell JM, Meyers RM. Carcinoma of the buccal mucosa and retromolar area. Otolaryngol Clin North Am 1972;5:327–331

24. Kraus DH, Vastola PA, Huvos AG, Spiro RH. Surgical management of squamous cell carcinoma of the tongue base. Am J Surg 1993;166:384–388

25. Krause C J. Personal communications, 1980.

26. Jackson SM, Hay JH, Flores AD, et al. Cancer of the tonsil: the results of ipsilateral radiation treatment. Radiother Oncol 1999;51:123–128

27. Lee JG. Resection margins of carcinoma of the oral cavity, oropharynx, hypopharynx, and larynx: a clinical study. Master's thesis, University of Iowa, 1973

28. Snow JB Jr, Gelber RD, Kramer S. Randomized preoperative and postoperative radiation therapy for patients with carcinoma of the head and neck: preliminary report. Laryngoscope 1980;90:930–945

29. Hinerman RW, Parsons JT, Mendenhall WM. External beam radiation irradiation alone or combined with neck dissection for base of tongue cancer: an alternative to primary surgery. Laryngoscope 1994;104:1466–1470

30. Schleuning AJ, Summers GW. Carcinoma of the tongue: review of 220 cases. Laryngoscope 1972;82:1446–1454

31. Renaud-Salis JL, Blanc-Vincent MP, Brugere J, et al. Standard, Options et Recommandations pour le prise en charge des patients; atteints de cancer epidermoide de l'oropharynx. Bull Cancer 1999;86:550–572

32. Del Campo JM, Felip E, Firaly J, et al. Preoperative simultaneous chemo-radiotherapy in locally advanced cancer of the oral cavity an orophar-ynx. Am J Clin Oncol 1997;20:97–100

33. Pfister DG, Harrison LB, Strong EW, et al. Organ preservation in ad-vanced oropharynx cancer: results with induction chemotherapy and radiation. J Clin Oncol 1995;13:671–680

34. Trible WM. Cancer of the oral cavity: five year end results in 237 pa-tients. Ann Otol Rhinol Laryngol 1969;78:716–724

35. Corsten M, Donald PJ. Unpublished data

36. Ash CL. Oral cancer: a twenty-five year study. Am J Roentgenol Radium Ther Nucl Med 1962;87:417–430

37. Russ JE, Applebaum EL, Sesson GA. Squamous cell carcinoma of the soft palate. Laryngoscope 1977;87:1151–1156

38. Fee WE Jr, Sonja LS, Rubenstein R, et al. Squamous cell carcinoma of the soft palate. Arch Otolaryngol 1979;105:710–718

39. Konrad HR, Canalis RF, Calcaterra TC. Epidermoid carcinoma of the pal-ate. Arch Otolaryngol 1978;104:208–212

40. Rider WD. Epithelial cancer of the tonsillar area. Radiology 1962;78:760–765

41. Fletcher GH, Jesse RH, Healey JE, et al. Oropharynx. In: MacComb WS, Fletcher GH, eds. Cancer of the Head and Neck. Baltimore: Williams & Wilkins; 1968:179

42. de Clercq LD, Chole RA. Retropharyngeal abscess in the adult. Otolaryn-gol Head Neck Surg 1980;88:684–689

43. Goss CM, ed. Gray's Anatomy. 29th ed. Philadelphia: Lea & Febiger; 1973:744–745

44. Rouviere H. Anatomie des lymphatiques de l'homme. Paris: Masson; 1932:37–38

45. Thawley SE, Sessions DG, Genden EM. Surgical therapy of hypopharyn-geal tumors. In: Thawley SE, Panje WR, Batsakis JG, Lindberg RD, eds. Comprehensive Management of Head and Neck Tumors. Vol 1. 2nd ed. Philadelphia: WB Saunders; 1999:910

46. Spiro RH, Kelly J, Vega AL, Harrison LB, Strong EW. Squamous carci-noma of the posterior pharyngeal wall. Am J Surg 1990;160:420–423

47. Moore DM, Calcaterra TC. Cancer of the tongue base treated by a transpharyngeal approach. Ann Otol Rhinol Laryngol 1990;99:300–303

48. Myers EN. Total glossectomy in cancer of the oral cavity. Otolaryngol Clin North Am 1972;5:343–355

49. Donald PJ. Resection of the pre-epiglottic space as a therapeutic option in vallecular invasion. In: Smee R, Bridger GP eds. Laryngeal Cancer. Amsterdam: Elsevier; 1994:489–493

50. Steiner W, Ambrosch P. Endoscopic Laser Surgery of the Upper Aerodi-gestive Tract. Stuttgart: Thieme; 2000:91–104

51. Panje WR, Little AG, Moran WJ, Ferguson M, Scher N. Immediate free gastro-omental flap reconstruction of the mouth and throat. Ann Otol Rhinol Laryngol 1987;96:15–21

52. Urken ML, Cheny ML. Free omentum and gastro-omentum. In: Urken ML, Cheney ML, Sullivan MJ, Biller HF, eds. Atlas of Regional and Free Flaps for Head and Neck Reconstruction. Philadelphia: Raven; 1995:321–329

3

Cancer of the Hypopharynx, Cervical Esophagus, and Mediastinum

Paul J. Donald

Squamous cell cancer, affecting the hypopharynx and the cervical esophagus, carries with it one of the most ominous prognoses of any site in the upper aerodigestive tract. As location of malignancy progresses downward from the oral cavity to the stomach, the 5-year survival rate falls accordingly. From the tip of the tongue to the oropharynx, the downswing of the survival curve is less steep; however, the curve plummets with progression through the hypopharynx and cervical esophagus. The aggressive biological activity of the lesions and the minimal symptoms experienced by patients through the early course of this disease are jointly responsible for this unfortunate circumstance.

Biologically, these lesions have a propensity for rapid local mucosal and submucosal spread and a proclivity for regional and even distant metastasis. So-called skip areas and multifocal disease are not uncommon in the piriform recesses and are almost the rule in cervical esophageal lesions. The rather localized nature of epidermoid tumors, so commonly observed in the rest of the head and neck region, is not a feature of hypopharyngeal and esophageal lesions.

The occult nature of the clinical presentation encountered in these neoplasms accounts for their large size when first seen. Often a cancerous cervical lymph node, indicating metastasis, is the only sign of trouble. The unfortunate stigma of a neck scar from a biopsy that should not have been done in a patient bearing the diagnosis of metastatic squamous cell carcinoma is a tragedy in the experience of most head and neck surgeons (**Fig. 3.1**). Most often a quick look with a laryngeal mirror reveals the source of the primary lesion. The symptom of mild dysphagia is commonly reported in a family practice setting, and fortunately hypopharyngeal and cervical esophageal tumors are rarely encountered in the experience of these practitioners. Only a chance pharyngoesophagogram will reveal the malignancy that may lurk there. Pain on swallowing, hoarseness, dyspnea, and hemoptysis are all late signs.

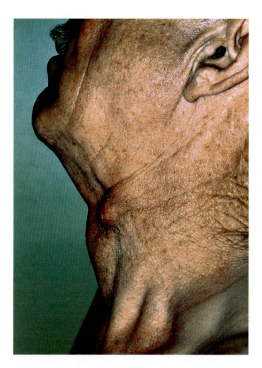

Fig. 3.1 Neck scar with tumor growing through it following a biopsy of a cancerous cervical lymph node metastatic from a pyriform sinus carcinoma.

◆ Anatomy

Hypopharynx

For the purpose of consistency, the start of the hypopharynx will be demarcated at the level of the valleculae and the lateral pharyngoepiglottic folds. The termination of this area inferiorly is at the level of the cricopharyngeus muscle (**Fig. 3.2**). Contained within the hypopharynx is, of course, the larynx, malignancies of which have an altogether different biological character from those of the pharynx. Once a tumor has migrated outside the confines of the larynx and has transgressed the hypopharynx, however, it assumes the more aggressive behavior of this latter region.

The hypopharynx includes both piriform fossae and an intervening area of pharynx directly posterior to the larynx; the anterior wall of this area is called the postcricoid area (**Fig. 3.2B**), and the posterior wall simply the posterior pharyngeal wall. Each piriform fossa is rimmed by the aryepiglottic fold medially, the lateral pharyngoepiglottic fold anterolaterally, and the lateral hypopharyngeal wall lateroposteriorly. The aryepiglottic fold is considered to be the medial wall of the piriform sinus. This fold is actually part of the larynx, but the medial wall of the piriform sinus begins 1 cm below the fold's superiormost extremity. This medial wall piriform mucosa is in continuity with that of its opposing side through the aforementioned postcricoid area. The lamina of the cricoid cartilage is the principal skeletal component supporting this latter region. The posterior cricoarytenoid muscles and a portion of the interarytenoid muscles intervene between the mucosa and the cartilage. The posterior surface of this—the posterior wall of the larynx—forms the postcricoid area, which also serves as the anterior wall of the posterior hypopharynx. At the inferior border of the cricoid the hypopharynx becomes the cervical esophagus. The posterior wall of the pharyngeal area is continuous with that of the oropharynx above and the cervical esophagus below.

The hypopharynx is composed of the middle and inferior constrictor muscles of the pharynx and their investing fascial layers. The loose areolar fascia between the buccopharyngeal fascia investing the muscular coats and the stout fascia of the prevertebral area exists in the same way that it does in the oropharynx and is called by some the alar fascia.

The pyriform fossae, except at their posterior extremities, are contained within the alae of the thyroid cartilage. Superiorly, the aryepiglottic and, slightly more inferiorly, the lateral cricoarytenoid muscles separate the fossae from the laryngeal lumen. The arytenoid cartilage composes part of this medial wall posteriorly. Inferiorly, the cricoid cartilage makes up this wall as the piriform progresses toward the cervical esophagus.

The lymphatics of the hypopharynx penetrate the thyrohyoid membrane to terminate in the nodes of the middle jugular chain. The drainage of the postcricoid area is less profuse than that of the piriform recesses, and the pattern of drainage is similar to that of the cervical esophagus.[1] The lymph nodes in which they terminate are grouped around the upper esophagus and trachea as well as in the supraclavicular fossa. The drainage from the posterior wall may ascend the lymphatic chain in the lateral and posterolateral neck, emptying into the midjugular chain, and may even reach the highest retropharyngeal node, the node of Rouvière (**Fig. 3.3**).[1,2]

Cervical Esophagus

The cervical esophagus is roughly the upper one third of that organ, but no precise demarcation exists. It begins at the level of the cricopharyngeus muscle opposite C6 and ends at the thoracic inlet. As the esophagus descends into the chest, it proceeds in a posterior direction carried by the trachea, which fronts it. The cervical tracheal membranous wall lies anteriorly to the esophagus and is separated from it by a flimsy layer of connective tissue. While in the neck, the trachea and esophagus deviate to the left ~0.5 cm from the midline of the spine. The cervical esophageal lumen measures ~2.3 by 1.7 cm and is somewhat flattened compared with its more rounded configuration in the chest. The relatively thin wall of the organ is responsible for its reputation as a delicate, poorly healing structure, and surgery to the esophagus has traditionally been

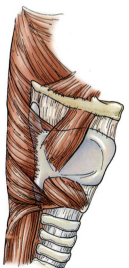
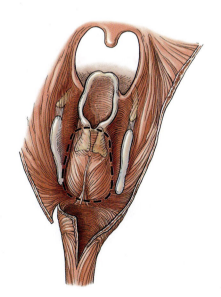

A **B**

Fig. 3.2 Anatomical boundaries of the hypopharynx: (**A**) External view. (**B**) Internal view.

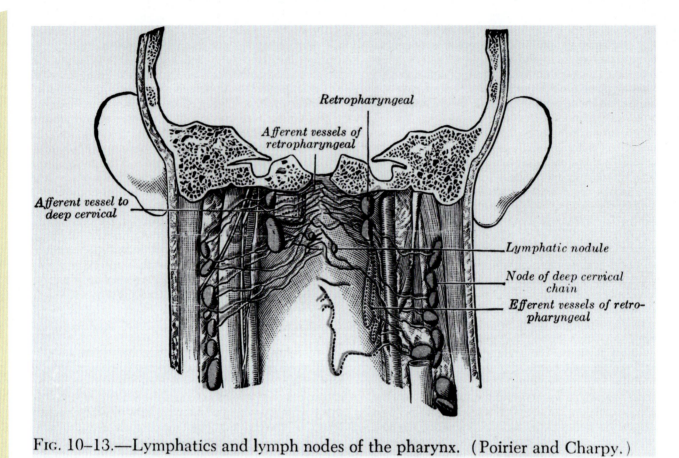

Fig. 10–13.—Lymphatics and lymph nodes of the pharynx. (Poirier and Charpy.)

Fig. 3.3 Illustration of the nodes draining the pharynx. Note the high retropharyneal nodes of Rouvière, which are inaccessible to the palpating finger. (Poirier and Charpy: from Goss CM, ed. Gray's Anatomy of the Human Body. 29th ed. Philadelphia: Lea & Febiger; 1975.)

fraught with misery because of its fragility. Compounding this problem is the extreme mobility of the esophagus. The prevertebral fascia that binds it to the prevertebral area is made up of loose areolar tissue, which permits the repetitive gliding traverse of the organ during swallowing. An excursion the distance of a vertebral body is common during the swallowing act, and such a degree of movement inevitably adds to the risk of any surgical procedure.

The major contributors to the blood supply of the cervical esophagus are the inferior thyroid arteries. Their twigs pierce the muscular coat in the ascending and descending course of each artery as well as near its termination. Minor contributions are also made directly from the subclavian, common carotid, vertebral, costocervical, superficial cervical, and even the superior thyroid arteries. A richer supply emanates from the right inferior thyroid artery than from the left; however, the overall circulation and nutrition do not differ between the sides.[3]

The lymphatic drainage described in 1932 by Rouvière,[4] based to a large degree on the work of Sakata,[5] has been little improved upon by the work of later investigators. A rich lymphatic network drains the mucosa and submucosa, and to a lesser degree the muscularis. These vessels are disposed in a longitudinal and transverse manner with the longitudinal vessels outnumbering the transverse by a ratio of 6:1.[5]

This, in part, probably accounts for the rapidity of submucosal spread that is characteristic of esophageal carcinoma. Connecting lymphatic vessels directly penetrate the muscular layer and terminate in adjacent thoracic nodes. The longitudinally disposed lymphatics of the thoracic esophagus run a particularly long course, with many of them reaching the neck, piercing the muscularis, and entering the cervical nodes (**Fig. 3.3**). Rouvière makes the point that the lymphatics of the upper two thirds of the esophagus have a great propensity to run superiorly and drain into these nodes. The lymph of the cervical esophagus drains directly into these nodes of the inferior neck (**Fig. 3.4**). These facts support the clinical findings that the inferior jugular aggregation of nodes is often involved in esophageal carcinoma in the neck and upper chest and that "skip areas," often of considerable separation from one another, are not uncommonly seen between cancers in the esophagus.

Mediastinum

The mediastinum is an extensive area located between the medial reflections of the pleurae; it houses the heart, great vessels, esophagus, trachea, and pulmonary hila. The portion of this region that principally concerns the head and neck surgeon is the superior compartment. The area is roofed an-

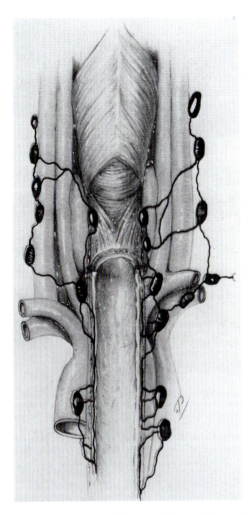

Fig. 3.4 Lymphatic drainage of the cervical esophagus and its integration with those of the hypopharynx. (From Postlethwair PW. Surgery of the Esophagus. New York: Appleton Century Crofts; 1979.)

teriorly by the manubrium sterni and the clavicular heads. A markedly thickened periosteal layer underlies the manubrium and during surgical dissection affords protection to the great vessels that lie underneath. Directly adjacent to this heavy fibrous layer is the thymus gland. It occupies a variable volume of the immediate lower neck and upper mediastinum, extending as far inferiorly as the fourth rib. The gland is relatively large at birth, reaching its maximum size at about the age of 2 years, but at puberty it begins to regress. In the adult, the gland involutes and is largely replaced by fat; the remainder measures 5 by 4 cm and is ~6 mm thick.

Intimately related to the deep surface of the thymus is the mediastinal fat pad. Numerous lymphatic channels and the pretracheal lymph nodes are found in this layer. The investing fascia of this pad also sheaths the great vessels as they cross the trachea. Near the inferior limit of the superior mediastinum, the aorta crosses the trachea from right to left. As it crosses, it gives off the right brachiocephalic artery, which, while crossing the trachea from left to right, may ascend into the lower neck. The left subclavian and left common carotid arteries emerge from the aorta on the left side of the trachea (**Fig. 3.5**). The left innominate vein crosses the trachea more superiorly than the aorta, obscuring a clear view of the trachea and lateral lymphatics. Both vagi as well as the right recurrent nerve are lateral to the trachea and deep to the vascular compartment. The width of the upper mediastinum varies with the patient's weight, measuring on the average between 5.6 and 7.4 cm (**Table 3.1**).

The lymphatics of the mediastinum that are surgically accessible are located in the pretracheal and paratracheal areas. As Sisson et al[6] have pointed out, no clearly established anatomical relationship has been elucidated between the cervical and mediastinal lymphatics. There is, however, the common finding that carcinoma involving lymphatics at the root of the neck remain stationary for a time and then spread to the mediastinum. The presumptive link between

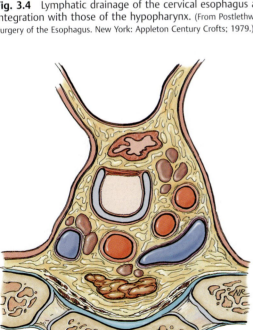

Fig. 3.5 Horizontal sectional view of the upper mediastinum taken at approximately the upper third of the manubrium sterni.

Table 3.1 Correlation of Cadaver Weight and Average Interpleural Distance

Cadaver Weight (kg)	Number of Cadavers	Average Distance between Pleural Reflections (cm)	Range (cm)
40–59	6	5.6	4.3–6.5
60–79	8	6.9	6.0–8.3
80–99	8	7.4	6.3–8.7

Source: From Carter DR. The anatomy of the mediastinum. Ear Nose Throat J 2982;60:157.

the two systems seems to be supported not only by this clinical correlate but also by the survival data in this patient group.[6] Although the nodes are not too plentiful, they are indeed present. In 20 fresh cadaver dissections, Mast and Jafek[7] found an average of three nodes in the pretracheal area, six in the right paratracheal area, and eight in the left paratracheal area. The ranges of these values are 0 to 8, 2 to 13, and 2 to 15, respectively.

◆ Pathophysiology

Squamous cell carcinomas of the hypopharynx may begin de novo or may spread from adjacent structures, especially the larynx and tongue base. Tumors with a geographic center on the aryepiglottic fold, lateral pharyngoepiglottic fold, and vallecula often involve the piriform sinus before they become symptomatic. However, these tumors are symptomatic much earlier than those that begin in the piriform recesses per se. This is some indication of the insidious nature of these neoplasms.

Most series of patients with primary tumors in this locale contain very few T1 lesions.[8] The symptoms of odynophagia, dysphagia, and voice change often do not appear until the lesion has attained massive proportions. Patients often present with weight loss and cervical adenopathy before developing symptoms referable to the hypopharynx. Moreover, hoarseness, hemoptysis, and airway obstruction generally do not ensue until there is laryngeal involvement. One patient in our own series did not seek attention until he developed intractable right heart failure secondary to upper airway obstruction caused by the large size of his tumor.

The rapid, aggressive spread of these carcinomas is in part due to the lack of restricting anatomical barriers in the hypopharynx.[9] The cervical esophagus harbors lesions that rapidly penetrate the mucosal walls to involve adjacent structures, and it has been postulated that this may be because of its lack of serosal covering.[10] The prevertebral fascia and the loose areolar fascia between it and the investing fascia of the muscular layers of the organ curiously provide a temporary but effective barrier to posterior spread of the cancer. The rich lymphatic network in the lamina propria and submucosa of the esophageal epithelium may explain the rapid longitudinal spread that is so commonplace with malignancies here (**Fig. 3.6**). The skip areas may be explained by the fact that the tumor cells embolize in the submucosal layer below the muscularis mucosae, travel a short distance longitudinally in this lamina, and then replicate and rupture

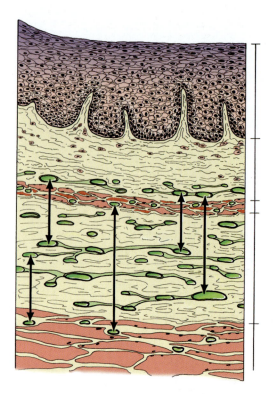

Fig. 3.6 Drawing of idealized photomicrograph illustrating the rich lymphatic network in the lamina propria and submucosal of the esophageal epithelium and its numerous interconnections, proving a possible explanation of the frequent finding of multifocal cancer in the esophagus. Epith, epithelium; LP, lamina propria; ME, esophageal muscle; MM, muscularis mucosae; SM, submucosal.

through the epithelial surface at a point some centimeters away from the original tumor.

That the hypopharynx has a lesser tendency to develop multiple tumor foci with intervening skip areas may be due to histological differences in its submucosal layer (**Fig. 3.7**). Instead of the thick submucosal layer and the well-developed muscularis mucosae characteristic of the esophagus, the pharynx possesses a dearth of the former and a replacement of the muscularis by a dense layer of elastic tissue. The pharyngeal mucosa is closely approximated to the longitudinal and circular muscle layers.[11] As the hypopharynx blends into the cervical esophagus, the thick elastic layer of the lamina propria becomes plusher and more richly endowed with lymphatics. The frequency of "multiple hypopharyngeal primaries" in this area as a possible manifestation of the multifocal cancer from a single tumor, in contrast to the rarity of this phenomenon elsewhere in the pharynx, may be explained on this basis; however, this finding is far less commonly seen in the hypopharynx than in the esophagus.

Carcinomas of the cervical esophagus commonly remain occult until they have reached considerable size. Dysphagia and odynophagia are not uncommonly preceded by a period of weight loss, the presentation of a lump in the neck, or symptoms of invasion of adjacent structures such as the larynx, the vagus and recurrent laryngeal nerves, or the cervical sympathetic trunk (**Fig. 3.8**). Symptoms of swallowing disturbance may also include the regurgitation of bloody material.

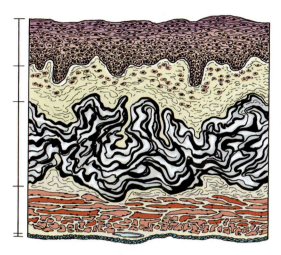
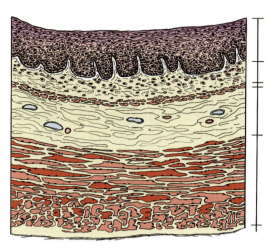

Fig. 3.7 Comparison of the submucosal layers of the oropharynx and the esophagus. The thick elastic layer of the oropharynx may provide a barrier to tumor penetration. No such barrier exists in the esophagus, and the mucosa is applied directly to the muscularis. The hypopharynx is a transitional zone regarding the elastic layer.

Here the elastic layer becomes attenuated, and the lamina propria possesses much loose connective tissue and is richly invested with lymphatics. Adv, adventitia; Ep, epithelium; Elas, elastic layer; LP, lamina propria; M, muscularis; ME, esophageal muscle; MM, muscularis mucosae; Ser, serosa; SM, submucosal.

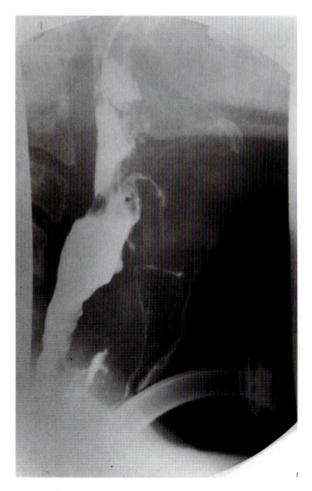

Fig. 3.8 Barium swallow of an elderly man with cervical esophageal carcinoma that had eroded through the entire wall of the esophagus and developed a sinus tract into the neck.

Rarely, a carcinoma may develop in a Zenker diverticulum (**Fig. 3.9**).[12] This alone is an excellent reason to perform esophagoscopy on every patient with this abnormality prior to its excision. The regurgitation characteristic of a pharyngoesophageal diverticulum is bloody only if a malignancy is present. Most patients with this cancer have prolonged histories of diverticula. Possibly the longstanding irritation of the mucosa secondary to stasis of food in the pouch may play a part in the initiation of such lesions.

A discussion of the lymphatic draining the hypopharynx would not be complete without a consideration of the retropharyngeal lymph nodes. In chapter 2 a discussion of the retropharyngeal lymph nodes refers to the paucity of nodes that exist at this site. Few as they may be, however, these nodes are occasionally the site of metastasis from carcinoma originating in the hypopharynx. The routine resection of these nodes during the radical procedure recommended by Bova et al.[13] may be in part at least the reason for his high 5-year tumor-free survival rates for this usually deadly tumor.

◆ Diagnosis

One of the most common presenting symptoms of all of these tumors is a lump in the neck (**Fig. 3.10**). This finding may be the only sign or symptom until indirect laryngoscopy or esophagoscopy reveals its primary source. It is not unusual for a patient with a painless, slowly growing neck mass to be treated with several courses of different antibiotics and occasionally have the misfortune to have a nodal biopsy before more skilled consultation is sought.

Unfortunately, sore throat, odynophagia, often with referred otalgia, dysphagia, hemoptysis, and hoarseness appear late in the course of these tumors. An early sign not uncommonly seen is the complaint of a sense of a foreign

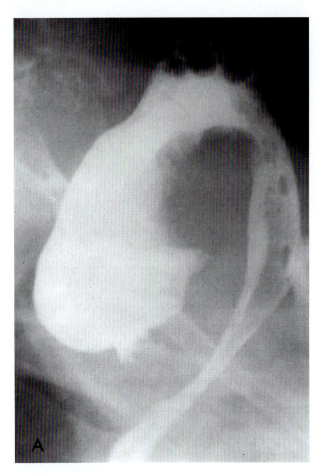

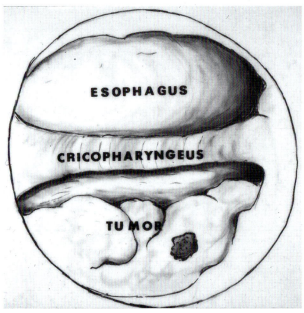

Fig. 3.9 A squamous cell carcinoma in the Zenker diverticulum. (**A**) Barium swallow showing irregular space-occupying lesion in the diverticulum. (**B**) Drawing of endoscopic view of tumor. (From Donald PJ, Huffman DI. Carcinoma in a Zenker's diverticulum. Journal of Head and Neck Surgery. 1979;2:71.)

body in the pharynx. This is, unfortunately, often dismissed by the primary care physician as globus hystericus. Very late symptoms such as severe restriction of swallowing and airway obstruction, which are often accompanied by significant weight loss of 20 lb or more, are often accompanied by bilateral lymphadenopathy are not uncommonly seen.

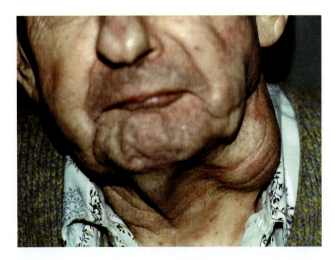

Fig. 3.10 Mass in the neck was the only symptom in this elderly man with a large pyriform sinus carcinoma.

A barium esophagogram followed by laryngoscopy and esophagoscopy is the standard diagnostic procedure for all of these lesions of the hypopharynx and cervical esophagus. The typical "apple core" appearance of esophageal cancers is pathognomonic (**Fig. 3.11 and Fig. 3.12**).

By far the most common hypopharyngeal lesion is that found in the piriform recesses. In Kirchner's series, 152 lesions were found in the piriform sinus, whereas only eight were seen in the postcricoid area and seven in the posterior pharyngeal wall.[14] In a series from the Mayo Clinic, 20 lesions were found in the posterior pharyngeal wall and only seven in the postcricoid area.[9] Som and Nussbaum[15] discuss the management of 61 large hypopharyngeal lesions that they described as postcricoid but which appear to have been large circumferential lesions whose precise geographic center was difficult to discern. The massive size of the lesions in their series is representative of most surgeons' experience. In our own early series only six of 37 piriform sinus tumors were T1 or T2 in size.[16] In the 20 years since that report over 200 additional pyriform carcinomas have been identified and only two of them have been T1 in size.

Although Conley[8] states that over 50% of patients with piriform sinus cancer have regional metastases when first diagnosed, Ogura et al[17] noticed cervical secondaries in 90% of his patients. Harwick[18] noted a 40% incidence of contralateral nodal involvement in his patients. In our series, 60% of patients had lymph node metastases, and in over half of these

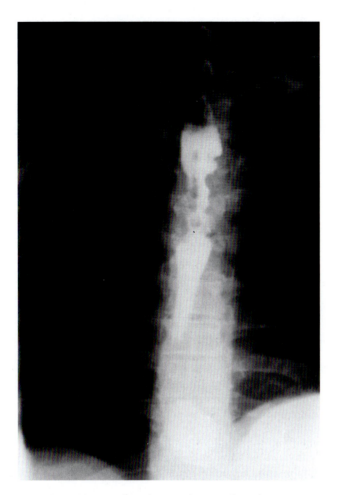

Fig. 3.11 Barium swallow showing the typical "apple core" appearance (*arrow*) of esophageal cancer.

cases the secondary lesions were N2 or N3 in extent. Kirchner[14] reports finding palpable adenopathy in 71% of his 116 cases, whereas Razack et al[19] note an incidence of 87.6%.

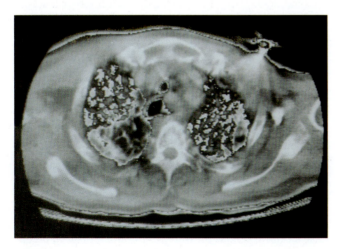

Fig. 3.12 Computed tomographic scan of the neck in horizontal section, showing the extraesophageal extent of carcinoma of the esophagus.

In cervical esophageal cancer, nodal metastases are also common. Postlethwait,[10] citing a growing trend toward routine use of scalene fat-pad biopsy for esophageal carcinoma in general, describes his own experience with 78 such biopsies, which revealed metastatic cancer in 40 cases. In Mustard's series,[20] a similar pattern was seen.

◆ Treatment

In the author's opinion, the most effective form of therapy for hypopharyngeal cancer is radical surgery that encompasses the entire tumor with a generous margin of healthy tissue followed by a full and timely course of irradiation therapy. The early results of the Veteran's Administration study on the treatment of advanced carcinoma of the larynx and hypopharynx with the chemotherapy/radiation therapy protocol has yet to have the absolute 5-year survival rates published. The early results show a slight survival advantage for the conventional treatment of surgery plus irradiation therapy, but the difference is not statistically significant. Failure at the local site was a common cause of death in the chemotherapy-radiation arm.[21] The experience of Som and Nussbaum[14] in which one patient out of 27 with hypopharyngeal cancer treated with primary irradiation therapy survived 5 years is echoed by others.[2,16,22–24] A recent report by Million and Cassisi[25] indicates a favorable prognosis when radiotherapy is used for very small lesions, but these diminutive lesions are unfortunately rare.

As has been noted, most often the lesions encountered are of substantial size, and radical excision with in-continuity radical neck dissection is generally the rule. We believe that there is good evidence to show that the use of postoperative irradiation therapy adds significantly to the survival rate.[16] In our own experience the survival rate has been better with postoperative rather than preoperative irradiation; this may be due to the fact that the shrinking effect on the tumor caused by preoperative irradiation makes it difficult to establish accurate resection margins at the time of surgery. In addition, the complication rate is much lower when the irradiation is used postoperatively.[23]

The approach to hypopharyngeal cancer treatment by the Brisbane group with laryngopharyngectomy and postoperative irradiation is even more radical than our own in that they almost always do a total pharyngectomy and reconstruction using a free flap of microvascularized tissue. Their 47% disease specific survival rate is excellent evidence of this modality of treatment.[21]

Wide extirpation of the lesion is the rule. Rarely, if ever, can the larynx be spared, because of the intimate relationship of the piriform sinus mucosa to the laryngeal skeleton (**Fig. 3.13**). A radical neck dissection is always done in the presence of cervical adenopathy. Occasionally the operation can be modified and the spinal accessory nerves spared but only if the nerve is distinctly separate from the metastasis. If the neck is clinically negative, a selective neck dissection is done that spares level 1 but includes level 4. If a positive node is discovered then a radical or modified radical neck dissection is done. Because of the frequency of bilateral metastasis,

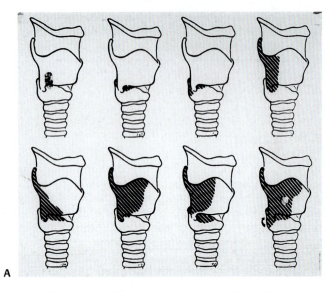

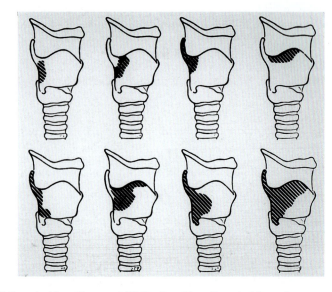

Fig. 3.13 Pattern of invasion of carcinoma of the pyriform sinus into (**A**) the cricoid cartilage and (**B**) the thyroid cartilage in 16 specimens. (From Kirchner JA. Pyriform sinus cancer: a clinical and laboratory study. Annals of Otolaryngology, Rhinology and Laryngology. 1975;83:793.)

if the contralateral neck is negative then a selective neck is done on that side. The issue of simultaneous bilateral neck dissections will be discussed in the next section.

The experience of Steiner and Ambrosch, Rudert, and others has shown that for lesions of the hypopharynx transoral laser microsurgical resection can effectively excise most hypopharyngeal lesions while at the same time preserve laryngeal function.[26,27] In their latest report in a series of 129 previously untreated patients with hypopharyngeal carcinoma with 98 cases being either T1 or T2, fifty-eight percent of patients had postoperative irradiation therapy. The local control rate was 87% and the 5-year overall (Kaplan-Meier) survival rate was 71% for stages I and II and 47% for stages III and IV tumors.[27]

Postoperative irradiation generally does a creditable job of eliminating occult cancer in lymphatics of the neck. It is not uncommon, however, to have to operate on a protein-depleted, asthenic patient who has been imbibing alcohol heavily and neglecting nutrition and is in a state of negative nitrogen balance. These individuals are at a high risk of developing a major postoperative complication that will necessitate a delay in radiation therapy. Unfortunately, once the "golden period" of 4 to 6 weeks has elapsed between surgery and irradiation, the efficacy of the latter modality rapidly diminishes. We have seen several patients develop neck metastases in the interim between surgery and the start of irradiation when dissection of the neck ipsilateral to the tumor was not done.

The addition of adjunctive chemotherapy in those patients with hypopharyngeal as well as other advanced head and neck carcinomas to the regimen of irradiation therapy has been shown to increase the local tumor-free control rate[28] by 10%. In this large cohort of patients they were at high risk by virtue of the presence of two or more positive cervical lymph nodes, extracapsular spread of nodal disease, or positive mucosal margins. The minimal follow-up was years, and

the average follow-up was over 45 months. It is important to note that the rate of adjunctive treatment-related severe complications was 34% in the postoperative radiotherapy alone group and 77% in those who had combined chemotherapy and postoperative irradiation. There were four chemotherapy-related deaths in the latter group. In more recent years we have adopted this postoperative combined radiation and chemotherapy strategy, and its efficacy will have to stand the test of time.

The problem cases of hypopharyngeal carcinoma involve those patients who have massive lesions, those with bilateral lymph node involvement, and those with lesions extending into the cervical esophagus.

Bilateral Neck Dissection

Bilateral adenopathy may be handled with either a staged neck dissection or a simultaneous bilateral neck dissection. Whether one procedure is superior to the other is not clear, but our preference with palpable bilateral nodes is to do a simultaneous dissection. A radical neck dissection is performed on the side of greatest pharyngeal tumor involvement, but the dissection on the contralateral side spares the internal jugular vein if possible. If both veins are to be sacrificed, certain precautions must be observed. Facial swelling and edema can be reduced if the patient's head is tipped up at a 30 degree angle during the surgery. In fact, if the head is flat or slightly dependent, the swelling can be so pronounced that it will produce exorbitism. Even with the head elevated, it is wise to tape the eyes securely shut, and place soft pads over the eyes then wrap the head with a cling dressing. Because of this slightly head-up position, the patient should have a central venous pressure (CVP) catheter placed preoperatively, so that in the event of an air embolism, the air may be easily withdrawn from the right atrium. A precordial Doppler scanner provides an excellent highly sensitive monitor in the event of this complication. The head is placed in a Mayfield headrest (Integra Lifesciences Corp., Plainsboro, NJ) without the cranial fixation pins. The horseshoe headrest is heavily padded and the head position frequently changed to prevent pressure necrosis of the scalp. About 10 mg of Decadron are given during the procedure, and the anesthesiologist is admonished to restrict intravenous fluids and replace lost blood with packed cells.

Once one jugular vein has been ligated, tremendous engorgement of the venous system on the contralateral side ensues. If the internal jugular vein must be taken on this side, blood loss will be reduced if its ligation is delayed until the end of the dissection of this neck. Careful hemostasis is essential as the dissection proceeds. Meticulous cross clamping of veins prior to cutting them supersedes the advantage of rapid dissection and clamping of vessels as they bleed because the increased venous pressure results in excessive blood loss with this latter method.

At the conclusion of the procedure the application of dermal grafts to the carotids provides excellent prophylaxis against the catastrophe of carotid blowout if the artery should become exposed in the postoperative period. The graft when exposed to air rapidly epithelializes and will not only cover the exposed artery but will spread to cover large raw areas that have become devoid of epithelium (**Fig. 3.14 and Fig. 3.15**).

There is much apprehension expressed in the literature regarding the hazard of simultaneous radical neck dissections.

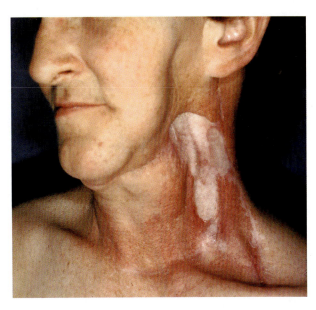

Fig. 3.15 Reepithelialization of large dehiscent area of neck by dermal graft on carotid artery.

Koch,[29] quoting Ahn et al,[48] mentions increased intracranial pressure, facial edema, blindness, and death as complications of simultaneous radical neck dissection. Suen and Stern[30] mention an overall eightfold increase in complications of bilateral neck dissection compared with unilateral. In an exhaustive review of 703 patients in the M.D. Anderson experience Ballantyne[31] reports on the results of 344 patients who had simultaneous bilateral neck dissections. Very few in the series had a simultaneous radical neck dissection; most had some form of a modified neck dissection on at least one side. There was a 6.1% postoperative mortality rate. This compared more favorably with the previously established rate by Sako[32] of 10%. The mortality in our group of simultaneous radical neck dissections was zero. Postoperative facial edema was common, but massive swelling was rare. The most serious complication was bilateral blindness that was attributed to massive fluid overload with consequent cerebral edema and exorbitism.

Total Laryngopharyngectomy

Total exenteration of the larynx and pharynx is often necessary in patients with large hypopharyngeal lesions. Preservation of a small strip of mucosa that can be only tightly approximated over a nasogastric tube is to be discouraged. Not only is the patient frequently troubled later by severe dysphagia, but also the cancer-excising potential of the operation is often compromised.

The surgery is approached through a modified H incision (**Fig. 3.16**). This provides optimal exposure and supplies ample opportunity for any necessary modification, should extension of the surgery be required. In addition, such exigencies as bilateral neck dissection or mediastinal resection can be easily provided for (**Fig. 3.17**).

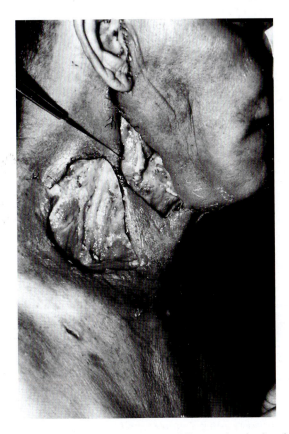

Fig. 3.14 Exposed carotid artery following slough of neck flaps.

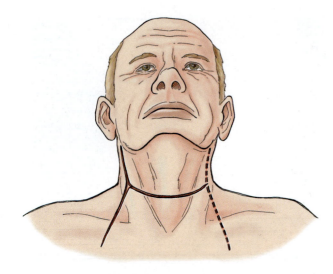

Fig. 3.16 Modified H incision. Dotted line represents extension into full H incision for bilateral neck dissection.

With lesions involving the posterior wall, preliminary endoscopic assessment of pharyngeal mobility must be confirmed at surgery. If mobility is not present, posterior pharyngeal wall transgression of tumor with fixation to the spine is suspected. If resectability is in doubt because of the suspicion of widespread spinal fixation of tumor, a small cutaneous incision in the line of the proposed neck dissection provides access to the normally easily dissectible retropharyngeal plane. Tumor penetration will be revealed by fixation of the pharyngeal wall to the prevertebral fascia. The pharynx in some instances may be separable from the spine, but firm dissection is required to do so. A whitish, plaquelike appearance of the muscular wall is usually encountered in this situation, indicating tumor penetration. Resections of

limited areas of the cervical spine are discussed in chapter 2. Fixation of tumor to the common carotid artery similarly indicates a poor prognosis. The artery may be resected and grafted, but the eventual survival rate is markedly reduced. In Kennedy's series[33] the 5-year tumor-free survival rate was no better than 10%. In our series published by Nayak et al[34] there was a 2-year and better survival rate of 20%.

If the pharynx is free of wide fixation, the radical neck dissection is then executed. Care is taken to ensure that the radical neck bloc is pedicled on the fascia connecting it to the pharynx. It is through this layer that the lymph vessels traverse. If one remembers that the carotid artery should be located deep to this connection, the continuity will be maintained. Lifting the bloc superiorly and using finger dissection anterior to the artery helps to preserve the en bloc nature of the dissection (**Fig. 3.18**).

Management of the thyroid gland in laryngectomy and even radical neck dissection is somewhat controversial. Standard practice is to remove any lobe of the gland that has a palpable mass. Local extension of neoplasm into the thyroid is not uncommon, and our practice in large, circumferential pharyngeal lesions is to take the entire gland. However, if the lobe on the side opposite the neck dissection is perfectly soft and that side of the neck is devoid of adenopathy, the lobe is saved.

The parathyroid glands are preserved when possible. When total thyroidectomy is done, postoperative vigilance for signs of hypercalcemia secondary to hypoparathyroidism is essential (**Fig. 3.19 and Fig. 3.20**). Even with preservation of one thyroid lobe, myxedema may occur because of diminished vascularity to the gland resulting from the neck dissection or from subsequent irradiation.[35] Postoperative T4

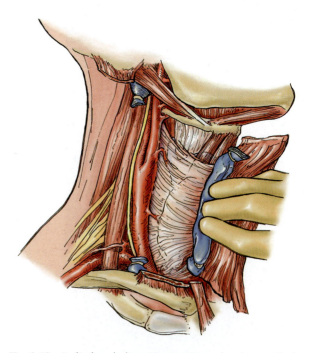

Fig. 3.18 Radical neck dissection specimen showing continuity throughout its length with the pharyngeal fascia, through which tumor may spread via the contained lymphatics.

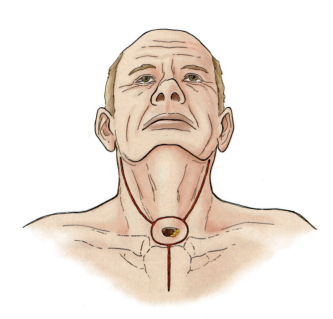

Fig. 3.17 Extension for mediastinal dissection.

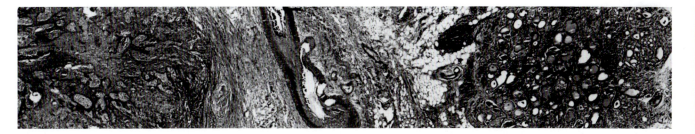

Fig. 3.19 Photomicrograph illustrating microinvasion of the thyroid gland by a hypopharyngeal carcinoma (H&E, ×130).

studies are important for early detection of hypothyroidism and subsequent thyroid hormone replacement.

As the superior margin of tumor resection is being delineated, the extent of involvement of the tongue base must be accurately assessed. A wide margin is necessary in instances of lingual involvement because of the pernicious nature of cancer once it invades this organ. If at all possible, the hypoglossal nerves are spared (**Fig. 3.21**); however, this must not be at the expense of adequate tumor resection. Often the nerves can be dissected from the surface of the mylohyoid muscle and retracted superiorly. A generous margin of tongue can then be excised without significantly compromising subsequent lingual function.

During the skeletonization of the larynx, the hypoglossal nerve on the side opposite the neck dissection is at risk because of its proximity to the greater cornu of the hyoid. The nerve can be protected by grasping this cornu with an Allis clamp, detaching the common tendon of the digastric muscle and the stylohyoid insertion, and then freeing up the cornu by dissection along its deep surface. The nerve may have to be taken as the subsequent excision proceeds, but this maneuver may prevent its needless sacrifice. The lower end of the laryngectomy is established on the basis of the inferior extent of the pharyngeal tumor and, if the cervical esophagus is involved, on whether it encroaches upon the anterior wall. Because the posterior wall of the trachea is so close to the anterior wall of the esophagus, it is necessary to take the trachea below the level of esophageal involvement. This is often a hard decision, for if the trachea must be taken low, excision of the manubrium is necessary for safe construction of the tracheostoma. In borderline situations in which the trachea is a bit short, but not so much as to mandate the excision of the manubrium, extra skin may be recruited by constructing an advancement flap of chest skin, which is then slid into the upper mediastinum (**Fig. 3.22**). One patient in our experience had a tracheal resection that left her with only 2.5 to 3.0 cm of residual trachea. Resection of the manubrium followed by advancement of chest skin and the use of a Silastic (Aisthetic Concepts, El Dorado Hills, CA) tube provided her with a clear airway.

Cervical esophageal involvement is usually an indication for mediastinal resection. Low hypopharyngeal malignancy involving the cricopharyngeus warrants an examination of the mediastinum. A computed tomographic (CT) scan of the medi-

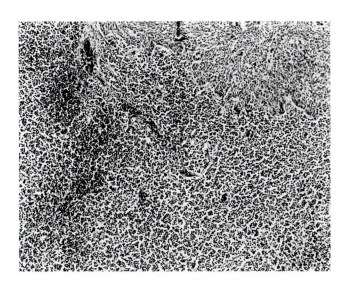

Fig. 3.20 Photomicrograph showing microinvasion of a parathyroid gland by a squamous cell carcinoma of the pyriform fossa (H&E, ×130).

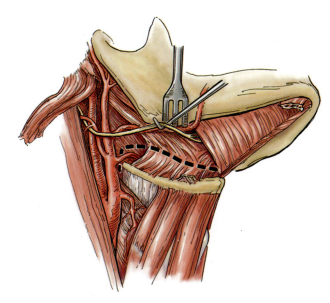

Fig. 3.21 Hypoglossal nerve may be dissected from the fascia of the lateral aspect of the pharyngeal constrictors if no tumor penetration exists.

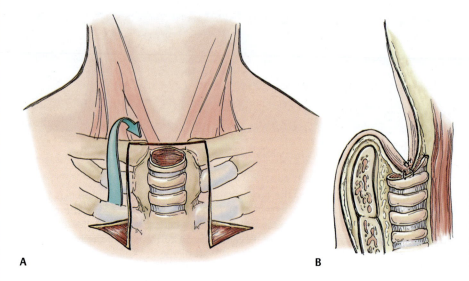

Fig. 3.22 How tracheal amputation can be occasionally handled by advancing a chest flap over the manubrium sterni into the upper mediastinum. (**A**) *Frontal view*, Advancement chest flap cut and Burow triangles excised to facilitate flap advancement to trachea. (**B**) *Lateral view*, Advancement flap sutured to anterior tracheal wall in upper mediastinum.

astinum and perhaps a positron emission tomographic (PET)-CT scan may provide some evidence of mediastinal spread. Mediastinoscopy will reveal evidence of nodal involvement of the anterior compartment. Large nodes usually bode ill, but microscopic adenopathy is potentially curable using a combination of resection and postoperative radiotherapy.

In some individuals with advanced tumors at these sites multiple levels in the hypopharynx, larynx, and oropharynx are involved with tumor, and the patient presents in a state of emaciation and general poor condition. It is important to perform a rapid resection and a quick closure. Reconstruction is delayed until a future time. Two stomas are then constructed,

an oropharyngostome and an esophagostome, with a bridge of skin over the paraspinous muscles and cervical spine.

The oropharyngostoma is best constructed by pulling down the upper skin flap like a curtain and making a transverse incision in the middle of it. The slit opens and the anterior margin is sewn to the base of the tongue and the walls of the pharynx to the posterior skin edge (**Fig. 3.23**). If a substantial tongue resection is necessary, the tongue and lateral pharynx may need to be sewn to the inferior edge of the upper flap. In this instance, if the lower flap cannot be advanced to the posterior pharyngeal wall, the gap is bridged with a skin graft (**Fig. 3.24**).

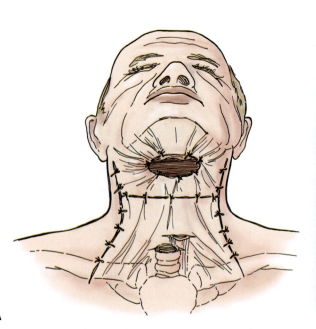
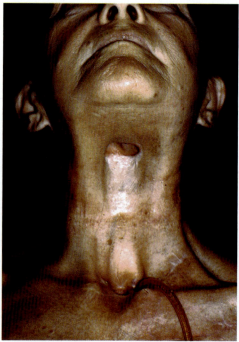

Fig. 3.23 (**A**) Pharyngostoma created by placing a slit in the upper flap of the modified H incision. (**B**) Healed pharyngostoma ready for pharyngoesophageal reconstruction.

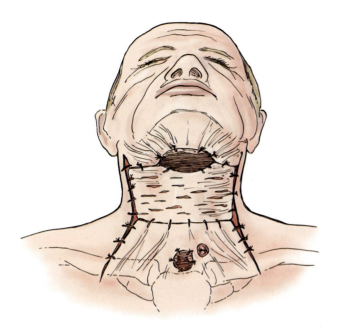

Fig. 3.24 When the upper flap is of insufficient length, the gap between the posterior pharyngeal wall and the lower skin flap is bridged with a skin graft. The esophagostoma is positioned laterally and when possible superiorly to the tracheostoma.

A nasogastric tube is placed into the esophagostoma for feeding. The oropharyngostoma is packed with iodoform-soaked gauze, dressed with fluffed gauze, and held in place with a Barton-type bandage. A nasal tube attached to continuous suction is placed in the oropharynx to evacuate saliva and reduce contamination of the wound edges. The nursing staff needs to be aware of the requirement for frequent dressing changes. This is essential to avoid aspiration and subsequent pneumonias as well as to prevent local infection. A nasogastric tube is used for feeding, or a feeding gastrostomy or jejunostomy is performed to eliminate the irritation of the nasogastric tube during the period of postoperative irradiation.

Reconstruction

Reconstruction may be either immediate or delayed. We tend to favor delay in debilitated patients with large tumors. Postoperative wound complications are not uncommon in this group of patients, and in these the safest and most expedient form of closure should be employed. A major wound breakdown may significantly delay the beginning of radiotherapy, and if longer than 6 weeks passes between the time of surgery and the onset of irradiation, the treatment will likely be of diminishing value as the delay progresses past this golden period. In addition, there is considerable reluctance on the part of many radiotherapists to irradiate a dehiscent wound; however, an established pharyngocutaneous fistula or granulating wound, in the face of irradiation, will usually continue to heal, albeit more slowly. New fistulae, wound infection, or massive skin flap loss may force a delay that could result in the appearance of a tumor nodule in the wound site or a metastasis in the unoperated neck. Early reconstruction

of the gullet, even with the institution of a "decompression" fistula, creates the potential for increased complications.

In most patients immediate reconstruction is done. The tubed thoracic skin flap described by Bakamjian[36,37] in 1965 was for the next 15 years the golden standard of pharyngeal reconstruction. There are still some cases in which this flap may be used but they are decidedly in the minority. The pectoralis major myocutaneous flap, or this flap used principally as a myogenous flap, with or without a covering with a skin graft or a free vascularized flap, is most commonly used. The advantages of the deltopectoral flap described by Bakamjian are its simplicity, rapidity of harvest, and thinness. The major drawbacks are the necessity of two separate operative stages, the sometimes-tenuous nature of the distal blood supply, and the occasional need for a delay to ensure satisfactory vascularity at the tip.[38] Despite these facts, for the sake of completeness I will include a brief description of the construction of the deltopectoral flap. This medially pedicled chest flap is based on the perforating branches of the internal mammary artery. Occasionally when there is a concern about the vascularity of the flap tip, a delay of 3 weeks is observed. Because of the exigencies of the tumor in many cases, this delay is often not possible. If a delay is an option, it is necessary to raise only the deltoid portion of skin and incise the flap's outline (**Fig. 3.25**).[29] In most instances, especially in an otherwise healthy patient, an immediately rotated flap survives without major complication.

The flap is elevated and tubed on itself with the cutaneous surface facing inside (**Fig. 3.26**). Interrupted, everting, absorbable sutures are used to tube the skin. A second layer in the subcutis is done using a vertical mattress suture tied loosely enough to avoid vascular compromise at the wound edges. The distal end of the skin tube is anastomosed end to end to the oropharyngostoma. A double layer of sutures will ensure a watertight closure. The esophagus is sutured into

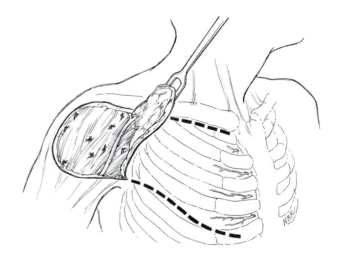

Fig. 3.25 In delaying the deltopectoral flap, only the portion of the flap over the deltoid muscle—that part that is supplied by the musculocutaneous perforators—need be elevated. The rest of the flap, which is supplied in the main by the perforating branches of the internal mammary arteries in the second, third, and fourth intercostal spaces, is simply outlined (*dashed line*).

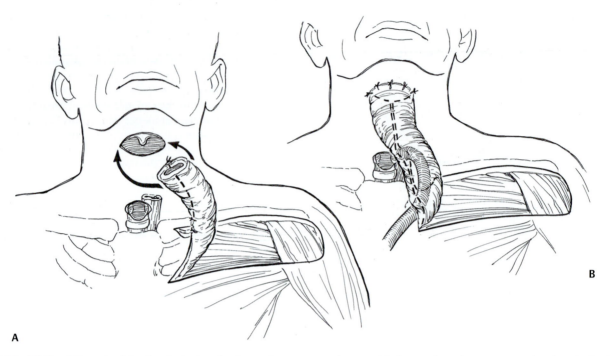

A

B

Fig. 3.26 **(A)** The deltopectoral flap is tubed using simple everting sutures. A watertight closure is accomplished with a second layer of loosely placed vertical mattress sutures in the subcutis. **(B)** The deltoid end of the tube is sutured end to end to the pharynx. The medial portion of the tube is anastomosed end to side to the esophagus, with the esophageal anastomosis placed in the back surface of the flap. The flap is tubed for a short distance beyond this anastomosis. The nasogastric tube is placed through the site, which also serves for decompression.

the back surface of the flap as an end-to-side anastomosis, and the flap is tubed for a short distance beyond this. The bottom end of the deltopectoral flap is left open and serves for decompression. The cervical skin flaps are closed over the reconstructed gullet, and the feeding tube is maintained through the enclosed aspect of the chest flap. Any exposed raw area is skin grafted.

As already mentioned, the deltopectoral flap is rarely used today. The pectoralis myocutaneous flap and either the anterolateral thigh or radial forearm free flaps are the most commonly employed. Although the pectoralis musculocutaneous flap has a vigorous blood supply the major drawback is its bulk. This is especially true in heavyset men and in women. A partial solution to this problem is the use of only the muscular part of the flap. This flap is especially important in women in whom the breast can be preserved and chest wall deformity diminished. The problem is to supply the lining to the inner surface of the flap to prevent contracture and subsequent stenosis. This can be provided by the application of a split-thickness skin graft.

The description of the elevation of the pectoralis major musculocutaneous flap is well presented in several articles[39,40] and texts.[41,42] Only a few salient points will be mentioned here. I think it is important to cut the flap full thickness, from skin through muscle, all at once over a length of ~4 cm at a time and then anchor the skin to the underlying muscle with sutures that will be removed at the time of the flap's inset. This will prevent shearing forces that may damage the perforating vessels going from the undersurface of the muscle to the cutaneous portion of the flap. Once the distal part of the flap skin is secured in such a manner, then the elevation of the flap from the chest wall is done. Once the insertions of the pectoralis muscle have been released from the chest wall, finger dissection will separate the remainder of the muscle up to its blood supply from the pectoral branch of the thoracoacromial artery exiting medial to the pectoralis minor muscle. The artery is easily found in the upper part of its course on the undersurface of the flap down to the level of the third rib, but more is obscure in the distal part. A random pattern extension may be fashioned at the distal part of the flap even over the inferior costal rim, but this should be minimized or avoided if possible because this paddle will slough in a significant number of cases. The pedicle may be tunneled under the upper chest skin, but no hesitation should be exercised in cutting the overlying skin if the slightest suspicion of subsequent pedicle compression exists. This is especially important if bilateral neck dissections have been done. Pressure at the pedicle may be relieved by the removal of the head and medial one fifth of the clavicle then insetting the flap in the notch. Similarly, if the flap is not easily covered by the neck skin once the flap is anastomosed to the pharynx and cervical esophagus, then the neck and chest skin incision is not closed over the area of tension and the pectoral muscle is covered by a split-thickness skin. The flap can even be employed as a pedicled flap rather then as an island flap, and the pedicle will be returned at a later date (**Fig. 3.27**). A watertight closure at the pharynx and esophagus with absorbable sutures is essential to a successful result.

The choice of free flap reconstruction is often between the anterolateral thigh and radial forearm flaps. The once popu-

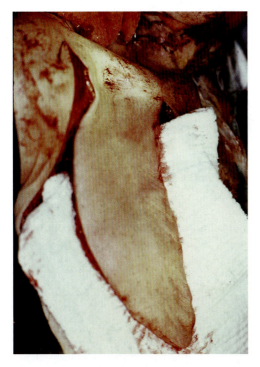

Fig. 3.27 Pectoralis major musculocutaneous flap used as a pedicled flap.

lar jejunal free flap has of late been abandoned in favor of the aforementioned cutaneous flaps. The reasons center around, first, the drawback of adding a laparotomy and its attendant potential complications to an already lengthy procedure for the ablation of the tumor. A straight-line flap is impossible to obtain because of the limitation inherent in the blood supply from the mesenteric arcade. The flap is often "C" or "S" shaped, sometimes resulting in difficulty in swallowing as well, making subsequent dilation of strictures at the site of the distal anastomosis troublesome. Additionally the copious mucous secretion interferes with the production of fistula speech and may be bothersome during swallowing. The advantages of the jejunal flap are that the flap is usually long enough to bridge the long gap that results from a hypopharyngeal and cervical esophageal resection and that it is mucous secreting. Its advantages are also its drawbacks in that the sufficient length required for maintaining the blood supply from its nutrient arcade also creates redundancy in many flaps, and the mucous secretion may be excessive.

The technique of harvest and inset of both the anterolateral thigh and radial forearm free flaps has been thoroughly described in the literature.[43] The disadvantages of the radial forearm free flap are usually the limitations imposed by flap length and the fact that the epithelium is without mucous glands. The other disadvantage is the necessity of placing a split-thickness skin graft at the donor site. The radial forearm flap has the advantages of ease and rapidity of harvest. The anterolateral thigh flap takes longer to elevate, has a shorter vascular pedicle, and is thicker and somewhat less pliable than the forearm flap. We prefer the radial forearm flap whenever

possible (**Fig. 3.28**). Both flaps stand up well to the rigors of irradiation therapy and have a very high success rate.

The recipient vessels are either the facial, superior thyroid, or lingual arteries and occasionally the stump of the external carotid and the external or internal jugular veins. Usually the patient with a hypopharyngeal or cervical esophageal carcinoma will need bilateral neck dissections. Often the neck on the side opposite the mucosal lesion will require either a selective or modified radical dissection in which the jugular veins on that side are preserved. In these instances the donor vessels are anastomosed to the jugular vein end to side. In those instances in which no vein is available in the neck, then a jump graft to a branch of the subclavian or axillary vein is done.

A watertight seal is essential for success. An obliquely oriented or irregular suture line at the site of the anastomosis of the flap to the pharynx and especially the cervical or upper thoracic esophagus is essential to prevent stenosis (**Fig. 3.29**). A monitoring skin paddle, in the case of the forearm flap, or of bowel, in the jejunal flap, aids in the periodic checks of the integrity of the microvascular anastomosis and the viability of the flap. Alternatively a Doppler can be utilized for flap monitoring.

In the delayed cases, it is very simple and convenient to employ the skin of the anterior neck for the inner lining. Despite the detrimental effects of radiation therapy, this skin stands up well to the demands of a pharyngoesophageal lining. The method used is based on the time-honored technique of Wookey.[44] The surgery is delayed until 4 to 6 weeks have passed from the time of cessation of radiotherapy. A flap is designed with its center in the midline of the neck (**Fig. 3.30**). It must be sufficiently wide when tubed so that it will give an internal diameter of adequate dimension. As the flap is elevated, greater length is generally taken on the side without the neck dissection. As the skin is peeled off the carotid artery on the neck-dissected side, the previously placed dermis graft will be seen to have become a layer of fibrous tissue. An easy dissection plane is generally found between this layer and the skin. Once the flaps have been elevated on either side, they are approximated one to the other. Special attention must be paid to the end near the tracheostoma where the skin edge must be elevated enough so

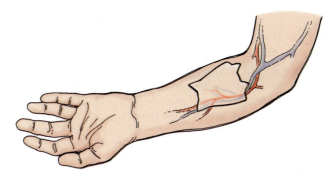

Fig. 3.28 Radial forearm free flap with vascular supply marked out.

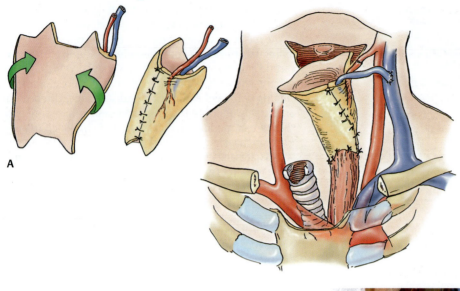

Fig. 3.29 (**A**) Radial forearm free flap harvested. (**B**) Flap tubed on itself. (**C**) Flap anastomosed to the cervical esophagus below and the oropharynx above.

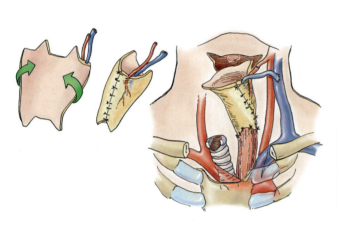

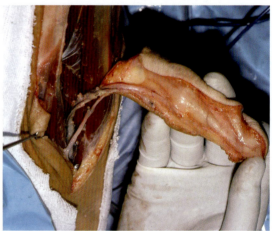

A

B

C

that the skin flap providing the outside layer can be approximated to the cutaneous tissue adjacent to the tracheostoma (**Fig. 3.30B**).

The outside lining utilizes a regional skin flap: either pectoralis major or nape of the neck (**Fig. 3.31**). The nape neck of flap is usually reserved for those unfortunate individuals who have previously lost one or both pectoralis flaps. It is used much less frequently now than in former years primarily because it is a staged procedure and requires extensive skin grafting over the posterior aspect of the shoulder that leaves a significant area of scarring (**Fig. 3.32**). It is an excellent alternative in women who wish to avoid any deformation of the breast. The nape-of-neck flap must be delayed in at least three stages (see chapter 1) because of the tenuous nature of its blood supply. The occipital arteries, the major nutrient vessels of this flap, can successfully supply a substantial flap of skin if the procedure is sufficiently delayed.

An advantage of this flap is that there is no necessity to return a pedicle because the flap slides around the neck like a scarf.

These reconstructed gullets serve as excellent food conduits and can be used for esophageal or fistula speech. The long-term complications include the occasional case of stricture and, in males, hirsutism (**Fig. 3.33**) of the flap lining. Hirsutism is a vexing problem and can be eventually eliminated by repeated mechanical epilation through a cervical esophagoscope and laser ablation of the hair follicles. A stricture is usually easily managed with bougienage and only rarely requires revision.

Management of Lesions of the Cervical Esophagus

A precise therapeutic approach to cervical esophageal carcinoma remains difficult to delineate. A large body of opinion

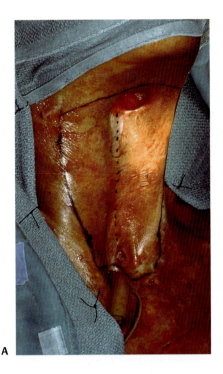
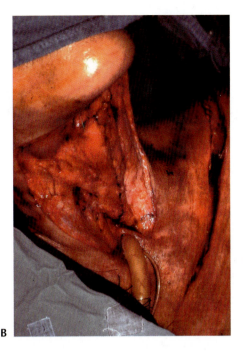

A   B

Fig. 3.30 Pharyngoesophageal reconstruction using a Wookey style flap of neck skin for internal lining and a deltopectoral flap for the outer. (**A**) Wookey flap outlined. (**B**) Flap elevated and approximated to itself to provide an inner lining.

concurs with that of Resano,[45] who believes that, whereas malignancies of the lower third of the esophagus are amenable to surgical extirpation, those in the cervical part are best managed by radiotherapy. The frequent problem of late diagnosis, with the tumor undetected until there is transmural penetration and it is already invading the larynx, trachea, carotid arteries, or spinal column, leaves only a few patients presenting with potentially resectable lesions. Tracheal and laryngeal penetration complicates the surgical attack and lowers the survival rate but does not render the lesion unresectable. Exophytic lesions tend to have a more favorable prognosis than endophytic ones. We heartily agree with the

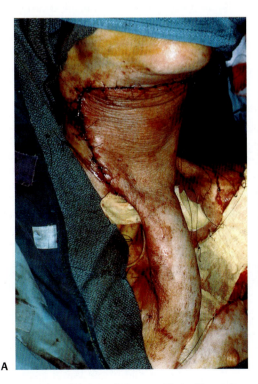
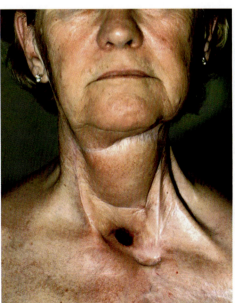

A   B

Fig. 3.31 (**A**) Outer lining provided with a deltopectoral flap. (**B**) Patient completely healed.

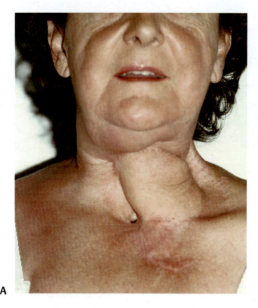
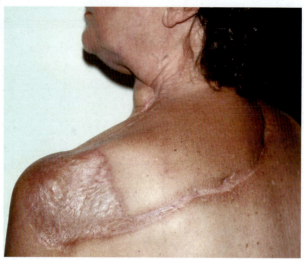

Fig. 3.32 (**A**) Patient with oro- and hypopharynx reconstructed with local Wookey flap and Zovikian flap. (**B**) Deformity from Zovikian flap.

comment of Parker[46] that a search for cure in those patients with potentially resectable lesions must not be abandoned because of the air of pessimism that commonly pervades the therapeutic considerations in these cases.

The 5-year cure rate of 25% following radical surgical extirpation is little improved since the report of Mustard[20] more than 45 years ago. Laryngopharyngocervical esophagectomy is the mainstay of treatment. The efficacy of postoperative irradiation has yet to stand the test of time. In the past, sporadic reports of a few random cases revealed no clear indication of its value.

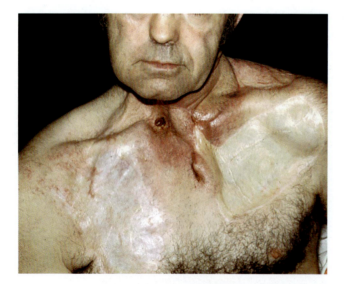

Fig. 3.33 Wookey flap reconstruction of pharynx covered with Zovikian flap. This patient was exceedingly hirsute, and the reconstructed pharynx was occasionally obstructed by hair, requiring depilation through an esophagoscope.

When the cervical esophagus is involved with tumor, the resection should extend into the upper thorax. Often this cannot be adequately achieved without exposure of the mediastinum. Tumor extension near the junction with the thoracic esophagus and beyond is best treated by total esophagectomy and gastric pull-up.

Total esophagectomy is a procedure of substantial magnitude that carries a significant mortality rate. It probably should not be undertaken in the elderly or debilitated patient or those with chronic pulmonary disease. Irradiation therapy in these individuals is probably the best choice despite the poor tumor control rate. However, the chronically starved, protein-depleted patient can be improved greatly with a high-calorie diet augmented by parenteral hyperalimentation.

Reconstruction often poses a problem because of the extensive distance a piece of gut must be transposed to achieve an upper anastomosis. The upper resection margin is often as high as the lower oropharynx. Several reconstructive options are available for reconstitution of the upper alimentary tract. Attempts to reestablish continuity by mobilizing the upper thoracic esophagus and possibly a small cervical esophageal remnant to obtain a primary anastomosis with the oropharynx should be assiduously avoided. The segmental blood supply to the esophagus is quickly devitalized by this maneuver resulting in slough at the anastomosis. An interposition of colon or jejunum may be done, but the limitation is again the vascular supply to the bowel flap. The most commonly employed flap is the gastric pull-up. The cardiac end of the stomach is mobilized by ligating the left gastroepiploic and left gastric arteries, then tubing this portion of the stomach, passing it up the mediastinum into the lower neck (**Fig. 3.34**).

If the terminal end of the bowel appears to have a precarious blood supply as it is brought into the neck it can

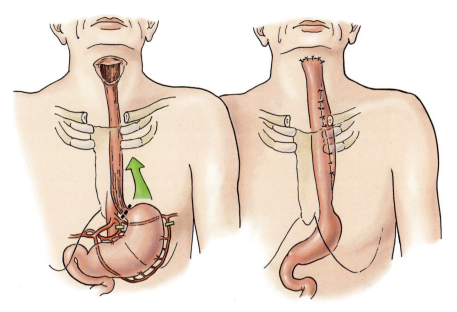

Fig. 3.34 Gastric pull-up.

be brought out into the neck or even onto the upper chest wall near the midline and a delayed closure done. A piece of gut, either colon or jejunum, must stretch from there to the stomach. A common problem is sloughing of the cervical end, which can be prevented by tubing the cardiac end of the stomach and either anastomosing it directly to the pharynx or bringing it out onto the chest. If the latter course is chosen, the cervical portion of the gullet can be reconstructed with a tubed deltopectoral or pectoralis flap (**Fig. 3.35A,B**). If the deltopectoral flap is used, at a second stage, the two tubes are hooked up and the patient is allowed to swallow when healing is complete, usually 10 days later (**Fig. 3.36A,B**). In any of these reconstructive procedures either to reconstruct

the hypopharynx or the entire esophagus it is often wise to excise the clavicular head on the side of the flap's passage. This prevents constriction of the flap as it passes over the clavicle with consequent vascular compromise. Removal of the head of the clavicle does not destabilize the shoulder and is of little functional consequence. The flap is inset into the gap left by the missing bone.

Mediastinal Resection

The extent of a mediastinal resection is predicated upon the degree of involvement of the trachea. If a cervical esophageal malignancy invades the overlying trachea and subglottic larynx,

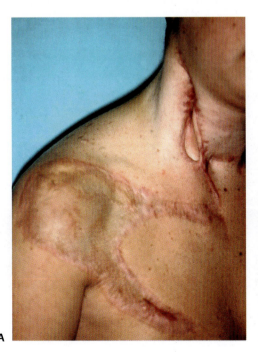

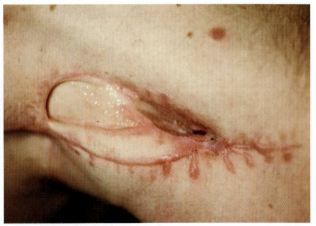

Fig. 3.35 This patient had a deltopectoral flap anastomosed to the upper oropharynx and a gastric pull-up. (**A**) Excision of the clavicular head avoids an acute angulation of the flap as it proceeds into the neck. (**B**) The cardiac end of the stomach was tubed and brought subcutaneously into close approximation with the sternal end of the deltopectoral flap.

A

B

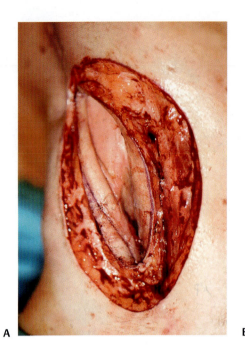

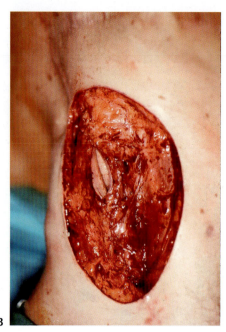

Fig. 3.36 (**A**) In the final stage, the skin bridge between the lower end of the deltopectoral flap and the transposed gastric tube is tubed on itself. (**B**) The skin tube is partially closed. The tube is subsequently completely closed, and the defect is covered with a local rotational flap.

the margin of resection necessitates a very low tracheostomy. For the amputated trachea to approximate the skin, a resection of a portion of manubrium is required. This resection differs from that used for a stomal recurrence following laryngectomy in that no skin is excised. The problem is that the trachea is too short to stretch over the manubrium to be sutured to the skin. An advancement flap on the chest can be made and slid into the uppermost mediastinum in the marginal case, but in most instances manubrial resection is necessary.

The problem with resecting the manubrium is the danger incurred by the subsequent proximity of the trachea to the innominate artery. The constant wearing away of the arterial wall by the trachea may result in a tracheoinnominate fistula or rupture of the artery into the mediastinal space. The frequency of this complication stimulated Sisson[33] to develop protection for the artery by the interposition of pectoralis major muscle flaps, and adoption of this step resulted in a vastly improved survival rate.

The incision extends vertically from the inferior limb of an apron flap (**Fig. 3.17**) or from the horizontal part of a modified H incision. The H incision is rarely used in this operation because most are done for tracheastomal recurrences of laryngeal cancer. It is usually reserved for those rare cases of tracheal carcinoma or aggressive malignancies of the thyroid in which the larynx can be preserved. The incision extends ~2 cm past the angle of Louis. Care is taken to identify and clamp the anterior jugular venous arch as it passes through the Burns space because it forms a ready source of air emboli.

The area of tumor involvement of the stoma, if a stomal recurrence is present, or of overlying skin in the case of pharyngeal tumor, is encircled by a wide margin of healthy skin (**Fig. 3.37**). In most cervical esophageal or subglottic cancers, skin penetration is uncommon. The superior margin of resection of the pharynx (if it is involved) is established and the bloc dissected inferiorly. Residual thyroid gland, if any, is included as the dissection plane carries down along the

plane of both carotid sheaths. Once dissection has proceeded as far into the root of the neck as possible, attention is turned to entering the mediastinum.

The periosteum is cut in the midsternal line to the required level of bony resection (**Fig. 3.38A**). Unlike the mediastinal resection for thyroid cancer, the manubrium is not simply split, but removed, to get the necessary prolapse of skin down to the trachea. The periosteal incision in the midline of the sternum is performed laterally over the sternoclavicular joints across the clavicular heads and about a quarter of the way along the anterior surface of the medial aspect of the bone. The greatest hazard in the clavicular resection is inadvertent rupture of the subclavian vessels lying just deep to

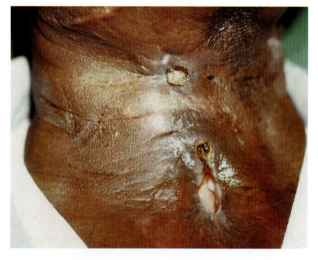

Fig. 3.37 Patient with a stomal recurrence following laryngectomy. In this case the tumor invaded the underlying esophagus, necessitating pharyngocervical esophagectomy.

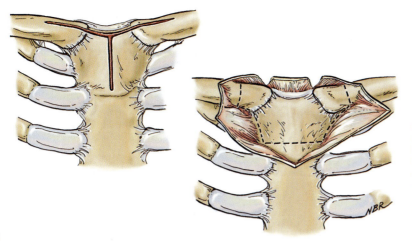

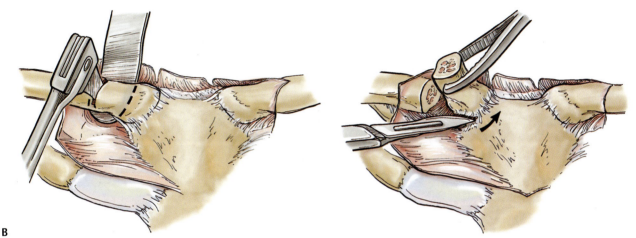

Fig. 3.38 Mediastinal resection. (**A**) The periosteum of the manubrium and clavicular heads is incised and dissected widely. Dashed line represents the proposed bony resection. (**B**) A malleable retractor is inserted under the clavicular periosteum to prevent damage to the underlying vessels. (**C**) The clavicle is grasped with bone-holding forceps and the sternoclavicular joint is separated by sharp dissection.

A

B

C

the bone. The most effective safeguard in preventing this is preservation of the clavicular periosteum. Some time should be spent in careful dissection of this layer on the bone's deep surface, creating a wide tunnel to insert a malleable retractor (**Fig. 3.38B**). A power saw is used to sever the bone up to the last few millimeters of the deep cortical surface, which is then finished off with an osteotome. The cut surface is grasped with bone-holding forceps, the remaining deep periosteum stripped, and the sternoclavicular joint separated (**Fig. 3.38C**).

Once both clavicular heads have been removed, the heavy layer of periosteum on the deep surface of the manubrium is dissected. As previously mentioned, as the manubrium is being cut, this stout layer provides protection for the underlying great vessels. A malleable retractor is slid between this layer and the overlying bone while the power saw is used to excise the manubrium from the first rib and the remaining sternum (**Fig. 3.38D**). Once the bone is removed, this fascial layer is excised en bloc with the underlying fat, thymus, and mediastinal lymphatics (**Fig. 3.38E**).

As the dissection proceeds more deeply, the left innominate vein is often seen crossing the field from left to right, obscuring the dissection. It is cross-clamped with Mixter clamps, divided, and suture ligated (**Fig. 3.38F**). Some postoperative swelling of the left arm is anticipated, but this dissi-

pates somewhat with time. Soft tissue is stripped superiorly off the trachea, with care taken not to penetrate the pleurae on the lateral boundaries of the mediastinal space. Bleeding must be meticulously controlled by ligature or cautery, as a mediastinal collection of blood will often be substantial before it produces sufficient symptoms for detection. Subsequent infection of a mediastinal collection is disastrous.

The dissection continues until the site for the establishment of the inferior resection margin is delineated. The trachea and esophagus are then amputated, and the bloc is stripped superiorly and then removed.

The reconstructive problems include (1) the necessity to fill in the potential dead space in the mediastinum, (2) the problem of a short trachea, (3) the need to reestablish the gullet, (4) the requirement to interpose soft tissue between the innominate artery and the trachea, and (5) the need to supply skin at the resection site of the stomal recurrence. The problem of reestablish the alimentary tract is usually solved by the use of the gastric pull-up. If prior gastric surgery precludes this option then a jejeunal interposition or a colonic flap is used. For short defects a radial forearm free flap or a free flap of jejunum can be employed (**Fig. 3.39**). The pectoralis myocutaneous flap satisfies the rest of the requirements mandated by the resection of the mediastinum. The skin paddle replaces the resected skin and provides an

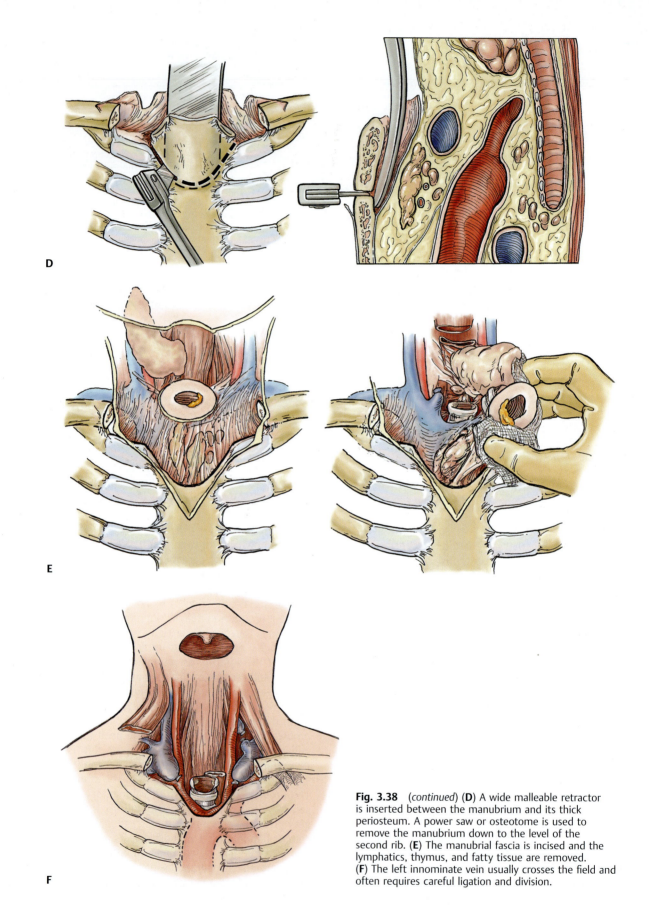

D

E

F

Fig. 3.38 (*continued*) (**D**) A wide malleable retractor is inserted between the manubrium and its thick periosteum. A power saw or osteotome is used to remove the manubrium down to the level of the second rib. (**E**) The manubrial fascia is incised and the lymphatics, thymus, and fatty tissue are removed. (**F**) The left innominate vein usually crosses the field and often requires careful ligation and division.

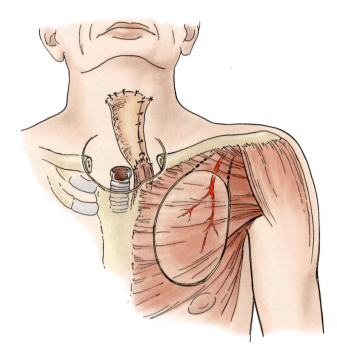

Fig. 3.39 Short length of resected cervical esophagus and hypopharynx replaced by free flap. Pectoralis major musculocutaneous flap being prepared for skin replacement of resected stomal area.

anchor for the shortened trachea. The muscle and fat protect the innominate artery and fill in the dead space in the mediastinum. The gastric pull-up has already been discussed, but some elements of the employment of the myocutaneous flap will be outlined.

The pectoralis flap has been a significant advance in the management of the defect after mediastinal dissection. In the original description of the procedure by Sisson,[47] a two-staged operation was required. In the first stage it was necessary to transpose a protective pad of pectoralis muscle, anchor it in place to the trachea, then at a second stage, remove the tumor and cover the resection defect with a bipedicled flap of thoracic skin. With the pectoralis flap only one stage is required. The flap is harvested taking care to maintain a wide paddle of skin not only to allow for the replacement of the resected cervical tissue but also to provide enough skin to invert through the tracheostoma and provide a tension-free closure with the tracheal stump. The thicker the patient's chest wall the wider the cutaneous part of the flap will need to be. In addition there needs to be enough muscle and fat to fill the resected mediastinum and avoid dead space.

Once the resection is complete, the pectoralis flap is elevated. A central slit is made in the flap that is wide enough to accommodate the thickness of the chest skin and the width of the amputated trachea. The slit is made in the axis of the nutrient vessels (**Fig. 3.40**). Sufficient elevation is made under the skin surrounding the slit to allow the skin to reach the trachea, which will be partially pulled up into the flap (**Fig. 3.41**). All of the sutures are placed, in circumferential fashion, left long, and tagged. Once placed, the sutures are tightened and the trachea is parachuted into the flap (**Fig. 3.42**). The cutaneous part of the flap is sutured into the defect left by removal of the generous skin margin around the stomal tumor (**Fig. 3.43**). The suture ends are left long and taped to the adjacent skin to aid in removal, which is typically done on the tenth to fourteenth day. A soft Silastic tube is placed in the tracheostome to keep the airway open.

Postoperatively the patient must be carefully observed for signs of hypoparathyroidism, and daily serum calcium levels are drawn. The patient is routinely placed on thyroid replacement because of the usual practice of taking the entire thyroid gland due to its proximity to the tumor. Due to the fact that the trachea has been considerably shortened the patient must have continuous mist by cupola and the intermit-

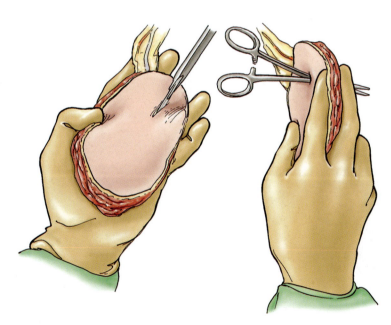

Fig. 3.40 Horizontal slit in skin of flap placed in the axis of the nutrient vessels. Blunt penetration in axis of vessels done large enough to accommodate the diameter of the transected trachea.

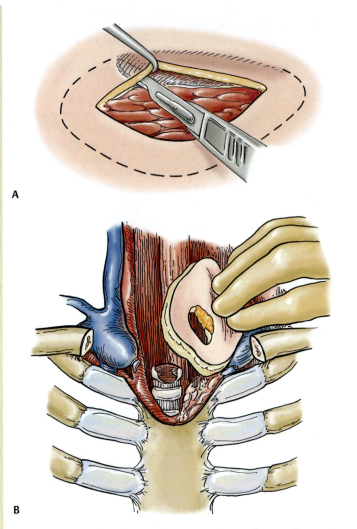

A

B

Fig. 3.41 **(A)** Skin elevation done circumferentially around central skin incision in flap to allow approximation of the trachea to the skin devoid of tension on the suture line. **(B)** Flap ready to be sutured to tracheal stump.

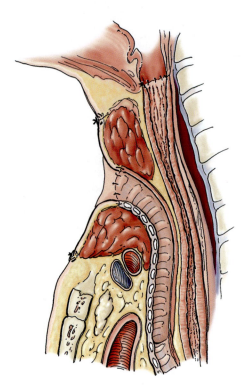

Fig. 3.43 Lateral view sagittal plane skin of flap periphery sutured to recipient defect in neck and lower chest.

tent administration of small amounts of saline to mobilize secretions and prevent dryness. Almost all patients will need to have a permanently placed soft plastic sort laryngectomy tube, preferably of Silastic, to maintain an adequate tracheal lumen. With proper care patients can be maintained with a remarkably foreshortened trachea as exemplified in case 2 (see below).

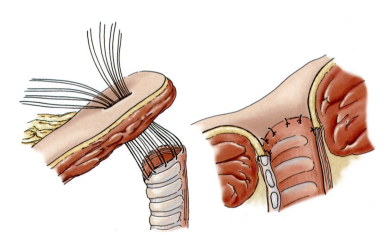

Fig. 3.42 Multiple sutures are placed loosely and then simultaneously tightened to allow the trachea to parachute through the pectoralis major flap.

Case 1

R.A.D. was a 57-year-old male when he first presented to us with a history of a mass in the left neck for a couple of months. He also had a minor left-sided sore throat and a foreign body sensation in his pharynx for many months. On examination he had a 2.5 cm hard mass in the left neck at the area of the jugulodigastric lymph node. Examination of the larynx and hypopharynx revealed a pyriform fossa carcinoma extending to the aryepiglottic fold and false vocal fold. After a panendoscopic examination, a transoral microsurgical laser resection was undertaken and the medial and anterior pyriform fossa, adjacent aryepiglottic fold and false vocal cord, as well as the lateral portion of the epiglottis were excised. No tracheotomy was required or nasogastric tube placed. The patient was discharged the following day on a soft diet with only minor discomfort and a hoarse voice. A modified radical neck dissection was done 1 week later as well as a revision of the laser resection because of a positive margin on the fixed sections of the previous laser excision. There was no tumor in the laser revision but three positive nodes in the neck dissection specimen. He began a full course of postoperative irradiation 4 weeks later. He is now over 3 years posttreatment and tumor free. He has occasional mild hoarseness, normal swallowing, and no residual pain.

This case report illustrates the efficacy of laser resection of selected hypopharyngeal lesions. Prior to laser microsurgery the patient's options would be either laryngectomy, neck dissection, and postoperative radiation therapy or combined chemotherapy and irradiation and staged neck dissection.

Discussion

The organ-sparing advantage of laser resection without the necessity of the tracheostomy often required during combined chemoradiation, or permanent, as in the case of laryngectomy as well as no need for a nasogastric or gastrostomy tube is clearly illustrated in this case. In our experience with laser hypopharyngectomy for carcinoma this scenario is the rule rather than the exception. At this point in time, however, I avoid laser excision when there is radiographic evidence of cartilage erosion.

Case 2 (Fig. 3.44–Fig. 3.46, p. 100)

J.H. was a 34-year-old male when first seen in the Department of Otolaryngology–Head and Neck Surgery at the University of California at Davis in 1979. He presented with hoarseness and a long history of alcohol and tobacco abuse. On laryngeal mirror examination a T1N0M0 squamous cell carcinoma of the right true vocal fold was seen. Panendoscopy and biopsy confirmed the diagnosis. A hemilaryngectomy was done on April 1979.

He remained disease free for 9 years and then presented in 1988 with a new primary in the right vocal cord and a 2 cm diameter lymph node in the right neck. A total laryngectomy without and a right modified radical neck dissection were done. He received then a full course of irradiation therapy.

He was disease free for 7 years; then he presented with a mass at the superior part of the trachea stoma (**Fig. 3.44**). Biopsy showed squamous cell carcinoma. A CT scan revealed no evidence of spread to the surrounding tissues such as the subclavian vessels and no additional adenopathy but was unclear as to invasion of the underlying esophagus. At surgery the classic resection of the skin surrounding the stoma with about a 3 cm margin of healthy tissue was done (**Fig. 3.45**). The manubrium steri was resected, as were the heads of the clavicles. The sternal excision was carried down to the angle of Louis. Periosteum deep to the sternum was incised and the resection carried down to the level of the trachea and included the thymus gland, the fat, and the lymphatics of the anterior mediastinum. The trachea was excised two rings below the stoma and the dissection carried up to the party wall between the cervical and upper esophagus (**Fig. 3.46**). He healed without complication.

Discussion

This exemplifies the most favorable situation regarding stomal recurrence. The lesion was situated above the equator of the stoma, and this site carries the best prognosis. The cervical esophagus was not invaded by tumor nor were any of the great vessels. In addition there was no gross adenopathy in the mediastinum and no tumor in the nodes examined. The biggest casualty of the procedure was the loss of the excellent esophageal speech he possessed prior to the surgery. He now uses fistula speech through a Blom-Singer valve (Forth Medical, London). He is now 12 years postoperative and free of disease.

Case 3 (Fig. 3.47–Fig. 3.52, pp. 101–102)

Mrs. E was a 65-year-old woman who had a laryngectomy at an outside facility 12 months prior to presentation for carcinoma of the larynx with subglottic spread. The margins of resection were close, and she received postoperative irradiation therapy. She noticed a mass adjacent to her stoma that was eroding through the skin of the neck, extending into the trachea to the level of about the sixth or seventh ring and into the anterior mediastinum. There was considerable erythema around the stoma and a fresh suture line from an attempt at resection of the stomal recurrence (**Fig. 3.47**). The tumor invaded the apical pleura of the left lung but did not involve the parenchyma. A CT scan showed evidence of erosion into the esophagus. No neck nodes were palpable.

Case Reports (*continued*)

A stomal resection was done including a wide field excision of skin. The heads of the clavicles and the manubrium sterni were removed to gain exposure (**Fig. 3.48**). After a dissection of the thymus, mediastinal lymphatics, and fat, access to the tumor extension in the trachea was gained. Amputation of the trachea left ~3.5 cm of trachea above the carina (**Fig. 3.49**). A segment of apical parietal pleura and attached first rib were resected (**Fig. 3.50**) A total esophagectomy was performed because of tumor extent into the upper thoracic esophagus. The continuity of the gut was reconstructed with a gastric pull-up (**Fig. 3.51**). All resection margins were histologically negative.

Reconstruction of the lost skin was done with a large pectoralis major flap (**Fig. 3.52A**). The short tracheal stump was pulled up into the flap and approximated to the skin (**Fig. 3.52B**). The stoma was stented with a long Silastic tube (**Fig. 3.52C**). Frequent moisturization of the tracheal-bronchial tree was done using frequent small aliquots of saline through the stoma. Following hospitalization for 6 weeks, the patient was able to resume most of her premorbid activities, such as bowling. She unfortunately succumbed to metastatic disease in the lungs 10 months later.

Discussion

Despite the eventual tragic outcome of this case, the patient led a relatively normal life until shortly before her death. Several important lessons were learned. A patient can survive despite a relatively short trachea. It is not necessary to mobilize the hilum of the lung or trachealize the right main stem bronchus to approximate the trachea to the skin. The skin of a pectoralis musculocutaneous flap can be advanced into the chest to achieve good tracheal to cutaneous tissue approximation. It is, however, important to resect sufficient sternum to facilitate this approximation.

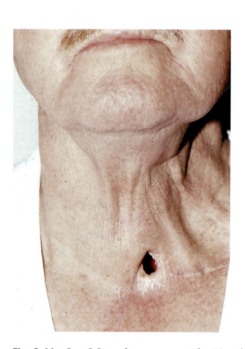

Fig. 3.44 *Case 2* Stomal recurrence at the 12 o'clock position.

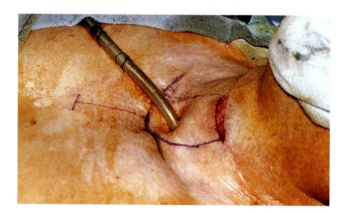

Fig. 3.45 *Case 2* Skin resection outlined.

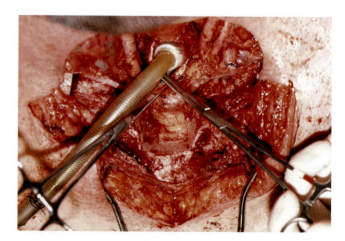

Fig. 3.46 *Case 2* Resection completed. Note the proximity of the innominate artery to the residual trachea.

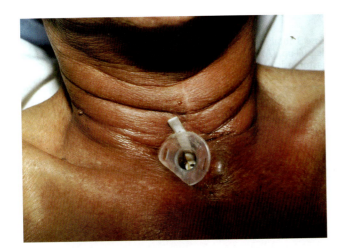

Fig. 3.47 *Case 3* Obvious stomal recurrence. Note erythema from recent previous surgery and subcutaneous tumor spread.

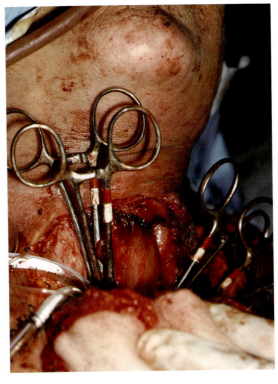

Fig. 3.49 *Case 3* Mediastinal resection and tracheal amputation done. Babcock clamps are placed on the tracheal stump deep in the mediastinum.

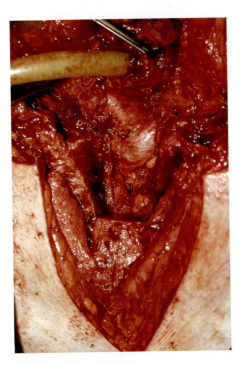

Fig. 3.48 *Case 3* Mediastinal exposure after removal of clavicular head and manubrium sterni.

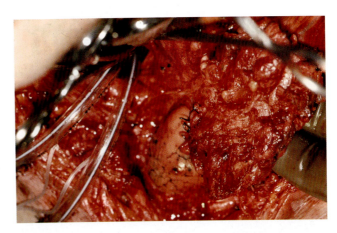

Fig. 3.50 *Case 3* Resection of anterior chest wall and anterior aspect of first rib as well as the parietal pleura. Note the dual endotracheal tubes. The one on the patient's left is endobronchial. Note the exposed apex of the left lung.

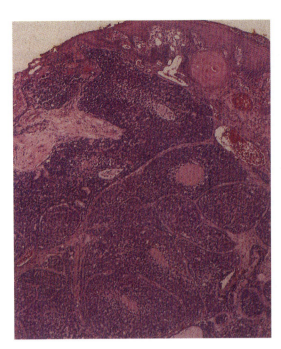

Fig. 4.6 Basaloid carcinoma of the larynx.

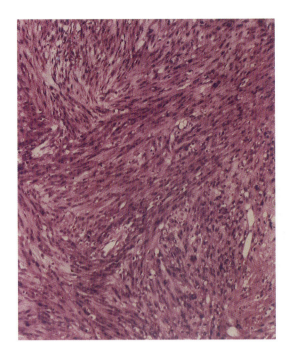

Fig. 4.7 Spindle cell carcinoma or carcinosarcoma.

Pseudosarcoma (Spindle Cell Carcinoma, Carcinosarcoma)

Biologically, there is nothing very "pseudo" about pseudosarcoma. This is a rare, high-grade malignancy, which typically presents in the larynx as a firm, gray, pedunculated or exophytic polypoid mass, sometimes with surface epithelial ulceration.[102] Other names in the literature are carcinosarcoma, spindle cell carcinoma, pleomorphic carcinoma, sarcomatoid carcinoma, or spindle cell sarcoma. Pseudosarcoma dates to a time when carcinosarcoma was considered a benign response of connective tissue to an adjacent squamous carcinoma. Spindle cell sarcoma was a recognition that the spindle cells were indeed malignant, but their epithelial origins were obscured.

Carcinosarcoma and *spindle cell carcinoma* are probably the most accurate terms because this tumor is now regarded as a sarcomatoid variant of epidermoid carcinoma. Both morphological components appear to be malignant (**Fig. 4.7**). The spindle cells have been shown to be immunoreactive to cytokeratin monoclonal antibodies, reflecting their epithelial origin. Vimentin can often be demonstrated, too, by immunofluorescence, indicating mesenchymal cell differentiation.[103] The cytology of carcinosarcoma is thought to arise by "divergent" metaplasia, in which a malignant mesenchymal morphology differentiates from what is fundamentally an epithelial carcinoma (most often a squamous cell carcinoma).[104,105] Sometimes a small, infiltrating, well-differentiated squamous cell carcinoma is associated with a large polypoid sarcomatous mass showing the histological features of a malignant giant cell tumor of soft parts.[106] Here again, both phenotypes are malignant. The spindle cell morphology of the neck metastases can be particularly vexing. Osseous components,[107] or fibrosarcomatous changes, or chondrosarcomatous elements (**Fig. 4.8**),[108] or myosarcomatous appear-

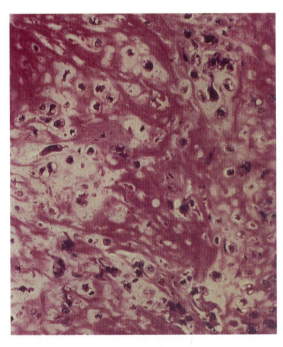

Fig. 4.8 Heterologous elements can be seen in spindle cell carcinoma, including this focus of osteosarcoma.

ances[109] have all been reported to occur. Clinically, the pattern of metastasis and survival of carcinosarcoma seems to parallel squamous cell carcinoma of the larynx. Thus treatment considerations run parallel and depend on the extent of the cancer.[110]

References

1. McComb WS, Healey JE, McGraw JP, et al. Hypopharynx and cervical esophagus. In: McComb WS, Fletcher GH, eds. Cancer of the Head and Neck. Baltimore: Williams & Wilkins; 1967:213–240

2. Gray H. Anatomy of the human body. In: Goss CM, ed. The Lymphatic System. 29th ed. Philadelphia: Lea & Febiger; 1975:744–745

3. Postlethwait PW. Surgery of the Esophagus. New York: Appleton-Century-Crofts; 1979:554–580

4. Rouvière H. Anatomie des lymphatiques de l'homme. Paris: Masson et Cie; 1932:115

5. Sakata K. On the lymphatics of the esophagus and on the regional lymph nodes with consideration of metastasis of the carcinoma. Mitt Grenzgeb Med Chir 1903;11:634

6. Sisson GA, Bytell DE, Becker SP. Mediastinal dissection—1976: indications and newer techniques. Laryngoscope 1977;87:751–759

7. Mast WR, Jafek BW. Mediastinal anatomy for the endoscopist. Arch Otolaryngol 1975;101:596–599

8. Conley J. Cancer of the pharynx. In: Concepts in Head and Neck Surgery. New York: Grune & Stratton; 1970:112–114

9. Soule HE. Tumors of the hypopharynx and parapharyngeal area. In: Dockerty MB, Parkhill EM, Dahlin DC, et al, eds. Tumors of the Oral Cavity and Pharynx. Washington, DC: Armed Forces Institute of Pathology; 1968:167–242

10. Postlethwait PW. Surgery of the Esophagus. New York: Appleton-Century-Crofts; 1979:341–414

11. Bloom W, Fawcett DW. Oral cavity and associated glands. In: A Textbook of Histology. 10th ed. Philadelphia: WB Saunders; 1975:617–618

12. Donald PJ, Huffman DI. Carcinoma in a Zenker's diverticulum. Head Neck Surg 1979;2:71–75

13. Bova R, Goh R, Poulson M, Coman WB. Pharyngolaryngectomy for squamous cell carcinoma of the hypopharynx: a review. Laryngoscope 2005;115:864–869

14. Kirchner JA. Pyriform sinus cancer: a clinical and laboratory study. Ann Otol Rhinol Laryngol 1975;84:793–803

15. Som ML, Nussbaum M. Surgical therapy of carcinoma of the hypopharynx and cervical esophagus. Otolaryngol Clin North Am 1969;2:631–640

16. Donald PJ, Hayes RH, Dhaliwal R. Combined Rx for pyriform sinus cancer using postoperative irradiation. Otolaryngol Head Neck Surg 1980;88:738

17. Ogura JH, Saltzstein SL, Spjut HJ. Experiences with conservation surgery in laryngeal and pharyngeal carcinoma. Laryngoscope 1961;71:258

18. Harwick RD. Carcinoma of the pyriform sinus. Am J Surg 1975;130:493

19. Razack MS, Sako K, Kalnis I. Squamous cell carcinoma of the pyriform sinus. Head Neck Surg 1978;1:31

20. Mustard RA. The use of the Wookey operation for carcinoma of the hypopharynx and cervical esophagus. Surg Gynecol Obstet 1960;111:577

21. Induction chemotherapy plus radiation compared with surgery plus radiation in patients with advanced laryngeal cancer. The Department of Veteran's Affairs Laryngeal Study Group. N Engl J Med 1991;324:1685–1690

22. Silver CE. Surgical management of neoplasms of the larynx, hypopharynx and cervical esophagus. Curr Probl Surg 1977;14:2–69

23. Donald PJ. Complications of combined therapy in head and neck carcinomas. Arch Otolaryngol 1978;104:329–332

24. Goepfert H. Carcinoma of the hypopharynx and cervical esophagus. In: Suen JY, Meyers EN, eds. Cancer of the Head and Neck. New York: Churchill Livingstone; 1981:415–433

25. Million RR, Cassisi MJ. Radical irradiation for carcinoma of the pyriform sinus. Laryngoscope 1981;91:439–450

26. Steiner W, Ambrosch P, Hess CF, Fron M. Organ preservation by transoral microsurgery in pyriform sinus carcinoma. Otolaryngol Head Neck Surg 2001;124:58–67

27. Steiner W, Stenglein C, Fietkau R, Sauerbrei W. Therapy of hypopharyngeal cancer, IV: Long-term results of transoral laser microsurgery of hypopharyngeal cancer. HNO 1995;43:133–146

28. Cooper JS, Forastiere AA, Jacobs J, et al. Postoperative concurrent radiotherapy and chemotherapy for high-risk squamous cell carcinoma of the head and neck. N Engl J Med 2004;350:1937–1944

29. Koch WM. Complications of surgery of the neck. In: Eisele D, ed. Complications of Head and Neck Surgery. St. Louis: Mosby; 1993:393–413

30. Suen JY, Stern SJ. Cancer of the neck. In: Suen JY, Myers EN, eds. Cancer of the Head and Neck. 3rd ed. Philadelphia: WB Saunders; 1996:471

31. Ballantyne A. Synchronous bilateral neck dissection. In: Larson DL, Ballantyne AJ, Guillamondegui OM, eds. Cancer in the Neck: Evaluation and Treatment. New York: Macmillan; 1986:153–182

32. Sako K. Simultaneous bilateral radical neck dissection. In: Chretian PB, Johns ME, Shedd DP, Strong EW, Ward PH, eds. Head and Neck Cancer. Vol 1. Philadelphia: BC Decker; 1985:166–168

33. Kennedy JA. Personal communication (unpublished data), 1973

34. Nayak UK, Donald PJ, Stevens D. Internal carotid artery resection for invasion of malignant tumors. Arch Otolaryngol Head Neck Surg 1995;121:1029–1033

35. Alexander MV, Zajtchuk JJ, Henderson RL. Hypothyroidism and wound healing: occurrence after head and neck surgery. Arch Otolaryngol 1982;108:289–291

36. Bakamjian VY. A two-stage method for pharyngoesophageal reconstruction with primary pectoral skin flap. Plast Reconstr Surg 1965;36:173–184

37. Bakamjian VY. Total reconstruction of pharynx with medially based deltopectoral skin flap. N Y State J Med 1968;68:2771–2778

38. Daniel RK, Cunningham DM, Taylor GI. The deltopectoral flap: an anatomical and hemodynamic approach. Plast Reconstr Surg 1975;55:275–282

39. Ariyan S. The pectoralis major musculocutaneous flap. Plast Reconstr Surg 1979;63:73–81

40. Ariyan S. Further experiences with the pectoralis major musculocutaneous flap for the immediate repair of defects from excision of head and neck cancer. Plast Reconstr Surg 1979;64:605–612

41. Pectoralis musculocutaneous flap. In: Panje WR, Schuller DE, Shagets FW, eds. Musculocutaneous Flap Reconstruction of the Head and Neck. Vol 2. New York: Raven; 1989:14–24

42. Pectoralis. In: McCraw JB, Arnold PG eds. McCraws and Arnolds Atlas of Muscle and Musculocutaneous Flaps: Head and Neck Reconstruction. Vol 6. Norfolk, VA: Hampton Press; 1988:127–165

43. Radial forearm free flap and anterolateral thigh flap

44. Wookey H. The surgical treatment of carcinoma of the pharynx and upper esophagus. Surg Gynecol Obstet 1949;75:499

45. Resano JH. Treatment of cancer of the esophagus. Bull Soc Int Chir 1975;6:311

46. Parker EF. Editorial: carcinoma of the esophagus. Ann Thorac Surg 1977;23:391

47. Sisson GA. Extended radical surgery for cancer of the head and neck – mediastinal resection for stomal recurrences. Otolaryngol Clin North Am 1969;2:617

48. Ahn C, Sindelar WF. Bilateral neck dissection: Report of results in 55 patients. J Surg Oncol 1989;40:252–255

4

Cancer of the Larynx

Bruce W. Pearson and Paul J. Donald

The greater part of this book is devoted to the management of large tumors that are difficult to treat. Function and form are often severely distorted, and the prognosis in many of the sites is only fair. Lesions of the larynx are different. Function is usually preserved, albeit with some compromise, and the prognosis for survival is excellent. The 5-year overall survival rate of 84% described by Thomas[1] is typical of the results of conservation laryngeal surgery. The five-year local control rate was 93% in the same report.

Every management model must accommodate *two key aspects* of laryngeal cancer: (1) laryngeal cancers are widely dissimilar, (2) no single treatment can provide the optimal management for all cases.

Within the same histological diagnosis (squamous cell cancer being the dominant player), the variations are huge. Prominent differences by site and stage yield distinctly dissimilar subtypes. Some presentations threaten voice early, some late, and others not at all. Nodes are no factor in some cases, the most critical factor in others. Small glottic cancers should kill almost no one. Large subglottic cancers lead to death in over half of those afflicted.

If one treatment was universally applied, small cancers would be grossly overtreated. This would guarantee excessive disability. Larger cancers would inevitably be undertreated. Undertreatment would lead to recurrence. Thus a "one size fits all" paradigm invites morbidity, late retreatment, and mortality. For laryngeal cancer, no single treatment can exist to the exclusion of all others.

This is primarily a chapter on the management of the local cancer. The terms *early* and *advanced* will refer to the local disease, not the staging (where neck factors dominate). Also, although the larynx is the theme, occasional references to cancers that arise in the hypopharynx will be unavoidable.

◆ Advances in Surgery for Laryngeal Cancer

At the middle of the twentieth century, all laryngeal cancer could be managed with three simple operations:

1. Direct laryngoscopy and excisional biopsy
2. Laryngofissure with cordectomy
3. Total laryngectomy

The history of laryngeal cancer surgery over the second half of the twentieth century was primarily devoted to adding more options between the second and third.

Suspension microlaryngoscopy and the laser refined direct laryngoscopy and excisional biopsy. Hemilaryngectomy and vertical partial laryngectomy succeeded laryngofissure and cordectomy. Supraglottic laryngectomy conserved voice and nasal breathing for patients formerly consigned to total laryngectomy. Supra*cricoid* laryngectomy rescued patients denied conservation surgery by horseshoe involvement of the anterior commissure. Patients receiving total laryngectomy because of lateralized cancers with cord fixation could achieve a lung-powered voice with near-total laryngectomy. Even total laryngectomy received an upgrade—tracheoesophageal puncture, a reliable means of reclaiming a voice.

By 1987, the panel of accepted procedures for laryngeal cancers looked more like this:

1. Direct microlaryngoscopy and laser excision[2,3]
2. Vertical ("hemi-")[4] or horizontal ("supraglottic")[5,6] partial laryngectomy
3. Supracricoid partial laryngectomy[7]
4. Near-total laryngectomy[8]
5. Total laryngectomy and primary tracheo-esophageal puncture (TEP)[9,10]

Since that time, we find more technology has accrued to support TEP rehabilitation,[11–13] expected gains in chemotherapy for squamous carcinoma have failed to materialize,[14–19] and more is known about swallowing,[20,21] quality of life,[22–24] and cost.[25–27] But the biggest trend in local tumor control has been the elaboration of transoral laser microresection.[28–35] This may replace the classic open conservation operations soon and extend to even more extensive disease.

◆ Advances in Radiation for Laryngeal Cancer

Radiation therapy is based on better planning now. Chemotherapy may be developing a role as a pretest of radiosensitivity (see later discussion). The precision of treatment alignment has improved as faster computed tomographic (CT) acquisition times have nearly eliminated motion artifacts. Surface coil technology has extended image accuracy in the neck even further. We are fast approaching the time when alternate plane reconstructions will be just as accurate as the primary (axial) images of the larynx. Patients receive better nutrition during therapy now because of percutaneous gastrostomies and better medications against mucositis. When the morbidity of radiotherapy is reduced, the dose can be higher, and with higher doses come more cures.

◆ Treatment Philosophies

Laryngeal cancer demands treatment. Even though our knowledge is incomplete, clinicians must act. At various times and in various centers, different leaders have adopted different approaches ("philosophies"). Here are some notable examples, subclassified into those for smaller laryngeal cancers and those for larger ones.

Smaller Laryngeal Cancers

◆ **1. Irradiate all new cases. Salvage any failures with conservation surgery.** Data from the national practitioners databank indicate only 15% of reported North American laryngeal cancer patients received surgery as primary treatment in the years 1990 to 1992.[36] This suggests a widespread belief that all new cases are radiotherapy candidates. In a busy office practice, and a complex world of choices, this concept has appeal for the caregiver. It would instantly streamline decision making—topognostic diagnosis would almost be superfluous. What difference will the exact site of a cancer make if all patients will receive the same treatment?

In the "biopsy and radiate" treatment paradigm, the place of conservation operations is to salvage failures.[37] Salvage

surgeons have little data with which to challenge the primary irradiation philosophy. They can't know if an early cancer was "resistant" or understaged. Nor can they know if the failures referred to their practices are a high or low proportion of the at-risk population. The surgeon sees the numerator, not the denominator. What can be seen is a low incidence of failure quoted in the general literature.[38] The actual incidence in their own region is unpublished.

Patients with T1 glottic cancer who fail to be cured by radiotherapy often tell their surgeon they were quoted a 95% chance of cure. Ninety-five percent was the "corrected 5-year tumor-free actuarial survival" for previously untreated patients with T1 glottic cancer treated first (but not solely) with radiotherapy.[38] In Harwood's data, it meant five of a hundred patients with the most favorable cancer in laryngology died of it—despite any follow-up treatment (surgery). Later data from Fein et al.[39] gave a 95% "5-year local control rate." But this was calculated from a patient base with a "minimum 2-year follow-up."

Hearing this statistic repeatedly, some laryngologists refer to "the 95% myth." Hawkins's[40] report from Princess Margaret Hospital is instructive. He found it necessary to start with ~120 T1 glottic cancer patients to ensure that 100 would be *expected* to be alive at the end of a 5-year study period. (A typical cohort of patients with early laryngeal cancer have comorbidities that include other cancers, heart disease, emphysema, stroke, advanced age, and more—not all cured patients survive the 5 years necessary to validate their result). With radiation as initial therapy, 92 *were* actually alive at 5 years. Eight (including four of the deaths) had required a salvage laryngectomy to get there. (With a specimen in hand, some were reclassified to higher T stages). Eighty-eight kept their larynx (and their life)—a respectable number. But six had not been cured by the radiotherapy—they had undergone a partial laryngectomy. This would reduce the "cured by radiotherapy" group to 82 patients (of the 100 expected to live). But were all these patients actually cured by radiotherapy? Sometimes a T1a glottic cancer is completely removed by the biopsy. This has been estimated from cordectomy specimens to be one in 10, even more in exophytic midcordal lesions.[41] If 10 patients were sent for radiotherapy who never had cancer, and eight were in the evaluable group, all would be cures.

Thus one could argue, in 1975, only 74 of the 100 patients with T1N0M0 glottic cancer were cured *because of the radiotherapy*. T1 glottic cancer is the most radiocurable cancer discussed in this entire book. Where this analysis still holds true, if radiotherapy is the sole treatment, the highest cure rate achievable would be ~75%, not 95%.

◆ **2. For T1a glottic cancer, excisional biopsy. For T1b glottic and localized supraglottic cancers, open conservation surgery** Primary excision might well be the optimum initial treatment for all early laryngeal cancers. Radiation overtreats the smallest cancers and undertreats some slightly larger ones. This philosophy holds that a few *very* early cancers can be treated endoscopically, but en bloc, and only a few. The majority are treated by selected formal open conservation operations, operations so well authenticated over time that their indications are well known, their techniques well established, and their functional and oncological results are plainly predictable—in expert hands.

Endoscopic resection of early laryngeal cancer has been practiced since the turn of the twentieth century. As recently as 1973, Lillie and DeSanto reaffirmed that suspension laryngoscopy, a margin-negative forceps-resection, and diathermy of the base is highly effective treatment for exophytic tumors on a mobile cord.[42] The cord had to be mobile, of course. A reliable frozen section laboratory was essential. Of all T1 glottic cancers presenting to Lillie and his colleagues for treatment, one third were suitable for suspension laryngoscopy and removal. The others received radiotherapy or open laryngofissure/cordectomy). Lillie reported 104 patients treated this way, 57 with T1 glottic ca and 47 with cancer in situ. Not one died of laryngeal cancer! Four required retreatment (again by endoscopic means). One required a laryngectomy—eight years after initial treatment.

The secret of success in Lillie's estimation was patient selection and complete endoscopic exposure. (Initially, this did not change when laryngologists substituted the CO_2 laser for diathermy.)[3] Lillie's indications for transoral resection were as follows:

1. Endoscopic exposure within one field of view—for bloc excision.
2. No previous treatment (especially stripping or biopsy)—the integrity of the cancer had to be obvious.
3. The anterior commissure had to be free of cancer. This kept the surgery away from the hardest area to expose and the hardest area to evaluate and guaranteed an excellent vocal result.

For cancers beyond Lillie's criteria, the range and coverage of the open conservation operations are astonishing. Open surgery demonstrates the exact extent of the cancer—no mistakes based on faulty staging (and no databank built on clinical staging mistakes). Excellent local control follows a margin-free operation. Voice is impaired but restored. Nasal breathing remains—no permanent stoma. Swallowing is impaired, but again, eventually restored. Eating continues with normal lubrication and normal taste. Open surgery overcomes the limitations of bloc endoscopic surgery: the entire lesion does not have to be exposed in one field of view. An involved anterior commissure or an arytenoid may very well be controlled. A patient can be cured with an artfully selected and skillfully performed conservation operation in days, not weeks. And conservation surgery preserves radiotherapy, valuable if a second primary ever emerges in the future.

Most surgeons believe that conservation surgery provides the optimum chance of cure with only *one* treatment. Opponents cite functional costs. Of course, the voice may be worse after a vertical partial laryngectomy than after radiotherapy—if the radiotherapy works. But it's certainly better

than what will later be obtained if radiotherapy fails. Long-established strategies to improve the quality of function after conservation surgery seem unfamiliar to many radiotherapists. Muscle flap reconstructions to improve voice volume in frontolateral partial laryngectomies have been available for 30 years.[43] Pull-down epiglottoplasty to enhance the airway result in frontoanterior vertical partial laryngectomy[44] is almost as venerable.

◆ **3. Microlaryngoscopy and transoral laser microsurgery**
Transoral laser microsurgery (TLM) is the natural child of transoral laser excision (TLE). TLE was pioneered by the Boston University school in the 1970s. Jako,[2] Strong,[3] Vaughan,[45] Davis et al,[46] Shapshay,[47] and Blakeslee et al[48] clearly established the principle that transoral laser excision could safely duplicate the bloc cancer excisions already known, with minimal morbidity and outstanding oncological and functional results. TLM carried the concept an important step further by incorporating transection of tumors in situ (by laser). This allowed multibloc excision, so the convenience, safety, cure rate, and functional advantages could be extended to many more (and larger) laryngeal cancers.[30,31,49–51] Almost every T1 or T2 squamous cell cancer of the larynx now has an integrated transoral surgical treatment, based on the availability of modern CO_2 lasers, microspot micromanipulators, special endoscopes adapted for laser surgery (and difficult exposures), and our detailed knowledge of how cancer spreads within the larynx, developed over decades of study. Treatment-related morbidity is significantly reduced over an open conservation operation, with equal or better oncological results, less cost, and equal or better function, especially long term.

When Vaughan, Strong, and Jako[28] reported on their experiences with transoral CO_2 laser resection of laryngeal carcinoma in 1978, it was polite to consider their report a wonderful illustration of the feasibility of TLE, but not a compelling demonstration of its significance. Transoral resection of T1a glottic cancers was already well known. The only increment in concept, marginal at that, seemed to be the use of an expensive high-tech "cooking" tool, the laser, which brought new problems, like evaporation of the pathology specimen, or fire in the airway. There were new regulations, too, like goggles in the operating room (OR). And unfamiliar modifications of the instruments, for plume evacuation. Many otolaryngologists had only recently become proficient with suspension microlaryngoscopy in 1978. Now there would be new balance issues, equipment developments, and expenses.

The narrow exposure of conventional laryngoscopes promised to restrict TLE to early disease—for which radiotherapy was already widely available, conventional, and competitive. The early pioneers themselves cited limits,[46] caution,[52] and ancillary roles, like diagnosing the depth of spread into the preepiglottic space (PES),[53] isolating the anterior glottis,[54] debulking a mass of tumor prior to elective radiation and/or chemotherapy,[55] and reestablishing an airway after blockage with tumor.[56] Many surgeons (including the authors) failed to appreciate the Boston group's advocacy of laser microresection as a primary mode of therapy, one that allowed most patients to return home the first postoperative day—eating, speaking, and tracheotomy free.

In Germany, several leading surgeons, most prominently Steiner and Rudert and their colleagues, did recognize the challenge, and they ran with it. Over 2 decades, the schools in Erlangen and Göttingen (Steiner), Kiel (Rudert and now Ambrosch), Cologne (Eckel), and Homburg (Iro) coordinated substantial upgrades in laser technology with an improved understanding of the indications and techniques for very early, early, and intermediate laryngeal cancers. They carefully documented their patients,[33,34,57-59] published their clinical results, and advocated the technology to their friends.

At the present time, transoral laser resection has emerged as a highly competitive treatment option in the centers with laryngologic experience. A steady flow of improvements in examining equipment, laser sources, distending laryngoscopes, micromanipulators, grasping forceps, insulated suction cauteries, and endoscopic training have brought laser excision within easy reach for the latecomers. This theme will be expanded below, along with clinical and technical details.

◆ **4. The selective approach: transoral laser microsurgery, open conservation surgery, or radiotherapy, depending on individual criteria** Doctors are never confronted with an early laryngeal cancer *alone*. The cancer comes in a patient—with goals, fears, preferences, and comorbidities, and strongly dissimilar expectations. Patient factors powerfully influence treatment selection. And so they should.

The task of the doctor is to evaluate both the tumor factors and the patient factors while considering the people and the tools reasonably accessible to the patient, and then to make a recommendation for treatment. The patient and relatives need a lot of information. They need help in understanding the applicable options, and a reasonable explanation of the prognosis that attends each option. Because neither the doctor nor the patient can control every factor that affects the prognosis, there are always imponderables as well.

The selective approach refers to the common observation that identical cancers can be treated in differing ways *for valid medical reasons*. There is no "treatment of choice" for a given cancer, but rather a choice of treatments (Ferlito).[60]

In the selective approach, it is perfectly OK that tumors within a uniform stage receive radiotherapy (± radiation response modifiers), open classic conservation surgery, or TLM. Patients suitable for frontolateral partial laryngectomy may prefer the opportunity to restore their most natural voice with radiotherapy. A tumor may be suitable for laser resection, but some patients may undergo an open conservation operation because of anatomical problems with exposure. Others will undergo TLM not because radiation or open surgery lack merit but because the tumor is accessible, and the patient's priorities are the time, the cost, long-term swallowing, and cosmesis.

Larger Laryngeal Cancers

◆ **5. Radical radiation and surgical salvage where salvage means total laryngectomy** To improve the cure rates for

T3 and T4 laryngeal cancers, in the mid-1960s, "combined therapy" (irradiation then surgery) was advocated over total laryngectomy alone. But Bryce and Ryder found that half of the larynges removed under the combined therapy protocol contained no detectable residual. In their hands, combined therapy produced no more cures than radiation followed by surgical salvage.[61] In fact, if the radiotherapy was "radical," a few patients with clinically advanced laryngeal cancer were actually cured by the radiotherapy alone. They could keep their larynx, defying predictions of loss.

In the 1970s and 1980s, radical radiation and surgical salvage (RRSS) became a widely practiced treatment philosophy for advanced laryngeal cancer.[62] Because patients would consent to radiation *and* surgery, there was no such thing as "radiation failure." Radiation and surgery were part of the program—it was just that some patients were excused from the second leg (laryngectomy) by virtue of their complete response to the first. Nonresponders at least had received their chance to avoid a total laryngectomy. The necessity for "radical surgery" was obvious after cancer persisted, and perhaps its acceptance was fortified.

By today's standards, RRSS protocols have included several more favorable patients to whom partial laryngectomy advances could have been applied up front, rather than the total laryngectomies then thought to be indicated. In the heyday of RRSS, loss of cord mobility was widely seen as a contraindication to conservation surgery. This was a belief that did much to ensure its own veracity because once the experience required to deliver conservation surgery had been deeply eroded by disuse, all that was left was radicalism.

Note that in RRSS philosophy, all candidates for surgery were, in fact, status postradiotherapy. They probably *did* require a total laryngectomy for salvage. Radiation contraindicates conservation surgery in many instances. When a cancer (originally advanced) persists or recurs despite radiotherapy, the margins are unpredictable, and the quality of healing is imperiled. In the RRSS scenario, cure and function after conservation surgery would rely on tissues that have been radiated to full dosages. Poor results would appear to be complications of surgery. Often enough, even patients with total laryngectomy would fail to be cured of their disease. This depressing result could only further reinforce the bias against surgery when laryngeal cancer was advanced. No wonder the search for cytotoxic chemotherapy intensified among the advocates of RRSS—surgery was obviously quite futile.

RRSS did preserve some larynges in advanced laryngeal cancer, irradiated larynges, which of course are not "normal." Swallowing symptoms are annoying, persistent, and sometimes severe in the irradiated patient. Note that everyone in the program received radiation to the pharynx because of its proximity to the larynx. This drawback was not limited by dose reduction—it was only early glottic cancer that was cured by 55 cGy over a 5 cm^2 field. Advanced cases required wider windows and typically received 60 to 70 cGy.

Under RRSS, two thirds of the patients required both treatments—radiation and surgery. And half of the patients (one third of the total) underwent both treatments and failed! The surgery that was performed was delayed by this (compared with up-front use, as in "combined" therapy, or as in surgery alone). A complete response at the end of the radiotherapy arm contraindicated surgery in the RRSS program, so laryngectomy was not allowed until it was clear the response would not be sustained.

RRSS has been thoroughly tested now. It is clear that some larynges are saved. None would remain had total laryngectomy been offered up front to the same patients. What is less clear is whether more *voices* have been saved. And worse, whether more *lives* are not ultimately lost. Some began to speculate that the delay in obtaining local control (surgery was withheld until the radiation had been proven unsuccessful) gave laryngeal cancers more time to entrench and to metastasize. DeSanto produced data to suggest that the complications of radiation and surgery were additive, but the benefits and cure rates were not.[63] RRSS produced fewer local cures, fewer overall cures, and shorter average survivals than what it had really been designed to replace, up-front total laryngectomy. The only benefit of RRSS over up-front surgery was the preservation of more larynges in the RRSS group.[64] But larynx preservation was not the same as voice preservation. With the advent of tracheoesophageal puncture and prosthesis technology, 85% of patients with no larynx can talk—all the more so if they have never been irradiated.

The prospects for voice in advanced disease are actually quite excellent now if surgery is performed without radiotherapy. This is due to the widespread use of primary tracheoesophageal puncture prostheses in patients who truly do need a total laryngectomy as primary treatment.

◆ **6. Chemoradiation and surgical salvage, with primary total laryngectomy for initial chemononresponders and secondary total laryngectomy for later chemoradiation recurrences ("organ preservation")** The principal weakness of RRSS was its inability to identify patients (a majority) who were destined to require the surgical component. Much better to spare the expense and morbidity of presurgical radiotherapy if we could know it wasn't going to work. In the 1980s, chemotherapy had been shown to produce partial or complete responses in as many as half of the squamous carcinomas treated in palliative protocols. Two facts became obvious as these experiences accumulated.

1. The main predictor of a poor response to chemotherapy was previous radiotherapy.
2. A good response to chemotherapy never seemed to lead, on its own, to a cure.

Physicians reasoned that susceptibility to cytotoxic agents might be an intrinsic characteristic of the tumor itself. And it might not be that dependent on which cytotoxic agent—chemotherapy *or radiotherapy*. A susceptibility to chemotherapy might signal sensitivity to radiotherapy. If so, chemotherapy could be used as a test. A favorable response might support a trial of radiotherapy when otherwise a total laryngectomy would be selected.[65,66]

To test this proposition, new protocols were designed for advanced laryngeal cancer in which chemotherapy was given first, to "pretest" for radiosusceptibility.[67–69] Two new catchphrases appeared to designate this strategy, *organ preservation*[70–72] and *chemoradiation*.[73,74] Organ preservation certainly cast chemotesting for radiosusceptibility in a favorable public light. The most fearful public image of head and neck cancer, a hole in the neck, (from total laryngectomy) was finally under attack. And all the negative associations of a tracheotomy—cough, communicative isolation, contamination, and unemployability might now at last be vanquished. Chemoradiation carried a connotation of interspecialty collaboration in the major health centers, and the hope for advances through synergy. The interests of patients and primary physicians were strongly and publicly affirmed by this language, but the reality was somewhat less gratifying.

Quite a few organs were not spared. A patient whose tumor showed little or no response to the test dose of chemotherapy was advanced directly past chemoradiation to laryngectomy—total laryngectomy. Patients were laryngectomized according to protocol even as they remained part of the "organ sparing" study cohort, a fact that must have seemed particularly ironic during further follow-up. That is, for nonresponding enrollees, the option of radiotherapy as a trial was foreclosed and so was the low but finite chance of a less-than-total laryngectomy. Poor responders were considered resistant to radiotherapy on the *assumption* chemoresistance was a valid indicator—even though this remains, to this day, a hypothesis.

Patients with chemoresponsive tumors received ionizing radiation (and, just in case, more chemotherapy). But for many, not even this would achieve organ preservation. If radiotherapy failed, which it did about half the time, these patients were operated. The protocol guaranteed that all patients treated by secondary surgery lost their larynx. Primary conservation surgery now seemed to be lacking any indication whatsoever. Some surgeons began referring to supracricoid laryngectomy and/or near-total laryngectomy as organ-sparing operations, as if to reclaim lost ground.

Unnoticed (by the lay press) in the early published reports, was the fact that no one could demonstrate any measurable survival benefit. Nor did there seem to be any improvement in locoregional control.[75,76] Ironically, by the early 1990s, even as the protocols were being abandoned or revised, chemoradiation was out in the community.

◆ **7. Selective surgery up front; a total laryngectomy, a near-total laryngectomy, or a supracricoid laryngectomy, as appropriate. Advanced transoral laser microsurgery when superior. Adjuvant radiotherapy for neck indications** The application of standardized treatment plans to advanced laryngeal cancer is undermined by the fact that laryngeal cancer is not one disease but several very different diseases, depending on site and stage, occurring in an equally complex variety of hosts.

There are at least five variations of T3 glottic disease alone. A chemoradiation-based treatment plan for T3 glottic cancer would be bound to overtreat some patients and undertreat others. The patients are also diverse. Invasive T3N0 glottic cancer in a diabetic attorney on chemotherapy for bladder cancer is not amenable to chemoradiation. An identical newly discovered T3N0 vocal fold cancer in a healthy young housewife with no other risk factors might be. But no single treatment protocol is universally applicable. No common plan is exclusive. The knowledge and objectivity of the oncologist, the training and interest of the radiotherapist, the judgment and experience of the surgeon, the patient's cooperation and expectations, and many more patient factors must be considered—independent of the tumor. Hence, selection and judgment are paramount.

Again, quoting Ferlito, there is no "treatment of choice," but rather a choice of treatments. In the selective approach, the options to be considered for treatment of advanced cancer (depending on the definition of advanced) include TLM, radiotherapy (± radiation response modifiers), all the advanced conservation and reconstructive procedures, the radical operations, their reconstructive techniques, and the various prosthetic devices. At the same time, one must anticipate the adjuvant roles of chemotherapy; "second look" microlaryngoscopy; airway safety precautions before, during, and after treatment; swallowing and nutrition programs; and glottic, neoglottic, prosthetic, or alaryngeal vocal rehabilitation.

Every choice will precondition the plans (by limiting the options) for future management. A choice for radiotherapy now will strongly impact the management of local failure in the future,[77] of neck node issues, the follow-up examinations, the treatment of complications, and the discovery and treatment of a second primary. This constitutes another layer in the selective approach. All the comorbidities must be factored in, including those the treatment might precipitate.

In advanced laryngeal cancer, cure by radiation is unlikely. Radiation is often prescribed, however, to improve survival or possibly avoid total laryngectomy. But when advanced cancer recurs, it has had extra time to metastasize. Without the delays imposed by the "radiotherapy-first" philosophy, without the margin obfuscations, the tissue devitalization—open operations are usually predictable and successful for advanced laryngeal cancer. Moreover, when open operations are done first, they are often not total laryngectomies. Supracricoid partial laryngectomy (SCPL) and near-total laryngectomy preserve high rates of local cure, in properly selected cases previously considered total laryngectomy candidates. The nontotal surgery techniques reach the necessary levels of sophistication and reliability in centers where they can be offered primarily, before radiotherapy has failed. Why not use them this way given that radiotherapy can be added *after* surgery. Total laryngectomy can be limited to the worst cases.

In the surgery-first paradigm, total laryngectomy is rare. Radiotherapy remains an optional modality but usually as a sequel to surgery, with neck indications guiding the choice. The supracricoid and near-total operations seem much more manageable when patients are not exhausted by the failure of previous treatments. Even after total laryngectomy, speech therapy programs and rehabilitative prostheses meet with general success—especially in the unirradiated patient.

◆ Epidemiology of Larynx Cancer

Pseudoepitheliomatous Hyperplasia and Cancer

Pseudoepitheliomatous hyperplasia is a benign lesion that mimics squamous cell carcinoma on histopathologic examination. It occurs in association with lesions that bear clinical resemblances to cancer as well. It is actually a reactive process to an underlying mesenchymal disease—typically blastomycosis,[78] aspergillosis,[79] tuberculosis,[80] or benign granular cell tumor[81] (granular cell myoblastoma in the older literature). Fungal entities are detected in biopsy specimens by immunofluorescence studies. Tuberculosis (TB) is characterized by granulomatous inflammation, caseating granulomas, and acid-fast bacilli. Granular cell tumors appear as glottic nodules, classically in the posterior glottis, where they are distinguished by their bland uniform histology and by cells with abundant eosinophilic cytoplasm and characteristic granules believed to represent lysosomes in varying stages of fragmentation. The danger, of course, in all of these cases is misidentification as a low-grade cancer when the patient has, in fact, a specific infectious disease that would respond to antifungal therapies like ketoconazole, fluconazole, or amphotericin, or to antituberculous medications, or in the case of a benign granular cell tumor, to simple transoral removal.

Papilloma and Cancer

Clinically, papillomas are usually found in children and present no diagnostic confusion. Their appearance is one of multiple soft confluent minipolyps, almost with a tapioca-like quality because each individual papilloma is slightly translucent with a darker vascular tuft in its core. Their development is connected with the papilloma virus, especially human papilloma virus (HPV) types 6 and 11. Sometimes they coexist with warts in other unexpected parts of the body.

Papillomas are also encountered in adults, as a continuation of the juvenile form or de novo. Interestingly, viral inclusion bodies similar to those found in benign laryngeal papilloma can sometimes be found in laryngeal cancer. Uncommonly, a patient with laryngeal papilloma develops well-differentiated laryngeal cancer, within the papillomatous field. Smoking seems to potentiate this risk.

Epithelial Cancer

The epithelial abnormalities confronting the pathologist (and the patient and the laryngologist) are not a simple dichotomy (i.e., "benign" versus "malignant"). Diagnoses on the vocal fold are rather a continuous spectrum, and the lesion can even be a mosaic.

◆ **Epithelial Dysplasia** The spectrum of hyperplastic epithelial diseases in the larynx reads as follows:

1. Benign normal squamous epithelium

2. Hyperplasia
   a. Primary
   b. Secondary (e.g., pseudoepitheliomatous hyperplasia)
3. Squamous hyperplasia (acanthosis) with reactive ("functional") keratosis. Smoking cessation and the aggressive treatment of laryngopharyngeal reflux (LPR) is sometimes successful in arresting this process.
4. Primary keratosis, with or without dysplasia ("atypia") (**Fig. 4.1**). Dysplasia ("atypia") is an abnormality of maturation, thus a foretaste of neoplasia. It can be

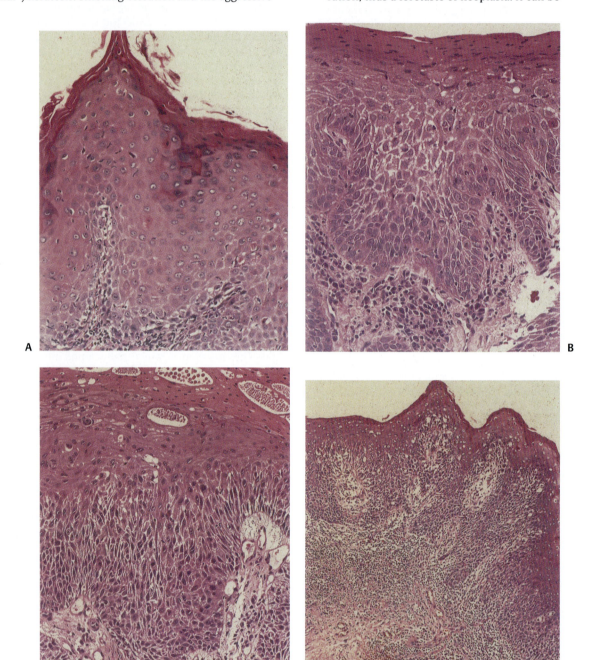

Fig. 4.1 (**A**) Laryngeal keratosis, with epithelial hyperplasia without dysplasia. (**B**) Laryngeal biopsy specimen, showing a flat type of keratosis with epithelial hyperplasia and mild dysplasia limited to the basal zone area, characterized by loss of cellular polarity, increase in nuclear size relative to the cytoplasm, and slight increase in the nuclear chromatin. (**C**) Laryngeal biopsy specimen, showing keratosis with moderate dysplasia involving up to two thirds of the thickness of the epithelium; note incidental finding of intraepithelial eosinophilic pooling. (**D**) Laryngeal biopsy specimen with keratosis and severe dysplasia; although the dysplasia does not involve two thirds or greater of the epithelial surface, this biopsy specimen qualifies as severe dysplasia, given the downward growth of the epithelium, which manifests marked dysplastic changes. This biopsy specimen borders on superficially invasive squamous cell carcinoma.

a. Mild
b. Moderate
c. Marked

Keratosis *with* atypia is a persistent cause of leukoplakia in the larynx. The risk of malignancy is higher than the risk for oral leukoplakia.

5. Carcinoma in situ
6. Invasive carcinoma

One can treat the first three diagnoses as if they were "benign." The second three should always be treated like cancer. The entire patch—all the abnormal epithelium—should be removed and studied for histopathology. The proper attitude in treating localized dysplastic lesions of the vocal cord is to achieve a complete excision and never settle for a mere biopsy.

Some patients with leukoplakia are elderly or otherwise considered high-risk patients for biopsy. High-dose retinyl palmitate has been studied as a medical alternative for laryngeal leukoplakia with (so far) impractical limitations. Issing et al treated 20 patients with induction doses of 300,000 IU/day for a week, escalating up to 1,500,000 IU/day by the fifth week in patients with resistant lesions.[82] Patients whose lesions regressed or remained stable were assigned a maintenance therapy of 150,000 IU/day. Patients whose lesions progressed were withdrawn. He observed complete remission in 15 patients, and a partial response in the remaining five, with three of the patients relapsing. The duration of treatment and follow-up was between 12 and 24 months.

Regression or progression, are both subtle and insidious, especially in recurrent leukoplakia after previous dysplasia. Laryngeal videophotography plays an important role in longitudinal diagnosis and follow-up. The comparison of small changes on separate print images from rigid videolaryngoscopy 8 to 16 weeks apart helps make up for deficiencies in note taking and paper diagrams.

◆ **Carcinoma in Situ** Carcinoma in situ (CIS) is a term borrowed from gynecologic pathology. For laryngeal CIS, the rule of full-thickness involvement does not apply. CIS means intraepithelial cancer; the cytology is neoplastic, and the basement membrane is intact (**Fig. 4.2**). Fechner emphasized that a pathologist cannot unequivocally identify a malignant cell *that is still confined to the epithelium*. Subjectivity does influence the interpretation of cytopathology. He preferred the designation "severe atypia" to carcinoma in situ.

Hypothetically, the treatment of carcinoma in situ is "stripping." Subepithelial removal of a clean laryngeal specimen should allow step sections to reveal the diagnosis (carcinoma in situ), and the prognosis (cure if normal margins). The basic ingredients for success are:

1. Selection—restrict stripping to sharply localized lesions on the membranous cord
2. Precision—generate an intact specimen and keep it oriented

To verify the virginity of the lamina propria, under the microscope, hydroinflate the subepithelial layer with injectable saline. Note that stripping has to be done with the biopsy,

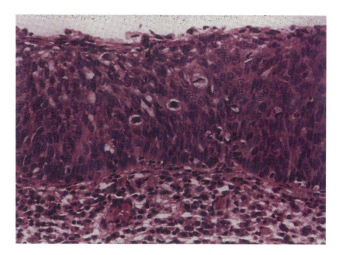

Fig. 4.2 Laryngeal carcinoma in situ, characterized by a dysplastic process involving the entire thickness of the squamous epithelium with loss of cellular maturation and polarity, an increase in the nuclear:cytoplasmic ratio, and mitoses scattered throughout all layers of the epithelium; the squamous epithelium is not thickened.

not as a follow-up procedure. Once the diseased site is incised, the basement membrane broken, stripping is jeopardized. Even the interpretation is compromised. Biopsy without these considerations greatly increases the chance that radiotherapy will be recommended in a patient who could otherwise have avoided it.

Verrucous Carcinoma

Verrucous carcinoma, or Ackerman tumor, is a very well differentiated squamous cell carcinoma with minimal cytologic atypia. Characteristically, the surface shows papillary fronds with prominent hyperkeratosis, and the depths of the tumor look benign (**Fig. 4.3**). This histological appearance makes diagnosis difficult, as the famous case of Frederick III (crown prince of Prussia, and emperor of Germany) shows. Treatment of this disease is often delayed until it is nearly incurable.

Verrucous carcinoma of the larynx should probably be treated by conservative surgical resection when possible, but radiotherapy can certainly be effectively used for disease that cannot be resected with preservation of laryngeal function. Total laryngectomy should probably be reserved for recurrent disease or the rare case of anaplastic transformation. McCaffrey et al reported on 52 histologically confirmed cases of verrucous carcinoma of the larynx treated at the Mayo Clinic between 1960 and 1987. Two patients died, both with a high-grade carcinoma recurrence in the larynx, which was histologically distinct from the original verrucous carcinoma. Four patients were treated with radiotherapy with three successes. In each case, the radiotherapy was given to control residual disease. None of the irradiated tumors in this series showed anaplastic dedifferentiation, and none of the irradiated patients died of uncontrolled local or regional disease.[83]

TLM in combination with a meticulous follow-up for early recognition of local recurrence would seem to be the optimal treatment option for early, very early, and perhaps some intermediate verrucous carcinomas at the present time. Damm

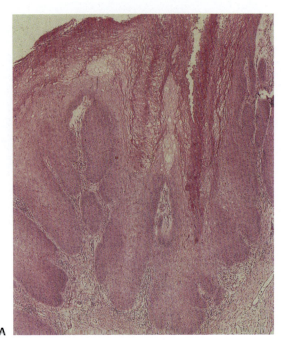

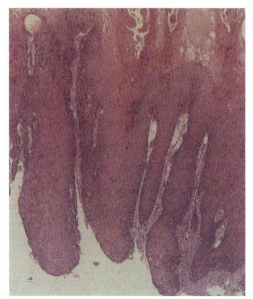

Fig. 4.3 (**A**) Histological appearance of verrucous carcinoma includes marked surface keratinization ("church-spire" keratosis), bulbous rete pegs "pushing" into the underlying stroma, absence of cellular atypia, and a mixed chronic inflammatory cell infiltrate. (**B**) This biopsy specimen shows the difficulty confronting the pathologist in the diagnosis of verrucous carcinoma, in that the

features of verrucous carcinoma are present; however, the absence of an adequate stromal component without a good epithelial—connective tissue interface precludes a definitive diagnosis of verrucous carcinoma. In this situation, additional (deeper) biopsy specimens would be necessary before definitively diagnosing a verrucous carcinoma.

et al reported 21 patients treated with transoral carbon dioxide laser surgery from 1986 to 1995. Fourteen had T1 lesions. Laser-cordectomy accomplished a complete removal in 10 cases. Extended laser cordectomy did likewise for the remaining four. Seven patients suffered from T2 verrucous carcinoma. Laser vertical partial laryngectomy was used to encompass their cancers. There were no tumor-related deaths in this series, no one received radiotherapy, and no patient required a laryngectomy.[84]

Invasive Squamous Cell Carcinoma

Some carcinomas, like verrucous, are locally invasive, but they invade so slowly and appear so well differentiated they are easily misread as benign. Others, like microinvasive carcinoma (**Fig. 4.4**), require very close scrutiny to find a site where the basement membrane is clearly penetrated. Invasive squamous cell carcinoma shows all the features of neoplasia—atypia (nuclear aberrations like pleomorphism

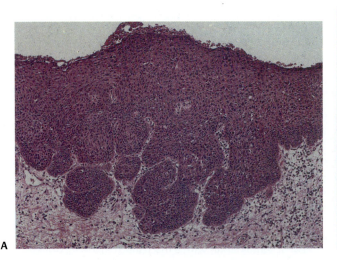

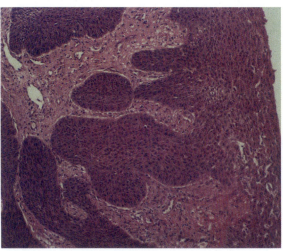

Fig. 4.4 (**A**) Superficially invasive (microinvasive) carcinoma developing as a continuum of carcinoma in situ, seen in the overlying epithelial component. (**B**) Superficially invasive (microinvasive) carcinoma developing from an epithelium without evidence of carcinoma in situ (full-thickness dysplasia).

and abnormal mitotic activity), disorderly maturation, deep elongation of rete processes into the stroma with branching off and island formation, and obvious invasion of mature tissues like muscle, cartilage, and bone (**Fig. 4.5**).

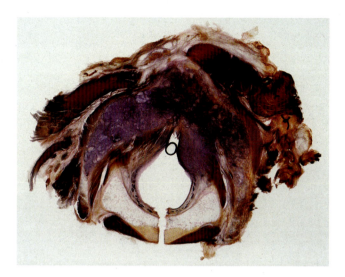

Fig. 4.5 Photomicrograph of squamous cell carcinoma of the pyriform fossa invading thyroid cartilage. (H & E ×)

Head and neck neoplasms are 5 to 8% of all cancers. Over one third occur in the larynx—up to half when one includes hypopharynx invading the larynx. The U.S. census reported 281,421,906 Americans in 2000. If the incidence of laryngeal carcinoma is five new cases per 100,000 per year, we could expect 14,000 new patients yearly. Some countries report 10 per 100,000. The highest urban rates come from São Paulo, Bombay, and Bangkok. The female to male ratio, once 1:11, has risen with the rising incidence of lung cancer in women.[85] This probably reflects tobacco's influence. Women get disproportionately more supraglottic cancer.[86] Most patients are older than 35. The peak incidence is between 60 and 75. African Americans have slightly more laryngeal cancer than Caucasian Americans.

In the United States, ~57% of laryngeal cancer is glottic, and 32% supraglottic. Perhaps 1% is truly subglottic cancer. Ten percent is sufficiently pervasive or transglottic or multicentric that the reported site of origin is disputable. Thirty percent of patients present with neck metastases. Second primary cancers are very frequent in patients with laryngeal carcinoma, 7 to 15% in glottic carcinoma, and up to *three* times higher in supraglottic cancer! These figures depend upon how long patients are followed. About one patient in a hundred has an occult synchronous smoking-related cancer (mouth, pharynx, bronchus, lung, or esophagus) at the time of presentation. This deadly incidence repeats itself every year thereafter and constitutes an important reason to follow patients even after the standard 5-year follow-up period.

Ninety to 95% of patients with laryngeal carcinoma smoked tobacco. (Many still do.) The agent of addiction is nicotine. The agent of carcinogenesis is the tobacco-related nitrosamines. Considerable data suggest smoking and alcohol abuse in combination have a synergic effect.[87] Other risk factors have also been suggested for laryngeal cancer too: toxic hydrocarbons in the oil and gas industry, inhaled irritants from cement dust[88] or asbestos,[89] formaldehyde,[90] dietary factors,[91] irradiation, papilloma virus infection,[92–94] and laryngopharyngeal reflux.[95,96] What makes these agents or cofactors difficult to incriminate is that so many people in the exposed populations also smoke.[97] It may be that different agents operate in glottic cancer versus supraglottic cancer versus hypopharyngeal cancer. Inhaled carcinogens presented to the larynx *from the lungs* (by mucociliary clearance from the bronchi and trachea) preferentially rise into the anterior glottis and the anterior commissure (and linger because the glottis is not ciliated). Carcinogens in the secretions from the mouth, nose, pharynx, and stomach bathe the supraglottic larynx. Inflammatory changes from LPR may increase local susceptibilities. Plummer-Vinson syndrome seems to put the postcricoid hypopharynx at more risk.

The significance of histological grade is uncertain. The tumor, nodes, metastasis (TNM) classification records three species, well-differentiated, moderately differentiated, and poorly differentiated. More important attributes are probably lymphatic vessel invasion and venous invasion (L and V in the TNM system). For L, the possibilities are two: no lymphatic vessel invasion, or lymphatic vessel invasion. For V, they include three: no venous invasion, microscopic venous invasion, and macroscopic venous invasion. Kupisz and Chibowski studied tumor angiogenesis in 60 patients with primary laryngeal cancer by quantitating the microvessel density with antibodies against factor VIII. A direct correlation was found between increased tumor angiogenesis and T stage, histological grade, and a shorter survival.[98]

Basaloid Squamous Carcinoma

Basaloid squamous carcinoma (BSC), first described by Wain et al in 1986,[99] is a pleomorphic epithelial cancer characterized by solid lobules and nests of basaloid cells and concomitant squamous cell carcinoma. Comedonecrosis and hyalinosis are frequent, as are cribriform features that need to be differentiated from adenoid cystic carcinoma.[100] The cytologic appearances (scanty cytoplasm and hyperchromatic nuclei) bear certain similarities to small cell carcinoma and the other neuroendocrine cancers, but BSC can usually be recognized on hematoxylin-eosin (H&E) section, and it lacks reactivity to neuroendocrine markers like chromogranin and synaptophysin, and has only very weak reactivity to neuron-specific enolase. BSC is positive for cytokeratins and negative for in situ hybridization to HPV (**Fig. 4.6**).

In the head and neck, BSC is a high-grade cancer with a predilection for the base of tongue, floor of mouth, pyriform sinus, and supraglottic larynx.[101] It behaves like an overly aggressive squamous cell cancer. Surgery to the primary is often not enough. Elective neck dissection and postoperative radiotherapy are usually recommended as well.

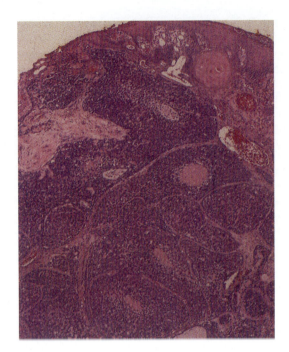

Fig. 4.6 Basaloid carcinoma of the larynx.

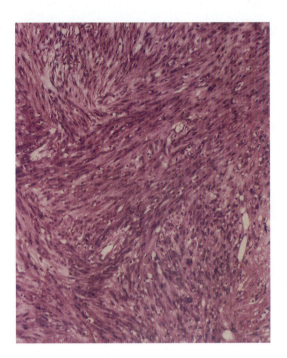

Fig. 4.7 Spindle cell carcinoma or carcinosarcoma.

Pseudosarcoma (Spindle Cell Carcinoma, Carcinosarcoma)

Biologically, there is nothing very "pseudo" about pseudosarcoma. This is a rare, high-grade malignancy, which typically presents in the larynx as a firm, gray, pedunculated or exophytic polypoid mass, sometimes with surface epithelial ulceration.[102] Other names in the literature are carcinosarcoma, spindle cell carcinoma, pleomorphic carcinoma, sarcomatoid carcinoma, or spindle cell sarcoma. Pseudosarcoma dates to a time when carcinosarcoma was considered a benign response of connective tissue to an adjacent squamous carcinoma. Spindle cell sarcoma was a recognition that the spindle cells were indeed malignant, but their epithelial origins were obscured.

Carcinosarcoma and *spindle cell carcinoma* are probably the most accurate terms because this tumor is now regarded as a sarcomatoid variant of epidermoid carcinoma. Both morphological components appear to be malignant (**Fig. 4.7**). The spindle cells have been shown to be immunoreactive to cytokeratin monoclonal antibodies, reflecting their epithelial origin. Vimentin can often be demonstrated, too, by immunofluorescence, indicating mesenchymal cell differentiation.[103] The cytology of carcinosarcoma is thought to arise by "divergent" metaplasia, in which a malignant mesenchymal morphology differentiates from what is fundamentally an epithelial carcinoma (most often a squamous cell carcinoma).[104,105] Sometimes a small, infiltrating, well-differentiated squamous cell carcinoma is associated with a large polypoid sarcomatous mass showing the histological features of a malignant giant cell tumor of soft parts.[106] Here again, both phenotypes are malignant. The spindle cell morphology of the neck metastases can be particularly vexing. Osseous components,[107] or fibrosarcomatous changes, or chondrosarcomatous elements (**Fig. 4.8**),[108] or myosarcomatous appear-

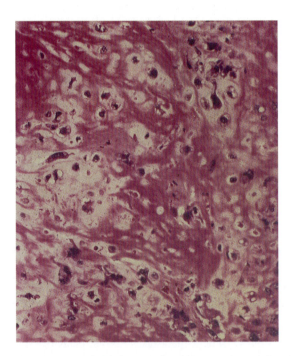

Fig. 4.8 Heterologous elements can be seen in spindle cell carcinoma, including this focus of osteosarcoma.

ances[109] have all been reported to occur. Clinically, the pattern of metastasis and survival of carcinosarcoma seems to parallel squamous cell carcinoma of the larynx. Thus treatment considerations run parallel and depend on the extent of the cancer.[110]

Neuroendocrine Tumors of the Larynx

Neuroendocrine cells are inconspicuous in the larynx, but both types are present—epithelial neuroendocrine cells (Kulchitsky cells), which can generate carcinoid tumors, and neural neuroendocrine cells (paraganglion cells), which can give origin to laryngeal paragangliomas. Neuroendocrine neoplasms are a very small proportion (0.5%) of laryngeal cancer, but it is so important to recognize them and distinguish them from squamous cell carcinoma (and from each other) that their story deserves our attention.

Neuroendocrine cells belong to the amine precursor uptake and decarboxylation (APUD) system.[111] They all contain secretory granules and have the capacity to synthesize precursors of biogenic amines such as serotonin (5-hydroxytryptamine), 5-hydroxytryptophan, adrenocorticotropic hormone (ACTH), norepinephrine, bombesin, calcitonin, antidiuretic hormone (ADH), and bradykinin. Related cells occur in the pituitary gland, thyroid gland, lungs, pancreas, gastrointestinal tract, adrenal medulla, sympathetic ganglia, paraganglia, thymus, and chemoreceptor systems. They secrete similar polypeptides and share common cytochemical and ultrastructural characteristics. They derive at least some of their constituent cells from the neural crest, many appear to receive cholinergic nerve endings, some react to changes in gas composition or neural transmitters, and all exhibit special staining characteristics attributable to their neurosecretory granules. A unique concept of dysplasia of the neuronal ectoderm has been proposed to explain the occurrence of multiple endocrine neoplasia and the multipotentiality of neoplastic cells derived from the APUD system to produce a variety of peptide hormones.

Clinically, four tumors arise from the laryngeal neuroepithelial cells, three from the epithelial (Kulchitsky[112,113]) variety (endocrinomas[114]), and one from the neural (paraganglionic) subtype. The epithelial derivatives, in ascending order of aggression, best to worst, are carcinoid tumor, atypical carcinoid tumor, and anaplastic small cell carcinoma. Wenig made a good case that these should be called well, moderately, and poorly differentiated neuroendocrine carcinoma of the larynx, reflecting the wide spectrum of behaviors but their close relations with each other.[115] Oat cell or small cell carcinoma (OCC or SCC) is not an unrelated entity, and "atypical" is more common in the larynx than the so-called typical carcinoids, which is contrary to most other sites. The neural (paraganglionic) neuroendocrine cells produce just one neoplasm, the paraganglioma. It behaves worse than a carcinoid tumor but much better than a small cell cancer.

Nicholas Kulchitsky (1856–1925) first identified the cells that bear his name by their special staining reactions. Chromaffin cells (react with chromium salts) typically occur in the adrenal medulla. Kulchitsky cells could better be shown by their ability to reduce silver salts (argentaffin reaction, and the term *argentaffinoma* has been used to describe a tumor derived from these cells, the carcinoid tumor). Clusters of 80 to 100 argentaffin cells in the basal layer of gastrointestinal and respiratory epithelium, in the crypts of Lieberkühn of the small intestine, or in the basal aspect of the ductal epithelium of bronchial mucus glands was an unexpected observation. Pesce et al[111] described their occurrence in the larynx, where they appear to receive an extra blood supply and cholinergic nerve endings, and the neurosecretory granules are present. The purpose of neuroepithelial cells in the larynx remains unclear. Maybe they just exist as stragglers, leftover remnants from the neural crest. Like melanocytes, they appear in the larynx, but they have no particular function that we recognize, except to intrigue the histologists.

Carcinoids in the larynx are Kulchitsky cell carcinomas (**Fig. 4.9**). So are the more aggressive atypical carcinoids, and, as in the lung, so are the highly anaplastic OCCs.[116] These are known by their immunohistochemistry. Investigators find panneuroendocrine markers (chromogranin, synaptophysin, neurofilament, NSE, LEU 7), and epithelial markers (pankeratin, AE1/AE3, cam 5.2), and specific hormonal markers (ACTH, calcitonin, insulin, etc.).[117–119] Carcinoid tumors share histological similarities with pancreatic islet cell tumors and medullary carcinomas of the thyroid, and they may coexist with other endocrine tumors. Most carcinoid tumors do not occur in association with other endocrine neoplasms, and they usually do not secrete hormones normally produced by cells other than enterochromaffin cells.

◆ **Carcinoid Tumor** Classic or typical carcinoid tumors in the larynx are slow growing, with an excellent prognosis (after complete resection, using conservation principles).[120] Some have discouraged endoscopic removal on the basis that carcinoid tumors are very vascular lesions. In our estimation, however, transoral laser microsurgery has reached the point where this feature is a caution, not a contraindication. Preoperative angiography and embolization seem unnecessary and risky. If open surgery is undertaken, the superior thyroid artery can be ligated en route to the tumor. Lymph node metastases are rare, to the point that neck dissection is virtually never required. Radiation and chemotherapy are considered ineffective for well-differentiated carcinoid tumors.[121]

◆ **Atypical Carcinoid Tumor** Atypical carcinoids are moderately differentiated neuroendocrine carcinomas seen more commonly than classic carcinoid tumors in the larynx. These lesions have higher mitotic activity and a propensity for perineural spread beyond their obvious boundaries, and they sometimes contain areas of necrosis. The pathologist's challenge may be to distinguish atypical carcinoids from medullary carcinoma, squamous cancer, acinic cell carcinoma, metastatic melanoma, or a paraganglioma. Carcinoids with atypical histological features have a much higher malignant potential and a higher rate of local and regional recurrence than the well-differentiated carcinoids.[122]

The mainstay of treatment is wide local resection. Radiotherapy can be very helpful (Logue et al found the reputation of atypical carcinoids for radioresistance is overblown[123]). Lymph node metastases occur in ~50% of patients, and these in turn have a high likelihood for developing systemic metastases and have a significantly worse prognosis. Elective neck dissection is encouraged for patients with atypical carcinoids because the likelihood of cervical lymph node metastases is so high. Adjuvant chemotherapy is used in patients with systemic metastases. Ferlito found a survival rate of 48%

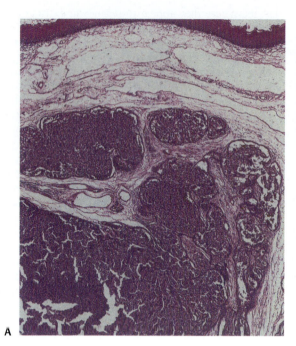 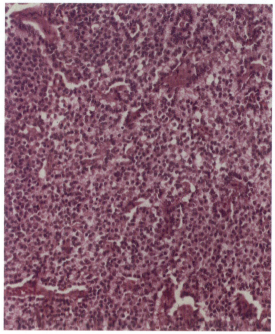

Fig. 4.9 (**A**) Laryngeal well-differentiated neuroendocrine carcinoma (carcinoid tumor): submucosal cellular neoplasm with lobular and solid growth patterns associated with a fibrovascular stroma. (**B**) Glandular differentiation may be seen in carcinoid tumors that are composed of uniform cells with centrally located round nuclei, vesicular chromatin, and eosinophilic cytoplasm.

at 5 years and 30% at 10 years for patients with atypical carcinoids.[121]

◆ **Small Cell Carcinoma (Oat Cell Carcinoma)** The first recognized case of anaplastic SCC, the most poorly differentiated neuroendocrine carcinoma, was reported by Olofsson and van Nostrand in 1972.[124] Poorly differentiated neuroendocrine carcinomas parallel SCCs/OCCs of the lung in every way—the same highly aggressive behavior in spite of treatment in a male with a heavy smoking history, metastases developing early, occasionally a paraneoplastic syndrome,[125] and very poor 5-year survival rates. Aguilar et al[126] report that 35% of primary OCCs in the larynx are transglottic, and 27% are supraglottic. Fifty-four percent of patients have regional metastases at initial presentation, and 17.6% have distant metastases. The median survival is 10 months and the 2- and 5-year overall survival rates are 16% and 5%, respectively.[127]

SCCs of the larynx should be managed as a systemic disease.[128] Surgery has not been effective in the treatment of these poorly differentiated tumors, partly because they seem to be disseminated at the time of diagnosis. Ferlito et al found 2- and 5-year survivals of 16 and 5%.[121] Patients who were treated with chemotherapy with or without other modalities had a 2-year survival rate of 52.2%. Forty-one percent of patients had regional recurrence only, 12.5% had regional recurrence and distant metastases, and 2% developed only distant metastases. Chemotherapy and radiotherapy to the neck currently appear to offer the least disabling and most effective forms of therapy. Laryngectomy followed by adju-

vant chemotherapy and radiotherapy may be indicated for cure in cases without metastases, but the detection of regional metastases suggests hematogenous spread, and this should usually restrict treatment to chemotherapy and radiotherapy.

◆ **Paraganglioma ("Glomus" Tumor)** The fourth type of neuroendocrine tumor in the larynx is the laryngeal paraganglioma. This cancer arises from neural crest cells [as opposed to the epithelial (Kulchitsky) cell origins just described for the carcinoid family], which also belong to the APUD system. Laryngeal paragangliomas are the laryngeal analogues of the more familiar paragangliomas we know in the neck (carotid body tumor, glomus vagale) or the ear (glomus jugulare, glomus tympanicum). The laryngeal paraganglia themselves are described by Lawson and Zak[129] in association with the superior laryngeal nerve just inside the supraglottic larynx and the recurrent laryngeal nerve just behind the cricothyroid joint. Thus, like the paraganglia elsewhere in the head and neck, all seem related to the branchial arch system and its blood vessels and autonomic nerves. Although carotid body cells react to changes in gas composition we are not aware of this for the paraganglion cells in the larynx, so *chemodectomas* is not an appropriate term. We know that catecholamines can be oxidized by chromic acid solutions to form brown polymers—the chromaffin reaction—used for years for adrenal gland and pheochromocytomas. But extraadrenal paraganglionic tissue does not have enough to stain. Therefore, it was called nonchromaffin paraganglioma tissue, but this, too, is an outdated term because now we know paraganglion cells, including those in the larynx, do have catecholamines. Finally, *glomus tumor* is not an appropriate term, either, because glomi are recognized structures in the skin, and these are not the origin of laryngeal paragangliomas (or, for that matter, so-called glomus tumors of the vagus, jugular region, or tympanum).

Clinically, the typical laryngeal paraganglioma is a small, smooth, red, supraglottic tumor, and sometimes painful. It is locally invasive but rarely metastatic. It is the only laryngeal neuroendocrine neoplasm with a female preponderance (3:1). Confusion with atypical carcinoid has led to incorrect diagnosis, inappropriate classification schemes, and overly aggressive treatment. Wide local excision (conservative surgery) is usually all these patients will require; elective neck dissection is not necessary, and the overall prognosis is excellent.

Melanoma

Sometimes primary mucosal melanoma appears to be pedunculated. The surface is bluish. Spindle cells are common, S-100 and vimentin immunofluorescence tests are positive, cytokeratin and iron are negative. The most important prognostic feature, as with cutaneous melanoma, may be depth of invasion. Prasad et al[130] graded mucosal melanomas in the head and neck according to depth as follows:

1. Melanoma in situ
2. Penetration into the lamina propria
3. Invasion into the deeper tissues—muscle, cartilage, etc.

The treatment, when possible, is surgery, including neck dissection(s). Radiation is also recommended, but radiotherapy *alone* is ineffective.[131]

Nonepidermoid Cancer

Nonepidermoid cancer of the larynx represents an extremely diverse group of diseases with differing prognoses and rationales of management. Diagnosis is dependent on a high index of suspicion by the clinician and accurate consulting in histopathology. These neoplasms can be grouped according to cells with secretory, connective tissue, lymphoreticular, or metastatic origins.[132]

Adenocarcinoma (Secretory Neoplasms)

Secretory neoplasms are also known as adenocarcinomas, glandular cancers, or malignant sialogenic tumors. They are rare in the larynx, but expected. Seromucinous glands are especially prevalent in the submucosa of the vestibular folds and the subglottis.

Adenoid Cystic Carcinoma

Adenoid cystic carcinoma presents a similar problem in the larynx as elsewhere in the head and neck—slow but relentless growth and a tendency for recurrence even after a long period clinically free of symptoms (**Fig. 4.10**). Typically, the patient with laryngeal adenoid cystic cancer is misdiagnosed as asthma. This reflects its salient characteristics—slow

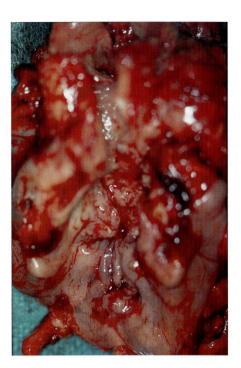

Fig. 4.10 Adenoid cystic carcinoma of the larynx. Present for 7 years until patient finally consented to have laryngectomy.

growth in an occult location—the subglottis or the upper trachea. The early age of onset, absent risk factors, normal voice, and slight female preponderance also divert the clinician's attention from a diagnosis of cancer. An aryepiglottic origin is also submucosal and silent. Ulceration is absent. Imaging and endoscopy famously underestimate adenoid cystic cancer, perhaps because of perineural spread. In other locations, this can be discontinuous, so the larynx is probably no exception. The prognosis is grave. The latency for the appearance of pulmonary metastases averages 4 years. About half the patients with adenoid cystic cancer are dead of disease within 5 years of recognition. Lifelong follow-up is essential for the survivors.

Mucoepidermoid Carcinoma

Mucoepidermoid carcinoma is slightly less common than adenoid cystic cancer in the larynx, perhaps because high-grade mucoepidermoid (so called adenosquamous) carcinoma is prone to be misdiagnosed as squamous cell carcinoma in this location. The male predominance may reflect its squamous associations. Well-differentiated mucoepidermoid carcinoma tends to respond favorably to primary surgery, neck dissection(s), and radiotherapy. High-grade (poorly differentiated) mucoepidermoid adenocarcinoma fares much worse.

Poorly Differentiated Adenocarcinoma

Mahlstedt et al[133] cited an incidence of 25% in a series of 15 malignant salivary gland cancers of the larynx, and a survival of 25%; the worst of this series compared with adenoid cystic and mucoepidermoid carcinomas. The prognosis for poorly differentiated adenocarcinoma was poorer than for squamous carcinoma of the same site and stage.

Mesenchymal Neoplasms (Sarcomas)

◆ **Chondrosarcoma** The most common sarcoma is laryngeal chondrosarcoma. The principle issue is how aggressive one might be. Well differentiated under the microscope, they are nevertheless locally invasive at surgery, and the gross and microscopic margins can be indistinct.

Chondrosarcoma is a slow-growing indolent tumor found predominantly in the lower skeleton in adult men. Ten percent occur in the head and neck, mostly in the maxilla or the larynx, and low-grade chondrosarcoma is the most frequently encountered mesenchymal tumor in the larynx. Among cartilage tumors in the larynx, more than 90% are chondrosarcomas, and 70% arise in the cricoid ring where they defy early

detection. With cricoarytenoid joint deformation, the cord is eventually immobilized, leading to a mistaken diagnosis of unilateral vocal cord paralysis. Chondrosarcoma also occurs in the thyroid cartilage (20%) and the arytenoid (10%).[134] The typical radiological appearance of chondrosarcoma is one of stippled calcification in a destructive mass. The differential diagnosis includes chondroma, chondrometaplasia (elastic cartilage in the glottis without nuclear atypia or invasion), dedifferentiated chondrosarcoma, tracheopathia osteoplastica, laryngeal osteosarcoma, and benign mixed tumor (ductal structures and myoepithelial cells in a chondroid stroma).

Laryngeal chondrosarcoma exhibits a lobular pattern on low magnification, increased nuclear cellularity and atypia, increased mitotic activity, prominent binucleate tumor cells, and the incomplete presence of a pseudocapsule (**Fig. 4.11**). A biopsy is valuable for histological grading (a prognostic factor for survival), but challenging because the mass is hard, and covered by normal-looking mucosa. Lower-grade chondrosarcoma can

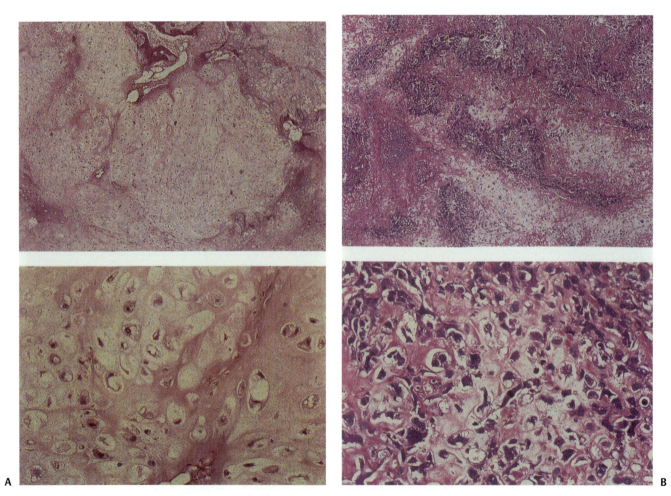

A   B

Fig. 4.11 Low-grade laryngeal chondrosarcoma. (**Top**) Lobulated cellular neoplasm. (**Bottom**) The tumor is composed of enlarged chondrocytes with hyperchromatic, pleomorphic nuclei, prominent nucleoli, and binucleate cells.

often be misinterpreted as chondroma. Higher grades of chondrosarcoma have a greater tendency to recur and metastasize.[135]

The main modality of treatment for low-grade laryngeal chondrosarcoma is conservation surgery. This applies even for recurrent disease. At the Mayo Clinic, in Rochester, MN, patients treated surgically and followed closely achieved a 5-year survival similar to that of age-matched controls.[136] Note that chondrosarcomas in other areas of the body are radiosensitive. Perhaps radiotherapy should play a more prominent role, especially where laryngeal surgery is excluded by patient preference or surgical contraindications and comorbidities.

◆ **Osteogenic Sarcoma** Laryngeal osteosarcoma, much rarer than laryngeal chondrosarcoma, presents with a rapid onset of symptoms because of the speedy growth of the tumor. Histologically, osteosarcoma is a high-grade neoplasm with a fibrosarcomatous or osteoblastic osteosarcomatous appearance and osteoclastic multinucleated giant cells. If a chondroblastic lesion contains malignant osteoid, it is referred to as a chondroblastic osteogenic sarcoma. Treatment is aggressive surgery to reduce the high morbidity and poor prognosis expected with laryngeal osteosarcoma.

◆ **Kaposi Sarcoma** Kaposi sarcoma is a vascular cancer characterized by soft violaceous macules that typically begin in the lower extremities in immunocompromised patients. It is most commonly found in patients with acquired immunodeficiency syndrome (AIDS). When it occurs in the larynx, treatment depends on the comorbidities and airway effects. Bleeding is a serious threat at biopsy or tracheotomy.[137] Various treatments described have included laser resection,[138] radiotherapy,[137] intralesional vincristine injection,[139] and low-dose α-2b interferon.[140] Because AIDS patients suffer from immunosuppression, several other tumors may occur. Squamous cell cancer of the larynx has been described, at a younger age than normal, and T cell lymphomas have also occurred. The differential diagnosis of opportunistic infections that appear in the immunocompromised larynx includes cryptococcosis, cytomegalovirus (CMV) laryngitis, laryngeal candidiasis, herpes simplex, and tuberculosis of the larynx.[141] Thus cervical adenopathy may be neoplastic or inflammatory.

◆ **Other True Sarcomas** Among the possibilities are several very rare sarcomas. Most information is based on anecdotal case reports. Examples include the following:

- Synovial cell carcinoma
- Leiomyosarcoma—coexpress vimentin and actin
- Rhabdomyosarcoma
- Fibrosarcoma
- Liposarcoma
- Malignant fibrous histiocytoma

Lymphoreticular Neoplasms

Lymphoreticular cancers are extremely rare in the larynx. Extramedullary plasmacytomas have been described. The issue is whether they are part of the broader disease process,

multiple myeloma. Non–Hodgkins lymphomas are reported in the larynx. In all hematopoietic neoplasms, surgery is for either or both biopsy and the relief of airway obstruction. The definitive treatments are nonsurgical.

Metastases to the Larynx

Freeland and Van Nostrand believed that the frequency of hematogenous and lymphogenous metastasis to the larynx is probably underestimated.[142] They described four patients, ages 43 to 57, with metastases from cutaneous melanoma, ovarian cystadenocarcinoma, nasopharyngeal carcinoma, and myeloblastic leukemia. Three of the four offered no laryngeal symptoms (although all could have been detected by indirect laryngoscopy). Nicolai et al reviewed the published reports up to 1996 and added three more sources to this list—renal carcinoma, lung adenocarcinoma, and colonic adenocarcinoma.[143]

◆ **Local Invasion from Regional Thyroid Cancer** Well-differentiated thyroid carcinoma sometimes invades the upper aerodigestive tract structures. The most common structures invaded are the recurrent laryngeal nerves, larynx, pharynx, and esophagus. The symptoms of invasion include airway insufficiency, dysphagia, and hemoptysis.[144] Lipton found age at diagnosis to be a negative prognostic factor and duration of disease before invasion to be a positive prognostic factor.[145] Later McCaffrey showed the site invaded will influence survival, with trachea and esophagus the worst. Muscle invasion, laryngeal invasion, and recurrent laryngeal nerve invasion had no significant independent influence on survival.[146]

Basically, three types of surgery can be performed when thyroid cancer invades the larynx: complete tumor removal, "shave" excision, and incomplete tumor excision. Radical surgery and adjuvant therapy provided no improvement in survival over treatment with near-total (skeletonizing) excisions combined with adjuvant therapy in McCaffrey's analysis. And patients treated with grossly incomplete debulking procedures, with or without tracheotomy, eventually died from their disease. If the tumor involves only the wall of the larynx or trachea, without intralumenal extension, "shaving" the tumor and the outermost anatomical layer from the trachea or larynx will produce local control rates comparable to more radical and destructive procedures.[144] Intralumenal extension is a more serious problem that generally requires full-thickness resection of a portion of the aerodigestive tract. Even here, conservation resections are preferable. In essence, when the lumen is not involved, "shaving" tumor from airway or esophagus is an acceptable treatment with a similar locoregional control rate and minimal morbidity when compared with definitive aerodigestive tract resection. When the lumen is involved, invasive thyroid carcinoma requires definitive resection of the affected portion of the larynx, hypopharynx, trachea, or esophagus to remove all gross disease, combined with the applicable surgical reconstruction.[147] Adjuvant therapy using radioiodine or external beam radiotherapy should be considered an integral part of any treatment plan for these tumors.[146]

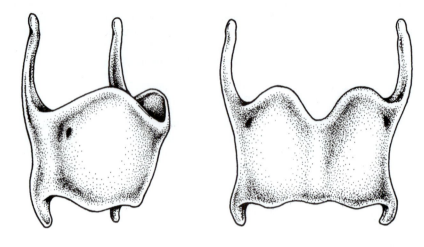

Fig. 4.12 Cricoid cartilage.

◆ Surgical Anatomy of Larynx Cancer

The Laryngeal Framework

The framework comprises nine cartilages, three unpaired (thyroid, cricoid, epiglottis) and three paired (arytenoids, corniculates, cuneiforms), and four membranes, two unpaired, the hyoepiglottic "ligament" and the thyrohyoid membrane, and two paired, the triangular membranes and the quadrangular membranes.

The thyroid cartilage alae join at the angle (**Fig. 4.12**). The upper end of the angle is the "Adam's apple." The angle is like the spine of a book—the right and left alae are the covers. The right and left fibroelastic membranes are like two pages inside the covers. Each page is split into an upper and a lower part, by a ventricle. The top part is the quadrangular membrane, the bottom part is the triangular membrane. Anteriorly, the triangular membranes fuse in the midline and the extension of this fusion down beyond the thyroid angle to the cricoid is the cricothyroid ligament. The Broyle ligament anchors the top of the dual triangular ligaments to the inner side of the angle a few millimeters below the thyroid notch. Because the free upper margins of the triangular membranes are also the vocal ligaments, the Broyle ligament[148] is the anterior attachment of the glottis. The lateral fibers of the thyroepiglottic ligament anchor the bottom of the dual quadrangular ligaments to the inner side of the angle, just below the thyroid notch, and the central portion of the thyroepiglottic ligament binds the lower end of the epiglottis to the angle. Because the free lower margins of the quadrangular membranes are the vestibular ligaments, and the lower end of the epiglottis is the petiole, the thyroepiglottic ligament is one anterior attachment of the supraglottis. The other is the hyoepiglottic ligament, which takes its origin on the uppermost inner edge of the hyoid body. The thyroid alae extend so far back they embrace the pyriforms. The superior cornua of the thyroid cartilage run posteriorly more than upward, they often hook medially to impress the mucosa of the *pharynx*, and from inside the larynx (e.g., transoral laser microsurgery), their distinction from the greater horns of the hyoid, which they nearly parallel, can be challenging. The superior laryngeal artery and nerve usually penetrate into

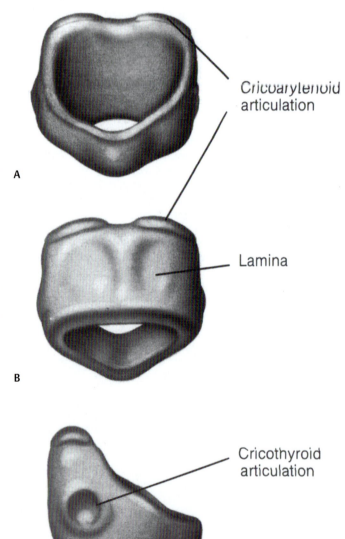

A

Cricoarytenoid articulation

Lamina

B

Cricothyroid articulation

C

Fig. 4.13 (**A**) Anterior view. (**B**) Posterior view. (**C**) Right lateral view. The thyroid cartilage includes the notch superiorly, the oblique line, two inferior cornua, two superior cornua, and occasional fenestrations.

the larynx through the thyrohyoid membrane to reach the paraglottic space (PGS). But sometimes they enter through a foramen in the thyroid ala instead. The thyroid cartilage begins to ossify in one's midtwenties, from the inferior margin upward. Cancer preferentially invades ossified cartilage because native cartilage lacks the preformed vascular pathways around which the initial calcification occurs.

The cricoid ring is the only complete ring in the airway (given that tracheal "rings" are arches) (**Fig. 4.13**). The cricoid is the foundation of the larynx: braces it open, bears its muscles, and gives rise to the conus elasticus. *Conus* is an inclusive name for the right and left triangular membranes and the cricothyroid ligament (their fusion anteriorly). The cricoid gives origin to all the intrinsic muscles of the larynx except the thyroarytenoids, which flow back from the inner aspect of the thyroid angle, outside the upper half of the conus. The steeply sloping upper border of the cricoid causes a signet ring configuration, and the greater mass of the ring, the posterior plate, bears the posterior cricoarytenoid muscles on its dorsal surface. Ossification proceeds from the upper margin down and lags behind the thyroid cartilage.

The epiglottis is a perforated leaflet of noncalcifying elastic cartilage projected up from the petiole and supported forward at its midlevel by the hyoepiglottic "ligament," a broad fibroelastic membrane from the hyoid (**Fig. 4.14**). This design encourages the epiglottis to fold back at its halfway line in the presence of a solid object (like a direct laryngoscope). The suprahyoid portion can cover the introitus quickly and passively, "breaking" at the attachment line of the hyoepiglottic ligament. It can also spring back with minimal assistance from the muscles of the supraglottis. In fact it is remarkable how little intrinsic muscle tissue is actually present in the false cords and preepiglottic tissues, considering how important is the function of the larynx in guarding the entrance to

the lungs. The suprahyoid epiglottis bears loose mucosa on its lingual aspect and tight mucosa on its laryngeal surface. The infrahyoid portion forms one wall of the triangular enclosure for the preepiglottic fat pad, the other two being the thyrohyoid membrane and the hyoepiglottic ligament.

We have already noted that the conus elasticus projects upward from the cricoid, and, after a short break (for the ventricle), the same "page" of fibroelastic tissue rises even higher, to the aryepiglottic fold, as the quadrangular membrane. These membranes play important roles in voice, swallow, airway, and the spread of laryngeal cancer. The vocal ligament is simply the thickened superior margin of the conus. The quadrangular membrane is the fibroelastic "skeleton" of the false cord. The epiglottis in front and the arytenoid/corniculate complex behind hold up the quadrangular membrane like two masts supporting a sheet. Between the mast ahead (epiglottis) and the masts behind (two arytenoids), and the membranes they support, the aryepiglottic folds laterally and the interarytenoid tissues behind, the airway is projected upward out of the floor of the pharynx, out of the secretions, and up into clear air. If the quadrangular membrane was a mainsail, the cuneiform would be a batten stiffening its leach (free edge). The whole idea is to project the airway up for breathing and to resist aspiration. The normal supraglottis can brace open for air, strike down instantly to protect the airway from food, then resurrect to its open mode immediately again for breathing.

The three "small" paired cartilages of the framework are as follows:

- The corniculates (cartilages of Santorini) capping the arytenoids
- The cuneiforms (cartilages of Wrisberg) stiffening the aryepiglottic folds

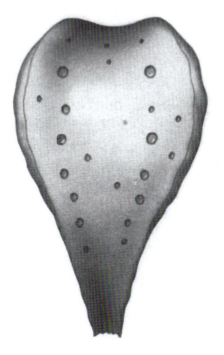
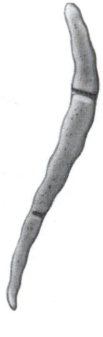

Fig. 4.14 Epiglottic cartilage. Note the perforations.

- The arytenoids, larger than expected, surmounting the cricoid. Because the vocal ligament occupies the vocal process and the cricoarytenoid muscles take up the muscular process, the thyroarytenoid and the vestibular ligament have no process of their own. The thyroarytenoid muscle spreads out in the lower depression on the anterolateral surface, the oblong fossa. The vestibular ligament gets a higher anchorage, the triangular fossa (**Fig. 4.15**).
- Perhaps a distant fourth set of paired cartilages might be the triciates, in the ligamentous posterior margins of the thyrohyoid membranes. The ligament connects the superior cornua of the thyroid cartilage with the greater horns of the hyoid bone.

Laryngeal Soft Tissues

The glottis is the triangle formed by the vocal folds and the commissures (**Fig. 4.16**). There is no lower anatomical limit. The glottis is smoothly continuous with the subglottis inferiorly. Some give a measurement to the height of the glottis, variously 5 or 10 mm. Others cite the histology, claiming the transition from squamous to respiratory mucosa marks the transition from glottis to subglottis. But from a surgeon's or an anatomist's perspective, it would be more accurate to refer to *two levels* in the anterior larynx, not three. The glottis–subglottis would be one level, and the supraglottis would be the second.[149]

The vocal fold is a layered structure (**Fig. 4.17**). The epithelial layer or contact mucosa is nonkeratinizing squamous epithelium and the source of glottic cancers. The lamina propria under the epithelium (submucosa) is loose areolar and myxoid tissue, also referred to as the Reinke space. Stiffness in this layer destroys the glottic wave and causes hoarseness.[150] Under the myxoid layer is the vocal ligament—the free edge of the conus elasticus. The muscle layer is next, and it is all thyroarytenoid muscle. Notice that there are too many muscle fibers to span between the anterior commissure and the vocal process. Most thyroarytenoid muscle fibers run an oblique course, from low anterior (their origins inside the lower half of the angle of the thyroid cartilage) to high posterior (their insertions on the anterolateral depression on the body of the arytenoid). The ventricles run up against the medial aspect of those fibers that slant higher than the plane of the vocal folds. The little bit that herniates over the top of the thyroarytenoid to nearly contact the ala is the saccule. The vocalis muscles are the medial horizontal muscle fibers, which do manage to form an intimate connection with the ligament.

The false "cords" consist of the ventricular band, the false cord itself, and the aryepiglottic (AE) fold. Some muscle fibers in the AE fold are parts of a long muscular sling that

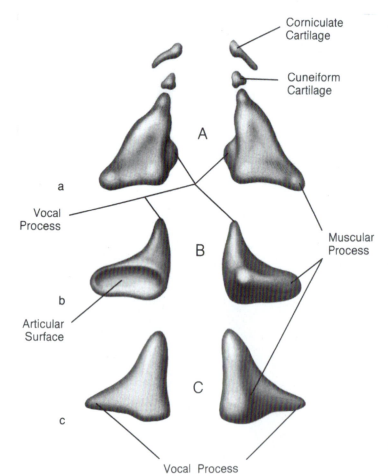

Fig. 4.15 Arytenoid cartilages. (**A**) Posterior view with cuneiform and corniculate cartilages above. (**B**) Inferior view (left), superior view (right). (**C**) Anterior view.

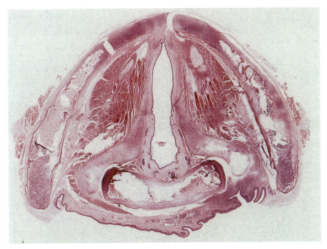

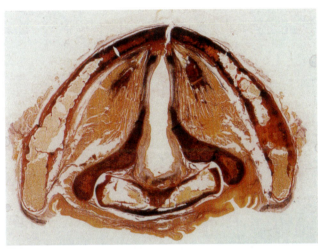

Fig. 4.16 (**A**) Horizontal section at the glottis. (**B**) Adult glottis.

ADULT

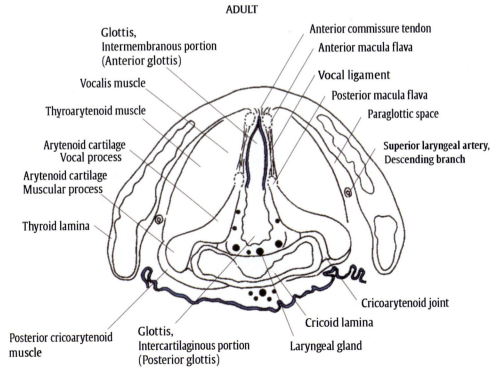

Glottis,
Intermembranous portion
(Anterior glottis)

Vocalis muscle

Thyroarytenoid muscle

Arytenoid cartilage
Vocal process

Arytenoid cartilage
Muscular process

Thyroid lamina

Posterior cricoarytenoid
muscle

Anterior commissure tendon

Anterior macula flava

Vocal ligament

Posterior macula flava

Paraglottic space

**Superior laryngeal artery,
Descending branch**

Cricoarytenoid joint

Cricoid lamina

Laryngeal gland

Glottis,
Intercartilaginous portion
(Posterior glottis)

B

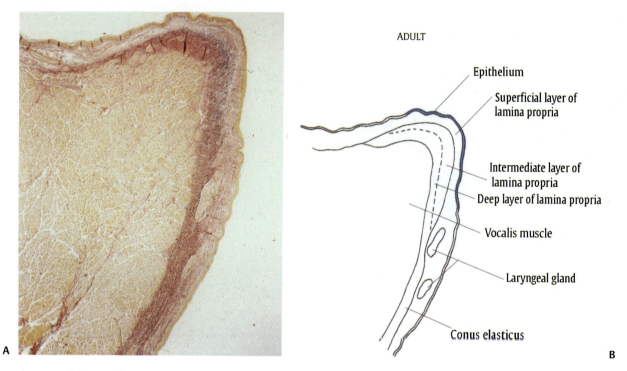

Fig. 4.17 (**A**) Coronal section of the midportion of the membranous vocal fold. (**B**) Adult midportion of the membranous vocal fold.

starts from the pharynx and flows downward, in the medial pyriform walls to unite behind the arytenoids at its lowest extent. A few of these fibers decussate in the interarytenoid region to insert low on the opposite arytenoid. Others form a thick band between the cartilages (the interarytenoid muscle). The continuous fibers seem to embrace the concavity on the posterior aspect of the two arytenoids, whereas the corniculates recurve back over them and "hook" down the muscles to ensure their support. Adduction wrinkles up the interarytenoid mucosa in the posterior commissure to assist in sealing out aspiration. The thin tight mucosa on the medial face of each arytenoid is also the blood supply to the avascular cartilage. No wonder ulceration sets up a granulating wound (a "contact granuloma") that proves slow to heal.

Paraglottic Space

The paraglottic "space" (PGS) (**Fig. 4.18**) is the connective tissue compartment containing the vascular supply, nerve fibers, and fibrofatty soft tissues between the thyroid ala and the intrinsic muscles and glands and ventricle of the larynx originally distinguished by Tucker and Smith[151] in 1962. The upper limit of the PGS is the lateral pharyngoepiglottic fold; the lower limit is the sloping upper margin of the cricoid. The conus elasticus directs the lower end of the PGS laterally as it descends, and thus it spills out over the cricoid cartilage.[152] The dorsal margin is the floor of the pyriform sinus. The dorsomedial adipose tissues extend toward the cricoarytenoid joint. Forward and medially, the PGS links with the preepiglottic (better "periepiglottic"[153]) space (**Fig. 4.19**). In some cases, the

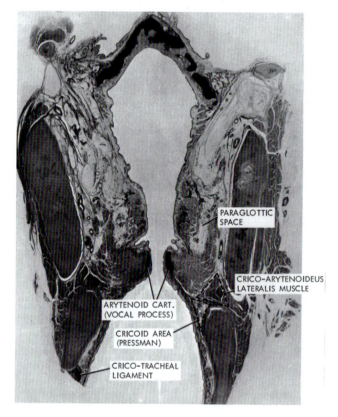

Fig. 4.18 Paraglottic space. (From Tucker G. Human Larynx Coronal Section Atlas, Armed Forces Institute of Pathology, Section 828 Pg. 24R. Reprinted with permission.)

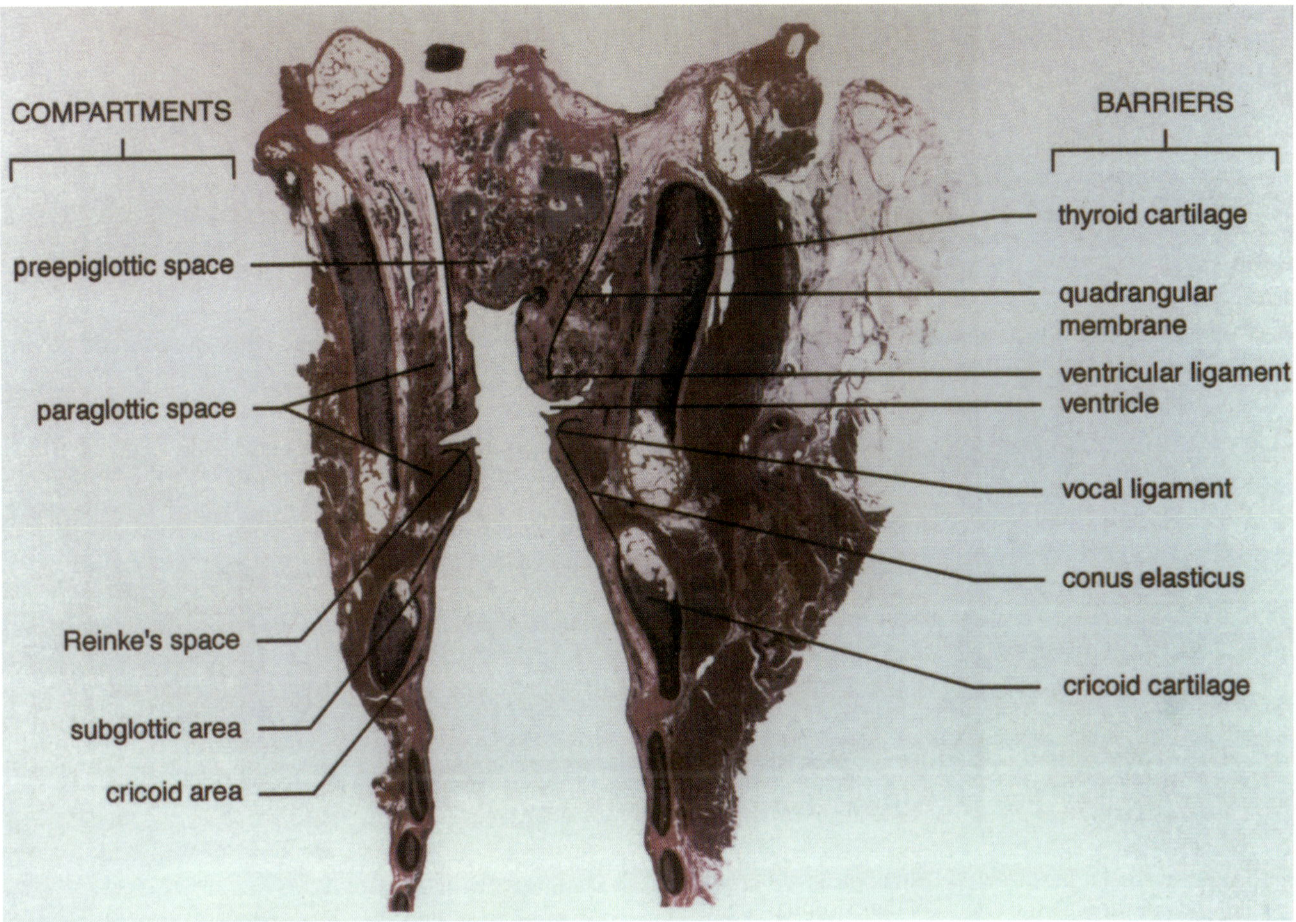

Fig. 4.19 The barriers and compartments of the larynx. Note continuity of paraglottic space to preepiglottic space.

PGS and the PES are completely separated from each other by a conspicuous collagenous fiber septum. Medially, small projections of the paraglottic adipose tissue extend between the fibers of the thyroarytenoid muscle. Anteriorly, at the lower margin of the thyroid cartilage, vessels in the paraglottic "space" exit the larynx through the "cricothyroid triangle." Laterally, at the lower margin of the thyroid cartilage, the soft tissues in the paraglottic "space" exit the larynx through the "cricothyroid interval." There is no cricothyroid membrane: only the soft cricothyroid muscle lies between the lower end of the PGS and the deep surface of the thyroid gland.[154,155]

If a probe is passed into the larynx through the cricothyroid triangle (below the thyroid cartilage), and passed upward on the inner perichondrium of the thyroid ala to the thyrohyoid membrane (above the thyroid cartilage), it will emerge near the superior laryngeal foramen. The probe lies in the PGS. The superior laryngeal artery descends in the PGS in parallel to the probe. It runs deep to the thyroid ala, to emerge through the cricothyroid triangle.[156] Actually, what emerges is the anterior branch and venae commitantes of the superior laryngeal artery. This comes down in the PGS lateral to the ventricle and thyroarytenoid fibers and exits the larynx to link with the cricothyroid artery in the prelaryngeal fibrofatty tissues that harbor the Delphian lymph node. Meanwhile, back inside the PGS, a posterior branch of the superior laryngeal artery was formed. This and its venae commitantes also descend but in the posterior part of the PGS—under the floor of the pyriform—to unite with the inferior laryngeal artery behind the cricothyroid joint. The Galen anastomosis, between the recurrent laryngeal nerve (same as the inferior laryngeal) and the superior laryngeal nerve, for the most part parallels the posterior circulation.

When transglottic cancer crosses the ventricle and involves both the vestibular and vocal folds, it does so within the PGS. Lymphatics drain each PGS (i.e., drain the larynx itself) through the same three exit points that admit the vessels and nerves (six in total, three per side) (**Fig. 4.20**). These again include the following:

- The superior laryngeal foramen, in the thyrohyoid membrane. Lymphatics exit here to level 2a and level 3 lymph nodes in the neck, including the jugulodigastric nodes.
- The cricothyroid triangle—bounded by
  - the lower edge of the thyroid ala
  - the lateral margin of the cricothyroid ligament
  - the anterior fibers of the cricothyroid muscle
- Lymphatics exiting the cricothyroid triangle are destined for the Delphian node, then either side of the neck.

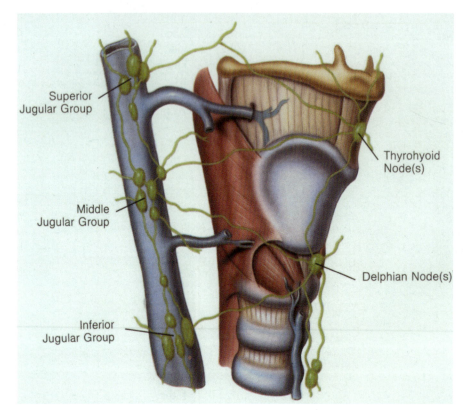

Fig. 4.20 Lymphatic drainage of larynx.

- The neurovascular passageways behind the cricothyroid joint and out through the origins of the cricopharyngeus muscle. These lymphatics target the paratracheal lymph nodes.

We consider the cricothyroid triangle[156] to be an important anatomical feature of the larynx because it serves as a route of connection between the anterior PGS and the extralaryngeal soft tissues, including the Delphian node. When anterior glottic/anterior commissure cancer spills over the conus elasticus into the muscles in the PGS anteriorly, it gains easy access through the cricothyroid triangle (direct or lymphatic) to the extralaryngeal lymph nodes and soft tissues. Because an extraconus pattern of descent (as opposed to submucosal) may *not* distort the appearance of the subglottis, subglottic spread goes unrecognized. Impaired motion may be subtle, late, and the first suggestive clinical clue. T2b glottic cancer is known to behave very badly, more like T3 than T2. One factor may be the anatomy.

Anterior Commissure, Conus Elasticus

The conus elasticus arises from the sloping cranial margin of the cricoid cartilage and ascends to end as two free horizontal cranial margins, the vocal folds (**Fig. 4.21**). The thickened anterior attachment is a Y-shaped structure, the Broyle ligament. Broyle himself used the term *Broyle's tendon,*[150] but tendons join muscle to skeleton, so ligament is more accurate. The Broyle ligament is not just the attachment of the vocal ligaments: it is the upper anchor point of the whole conus elasticus to the thyroid cartilage. Broyle anterior filaments penetrate like Sharpey fibers into the micropits on the inner

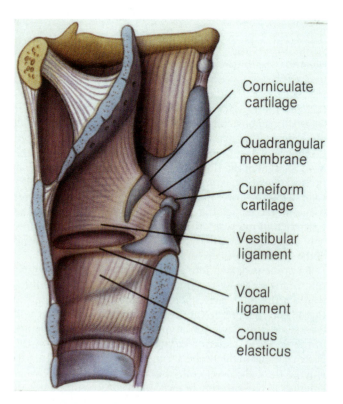

Fig. 4.21 Midsagittal section larynx illustrating the fibroelastic membranes that line the interior of the larynx: the conus elasticus inferior to the laryngeal ventricle and the quadrangular membrane superiorly.

aspect of the angle of the thyroid cartilage about halfway up. Anterior commissure cancer can penetrate here also. A small nodule of nearly pure elastic tissue normally lies in the anterior portion of the vocal ligament, the macula flava.

If the conus was sectioned at the cricoid it would look like a horseshoe—higher up it would be an A-frame. The feet taper to points under the arytenoids. The anterior edges of the right and left triangular sheets fuse to form the cricothyroid ligament. The cricothyroid ligament ascends to and beyond the lower margin of the thyroid cartilage. Inside the angle, inner fibers continue to the anterior commissure. When the folds adduct, the conus shapes the subglottic air column into a mitered cap. All the energy of exhalation is focused on the narrow glottic slit. Voice shunts try to re-create this shape—open below, narrow above.

The conus and the cricoid envelop two layers of continuous tissue, the glandular submucosa and the respiratory mucosa. These layers continue from the vocal folds to the trachea with no natural impediment to the descent of mucosal cancer from the anterior glottis right down to and *beyond* the cricoid. In the upper level of the subglottis, the thyroarytenoid muscles live outside the conus and narrow it, as the muscles are confined inside the enclosure of the thyroid cartilage. In the second level, the cricothyroid interval, the ligament rises vertically, and the rest of the conus is lightly impressed side to side by the cricothyroid muscles. At the lowest level, inside the cricoid cartilage itself, the lumen is circular and the conus runs out.

Subglottis

Technically, the subglottis extends from the lower squamocolumnar junction of the vocal cord to the plane of the inferior margin of the cricoid. The position of the squamocolumnar junction varies. It is histologically distinct but not clearly visible to gross clinical examination. The inferior margin is also a bit obscure, viewed from inside the larynx because the junction between the cricoid and the first tracheal arch (not ring) is indistinct. Sometimes, in fact, they are fused.

Within the subglottis, anatomists distinguish four zones. The first three are evident anteriorly—an upper zone (within the lower thyroid cartilage), a middle zone (thyroid to cricoid), and the lower zone (within the cricoid). Relying as they do on extraluminal landmarks, these zones are indistinct when viewed from the luminal side. The cricothyroid membrane gradually tapers to a point as we move posteriorly. The lowest level of the subglottis (the cricoid arch) expands to the full height of the cricoid plate posteriorly. Therefore the posterior subglottis, within the cricoid plate, is considered a fourth and independent zone.[157]

T1 vocal cord cancer is often reported without the lower margin of the tumor being directly observed. A clear definition of what constitutes the lower margin of the glottis (the upper margin of the subglottis) is also not always clearly specified. Some consider the glottic region 5 mm high, others 10 mm,[158] and others set different standards at different points along the cord. How far a glottic tumor extends below the plane of the upper surface of the vocal cord is often not precisely visualized. If it was it would be recorded in millimeters.

Cancer is rarely primary in the subglottis, but glottic cancer commonly hides in the subglottic concavity anteriorly (the upper anterior subglottis) where it is poorly and tangentially visualized. Anterior commissure cancer spreads down into the midsubglottic zone (cricothyroid level), and in T1b glottic carcinoma, subglottic invasion is the putative limit on conservation surgery. Failures of radiotherapy for "T1a" vocal fold cancer are sometimes attributed to understaging in the subglottis. Disciplined use of the 70-degree laryngeal telescope at direct laryngoscopy would probably do much to eliminate confusion.

Cricoarytenoid Unit

If we subdivide the cricoid ring into six segments, the anterior two, from 10 o'clock to 2, would be a simple arch. The lateral two (8 o'clock to 10 on the left, and 2 o'clock to 4 on the right) would feature the tiny lateral cricoarytenoid muscles on their upper margins. The posterior two, 4 o'clock to 8, would constitute the posterior cricoid plate, covered with the posterior cricoarytenoid muscle fibers. At the junction of the lateral and the posterior elements of this model (4 and 8 o'clock), we would find two cricoarytenoid joints, smooth ovals, oriented to the circumference of the ring, and slanted with the slope of the ring. Perched on these sloping ovals by their crosswise radial joint faces would be the two arytenoid cartilages, stabilized by their supporting ligaments and the joint capsule, and positioned by several muscles, all the ones ending with –*arytenoid*. Each arytenoid cartilage and its supporting cast of movers and shakers is a unit of vital infrastructure—the cricoarytenoid unit (**Fig. 4.22**). Injure this, and most patients will aspirate to some degree. Destruction of the cricoarytenoid complex "dismasts" the supraglottis on one side. This severely impairs a patient's capacity to resist aspiration—much more so than does loss of the epiglottis.

We need to school ourselves to describe the arytenoid's movements separately from those of the cord. Otolaryngologists appreciate the importance of cord mobility in diagnosing invasion by cancer, but the subtleties deserve further scrutiny. Brasnu et al found that *simultaneous* immobility of the vocal cord and the arytenoid was associated with tumor infiltration into the cricoarytenoid muscles in 33% of endolaryngeal tumors (and 66% of hypopharynx and aryepiglottic carcinomas). An arytenoid cartilage can be immobilized by the mass of a tumor on top of the arytenoid, usually from the hypopharynx. Vocal cord mobility may be preserved in the same case, by the absence of any extension into the cricoarytenoid muscles.[159]

Supraglottis

The epiglottis can be omega shaped and interfere with clinical visibility of the glottis. The petiole is attached to the thyroid cartilage just inside the notch. The periepiglottic "space" (**Fig. 4.18 and Fig. 4.23**) (the fibrofatty tissue of the PES) was so named by Reidenbach to acknowledge the fact that the infrahyoid epiglottis is too narrow to contain this tissue.[153] Reidenbach found the two-dimensional concept of a ball of preepiglottic fat bounded by the thyrohyoid membrane in

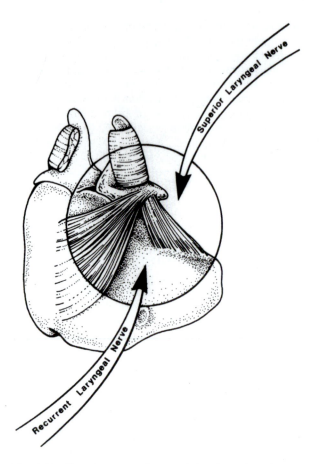

Fig. 4.22 The cricoarytenoid unit includes the ipsilateral arytenoids cartilage, the cricoid cartilage, the cricoarytenoid musculature, and the associated superior and recurrent laryngeal nerves.

front, the hyoepiglottic ligament above, and the epiglottic cartilage behind to be too simplistic. The upper part of the PES *is* filled with adipose tissue, but it extends *around* the epiglottis, in a horseshoe fashion. *Periepiglottic* is a more accurate term.

The lower part of the PES is subdivided by two paramedian sagittal collagenous septa, the quadrangular "ligaments" (membranes). The medial compartment bordered by these ligaments is closed posteriorly by the infrahyoid epiglottis and inferiorly by the thyroepiglottic ligament. The quadrangular membranes continue back past the epiglottis toward the cuneiforms and the arytenoids. The glands of the vestibular folds lie medial to the quadrangular membranes. The thyroarytenoid muscles, rising to gain attachment to the oblong fossa on each arytenoid, eventually lie on the posterolateral aspects of the quadrangular membranes.

The further a quadrangular membrane proceeds away from its origins on the inner aspect of the thyroid cartilage, the more it loses its definition and continuity. Reidenbach described devolution into several layers, with multiple dehiscences, and eventual dissipation in the aryepiglottic folds.[160]

The upper layers enclosing the PES include a ligament and a membrane. The hyoepiglottic *ligament* consists of a cranial fiber layer, anchored within the lingual muscles, and a caudal layer attached to the hyoid bone itself. Both layers fuse to form a dense collagenous mass anterior to the lingual surface of the epiglottis. Above this tissue, Reidenbach identifies a hyoepiglottic *membrane*, which extends between the epiglottis and the tongue.[153]

The main structure limiting the PES anteriorly is the thyrohyoid membrane. This passes upward to an attachment on the inner *upper* margin of the hyoid, leaving space for a small midline bursa between the membrane and the bone. By releasing this attachment on bone, the preepiglottic unit can be kept entirely intact (en bloc) in a supracricoid laryngectomy for supraglottic disease. From the outer aspect of the thyrohyoid membrane, numerous collagenous septa radiate directly into the infrahyoid muscles. On the inner aspect, the periepiglottic adipose tissue is not connected to the thyrohyoid membrane. The functionally important (to swallowing) strap muscles are visualized and preserved in a laser supraglottic laryngectomy because swallowing restoration requires this functionality.

It is widely stated that tumor invasion of the PES has a significant prognostic importance in supraglottic laryngeal carcinomas. The lymphatics drain to cervical lymph nodes from the PES, and tumors with PES invasion are still considered T3 in the American Joint Committee on Cancer (AJCC) staging system. Dursun et al[161] showed that PES invasion should not be considered such a significant prognostic factor because the majority of the supraglottic lesions already demonstrate PES invasion. This would not be surprising to an anatomist. The epiglottis is studded with multiple glandular pits on its laryngeal surface, and most of them are perforated into the PES at their base.

The epiglottis is rich in sensory innervation via the internal branch of the superior laryngeal nerve. Throat clearing and referred otalgia are frequent presenting signs in supraglottic cancer. Voice disturbance requires spread to the glottis and thus appears late, if at all, and usually from an infrahyoid tumor.

Lined by lubricating glands, the ventricle and saccule normally serve as the "oil cans" of the voice. The space created by the ventricles is probably more responsible than the embryology for the reputation supraglottic cancer has gained for sparing the glottis. Tumors usually have to grow in front of them (at the petiole), around them (in the PGS), or behind them (at the arytenoid) to affect both levels.[162] Ventricular cancer becomes "transglottic" early by these routes. An actual anatomical structure that might act as a barrier between the glottic and supraglottic areas has never been demonstrated in whole organ serial section studies. Nevertheless, most squamous cell carcinomas arising on the supraglottic mucosa do remain confined above the ventricle,[163] and this fact is reflected in the high rate of local control obtained by surgeons performing horizontal supraglottic laryngectomy: 80.6% to 98%.

Hypopharynx

Cancer of the hypopharynx is often considered separately from larynx disease. Some think mixing the two might breed confusion, but clinically the opposite is true. The division be-

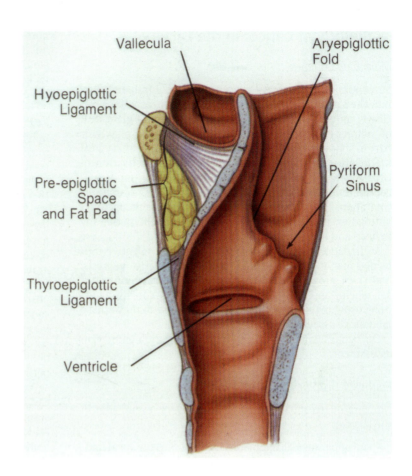

Fig. 4.23 Midsagittal section larynx: note the preepiglottic space.

Labels in figure: Vallecula, Aryepiglottic Fold, Hyoepiglottic Ligament, Pre-epiglottic Space and Fat Pad, Pyriform Sinus, Thyroepiglottic Ligament, Ventricle

tween larynx and pharynx is a longstanding tradition in the TNM staging system. But one cannot omit the hypopharynx and still provide a rational model for the diagnosis, staging, and treatment of larynx cancer. The thyroid ala (larynx) embraces the pyriform sinus (hypopharynx) on one side, and the supraglottic larynx on the other. The inferior pharyngeal constrictor (hypopharynx) takes origin from the larynx. The back of the cricoid (larynx) is the front of the hypopharynx. The posterior cricoarytenoid muscles responsible for the laryngeal airway are on the hypopharyngeal side of the cricoid! Facing a laryngectomy for hypopharyngeal cancer, any distinction between larynx cancers and pharynx cancers seems especially artificial to the patient. The treatment of most laryngeal cancer has important implications for pharyngeal swallowing. For treatment and nodal risk and prognosis, it might be just as valid to group supraglottic cancer with hypopharyngeal disease as with glottic and subglottic carcinoma.

Neighboring Structures in the Laryngeal Region

The outer (longitudinal) coat of muscle fibers in the cervical esophagus rises and converges to insert on the median tubercle on the posterior plate of the cricoid (between the posterior cricoarytenoid muscles). The esophagus usually deviates left in the neck. Therefore, a tracheoesophageal puncture tract also often deviates left.

The tongue is a fluid and is thus deformable but incompressible and is confined within the arch of the mandible. The mandibular arch extends from the base of the skull like a rigid chinstrap, and how much space exists within the arch to accommodate the incompressible tongue is a critical factor in the ease of endolaryngeal access. Glossopharyngeal sensory elements in the base of the tongue trigger reflex laryngeal elevation and closure during swallowing. After a supracricoid laryngectomy, the arytenoids must rise to appose the tongue base surface during a swallow.

The pyramidal lobe of the thyroid gland lies on the laryngeal framework just off the midline. The upper borders of the thyroid gland overlie the cricothyroid muscles. The two lobes cover the recurrent laryngeal motor nerves. They also grip and impress the cricopharyngeal region of the hypopharynx. Because the sternothyroid muscles insert on the oblique line of the thyroid cartilage and restrict upward development, an enlarging thyroid expands downward into the superior mediastinum. When the larynx is irradiated, the thyroid is unavoidably treated, too. Hypothyroidism is a common delayed complication of laryngeal radiotherapy.

In the capsular tissues behind the thyroid and in the fat between the trachea and the carotid arteries lie the parathyroid glands. Here they are vulnerable to interruption of the blood supply (the inferior thyroid arteries) during laryngeal surgery, and to direct resection in paratracheal node dissection and/or laryngopharyngoesophagectomy.

◆ Biology of Cancer in the Larynx

Molecular Genetics

Susceptibility to laryngeal cancer is probably influenced by inherited genetic factors. Tobacco-related nitrosamines can clearly induce epithelial neoplasia, but there is a great deal of indirect evidence that genes set the stage (and play their part in sporadic cases). Epigenetic processes such as atypical methylation of gene promoter regions, the inactivation of DNA-repair genes, and more direct mutations of tumor-susceptibility genes may predispose to cancer. p53 alterations (mutations, allelic losses at p53 locus, and plasma anti-p53 antibodies) predict resistance to neoadjuvant chemotherapy in head and neck squamous cell carcinoma.[164]

Methylation changes constitute potentially sensitive molecular markers to define risk status, achieve early diagnosis, and track prognosis for recurrence. High-throughput DNA sequencing approaches and differential gene expression profiling using high-density microarrays promise to make these laboratory assays a bedside reality.

Oncogenes will be discussed under the section on margin assessment.

Epithelial Histology

Nonkeratinized squamous epithelium covers several sites in the larynx:

- The upper medial and medial edges of the true vocal fold
- The posterior surface of the epiglottis
- The aryepiglottic folds

Keratinization of laryngeal squamous epithelium is pathological.

Pseudostratified ciliated epithelium covers the rest of the laryngeal surfaces, including the ventricle. Numerous seromucinous glands lie in the adipose submucous stroma of the ventricular band and the roof of the ventricle.

◆ Introduction to a Clinical Classification of Laryngeal Cancer to Support Treatment Selection

The initial selection of therapy for laryngeal cancer is not a minor responsibility. Patients need relevant information and concrete guidance, not deference to the least alarming treatment option. The best opportunity to initiate good decision making is the physician's initial encounter with the disease. The cure of cancer and the quality of life are forever conditioned by the choices made initially. At the beginning, the choices will never be broader, the impact of minor mistakes will never be greater, and the cost of proceeding along the wrong path will never be more exorbitant. Once laryngeal cancer is recurrent and out of the box, it's hard to play "catch-up."

Sooner or later the weight of the responsibility for guiding patients impels thoughtful physicians to reexamine their classifications for treatment. Working classifications in support of active decision making are personal constructions—no two institutions precisely agree on one, and they are simply too subjective for broad acceptance in our literature. As knowledge and technologies advance, decision pathways need to keep pace. At a national level, we settle for something formal, such as the anatomically based TNM staging system. Face to face with the individual patient, however, we need a much more practical classification, one that relates options to consequences and individual presentations to individual treatment choices.

This chapter provides a classification of laryngeal cancer that will fit the latter description. It is not the TNM system. The TNM classification has so deeply embedded itself into our literature that we sometimes fail to notice how ill-adapted it has become for prescribing therapy, particularly with the tremendous growth in diagnostic technology and new options available for treatment. This chapter incorporates what we have learned from successful and unsuccessful experiences of *treatment*. We have come to acknowledge that laryngeal cancer is diverse but not undecipherable. It can be classified into six distinct categories by its recommended surgery—by six well-known anatomicopathological "tissue blocks," each one producing a known defect, and a known prognosis for both cure and function.

Previously, we had resisted the notion of a "clinical-surgical" classification for two reasons. First, for two of the main surgical concepts (supracricoid laryngectomy and near-total laryngectomy) we had insufficient independent confirmation of the expected outcomes. Therefore, it was not yet clear to us where these concepts would fit. Second, in an ideal world, multidisciplinary treatment paradigms should rest on the basic knowledge equally known in all disciplines. Anatomy formed the foundation of the TNM classification, for example—at least until most recently. A paradigm based on surgery might only inform surgeons. Nonsurgeons would have to incorporate new knowledge—the surgical anatomy relevant to laryngeal cancer patients. Otherwise they would stand on unfamiliar territory when treatment selection was to be discussed.

In practice, clinicians readily differentiate six different "severities" of disease. Six separate cohorts of patients "fit" in these categories, with no one left over. Each can be ranked according to their prognosis for cure and function, *should surgery be advised for treatment.*

Briefly, the six major categories, identified with their core operation, are as follows:

1. Patients locally curable by **transoral biopsy-resection**
2. Patients locally curable by **classic partial laryngectomy (vertical or horizontal)**
3. Patients locally curable by **supracricoid resection**
4. Patients locally curable by **near-total laryngectomy**
5. Patients locally curable by **total laryngectomy**
6. Patients requiring **more than a total laryngectomy** for local cure

Note that *classifying a patient into a clinical surgical category* is not the same as *advocating surgery*. The classification only helps suggest *which* surgery would be appropriate, if the surgical option were to be selected. Other factors, particularly patient factors, must be considered to support an actual choice. Assuming no prior treatment, radiation is *feasible* whatever the tumor's presenting pattern of invasion and extent. So is chemotherapy. What needs to be specified *just to make an informed decision on therapy* is the expected outcome of each modality, especially the predictable *functional* impairment to be expected from a cure by surgery.

Treatment recommendations need to be based on sophisticated knowledge of laryngeal surgery *even if surgery is deferred*. One needs to ask what established operation would this particular tumor require, and one needs to know why the next surgery up is too much, why the next one down is too little, and how far up the scale the patient is propelled if initial nonsurgical therapy fails. Arguably, no one can explain to a patient the critical comparisons between surgery and nonsurgical treatment *unless they can accurately determine which operation the patient would need*.

Note that the classification we use aligns itself remarkably well with six separate categories of expectation for rehabilitation:

1. Transoral biopsy-resection provides nearly certain cure and a near normal voice.
2. Classic partial laryngectomy increases the stress on voice (vertical partial laryngectomy) or swallowing (horizontal supraglottic laryngectomy), but nasal breathing is preserved.
3. Supracricoid resection carries the voice and swallow components to their maximum physiological consequences without loss of nasal breathing.
4. Near-total laryngectomy is the first level to compel acceptance of a permanent stoma.
5. Total laryngectomy is the first level to require a prosthesis for lung-powered voice.
6. Beyond total, patients acquire more dysphagia (flaps), worse voice (often an electromechanical device), stomal dependency, and much more uncertainty as regards local control (recurrence).

◆ AJCC Laryngeal Carcinoma Staging (TNM)

The TNM classification is a low-level aid in predicting prognosis, and it is a useful document in holding to a uniform curriculum while teaching students different cancers within the same organ. It is also a SEER requirement for tumor board certification.[165] The American College of Surgeons requires proof of TNM-compliant tumor board activity for accreditation as a cancer center. All authors submitting treatment results for peer-reviewed publication are expected to stage their clinical material according to the TNM classification. But most authors then go on to explain obvious incongruencies between the TNM stages and their treatment categories.

Table 4.1 presents for reference the AJCC 2002 TNM staging system[166]:
The TNM staging system is a time-honored reporting system, but it does not correlate well with prognosis. Hermans

noted that the degree of involvement of the PGS (at the level of the true vocal cord) and the degree of infiltration of the PES was more strongly linked to the prospect of local control than was the clinical T-classification.[167] Several authors who have used a summation-of-areas technique on their patients' CT scans have found volume is more important than stage in predicting the response to irradiation.[168] Six cubic cm (~18 mm × 19 mm × 18 mm) has been the practical dividing line found useful in one institution. Laboratory studies on the patient [e.g., human immunodeficiency virus (HIV) status], and the specimen (e.g., immunohistopathologic staining) are emerging now as important clinical tools, too. Absent from the staging system, but not our management planning, they represent further enhancements of our ability to customize treatment, and thus to improve our results.

The TNM staging system also correlates poorly with treatment. Almost any paper reporting on a specific operation, for example, will cite results across several different T stages, all of which were selected for that treatment. And any paper reporting on a specific site and T stage will describe the outcome for several different treatments, all selected for that particular stage. Terms like *advanced* and *locally advanced* get used as if they were the same. For example, a T2N1M0 laryngeal cancer is classified "advanced" (stage III). But radical surgery is illogical for T2 cancer. When it comes to choosing treatment, the primary and the neck are in many ways separate entities. Either can be early or advanced, independent of the other. In fact, supraglottic cancers can be invisible at their primary site and their *only* clinical manifestation may be a cervical lymph node (the undiscovered primary).

TNM reporting is specific in theory but modestly inaccurate in practice. Many of the staging forms that feed national surveillance and epidemiology databases were transcribed after hours by an overworked doctor and an underpaid registrar poring over a tall stack of charts in a lonely medical records department. Records can be hard to decipher. Diagrams can defy interpretation. Clinical and operative notes can disagree. Imaging reports and pathology reports can diverge. Small tumors may have been distorted by a biopsy. Large tumors may have required speculation regarding their site of origin. Palpating a node may jump the patient an entire stage. A node missed in the office may be obvious at a "staging neck dissection," so the clinical and pathological stages disagree. Clinical staging *should* be done before surgery, but different specialists examining the same patient can still disagree on the stage. And as the tools change, so do the diagnoses. Unfortunately, it is hard to remember all the official subtleties when we stage our cases. And the TNM system periodically changes, as does the judgment of the examiners.

Clinical-Surgical Classification

Throughout this chapter, we make a determined effort to completely separate in our minds the act of staging a patient and the act of determining the treatment of a patient. We acknowledge the TNM system at the time of *diagnosis*, but as soon as we consider the selection of *treatment*, we shift to the clinical classification introduced earlier. This is grounded in something completely different: surgical anatomy. Nonsur-

Table 4.1 The 2002 AJCC 2002 TNM Staging System

TX: cannot assess the primary
T0: no evidence of the primary
Tis: ca in situ
STAGE 0 = TisN0M0

Supraglottis (the subsites are the suprahyoid epiglottis, infrahyoid epiglottis, laryngeal aspect of the aryepiglottic folds, arytenoids, and ventricular bands)

T1: Tumor limited to one subsite, and normal mobility
STAGE 1 SUPRAGLOTTIC CA means T1
T2: Tumor invades more than one subsite (or an adjacent site—glottis, base of tongue, vallecula, medial pyriform wall, without fixation of the larynx
STAGE 2 SUPRAGLOTTIC CA means T2
T3: Tumor with vocal cord fixation or invades postcricoid, preepiglottic space, paraglottic space, thyroid cartilage inner cortex
STAGE 3 SUPRAGLOTTIC CA means T3 or any N1
T4a: Tumor invades through thyroid cartilage, or beyond larynx—trachea, soft tissues of neck including deep extrinsic muscles of tongue, strap muscles, thyroid gland, or esophagus
STAGE 4A SUPRAGLOTTIC CA means T4a or any N2
T4b: Tumor invades prevertebral space, encases carotid artery, or invades mediastinal structures
STAGE 4B SUPRAGLOTTIC CA means T4b or any N3
STAGE 4C SUPRAGLOTTIC CA means M1

Glottis (the subsites are the true vocal folds, including the anterior and posterior commissures)

T1: Tumor limited to the vocal cord(s) (may involve anterior or posterior commissure with normal mobility)
T1a: limited to one cord
T1b: involves both cords
STAGE 1 GLOTTIC CA means T1
T2: Tumor extends to supraglottis and/or subglottis OR with impaired mobility of the vocal cord
STAGE 2 GLOTTIC CA means T2
T3: Tumor limited to larynx with vocal cord fixation, and/or invades paraglottic space, and/or thyroid cartilage inner cortex erosion
STAGE 3 GLOTTIC CA means T3 or any N1
T4a: Tumor invades through thyroid cartilage, and/or beyond larynx—trachea, soft tissues of neck including deep extrinsic muscles of tongue, strap muscles, thyroid gland, or esophagus
STAGE 4A GLOTTIC CA means T4a or any N2
T4b: Tumor invades prevertebral space, encases carotid artery, or invades mediastinal structures
STAGE 4B GLOTTIC CA means T4b or any N3
STAGE 4C GLOTTIC CA means any M1

Subglottis (is all one subsite)

T1: Tumor limited to the subglottis
STAGE 1 SUBGLOTTIC CA means T1
T2: Tumor extends to vocal cord(s) with normal or impaired mobility of the vocal cord
STAGE 2 SUBGLOTTIC CA means T2
T3: Tumor limited to larynx with vocal cord fixation
STAGE 3 SUBGLOTTIC CA means T3 or any N1
T4a: Tumor invades cricoid or thyroid cartilage, and/or invades tissues beyond larynx—trachea, soft tissues of neck, including deep extrinsic muscles of tongue, strap muscles, thyroid gland, or esophagus
STAGE 4A SUBGLOTTIC CA means T4a, or any N2
T4b: Tumor invades prevertebral space, encases carotid artery, or invades mediastinal structures
STAGE 4B SUBGLOTTIC CA means T4b, or any N3
STAGE 4C SUBGLOTTIC CA means any M1

Key
Regional Nodes (N)
Nx: Regional nodes cannot be assessed
N0: No regional lymph node metastasis
N1: Single ipsilateral node under 3 cm
N2a: Single ipsilateral node > 3 cm, < 6 cm
N2b: Multiple ipsilateral nodes, < 6 cm
N3: Node > 6 cm

Distant Metastases
Mx: Distant nodes cannot be assessed
M0: No distant metastasis
M1: Distant metastasis (biopsy proven, Y, N)

Histological Grade (G)
Gx: Grade cannot be assessed
G1: Well differentiated
G2: Moderately differentiated
G3: Poorly differentiated

Residual Tumor (R)
Rx: Presence of residual tumor cannot be assessed
R0: No residual tumor
R1: Microscopic residual tumor
R2: Macroscopic residual tumor

Additional Descriptors
m: Suffix multiple tumors in a single site
y: Prefix classified after initial multimodality therapy
r: Prefix recurrent after a disease-free interval
a: Prefix stage determined at autopsy

Lymphatic Vessel Invasion (L)
Lx: Lymphatic vessel invasion cannot be assessed
L0: No lymphatic vessel invasion
L1: Lymphatic vessel invasion

Venous Invasion (V)
Vx: Venous invasion cannot be assessed
V0: No venous invasion
V1: Microscopic venous invasion
V2: Macroscopic venous invasion

gical treatment options can then be tested against a needed benchmark—that specific patient's best surgical option.

We believe all new patients with laryngeal cancer can be subcategorized into six separate and definable surgical categories, at the initial encounter. Each category has predictive value. Each has an enormous knowledge base, the history, the core operation associated with the category, its indications, limitations, anatomical extent, application, and reported outcome expectations, in terms of local cure, disability, and risk. This classification incorporates much more clinical information than the three points of a physical exam seen in the TNM, and, being interesting, it is easier to remember.

Plain English designations like "early" and "advanced" can be used, and they already enjoy widespread use in clinical practice. Authorized definitions are lacking, but they can be assigned. We can also designate the cases in between as "intermediate," and add "very" to the extreme examples at either end. All new "normal" laryngeal primaries can be assigned to one of five categories. Then a sixth category ("extreme") can be added to accommodate the cases that will always be above and beyond the conventional. A working classification of all new laryngeal cancers can be proposed that places every single primary into one of six clinical categories, each to be distinguished by a specific anatomical extent; a common general clinical prognosis; a well-known surgical strategy if surgery were to be chosen for treatment; and an expected outcome in terms of voice, swallow, and airway if surgery was successfully applied.

I. Very early laryngeal cancer. "Very early" would be an especially favorable subset of early cancers that can be cured by little more than a biopsy. Small, localized, exophytic, midcordal glottic cancer on one fully mobile vocal cord would be the principal example. The entire tumor can be completely exposed in one direct laryngoscopic view. A total transoral resection can be safely accomplished without any damage to the anterior commissure or the arytenoid. The underlying glottic musculature will remain almost entirely undisturbed. The rare supraglottic representative in this category would be a small, localized, exophytic, epithelial cancer of the epiglottic rim. The entire tumor can be completely exposed in one direct laryngoscopic view. A total transoral resection can be safely accomplished without any damage to the false cord, the medial pyriform wall, or the infrahyoid epiglottis, and without penetrating the hyoepiglottic ligament, the fibrofatty tissues of the PES, or any musculature of the supraglottic larynx.

II. Early laryngeal cancer. "Early" laryngeal cancer generally means mobile cords, with an implication of favorable disease. "Early" glottic in this classification means superficial glottic cancer that fits safely within the confines of a vertical partial laryngectomy (e.g., the block described as a vertical frontolateral partial laryngectomy[169] or a hemilaryngectomy. "Early" glottic cancer will typically involve the anterior commissure or one arytenoid, but mobility of the vocal cord is completely preserved. Early supraglottic cancer fits safely within the block described as a classic horizontal supraglottic

partial laryngectomy. It may penetrate the epiglottis to involve the PES, but the mobility of the supraglottic larynx is completely preserved.

III. Intermediate laryngeal cancer. Inevitably, some cases will fall *between* "early" and "advanced" because they are too big for the classic conservation operations like supraglottic laryngectomy or vertical partial laryngectomy, but they seem too little for the cricoid-resecting, stoma-requiring operations like total and near-total laryngectomy. "Intermediate" is a suitable designation for these.

IV. Advanced laryngeal cancer. "Advanced" laryngeal cancer means fixed cords, implying deep invasion, thus unfavorable disease. Some of these have surgical options below a near-total laryngectomy for example. But a formidable subset always remains for which total laryngectomy will prove necessary.

V. Very advanced laryngeal cancer. "Very advanced" might better describe the subgroup of advanced for whom nothing less than a total laryngectomy will do. Subglottic primaries, advanced invasive bilateral cancers, and a few others are included.

VI. Extremely advanced laryngeal cancer. We need a category called "Extremely advanced" to recognize that not even a total laryngectomy will encompass spread beyond the larynx and one pyriform, and flap reconstructions will be the minimum requirement for the hypopharynx.

Note that a special classification tied to "surgical" categories is actually quite intuitive in practice. It is vulnerable on theoretic grounds to the charge that procedural concepts are always changing, and, by comparison, the bedrock of the TNM system is anatomy. New treatments (e.g., laser excision) are changing the functional prognosis unevenly across TNM groups. This classification, based on "surgical" categories, *is* more dynamic, and more suited to capturing these changes. Besides, enough time has now elapsed that the surgical categories are historic. Thus they are stable, just as they are distinct.

Another convention challenged is the rigid separation between laryngeal cancer and hypopharyngeal cancer. Every day, we see that patients are more likely to lose their larynx with *hypopharyngeal* cancer than with *laryngeal* cancer. Why should hypopharyngeal cancer be split off into a parallel universe from the larynx? Every radiotherapeutic and surgical treatment program we know for advanced laryngeal cancer impacts upon the function of the hypopharynx and vice versa. For some, pharyngeal dysphagia is the *major* impact.

◆ Diagnostic Evaluation

Clinical

Voluntary vocal fold motion may be normal, impaired, or fixed. The main cause of fixation is muscle replacement by cancer, but tumor bulk, joint invasion, nerve destruction, and direct extension of mucosal cancer cord to the cartilaginous framework of the larynx are sometimes contributory causes. The membranous cords may participate while the arytenoids still move. The false cords may exhibit impairment or fixation as well. Mobility can be transmitted from the pharynx. It can be imparted by airflow (paradoxical adduction on inspiration instead of active abduction). And immobility is not always abnormal. Some points, like the anterior commissure, are normally fixed.

Imaging

Ultrasound

For the larynx itself, the primary site, B-mode ultrasonography is probably not as helpful as a plain soft tissue x-ray of the neck. It provides a low-quality image determined by the air–mucous membrane boundary and the (ossified) cartilaginous skeleton of the larynx. Ultrasonography may be useful in the neck, or occasionally for a larger laryngeal lesion, but there is no advantage in the detection of small or intermediate processes.[170] Ultrasound scanning has been recommended for the liver for all hypopharyngeal tumors, for laryngeal cancer patients with large cervical adenopathy (N2 or N3), and for poorly differentiated cancer wherever the site of the primary.[171] But now this is probably superseded by the advent of the positron emission tomographic (PET) scan. Kau et al found an accuracy of 89% for ultrasound-guided fine-needle aspiration cytology in the neck.[172] Again, this falls in the same range as PET, 90.5%.

Computed Tomography

Pretherapeutic staging for local extension of laryngeal carcinoma can be assisted by CT of the vocal muscle tissues, the PGSs, and the laryngeal commissures.[173] The ability of CT imaging to reveal pathological conditions that are undetectable by palpation or endoscopy will ensure its continuing value in laryngeal cancer patients. It has been especially cited for its service in cases with neoplastic cartilage invasion, where its high negative predictive value has been repeatedly affirmed. (False-positive results occur because reactive inflammation may lead to overestimation of neoplastic cartilage invasion.)

CT is better than PET to monitor size and structural changes in tumors and lymph nodes, but not as good for screening, posttherapeutic monitoring, or the early detection of local recurrence. A recurrence can best be diagnosed by CT if a baseline study has been performed after the end of therapy.[174] Sometimes tumor perfusion can be roughly determined (~15% do not absorb any contrast medium).

CT is especially competitive with MRI because modern multilayer (multidetector) spiral CT scans produce thinner (submillimeter) collimations of sections in shorter examination times than are possible with magnetic resonance imaging (MRI).[175] Localized disease of the larynx can more effectively be assessed with low-artifact CT than with MRI. The choice between CT and MRI is probably determined by one's experience with these modalities.[176] The resolution is sharpest with CT, but MRI shows more soft tissue contrast.

The limitations of laryngeal CT are common to its limitations in other systems. The number of planes is limited. Me-

tallic artifacts occasionally come into play. Respiration and swallowing can cause motion artifacts (spiral CT less so than conventional CT). The principal limitation in laryngeal cancer is that conventional CT does not differentiate residual or recurrent tumor from posttreatment inflammation, fibrosis, edema, or scarring. MRI has the same shortcoming.

"Virtual laryngoscopy" is a newly publicized CT technique that uses three-dimensional reconstruction of two-dimensional CT images to yield a three-dimensional view of the relationships between a tumor and the cartilaginous structures of the larynx.[177] It does not require general anesthesia, it allows three-dimensional visualization of the airway *beyond* areas of narrowing, and it gives a moderately accurate representation of vocal cord lesions, in terms of both definition and spatial representation. It does, however, require an air–mucosa interface to produce an image, it does not identify functional lesions of the vocal cords, and it cannot provide the histology, so direct laryngoscopy is still required.

Magnetic Resonance Imaging

MRI is possibly the optimal method of examination in cooperative patients.[178] It is widely used now for the detection of neoplastic invasion of the PES, the PGS, the subglottic region, and cartilage. Glottic squamous cell carcinoma usually demonstrates increased signal intensity on T2-weighted MRI (higher water content).[179] Basaloid carcinoma displays a distinct lobulated enhancement pattern on contrast-enhanced T1-weighted images.[180] MRI makes it possible to directly acquire images in any number of planes. In contrast to CT, metallic artifacts hardly come into play.[181]

The highest accuracy of MRI has been found in the detection of invasion to the prelaryngeal soft tissue (92%).[182] MRI can correctly depict invasion of the PES, PGS, and cartilage by laryngeal cancer *Li*, (1998). Berkiten et al found the accuracy of MRI to be 84% for the anterior commissure, 80% for vocal cords, 76% for the thyroid cartilage, and 72% for the pyriform sinus and the subglottic region.

Duflo et al and Castelijns et al found MRI to be slightly more sensitive than CT in detection of neoplastic cartilage invasion.[173,178] When Declercq et al's gadolinium-enhanced in vitro MRI of 10 total laryngectomy specimens was correlated with subsequent pathological examination, the authors showed MRI to be more sensitive than CT, but sometimes overestimated the degree of cartilage invasion.[183] False-positive results are inevitable because reactive inflammation and neoplastic cartilage invasion can have similar appearances.[184] DeClercq et al interpreted the absence of false-negatives in their study as proof that "cartilage invasion can be ruled out when a normal signal intensity is seen on in vitro MRI of the cartilage."[183] Atula et al on the other hand reported three false-negative (and three false-positive) MRI examinations for cartilage invasion in 18 patients who underwent total laryngectomy. They cautioned that false findings are not uncommon with MRI.[185] Surprisingly, Carriero et al found the sensitivity, specificity, and diagnostic accuracy of MRI in the larynx were unaffected by the use of contrast medium. In their opinion, routine use of contrast medium [gadolinium-diethylene-triaminepenta-acetic acid (Gd DTPA)] in laryngeal cancer cases is not justified.[186]

Murakami et al found that among 80 early glottic squamous cell carcinomas treated with radiation therapy for cure, 48 (60%) were detectable on MRI. MRI detectability (increased signal on T2-weighted images) was a significant predictor of poor outcome with radiotherapy.[179] Signs of cartilage involvement also have prognostic significance for the risk of tumor recurrence.[176] And tumor volume is very predictive for recurrence, too, if radiotherapy is used as the treatment.[178] MRI is probably indicated when there is uncertainty of the extent of the subglottic extension, or invasion of the cartilages, and some think these may be the only indications for MRI at the primary site.[187] Neither CT nor MRI shows mucosal detail, but both do help clarify the submucosal extent of disease.[188] The long examination time with MRI carries the risk of movement artifacts in the head and neck region.[181]

Clinical palpation of the neck is sometimes inaccurate. MRI examination is more accurate in detecting cervical lymph node metastasis and can certainly image occult lymph nodes, which are inaccessible on palpation.[189] The accuracy of MRI (85%) (and CT—84.9%) in the neck is superior to ultrasound (72.7%) and palpation (69.7%),[172] but not quite as sensitive as PET. MRI is better than PET to monitor size and structural changes in lymph nodes.

In 1998, Fried et al reported on the first image-guided biopsies on the head and neck performed in an MRI scanner.[190] Access to the patient, for both percutaneous and transoral approaches during imaging, occurred through the vertical space between the upright coils of the scanner (an investigational "open configuration" model). Fast image acquisition (up to 2 s/image) and general anesthesia or intravenous sedation were used. MRI provided the necessary anatomical information for safe needle placement. Open magnet MRI-guided biopsy of the head and neck was thus feasible but suffered obvious limitations. The scanner itself required a multimillion-dollar installation, and the need for nonmagnetic instruments and materials severely curtailed the use of available instrumentation.

◆ **Imaging Myths**

1. Endoscopic ultrasonography "improves the diagnostic workup in laryngeal cancer and its precursor lesions." Therefore, it should have an important influence on treatment. No one contends endoscopic ultrasound rules surgery in or out, or radiation. The notion that cartilage invasion determines which mode of treatment is used is false (see later discussion). Other factors determine the treatment mode.

   Once the mode is selected, ultrasound findings are superfluous. For radiation, the "depth" suggested by ultrasound will not control the dose, or the fields, or the fractionation schedule, or the addition or subtraction of chemotherapy. If open surgery is favored, patient factors, surgeon factors, and the clinical examination will determine which operation is selected. The CT or MRI findings, and especially the microlaryngoscopy and angled telescope examinations, will give better depth and distribution information than ultrasound. Laser microsurgery

will be informed by these same sources. Then, at the time of treatment, there will be further refinements. A laser surgeon *sees* the actual tumor depth, in situ, in real time, in three dimensions (by laser tumor transection under the microscope and by frozen section),[191] Depth estimates from an ultrasound examination will simply be overruled by the tangible surgical findings.

   There may be a role for ultrasound in the neck (non-endoscopic). But PET, CT, and MRI findings supersede ultrasound for decisions in the neck—the presence and contrast enhancement of nodes, for example.

2. We need to visualize cartilage invasion (with MRI, etc.) because cartilage invasion is a contraindication to radiation therapy. This issue is moot for most patients because people with cartilage invasion usually have more cogent contraindications to radiotherapy (most commonly, that they have already been radiated), and cartilage invasion is not an absolute contraindication to radiotherapy. For early anterior commissure disease with cartilage invasion, some therapists favor radiotherapy.[192] They just emphasize adequate fields and dosages and planning.

3. We need to visualize cartilage invasion (with MRI, etc.) because cartilage invasion is a contraindication to voice-sparing surgery. But cartilage invasion is not a contraindication to voice-sparing surgery. Supracricoid laryngectomy takes the entire thyroid cartilage, for example, and preserves a voice. Cartilage invasion just reaffirms that the surgeon needs to perform an adequate resection with a safe margin, including cartilage.

4. We need to visualize cartilage invasion (with MRI, etc.) because cartilage invasion is the key to staging (and, by inference, staging prescribes treatment). Of course stage does not prescribe therapy. Who would follow a plan based on a look-up table that ignored a patient's medical history, past history, social history, and the rest of the physical examination, the other images, the laboratory values, and the special tests? "Stage" is a reporting requirement, not a treatment directive. Stage is a derivative, not a prime driver, a very rough guide to prognosis, not at all a guide to treatment, not even the treatment mode gets determined by stage. The idea that a "stage = treatment" look-up table is even a desirable thing is addressed elsewhere in this chapter (and, it is hoped, convincingly refuted).

5. Partial surgery requires an accurate diagnosis of subglottic extent. MRI is useful to diagnose subglottic extent. Therefore partial laryngectomy requires an MRI. MRI is unable to "see" mucosal margins. This is a job for microlaryngoscopy and the angle degree laryngeal telescopes. Extended transoral laser resections and near-total laryngectomies do encompass subglottic extension, and they qualify as "partials."

6. *The initial treatment of early-stage laryngeal cancer is radiation therapy, with surgery reserved for salvage therapy.* This of course is demonstrably untrue. Very early glottic cancer is cured by transoral resectional biopsy. Early laryngeal cancer can be cured by transoral laser microresection or open surgery, and the cure rates equal

or exceed those obtained by radiotherapy. Intermediate cancer is more likely to be cured by supracricoid partial laryngectomy than radiotherapy. The idea that imaging helps to identify exceptions to the "radiate first" rule is clearly faulty because no such rule exists.

7. The initial treatment of early-stage laryngeal cancer should be radiation therapy because failures will show up earlier now, with PET scanning. The patient will be rescued in time, plenty of time for successful salvage surgery. Recurrences would have to be detected before growing beyond their presenting dimensions, and local healing and function would have to be unimpaired by radiotherapy. In practice, neither of these happens. Also, PET scanning would have to become much more sensitive to tiny foci, and patients would come in for PET scanning much more frequently. These have not yet occurred. If they do, insurance companies will surely object.

8. Their special knowledge of the surgical options enables radiologists to appreciate that tumor volume; cartilaginous invasion; spread across supraglottic-glottic-subglottic boundaries; infiltration of preepiglottic, paraglottic, and pharyngeal planes; and nodal disease are critical factors in the selection of therapy.[175] It seems unreasonable to expect the average radiologist to develop insight into transoral laser microresection, supracricoid laryngectomy, near-total laryngectomy, TEP technology, and all the new concepts on voice and swallowing physiology when otolaryngologists themselves are struggling to master these concepts. Surgeons respect the anatomicopathological consultation they receive from diagnostic radiology. In fact they often marvel at it. But the radiologist's knowledge of surgical indications repeats questionable concepts and inaccuracies now persisting in our own surgical-oncological literature. We have to clarify the questions we have for radiology. Otherwise we will just get the answers they find instead of the answers that would be important.

Nuclear Medicine: Positron Emission Tomography

18-fluorodeoxyglucose positron emission tomography (FDG-PET) is a functional imaging method based on the high rate of glycolysis in different types of cancer cells. It is becoming increasingly valued for its technical efficacy in the detection of residual tumor[193] or recurrent laryngeal cancer after radiotherapy.[194] Brouwer et al claimed a sensitivity of 100%, a specificity of 85%, a positive predictive value (PPV) of 87%, and a negative predictive value (NPV) NPV of 100%.[195] De Boer et al reported similar experiences.[196] Dietz et al felt these reports were a little too optimistic, at least for patients undergoing chemoradiation for larynx organ preservation. They reported three false-negatives among 20 cases. One case was due to an increased glucose value (203 mg%). The authors called for further trials to optimize the calculation integrating blood sugar and tumor glycolysis with the aim of improving sensitivity and specificity.[197] Pretreatment uptake of FDG using tumor to cerebellar ratio parameters was significantly related to the histological grade of squamous cancer ($p = 0.04$) in studies by Nowak et al[198] and Slevin et al but not to tumor type.[199]

Terhaard et al tried to determine whether PET could differentiate between local recurrence and late radiation effects after radiotherapy for laryngeal/pharyngeal cancer.[200] In 27 (all) of the patients with negative initial FDG scans, biopsies taken at the same time were negative, and no recurrence was seen for at least 1 year. In 34 of 48 patients, the first FDG scan was a true positive. In 12 of the 14 patients with false-positive results, FDG scans were repeated and a decreased FDG uptake was found in nine of the 12. The sensitivity and specificity of the first scan were 92% and 63%, respectively; including subsequent FDG scans, the rates were 97% and 82%, respectively. Terhaard et al concluded that when a local recurrence is suspected after radiotherapy for cancer of the larynx/pharynx, an FDG-PET scan should be the first diagnostic step. No biopsy is needed if the scan is negative. If the scan is positive and the biopsy negative, a decreased FDG uptake measured in a follow-up scan indicates that a local recurrence is unlikely.

Given PET scanning's low specificity, lack of anatomical resolution, and high cost (especially cost) some authors have naturally raised questions about recommending this study for routine screening.[193] Bongers et al determined the actual cost comparisons of detecting recurrent or residual disease by PET scanning (versus laryngoscopy and biopsy) and concluded the cost-effectiveness ratio lay well within an acceptable range. The cost per patient for an ^{18}F-FDG-PET scan was 682 euros. The saved costs from reducing CT scans and panendoscopies were 618 euros.[201] Bongers et al detailed the potential improvement in quality of life due to early detection of recurrent disease,[201] and Kim et al noted that a prompt early diagnosis of failure of radiotherapy should lead to less radical salvage surgery.[202] PET scanning would avoid panendoscopy-related complications. Note that repeated biopsies in irradiated tissue may initiate infection, further edema, and failure to heal, and repeated negative biopsies do not exclude the presence of viable tumor.[195]

Endoscopy

◆ **Microlaryngoscopy and Biopsy** Direct laryngoscopic visualization and exposure is an underreported technical variable in endoscopic diagnosis (and treatment). Exposure is determined by the experience of the clinician, the availability of equipment, the anatomy of the patient, the depth of anesthesia, the degree of muscular blockade, and the caliber of the endotracheal tube.

◆ **Anesthesia** Beware the patient with stridor: anticipate a tracheotomy. Instrumentation of the difficult larynx can quickly deteriorate to airway obstruction. An orderly tracheotomy under local anesthesia is preferable. Stridor should always suggest this plan.

General anesthesia by oral intubation is usually perfectly fine for adult laryngoscopies—a small tube (# 5.5 or 6 ID) between the arytenoids. The tube lies in the posterior commissure and serves to separate the cords. It provides posterior countertraction (against the anterior lift of the laryngoscope tip at the petiole). If the tube is small (5.5), the entire membranous vocal folds are completely accessible. Displace the tube into the anterior commissure with the blade, and the posterior commissure is completely accessible.

◆ **Anterior Laryngeal Access**   In a general sense, a difficult mirror exam predicts a difficult direct laryngoscopy (and intubation). The most important determinants are the presence of teeth, the bulk of the tongue, and the opening capacity of the mouth. The teeth project forward, so they lever a laryngoscope backward. The mandible and the stylohyoid complex, unyielding, suspended from the skull base, kink the airway above the larynx, opposing linear access. The tongue fills the major part of this fixed ring, the tongue is a fluid—displaceable but incompressible, so a bulky tongue severely obstructs straight-line access, especially to the anterior commissure. The advantage of a narrow-bodied endoscope (like the Hollinger laryngoscope) is that it can sink into the tongue and tongue base more deeply than the wider-bodied instruments—or flank the tongue base by side access over the molar region. Its narrowness makes it monocular (no microscope). Laryngeal telescopes come to the rescue, but telescopes impede instrumental and operative access. It takes escalation to a Dedo laryngoscope (20 mm wide) to achieve binocular microscopic vision. Other instrumental solutions to anterior commissure access are the Zeitels Universal Modular Glottiscope System (Endocraft LLC, Providence, RI)[203] (to hold the false cords aside), or a long (20 cm) flat-bodied 8661E laryngoscope (Karl Storz Endoscopy-America, Inc., Culver City, CA) if the only route of approach is over the incisor teeth.

◆ **General Access**   A square-tipped blade (as opposed to a round one) fits the vallecula. A vallecular endoscope like the Lindholm laryngoscope elevates the tongue base, which in turn supplies excellent exposure of the supraglottis, without actually risking contact with the laryngeal interior. The exaggerated upturn of the tip lets the body remain aligned with the larynx. Thus telescopes can be passed to inspect the entire interior of the larynx.

Standard round-tipped instruments like the (Storz) 8661 CN laryngoscope (18 cm long, half-dome cross section) are designed to bypass the supraglottis and proceed directly to the glottis. Don't forget your checklist on the way in: posterior pharyngeal wall, tongue base, vallecula, pyriforms, postcricoid region, arytenoids, AE folds, false cords, epiglottis, and ventricles. A longer, thinner laryngoscope like the 19 cm 8661 DN (Storz) is better to view the subglottic larynx and upper trachea. Unfortunately, the cutoff bevel of the tip of most laryngoscope blades is overly slanted, presumably to reduce the risk of trauma to the posterior hypopharyngeal wall, during insertion. At the glottic level, however, the slant lets the false cords fall into view. Advance further to muscle them aside, and you cover up the anterior commissure. The Zeitels glottiscope[203] overcomes this disadvantage at the cost of being perilously blunt.

"Sniffing the morning air" describes the optimum patient posture: head extended on the atlantooccipital joints, neck *flexed* gently on the thorax. Lubricate the scope and the lips. Protect the upper teeth with a custom-made thermoplastic splint, to dissipate the fulcrum pressure. (We mold Aquaplast (WFR/Aquaplast Corp., Wyckoff, NJ) in situ, at the commencement.)

Direct laryngoscopy is primarily a handheld diagnostic examination, after which suspension provides the stability required by a microscope. The microscope provides magnification, illumination, and stereoscopic vision. Microlaryngoscopy includes additional diagnostic advantages. Fine vascular patterns emerge. Subtle tissue textures become obvious. Margins look more apparent, as do the nuances of the pathology. The image is visible to the assistants and students via the video camera. Modern chest supports no longer immobilize the chest brace. The Göttingen 8585G (Karl Storz Endoscopy-America, Inc., Culver City, CA) features a supporting table that slides right and left, swivels toward the head or the foot, and raises up or down on a rack and pinion column. During an operative microlaryngoscopy, frequent readjustments overcome limits on access.

Handheld instruments are available to palpate, displace, and even spread the cords during a direct microlaryngoscopy. The lengthy trajectory (400 mm) to the pathology amplifies a surgeon's involuntary hand movements. A special chair, with arm and hand rests, provides more purposeful control and enhances fine movement of the joystick on a laser micromanipulator. A 400 mm objective lens is an essential accessory for the microscope. Anything less and the microscope body sets up too close to the laryngoscope. Instruments cannot be aligned inside the laryngoscope if they bump into the microscope body. Slots in the sides of a laryngoscope can further defeat this alignment problem (again, the Zeitels glottiscope[203] solves this problem).

Rigid laryngeal telescopes add angled viewing capabilities and extreme depth of field to microlaryngoscopy. To overview the larynx without a laryngoscope in the lumen, elevate the vallecula/tongue base with a Lindholm laryngoscope (Karl Story), and view the interior with a 30 degree laryngeal telescope. With a 70 degree telescope, the view of the anterior commissure and the ventricles is spectacular. Either instrument is invaluable to look past a bulky supraglottic lesion to the glottis. And for laryngeal photography, the deep fields of view are advantageous.

Endoscopic Imaging Techniques

Endoscopic imaging techniques mean those that might be used during microlaryngoscopy to get further information about tumor extension and differentiation.

◆ **High-Frequency Ultrasound**   Arens et al has demonstrated the feasibility of using a small flexible endolumenal ultrasound transducer to obtain real-time imaging in the larynx. Using a high-frequency (10 and 20 MHz) probe, and flooding the larynx with 0.9% saline, he could obtain 360 degree cross sections of anatomical structures up to a depth of 2 cm. The potential value, he judged, would be that thyroid cartilage invasion could be visualized.[204] To the trained observer, ultrasonography *can* provide information on depth. But it cannot disclose surface extent. Therefore, in precancerous lesions and microinvasive cancer, ultrasonography adds no additional information to what the microlaryngoscopy alone can furnish.[205]

◆ **Autofluorescence** Using blue filtered light at 380 to 460 nm or from a helium-cadmium laser to enhance the visible demarcation of dysplastic or neoplastic mucosa from normal mucosa is called autofluorescence endoscopy. Fluorescence is captured by an image-intensified camera and displayed on a video monitor after previous computerization. Precancerous and cancerous lesions show a faint red to violet fluorescence. Normal mucosa and hyperplastic hyperkeratotic epithelium exhibit a light greenish autofluorescence. Proponents advocate autofluorescence to help differentiate dysplasia, carcinoma in situ, and microinvasive lesions, and to help in the surface evaluation of laryngeal tumor margins.[206,207]

◆ **Contact Endoscopy** Contact endoscopy is performed with two different endoscopic telescopes of 60 × and 150 × magnification after staining the laryngeal mucosa with 1% methylene blue. When the telescope is directly applied to the tissue, one can observe cells, mainly by their nuclei, and infer their different grades of abnormality in situ. A xenon light source provides the necessary illumination.[208,209]

Biopsy and Histopathology

In the larynx, most destructive or proliferative lesions that look like cancer are cancer. It must be remembered, however, that misdiagnosis is always a possibility. Each biopsy report should be discussed with the pathologist in depth. Histoplasmosis,[210] leishmaniasis,[211] radionecrosis,[212–214] tuberculosis,[80,215] leprosy,[216] Wegener granulomatosis,[217,218] and polymorphic reticulosis[219] can all look like cancer in the office. Furthermore, pseudoepitheliomatous hyperplasia over a myoblastoma[81] or blastomycosis[220,221] can be misinterpreted by the pathologist as cancer. Pseudosarcoma[105,222] may harbor an associated squamous carcinoma. Verrucous cancer[83,223] is so benign in its microscopic appearance that a little clinical prompting may be an important ingredient in the diagnosis. A few dangerous malignancies other than squamous cell cancer occasionally turn up in the larynx also, such as SCC,[123,224] atypical carcinoid,[225] adenocarcinoma,[133,224,226,227] melanoma,[228,229] metastatic cancer,[142] and local invasion from the thyroid.[230] The option must always be kept open that laryngoscopy may terminate with the biopsy.

Assessment of Margins

Lee[231] confirmed the impression that is basic to our understanding of the principles of cancer surgery in general, which is that positive resection margins are accompanied by a high local recurrence rate. DiNicola and Resta studied recurrence in relation to the histopathological diagnosis of the resection margin in 564 patients who underwent open surgery for laryngeal carcinoma.[232] When a marginal biopsy was shown to be positive for neoplasm, the incidence of local recurrence was 36.4% (versus 10.1% overall in the cases studied). For patients treated with partial laryngectomy, 46.2% recurred with positive margins versus a 3% recurrence rate with negative margins. Obviously, quality control in a partial laryngectomy is highly related to communications between the pathologist and the surgeon. How they evaluate margins, and how well, has vital implications for the results.

Light microscopy is the principal tool for margin evaluation today, but this may be changed in the future. The proto-oncogene eIF4E is elevated in head and neck squamous cell carcinomas, and eIF4E in the surgical margins may be an independent prognostic factor. Overexpression of eIF4E, detected by Western blot analysis, in histologically normal surgical margins correlated with an increased local-regional recurrence rate in a study by Franklin et al.[233] Mutation of the p53 tumor-suppressor gene is the most common genetic alteration identified thus far in human laryngeal carcinoma. p53 plays a crucial role in cell cycle control and apoptosis in response to DNA damages. Mutations and allelic losses at 17p are among the commoner genetic alterations in primary head and neck squamous cell carcinoma. In the Department of Veterans Affairs Laryngeal Cancer Cooperative Study, Bradford et al initially found larynx preservation (but not survival) to be higher in patients whose tumors overexpressed p53.[72] They later concluded the presence of a p53 mutation was associated with decreased patient survival.[234] Narayana et al's studies suggested p53 mutation was an independent adverse prognostic factor in patients with early-stage glottic carcinoma.[235] Golusinski et al studied p53, Ki67, proliferating cell nuclear antigen (PCNA), DNA ploidy, and cell proliferating activity, as well as the degree of morphological differentiation and ultrastructural cell maturity in 120 patients with laryngeal cancers.[236] They correlated their findings with data obtained from follow-up examinations and the clinical course of the disease. On the basis of the results, they suggested the pathologist's morphological and biological evaluation of neoplastic cells in cancer of the larynx should include grade, DNA flow cytometry, and the occurrence of oncoprotein p53 and nuclear antigen Ki67. Krecicki et al, on the other hand, could not show any correlation between Ki-67 antibody immunostaining and prognosis in 154 laryngeal cancers.[237]

The surgeon's goal should be that no patient leaves the operating room with a positive margin. If, on permanent section, a negative frozen-section was reversed, the patient could be offered shorter follow-up intervals. Another recourse might be supplementary radiation therapy, but more intensive follow-up, perhaps including elective laryngoscopy and PET scanning, would still be advisable.

◆ Treatment of Early Laryngeal Cancer (Species I and II with CO_2 Lasers)

Because this book is directed to managing the difficult case, the treatment of early lesions (with the exception of transoral laser microsurgery) is bypassed to concentrate on the problem cases. The exception to this is the use of the CO_2 laser in the removal of early-stage lesions.

Transligamental Laser Cordectomy

Transligamental resections also use very low power (1 W), but they proceed through the plane between ligament and muscle, and thus offer the prospect of more damage to the mucosal wave. Voice becomes the reason to distinguish among these procedures, but all produce a very serviceable voice. The opposite vocal fold retains normal viscoelastic properties and normal lubrication, and this is the source of the main mucosal wave in the higher cordectomies.

Transmuscular Laser Cordectomy

◆ **Preoperative Considerations** Laser microresection is a subset of surgery, not a separate treatment. It yields the cure rates of surgery, but open surgery is ablation by mechanical energy supported by thermal cautery with the inferred disadvantage of an inferior functional result. Magnano et al reported that for T1a glottic cancer, open surgery, laser resection, and radiotherapy give comparable survivals, open surgery yields the worst functional outcome, and radiotherapy and laser resection were comparable. If laser resection and radiotherapy yield similar functional *and* curative outcomes, the secondary morbidity and cost of radiotherapy would favor laser resection as optimal treatment.[238]

A CO_2 laser generates invisible coherent light at a wavelength of 10,600 nanometers (far infrared). A superimposed red helium neon (HeNe) beam renders visible its focus and location. We use a Sharplan Acuspot 712 (Sharplan Lasers, Inc., Allendale, NJ) micromanipulator to control the spot size, focus, and position of the beam. The mounting frame is the same width as the microscope body—narrow enough to avoid adding any impediment to the introduction of long instruments.

◆ **Surgical Technique** Laser procedures never start until the focal point of the laser beam and the operator's vision coincide at all magnifications. Because the steps to ensure this are critical, here are the practical details.

- Turn the microscope *eyepieces* to 0 diopters each (0–0).
- Dial the highest *objective* magnification.
- Bring the visible surface of a test target (like a tongue depressor) into crystal clear focus and snug up the lock knobs on the microscope arms so the body of the microscope will stay exactly where it is for the rest of the setup.
- Unlock the focus ring on the *micromanipulator* and dial the HeNe beam into its sharpest focus on the target you already have in visual focus. When the visible red dot is as tight as possible, lock the laser micromanipulator focus ring. Now the laser and the target are in focus together, at least at high power.
- Without *any* movement of the microscope body, or the target, dial in the *minimum* magnification. The target now appears farther away and usually (unless your eyes are perfect) out of focus. The laser spot appears equally out of focus, but with respect to the target, the original

adjustment is unchanged. The laser beam reflects off the micromanipulator mirror. None of this was changed by dialing in a lower visual magnification.
- Adjust the eyepieces (only) now: bring the low-power view into focus.
- As the target comes into focus with the eyepiece diopter rings, the target surface *and* the HeNe spot will once again appear sharp. The microscope viewing optics are now parfocal, and the laser is focused accurately on the specimen at *each* magnification, not just high power.

The laser has two "modes": continuous stream and micropulsed.

Continuous mode shines a steady beam of infrared energy on the target and provides the least opportunity for heat dissipation ("thermal relaxation"). This produces the most coagulation, the least bleeding, the most char, and the greatest thermal artifact for histopathology.

Micropulsing is a way to produce less char and better cutting—at the cost of reduced coagulation. So long as bleeding does not interfere with vision and cutting, cancer and normal tissue types can be grossly differentiated in situ. The micropulse modes preserve the fine features of a cut surface with almost no char.

Muscle is soft with a striated architecture. Glandular tissue has a vascular micronodular character. Fat is oily-wet and lobulated. It seems to produce a heavier plume. The domino-like black and white pattern of calcified cartilage or bone helps announce it on minimal early exposure. The most heterogeneous tissue is squamous carcinoma itself—firmer than normal or mealy and friable, paler than normal yet prone to bleed, structureless, microexudative, ugly, and certainly less attractive than its neighbors, in which it is mired and merged.

The micropulsed modes (e.g., Clearpulse, Laserscope, San Jose, CA) produce less collateral thermal coagulation to degrade the pathology margins, when that is important. But they also do less to prevent small vessel hemorrhage, so the need for a suction coagulator is more frequent. They provide wonderful precision for the mucosal cuts on a vocal cord, tightly focused around 1 to 3 W. For pharyngeal mucosa, which exhibits a greater tendency to bleed, the continuous mode works best. Micropulsing can be adjusted (on–off cycle and waveform) to secure more or less cautery, to further enhance control. Continuous mode coagulation can be increased too, by defocusing the beam. Because vaporization depends on the power *density* of a laser beam, as the beam is defocused (spot size increased) wattage must usually be increased.

◆ **Results** The micropulsed modes provide everything a patient with a T1 glottic tumor requires—the sharpest incisions and the least thermal injury. Bleeding is not a big factor in very early cancer. A good voice result requires mucosal preservation. Collateral thermal damage is minimal beyond the exact laser cut with micropulsed laser incisions, and the pathology specimen exhibits the least thermal artifact at the margins.

Laser Total Cordectomy

◆ **Preoperative Considerations** The first priority is to optimize the exposure. There are three movable elements to arrange: the laryngoscope, the patient (table), and the operator.

Before you settle on a fixed position of the laryngoscope, study the tumor with laryngeal telescopes. Use an angled telescope (30 to 70 degrees). Look in the ventricle. Spread the anterior commissure. Reach beyond the tumor and study the subglottis. Then finalize which laser laryngoscope to use, how far to advance it, and the ancillary issues of endoscopic exposure. The angle of approach will be midline or paralingual. The angle of the head will be straight or slightly turned. In the offset mode, the scope passes across the premolar teeth.

Finalize the setup by raising the table to a comfortable height for the operator. Align the optical axis of the microscope with the operative lumen of the microscope. Confirm a true stereo three-dimensional view, and then carefully plan the sequence of the excision.

◆ **Surgical Techniques** For vocal fold mucosa, start in a micropulsed mode at 1.5 W power (safe, but weak). Draw a line around the tumor at a carefully surveyed margin of at least 2 mm. A continuous line is efficient but you can slow the tempo by substituting adjoining "spot-welds" if necessary. Imagine you will be determining the mucosal margin, and the pathologist will help with only the deep margin. Select the appropriate depth by observing the microarchitecture of the cord. Micropulsed modes provide a char-free trough about 0.5 mm wide through which the layered anatomy of the underlying tissue is obvious. Manipulate the target with suction-retractors. This offsets one of the limitations of laser excision—the straight-line inflexibility of the laser beam. It also assists in evacuating the plume.

Once the front mucosal cut is made, anterior to the cancer, and the longitudinal incision is complete, lateral to it, grasp the posterior tip of the specimen with microcup forceps and laser-dissect it forward and toward you, under traction. To visualize the lower edge of the tumor as you go, roll the specimen laterally. Laser-dissect to the anterior cut, and you will have freed up the specimen completely.

If the depth of a lesion is in doubt, make the same mucosal outline but then transect the cancer in two. Visualize normal tissue in the base of this laser wound and in this way determine the depth. Now with the laser remove the anterior specimen. Next the posterior specimen is removed in a similar fashion.

Keep each vocal fold specimen oriented. Ink the deep margin and tease out the bloc on a Gelfoam (Pfizer Inc., New York, NY) pad marked anterior and posterior. Ask the technician for *transverse step sections*. Each section will reveal an upper and lower mucosal margin and an inked base.

◆ **Results** Cordectomy ought to create a gap in the glottis and reduce the power of the voice. Cicatricial stiffness at the resection site should also produce hoarseness. In practice, the effects on the voice are nominal. The expected reduction in the power of the voice is offset by the neocord that regenerates. Hoarseness is reduced by the pliability of the

remaining vocal fold, and the fact that the glottis is lubricated by two normal ventricles. Over time, all these features persist because there is no ionizing radiation effect to induce atrophy.

Voice aside, in the author's opinion, patients with very early laryngeal cancer suffer arguably less morbidity from transoral surgery (laser or conventional) than radiation. Both treatments require a direct laryngoscopy and biopsy under a general anesthetic. In the laser surgery paradigm, the treatment is done—microsurgical cordectomy and the biopsy are one and the same operation. In the radiation-based strategy, after the laryngoscopy, the patient requires another consultant and 6 more weeks of radiotherapy. If radiation dries up the pharynx, the patient will develop annoying swallowing symptoms laser resection will never produce. If radiation plays any role in the induction of cancer, and given the high incidence of second primaries among these patients, obviously avoiding radiation is desirable. No point wasting radiotherapy on very early glottic carcinoma: the patient's advantage is better served by preserving this option for the future.

Treatment of Very Early Supraglottic Cancer

A tiny exophytic cancer on the suprahyoid epiglottic margin (laryngeal side) is extremely rare, and because it produces no symptoms at such an early stage, diagnosis requires luck: the patient was undergoing a laryngoscopy for something else. The author cannot recall seeing one presenting in the undiscovered primary scenario. Presumably, if that were to occur, the primary would be found to extend off the laryngeal surface of the epiglottic tip to involve something with richer lymphatics—the AE fold or PES, for example.

Endoscopic biopsy *and radiotherapy* seems overtreatment for such a localized cancer. The same would be true of endoscopic biopsy and open conservation surgery (i.e., transhyoid pharyngotomy and epiglottectomy). The exceptions might be inability to expose, but this seems unlikely, too, given a high epiglottic location.

The ideal treatment would be laser epiglottectomy. This would combine the biopsy, a chance to confirm the suspected limited extent, and the complete excision into one outpatient intervention. Zeitels et al noted some epiglottic cancers invade the PES with no detectable signs on MRI or CT scanning, or preoperative clinical examination.[239] Laser epiglottectomy provides an opportunity to rule out this possibility by histology, or to diagnose and treat it if present. Laser epiglottectomy causes no significant problems with postoperative swallowing, airway, or voice. More important, the biggest threat to the patient with very early supraglottic cancer is probably the high incidence of second primaries. Transoral laser resection preserves every possible treatment option, including the option of further laser surgery.

◆ Treatment of Early Laryngeal Cancer (Species II)

Limited or "early" laryngeal cancers are those discovered when *the movable components of the larynx (folds, aryten-*

oids) remain *mobile*. Mobility suggests the depth of the cancer is limited. The muscles still work. Movement encourages two hopeful possibilities: cure with function and restricted access to intralaryngeal lymphatics. "Early" cases account for more than half of laryngeal cancer overall. This is one reason the general prognosis for laryngeal cancer is favorable.

In the TNM system, this important distinction (mobility) is diminished by a lack of uniformity in application. Freely mobile tumors receive the following designations:

- *Glottic cancer:* T1 and T2a are freely mobile; impaired mobility is T2b.
- *Supraglottic cancer:* T1 *and* T2 are freely mobile; there are no a/b subcategories. T3 is a true cord fixation.
- *Subglottic cancer:* Only in T1 are the cords freely mobile.

The management of limited laryngeal cancers is possibly the greatest area of persistent controversy between radiotherapists and head and neck surgeons. Both claim good success because *whichever* treatment strategy is chosen, patients usually do survive with *early* laryngeal cancer. This points up a common fallacy: that the treatment strategy for early laryngeal cancer should be built upon *survival figures*. In fact, functional metrics deserve heightened attention in decision making if survival figures are similar: the voice, aspiration, and swallowing.

In 1999, DiNardo and Kaylie studied current treatment practices for early laryngeal cancer among 1000 members of the American Academy of Otolaryngology–Head and Neck Surgery. For early glottic cancers, 37.1% recommended hemilaryngectomy, 8.1% favored radiation therapy, and 50.4% favored "patient choice." For early supraglottic cancer, conservation surgery was advocated by 41.6% and radiation therapy by 5.3%, and 48.3% felt the patient could decide the therapy after an explanation of the treatment options. When patients were left to "weigh" the treatment options on their own, surgery was much less likely to be chosen. Interestingly, practice region and setting did not correlate strongly with physician recommendations. The date of residency completion and rating of available radiation oncology services were more significant factors. A stronger reliance was placed on "patient choice" among younger physicians.[240] Older physicians felt a stronger need to be directive, perhaps because they were more aware that some patients do die from what begins as an early laryngeal cancer. Perhaps "potentially fatal" seems an overreaction to small cancers when they first appear. Perhaps radiotherapy, or a small operation, have equal appeal, whichever the patient might judge "the least radical." But stronger physician direction is needed to avert a tragic misstep in early laryngeal cancer, *undertreatment*. When "noninvasive" treatment fails, patients may face giving up their larynx to save their life. This is a preventable tragedy. The tumor burden at initial diagnosis is minuscule in early laryngeal cancer. And the instruments available for treatment are very powerful.

Nonsurgical Treatments for Early Glottic Cancer

History

Vertical and horizontal partial resections and reconstructions have been thoroughly refined by years of experience. We know their limits, risks, advantages, shortcomings, indications, and results well. The classic open "conventional" conservation operations for limited glottic and supraglottic cancers are as follows:

- Vertical partial laryngectomy (a family of procedures from frontolateral partial laryngectomy to hemilaryngectomy)
- Horizontal partial laryngectomy (supraglottic laryngectomy)

All members of this class of operation preserve a cricoid ring, lined with mucosa. This will support the airway and spare the patient the inconvenience of a permanent tracheostomy.

The patient always retains an innervated muscular glottic valve for voice. In the closed position, the valve prevents aspiration from the pharynx to the trachea. Most patients keep two (at least one) fully functional "cricoarytenoid units."

The indications for conservation laryngectomy are conveyed in a mixture of terms in the literature. Surgeons usually refer to the anatomy, nonsurgeons to the staging.

Hemilaryngectomy is offered for lateralized T1 and T2a glottic cancers. Early T1s are excluded by their suitability for transoral removal. T2as are sometimes excluded by their inferior extent—violation of the cricoid ring is a clear and dangerous contraindication.

We have all learned to be very cautious about T2bs. Limitations of motion suggest cancerous penetration *outside* the conus elasticus, in the muscular tissues, and the surface appearance is a poor indication of extent.

The anterior commissure is a fixed point, the cartilage is close at hand, and the distinction between T1 anterior commissure (AC) cancer and T3 can be treacherous. Subtotal laryngectomies with a pull-down epiglottoplasty are curative for T1/T2 AC cancer, but not T3.

If a glottic cancer is fixed, a hemilaryngectomy is usually not safe. The PGS is involved, and hemilaryngectomy does not remove the necessary "bloc."

Supraglottic laryngectomy is effective for anterior T1 supraglottic lesions because the ventricle keeps them off the glottis, even the bulky ones originating in the infrahyoid region. Inferior spread beyond the supraglottis (T2) usually occurs by flanking the ventricle. Anteriorly, this places the cancer beyond what a supraglottic laryngectomy can encompass. Posteriorly it sets up aspiration. (The cricoarytenoid unit will be lost.)

Always listen to the voice in supraglottic cancer. If the voice sounds normal, anterior-inferior spread is usually absent. A supraglottic laryngectomy will probably be possible. If the voice sounds hoarse, anterior glottic involvement is likely. Supraglottic laryngectomy will probably not be possible.

A patient's *pulmonary status* might contraindicate a supraglottic laryngectomy. Aspiration after surgery can push patients with severe lung disease beyond their capacity to compensate. Then the only way to stop the aspiration will be to separate the airway and the pharynx. One has, in effect, taken two operations to achieve the status of a total laryngectomy. And the laryngectomy was performed on a very sick patient.

After supraglottic laryngectomy, neck dissection and radiation cause impressive arytenoid edema and pharyngeal dysphagia. This can thoroughly sidetrack a patient's recovery. If the only way to overcome the airway obstruction is a tracheotomy, and the only way to control the cough is a cuffed tube, once again the voice and airway benefits of supraglottic laryngectomy are lost.

Radiotherapy

Early laryngeal cancer includes several T subtypes. A whole family of conservation procedures has gradually been developed to deal with them. Considered separately, each "organ-sparing" operation is rather uncommon itself. Thus a general otolaryngologic practice provides limited experience with open frontoanterior vertical partial laryngectomy for T1b glottic carcinoma, or transoral laser microresection for T2a AC cancer. For patients with these diseases, just the unspecialized expertise to select surgical treatment is often a distance away. So is the actual treatment program, and the personnel skilled in aftercare and rehabilitation. Laryngoscopy and biopsy are always available locally and will confirm the tissue diagnosis. This will diagnose the actual clinical stage. In other words, all one needs to select radiotherapy is readily at hand. What then is the appeal of an unheard of operation at a distant treatment facility when the regional radiotherapy center offers a bloodless treatment claiming better voice results? This is the organ of voice. Surely it is better to submit to a beam passing painlessly through the skin than the obvious dangers of a knife.

Is the advantage of radiotherapy over surgery actually the quality of the voice? Probably not for T1a glottic cancer—probably yes for T1b, where resection has to include the AC. But T1bs are the cases that fail with radiotherapy—patients with AC disease.

Maheshwar and Gaffney[241] reviewed all patients treated with radical radiotherapy for T1 glottic carcinoma in a British head and neck cancer unit between 1989 and 1996. Despite steps to ensure an adequate dose of radiation to the region, 57.1% of the tumors involving the AC recurred at the primary site! In 1996, Hirota et al[242] reported on 184 patients with T1 and T2 laryngeal glottic cancer, all of whom were treated by primary radiotherapy. Without anterior commissure involvement, the 5-year recurrence-free survival was 89.9%. With AC involvement, it was only 57.6%. And the dose necessary to control AC involvement was at least 70 Gy. 70 Gy carries consequences for voice; atrophy, desication, and chronic laryngitis. In one more large radiotherapy series, Burke et al[243] found AC involvement doubled the risk of failure. The 5-year local recurrence rate for T1a glottic cancer was a respectable 8%; but for T1b, it was 20%. In this same report, decreased mobility quadrupled the rate of failure; 77% of the T2b patients recurred after primary radiotherapy.

After radiotherapy for early glottic carcinoma, Rodriguez-Cuevas et al[77] reported that 13 to 24% of patients required salvage surgery. The median time to recurrence was 14.5 months. Half could have a partial laryngectomy for salvage; half required a total laryngectomy.

Spector et al provided comprehensive outcomes data on 659 patients with T1 glottic carcinoma.[244] Similar rates of *disease-specific survival* (95%) followed all treatments studied, but unaided laryngeal voice preservation and actuarial survival were poorest in the low-dose radiation therapy group. Initial local control was slightly better for open conservation surgery—92% for surgery, 89% with high dose (67.5 to 70 Gy) radiotherapy. For ultimate local control, *salvage treatment* erased significant differences. Unaided laryngeal voice preservation was best for

conservation surgery (93%), fair for high-dose radiation (89%), and poor for low-dose radiation (80%). The same investigators also reported on 134 patients with T2N0 glottic carcinomas roughly divided equally for treatment modality.[245] Radiotherapy failed to achieve local control in 15%. So did *open* surgery (no laser, no microscope). The 5-year actuarial and disease-specific survivals were 81.5% and 92%. There were no statistical differences in 5-year local control, voice preservation, or 5-year actuarial and disease-specific cure rates favoring one modality. (Transoral microresection was not evaluated.) An incidence of 10.4% regional metastases, 2.2% distant metastases, and 6% second primary tumors was documented.

One interpretation of these results would be that if radiotherapy is given in the treatment of early glottic cancer, most surviving patients will experience the swallowing complications and side effects of heavy dosage. Of 20 irradiated patients, two to four will require salvage surgery. Five (25%) will die during follow-up, two from the cancer, three from other causes. Maybe the successfully radiated cases will have better voices. This is not documented.

If open conservation surgery (as used by the authors 12 to 30 years ago) was chosen, no patients would experience the swallowing complications and side effects of heavy radiation. Two to four would require further treatment for recurrence but all options would be open. Five of the 20 would die during follow-up, two from the cancer, and three from other causes, just as already described. The successfully operated cases might have hoarse voices. Again, this was not documented.

Whichever treatment is elected, one to two of 20 patients get a second primary in the region. The difference would be the presence or absence of prior radiotherapy, and the limits this would impose on the treatment. Two will get regional metastases, pointing up the importance of considering the neck in the management of early (but not very early) disease. Surgery has the advantage of diagnosing the Delphian node. Radiation has the advantage of treating the neck concurrently. The carotid arteries would have to be included in the fields, unfortunately.

Magnano et al[238] reviewed 196 cases of T1–T2/N0 cancers of the glottic larynx and teased out the figures for the T2N0 cases, where a difference by modality seemed evident. The "no evidence of disease" (NED) survival of patients who underwent partial laryngectomies (90% of cases) was significantly better ($p = 0.05$) than the survival of patients given radiotherapy (73%). Involvement of the AC seemed to expose patients to a greater risk of recurrence when radiotherapy alone was used (five out of 23 cases, 21.7%, compared with three out of 52 cases, 5.7%, among the surgically treated patients).

Hamoir et al[246] reported their median 44-month follow-up data on 118 T1/T2 laryngeal cancers (84 glottic, 34 supraglottic), and 23 mostly T1 hypopharyngeal cancers, all of whom received a voice-sparing external partial laryngectomy. Overall survival rates for T1–T2 glottic cancer at 3, 5, and 10 years were 90, 90, and 78%, respectively. For patients treated for T1–T2 supraglottic cancer, overall survival at 3, 5, and 10 years was 73, 68, and 48%. T1–T2 hypopharyngeal cancer survival rates at 3 and 5 years were 74 and 37%, respectively.

Results like these are helpful in counseling a patient with "early" glottic cancer but are inconclusive. Radiotherapy reports typically commingle "very early"—easily treated through the mouth—and "early"—vertical partial candidates, into one group, T1 (a and b). Surgical reports on vertical partial laryngectomy are preselected to exclude T1a. T1a never needs that big an operation. And they typically *include* T2a. T2a cancers are still early. They are still good candidates for vertical partial laryngectomy. The *exclusion* of favorable cases (T1a) *and* the *inclusion* of less favorable cancers (T2a) will predictably worsen the results of partial laryngectomy. The problem is, staging numbers popular among results analysts (T1 and T2) group very dissimilar entities from every other standpoint—histopathologic extent, surgical indications, potential disability, and functional and oncological results. Virtually every analysis shows T2b has much more in common with T3 than T2a, and so on. A lot of data are published and the TNM reporting requirements are satisfied. But no valid reference data are created for "early" glottic cancer, except what we can infer from the literature by careful dissection of the results.

If all surgery could do was equal the cure rate of radiotherapy, the functional appeal of radiotherapy would win out. Patients would be better served by the preclusion of a temporary tracheostomy, the avoidance of open surgical intervention, and a superior quality of voice. In practice, the main deterrent to universal radiation is the complicated problem of tumor persistence and insidious progression. Schwaab et al reported on 259 early glottic cancers irradiated for cure at the Institut Gustave-Roussy.[247] The local failure rates were 16% for T1b and 36% for T2a. Persky et al[248] reviewed 34 patients undergoing primary radiotherapy for early carcinoma of the anterior commissure. There were five T2a lesions. Within 3 years of treatment, two had recurred locally and both required total laryngectomy for salvage. Ton-Van and Lefebvre[249] reported a 28% recurrence rate in 64 early glottic cancer patients (*including T1a*) treated with radiotherapy. Rodriguez-Cuevas et al[77] found that after radiotherapy for early glottic carcinoma, 13 to 24% of patients require salvage surgery. The median time to recurrence was 14.5 months. Half could have a partial laryngectomy for salvage but half required a total laryngectomy.

We know that the greater the tumor volume, the more likely a cancer will recur, that men fare worse than women, and that field size and dose are important. Usually, however, the reasons for unexpected failure are obscure. Even when tumor has disappeared from the surface of the larynx, occult submucosal disease may infiltrate far beyond the confines of the original lesion before detection. Clinical reports[63] and whole organ serial section studies[250,251] have clearly shown this to be an intrinsic peril of radio-recurrent cancer, not just a problem of improper follow-up or cursory examination. In glottic tumors, the only indication of recurrent disease may be subtle fixation of a previously mobile cord. Options available to rescue failures are limited by the fact that radiotherapy can only be used once. If a conservation operation *could* have encompassed the disease, it will rarely suffice at the time of retreatment.

Once a recurrence is recognized, the patient confronts two foes, a more disabling operation, and a lower chance of cancer control. Conservation operations may or may not apply. A tumor with indistinct borders lies situated in tissues less tolerant of a wound. Delays in stomal healing and complicated vocal shunt recovery limit their prospect of functional success. A fistula complicating what is now the second major

treatment for the cancer may greatly prolong the need for enteral nutrition. This means further hospitalization and expense. Salvage surgery may preserve the patient's survival after failed radiotherapy but devastate employment, social acceptance, and self-esteem.

Some degree of long-term hoarseness and a dry throat seem a reasonable price to pay when radiation does succeed. But what about persistent laryngeal edema or pain, a serious diagnostic dilemma when it occurs? Ward et al[252] found persisting cancer to be frequent (53%) in those in whom edema persisted over 6 months after therapy. The most tragic statistic was the low surgical salvage rate, 26%. These lesions were T1 or T2N0M0 at presentation, and not expected to fail.

The long-term carcinogenic effects of radiation create another level of concern. Patients cured of their early larynx cancer by radiotherapy are *not* cured of their propensity to grow *second primaries* in the neighboring tobacco-exposed mucosa. In the younger individual, whose life expectancy might be another 35 or 40 years, the long-term possibility that a new malignancy will be promoted is probably very real. Continuous evidence from the atomic bombing of Hiroshima and Nagasaki, the effect on children exposed to radiation during the above-ground nuclear tests in the western U.S. desert, and finally the elevated incidence of thyroid cancer in individuals exposed to thymic irradiation in infancy and cerebral malignancy in those treated in early life for retinoblastoma provide startling corroborative evidence to support this concern. And thanks to the aging population phenomenon, some 70-year-olds are now destined to live with this propensity for another 20 or even 30 years. Harwood et al[38] examined the prospect of malignancy from small doses of radiation during the period from 5 to 10 years after treatment and calculated a risk as small as 2%. Lawson and Som[253] offered one closer to 10. About 6% of surviving patients will require treatment for a second primary in the head and neck. Surgery will be necessary: radiotherapy will not be available. Wound healing will be compromised. Late effects of radiotherapy on the carotid arteries will raise the stroke risk for surgery. Extensive neck metastases will only have surgery for their control.

In short, the decision to irradiate someone with "early" glottic cancer may be a long-term strategic mistake. Radiotherapy is overtreatment for a cancer that can be simply excised—too toxic for a patient with a 20- or 30-year future, too precious to waste on a simple surgical cancer, and too ineffective if one patient in every four or five will have to be treated again.

Radiation oncologists are among the strongest advocates of partial laryngectomy—in the role of a salvage operation. Partial laryngectomy has the potential to avert the disaster of a total laryngectomy if radiation fails to cure early glottic cancer. Watters et al studied 33 patients in exactly this position.[254] (Sixteen started as T1 lesions, and 15 as T2. Thus transoral laser excision must have been a plausible option at the time of their initial presentation.) The interval from radiotherapy to salvage surgery ranged from 2 to 188 months (median 10). Surgery consisted of 25 vertical partial laryngectomies, six supraglottic laryngectomies, and two endoscopic laser resections. This approach generated seven further recurrences, thus seven total laryngectomies, of which six were successful. There were two pharyngocutaneous fistulae and three laryngotracheal stenoses requiring further surgery, thus a 15% major postoperative complication rate.

Overall, for 33 patients hoping radical radiotherapy would secure all four assets—voice, cure, one treatment, and no surgery—30 were potentially laser-resectable at their biopsy; 76 treatments were required. Forty-three were unplanned surgical treatments, eight being total laryngectomies. Ultimately (except that follow-ups ranged as low as 12 months) this tenacious program did save the life of 32 of the 33 patients. And only eight (24%) lost satisfactory speech and swallowing. For a reader who believes the patient's prior alternative was a total laryngectomy, or a risky mutilating operation, these are good results. For someone who believes almost all of these patients could have been cured the first time around with endoscopic laser surgery, the clinical interpretation would be quite different.

Chemotherapy

Platinum-based induction chemotherapy regimens are sometimes offered to patients with *intermediate* or *advanced,* and sometimes *very advanced* laryngeal cancer. Should it be offered in *early* disease? We know early visible cancer *can* disappear (called a "complete response") with chemotherapy. Does that mean it is just hiding and waiting to recur? Or is it sometimes cured? In intermediate cancer, Kies et al[255] sometimes observed complete clinical remission, including negative biopsies. However, the cancer typically recurred—unless the patient was then treated with radiotherapy, or surgery, or both.[256] Long-term studies seem consistent with the proposition that, for most patients, the final results are what would have been expected from the radiation or surgery alone.[257]

But is the transient nature of the response to chemotherapy we observe in advanced disease true for early cancer?[258] From 58 patients with early glottic cancer and a "complete response" (to cisplatin-fluorouracil) Laccourreye and Brasnu[258] described 21 who opted for no additional treatment, just monthly follow-up. Of these highly selected patients, 14 (70%) appeared to maintain their response (in the larynx). The remaining seven were salvaged with conventional treatments, which never included a total laryngectomy. In another publication,[259] the senior Laccourreye described an earlier cohort of 25 patients who also received no further treatment after a complete response to cisplatin-fluorouracil chemotherapy. Seventeen recurred locally (and five developed a metachronous second primary), but partial laryngeal surgery or radiation therapy salvaged all 17 local recurrences.

These reports suggested that some patients, patients with the most favorable of cancers—namely early glottic carcinoma with no nodes and a complete response to chemotherapy—may be cured! Complete responders made up about one quarter of the early glottic lesions treated by Laccourreye. He gave a figure of 24% in his 1999 report on T2 glottic cancers undergoing multimodal therapy.[260] So if 100 patients with early glottic cancer received chemotherapy, and cooperated fully with follow-up, we could postulate about 75 would be found to show persistent disease. All these would require the surgery or radiation which chemotherapy had temporarily deferred. Of the 25 patients without visible cancer (the

"complete responders"), glottic cancer would reappear in about 10 to 15. Detected in time, they too would require surgery or radiation therapy as treatment. This leaves 10 to 15 patients, perhaps one in eight of the original cancer sufferers, who might be classified as "cured". Their only interventions would have been their original biopsy and the course of chemotherapy. Keep in mind when treatment was selected for these patients initially, the small cohort of eventual cures could not be distinguished from the 85 to 90 patients who received chemotherapy without benefit. Further, all patients who failed to be cured by chemotherapy started with favorable clinical disease—that is, all patients had T1 or T2 invasive squamous cell carcinoma of the glottis, so almost none would have had cancer in the neck nodes at the time of their initial presentation.

One explanation for these hopeful observations would be that cisplatin-fluorouracil does cure early glottic cancer one eighth of the time. Another explanation would be that some patients were already cured when the chemotherapy began—because their biopsy was, in fact, a complete excision of the tumor. Complete removal by "biopsy" has certainly been seen to occur in T1a glottic cancer confined to one mobile cord. On the other hand, any study examining patients selected for the disappearance of their lesion after biopsy and chemotherapy ("complete responders") would include *all of those patients who lost their tiny well localized cordal cancer to the biopsy*. Perhaps both explanations play a role.

In Laccourreye et al's 1996 report,[258] one third *of the complete responders* were unable to translate their favorable chemosensitivity into an actual clinical cure. But still, they were followed closely, detected early, and salvaged completely. So one could argue that by following (only) the complete responders, nothing was lost. But is this true? One would have to be certain that the extent of their surgery was not increased—from laser cordectomy to supracricoid partial laryngectomy, for example. One would also need to calculate the additional economic costs, especially the costs of the chemotherapy program, including the chemotherapy given to partial and nonresponders, for example, and the cost of treating most patients twice where one treatment might have produced the same outcome. Are there any other gains that only chemotherapy would produce for patients with early glottic cancer? How about reduction of the carcinogenic potential of all the "condemned mucosa" thought to be present in the region. Unfortunately, the rate of metachronous second primaries was 14.3% in Laccourreye et al's 1996 report. It therefore seems probable that the risk of a second cancer continues undiminished, even in "complete responders," just as it is known to do after radiotherapy.

If chemotherapy alone can cure a few patients, but mostly does not, does it have a role as an induction modality for patients we already plan to treat with a conventional therapy? Laccourreye's extensive work also speaks to this issue. In a nonrandomized retrospective study of 100 patients with T2 squamous cell carcinoma of the glottis followed a minimum of 3 years, all patients received platinum-based induction chemotherapy *and* open partial laryngeal surgery.[260] Seventy-six retained visible cancer after chemotherapy (fifty-eight had shown a partial response). Twenty-four patients had a complete clinical response. Interestingly, the pathologist could not identify histological evidence of cancer in the surgical specimens of 31 patients (most of them the complete responders). The 5-year actuarial local control estimate for this dual modality program was 95.7%. It was 97.7% if the vocal cord was mobile and 93.8% if the motion of the vocal cord was impaired. Salvage treatment resulted in local control in all but one patient (99%) and a 95% rate of laryngeal preservation. These results for T2 glottic cancer represent a unique 10-year experience. They rival those obtained in other large series for T1 glottic disease.

Earlier in the 1990s, Wolf and Hong[18] had *considered* using induction chemotherapy for early laryngeal cancer. But the outcome of conventional treatments seemed too good, in terms of survival and function, to justify the additional toxicity. On the basis of the experiences cited earlier, Laccourreye et al concluded that in patients with early or intermediate invasive glottic carcinoma, platinum-based induction chemotherapy prior to conservation surgery may well merit further scientific scrutiny.[260]

What is the practicing laryngologist to do? At the present time, many do not offer chemotherapy for early (or intermediate) laryngeal cancer? Conservation surgery is "organ sparing" itself, without chemotherapy. So any rationale tied to the characterization of chemotherapy as "organ sparing" simply disappears. Among all the patients who first present with glottic cancer, there will be nonresponders. They will need conventional therapy. There will be partial responders. They will also need further treatment by some nonchemotherapeutic modality. There may be complete responders, but as we have seen, some of these will recur. Because all these patients will need salvage treatment by radiation, surgery, or both, why not do it now? If the cancer has spread to extraglottic sites, like the supraglottis, the likelihood of needing conventional treatment is even greater. And for patients with adenopathy, no one will escape the need to proceed to radiation or surgery or both. If chemotherapy *is* given, what about its systemic toxicities, its effects on wound healing, and its cost?

Other physicians opt to follow the lead of those studying more advanced disease. *Don't offer chemotherapy as a cure, but do use the response to chemotherapy to help select the treatment.* But what treatment goes with what response? Some might assert that incomplete responders must have the worse disease, so they should have the more aggressive treatment (open surgery, for example). Complete responders are considered to have more favorable disease, so they could be "rewarded" with radiotherapy, or a less invasive operation (laser resection perhaps). But this entire rationalization may be backward. The partial responders are the only patients with a lesional target still visible. Laser excisions are designed to "follow the tumor," so partial responders would actually be the ones more suited to laser microresection. Open formal operations, like vertical partial laryngectomy (VPL), are also dependent on a visible tumor but laryngeal landmarks can guide the excision if the selection is expert and the patient was laryngoscoped by the surgeon before chemotherapy. One "dividend" for a complete response might be a lessened risk of tumor implantation in the broader field the open operation would require.

Another rationale for chemotherapy would be to use it as a prelude to radiotherapy. Many patients with early glottic cancer choose radiotherapy as their primary treatment, but the dosage is limited by its toxicities, especially its long-term degenerative effects. And failure of radiotherapy usually leads to more radical surgery for salvage. If chemotherapy could provide a synergy with radiotherapy, perhaps it might increase the chance of cure. If the dose of radiation could be reduced, perhaps we could decrease the incidence of side effects. Unfortunately, this rationale has much more theoretic appeal than it has support in the literature or in practice. The principal limitation of radiotherapy is not its power but its small therapeutic ratio. And platin-fluorouracil-based chemotherapy potentiates the toxicity of radiotherapy and does not improve on the ratio.

Another appealing rationale would be to cast chemotherapy in the role of a prelude to surgery, something that could shrink the tumor, demote it in some way, or otherwise impair its vitality. If cytotoxic drugs can degrade the malignant potential of a cancer cell, perhaps in the role of pretreatment, why wouldn't a partial or a complete response enfeeble the whole tumor? The goal would be to diminish the cancer's ability to disseminate a viable clone of implants during the manipulations of surgery. Clinically, tumors do look more subdued after a partial response, and this may be a valid rationale. But maybe preoperative radiotherapy could produce all of the advantages mentioned earlier for chemotherapy. Especially if the dose was kept so low that less than half the recipients had a complete response (as we seem to accept in chemotherapy). The advantage of chemotherapy over radiotherapy in this paradigm might only be that we can repeat chemotherapy—it has an advantage over radiotherapy in that it does not seem to prejudice the treatment of a second primary cancer.

One of the unsolved dilemmas in early glottic cancer is what to do with the discovery of a positive Delphian node. This would normally signal the need for additional treatment in the neck, but what? Maybe pretreatment chemotherapy (so-called induction chemotherapy) could play a role as a test. If the primary had been shown to be resistant to pretreatment (induction) chemotherapy, we might place more confidence in surgery to treat the necks. A complete response by the primary on the other hand may tip the physician toward postsurgical (adjuvant) radiotherapy. What this would require is evidence of the following:

- Chemotherapy can predict radiocurability.
- Chemoresistance foreshadows radioresistance.
- The delay giving chemotherapy was not unsafe for the patient.

In considering what we are actually achieving today with chemotherapy, I find it hard to escape the conclusion that before real progress is made, we will need agents with more power and more specificity against neoplastic squamous cells, and our patients need more accurate and pragmatic terminology. A "partial response" defines an interesting observation for an investigator, but not some clinical benefit for the patient. A "complete response" from the doctor's perspective may prove incomplete from the patient's standpoint. We actually have to kill or remove every last cancer cell. Anything less will fall short. Squamous cell cancer is cured or not.

A clinically evident squamous carcinoma contains 10 billion cells (10^{10}). One hundred million cells (10^8) are too few to produce a visible mass. A "partial response" is a reduction in local tumor burden from 10^{10} to ~10^9 cells, a heartening shrinkage maybe, but not a disappearance. Partial removal by a cauterization might reduce the "local tumor burden" to 10^9 cells too, and in less time, at lower cost. But unless shrinkage improves surgical access to the residual cancer, or reduces the residual cancer's viability (capacity for implantation at surgery), or increases its susceptibility to radiotherapy, the advantage to the patient is nil.

A "complete response" might simply be the reduction of 10^{10} cancer cells (visible) to 10^8 cancer cells (invisible). At a million cells, even the pathologist might miss the evidence. A complete response might just be another form of incomplete removal—no cure, no increase in length of survival, no extra time before the reappearance of symptoms. At the time of this writing, chemotherapy outside peer-reviewed protocols has yet to become an orthodox option for early and intermediate laryngeal cancer. While studies are ongoing, the basis for patient treatment must be the reality of what we know, not the promise of what we hope.

Classic Conservation Surgery for Early Glottic Cancer

A comprehensive selection of "conservation" operations, have been developed to deal with the diverse presentations of early glottic cancer. These include the frontolateral partial laryngectomies (up to "three-quarter" laryngectomy), frontoanterior partial laryngectomy, and all of their various reconstructions. The very diversity of these operations presents a serious challenge for surgeons, the challenge to acquire sufficient experience. But good surgical teams and medical facilities do this work. For patients, the problem is to access them.

Conservation operations are very formal and specific. Small details have big consequences. All aspects are complex; patient selection, preoperative counseling, minimizing the impact of comorbidities like prior radiotherapy, the care of complications, postoperative treatment, predismissal patient education, and optimizing the functional prognosis. From the patient's point of view, a source of open conservation surgery may well be distant. A source of radiotherapy equipment (not to be confused with radiotherapy *expertise* in laryngologic cancer) may be close at hand. Convincing retrospective *survival* data can be cited to justify either radiation or surgery in the treatment of early laryngeal cancer (but not medium or advanced laryngeal cancer, to be discussed later). The whole area is perhaps the greatest controversy between good radiotherapists and good conservation surgeons. In recent years, transoral laser microsurgery has swung the pendulum of "indications" strongly toward the side of conservation surgery. But as with the open operations, access remains problematic for the patient. Important limits on the distribution of necessary skills and equipment restrict the availability of these procedures. At the time of this writing, the essential ingredients of management in early laryngeal cancer include an accountable specialist, an appreciation of the nature and extent of early laryngeal cancer, careful study of the needs and possibilities of the particular patient, the skill to manage the technology eventually selected, and the

willingness and ability to provide follow-up of the patients. If cure rates are deemed uniform among one modality versus another, functional disability (and, increasingly, cost) may be the critical issues in treatment selection. Here, we will try to highlight some genuine differences.

Frontolateral Vertical Partial Laryngectomy

VPL was designed for glottic cancers with mobile vocal folds too big for transoral removal (**Fig. 4.24**). Most involved the AC. The ideal case was primary but many were postirradiated. Surgeons liked these operations for their functional elegance and their power to cure patients of doubtful radiocurability (the bulky glottic cancer involving the AC), without a permanent stoma, and without the loss of the voice. Radiotherapists liked these operations, too, *but as salvage surgery*. The indications for radiotherapy could be liberalized perhaps if failures of treatment could be rescued by something *less* than the dreaded total laryngectomy. Several papers soon appeared to assert that VPL was as trouble free *after radiotherapy as before, but for salvage procedure*.

◆ **Patient Selection** Frontolateral VPL targets glottic lesions with anterior (commissure) glottic region invasion. Suitable cancers extend from one true cord across the AC to involve the opposite cord a distance of no more than one third of its anterior length.

The most critical limitation is subglottic extension. Mucosal cancer will usually extend ~2 to 3 mm beyond visible tumor in early laryngeal disease. Just as attempts at hemilaryngectomy were said to be ill advised if the visible neoplasm extended any more inferiorly than 5 mm below the free edge of the true cord, the same is true for unmodified frontolateral VPL. Actually extended techniques have emerged to shave off increasing amounts of the cricoid ring. They will be mentioned below.

Posterior involvement was also an issue: what constituted adequate surgical excision of the intrinsic laryngeal muscles attached to the arytenoid. Visible extension to the vocal process requires excision of nearly the entire arytenoid (to capture the entire mucosal cover and all the thyroarytenoid muscular attachments, which spread over its anterior and lateral surfaces).

The authors believe VPL works best as a primary operation. Several papers suggest VPL is nearly as good after radiotherapy. We suspect the complications are underreported: we all have a tendency to identify success and underreport failure. Lydiatt et al challenged reports of an increased complication rate with partial laryngectomy in previously irradiated patients. For 68 VPL patients with adequate follow-up over a 10-year period, they found wound complications, time to decannulation, length of hospitalization, or ability to swallow was no worse in the previously irradiated VPL patient group than those treated with primary VPL. When surgical salvage was included, the local control rates were 93% for previously treated patients and 98% for unpretreated cases in their series. But overall 5-year survival rates were 79% for previously treated VPL patients and 95% for primary VPL.[37]

◆ **Preoperative Considerations** Age is probably a legitimate factor in deciding upon any patient's suitability for surgery; typically we will consider the patient's physiological age to

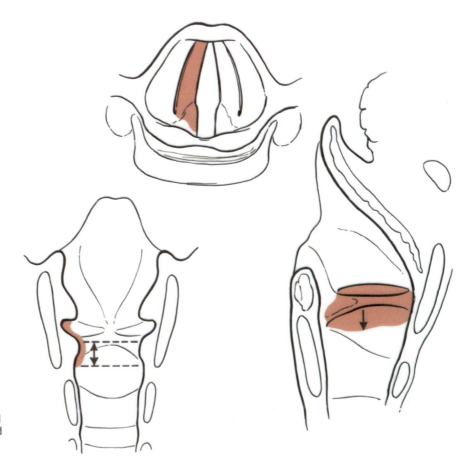

Fig. 4.24 The limits of tumor extension for resection of laryngeal cancer by vertical hemilaryngectomy in superior, coronal, and sagittal views. Subglottic extension should be no greater than 5 mm.

be much more relevant than the chronological. However, a septuagenarian may appear robust and healthy but lack the flexibility of mind or habit to adjust to the alterations of voice, swallowing, and airway that may follow cordectomy or hemilaryngectomy. A 72-year-old vigorous, healthy patient in my experience (PJD) had a small cordal lesion that failed to be cured with radiotherapy. A hemilaryngectomy with an otherwise uneventful postoperative course was marred by the patient's insistence that he could not swallow or breathe, despite the fact that when observed he could swallow without apparent obstruction, pain, or aspiration, and had a clear airway, albeit a hoarse voice. This finding was supported by fluorographic studies. The patient was so insistent on his disability that he required periodic admissions to the hospital because of inanition. A more thorough preoperative investigation into his psychological status might have revealed some clue to his rigidity and lack of adaptability. However, this exemplifies the problems with partial laryngectomy in the elderly.

◆ **Surgical Resection** Hemilaryngectomy is performed following a tracheostomy done under local anesthesia. After sterile preparation, a flexible endotracheal tube is placed through the tracheostomy site and sutured in place.

A horizontal incision is made in a skin crease at the level of the cricothyroid membrane (**Fig. 4.25A**). Rarely is a neck dissection required, but if it is, a modified H incision may be used (**Fig. 4.25B**). Skin flaps are elevated superiorly and inferiorly on the plane of the strap muscles (not the subplatysmal plane). The hyoid bone is the upper limit, and the first tracheal ring is the lower. A self-retaining retractor is installed.

On the side of the tumor, the sternohyoid and thyrohyoid muscles are incised from their origin on the hyoid bone (**Fig. 4.26**). A clean incision down to bare bone permits the dissection of some periosteum along with the attached muscle, which facilitates suturing in the reconstruction of the neocord later on.

The thyroid perichondrium is incised along the superior border of the thyroid cartilage the entire length of the affected side, and on the opposite side a sufficient distance to give adequate exposure for the cartilage cuts. The prelaryngeal fascia and its lymph node are peeled off the larynx to the first tracheal ring and sent to the histopathologist. A vertical incision is made through the external perichondrium in the midline, from top to bottom. The perichondrium is carefully dissected away from the entire thyroid lamina of the affected side, from the midline to the posterior limit.

145

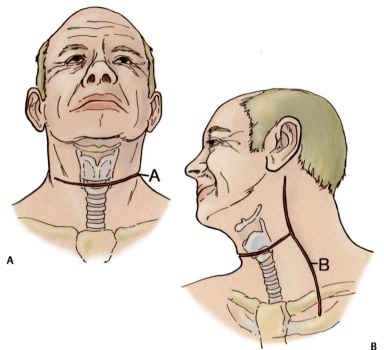

Fig. 4.25 Incisions for partial laryngectomy. (**A**) For hemilaryngectomy. (**B**) For radical neck dissection, when required.

The cartilage cuts may be marked with dye, using a nonsiliconized needle. The markings go vertically through the midline of the thyroid cartilage and near the posterior border, with a connecting rim of cartilage left between the superior and inferior cornua, 3 to 4 mm in width (**Fig. 4.27**). Because this cartilage strip is primarily pharyngeal (it is part of the lateral wall of the piriform fossa), it can safely be left behind, when the AC is involved, and marking extends ~4 mm lateral to the midline.

A sagittal saw is used to make the cartilage cuts, stopping just short of the internal perichondrium. The perichondrium is approached with great care to avoid damage by the saw. A horizontal incision is made with a scalpel in the cricothyroid membrane on the superior surface of the cricoid arch (**Fig. 4.28**). Bleeding from the cricothyroid artery, which crosses the cricothyroid membrane, is controlled by cautery.

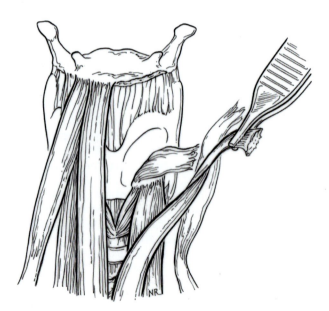

Fig. 4.26 Hemilaryngectomy. Strap muscles are excised from hyoid bone, taking a little hyoid periosteum.

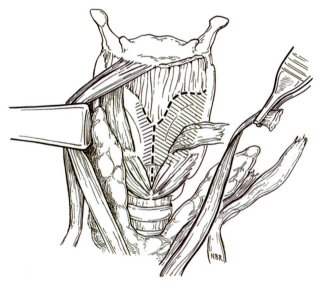

Fig. 4.27 Hemilaryngectomy. Perichondral incision over the superior aspect of the ipsilateral thyroid ala, splitting the perichondrium in the midline to the cricothyroid membrane. The incision extends superiorly 3 to 5 mm onto the other side. Crosshatched area represents the amount of perichondrial elevation.

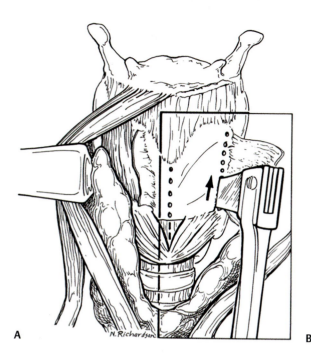
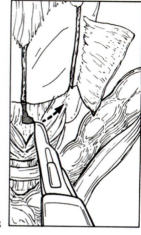

Fig. 4.28 Hemilaryngectomy. (**A**) With the strap muscles of the opposing side retracted, the cartilage cuts are made with the oscillating saw: one in the midline and the second laterally, sparing a 3 to 4 mm strip of thyroid ala. (**B**) Cartilage cuts completed. An incision is made through the cricothyroid membrane with the blade hugging the superior surface of the cricoid cartilage.

The patient's head is further extended and the surgeon dons a headlight. With the cricothyroid membrane incision retracted with small skin hooks, the subglottic surface of the glottis is visualized. If the tumor extends to the sloping upper margin of the cricoid, the superior half of the cricoid cartilage should be included in the specimen. Any further subglottic extension should be managed by near-total laryngectomy.

An incision in the midline is carried from the cricothyroid membrane to just under the AC, through the internal perichondrium and endolaryngeal mucosa. If the lesion is limited to one side, the scalpel with a no. 15 blade is gently inserted between the cords and firmly cut anteriorly so that a perfect bifurcation of the glottis is achieved through the center of the AC (**Fig. 4.29**). This incision is extended superiorly into the petiolus of the epiglottis.

When the lesion extends across the AC, the cords are pulled apart by hooks, and the AC as well as a 2 mm margin of involved contralateral vocal cord is included in the specimen.

The petiolus of the epiglottis is detached from its insertion into the thyroid ala. The thyroid alae can now be pulled widely apart and the tumor viewed (**Fig. 4.30**). Excision of the cancer is accomplished inferiorly with scissors by placing one blade inside the laryngeal lumen and the other along the upper margin of the cricoid (or lower, to include an upper margin of cricoid ring, if necessary). As the arch of the cricoid sweeps toward the posterior laminae (**Fig. 4.31**), the cricoarytenoid joint is entered. The posterior margin of the resection is delineated with the angled (Panzer's) gallbladder scissors, with care taken to achieve an optimum margin without excising too much mucosa. Some of the arytenoid and AE fold epithelium will be important in the reconstruction.

The final mucosal incision follows the apex of the AE fold and connects the release of the arytenoid body to the cut through the epiglottic petiolus. This resection develops a specimen that is comparable in many ways to a cordectomy, but its volume is large inferiorly and superiorly and the arytenoid body and thyroid ala are included. A reasonable neocord regenerates without reconstruction following a cordectomy, provided the arytenoid remains. In the more extensive resection that we have chosen to call hemilaryngectomy, an attempt at glottic reconstruction is worthwhile. Glottic reconstruction is indicated to avoid a very breathy voice. On

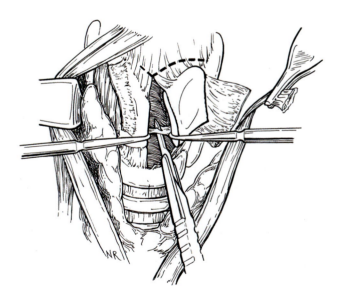

Fig. 4.29 Hemilaryngectomy. The thyroid alae are held apart with hooks, and care is taken to split the anterior commissure precisely in the midline with a no. 15 scalpel blade. The incision need not clear the tumor by more than 1 mm.

◆ **Surgical Technique** Perform a tracheostomy under local anesthesia. Induce general anesthesia. Suture the flexible endotracheal "J" tube into place to prevent distal migration toward the right main bronchus. If you need to revisit the endolaryngeal appearances (with no tube in the way), cover the tracheotomy site with adhesive Tegaderm (3M, St. Paul, MN) and perform a direct laryngoscopy. Carefully inspect the tumor limits with the 30 degree laryngeal telescope.

Make a horizontal skin incision in a crease at the level of the cricothyroid membrane. Elevate flaps superiorly to the hyoid and inferiorly to the first tracheal ring. Follow the plane of the strap muscles (deeper than the subplatysmal plane). Maintain the exposure with a self-retaining retractor like the May-Horner thyroid frame (Ethicon Surgery Company).

Release the sternohyoid muscle partially from its medial attachment on the side of least involvement or retract it to maximize the exposure. Leave the prelaryngeal fascia in place and make note of the status of the Delphian node in front of the cricothyroid ligament. Situate the vertical cartilage cut on this side (the good side) about one third the distance from the midline to the posterior limit of the ala.

Enter the laryngeal lumen at the site planned at the time of the laryngoscopy. Clear the tumor by a 2 mm margin or so on the side of least involvement. The shortened cord retracts toward the arytenoid. Place a 5–0 Monocryl mattress suture (Ethicon, Inc., Somerville, NJ) through the remaining thyroid ala, and anchor this cord as far anteriorly as possible (**Fig. 4.35**).

On the side of greater involvement, perform a similar resection, but this time with the advantage of having the tumor under direct vision. Consider reconstructing the missing cord on the more involved side with a sternohyoid muscle flap (**Fig. 4.36**).

◆ **Reconstruction**

Stenting Insert an Eliachar Laryngeal Stent (Hood Laboratories, Pembroke, MA) for 3 weeks to improve the shape and function of the glottic aperture after these maneuvers. Incise a small trapdoor flap in the top of the stent to dissipate the force of a cough. The stent will minimize the accretion of glottic adhesions and produce a better result than a keel.

Epiglottic Laryngoplasty Frontoanterior VPL fits the "horseshoe" AC cancers where cordal involvement is nearly symmetric. Some glottic cancers extend all the way around the glottis to (barely) the vocal process of the arytenoid cartilage of the least-involved side (**Fig. 4.37**). Epiglottic laryngoplasty (the Kambic-Sedlacek reconstruction[266,267]) provides a valuable reconstructive option to closure around a keel.

VPL with epiglottic reconstruction (VPLER) is an open operation for early anterior glottic region ("anterior commissure") carcinoma described by Sedlacek in 1965,[268] Kambic et al in 1976,[266] and Tucker et al in 1979.[269] The hallmark of this approach is the reconstruction. The surgeon repairs the site of the anterior laryngeal tissue loss with a pull-down sliding epiglottic advancement flap. The anterior glottic complex lost by the excision is supplanted by the epiglottis and the newly redundant AE and false vocal cords as the epiglottis is brought into the supportive framework of the larynx. Indications are limited because there must be no epiglottic or extensive ventricular involvement. The reconstruction uses the epiglottis to provide support and adequate mucosa for glottic competence. Cure rates are excellent with careful selection, and patients are generally able to swallow by the tenth postoperative day. The phonatory results are usually poor. Nowadays, transoral laser surgery, frontolateral partial

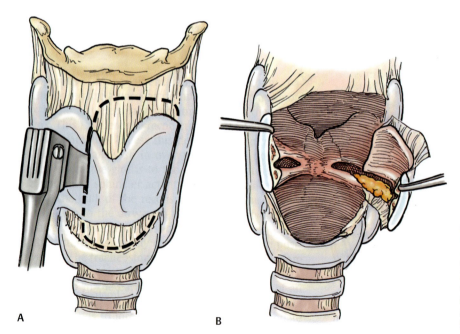

A   B

Fig. 4.35 Frontolateral partial laryngectomy. (**A**) The medial cartilage incision extends beyond the midline to the thyroid cartilage so that an incision through it will clear the tumor on the underlying vocal cord. (**B**) The larynx is opened and tumor extent visualized. The tumor on the cord of least involvement is cleared by a 1 to 2 mm margin of healthy tissue.

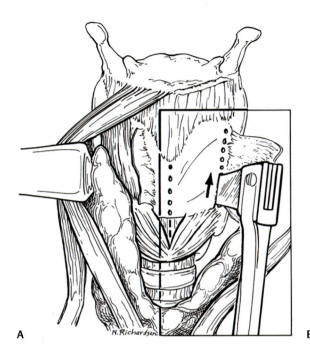
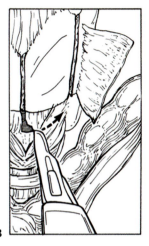

Fig. 4.28 Hemilaryngectomy. (**A**) With the strap muscles of the opposing side retracted, the cartilage cuts are made with the oscillating saw: one in the midline and the second laterally, sparing a 3 to 4 mm strip of thyroid ala. (**B**) Cartilage cuts completed. An incision is made through the cricothyroid membrane with the blade hugging the superior surface of the cricoid cartilage.

The patient's head is further extended and the surgeon dons a headlight. With the cricothyroid membrane incision retracted with small skin hooks, the subglottic surface of the glottis is visualized. If the tumor extends to the sloping upper margin of the cricoid, the superior half of the cricoid cartilage should be included in the specimen. Any further subglottic extension should be managed by near-total laryngectomy.

An incision in the midline is carried from the cricothyroid membrane to just under the AC, through the internal perichondrium and endolaryngeal mucosa. If the lesion is limited to one side, the scalpel with a no. 15 blade is gently inserted between the cords and firmly cut anteriorly so that a perfect bifurcation of the glottis is achieved through the center of the AC (**Fig. 4.29**). This incision is extended superiorly into the petiolus of the epiglottis.

When the lesion extends across the AC, the cords are pulled apart by hooks, and the AC as well as a 2 mm margin of involved contralateral vocal cord is included in the specimen.

The petiolus of the epiglottis is detached from its insertion into the thyroid ala. The thyroid alae can now be pulled widely apart and the tumor viewed (**Fig. 4.30**). Excision of the cancer is accomplished inferiorly with scissors by placing one blade inside the laryngeal lumen and the other along the upper margin of the cricoid (or lower, to include an upper margin of cricoid ring, if necessary). As the arch of the cricoid sweeps toward the posterior laminae (**Fig. 4.31**), the cricoarytenoid joint is entered. The posterior margin of the resection is delineated with the angled (Panzer's) gallbladder scissors, with care taken to achieve an optimum margin without excising too much mucosa. Some of the arytenoid and AE fold epithelium will be important in the reconstruction.

The final mucosal incision follows the apex of the AE fold and connects the release of the arytenoid body to the cut through the epiglottic petiolus. This resection develops a specimen that is comparable in many ways to a cordectomy, but its volume is large inferiorly and superiorly and the arytenoid body and thyroid ala are included. A reasonable neocord regenerates without reconstruction following a cordectomy, provided the arytenoid remains. In the more extensive resection that we have chosen to call hemilaryngectomy, an attempt at glottic reconstruction is worthwhile. Glottic reconstruction is indicated to avoid a very breathy voice. On

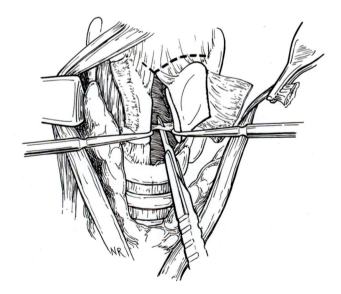

Fig. 4.29 Hemilaryngectomy. The thyroid alae are held apart with hooks, and care is taken to split the anterior commissure precisely in the midline with a no. 15 scalpel blade. The incision need not clear the tumor by more than 1 mm.

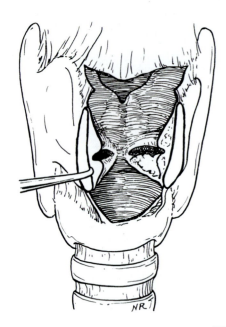

Fig. 4.30 Hemilaryngectomy. The thyroid alae are held apart and the tumor extent is visualized. An incision through the thyrohyoid membrane extends into the laryngeal lumen, separating the epiglottis from the rest of the larynx.

the other hand, it carries with it the danger of postoperative airway obstruction. The surgeon ought to be a little less eager to discontinue the hemilaryngectomized patient's tracheotomy than might be the case for a laryngofissure and cordectomy.

◆ **Reconstruction**

Imbrication One way to reduce the open void on the major side is to reconstruct a neocord by imbricating two preserved upper and lower thyroid cartilage strips and covering them with a false vocal fold flap.[261] Har-El et al judged voice quality

as good or excellent in 100% of the patients who underwent imbrication laryngoplasty, certainly better than the typical voice after hemilaryngectomy.[261] However, only a handful of patients would have an early glottic cancer big enough to justify a VPL yet limited enough to preserve the requisite horizontal strips of thyroid ala, particularly the inferior one, and the necessary tissues of the false cord. The resection described for partial laryngectomy and imbrication laryngoplasty was "the entire vocal fold, with its ligament, muscle, adjacent paraglottic tissues, and the adjacent block of thyroid cartilage." When VPLs have been reported to fail, they have done so at the subglottic margin. The resection described then sounds too limited to guard against this risk, and therefore, too limited to be considered with most patients who would be considered "early glottic carcinoma" in the classification we follow.

Reconstruction with Cervical Fascia Krajina and his colleagues at Zagreb University used a pedicled flap of deep cervical fascia in the reconstruction of laryngeal defects, especially after a partial vertical laryngectomy.[262,263] He approached the larynx through a classic U-shaped Gluck-Sorensen incision, with its base below the mandible, then raised a cervical flap in the subplatysmal plane. The superficial and middle cervical fascia would be incised immediately above the tracheal stoma, then out and up along the lateral border of one omohyoid muscle. A fascial flap could then be carefully elevated up to the hyoid bone.

Depending on the place and size of the laryngeal defect, the base of the flap could be positioned cranially, based on the hyoid bone. (In some cases it could be based laterally, on the omohyoid muscle.) Once the flap was elevated and protected, the bare sternohyoid muscle on the tumor side could be released, just below the hyoid (and below the base of the flap). This would expose the main ala for the resection and provide an inferiorly pedicled muscle flap for later placement on the *outside* of the fascia flap.

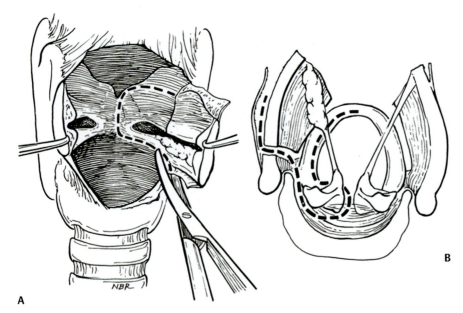

Fig. 4.31 Hemilaryngectomy. **(A)** The scissors hug the superior surface of the cricoid cartilage, excising the hemilarynx up to the posterior commissure. The dashed line represents the line of incision. **(B)** The dashed line represents the intraluminal and extraluminal extent of resection.

A

After carrying out the partial laryngectomy in the usual fashion and observing the size of the cartilage and soft tissue resections, the surgeon could tailor the fascial flap to exceed the defect, anticipating 10 to 15% shrinkage of the flap. Then the flap would simply be contoured into the defect (with no tension) and sewn to its mucosal edges with fine (4–0 or 5–0) interrupted absorbable sutures. The outer surface of the flap would be sutured to a repositioned sternohyoid muscle for backing and support.

Experience with this technique showed it was probably only valid for two-dimensional defects. Complex reconstructions like those required after partial pharyngectomy needed complex conventional flaps. Complications were those one might expect: granulations, partial flap necrosis or complete necrosis, edema with delayed decannulation (especially in salvage cases), or swallowing and aspiration difficulties. Granulations or necrosis would require endoscopic debridement.

Cervical fascia is a thin, firm sheet of fairly elastic, living mesenchymal tissue with low metabolism and sufficient resistance to saliva, infection, motion, and irradiation that its use as a conforming "patch" is quite acceptable. Not being skin, there is no hair growth, keratosis, or epithelial desquamation. Its disadvantages are that it is not epithelialized, it provides no framework to maintain the airway, and its blood supply is limited. Granulation tissue grows on the exposed surface of a fascial flap and extends the time required for epithelialization; this in turn causes fibrosis and more wound contraction. Thus results depend on local vascularity, antisepsis, and, when necessary, debridement. Krajina felt an important advantage to cervical fascial flap reconstruction was preservation of the laryngeal lumen after partial laryngectomy.

Bipedicled Sternohyoid Muscle Flap   Bailey presented an innovative technique for glottic reconstruction after VPL using a bipedicled sternohyoid muscle/perichondrial flap. This expanded the scope of VPL for early cancer by improving the patient's tolerance for extended resections of the posterior glottis. The transposed soft tissues tend to partially compensate for the loss of the arytenoid mass. Meanwhile, the preservation and direction of the pedicles limit the encroachment of the reconstruction on the airway[43] (**Fig. 4.32A,B,C and Fig. 4.33**).

Muscle had a better blood supply than fascia, hence a greater potential for healing. This feature would be especially attractive in radiotherapy failures. The flap was simply transposed deep to the mobilized ala of the thyroid cartilage (which was hinged posteriorly on the inferior constrictor muscle after the thyrotomy). This served as the lever to medialize the flap. Bailey preserved the external alar perichondrium on the deep surface of the muscle. If the ala was more extensively removed, the external alar perichondrium itself could do this task (i.e., draw in the muscle flap).

Bailey noted a muscle flap was *not* needed when all that had been resected was a vocal fold. But when a larger posterior defect was created, by resection of most or all of the arytenoid, a muscle flap was very helpful. Its bulk would reduce air wastage: the patient could sustain voice and not run out of air before completing a sentence. The superior vector renewed support of the false cord and AE fold, which facilitated swallowing. The lateral pull helped the patient to open the airway for breathing. Disadvantages could be overcome by technical steps, or they faded with time. The taut lateral pull sometimes required relief through partial release of the inferior muscle pedicle. Right after surgery, the flap would

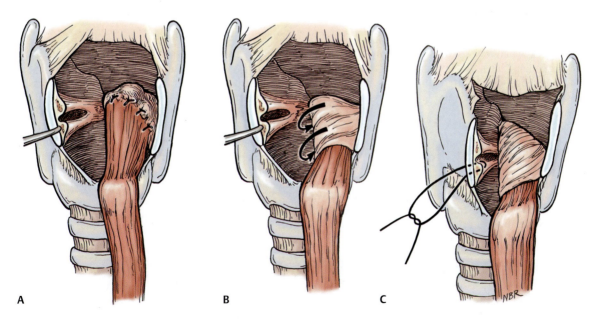

Fig. 4.32   "Reconstruction modified after Bailey." Hemilaryngectomy. (**A**) The larynx is reconstructed by bringing in a muscular flap of sternothyroid and sternohyoid muscle, then suturing it to any residual arytenoid cartilage or to the raw bed over the lamina of the cricoid cartilage. (**B**) A mucosal flap of aryepiglottic fold is folded over the muscle to reconstruct the "neocord." Size 4-0 absorbable sutures secure this mucosa to the subglottic mucosa. (**C**) An anchoring suture draws the uninvolved vocal fold to the anterior of the larynx. The suture is secured by passing it through the two holes in the anterior extremity of the residual thyroid ala.

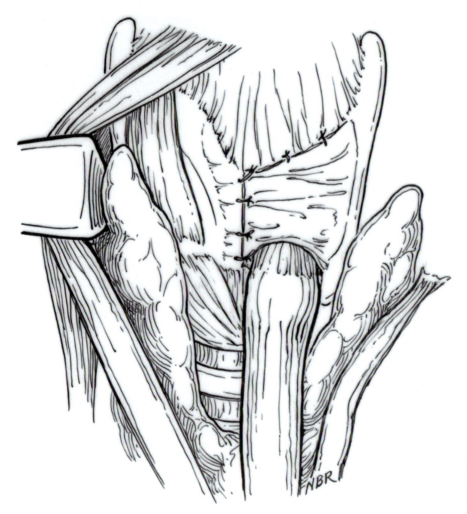

Fig. 4.33 Hemilaryngectomy. The thyroid perichondrium is sutured closed, but no actual sutures are placed between it and the bulk of the muscle flap.

swell and obstruct the airway, so the tracheotomy might last a few days longer. Long term, the neocord was a "pad" shape and slightly foreshortened. It often functioned against the remaining false cord (not the true) for voice. Thus the tone of the voice would be hoarse.

♦ **Postoperative Management** Hemilaryngectomy patients usually require a nasogastric tube. The cricoarytenoid complex is the key. Hemilaryngectomy dismasts the posterior larynx. This is where the reconstructive creativity of the surgeon is paramount. Unless this defect is recognized and addressed, saliva can wash in over the side and down the companionway of the glottis to the lower respiratory tract. There is not much sphincter activity left at the glottic level to resist it. The bulk of the reconstruction and the upward vector it applies to the airway in the cricoarytenoid region are the factors the surgeon must optimize.

Oral alimentation is usually delayed until the tenth postoperative day. The tracheostomy is usually not corked before this date. A balance exists between voice and airway. A voice that is too good in the early phases often forewarns of an inadequate airway later. Over a period of several months, the operated side tends to foreshorten. Some patients phonate

against their reconstruction with the false cord of the good side instead of their true vocal fold. If the glottic chink is too short, especially after contralateral anterior cordal resection, it can sometimes be lengthened by a secondary laryngotomy and insertion of a keel. Breathy dysphonia can be slightly improved with implantation techniques (e.g., Gore-Tex, W. L. Gore and Associates, Inc., Flagstaff, AZ) to reduce a gap. But vocal results for "phonosurgery" following hemilaryngectomy are poor in general because the soft pliability of the phonatory tissues does not return. The neocord is more fibrous than normal, and the mucosal wave is almost entirely dependent on what can be achieved by the lamina propria on the remaining good side. The best policy is to make sure the patient's expectations for voice quality are realistic before the surgery is performed. Unfortunately, prior radiotherapy is an important diminishing factor.

Speaking is discouraged for 10 to 14 days, and decannulation weaning is begun at this time. Oral feeding is delayed for the same span of time. Aspiration is not much of a problem, and decannulation is usually successfully achieved.

♦ **Results** Conservation surgery is usually curative—*if negative margins are achieved*. Technical expertise in the performance is important and so is reliable immediate frozen-section histopathology. Sheen et al[264] found seven recurrences in the larynx in 49 partial vertical laryngectomies. Two occurred beyond 5 years. The recurrence rate was 14% if the two cases beyond 5 years are considered second primaries. Five of six patients were successfully salvaged with total laryngectomy. The seventh patient survived 4.5 years after cisplatin-based chemotherapy. The actuarial 5-year survival rate was 97.4%. The larynx preservation rate was 88%. The quality of voice was considered worse than what successful radiotherapy might have produced. The question would be whether radiation could produce 44 patients with no recurrence on 5-year follow-up, and whether salvage surgery could produce such a high rate of success (86%) if the tumors were radiorecurrent cancers.

Among patients with stage I to II glottic carcinoma managed with VPL, local recurrence results in a reduced rate of survival and a high rate of necessity for salvage total laryngectomy. That is, the consequences of failure to achieve local control with the initial surgery are severe, and surgeons who undertake conservation laryngeal operations like VPL carry a very high responsibility for initial cure.

Laccourreye et al compared 103 patients who had local recurrence with 311 patients who achieved local control after VPL for stage I to II glottic carcinoma.[265] All except eight were followed until death or for a minimum of 10 years. The 10-year actuarial survival estimate was 63.1% for the "successful local control" patients and only 30.8% for "local recurrence" patients. Of the local recurrence group, 44.6% died *of their initial disease* compared with only 6.3% in the local control group. The 10-year actuarial lymph node control estimate was 96.1% for patients achieving local control with their first operation and 70.2% for those failing initial local control. Of patients experiencing local control with their initial surgery 96.7% never experienced metastases, a figure that dropped to 80.2% for patients who did experience local recurrence. Salvage treatment was unsuitable for 4.7% of patients with local recurrence. For those in whom it could be applied it yielded an 86.7% local control rate, a 21.4% laryngeal preservation rate, a 4.5% death rate, and an 11.2% rate of incidence of severe complications.

Frontoanterior Vertical Partial Laryngectomy

◆ **Patient Selection**   The classic indication for frontoanterior VPL was an early anterior glottic cancer that

- involved the AC, the anterior third of one vocal cord, and the anterior half of the other.
- exhibited unimpeded vocal fold mobility—T2a but not T2b.
- had no more than 10 mm of subglottic extension (presumably keeping the cancer high enough—within the embrace of the thyroid cartilage, and safely above the upper margin of the cricoid). The surgeon should recognize the potential of T2 anterior glottic cancers for anterior inferior submucosal spread.
- did not threaten either arytenoid (raising the requirement for a fronto*lateral* VPL).
- remained confined within the larynx—no extra-laryngeal spread (**Fig. 4.34**).

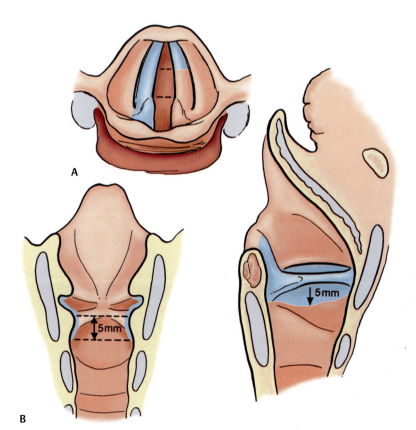

Fig. 4.34   The limits of tumor extension for resection of laryngeal cancer by frontolateral vertical hemilaryngectomy in (**A**) superior, (**B**) coronal, and sagittal views.

◆ **Surgical Technique** Perform a tracheostomy under local anesthesia. Induce general anesthesia. Suture the flexible endotracheal "J" tube into place to prevent distal migration toward the right main bronchus. If you need to revisit the endolaryngeal appearances (with no tube in the way), cover the tracheotomy site with adhesive Tegaderm (3M, St. Paul, MN) and perform a direct laryngoscopy. Carefully inspect the tumor limits with the 30 degree laryngeal telescope.

Make a horizontal skin incision in a crease at the level of the cricothyroid membrane. Elevate flaps superiorly to the hyoid and inferiorly to the first tracheal ring. Follow the plane of the strap muscles (deeper than the subplatysmal plane). Maintain the exposure with a self-retaining retractor like the May-Horner thyroid frame (Ethicon Surgery Company).

Release the sternohyoid muscle partially from its medial attachment on the side of least involvement or retract it to maximize the exposure. Leave the prelaryngeal fascia in place and make note of the status of the Delphian node in front of the cricothyroid ligament. Situate the vertical cartilage cut on this side (the good side) about one third the distance from the midline to the posterior limit of the ala.

Enter the laryngeal lumen at the site planned at the time of the laryngoscopy. Clear the tumor by a 2 mm margin or so on the side of least involvement. The shortened cord retracts toward the arytenoid. Place a 5–0 Monocryl mattress suture (Ethicon, Inc., Somerville, NJ) through the remaining thyroid ala, and anchor this cord as far anteriorly as possible (**Fig. 4.35**).

On the side of greater involvement, perform a similar resection, but this time with the advantage of having the tumor under direct vision. Consider reconstructing the missing cord on the more involved side with a sternohyoid muscle flap (**Fig. 4.36**).

◆ **Reconstruction**

Stenting Insert an Eliachar Laryngeal Stent (Hood Laboratories, Pembroke, MA) for 3 weeks to improve the shape and function of the glottic aperture after these maneuvers. Incise a small trapdoor flap in the top of the stent to dissipate the force of a cough. The stent will minimize the accretion of glottic adhesions and produce a better result than a keel.

Epiglottic Laryngoplasty Frontoanterior VPL fits the "horseshoe" AC cancers where cordal involvement is nearly symmetric. Some glottic cancers extend all the way around the glottis to (barely) the vocal process of the arytenoid cartilage of the least-involved side (**Fig. 4.37**). Epiglottic laryngoplasty (the Kambic-Sedlacek reconstruction[266,267]) provides a valuable reconstructive option to closure around a keel.

VPL with epiglottic reconstruction (VPLER) is an open operation for early anterior glottic region ("anterior commissure") carcinoma described by Sedlacek in 1965,[268] Kambic et al in 1976,[266] and Tucker et al in 1979.[269] The hallmark of this approach is the reconstruction. The surgeon repairs the site of the anterior laryngeal tissue loss with a pull-down sliding epiglottic advancement flap. The anterior glottic complex lost by the excision is supplanted by the epiglottis and the newly redundant AE and false vocal cords as the epiglottis is brought into the supportive framework of the larynx. Indications are limited because there must be no epiglottic or extensive ventricular involvement. The reconstruction uses the epiglottis to provide support and adequate mucosa for glottic competence. Cure rates are excellent with careful selection, and patients are generally able to swallow by the tenth postoperative day. The phonatory results are usually poor. Nowadays, transoral laser surgery, frontolateral partial

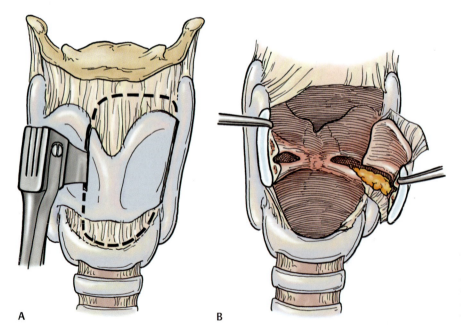

A　　　　　　　　　　　B

Fig. 4.35 Frontolateral partial laryngectomy. (**A**) The medial cartilage incision extends beyond the midline to the thyroid cartilage so that an incision through it will clear the tumor on the underlying vocal cord. (**B**) The larynx is opened and tumor extent visualized. The tumor on the cord of least involvement is cleared by a 1 to 2 mm margin of healthy tissue.

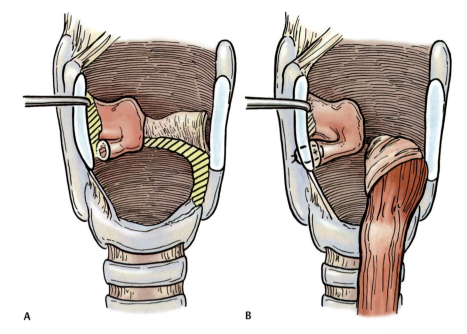

Fig. 4.36 Frontolateral partial laryngectomy. (**A**) Defect following resection. The tumor on the cord of least involvement is cleared by a 1 to 2 mm margin of healthy tissue. The resection of the cord of greatest involvement is similar to that for a standard hemilaryngectomy. (**B**) The resected cord is reconstructed with a sternohyoid muscle flap. An anchoring suture fixes the residual cord to the remaining thyroid ala.

A

B

laryngectomy, or radiotherapy are all more commonly offered for early cancers at the AC site. Eckel[270] found VPLER useful for local recurrences following failed endoscopic laser resection and in selected patients with recurrence following radiotherapy. It is also an important operation for primary

tumors at the AC presenting with overriding problems with exposure—transoral laser surgery would be contraindicated by this finding.

The approach is identical to that for a frontolateral VPL. The perichondrium is split in the midline and incised both supe-

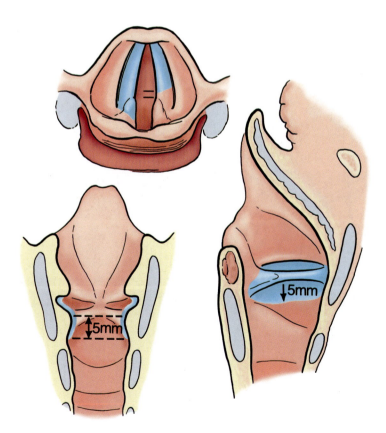

Fig. 4.37 The limits of tumor extension for resection of laryngeal cancer by the extended hemilaryngectomy operation with epiglottic laryngoplasty (Kambic-Sedlacek-Tucker procedure).

riorly and inferiorly throughout its length (**Fig. 4.38**). The cartilage cut on the most affected side is unchanged and on the least involved side is carried around almost to the same extent (**Fig. 4.39**). Superiorly, an incision is made in the inferior aspect of the thyrohyoid membrane, completely separating the insertion of the epiglottis from the thyroid cartilage. Inferiorly the cricothyroid membrane is incised horizontally (**Fig. 4.40**). Using this incision, the most involved site is cut with scissors along the cricoid arch, through the cricoarytenoid joint and the interarytenoid area.

On the side of least involvement the cricoid is again hugged with the scissors, and an incision across the cord is made 1 to 2 mm beyond the lesion. The specimen is removed, and it is obvious that most of the thyroid cartilage has been excised (**Fig. 4.41**). No attempt is made to turn muscle flaps for the reconstruction of each individual cord. The petiolus of the epiglottis is grasped with a tenaculum and retracted inferiorly. Dissection on the anterior surface of the epiglottis into the PES is done. This is a simple maneuver. Scissors dissection proceeds until the epiglottis is pulled with ease into the defect left by the thyroid cartilage excision. As the epiglottis prolapses into the gap, it pulls with it the false cords and the AE fold mucosa, which become folded upon themselves (**Fig. 4.42**). This redundant mucosa compensates for the lost cords, and the epiglottis for the lost structural component. The epiglottis is sewn in place with long-lasting suture such as Monocryl (**Fig. 4.43**). The thyroid perichondrium is approximated (**Fig. 4.44 and Fig. 4.45**), the strap muscles are returned, the wound is drained, and the skin is closed (**Fig. 4.46**).

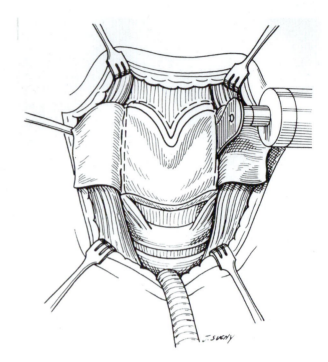

Fig. 4.39 Cartilage cuts being made with saw. (From Tucker HM, Wood BG, Levine H, et al. Glottic reconstruction after near total laryngectomy. Laryngoscope 1979;89:609. Reprinted with permission.)

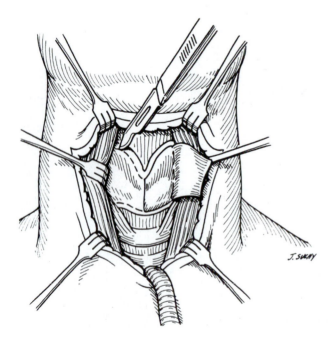

Fig. 4.38 Strap muscles retracted and perichondrial cuts being made. (From Tucker HM, Wood BG, Levine H, et al. Glottic reconstruction after near total laryngectomy. Laryngoscope 1979;89:609. Reprinted with permission.)

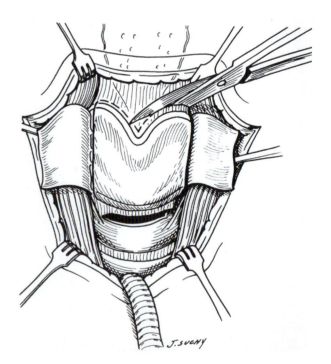

Fig. 4.40 Cricothyroid membrane incised and left thyrohyoid membrane being cut with scissors. (From Tucker HM, Wood BG, Levine H, et al. Glottic reconstruction after near total laryngectomy. Laryngoscope 1979;89:609. Reprinted with permission.)

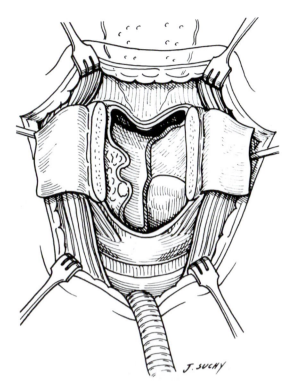

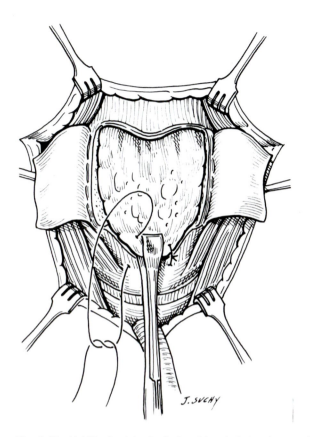

Fig. 4.41 Surgical defect after completion of near-total laryngectomy. (From Tucker HM, Wood BG, Levine H, et al. Glottic reconstruction after near total laryngectomy. Laryngoscope 1979;89:609. Reprinted with permission.)

Fig. 4.42 (**A**) Base of epiglottis being grasped with tenaculum and preepiglottic space contents being dissected away with scissors. (**B**) Lateral view of preepiglottic space contents being dissected away from anterior surface of epiglottis. (From Tucker HM, Wood BG, Levine H, et al. Glottic reconstruction after near total laryngectomy. Laryngoscope 1979;89:609. Reprinted with permission.)

Fig. 4.43 Mobilized epiglottis displaced interiorly into laryngeal defect and base being sutured to cricothyroid membrane. (From Tucker HM, Wood BG, Levine H, et al. Glottic reconstruction after near total laryngectomy. Laryngoscope 1979;89:609. Reprinted with permission.)

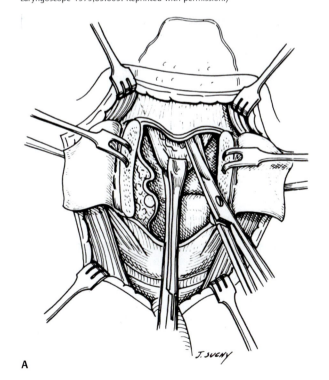

A

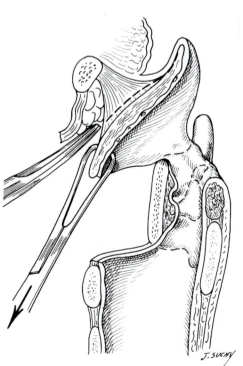

B

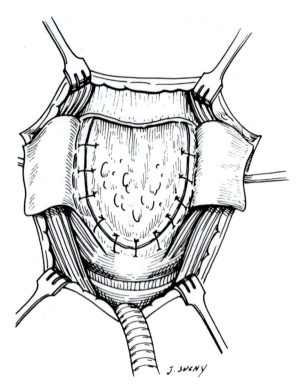

Fig. 4.44 Epiglottis sutured to thyroid ala remnants and cricothyroid membrane (complete). (From Tucker HM, Wood BG, Levine H, et al. Glottic reconstruction after near total laryngectomy. Laryngoscope 1979;89:609. Reprinted with permission.)

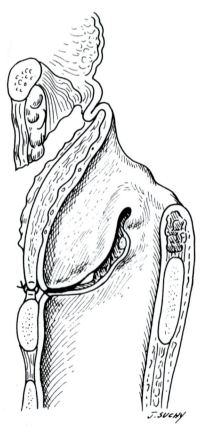

Fig. 4.45 Lateral view of epiglottis sutured to cricothyroid membrane in a submucosal fashion. Also depicts close proximity of endolaryngeal mucosa, which is not sutured. (From Tucker HM, Wood BG, Levine H, et al. Glottic reconstruction after near total laryngectomy. Laryngoscope 1979;89:609. Reprinted with permission.)

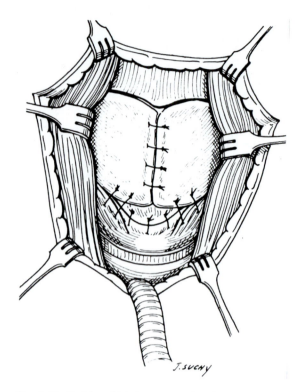

Fig. 4.46 Perichondrial closure completed.

◆ **Postoperative Management**　Speaking is discouraged for 10 to 14 days, and decannulation weaning is begun at this time. Oral feeding is delayed for the same span of time. Fortunately, aspiration is not much of a problem, and decannulation is usually successfully achieved.

◆ **Results**　Lelievre et al reported on 18 partial vertical reconstructive laryngectomies with epiglottoplasty in which he always preserved both arytenoids and usually more thyroid cartilage than Tucker described. Decannulation was achieved on the thirteenth day, and the mean hospital stay was 22 days. One patient developed a swinging epiglottis after 2 years.[271]

Three-Quarter Laryngectomy

The appropriate place to discuss a much less common and not very frequently performed inferior extension ("three-quarter laryngectomy") is probably here.

◆ **Patient Selection**　In selected patients with a cancer involving both the ventricular fold and the true cord, some surgeons have advocated a so-called extended (three-quarter) supraglottic laryngectomy technique (**Fig. 4.47**). This seems to be an attempt to combine a supraglottic resection and a hemilaryngectomy (**Fig. 4.48**). Three-quarter laryngectomy creates a significant aspiration problem. In a standard supraglottic laryngectomy the only protective sphincter remaining in the upper airway is that of the intact mobile true vocal cords. In the extended procedure this last guardian of the airway is compromised by the removal of one

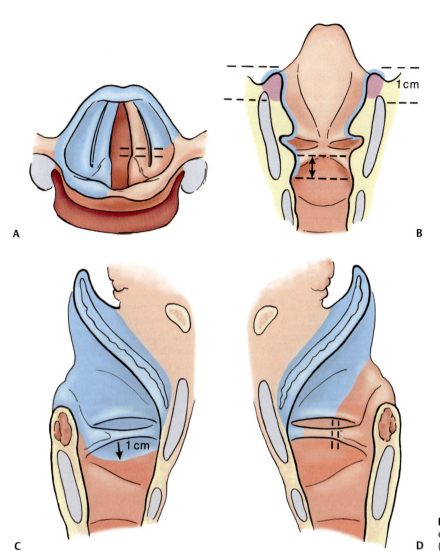

A

B

C

D

Fig. 4.47 Limits of tumor extension resectable by extended supraglottic laryngectomy. (**A**) Superior, (**B**) coronal, and (**C**) and (**D**) opposing sagittal views.

cord. The neocord replacing it must be substantial in size and the remaining cord fully mobile to avoid aspiration. It is said to be possible to resect the anterior one third of the contralateral cord, but some of these patients cannot be safely decannulated.

Surgical Techniques   The skin incision is the same as that for a supraglottic laryngectomy (**Fig. 4.25A**), and a radical neck dissection is usually required. Split the thyroid perichondrium in the midline and widely elevate the perichondrial layer back to the inferior constrictor, from top to bottom and side to side. The cartilage cuts anticipate removal of the entire lamina on the most involved side, and the upper half on the opposing side (by means of an oblique cut, angling to the superior cornu). Enter the hypopharynx through the vallecula. Transect the supraglottic mucosa on the least involved side as if you are performing a supraglottic laryngectomy—cross the false cord in front of the arytenoid, and enter the ventricle above the true cord. At the midline, bisect the AC with the scalpel and drop down to the cricothyroid membrane. Continue back and up with scissors. Follow the superior rim of the cricoid cartilage back and up to the cricoarytenoid joint. Then rise

across the interarytenoid muscles and remove the specimen (**Fig. 4.49**).

Repair the defect left behind after a three-fourths laryngectomy with an osteomuscular flap.[272] Release the mylohyoid muscle at the upper border of the body of the hyoid bone and free a small piece (~5 mm), pedicled on its attached strap muscles. Turn the muscles in 90 degrees toward the laryngeal cavity. Substitute the hyoid bone for the removed arytenoid and use the muscles to bridge over the laryngeal hemilumen as a glottic replacement. Advance the postcricoid mucosa to cover the transplanted hyoid bone or it will never survive. Lift the cut edge of the thyroid cartilage up to the base of the tongue. Suture them together with 2–0 Monocryl to close the wound and maintain essential elevation (to swallow) (**Fig. 4.50**).

◆ **Results**   Tu et al reported 108 cases treated within a period of 12 years (1979 to 1990).[272] Three-year survival rates for 66 supraglottic cases ranged from 78.6% for stage II to 66.7% for stage IV; for 42 stage II glottic cases, 79.3%. The decannulation rate was 80%, a socially acceptable voice was achieved by 80% of the patients, and all cases resumed oral food ingestion.

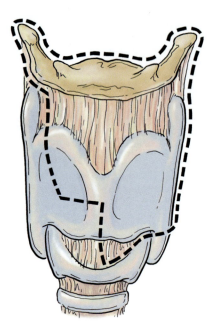

Fig. 4.48 Suprahemilaryngectomy. Almost the entire thyroid external perichondrium is elevated. Cartilage incisions require the excision of most of the thyroid lamina on the side of greatest involvement, leaving only a vertical 3 mm cartilage posterior strip between the superior and inferior thyroid cornua. The contralateral ala is incised horizontally to its midportion, then inclined obliquely upward. The thyroid cartilage is also cut in the midline from top to bottom, to facilitate dissection.

Transoral Laser Microresection for Early Glottic Cancer

Of the various therapeutic strategies discussed in this monograph, TLM is probably the one that has undergone the greatest expansion[273] since the original publication of *Management of the Difficult Case* in 1986. Since then, most of the otolaryngology community has accepted the idea that endoscopic laryngeal surgery is feasible and that early cancers are potential candidates. What is currently gaining interest is the mounting evidence that

- the perioperative morbidity is less than the oncologically equivalent open approaches.
- the long-term outcomes of oncologically equivalent procedures are equal to, or better than, outcomes with the open approach.
- costs are much lower.

TLM is characterized by a low complication rate, rare use of a tracheotomy, decreased stays in hospital, and apparent improvements in swallowing. In true vocal cord lesions, voice outcomes can be equivalent to radiation with less treatment morbidity. Local recurrence, distant spread, and survival all compare favorably with open approaches and even more so with radiotherapy.

Unfortunately, the name *minimally invasive transoral laser-assisted microsurgical resection* fails to convey the concept. Minimally invasive transoral resection is often neither "minimally invasive" nor completely "transoral." The pressure of the instrumentation can disable the tongue, and the surgery can divide arteries and extend out to the inner aspect of the strap muscles. It can necessitate open neck dissections, feeding gastrostomies, selected tracheotomies, or combined through and through excisions where the neck dissection becomes confluent with the laser wound. Transoral "laser" surgery is also transoral cautery and transoral forceps surgery. A laser is necessary for TLM, but insufficient. Safe endoscopic laser resections cannot be done without specialized forceps for grasping and manipulating the specimen and insulated suction cauteries with or without microclips for hemostatic vascular control. *Microsurgery* suggests the microscope but overlooks the essential specialized laser-endoscopes, the very helpful endolaryngeal telescopes, and the requirements for suspension and video. The associated neck

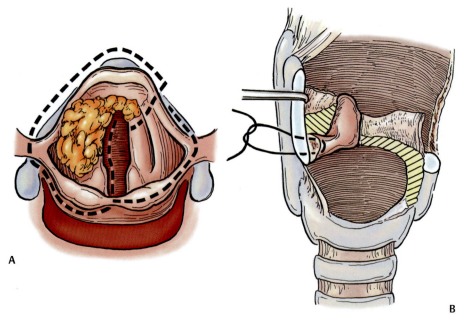

A

B

Fig. 4.49 Suprahemilaryngectomy. (**A**) On the side in which the vocal cord is not involved with tumor, the incision is made similarly to the supraglottic laryngectomy cut on the side of least involvement. When the anterior commissure is reached, it is bisected and the membranous incision is carried through to the cricothyroid membrane. The superior surface of the cricoid is hugged with the scissors, but now the outer blade cuts through the medial wall of the pyriform sinus at the level of the cricoid. In the hypopharynx, a vertical incision connects the one through the vallecula with the one previously mentioned in the medial pyriform wall. This connecting incision usually runs through the lateral pharyngoepiglottic fold and anterior pyriform fossa apex. (**B**) Larynx with residual cord following extended supraglottic laryngectomy.

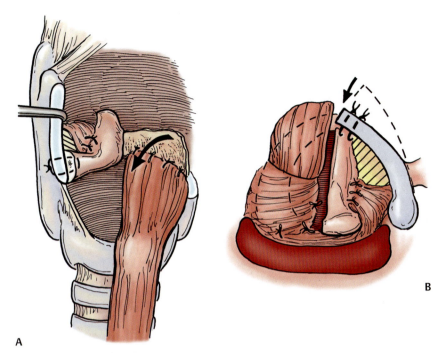

Fig. 4.50 Suprahemilaryngectomy. (**A**) A large neocord fashioned from as bulky a flap of strap musculature as possible is sutured into the defect created by the excision on the side of greatest involvement. It is sutured posteriorly as closely as possible to the remaining cord. (**B**) A flap of pyriform fossa and postcricoid area mucosa is sutured over the neocord.

operations are not "micro." Resection is the dominant curative agent but it is not the only use of the laser. Sometimes we use vaporization to produce central tumor reduction or distal margin advancement. Sometimes the narrow cutting beam is defocused and broadened for microcauterization.

Open conservation surgery, carefully selected, offers cure—at a price. Consider the conduct of the procedure itself. After an endoscopy and biopsy, we open the neck. Then we disassemble the muscles, nerves, and vascular structures in the neck and expose the larynx for resection. We cannot *see* the cancer at this point: we approach it on its deep surface ("blind" side). We enter the aerodigestive tract, restudy the field we have now distorted, and remove all the tissue judged to contain the cancer, plus a safety zone of surrounding normal tissue; all this without the magnification or stability of an operating microscope. The specimen must come out in one piece (Halsted's en bloc principle). When bleeding is cauterized, and the margins reported free, we advance the edges of the defect. More tissue is mobilized and sutured to separate the closure site from the neck. Then we reassemble the remaining layers over a drain, close the skin wound, and perform a tracheotomy. A feeding tube is placed in the stomach.

Contrast this with "minimally invasive" TLM to accomplish the same thing, through the natural passageway, the mouth. Specialized laryngoscopes expose the cancer right away: the actual mucosal margins are visible even before the first incision. A finely adjusted CO_2 laser-cutting beam is directed with a micromanipulator under microscopic magnification and high-intensity illumination. The tumor is drawn one way or another to suit the linear orientation of the cutting beam. The surgery follows the actual tumor, not some standardized bloc determined without the diagnostic guidance the operation itself is providing. No need to duplicate "standard" operations. The mucosal margin is obvious. The deep margin is clearly demonstrated by laser-dividing the tumor right through its center, all the way to normal underlying tissue. The tumor can be subdivided into manageable units because, unlike a steel instrument, a beam of light can transect cancer without physical transplantation of viable cancer cells from one location to another. Each can be exposed and removed step by step, improving exposure and diagnosis, until the cancer is completely excised. The safety margin of normal surrounding tissue is individualized—the least chance of overtreatment, the best chance of complete removal. Once the margins are negative, the operation is done. There is no attempt to close the gap or mobilize tissues in the area. And with no opening in the neck, we have eliminated the risk of a fistula.

If the original findings so indicate, a second-look microlaryngoscopy can be performed several weeks later. Because the primary wound was never closed, granulation can be removed and submitted for biopsy, a measure of quality control that closed operations cannot duplicate. A second look can provide the earliest possible detection of persistence at the primary site. Limited recurrence can be removed with a laser. Radiotherapy remains an option. The local microcirculation has not been disturbed by the endoscopic approach. Open conservation surgery remains available as well. However, reports of salvage surgery are a rarity, possibly due to the initial success of TLM in achieving local control.

If an elective neck dissection is indicated, a second look is a good time to do it. There is no communication into the aerodigestive tract, so the neck dissection is sterile. Air cannot enter the neck from a cough. Blood cannot enter the airway from the neck. Under these conditions, neck dissection is a more predictable operation, with an expected hospitalization of only 3 to 4 days.

TLM is now well described, including in English, and can no longer be considered an unconventional option for treatment.

Laser Extended Cordectomy (Includes Anterior Commissure), or Laser Frontolateral Partial Laryngectomy

◆ **Patient Selection** In our practice, this operation is the "vertical partial laryngectomy" of choice. Inability to expose might be the only contraindication. Because it carries such a strong diagnostic component and is such a rational approach—customized to every patient—transoral laser frontolateral partial laryngectomy supersedes the open operations.

◆ **Preoperative Considerations** TLM requires a personal apprenticeship, a patient with realistic expectations, a stable microscope, a reliable CO_2 laser, an extensive array of well maintained laser and microlaryngeal equipment, special endoscopes, hand instruments, cautery, plume suction, and a willing able frozen section histopathologist. The cords must be mobile.

◆ **Surgical Techniques** Much more in the way of detailed intraoperative instruction is provided elsewhere in this chapter. Pertinent to early glottic disease is the issue of AC involvement.

Zeitels described a satisfactory technical sequence to determine whether a glottic cancer has invaded the thyroid lamina anteriorly *before* the surgeon disturbs the structural integrity of the Broyle ligament. Begin by lifting the larynx with the blade and distal tip of the laryngoscope ("elevated vector suspension")[54] and transecting the anterior vestibular folds and the thyroepiglottic ligament with the laser. This provides an avenue to approach the superior inner aspect of the angle of the thyroid cartilage *and* the superior surface of the AC. Using increased external counterpressure on the thyroid cartilage to tip the larynx, observe the actual insertion of the Broyle ligament into the cartilage. If the carcinoma requires it, this exposure will allow complete endoscopic resection of the AC and even the associated cartilaginous framework. By following a plane down on the deep surface of the strap muscles, you can even include the cricothyroid ligament and the Delphian lymph node. A negative anterior infrapetiolar supraglottic exploration justifies judicious preservation of the AC anatomy. This in turn improves the prospects for a good voice.

Laser excision can be expanded to beyond the vocal ligament into the PGS laterally, onto or including the AC anteriorly, or below into the subglottis as well as superiorly into the supraglottis. The limitations, as far as one author of this chapter is concerned (PJD), is invasion of cartilage. These patients will require open partial or, more safely, total laryngectomy.

Local Control after Transoral Laser Microsurgery

Between 1979 and 1991, Steiner treated more than 1200 patients with malignant tumors of the upper-aerodigestive tract transorally using laser microsurgery with curative, palliative, or symptomatic intention. In 1993, he reported 240 patients without prior treatment, treated before 1985 with curative intention for cancer of the larynx.[30] He excluded patients with simultaneous second primaries and/or distant metastases. No patient had N3 (UICC 1987) neck metastases, but the series otherwise included all stages of disease (pTis-pT4 (p)N0-pN2c). He divided his patients into two groups. Group A (*n* = 159) included very early and early glottic cancers. All patients were treated by laser microsurgery. Six percent developed local recurrences and only one patient required a total laryngectomy. The overall 5-year survival rate (Kaplan-Meier) was 86.5%. The adjusted 5-year survival rate was 100%.

In a retrospective study of 160 patients with very early and early laryngeal cancer treated by laser endoscopic microsurgery from 1988 to 1996, Moreau[274] reported a corrected actuarial survival at 5 years of 97% for the 98 infiltrative glottic tumors and 100% for the 18 infiltrative supraglottic and 27 in situ carcinomas. No local recurrences were noted, in either the 118 infiltrating cancers (in whom two precancerous lesions were treated with a further laser excision), or in the 27 in situ carcinomas. Thus local control was 100%. One patient died of his cancer, with lung metastases after neck recurrence. The authors credited strict case selection, as in cases with significant involvement of the AC, for their excellent results.

Eckel et al[275] reported 85.8% local control for all patients with glottic carcinoma, stages I and II, treated with laser surgery (*n* = 202) from 1986 to 1994. Their cause-specific survival was 96.7%. They considered laser microresection to be superior to radiotherapy in its ability to produce cure more quickly, more safely, and at less cost.

In 1996, Steiner and Ambrosch updated their TLM results for 271 patients with very early and early (T1a,T1b,T2a) glottic cancer.[276] The treatment was laser microresection only, and they reported 29 patients with Tis, 151 with T1 cancers, and 81 with T2a (i.e., vocal cord mobility was okay). Cancer involved the AC in 42% of their patients. The incidence of local recurrence was 8%. Three patients received a total laryngectomy. The incidence of voice preservation was 99%. Two patients died of the cancer but not from local disease. Intercurrent deaths from other causes were as follows: from second primaries, 4.4%; from other intercurrent diseases, 20%; and from cause unknown, two cases. The overall 5-year (Kaplan-Meier) survival rate was 85%, nearly identical to their earlier report.

Voice Results after Transoral Laser Microsurgery

Sittel et al studied voice results in eighty patients after TLM of T1 or T2 glottic cancers. Resection or preservation of the AC played a key role, whereas the amount of tissue removed bore little relation to voice quality. Glottic voice production mechanisms yielded better results than supraglottic substitute phonation.[277]

Rosier et al found that for 81 T1a and 25 T1b glottic carcinomas treated between 1979 and 1995, radiotherapy and laser yielded similar oncological and functional outcomes.[278]

(Open partial laryngectomy was also effective for cure but not as successful for voice quality.) With a median follow-up time of 63.5 months, the 5- and 10-year locoregional control was 91 and 87%, respectively, whichever treatment was selected. Because laser excision and radiation therapy (RT) produced identical cure rates and equally satisfactory voice outcomes, laser excision was the preferable treatment based on the issues of cost and future second primaries. The actuarial incidence of a second primary reached 19% at 10 years in this series, and of course the adverse impact of prior radiotherapy on the treatment of the second primary was never a feature for patients who had been treated with the laser.

Cost of Transoral Laser Microsurgery

In a cost analysis and comparison between laser cordotomy and external beam radiation for early glottic carcinoma, Brandenburg found that laser surgery was much less expensive.[25] "Lost time from work," a factor that would have made the differences even larger, was excluded. The cure rates were equivalent, and the voice quality after laser cordotomy was comparable to the voice obtained after radiation.

Treatment of Early Supraglottic Cancer

Radiotherapy

Freeman and Mancuso found that the likelihood of local control after radiotherapy was related to primary tumor volume. An adequate estimate of the volume could be obtained through CT. For supraglottic cancer, favorable tumors were those less than 6 cubic centimeters in volume.[168]

By 1987, supraglottic laryngectomy and bilateral conservation neck dissection had long proven its value for early supraglottic disease. Whenever the neck was positive, however, it became common to add high-dose radiotherapy to the program. This undermined the functional rehabilitation achieved. So supraglottic laryngectomy, at the height of its powers in terms of exceptional local control, became controversial again. Radiation alone or total laryngectomy enjoyed a resurgent advocacy, not because of the unsuitability of a particular supraglottic cancer for a partial laryngectomy, but for the prognosis after treatment in the neck.

Patients with small supraglottic lesions usually retain a normal voice whether irradiated or operated. With both treatments there is some difficulty in swallowing. Radiation damages the lubrication. Surgery alters the mechanics. Unirradiated patients are probably in a better position to deal with a second primary cancer in the head and neck. This is a slightly more frequent problem in supraglottic than in glottic cancer.[279]

Irradiation alone is frequently successful in controlling lesions that involve more than half of the PES. Thus radiotherapy is a logical first choice if a total laryngectomy is deemed the only other treatment option. However, where near-total laryngectomy or a supracricoid partial laryngectomy is available, a total laryngectomy is almost never "the only other treatment option." Lee et al,[280] from the M.D. Anderson Cancer Center, reported good results with combined supraglottic laryngectomy and postoperative irradiation for patients with moderately advanced lesions. But Pinilla et al found a significant reduction in survival in patients who failed irradiation as initial treatment for their supraglottic tumors compared with the minimal influence of failed radiation on overall survival in glottic tumors.[281] Glottic cases can usually be salvaged after failed irradiation, possibly because the problem remains local. Supraglottic cancer is more prone to extend to involve the neck during the extra time afforded to it by the failure of initial treatment.

These data raise special concern about the cases in which radiotherapy failed locally. Radiorecurrent supraglottic cancer does usually necessitate a laryngectomy. If the neck was involved, bilateral neck dissections would not be uncommon as well. Total laryngectomy and bilateral neck dissections carry a significant risk of major morbidity (fistulae, pharyngeal stenosis, etc.) after high-dose radiation.

If a supraglottic laryngectomy failed locally, an attempt to salvage the patient with radiotherapy alone would be uncommon because the success rate would be low. But radiotherapy would not be the only option. Total laryngectomy and bilateral neck dissection would usually be possible and advisable. In an unirradiated neck, the risk of a total laryngectomy and bilateral neck dissection is low. Surgery also yields a specimen. If the histopathology so indicated, high-dose salvage radiotherapy could be added to follow the surgery. This would not be an impediment to future surgery—the maximum surgery would already have been completed.

Supraglottic cancer metastasizes to the neck. Even small primaries are known to be dangerous in this manner. The PES is essentially a midline structure. Cancer metastasizing from the supraglottis puts both sides of the neck at risk. The lymphatics of the supraglottic larynx drain to cervical lymph nodes via the PES. Tumors with PES invasion are already considered to be T3 in TNM staging.[161] Neck metastases often lead to radiotherapy. Neck radiotherapy includes radiotherapy to the primary site, especially if both necks are targeted. Surgery in the neck affects the primary site, too. Neck dissections necessarily impair lymphatic drainage from the primary site.

Radiotherapy and supraglottic laryngectomy (or supracricoid laryngectomy) are a very poor combination. Given before surgery, radiation treatment increases the chance a supraglottic laryngectomy will be a wrong choice of procedure. Usually, it will be an underestimate. Prior radiotherapy increases the likelihood a surgeon performing a supraglottic laryngectomy will misjudge margins. When patients undergoing near-total laryngectomy for advanced supraglottic cancer had received prior radiotherapy, the local failure rate was over 15 times the rate observed in patients who had not previously been irradiated.

In an N0 neck, if no cancer is present, irradiation will obviously "succeed." This provides padded statistics for therapy, and no information on prognosis. If cancer was present but occult, a neck dissection, which need not be radical, removes cancer earlier and identifies its presence. This may influence the approach to the opposite neck, or to the follow-up. It educates the investigator who, after successful irradiation, will always remain in doubt about the validity of the treatment, having no information as to the true status of the neck. Sometimes either treatment fails in an N0 neck. If it was dissected, the information gained at surgery (e.g., carotid involvement or extracapsular node invasion) may provide the critical justification needed to recommend additional treatment. If it was irradiated, everything in the neck will get firm, and by the time the failure is obvious to palpation, the time for a successful salvage operation will have passed.

At the editor's (PJD) institution, prophylactic irradiation appears to be as effective as radical neck dissection in eliminating microscopic neck disease and equal or even superior to conservation neck dissection. Unfortunately, the irradiation induces a good deal of laryngeal edema that interferes with the early acquisition of swallowing and airway competence. However, when the lesion invades the tongue base or has an appreciable extension over the so-called marginal area, the addition of postoperative irradiation adds a margin of insurance.

The temptation to turn to prophylactic postoperative irradiation, which has been claimed to be a serious competitor of block dissection in eliminating microscopic cancer in the neck,[282] is not justified by our own experience. After a supraglottic laryngectomy, radiation induces a persistent glottic edema that interferes with the timely acquisition of a safe airway. Operative impairment of the regional lymph drainage in the neck might contribute. A tracheotomy will manage this problem, but now the patient acquires the most objectionable part of a *total* laryngectomy. The tracheotomy is likely to be long-standing, quite possibly permanent. The main advantage of conservation surgery is lost. The patient required two major treatments and secured less of a chance to achieve a local cure with no aspiration. A total laryngectomy up front might have been a better choice; or a near-total laryngectomy. A near-total laryngectomy would not have avoided a tracheotomy, but it would have established it primarily, with greater safety, with consent. And it likely would have preserved a lung-powered, nonprosthesis-dependent voice.

Perhaps when the cancer invades the tongue base, or is poorly differentiated, or is associated with multiple nodes with extracapsular invasion, the addition of postoperative radiation contributes hope. But it should never be relied upon to sterilize margin-positive residual disease at the primary site, or to compensate for optimistic conservatism in the neck.[283] Steiniger et al reported 29 patients undergoing supraglottic laryngectomy. Seventeen received postoperative radiotherapy, and 12 did not. Irradiated patients had a higher incidence of lifelong gastrostomy dependency (35% vs 0%; $p = 0.03$) and acute upper airway obstruction (29% vs 0%; $p = 0.05$). There was a trend toward greater tracheotomy dependency (24% vs 0%), aspiration pneumonia (35% vs 9%), and delayed independent swallowing (34.8 weeks vs 7.8 weeks). Overall survival was equal in both groups.[283]

Mendenhall et al[284] summarize a list of important reasons for postoperative irradiation when supraglottic cancer is treated surgically: positive or close margins, subglottic extension, thyroid cartilage invasion, extension of the primary tumor to the soft tissues of the neck, perineural invasion, vascular space invasion, two or more positive nodes, and extracapsular extension. They preferred to avoid routine high-dose preoperative or postoperative irradiation in supraglottic laryngectomy.

Unfortunately, chronic obstructive pulmonary disease (COPD) is commonly present in patients with laryngeal cancer. The addiction to cigarette smoking that is at least partly responsible for the genesis of the neoplasm is also integral to the development of this respiratory ailment. Leonard and Litton[285] showed that at least 66% of their postoperative supraglottic patients demonstrated cineradiographic evidence of aspiration. They had to convert 12% of their patients to a total laryngectomy for this reason. Predicting how well an individual with mild to moderate COPD will do with a supraglottic laryngectomy is most difficult. The patient with dyspnea at rest or on slight exertion is definitely not a candidate for this operation. Pulmonary function indices such as the forced expiratory volume in 1 second (FEV_1) are helpful to assess obstructive and restrictive pulmonary disease. Hypoxemia indicates the seriousness of a ventilation-perfusion mismatch. The old-fashioned "two-flight test" is still a good predictor, too. A patient that can climb two flights of stairs without being unduly short of breath will most likely tolerate a supraglottic laryngectomy without significant respiratory trouble.

Smoking suspension and intensive follow-up screening, especially for pulmonary cancer, may be the most important tools we have to reduce mortality in supraglottic cancer.[279] Wagenfeld et al found a second respiratory tract malignant neoplasm developed in 20 of 163 cases of supraglottic carcinoma. Using an actuarial method of calculation, they projected that 19% of survivors will experience a second respiratory tract malignant neoplasm within 5 years after the diagnosis of supraglottic carcinoma, which is three times the incidence in patients who survive glottic carcinoma and 14 times the incidence in the normal population. The death rate from intercurrent disease in patients with supraglottic carcinoma was twice that seen in the general population, and this difference was due almost entirely to second respiratory tract tumors. They pointed out that even if the cure rate of patients with primary supraglottic carcinoma was 100%, only half of these patients would actually be alive at 5 years, owing to deaths from intercurrent disease.[279]

Horizontal Supraglottic Laryngectomy for Early Supraglottic Cancer

The diagnosis of supraglottic cancer is often delayed until the volume is great. But supraglottic laryngectomy can deal with more extensive cancers than those usually treated by hemilaryngectomy. Supraglottic laryngectomy is usually combined with at least one neck dissection, and it produces a higher incidence of immediate and late postoperative complications than hemilaryngectomy. Our practice is to perform a modified neck dissection on the side of greatest involvement, for staging, exposure, and clearance. If the primary neck dissection is reported to be positive, at least a conservation neck dissection is performed on the opposite side. An aggressive policy with regard to the neck is essential in supraglottic cancer because this is the site most often responsible for failure.

Supraglottic laryngectomy has outstanding results for local control—with proper selection and expert performance. Until some nonsurgical cancer therapy emerges that is clearly superior in outcome, it will continue to merit our respect. But what proportion of patients should have a supraglottic laryngectomy? Some reviewers cite the variable incidence in one center versus another as evidence that performance depends upon referral patterns and the "philosophy" of the doctor, not the intrinsic merits of the operation. Others argue that the true proportion of *candidates* is an absolute, defined by tumor extent and pulmonary studies, but because every patient suitable for a supraglottic laryngectomy also has other choices, one would predict these differing proportions. Comorbidities play a role in treatment selection. So does experience, and experience is usually anecdotal. Patients have a say. So does the literature, although inconclusively—supraglottic cancer is a biological challenge, not an industrial model.

◆ **Patient Selection** Supraglottic laryngectomy works very well for cancers that "fit" within a particular laryngeal block: the anatomical supraglottic larynx (except for the arytenoids). Whenever supraglottic laryngectomy is extended *beyond* the supraglottis, patients experience too much aspiration. Therefore, the determination must be made, preoperatively, that a cancer fits within the supraglottic laryngectomy block (the "supraglottic supraglottis").

In the office, the lower margin is hard to see: the supraglottic cancer overhangs it. But the anterior lower clinical margin is probably the easiest one to assess by the voice. The AC has to be free, and if it is, the voice is usually normal.

Both the arytenoids should be free. So should the AE fold. The cuneiform cartilage is a typical guide to the posterior margin. Both false cords should exhibit normal movement. This is not a typical observation that laryngologists make. It must be made in supraglottic cancer, however, and in the office because direct laryngoscopy is too late. When motion is impaired, cancer probably invades the deep lateral margin (the PGS), and a *supraglottic* supraglottic laryngectomy will prove insufficient.

Whole organ sections of laryngectomy specimens suggest that a tumor situated above and below the glottic level may have arrived there not by crossing the ventricle but by encircling it. In so doing, part of the tumor is visible posterior to the ventricle (or on the arytenoid cartilage) This, then, is a finding that contraindicates supraglottic laryngectomy, with or without limited mobility of the true vocal cord.

Some patients are poorly suited to supraglottic laryngectomy. The primary cancer might fit the criteria, but the patient does not. A patient with marginally compensated pulmonary insufficiency can easily slip into pulmonary failure from intermittent aspiration after surgery. Approximately half the patients with lesions technically suitable for supraglottic laryngectomy were judged ineligible on this account, or due to other major medical problems, according to Mendenhall and Parsons[295]. Medical comorbidities are the best-known contraindications to supraglottic laryngectomy, but psychological factors deserve equal notice. Fear, unrelenting cough, sleep deprivation, and inability to talk after surgery render elderly patients prone to confusion. Depressed patients are passively uncooperative, thus unable to fully recover in the aftermath of surgery. Complications, which delay discharge, can precipitate withdrawal, depression, and disruptive psychosis after surgery. Just when you need to sustain a feeding tube, a tracheotomy, or a dressing, the patient loses heart.

The patient and family are often instrumental in making a decision to avoid surgery. Age and family reluctance are an important signal of caution, at least. This is sometimes stated in terms of their previous experiences with surgery or radiation therapy (which may or may not be a valid influence). More often it may reflect an unspoken fear by those who know the patient best. A deeply unmotivated patient becomes too burdensome to the family after surgery.

The difficulty is that none of these criteria are easily quantified. In the end, a badly based decision *not* to offer supraglottic laryngectomy can lead down the road to salvage surgery. Larger conservation operations are almost always contraindicated in that context. Even a total laryngectomy may fail to conjure up a cure.

◆ **Preoperative Considerations** According to Weinstein et al, CT and MRI offer valuable help in evaluating the tongue base, vallecula, hyoid bone, PES, and thyroid cartilage.[286] Others find CT is important to evaluate the neck, but it plays little role in determining the feasibility of supraglottic laryngectomy for supraglottic carcinoma. Maroldi et al[287] correlated their CT detection rates with surgical and pathological data for tumor spread to the glottis, the thyroid and arytenoid cartilages, the pyriform sinus, and the base of the tongue. Of 69 surgically treated patients with supraglottic laryngeal carcinoma, 31 had supraglottic laryngectomies, and 33 total laryngectomies. Preoperative CT correctly assessed the glottis (as negative or positive) in 52/69 (only 75.3%). In deciding the feasibility of supraglottic laryngectomy, endoscopy alone did not differ significantly from endoscopy plus CT. Basically, when the safety of a supraglottic laryngectomy was at issue, CT did not alter the decision made by endoscopic examination often enough to justify its routine use.

Painstaking preoperative counseling is absolutely essential before a supraglottic laryngectomy. All patients need to be apprised of certain possible eventualities. They will be sedated but awake for the temporary tracheostomy, then asleep for the rest of the surgery. The induction of general anesthesia will be safe, not compromised by the tumor, and the tumor itself will not be traumatized by intubation. We will restudy the tumor under magnification this way, in its pristine state, with no tubing in the way, nothing to interfere with endoscopy, or with the telescopes we intend to use to reconfirm that the tissues we intend to save are tumor free and safe to preserve.

The patient should be told to expect severe difficulty in swallowing, including the probability that a temporary gastrostomy will be required before swallowing is restored. A gastrostomy would be especially common and lasting if extension to the tongue base is found. The tumor may turn out to be more extensive than originally thought. A supracricoid laryngectomy may be necessary if the glottic level is involved. A near-total laryngectomy might be required if the PGS is invaded. Both will preserve communication, but the voice will be very different. There may be a need for a tracheostomy for a prolonged period of time (even if a supraglottic laryngectomy is done). This is especially true if radiation is added postoperatively. A near-total laryngectomy will necessitate the acceptance of a permanent tracheostomy. The knowledge that the voice is preserved, despite the presence of a tube, helps immeasurably in the encouragement of surgical patients.

◆ **Surgical Technique**   The anatomical limits of a supraglottic laryngectomy were discussed earlier (**Fig. 4.51**). As-

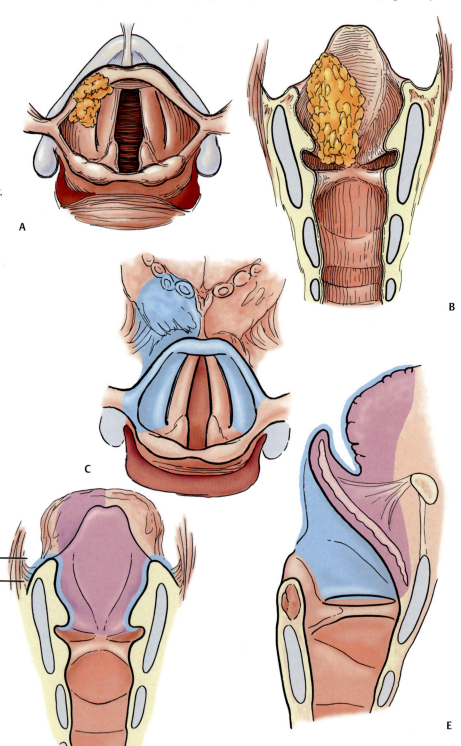

Fig. 4.51 Supraglottic laryngectomy. (**A,B**) Appearance of typical lesion; (**C**) superior, (**D**) coronal, and (**E**) parasagittal views of the limits of tumor extension for resection of laryngeal cancer by supraglottic laryngectomy.

suming, then, a policy of supraglottic laryngectomy plus unilateral or bilateral neck dissection for early supraglottic carcinomas, the open operation proceeds as follows.

A tracheostomy is sited below the thyroid isthmus and later kept out of communication with the operative field. It is usually performed under local anesthesia and intravenous sedation. A "J" tube, a wire-spiral reinforced endotracheal tube, is connected to the hose extensions supplied by anesthesia from the foot of the table and also a CO_2 sensing line. General anesthesia is induced, and the "J" tube is secured with a suture. In preparation for the endoscopic examination that follows, we cover the trache site with a sterile adhesive film (Tegaderm, 3M).

By lifting the epiglottis with a Lindholm laryngoscope (the square end fits into the vallecula and elevates the tongue base) we can achieve preliminary exposure of the larynx without touching or obscuring the supraglottis in any way. Rigid 30 and 70 degree laryngeal telescopes provide a panoramic view of the uninstrumented laryngeal interior. Bypass the lesion to obtain a view of the AC and the glottis. Examine the more distal features as well. Conclude the endoscopic examination (and biopsy if appropriate) with the passage of a nasogastric feeding tube.

Approach the cancer through a horizontal skin incision sited in the skin crease about the level of the cricothyroid ligament (**Fig. 4.52**). On the side of the associated neck dissection, extend the incision up the sternomastoid to the mastoid. Unless positive level 2 nodes are in contact with the accessory nerve as it travels between the skull base and the undersurface of the sternocleidomastoid muscle, it is not necessary to include the accessory nerve in the neck dissection. In a staging (N0) neck, the jugular vein and the sternomastoid muscle can also usually be spared. A more pressing consideration is the proximity of level 2 or 3 disease to the hypoglossal or vagus nerves.

Loss of either will have such a profound impact on swallowing as to make recovery from supraglottic laryngectomy almost untenable on functional grounds. With appropriate individualization to safeguard these nerves, an adequate dissection to remove all the lymph node–bearing tissues of the first neck needs to be accomplished.

In practice, we usually perform the neck dissection in a discontinuous manner, then turn our attention to the larynx. The pedicle of the neck specimen in continuity with the supraglottic specimen is quite small—only the omohyoid muscle and its fascia. There is little point obstructing access to the larynx by preserving it. During the supraglottic laryngectomy, the pathologist studies the neck. A positive frozen section report (on a neck we had judged N0 clinically) would favor a simultaneous conservation neck dissection on the other side, after the supraglottic resection was concluded.

The supraglottic laryngectomy itself begins with the exposure of the anterior aspect of the larynx. The object of the approach is threefold:

- Expose the upper two thirds of the thyroid laminae.
- Confirm that no carcinoma has infiltrated so far forward in the PES that the thyrohyoid membrane is compromised.
- Produce the inferiorly based muscle/perichondrial flap that will become the eventual closure between the glottic unit and the tongue base (**Fig. 4.53**).

Extend the field of exposure from the suprahyoid tissues to the bottom of the thyroid cartilage. Cleanly incise the strap muscles from the hyoid and reflect them downward *with the thyroid perichondrium* (**Fig. 4.54**). Take care to incise the

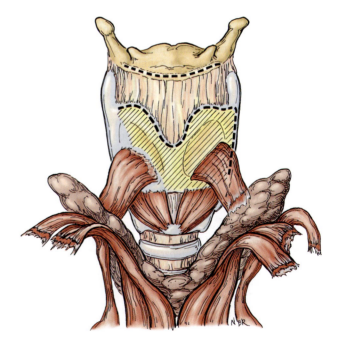

Fig. 4.53 Supraglottic laryngectomy. Strap muscles are dissected from the hyoid bone along with some hyoid periosteum (*upper dashed line incision*). Perichondrial incisions are outlined on the thyroid alae. Shaded area represents amount of perichondrial elevation.

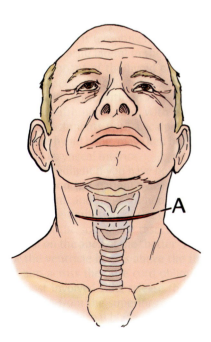

Fig. 4.52 Incisions for partial laryngectomy. For supraglottic laryngectomy.

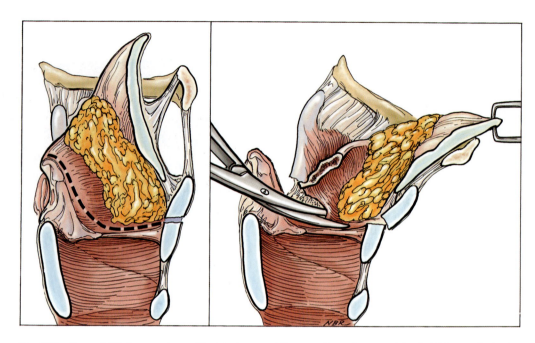

Fig. 4.58 Supraglottic laryngectomy. The intralaryngeal line goes from the aryepiglottic fold near the body of the arytenoids through to the apex of the ventricle, through the ventricle with one scissors blade and through the laryngeal soft tissues via the cartilage cut with the other blade.

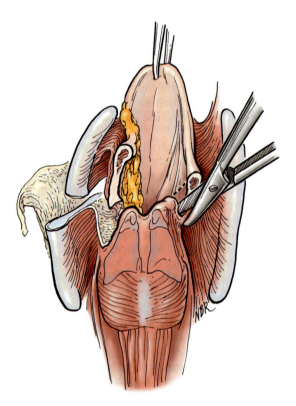

Fig. 4.59 Supraglottic laryngectomy. The scissors now engage the aryepiglottic fold on the least involved side. The start of this incision is usually further anteriorly on the fold than on the side of greatest tumor involvement. This facilitates the passage of the outer scissors blade through the more anteriorly placed cartilage cut of the least involved side. This incision meets that of the opposing side, and the tumor of the supraglottis is removed from the rest of the larynx.

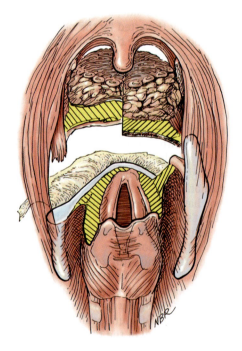

Fig. 4.60 Supraglottic laryngectomy. If the vallecula or tongue base is involved, a generous margin of healthy tongue is mandatory. Illustration shows defect remaining following supraglottic laryngectomy with substantial tongue base resection.

suming, then, a policy of supraglottic laryngectomy plus unilateral or bilateral neck dissection for early supraglottic carcinomas, the open operation proceeds as follows.

A tracheostomy is sited below the thyroid isthmus and later kept out of communication with the operative field. It is usually performed under local anesthesia and intravenous sedation. A "J" tube, a wire-spiral reinforced endotracheal tube, is connected to the hose extensions supplied by anesthesia from the foot of the table and also a CO_2 sensing line. General anesthesia is induced, and the "J" tube is secured with a suture. In preparation for the endoscopic examination that follows, we cover the trache site with a sterile adhesive film (Tegaderm, 3M).

By lifting the epiglottis with a Lindholm laryngoscope (the square end fits into the vallecula and elevates the tongue base) we can achieve preliminary exposure of the larynx without touching or obscuring the supraglottis in any way. Rigid 30 and 70 degree laryngeal telescopes provide a panoramic view of the uninstrumented laryngeal interior. Bypass the lesion to obtain a view of the AC and the glottis. Examine the more distal features as well. Conclude the endoscopic examination (and biopsy if appropriate) with the passage of a nasogastric feeding tube.

Approach the cancer through a horizontal skin incision sited in the skin crease about the level of the cricothyroid ligament (**Fig. 4.52**). On the side of the associated neck dissection, extend the incision up the sternomastoid to the mastoid. Unless positive level 2 nodes are in contact with the accessory nerve as it travels between the skull base and the undersurface of the sternocleidomastoid muscle, it is not necessary to include the accessory nerve in the neck dissection. In a staging (N0) neck, the jugular vein and the sternomastoid muscle can also usually be spared. A more pressing consideration is the proximity of level 2 or 3 disease to the hypoglossal or vagus nerves.

Loss of either will have such a profound impact on swallowing as to make recovery from supraglottic laryngectomy almost untenable on functional grounds. With appropriate individualization to safeguard these nerves, an adequate dissection to remove all the lymph node–bearing tissues of the first neck needs to be accomplished.

In practice, we usually perform the neck dissection in a discontinuous manner, then turn our attention to the larynx. The pedicle of the neck specimen in continuity with the supraglottic specimen is quite small—only the omohyoid muscle and its fascia. There is little point obstructing access to the larynx by preserving it. During the supraglottic laryngectomy, the pathologist studies the neck. A positive frozen section report (on a neck we had judged N0 clinically) would favor a simultaneous conservation neck dissection on the other side, after the supraglottic resection was concluded.

The supraglottic laryngectomy itself begins with the exposure of the anterior aspect of the larynx. The object of the approach is threefold:

- Expose the upper two thirds of the thyroid laminae.
- Confirm that no carcinoma has infiltrated so far forward in the PES that the thyrohyoid membrane is compromised.
- Produce the inferiorly based muscle/perichondrial flap that will become the eventual closure between the glottic unit and the tongue base (**Fig. 4.53**).

Extend the field of exposure from the suprahyoid tissues to the bottom of the thyroid cartilage. Cleanly incise the strap muscles from the hyoid and reflect them downward *with the thyroid perichondrium* (**Fig. 4.54**). Take care to incise the

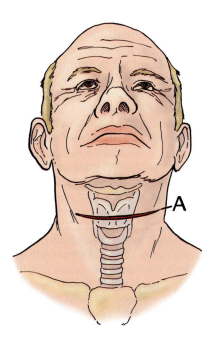

Fig. 4.52 Incisions for partial laryngectomy. For supraglottic laryngectomy.

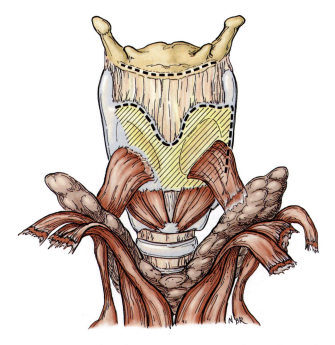

Fig. 4.53 Supraglottic laryngectomy. Strap muscles are dissected from the hyoid bone along with some hyoid periosteum (*upper dashed line incision*). Perichondrial incisions are outlined on the thyroid alae. Shaded area represents amount of perichondrial elevation.

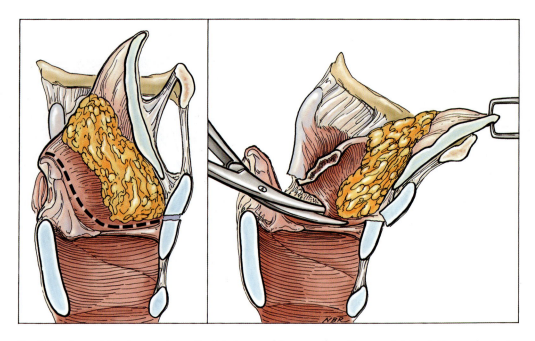

Fig. 4.58 Supraglottic laryngectomy. The intralaryngeal line goes from the aryepiglottic fold near the body of the arytenoids through to the apex of the ventricle, through the ventricle with one scissors blade and through the laryngeal soft tissues via the cartilage cut with the other blade.

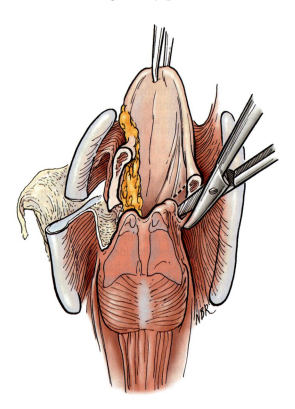

Fig. 4.59 Supraglottic laryngectomy. The scissors now engage the aryepiglottic fold on the least involved side. The start of this incision is usually further anteriorly on the fold than on the side of greatest tumor involvement. This facilitates the passage of the outer scissors blade through the more anteriorly placed cartilage cut of the least involved side. This incision meets that of the opposing side, and the tumor of the supraglottis is removed from the rest of the larynx.

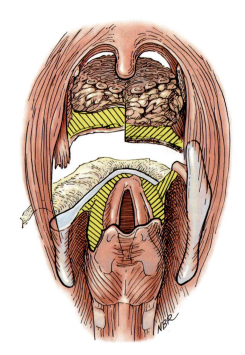

Fig. 4.60 Supraglottic laryngectomy. If the vallecula or tongue base is involved, a generous margin of healthy tongue is mandatory. Illustration shows defect remaining following supraglottic laryngectomy with substantial tongue base resection.

suming, then, a policy of supraglottic laryngectomy plus unilateral or bilateral neck dissection for early supraglottic carcinomas, the open operation proceeds as follows.

A tracheostomy is sited below the thyroid isthmus and later kept out of communication with the operative field. It is usually performed under local anesthesia and intravenous sedation. A "J" tube, a wire-spiral reinforced endotracheal tube, is connected to the hose extensions supplied by anesthesia from the foot of the table and also a CO_2 sensing line. General anesthesia is induced, and the "J" tube is secured with a suture. In preparation for the endoscopic examination that follows, we cover the trache site with a sterile adhesive film (Tegaderm, 3M).

By lifting the epiglottis with a Lindholm laryngoscope (the square end fits into the vallecula and elevates the tongue base) we can achieve preliminary exposure of the larynx without touching or obscuring the supraglottis in any way. Rigid 30 and 70 degree laryngeal telescopes provide a panoramic view of the uninstrumented laryngeal interior. Bypass the lesion to obtain a view of the AC and the glottis. Examine the more distal features as well. Conclude the endoscopic examination (and biopsy if appropriate) with the passage of a nasogastric feeding tube.

Approach the cancer through a horizontal skin incision sited in the skin crease about the level of the cricothyroid ligament (**Fig. 4.52**). On the side of the associated neck dissection, extend the incision up the sternomastoid to the mastoid. Unless positive level 2 nodes are in contact with the accessory nerve as it travels between the skull base and the undersurface of the sternocleidomastoid muscle, it is not necessary to include the accessory nerve in the neck dissection. In a staging (N0) neck, the jugular vein and the sternomastoid muscle can also usually be spared. A more pressing consideration is the proximity of level 2 or 3 disease to the hypoglossal or vagus nerves.

Loss of either will have such a profound impact on swallowing as to make recovery from supraglottic laryngectomy almost untenable on functional grounds. With appropriate individualization to safeguard these nerves, an adequate dissection to remove all the lymph node–bearing tissues of the first neck needs to be accomplished.

In practice, we usually perform the neck dissection in a discontinuous manner, then turn our attention to the larynx. The pedicle of the neck specimen in continuity with the supraglottic specimen is quite small—only the omohyoid muscle and its fascia. There is little point obstructing access to the larynx by preserving it. During the supraglottic laryngectomy, the pathologist studies the neck. A positive frozen section report (on a neck we had judged N0 clinically) would favor a simultaneous conservation neck dissection on the other side, after the supraglottic resection was concluded.

The supraglottic laryngectomy itself begins with the exposure of the anterior aspect of the larynx. The object of the approach is threefold:

- Expose the upper two thirds of the thyroid laminae.
- Confirm that no carcinoma has infiltrated so far forward in the PES that the thyrohyoid membrane is compromised.
- Produce the inferiorly based muscle/perichondrial flap that will become the eventual closure between the glottic unit and the tongue base (**Fig. 4.53**).

Extend the field of exposure from the suprahyoid tissues to the bottom of the thyroid cartilage. Cleanly incise the strap muscles from the hyoid and reflect them downward *with the thyroid perichondrium* (**Fig. 4.54**). Take care to incise the

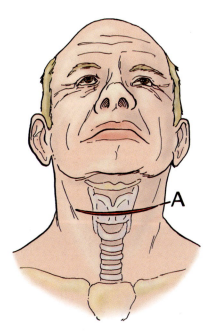

Fig. 4.52 Incisions for partial laryngectomy. For supraglottic laryngectomy.

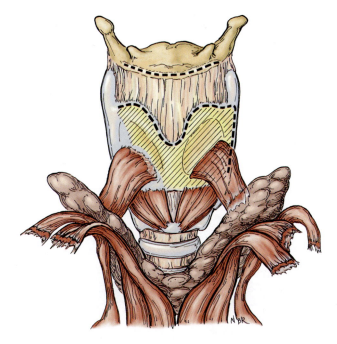

Fig. 4.53 Supraglottic laryngectomy. Strap muscles are dissected from the hyoid bone along with some hyoid periosteum (*upper dashed line incision*). Perichondrial incisions are outlined on the thyroid alae. Shaded area represents amount of perichondrial elevation.

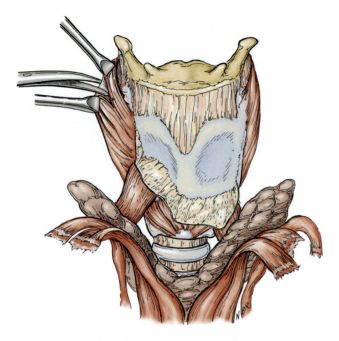

Fig. 4.54 Supraglottic laryngectomy. Perichondrium reflected.

perichondrium along the entire superior border of the thyroid cartilage to continue the reflection inferiorly.

Tattoo the cartilage cuts on the thyroid alae with a sharpened wooden Q-tip dipped in methylene blue. The proper level at the midline is just below the thyroid notch (**Fig. 4.55**). A good deal has been written about the level of the true vocal cords, the minuscule difference between males and females, and the division of the thyroid cartilage into fractions and

millimeters in the hope of guiding the surgeon.[288] From a practical standpoint, there are two crucial points:

- Take tremendous care not to injure the AC. Injure it and the patient may never swallow.
- Recognize that the level of the AC is nearly as high as the thyroid notch.

After a supraglottic laryngectomy, the patient depends on the competence of the glottis to protect the airway and allow swallowing. Low entry (seeking to avoid tumor) risks inadvertent damage to the AC tendon, or more accurately, its anchorage forward to the inside of the thyroid angle. The resulting loss of cord tension, quite apart from its effects on the voice, is a critical blow to deglutition. At least the lower three quarters of the angle of the thyroid cartilage should be preserved. Without this mooring point, the cords will bow, and aspiration will follow.

Use a Stryker saw to make the cartilage cuts down to the internal perichondrium. Carry the incision directly horizontally to the posterior border of the thyroid ala on the side of the greatest involvement. On the opposite side, the incision proceeds horizontally across the middle of the ala and then slants obliquely to the superior border, just ahead of the superior cornu. In preparation for the soft tissue resection, the patient should now be given a potent muscle relaxant in adequate dosage to assure complete relaxation of the vocal cords.

For a tumor limited to the supraglottic endolarynx, incise the suprahyoid musculature and enter the vallecula on the "better" side. If the vallecula might be involved, or worse, the tongue base, make your entrance through the opposite pyriform fossa (**Fig. 4.56**). Then make the suprahyoid cuts as the lingual extent of the tumor is directly visualized. Note that when the cancer extends above the supraglottis, the hyoid is not skeletonized.

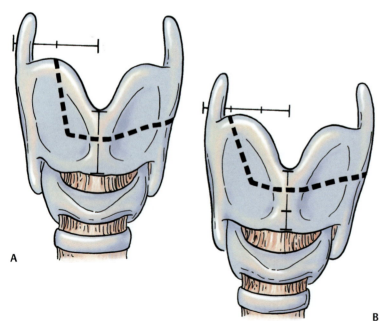

A

B

Fig. 4.55 Supraglottic laryngectomy. Cartilage cuts outlined in (**A**) male and (**B**) female.

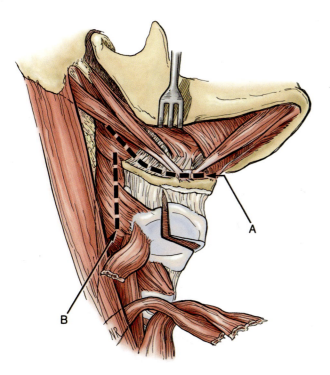

Fig. 4.56 Supraglottic laryngectomy. Line (A) represents a vallecular approach, used when the lesion does not extend onto the lingual aspect of the epiglottis. The pyriform fossa entrance (B) is used if there is lingular epiglottic, vallecular, or tongue base invasion.

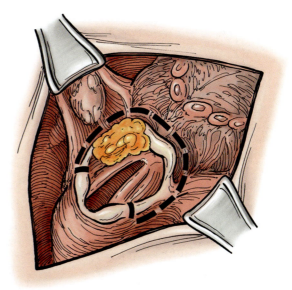

Fig. 4.57 Supraglottic laryngectomy. Resection proceeds superiorly, conserving pyriform sinus mucosa wherever possible. In lesions extending no further superiorly than the laryngeal surface of the epiglottis, the resection is carried just above the vallecula, with the tongue base musculature cut off at the level of the hyoid bone.

By careful dissection, it is usually possible to identify and preserve all of the superior laryngeal nerve on the less involved side. On the more involved side, an attempt to preserve this structure is usually thwarted by the need for an adequate deep margin, and in any case there is little sensory mucosa left to justify its preservation. On the side of least involvement, it is tempting to cut across the hyoid and leave the greater cornu lateral to the pyriform. However, in a slim neck, a remnant of the hyoid can feel like a palpable mass to the subsequent follow-up examiner. It is probably better to grasp the horn with an Allis clamp, carefully avoid the nearby twelfth nerve, and, with vigorous retraction, cut off all the attachments with a scalpel. The specimen, including the entire hyoid bone, may then be delivered forward to deal with the laryngeal interior.

Don a headlight if you have not already done so, and maximally extend the patient's head. Grasp the epiglottis with a tenaculum, and use skin hooks to retract the false cords. Confirm the limitation of the tumor to the supraglottic larynx. Begin the soft tissue resection with a limited mucosal incision on the apex of the "better" AE fold (**Fig. 4.57**). Notice that the ventricle begins above the tip of the vocal process, and aim across the false cord obliquely as if to reach it. On the most involved side, release the lateral wall of the pyriform fossa from the superior cornu of the thyroid cartilage. Position the internal blade of the scissors to cut sequentially across the cuneiform, down toward the vocal process at the level of the true cord, and forward to carry right on into the ventricle at its apex. Position the external blade to traverse

the medial pyriform sinus mucosa and follow a course across the anterior apex of the sinus (**Fig. 4.58**). At this point the external blade will continue out of the pharynx and into the soft tissue until it slips under the thyroid perichondrium into the cartilage cut (**Fig. 4.59**). Continue cutting, with one blade proceeding forward in the ventricle and the other in the horizontal cartilage cut.

Retract the supraglottis superiorly and unfold the specimen a bit. Pause to visualize the AC and the proximity of the cancer to the petiole. Extend the horizontal cut precisely above the commissure, crossing the midline to reach the anterior recess of the second ventricle. Direct the inner scissors blade within that ventricle and the outer scissors blade back up into the oblique cut made in the thyroid cartilage earlier. All this is on the remaining "better side." Transect the soft tissues carefully all the way back to the back of the ventricle. Then pass up through the AE fold and the pyriform to complete the release, again keeping a watchful distance from the posterior margin of the tumor. Inspect the specimen before you deliver it to the frozen section laboratory.

If the pyriform fossa was the site of entry to avoid vallecular disease, the superior release of the specimen remains to be accomplished. Turn the specimen up to avert the tongue base and proceed from the good side to the bad. Finish the final release through the lateral pharyngoepiglottic fold on the most involved side and deliver the specimen in one bloc (**Fig. 4.60**).

While the supraglottic laryngectomy specimen is undergoing quick-section analysis, don't forget to do a cricopharyngeal myotomy. Place an index finger in the pharynx, and continue down as far as the cervical esophagus. The lumen tightens up in the transitional zone, right behind the cri-

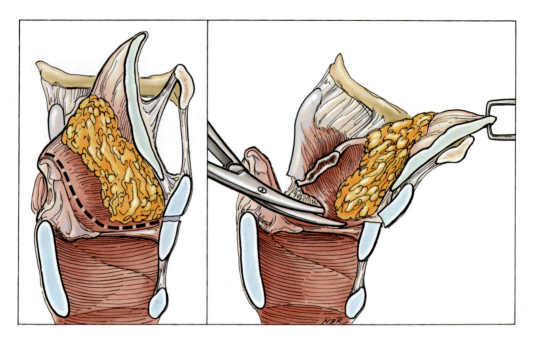

Fig. 4.58 Supraglottic laryngectomy. The intralaryngeal line goes from the aryepiglottic fold near the body of the arytenoids through to the apex of the ventricle, through the ventricle with one scissors blade and through the laryngeal soft tissues via the cartilage cut with the other blade.

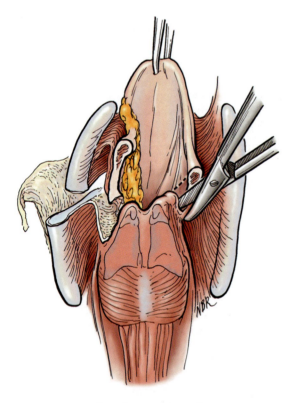

Fig. 4.59 Supraglottic laryngectomy. The scissors now engage the aryepiglottic fold on the least involved side. The start of this incision is usually further anteriorly on the fold than on the side of greatest tumor involvement. This facilitates the passage of the outer scissors blade through the more anteriorly placed cartilage cut of the least involved side. This incision meets that of the opposing side, and the tumor of the supraglottis is removed from the rest of the larynx.

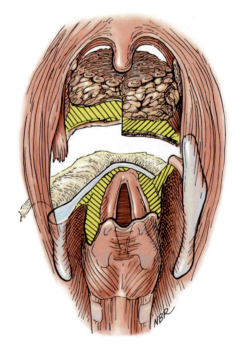

Fig. 4.60 Supraglottic laryngectomy. If the vallecula or tongue base is involved, a generous margin of healthy tongue is mandatory. Illustration shows defect remaining following supraglottic laryngectomy with substantial tongue base resection.

coid—the cricopharyngeus is simply that portion of the inferior constrictor that inserts on the cricoid. Close observation on the posterior surface of this zone reveals the horizontal striations of the muscle coat. Cut through the muscle (only) with a fresh scalpel, in the midline, to avoid the recurrent laryngeal nerves traversing the muscle, behind the cricothyroid joint, on their way to the glottic musculature. Safeguard the integrity of the mucosa by working in a dry field, seeing the muscle fibers part, and feeling the release of the constriction and the proximity of the blade edge to your finger. Cut ~2 cm, top to bottom. The remaining mucosa will appear perilously thin. It is durable, however, and it does not seem prone to spontaneous perforation.

Careful closure is the key to low fistulization rates and the successful rehabilitation of swallow. Mucosal approximation is not the object. The goal is to elevate the remaining larynx as high as possible and position the tongue base in an overhanging configuration. The primary closure is basically in one layer. Place all the sutures before any are tied. With the patient's head still in the extended position, begin the closure internally by suturing, for as far as possible, the medial pyriform mucosa to the residual arytenoid mucosa, using light catgut (**Fig. 4.61 and Fig. 4.62**). An unclosed area of considerable extent is left anteriorly to reepithelialize spontaneously. Continue with the external closure by suturing the thyroid perichondrial flap to the raw tongue base, using interrupted Monocryl mattress sutures. Tag the flap-to-tongue sutures (2–0 Monocryl) with mosquito hemostats while they wait to be tied. Each one penetrates raw tongue ~1 cm away from the cut edge of the mucosa. This will direct the cut surface of the tongue, not mucosa, to abut the raw surface of the

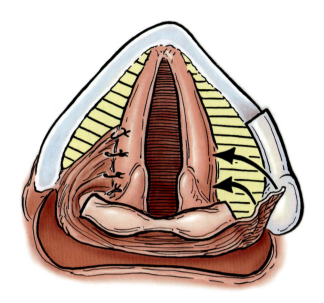

Fig. 4.62 Supraglottic laryngectomy. The medial pyriform sinus mucosa is elevated and approximated to the arytenoid and ventricular mucosa as far as possible without undue tension. The remaining area anteriorly is left raw.

excised false cord area (**Fig. 4.63A**). Approximate the lateral pharyngeal walls using 3–0 Monocryl.

Sharply flex the head and tie the sutures sequentially. Add as much of a second layer closure as possible with the strap muscles. Approximate them to the suprahyoid muscles with 3–0 Monocryl (**Fig. 4.63B**). This acts as an offset bed for the primary closure but it is not the *strength* of the repair. That resides in the perichondrial flap-base of the tongue closure. One might expect a partial dehiscence to lead to a fistula, but here it invites supraglottic stenosis. One way to offload some of the vertical tension is to place a 2–0 Monocryl suture through the cricothyroid ligament and snug it up toward the median mylohyoid raphe. Another is to release the sternothyroid muscle and eliminate its drag on the better side of the laryngeal unit. Drain the wound and close the skin. Some have proposed it may be helpful to keep the patient's head in the flexed position initially, and some surgeons have gone so far as to attach a wire to the mandible and secure it to the sternum during this period. We have not found that necessary. The low-pressure tracheotomy tube cuff should be inflated to prevent aspiration as the patient regains consciousness.

The excision of significant tongue base volume requires some type of flap reconstruction to preclude aspiration. A pectoralis or trapezius myocutaneous pedicled flap (**Fig. 4.64**) or a radial forearm free flap can be used. The deltopectoral flap was the workhorse flap for head and neck reconstruction for many years. Although it worked well, it has been replaced by these flaps that possess an island pedicle or are free vascularized tissue flaps, principally because it required a second operative stage to return the flap's pedicle to the chest. A gentle bulge of the flap into the hypopharynx can be created by sewing the flap's subepithelial tissue to itself. Oftentimes the actual bulk of a myocutaneous flap may not only preclude the need for these sutures, but in fact the

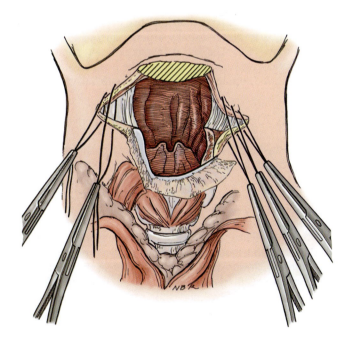

Fig. 4.61 Supraglottic laryngectomy. The pharyngeal closure is begun by inserting sutures in the lateral pharyngeal wall, approximating pyriform fossa mucosa to itself up the thyroid perichondrium.

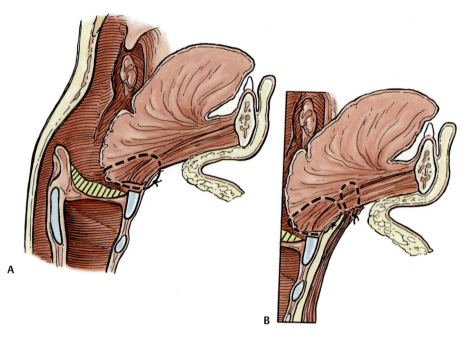

A

B

Fig. 4.63 Supraglottic laryngectomy. (**A**) The remaining closure is achieved by suturing the perichondrium to the tongue base. No attempt is made to achieve a mucosa-to-mucosa approximation. All sutures are placed, and then the head is flexed acutely forward and all the sutures are tied at once. Tongue base sutures must pass through mucosa and full-thickness muscle to securely anchor the laryngeal remnant. (**B**) A second layer consisting of strap muscles sutured to the tongue base musculature adds a little support.

flap may be too large. In time because of the lack of innervation to the muscle the flap will atrophy in time. On the other hand, a radial forearm free flap may need these sutures (**Fig. 4.65**).

◆ **Postoperative Management** Aspiration is an expected complication of supraglottic laryngectomy. Thin liquids are the most difficult to control. Patients usually do not begin swallowing until ~12 to 14 days. Soft, smooth-consistency foods such as applesauce or pudding should be used at the start.

Empathetic counseling and special instruction from a swallowing therapist (a speech pathologist familiar with laryngectomy patients and with swallowing problems in the neurologically impaired) are vital to success. Using half teaspoonfuls of food, one practice drill consists of the following:

- Inhale
- Hold your breath
- Swallow
- Swallow
- Cough
- Swallow
- Breathe

With assistance from the therapist, the patient corks the tracheostomy, clears the airway, places the food in the mouth, and initiates the drill. Therapists provide the time and encouragement necessary to shepherd a patient through a difficult rehabilitation. From pureed foods, the patient progresses to those with a more particulate consistency. Fluids, especially those with effervescence, are the most difficult to handle. Once swallowing with minimal aspiration is accomplished, the patient may abandon the drill in part, eventually discarding it entirely.

The presence of a tracheostomy after surgery makes swallowing more difficult. Here is the paradox. Successful deglu-

tition is sometimes delayed until the patient gets rid of the tracheostomy tube—but a tracheostomy tube with a cuff may be needed to prevent aspiration. Decannulation is impermissible until patients can swallow their secretions, but patients can't swallow their secretions until they are decannulated.

In the first few weeks after an open supraglottic laryngectomy, we delay full decannulation until after the larynx has passed inspection with a flexible transnasal endoscope. The patient should be able to demonstrate the ability to sleep in a recumbent position with the tube plugged. To shorten hospitalization, it is acceptable practice to go home with the feeding tube in place—usually a percutaneous endoscopic gastrostomy (PEG). The key is instruction and compliance. This practice can sometimes reduce the hospital stay for an uncomplicated supraglottic laryngectomy to 5 days.

◆ **Results** Ogura et al[289] reported on 263 patients with previously untreated squamous cell carcinoma of the supraglottic larynx treated at Washington University Medical Center in St. Louis between 1955 and 1971; 177 patients (67%) underwent a supraglottic laryngectomy. Lee et al reported on 404 patients who were treated for supraglottic cancer at the M.D. Anderson Cancer Center in Houston from 1974 to 1984.[280] Only 60 patients (15%) underwent conservation surgery. Fifty (83%) of 60 patients (thus almost everyone) who had surgery at the M.D. Anderson Cancer Center received postoperative radiotherapy. Presumably, almost everyone at the center had moderately advanced primary lesions or positive margins, and/or multiple positive nodes, or extracapsular extension. Early or intermediate primary lesions or patients without multiple positive nodes or extracapsular extension would not have had an indication for radiation. Finally, Weems et al[290] reported on 195 patients treated with either or both surgery and irradiation at the University of Florida between 1964 and 1984; 30 patients (15%) underwent a supraglottic

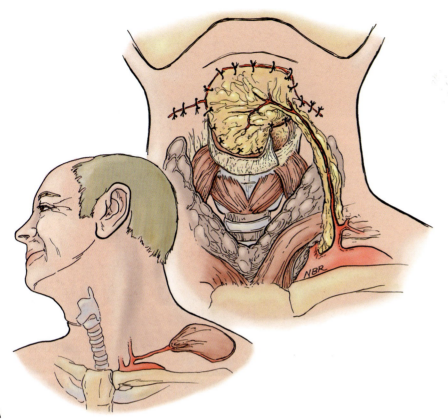

A

Fig. 4.64 Supraglottic laryngectomy. (**A**) A trapezius musculocutaneous flap is used to reconstruct the tongue base. (**B**) The flap is pedicled on the transverse cervical artery and rotated into position in a one-stage procedure. (**C**) Trapezius flap based on the transverse cervical vascular pedicle. (**D**) Flap rotated into place. Note the flap's bulge, which simulates the base of the tongue.

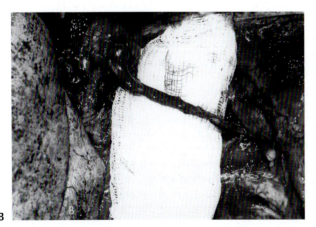

B

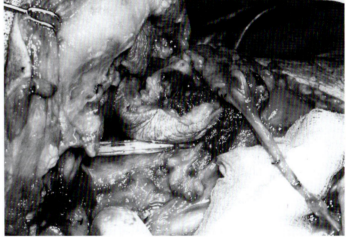

C

laryngectomy. Approximately half of the patients who underwent a supraglottic laryngectomy at the University of Florida received adjuvant irradiation.

Transoral Laser Microresection for Early Supraglottic Cancer

CO_2 Laser Supraglottic Laryngectomy

◆ **Surgical Techniques** Laser supraglottic laryngectomy begins with oral endotracheal intubation and general an-

esthesia. The intubating laryngoscope lifts the tongue, not the cancer. The ideal tube is laser shielded, with two cuffs, each inflated with saline.

With the exception of a Lindholm laryngoscope with extra suction tubes added, closed laryngoscopes are not suitable for this surgery. We prefer to operate through a bivalved distending supraglottiscope, such as the Storz 8588 E modification of the Weerda distending operating laryngoscope (Karl Storz Endoscopy-America, Inc.). The interior is matte to eliminate stray reflections. A mechanical table supports the suspension handle but maintains the freedom necessary

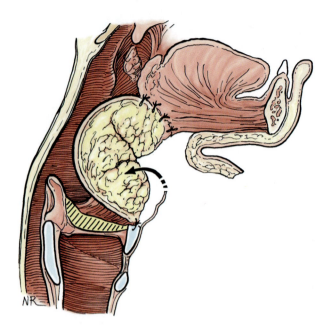

Fig. 4.65 Supraglottic laryngectomy. The flap is sutured to itself to produce a bulge to deflect the bolus during deglutition, which helps prevent aspiration. The distal flap is sutured to the cartilage remnant, with the perichondrium overlapping a portion of the new undersurface of the flap.

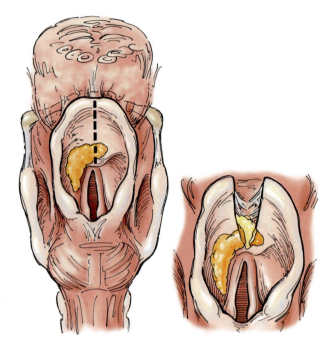

Fig. 4.66 Laser resection supraglottic carcinoma. Laser transects the epiglottis through the vallecula and hypoepiglottic ligament, bisecting the preepiglottic space, to the level of the hyoid bone. Tumor may be transected during this maneuver. The transection should be to the inferior limits of the tumor.

to readjust the view on a moment's notice. The nurse prepares four sets of suction tubes: one on the laryngoscope; one on the grasping forceps; one to the long, straight, insulated suction-cautery; and a spare. The microscope stand must be very stable. Fit the microscope body with a fine micromanipulator, like the Sharplan 712 Accuspot (Sharplan Lasers [UK] Limited), which is capable of producing a 0.25 to 0.3 mm spot size at 400 mm (objective lens). This permits a temperature gradient at the perimeter of the excision that is so sharp the zone of coagulation is only ~0.5 mm thick (i.e., the pathologist can evaluate the margin). Set the eyepieces at 0 and view a target at the highest magnification. Focus the red HeNe aiming beam (the CO_2 beam is invisible). Then personalize the eyepieces to be parfocal throughout the range of lower magnifications. Plan to cut, not vaporize. Most of the work is in continuous mode at ~4 to 8 watts.

Protect the teeth with a thermosetting hard plastic guard, the face with a moist towel, and the operating personnel with safety goggles (for the operator, the microscope fulfills this role). Place the upper blade of the endoscope in the vallecula and spread the blades to lift the base of the tongue and to expose the supraglottis. Reconfirm the tumor's dimensions and use angled laryngeal telescopes to reconfirm the distal margin.

1. Laser-divide the suprahyoid epiglottis in the midline—even if this divides some tumor. Carry this incision all the way down to the hyoid on the vallecular side. If possible, continue to the lower margin of the tumor on the laryngeal side (**Fig. 4.66**).
2. Starting from the hyoid region of the first incision, cut outward in the coronal plane, through the vallecula all

the way to the lateral pharyngoepiglottic fold (**Fig. 4.67**). Cross the fold to the beginning of the next mucosal incision, which will be from the termination of this latter incision across the medial wall of the pyriform sinus. Look for the superior laryngeal artery coming to supply the supraglottis. Coagulate it with an insulated alligator forceps, and *place at least one secure titanium hemaclip on the still viable main trunk* (**Fig. 4.68**).

3. Continue the mucosal incision in the upper part of the medial pyriform, and, depending on the extent of the tumor, include as much AE fold and ventricular fold as appropriate. Ultimately, you will cross below the tumor to join the lowest part of the initial vertical incision (**Fig. 4.69**). Notice that arytenoid resection would be an indication for a tracheotomy and a cuffed tube to preempt the inevitable aspiration this will produce in the postoperative period.
4. Approach the hyoid through the vallecular incision. Divide the hyoepiglottic ligament, if not already done so, at the hyoid to release the hemispecimen, and continue caudally to the upper margin of the thyroid cartilage. Note the inner aspect of the strap muscles, and stay in front of the PES. Out laterally, continue down on the inner aspect of the thyroid ala (**Fig. 4.70**). By careful observation through the vertical (initial) incision, two important points should be evident: (1) the lower limit of the infrahyoid cancer and (2) the upper limit of the AC.
5. Free the PES down to the petiole above the AC and remove the hemispecimen (sometimes removing the upper

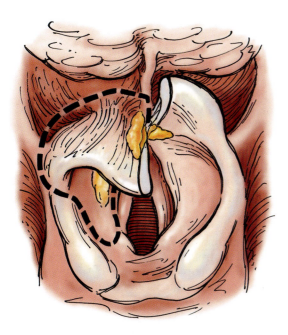

Fig. 4.67 Laser cut in the coronal plane laterally through the vallecula, hypoepiglottic and the fat of the preepiglottic space along the hyoid to the lateral pharyngoepiglottic fold. The resection should be to the inferior limit of the tumor. The anterior limit of the resection should be close to the thyrohyoid ligament superiorly and may extend inferiorly along the posterior surface of the thyroid cartilage as far as the insertion of the epiglottis on this cartilage.

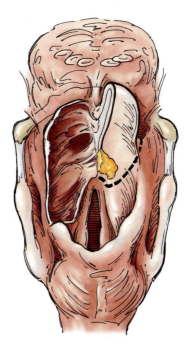

Fig. 4.69 The cut in the aryepiglottic fold or medial wall of the pyriform sinus is directed medially through the false vocal fold. It is extended anteriorly until it reaches the initial vertical cut in the epiglottis. All cuts must clear the mucosal and deep extent of the tumor.

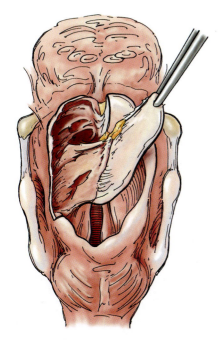

Fig. 4.68 The cut proceeds posteriorly across the pharyngoepiglottic fold onto the superior apex of the aryepiglottic fold, or if tumor is present more inferiorly through the medial wall of the pyriform sinus. Incision proceeds to the corniculate cartilage and crosses the superior laryngeal artery, which is clipped.

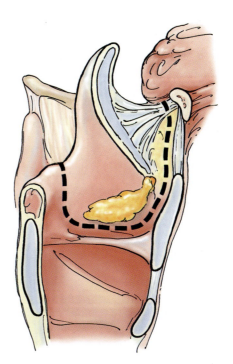

Fig. 4.70 If not already done at the beginning of the resection, the incision in the vallecula is extended through the hypoepiglottic ligament, which is now transected, and the incision is carried down to the upper level of the thyroid cartilage sticking to the anterior limit of the preepiglottic space and continuing down to the epiglottic petiole just superior to the Broyle ligament.

half, then the lower half, taking advantage of the laser's ability to subdivide a bulky specimen into more manageable subunits).

6. Tailor the laser excision of the opposite side in a similar fashion (**Fig. 4.71**).

7. Carefully confirm all margins with frozen section, and demonstrate absolute hemostasis with the telescopes and the microscope.

8. Place a nasogastric tube into the postcricoid lumen under direct vision, and plan to use it for about a week.

◆ **Postoperative Management** Most patients do not require a tracheostomy, but to pass on one is an individual clinical decision. Reasons for a tracheotomy might include a lengthy dissection with difficult access and tongue trauma. Here, a tracheotomy gets the intraoperative tubing out of the way and bypasses expected postop tongue swelling. Another might be risk of bleeding—no clip on the superior laryngeal artery or hypertension, or both, plus recent use of anticoagulants.

With intact strap muscles, no associated neck surgery, and no tracheotomy, the return of swallowing is faster than after open supraglottic laryngectomy. This is so even though there was no attempt at primary closure or glottic elevation at the time of the laser resection.

◆ **Results** The cure rates for early (and intermediate) supraglottic cancer using transoral carbon dioxide laser resection are comparable to the outcome after conventional open conservation resections. Iro et al reported 141 con-

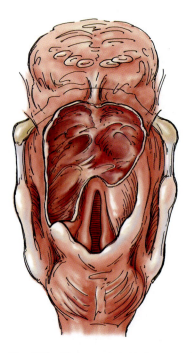

Fig. 4.71 The opposite side is resected tailoring it to tumor extent similarly to the first.

secutive patients with stage I to stage IV supraglottic carcinomas treated by TLM ± neck dissection ± radiotherapy between February 1979 and December 1993.[33] The 5-year recurrence-free survival rate for the 92 patients with UICC stage I, II, or III disease was 73.9%. What makes transoral carbon dioxide laser microresection a superior option to open supraglottic laryngectomy is the significantly lower morbidity. In Rudert et al's series,[58] with an overall 3-year survival for early stages of 88%, only seven of 34 patients, predominantly higher stages, required a tracheostomy.

Eckel and Schneider presented impressive data supporting their choice of TLM for early-stage supraglottic cancer.[275] Compared with radiotherapy it was safe, it saved time, and it was more cost-effective. Fifty-eight percent (290/504) of their consecutive institutional series of laryngeal cancer cases (all stages) from 1986 to 1994 were treated with this modality. Local control for all patients with stages I and II supraglottic carcinoma treated with laser surgery (n = 40) was 87.3%, and cause-specific survival was 78.6%. During the same period, total laryngectomy was performed in 130 patients (26%), conventional partial laryngectomies in 31 (6%), radiotherapy in 34 (7%), and 19 (4%) had no curative treatment.

The essential prerequisite for successful transoral carbon dioxide laser surgery in supraglottic cases is adequate resection technique. This means endoscopic access to the entire cancer. The limiting feature is exposure. Local control requires, first and foremost, clear resection margins.[33] It does not mean access all at once, or all the cancer in one field of view. The laryngoscope will be moved and repositioned during surgery. This is what allows the access to each margin in turn. Also it does not mean perfect exposure right away. The proximal supraglottis will be resected first. Then the distal margins will become accessible. In supraglottic cancer, in our experience, the "upper limit" of TLM depends not upon the bulk of the tumor but where and to what degree the tumor extends beyond the supraglottis, and, as in open surgery, the patient's comorbidities and physiological reserve. The question to ask is whether you can resect what you need to resect *without precipitating the need for open reconstruction.* Very early and early supraglottic cancers are almost always candidates for TLM because, strangely enough, no reconstruction, not even elevation of the larynx, is necessary. Perhaps the strap muscles (intact) provide the necessary vectors. Intermediate and advanced supraglottic cancers should only be considered candidates for TLM on a case-by-case basis.[33] Will the necessary resection destroy a cricothyroid unit? The cricoarytenoid unit consists of an arytenoid cartilage, the cricoid cartilage, and the associated musculature (and the superior and recurrent laryngeal nerves necessary for the reflex activity of that unit). Loss of the cricothyroid unit on one side doesn't just escalate the complexity and extent of the resection. Treacherously, it destroys the glottic mechanisms essential to protect against aspiration once the supraglottis is absent. Loss of the cricoid unit almost guarantees intolerable aspiration and dysphagia. Aspiration negates the goal of conservation. It usually necessitates secondary surgery.

Neck indications are a separate but important issue in supraglottic cancer treated by TLM. At least for N0 cases, selective, conservation, and bilateral neck dissections do not have to be performed at the same time as the transoral laser excision of the primary. After all, the neck is not being opened to access the primary. In some patients, especially the frail and elderly, staging may well improve the tolerance for supraglottic surgery. The patient can recover from the laser operation, regain swallowing, and then go on to have sterile (unconnected to an open pharynx) neck dissections at the second sitting.[276] The surgeon, informed by the final pathology report on the laser operation, can use this opportunity to undertake a "second look" direct laryngoscopy.

Management of the Neck in Early Supraglottic Cancer

Cervical metastases are much more likely in supraglottic cancer than in glottic or subglottic squamous cell carcinoma of the larynx, and prognosis is adversely affected by cervical metastases, the likelihood of which was increased in tumors with larger surface dimensions.[291] In Moe et al's study, the presence of three or more positive nodes predicted distant recurrence and decreased survival. So did level 1 and 5 involvement versus 2, 3, or 4. Age, sex, race, and tobacco or alcohol use were not associated with number or extent of regional metastases.[291] Macroscopic transcapsular spread is very strongly associated with neck node relapse. In a prospective study of 170 patients with squamous cell carcinoma of the larynx or the hypopharynx treated from 1981 to 1988, Brasilino de Carvalho found survival rates dropped from around 50% to 5.8% and 10.2%, respectively, when macroscopic transcapsular spread was present ($p < 0.0001$).[292] The risk of macroscopic extracapsular extension tracked the N category of the TNM classification and the diameter of any metastatic lymph node over 3 cm. *Microscopic* transcapsular spread of nodal carcinoma did *not* produce a statistically significant increase in recurrence or in death rates compared with the rates observed when metastatic disease was confined to the lymph nodes. Five-year global and disease-free actuarial survival rates were 56.8% and 52.0% in these categories.

In 1990, Lutz et al reported on 202 patients who underwent surgery for supraglottic cancer at the University of Pittsburgh School of Medicine between 1975 and 1986.[293] Just over one third (72 patients, 36%) received a supraglottic laryngectomy. A distinguishing characteristic of the overall group was the significant risk of recurrence in the undissected neck (despite adjuvant radiotherapy in many cases). Of 47 patients who developed recurrence (23% of the 202), 39 recurred in the neck, and of these, *35 were in the contralateral undissected neck.* Myers and Alvi[294] stated that since 1990, their policy has been to treat all patients with cancer of the supraglottic larynx with bilateral neck dissections. The indication for adjuvant radiation therapy has been the presence of extracapsular spread.

The indications for postoperative irradiation at University of Florida (UF) include close or positive margins, multiple positive nodes, and extracapsular extension.[16] Extracapsular extension is probably only meaningful when it is gross. Whenever the listed indications for postoperative irradiation include close or positive margins, one hopes this will not translate into a higher tolerance for close or positive margins. We do not trust radiotherapy to provide a reprieve. Supraglottic laryngectomy with close or positive margins should cause reflection on the root causes—patient selection or intercommunication impediments between the surgeon and the frozen section histopathologist.

In VPLs, supracricoids, near-totals, and totals, the selection of therapy at the primary site is based mainly on the primary tumor. It is little influenced by one's intentions toward the neck. Not so with supraglottic carcinoma. The treatment of the neck has a powerful bearing on the selection of treatment of the primary. Consider the case in which bilateral neck metastases are present. Unless the pattern of metastasis is such that both hypoglossal nerves, the suprahyoid elevators, and one jugular vein can be preserved, supraglottic laryngectomy is probably not advantageous. The supraglottis is a midline structure. Cancer cells entering lymphatic channels in the PES have access to both sides of the neck. Neck dissections remove lymphatic drainage routes. Two full radical neck dissections produce glottic/arytenoid edema. Swelling obstructs the airway. Submandibular triangle extirpations threaten the mylohyoid motor nerves from V3. This risks bilateral denervation of the mylohyoid and digastric muscles. Paralysis weakens elevation of the laryngeal remnant, required during swallowing. On the side of the greatest metastatic involvement, on the carotids, above the hyoid, the twelfth nerve lies at risk. In the absence of the supraglottis and with half the tongue and the thyrohyoid muscle paralyzed, aspiration can be intractable. In patients with bilateral neck disease, radiation therapy will often be instituted postoperatively. Arytenoid edema will increase. So will dysphagia. The priorities are airway, cure, swallow, and voice. Sometimes a supraglottic operation is incompatible with these goals when one considers its fate after neck treatment.

Early supraglottic cancer often presents itself with clinically negative neck nodes (N0) but still a high risk for occult bilateral neck disease. According to Mendenhall et al, these patients should be treated with radiation therapy because of the ease of bilateral elective neck irradiation.[295] Alternatively, patients with early supraglottic cancer but at high risk for occult bilateral neck disease would be candidates for supraglottic laryngectomy and bilateral conservation neck dissections. We start with the neck considered to be at highest risk. During the supraglottic surgery, we study it with frozen sections. If the first N0 neck proves negative, the likelihood of finding cancer in the other side (also N0) becomes minuscule. Surgery can be limited to the first side (and classified as a "staging conservation neck dissection"). If, on the other hand, the first side proves positive, conservation surgery is justified on the second side.

In this second scenario, at least one neck is positive. Thus the question will inevitably be asked, Is postoperative radiotherapy indicated? The answer depends on the answers to three subsidiary questions. How thorough and meticulous was the neck surgery? (It is hard to justify the permanent functional impairments associated with radiotherapy if the cancer has already been removed.) Did the surgeon look for and find macroscopic extracapsular extension? (Macroscopic extracapsular extension is the one evidence-based indication that the chance of recurrence is high. Unfortunately, it does not also indicate the responsiveness to radiotherapy is high.) Is there any finding other than extracapsular extension to favor radiotherapy versus simple vigilance in follow-up? (Macroscopic extracapsular extension is rare in the clinically and radiologically negative neck.)

For patients with early-stage primary lesions but *advanced* neck disease (N2B or N3), combined treatment is usually considered necessary to produce a high rate of control of the neck disease.[4] One strategy is to treat the primary lesion for cure by irradiation, then follow with bilateral neck dissections in the hope the primary is already controlled. If such a patient were treated by supraglottic laryngectomy and neck dissections *and postoperative irradiation*, the radiation therapy portals would almost invariably include the primary site. The morbidity from radiation to the larynx, a site that was probably already controlled by the surgery, tends to be high. Some consideration might be given to the proposition that if the indication for radiotherapy is the neck, the fields should reflect that fact and the laryngeal remnant should be spared.

Laryngeal cancer can appear, for the most part, in only three sites: the larynx, the lymph nodes, and the lungs. Lung metastases are late, extremely difficult to treat (even to palliate), and, fortunately, quite uncommon. A second cancer primary in the lung is more likely. The same risk factors pertain: inhaled carcinogens, susceptible genetics. The most important treatment of systemic metastases is to avoid them by controlling cancer at the primary site *with the first treatment.*

◆ Treatment of Intermediate Laryngeal Cancer (Species III)

Clinical concepts like "early" and "advanced" would not be very helpful if they overlapped. If *early* could be extended and still be "early," if *advanced* could be limited and still be "advanced," what would be the basis for classification? Some cancers do impair cord motion (suggesting "advanced") but also exhibit features favorable to conservation—a limited mucosal footprint, an exophytic morphology, a sharply demarcated margin. There *are* "in between" cases so there is an "intermediate" category. And embedded in the intermediate category can be sensed an operative strategy with a now well-established pedigree—supracricoid partial laryngectomy with reconstruction (cricohyoidoepiglottopexy [CHEP] or cricohyoidopexy [CHP]).

The classic partial laryngectomies (vertical hemilaryngectomy, horizontal supraglottic laryngectomy) are too little for intermediate laryngeal cancers. It is often possible of course to encompass intermediate cancers by *extending* a vertical hemilaryngectomy or *extending* a horizontal supraglottic laryngectomy. But extending the classic conservation procedures leads to unsatisfactory results. Local control is reduced. Swallowing is less predictable. The airway is compromised. The voice is disappointing. Near-total laryngectomy or total laryngectomy, the "advanced" surgical strategies, are too much for intermediate cancer. They impose a permanent tracheostomy, whereas radiotherapy does not (and neither does SCPL). Patients with intermediate cancer often do not actually hear of the appropriate surgical option—SCPL—because it is not offered everywhere. It is also the case that many physicians view "intermediate" cancer not as a distinct entity deserving of its own class, but as a quirky part of the "advanced" group. It is a favorable part, in the sense that the tumor volume is low (for an advanced cancer). This is taken to be an indication of radiosensitivity. Here is where the strategy of RRSS for T3 cancer *should* have the very best chance of succeeding. Here is where it might succeed *without* the "surgical salvage" component! In this paradigm, the place of "modern conservation surgery" is to salvage the occasional failure of radiotherapy. Radiate, because conservation surgery will preserve us all from the reason not to radiate (the dreaded total laryngectomy). As regards modern chemotherapy, perhaps neoadjuvant chemotherapy will further improve that chance of organ preservation.[260]

Intermediate laryngeal cancers extend across more than one region. For example, supraglottic cancer can, by descending to involve the vocal cords, exclude a supraglottic laryngectomy. And glottic cancer can, by its extent into the subglottis, undermine the support for a VPL. Some intermediate glottic cancers impair glottic motion (T2b). This is usually a sign of significant invasion into the muscle fibers, preferably in the anterior, not the posterior, reaches of the larynx. The cancer spares the arytenoid complex. The mobile tissues may be impaired, but they are not so pervaded as to be fixed. If these cancers were considered advanced, they do seem more favorable than what we typically mean by "advanced." Surgeons who do not see this as an invitation to RRSS are clearly tempted to modify the more invasive laryngectomies to treat the "not quite advanced" tumors. Critics will note that modifications of the higher end laryngeal excisions invite serious functional difficulties—aspiration, dysphagia, poor voice, and an unstable airway. But many times, modifying the classic operations (as primary treatment) has produced impressive benefits in intermediate cancer: a laryngeal voice, swallow without desiccation, breathing without a permanent tracheotomy, and cure without exhausting the treatment options for a second primary in the future. This is particularly true of supraglottic cancers that invade the PES *and* the glottic level. The rational surgical "bloc" to define this tumor is the SCPL with CHP. It is also well described for the "horseshoe" glottic cancers that may well extend to involve the thyroid cartilage and the subglottis. The rationale to define this cancer may well be the SCPL with CHEP.

These are the cases we refer to then as intermediate. "Early" conservation operations are not appropriate because they require unpredictable modifications and carry too high a risk for recurrence. "Advanced" operations are not appropriate because of doubts about their need and their morbidity. Intermediate cases do represent a distinctive clinical category, and when they present themselves in actual practice, appropriate strategies for their management should be offered. In a few pages, we will detail the features that distinguish the intermediate group, expand on this paradigm more formally, and focus our attention on the best developed surgical strategy we have to deal with this category—supracricoid partial laryngectomy.

Radiotherapy

◆ **Radiotherapy Alone for Intermediate Laryngeal Cancer**

What should we do about cancers too big for supraglottic laryngectomy? Operate? Radiate? It all depends on what "big" means. Parsons et al presented evidence that local tumor volume may be the most reliable predictor of control by radiotherapy.[296] They conceded that an infiltrative cancer filling more than 50% of the PES might be a *reason to select* supraglottic laryngectomy. But for supraglottic cancers *extending to the true vocal cords*, supraglottic laryngectomy wouldn't be possible. Thirty years ago, the surgical option was total laryngectomy. Because radiation can sometimes be curative in these cases, Mendenhall et al recommended we radiate all these patients primarily, to at least offer the possibility of saving their larynx.[284]

Of course radiotherapy is applied to intermediate laryngeal cancers, and sometimes it works. But often it fails, more often than in early laryngeal cancer. Authoritative figures are hard to extract because patients suitable for supracricoid laryngectomy are (as of this writing) *never* described in a separate cohort in papers on radiotherapy outcomes. Radiotherapy is often attempted in fact not because the odds favor cure but because of the inaccurate assumption that the patient's actual surgical option is total laryngectomy. This points up the advisability of always obtaining an expert surgical opinion before any treatment begins. It is unfair to expect a radiation oncologist to be knowledgeable about the applications of the specialized laryngeal surgical technologies today—particularly the supracricoid conservation operations, the near total operative strategies, the TLMs, and the numerous ancillary strategies in support of the restoration of function.

Unfortunately, recurrences after radiotherapy (if the original was intermediate) rarely come to the surgeon's attention in time for a partial laryngectomy. The treatment of recurrences by partial laryngectomy is hard: prior radiotherapy impairs wound healing and compromises the selection of surgical margins.[297] Of course, the treatment of recurrences after surgical treatment by SCPL and CHP is also difficult. However, this is very uncommon given that 3-year success rates are 95%.

◆ **Chemoradiation for Intermediate Laryngeal Cancer**

The so-called organ preservation protocols for advanced laryngeal cancer were predicated on the idea that if we could predict the poor responders *before* we gave radiation, unfavorable cases could proceed directly to surgery. (Clearly, we share an obligation to avoid the expense and morbidity of any program of therapy if we know it is destined to fail.) Patients were pretreated with chemotherapy, usually platinum-based, and nonresponders were exempted from radiotherapy and referred for total laryngectomy. But, in retrospect, it seems many were intermediate (T2) or advanced (T3) cancers at the time of presentation; therefore, total laryngectomy would not have been the optimum surgical option.

Patients who responded to "neoadjuvant" chemotherapy (many of them mobile glottic or supraglottic tumors into the AC) were irradiated in the chemoradiation protocols, presumably with an improved chance of cure. Because they responded to chemotherapy, this was usually repeated as well. The results of these trials will be further discussed in the section on advanced laryngeal cancer. Suffice it to say, the 1991 Department of Veterans Affairs Laryngeal Cancer Study Group trial demonstrated no significant advantage in survival in patients who received induction cisplatin/5-FU and radiotherapy versus total laryngectomy and postoperative radiotherapy,[69] and the original protocols have undergone redesign.[19] In the latest iteration, giving chemotherapy and radiation concurrently (versus sequentially) a small claimed benefit—a slight increase in 2-year locoregional control—came at the expense of increased toxicity. It is not clear that chemotherapy had any more impact than might have been obtained by simply increasing the radiotherapy dose. But there was a rise in high-grade toxicity (over sequential chemotherapy– radiotherapy trials) from 60 to 80%.[19]

With time, the original hypothesis (that chemosensitivity does predict radiocurability) has been called into question. Some patients predicted to do well with radiotherapy by their chemoresponsiveness did not do well. Some who were denied radiotherapy by their apparent chemoresistance may have done well, but we can never know. Now it emerges that we may be able to determine chemosensitivity (and thus select patients for radiotherapy) *without giving chemotherapy*. Cabelguenne et al have published a prospective study to show that p53 alterations (mutations, allelic losses at p53 locus, and plasma anti-p53 antibodies) predict nonresponse to neoadjuvant chemotherapy in head and neck squamous cell carcinoma.[164] Eschwege et al showed that a low T stage is an even better predictor of a good response.[17]

Cure by chemoradiation requires more than cytotoxicity, and more than just a response. Cure requires a *sustained, complete* response. The incidence of cancer-free survival in the "organ sparing" programs is similar to the results of radiotherapy alone. And radiotherapy is preeminently organ sparing. In the radiate-first treatment paradigm for intermediate supraglottic cancer, to achieve more cures and more voices may simply require that we improve our radiotherapy results. Maybe Mendenhall and Parsons[102] are right. Invest the patient's resources in one modality—radiation—and do it well. There is not enough advantage in chemoselection to justify the extra cost, the complications, or the delay.

By now, it should be evident that the assumptions underpinning primary radiation as a choice (actually, RRSS) are inaccurate. Even in the presence of gross pathological PES invasion, total laryngectomy is *not* the surgical treatment. And if it were, many of the patients (unirradiated patients) would speak. But SCPL and CHP constitute the surgical treatment for unirradiated intermediate supraglottic cancer that stops clearly short of the cricoid—as most do.[298] (And near-total laryngectomy is the surgical treatment for unirradiated advanced [meaning fixed, lateralized, perhaps involving the pyriform] supraglottic cancer, even if it involves the cricoid.) These operations (SCPL and near-total laryngectomy) have been practiced for 30 years. We have a lot of data regarding their outcome. Laccourreye presented 68 patients with squamous cell carcinoma of the supraglottis who underwent SCPL and CHP from 1974 through 1986. In all cases, a conventional horizontal supraglottic laryngectomy was contraindicated. All but three patients (95.4%) recovered physiological deglutition. None required a permanent tracheostomy. The 3-year actuarial survival rate was 71.4%, and *no local recurrences were encountered*.[299] Thus, done well, SCPL and CHP provide a reliable cure, a lung-powered voice, no stoma, and almost always pharyngeal swallowing, particularly when it is performed *before* radiation. Near-total laryngectomy provides cure and voice and swallow for the advanced cases, on the same basis, but it always accepts a permanent stoma.

Note that radiation would still be held in reserve in both these scenarios. It would be available for neck indications discovered at surgery, or for a second primary that could arise in the future. Ironically, in practices in which primary surgery is favored for intermediate (or advanced) supraglottic cancer, the commonest indication for total laryngectomy is *radiation failure*. The notes accompanying these patients often suggest that, at presentation, at the most, the patient had *early* or intermediate supraglottic disease. The patients usually declare that they and their doctors elected radiotherapy *to avoid total laryngectomy*. And that total laryngectomy is what had been offered to them as their surgical option. We can hope the day will come when it is recognized that total laryngectomy is best for very advanced disease, not for primary intermediate laryngeal cancer. Even if the results were not changed much by this information, at least the initial treatment selection will have been better informed and consented to.

Brasnu et al have drawn attention to a different possible role of preoperative chemotherapy. They have used it in the evaluation of arytenoid mobility, a crucial determinant in the supracricoid operations. Sometimes, after a partial response, the authors have observed that a "sticky" arytenoid became mobile. This may be an instance when SCPL is recognized to be feasible when an arytenoid is relieved of the "bulk" factor of a nearby tumor in the false cord.[159] Doing this with chemotherapy (instead of radiation) at least preserves the option of radiotherapy for future regional use.

Classic Conservation Operations for Intermediate Laryngeal Cancer

Supracricoid Partial Laryngectomy

SCPL is the largest open resection we can offer for laryngeal cancer yet still preserve nasal breathing (i.e., no permanent tracheotomy). It *can* achieve a biological voice, aspiration-free swallowing, and a cure, but a flawless technique is imperative. As with near-total laryngectomy, there is not much room for deviation from the method described by the developers. The only way to achieve reproducible results is to follow the guidelines precisely, and fortunately, in the period since 1986, the guidelines have been clearly delineated.

SCPL takes advantage of the fact that many intralaryngeal cancers arise in the anterior part of the larynx and obliterate the AC but spare the following:

1. The posterior laryngeal tissues (including both arytenoids)
2. The foundation of the laryngeal airway, the cricoid

When infiltrative *glottic* "horseshoe" lesions preclude a conventional VPL, sometimes the main objections would be overcome if the entire thyroid cartilage and the soft tissues it encloses anteriorly could be removed en bloc. When infrahyoid *supraglottic* cancers spread to the anterior glottis and preclude a supraglottic laryngectomy, there is often a large posterior and inferior subunit of the larynx with no cancer in it.

SCPL removes the entire thyroid cartilage and all the intrinsic laryngeal soft tissues the thyroid cartilage tends to enclose, back to, but not including, the arytenoids, up to, but not including, the hyoid, and down to, but not including, the cricoid. The SCPL resection bloc unit for *glottic* cancer consists of the following:

- The supraglottic larynx, except for the hyoid bone and the suprahyoid epiglottis, sparing both arytenoids
- The anterior glottis (bilaterally) as far back as necessary, sparing both arytenoids
- The subglottis down to the upper margin of the cricoid, sparing both arytenoids

Having emphasized otherwise, it may occasionally include the anterior part of one arytenoid.

The following structures are saved in a SCPL for intermediate glottic cancer:

- The suprahyoid epiglottis, usually
- At least one and a half (but generally both) arytenoids

Clearly, we have to perform an exceptionally careful clinical evaluation of the posterior larynx to determine the candidacy of a given patient for an SCPL. SCPL leaves a large vertical gap and a "sphincterless" larynx. Both can be rectified by the strategy of CHEP. A successful "pexy" will enable the patient to elevate the arytenoids to the tongue base during swallowing, to defend against aspiration. It will also provide for a mucosal wave, which is necessary for voice. The loose tissues over at least one corniculate will usually participate, along with any neighboring structures soft enough to oscillate, depending on the variables of the case. The substrate for nasal breathing, the cricoid, will also remain. (If the cricoid were violated, as it is in a near-total laryngectomy, the airway would be limited by malacia. And if it were lost, as it is in a total laryngectomy, it would be limited by intentional surgical separation of the airway and the foodway.) For all its functional compromises, supracricoid laryngectomy offers one powerful benefit over more extensive resections like near-total and total laryngectomy. The patient is free from permanent dependence on a hole in the neck to breathe.

At the time of this writing, SCPL is still treated as "new" technology in many American centers. Many discerning surgeons must have deemed it risky, dispensable, unphysiological. Aspiration is troublesome enough after removing just the supraglottic sphincter. Here the *glottic* sphincter would also be eliminated. Surely swallowing without aspiration would be impossible. Supraglottic laryngectomy produces a wound that can barely be closed. Wouldn't the vertical closure required for an SCPL be even more impossible? Laryngeal surgeons hesitate to cut across anatomical planes in cancer cases for fear of encountering cancer. It is not immediately apparent how the details of the reconstruction work—the tracheal releases, the innovative suturing. Nor is the special physiology obvious: elevation of the arytenoids to the tongue base for swallowing, generation of a mucosal wave for voice. Some say it took 20 years for SCPL to be appreciated in the United States (Lefebvre, 1974, to Weinstein and Laccourreye, 1994),[300] and before that it took 20 years in Europe (Meier and Reider in Austria in 1959 to Lefebvre in the 1970s).[301]

Supracricoid Partial Laryngectomy and Cricohyoidoepiglottopexy

SCPL and CHEP (Labayle subtotal laryngectomy[302]) evolved from a desire and indeed a need to extend the benefits of local resection and reconstruction to patients with just a little too much disease for a safe VPL. The gradual change to SCPL and to CHEP brought about an increase in long-term survival, local control, and laryngeal preservation rates when compared with historical controls using VPL or radiotherapy.

◆ **Patient Selection** Case selection is critical for SCPL—intermediate disease needs to be diagnosed and distinguished preoperatively. During the course of a classic (open) frontoanterior VPL, it will be far too late to upgrade to a supracricoid laryngectomy. The same is true with a supraglottic laryngectomy. Patients are ill-served by last-minute upgrades of the operations really designed for early laryngeal cancer. The tracheotomy has already been sited. The thyroid cartilage has already been cut. The principles of reconstruction will already have been violated. (These restrictions are *not* true of a transoral laser excision. Transoral laser operations *can* be upgraded.) The patient needs a doctor who will attach serious importance to differentiating "intermediate" cancer from "early" cancer before selecting the initial therapy. T2s have a local failure rate of 20 to 25% with classic partial laryngectomies (Weinstein[300]), whereas SCPL is almost always curative. Equally important is the distinction between "intermediate" laryngeal cancer and "advanced." SCPL can avoid a permanent tracheotomy; near-total laryngectomy never can.

The indications for SCPL and CHEP are carcinomas of the glottis that

- spread beyond the confines of the membranous portion of the true vocal cord; or
- present with limitation (but not fixation) of true vocal cord mobility.

The published contraindications to SCPL and CHEP[303] are the following:

- Arytenoid cartilage fixation
- Infraglottic extension to the superior cricoid border (less than 10 mm anteriorly, 5 mm posterolaterally)
- Cricoid invasion
- External thyroid cartilage perichondrium invasion
- Extralaryngeal spread
- Massive invasion of the PES (with possible hyoid involvement)

Note that invasion of the *inferior PGS* threatens the cricoid, and invasion of the *superior PGS* threatens the PES. In our practice, arytenoid cartilage fixation, invasion of the PGS, or threatened contact (on one side) with the cricoid, is usually an indication that if surgery is advised, the choice of operation will be a near-total laryngectomy, not a supracricoid partial. These are features of advanced cancer, not intermediate disease. As we have noted, inferior PGS disease can extend right on out through the interval between the cricoid and the thyroid cartilages. So we need a resection strategy that will include both cartilages, on the tumor side, and the overlying extralaryngeal soft tissues, like the strap muscles, their fascia, and the thyroid gland on that side. This is what near-total laryngectomy achieves.

Infraglottic extension to the superior cricoid border is even more serious. When it is anterior, it is usually superficial but bilateral. Near-total laryngectomy is for deep but lateralized disease and requires as much preservation of subglottic mucosa (almost all of it on the less involved side) as possible. Supracricoid laryngectomy requires that the intraoperative cricothyrotomy for the anesthesia tube be safe, that is, through healthy tissues in the cricothyroid interval. The presence and extent of subglottic cancer are critical determinations in the selection of surgical therapy. Infiltrative subglottic extension into the cricothyroid interval, that is, below the inferior border of the thyroid cartilage and thus below the lowest fibers of the thyroarytenoid musculature, will usually escalate curative surgical treatment to a total laryngectomy. This is probably what the phrase "significant subglottic disease" should mean. Not 5 mm, not 10 mm, but beyond the inferior border of the thyroid cartilage. The actual dimension would be different for men and women because the distance is different. More practically, it is hard to determine because the landmarks are not very prominent but smooth. A 70 degree laryngeal telescope is the best visualizing instrument. Incremental laser biopsy is probably the most accurate histological technique. But for now, our point is simply to clarify why and how anterior subglottic extension is a critical determination in laryngeal cancer. In brief, beyond the lower border of the thyroid cartilage, it becomes a feature of very advanced laryngeal cancer. Supracricoid operations are for intermediate laryngeal cancer, and near totals are for advanced, not very advanced, disease. Supracricoid operations are excluded by cricoid invasion (or *external* thyroid cartilage perichondrium invasion, or any extralaryngeal spread, or gross *PES* involvement with possible hyoid invasion). They are useful for the more symmetrical horseshoe lesions of the glottic larynx where both arytenoids are spared (and mobile). Near-total laryngectomy is for lateralized (paraglottic) disease, in which only the "good side" arytenoid remains spared and mobile, and half the cricoid must go. But neither operation can succeed if the anterior subglottis is involved to threaten the cricoid bilaterally. Both require subglottic mucosa to be spared, the entire circumference in the supracricoid operations and at least half the circumference in the case of near-total laryngectomy.

◆ **Preoperative Considerations** The planning for the reconstruction, the CHEP, has to begin right up front, before the resection, before the larynx is even exposed. A "normal" preliminary tracheotomy would compromise the strength and integrity in the anterior tracheal wall when later, at the time of the pexy, we face the need for mobilization and tracheal movement upward in the neck. A normal tracheotomy would also be situated way too high by the elevation, behind the submentocervical angle in fact. A temporary stoma will be needed for the postop recovery period, but the prospective site for this is relatively inaccessible behind the sternum at the beginning of the operation. Therefore the early intraoperative endotracheal intubation is to be accomplished at the upper margin of the cricoid.

◆ **Surgical Technique**[300,304,305] In the OR, post a video print of the endoscopic appearance and the notes. This will help inform anesthesia regarding the airway challenge. Also post the preop CT scan to clarify any questions the team may have about the neck—extralaryngeal disease, or the presence and laterality of nodes. Intubate the patient yourself, with a small endotracheal tube (over a stylet). Lead a double-length long circuit anesthesia tubing (and CO_2 tubing) from the oral endotracheal site down inside the right arm to the anesthesiologist at the patient's foot.

Perform a microlaryngoscopy and a microbiopsy. Use a vallecular laryngoscope like the Lindholm, at first, so you can study the untouched supraglottis with an angled telescope (30 degrees, then 70 degrees). Now decide on the safety and feasibility of suprahyoid epiglottic preservation (to clarify that the reconstruction *can* be a CHEP, not a CHP). Next take careful note of the extent of the tumor toward the arytenoids, to prove they can be safely preserved (both of them). Finally, use an angled telescope to clarify that the subglottic extent is sufficiently limited, that the cricothyroid interval is free of cancer, so that the cricothyrotomy will be safe. Pass a nasogastric (NG) tube, extend the neck with a shoulder roll, and drape out the field. Leave the tip of an endotracheal "J" tube and its cuff inflation tube exposed nearby to later be connected to the cricothyrotomy.

Create the skin incisions and elevate the flaps to visualize the strap muscles. We would usually perform a discontinuous conservation neck dissection for N1 glottic disease and follow the neck for most N0 patients. Then irrigate the wound, approach the larynx and locate the inferior margin of the hyoid bone. Standing on the more diseased side, begin the dissection on the "good" side. Transect the thyroid isthmus (respecting the Delphian node), to expose the trachea. Skeletonize the front of the trachea down to the carina, so later it can be elevated more easily.

Retract the insertion of the omohyoid muscle on the tumor side, and cut the *sterno*hyoid, then the *thyro*hyoid mus-

cles slightly above the palpable superior border of the thyroid cartilage. This will expose the thyrohyoid membrane (**Fig. 4.72**). Release the stylopharyngeus muscles descending into the upper border of the thyroid cartilage and the superior cornua. Repeat this on the other side. Then strip the superficial sternohyoid muscles down and cut the deeper sterno*thyroid* muscles over the thyroid gland. Now the entire thyroid cartilage is visible. With further retraction, the cricoid cartilage and cricothyroid membrane can be exposed.

Rotate the larynx with your fingers and sever the inferior constrictor muscle (and the perichondrium) from its origins along the posterior border of the thyroid cartilage. Do this on both sides (**Fig. 4.73**). Elevate both pyriforms on the inner surface of the thyroid alae with a Freer, perhaps a little more extensively on the "good" side. Carefully display the inferior cornua of the thyroid cartilage on each side and clear the notch in front of the base of the cornu on the tumor side with a small Farabouef elevator. Disarticulate the cricothyroid joint (**Fig. 4.74**). (The cornu may break, or you may cut it—the objective is to free the thyroid cartilage from the cricoid—without injuring the recurrent laryngeal nerve.) Repeat this disarticulation on the other side. Now the thyroid cartilage is free of both muscle attachments and cricoid attachments.

Hold up the upper cut ends of the sternohyoid/thyrohyoid muscles with Duval forceps and, working from below, skeletonize the *inner* aspect of the hyoid bone (never the outer!) with an elevator. Note that the suprahyoid soft tissues all remain intact, and all remain attached to the hyoid. Cut the thyrohyoid membrane and the preepiglottic tissue above the thyroid cartilage (leaving the upper epiglottis for a CHEP). Save the superior laryngeal nerves (no need to dissect them

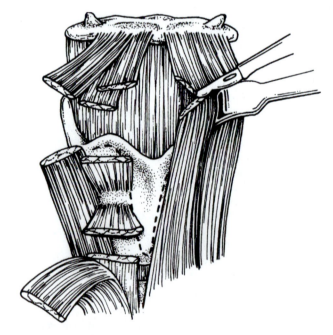

Fig. 4.72 Supracricoid partial laryngectomy with cricohyoidepiglottopexy. The strap muscles have been transected. The sternohyoid and thyrohyoid are cut at the top of the thyroid cartilage, and the sternothyroid is then transected. This is done bilaterally.

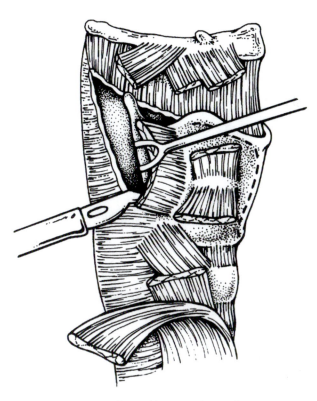

Fig. 4.73 Supracricoid partial laryngectomy with cricohyoidoepiglottopexy. A no. 15 blade is used to transect the constrictor muscles from the posterolateral aspect of the whole length of the thyroid cartilage. They are also cut from their point of attachment at the superolateral aspect of the cartilage.

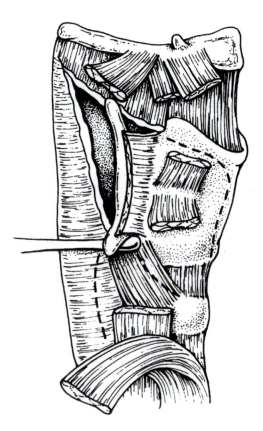

Fig. 4.74 Supracricoid partial laryngectomy with cricohyoido-epiglottopexy. A Freer elevator is utilized to disarticulate the cricothyroid joint. Care is taken not to damage the recurrent laryngeal nerves. The nerves are not identified at any point in the dissection.

out). Enter the laryngeal lumen, leaving the mobile unfettered epiglottic remnant *with* the patient, and notice the endotracheal tube in the lumen of the larynx (**Fig. 4.75**).

Interrupt the excision now to resituate the anesthetic tube. Cut a transverse anterior supracricoid cricothyrotomy right on the upper margin of the cricoid. This now becomes the lower margin between the surgical specimen and the new temporary intraoperative airway. Ask anesthesia to withdraw the oral endotracheal tube. Meanwhile, place the previously prepared "J" tube into the cricothyrotomy. Anesthesia can now reconnect the same double-length anesthesia tubing to maintain ventilation and pull it down at the foot. Note that this was a cricothyrotomy, not a tracheotomy. Tracheotomy is *not* an option. The trachea still lies at its normal level, not at the higher level it will rise to when it is mobilized and stretched superiorly by the closure.

Returning to the upper opening, retract the specimen down and forward. Notice the supraarytenoid mucosa (which includes the cuneiforms and the corniculates). This is the soft tissue that will generate the mucosal wave essential to voice. On the "good" side, transect the false cord and the true cord as far in front of the arytenoid as the tumor permits (**Fig. 4.76**). Continue to distract the thyroid cartilage forward, and carry the incision down to the cricoid. Angle forward on the upper surface of the cricoid to join the cricothyrotomy. Reflect the specimen forward. It is free now on the three sides (upper, lower, and "good"). Observe the cancer at the AC, and reconfirm especially the inferior extent of the lesion on the worst

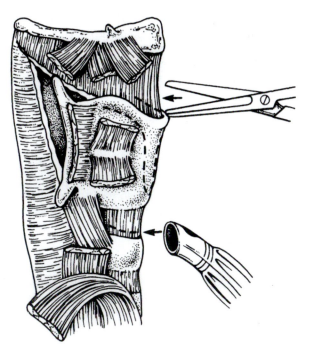

Fig. 4.75 Supracricoid partial laryngectomy with cricohyoido-epiglottopexy. A horizontal cricothyrotomy is performed, and the larynx is then entered from above via transection of the thyrohyoid membrane.

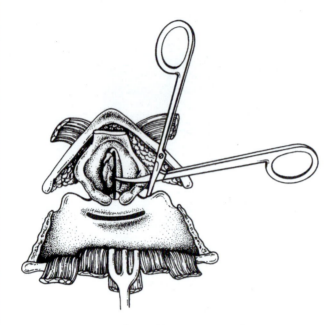

Fig. 4.76 Supracricoid partial laryngectomy with cricohyoidoepiglottopexy. The larynx is viewed from above, and the transection begins on the less involved side.

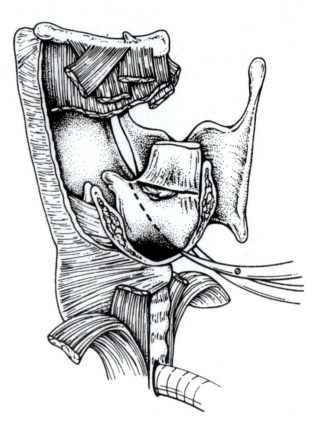

Fig. 4.77 Supracricoid partial laryngectomy with cricohyoidoepiglottopexy. The larynx is opened up like a book by cracking the thyroid cartilage on its anterior spine. The resection on the tumor-bearing side is done.

side. Gently crack the thyroid cartilage open at the angle (like a book) to see the "bad" side well. Continue the lower incision along under the cancer on the "bad" cord, keeping a safe distance from the tumor, and ascend to the upper laryngotomy (again keeping as much arytenoid as the tumor allows) to release the specimen (**Fig. 4.77**). Maintain orientation as the specimen is liberated and detached from the patient, then use frozen section reports on tiny slivers cut from either specimen or the patient to confirm the margins of the resection.

The specimen that is removed includes the entire thyroid cartilage and both sets of membranous cords (true and false). The respiratory passageway that remains is braced wide open by an incollapsible ring, the cricoid. To resist aspiration, the patient needs to be able to occlude the airway during swallowing. The minimal requirements for this task are a mobile "arytenoid mass" and sufficient tongue base and pharyngeal motor activity that the bolus is stripped from the pharynx *before* the airway opens and the patient inhales. Draw the arytenoids forward—to anything available—especially on the "good side," to oppose the posterior cricoarytenoid muscle (**Fig. 4.78**). Without some counterbalancing activity, an unopposed posterior crico arytenoid muscle (PCA) muscle will draw its arytenoid back *out* of the airway. To help retain arytenoid mobility, especially on the "bad side," where the front of the cartilage may be denuded, repair the overlying mucosa with 5–0 Monocryl. Generally, the patient will need the participation of both arytenoids for swallowing. The expected configuration for swallowing will be a "T" closure between two arytenoids and the epiglottic remnant.

Pharyngeal clearance mechanisms are enhanced by dealing with the pharyngeal musculature. During the resection, capture the middle of the cut ends of the inferior constrictor muscle with sutures, and do not cut them—leave them long. "Wing out" the pharynx, and trim any pharyngeal tissue you

think will be adynamic. (Because the sutures are left long, they can still be tied when flexion obscures the view.)

Now prepare to approximate the hyoid to the cricoid. Vertical closure of this lengthy wound (pexy) is a daunting task, and the following techniques are essential.

Capture the cricoid with 0 Vicryl (Ethicon, Inc., Somerville, NJ) on a curved needle that will be long enough to seize a huge bite of tongue base eventually. Pass it in well below the anterior cricoid arch, and exactly in the midline, to include some first tracheal ring for reinforcement. Run it up behind the anterior cricoid arch outside the inner perichondrium, ideally in a submucosal plane. Be certain you won't "saw through" the arch when the tension is applied.

Retrieve the needle in the operative defect. Pass it up into the tongue base in the midline. Take a short grip on the needle and slide along submucosally as high as you can go. Then rotate it and capture the needle tip when it becomes exposed in the suprahyoid muscles. You need to be well around the hyoid, and exactly in the midline. Midline placement is essential because any roll around the vertical axis will misalign the cricoid with the epiglottis or the tongue base. Capture a lot of tongue soft tissue. If necessary, come out temporarily in a layer between the soft tissue and the inside of the hyoid to regroup. Unlike a supraglottic laryngectomy, where you want "overhang," in this closure you would like mucosa-to-mucosa alignment.

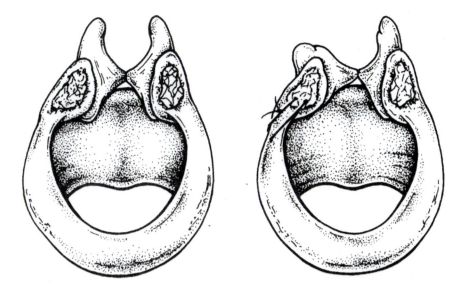

Fig. 4.78 Supracricoid partial laryngectomy with cricohyoidoepiglottopexy. A schematic of bilateral arytenoids. On the left is the arytenoid prior to suture placement; on the right the arytenoid has been positioned anteriorly.

Now pass two more 0 Vicryl sutures around the cricoid, submucosally again, ~6 mm *off* the midline. Include some first tracheal ring. Make very sure these sutures exactly parallel each other, and the midline suture, as they span the gap. Pass each one into the tongue and around the hyoid just the way you did for the midline suture (**Fig. 4.79**).

Distract the cricoid upward and release the lower trachea in the mediastinum with your fingers. Now do the "real" tracheotomy and replace the "J" endotracheal tube in the new location to get it out of the defect you are about to close. It may be helpful to leave two traction sutures on either side (like a pediatric case) for tube replacement.

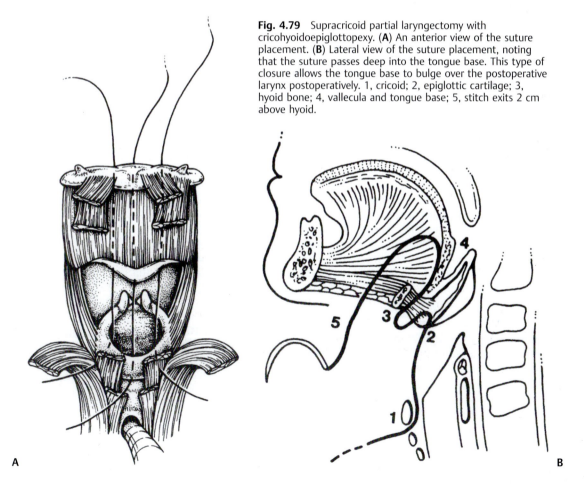

Fig. 4.79 Supracricoid partial laryngectomy with cricohyoidoepiglottopexy. (**A**) An anterior view of the suture placement. (**B**) Lateral view of the suture placement, noting that the suture passes deep into the tongue base. This type of closure allows the tongue base to bulge over the postoperative larynx postoperatively. 1, cricoid; 2, epiglottic cartilage; 3, hyoid bone; 4, vallecula and tongue base; 5, stitch exits 2 cm above hyoid.

A

B

Flex the head, and elevate the cricoid strongly. Snug up the 0 Vicryl closure sutures and tie them using forceps. Start with the midline suture and tie a "granny" knot, so it slides. Then put five knots (total) in each stitch to fix the pexy. The objective is complete cricohyoid impaction, and the cricoid *must align inside the hyoid*, not ride backward or forward. Flexion and vertical approximation obscure the pharynx. Now the previously placed traction sutures help with the pharyngeal closure. Use the sternohyoid muscles to assist the repair by suturing them up to the suprahyoid tissues.

Irrigate, cauterize any persistent bleeders, complete the sponge count and the needle count, and place a suction drain in the neck. Start the skin closure by placing 2–0 chromic interrupted subcutaneous sutures at the hatch marks to ensure alignment. Then run a second subcutaneous chromic closure to assure a watertight seal (so the suction drains work) and close the skin with surgical staples. Exchange the endotracheal "J" tube for a Xeroform-collared tracheostomy tube, to ensure the safety of the airway postoperatively. Dress the neck and affix the NG tube to the nose. A day or two later, the interventional radiologist will insert a PEG tube directly into the stomach for feeding. The purpose of the NG tube is to facilitate inflation of the stomach for this procedure. In general, the PEG tube will be used for feeding for about 1 month after a CHEP.

An SCPL and a CHEP are used for glottic cancer, so radiation is rarely given pre- or postop (no neck indications). Patients can talk on the phone and start deglutition training as soon as the tracheotomy is out (14 days in an uncomplicated case). At 6 months, according to Weinstein[300], the decannulation rate for SCPL is ~94%, and feeding tube removal rate is ~97%.

◆ **Complications** Naudo et al and Laccourreye et al reviewed the postoperative course, complications, and functional outcome of 190 patients consecutively treated with SCPL with CHEP. The average times until removal of the tracheostomy and NG feeding tubes were 9 and 16 days, respectively. The postoperative mortality rate was 1%. Major complications included pneumonia from aspiration 8.5%, cervical wound infection 4.2%, symptomatic laryngocele 3.1%, ruptured pexy 1%, laryngeal chondroradionecrosis 0.5%, and laryngeal stenosis 0.5%. Normal swallowing without gastrostomy, and respiration without tracheostomy were achieved by the first postoperative year in 187 of the 190 patients (98.4%). Completion total laryngectomy, permanent gastrostomy, and permanent tracheostomy were requested in 0.5% of the patients. SCPL with CHEP does not appear to result in an increased rate of postoperative complications compared with VPL.[306,307]

◆ **Results** Chevalier et al reported 5-year results for 90 patients with intermediate and 22 with advanced glottic carcinomas (112 total) consecutively treated with CHEP (SCPL and CHEP) from 1972 to 1989.[308] The Kaplan-Meier 5-year actuarial survival was 84.7%. Approximately one patient in 20 (5.4%) developed a local recurrence, 6.4% had nodal recurrences, and the rate of distant metastasis was 1.2%. All of these figures were less than the estimated incidence of a metachronous second primary tumor (10.8%).

Chevalier et al's 5-year absolute survival rates were 81.3% to 85.5% (depending on stage). The 5-year cause-specific survival rates were 94.1 to 96%. Five-year actuarial local control rates were 94.4 to 95.4%. The overall local control of 97.3% with a laryngeal preservation rate of 95.5% was a very clear improvement over the historical controls treated by VPL or radiotherapy. Local recurrence was statistically more likely in patients with positive margins ($p = 0.007$), and nodal recurrence was statistically more likely in patients with local recurrence ($p = 0.005$). Only two patients required a permanent tracheostomy. None needed a completion total laryngectomy or a permanent gastrostomy for aspiration.

Laccourreye et al confirmed Chevalier et al's outstanding results in a report of 62 patients with glottic carcinoma invading the AC, consecutively managed with SCPL and CHEP.[305] We caution that both reports include "early" glottic cancer cases, not just intermediate. But the challenge of determining depth of invasion in the anterior larynx, where the anatomy is more naturally fixed (AC), and the thyroid cartilage and perichondrium are accessible to silent invasion is simply a practical reality. SCPL protects these patients from the dangers of an inadequate frontoanterior partial laryngectomy while preserving the high cure rate of such an intervention. Laccourreye et al's 3-year actuarial survival estimate using the Kaplan-Meier life table method was 93.3%, and the 5-year actuarial survival estimate was 86.5%. The 5-year actuarial local control rate was 98.2% because only one patient developed a local recurrence (and he was successfully salvaged with RT, resulting in an overall 100% local control rate and laryngeal preservation rate!). No patient required a completion total laryngectomy (e.g., for aspiration), and no one was left with a permanent tracheostomy. One patient developed a nodal recurrence.

Supracricoid Partial Laryngectomy and Cricohyoidopexy

For many patients with supraglottic cancer, a supraglottic laryngectomy is insufficient cancer surgery. Some have T2 cancers that have drifted down from the supraglottic region anterior to the ventricles, and now they involve the AC and a cord. SCLP and CHP is an alternative to total laryngectomy, radiation and salvage surgery, or slightly extended horizontal supraglottic laryngectomy for patients with *supraglottic* carcinoma and anterior glottic extension (i.e., intermediate laryngeal cancer). The cords retain motion, indicating that the tumor does not permeate the PGS. (Slight impairment is permissible in selected instances, but complete fixation would imply permeation of the PGS, and removal of only the PGS, leaving its neighbors behind, would constitute a risk at the margins for the patient.)

SCLP and CHP (Mayer-Piquet subtotal laryngectomy) is a useful alternative to total laryngectomy, radiation therapy and surgical salvage, and extended supraglottic laryngectomy, in select cases of supraglottic carcinoma.[299] The relative indications include the following:

- Carcinomas of the supraglottis that involve the glottis and AC
- Carcinomas of the supraglottis that may invade both ventricles and threaten the glottis

- Transglottic carcinomas that present with incomplete vocal cord immobility, sparing the arytenoid
- Carcinomas of the supraglottis that invade the thyroid cartilage

Although these tumors do descend below the classic supraglottic block anteriorly, they should not compromise the motion of either arytenoid posteriorly. True arytenoid fixation would contraindicate SCPL by signaling involvement of the cricoarytenoid joint. (Brasnu[303] showed if the *bulk* of a supraglottic tumor immobilized the false cord, but the true cord was mobile, then the cricoarytenoid joint was okay.) Major PES invasion is a potential contraindication to SCPL if hyoid involvement is a risk. Outer thyroid perichondrium involvement is another contraindication. The reconstruction generally requires the preservation of perichondrial and strap muscle tissues that now might be compromised by cancer.

Hassmann and Skotnicka examined whole organ sections of 90 total laryngectomy specimens. Histologically, 22 (25%, mostly supraglottic tumors) could have been eradicated by SCPL. The sites of origin in this analysis were supraglottic (48), transglottic (22), and glottic (20). Several had been staged pT4.[309]

The incidence of nodal metastases is much higher in intermediate *supra*glottic carcinoma than it is in intermediate glottic cancer. Thus the chance is high (34% in Brasnu's[303] cases) there will be neck indications for radiotherapy *after* the SCPL and CHP are completed. The neck deserves radiotherapy if the nodes are guilty—of multinodal involvement or gross extracapsular spread, for example. But what may *not* be justified is the practice of equal punishment at the primary site, now an innocent (tumor-free) bystander trying to heal and function after an SCPL and CHP. The cancerous laryngeal tissues have already been interred. The radiotherapy is being imposed for a crime that the primary site did not commit. To us, it seems the very antithesis of a rehabilitative strategy to dose the reconstructive area above 4500 R.

◆ **Patient Selection** In general, the indications for SCPL have become more numerous since the first descriptions made by Majer, Labayle, and Piquet.[7,301] One reason is the discovery that supraglottic cancers could be operated, and epiglottic tip preservation was not mandatory. SCPL with CHP permits adequate phonation, respiration, and deglutition in "intermediate" cases of *supraglottic* carcinoma, which have heretofore been subjected to total laryngectomy.

◆ **Preoperative Considerations** SCPL and CHP will consist of resection of the entire thyroid cartilage and PGS, as well as the epiglottis and the whole PES. It will spare the immediate neighbors of the PGS, the cricoid cartilage, the hyoid bone, and usually two arytenoid cartilages.[299] The most important asset for success may well be a team of nurses and colleagues familiar with the postoperative care and rehabilitation of these patients. They will likely go home with a tracheotomy and a feeding tube still in place because functional recovery is prolonged.

◆ **Surgical Technique** The operation follows an identical format to the partial laryngectomy just described for intermediate *glottic* cancer. The main difference is the inclusion of the entire PES and the suprahyoid epiglottis in the specimen. This extends the block, but not the overall prognosis. The best guarantee of a local cure appears to be expert case selection and negative surgical margins. Unfortunately, pretreatment with neoadjuvant chemotherapy does not improve local control, and postoperative radiotherapy does not finesse positive margins.

Post the video prints and the CT scans. Intubate the patient and perform a careful microlaryngoscopy. Use a vallecular laryngoscope, like the Lindholm, to examine and not obscure the supraglottis. Use the angled telescopes. See the subglottis, the ventricles, the tumor margins. Palpate the vallecula, the false cords, the epiglottis. Make sure the hyoid itself is not likely threatened by cancer. Take microbiopsies, get frozen sections.

For N0 intermediate supraglottic cancer, raise the flaps and perform a (discontinuous) *staging* neck dissection. The most important indication that the other neck might need treatment, too—the discovery of positive nodes in the first neck.

Approach the thyrohyoid membrane through the straps, expose the anterior aspect of the larynx and trachea, and release the inferior constrictor from the posterior border of the thyroid (cartilage) (**Fig. 4.80A,B**). Elevate both pyriforms. Disarticulate the cricothyroid joints (**Fig. 4.81**). The thyroid cartilage is free of direct attachments now, both muscular and cricothyroid. What remains is to release the entire supraglottis, and simultaneously preserve the hyoid bone for the CHP (**Fig. 4.82**).

Hold up the upper cut ends of the sternohyoid/thyrohyoid muscles with Duval forceps and skeletonize the *inner* aspect of the hyoid bone (again, never the outer!). Note that resection of the entire supraglottis, en bloc, including the PES, is not incompatible with preservation of the hyoid bone.[163] Cut the *upper extremity of the thyrohyoid membrane* for a CHP. See the blue of the lateral vallecular mucosa. Always save as much superior laryngeal nerve as possible—again, don't dissect it out. Enter the oropharyngeal lumen at the vallecula. Notice the endotracheal tube in the interior of the pharynx.

This completes the upper opening. The lateral openings, the lower one (the cricothyrotomy), the removal of the specimen, and the subsequent tracheal mobilization and re-siting of the tracheotomy are all the same as they were for the SCPL and CHEP (**Fig. 4.83**). Bear in mind the patient will need two well-supported (forward) arytenoids for swallowing. A "T" closure of two arytenoids and the tongue base will be the expected configuration for swallowing.

Vertical closure of the excisional defect is again a challenging obligation. The three parallel vertical Vicryl sutures are critical. Capture the cricoid and some reinforcing tissue below the hyoid, and a lot of reinforcement above (**Fig. 4.84**). Use careful alignment to avoid any torsion around the vertical axis and aim for cricohyoid and mucosal alignment. Make sure the release of the trachea is complete. Flex the head and elevate the cricoid. Use forceps to tie a "granny" knot to slide. Then put four more knots in each stitch to fix the pexy in complete cricohyoid impaction.[310]

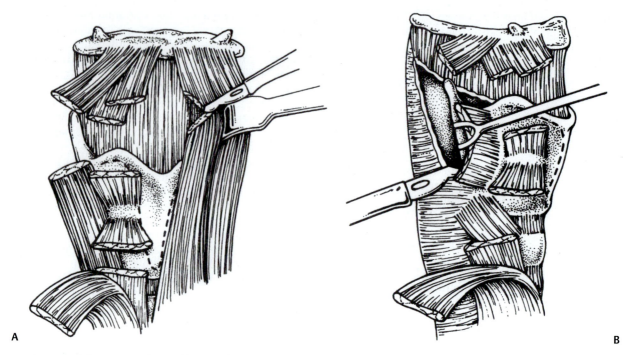

A   B

Fig. 4.80 **(A)** Supracricoid partial laryngectomy with cricohyoidoepiglottopexy. The strap muscles have been transected. The sternohyoid and thyrohyoid are cut at the top of the thyroid cartilage, and the sternothyroid is then transected. This is done bilaterally. **(B)** Supracricoid partial laryngectomy with cricohyoidoepiglottopexy: A no. 15 blade is used to transect the constrictor muscles from the posterolateral aspect of the whole length of the thyroid cartilage. They are also cut from their point of attachment at the superior lateral aspect of the cartilage.

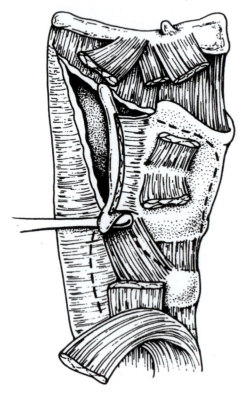

Fig. 4.81 Supracricoid partial laryngectomy with cricohyoido-epiglottopexy. A Freer elevator is utilized to disarticulate the cricothyroid joint. Care is taken not to damage the recurrent laryngeal nerves. The nerves are not identified at any point in the dissection.

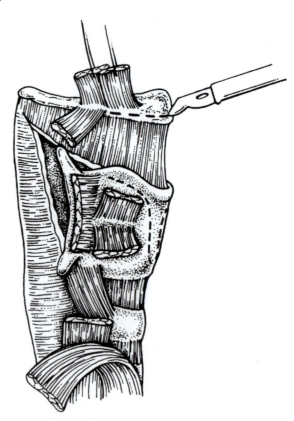

Fig. 4.82 Supracricoid partial laryngectomy with cricohyoido-epiglottopexy. A horizontal cricothyrotomy is performed, and the larynx is then entered just below the hyoid bone.

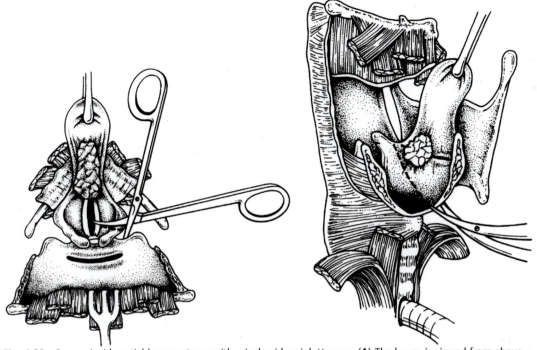

A
B

Fig. 4.83 Supracricoid partial laryngectomy with cricohyoidoepiglottopexy. (**A**) The larynx is viewed from above, and the transection begins on the less involved side. (**B**) The larynx is opened like a book by cracking the thyroid cartilage on its anterior spine.

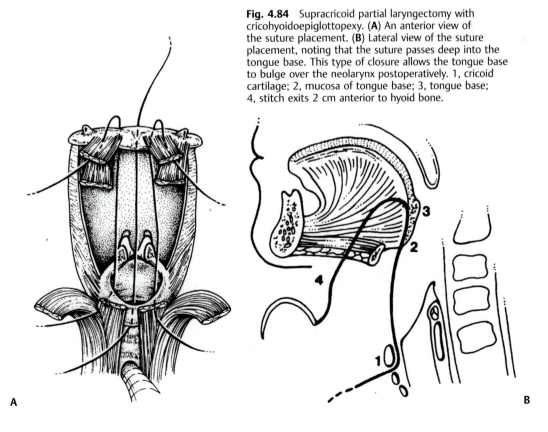

Fig. 4.84 Supracricoid partial laryngectomy with cricohyoidoepiglottopexy. (**A**) An anterior view of the suture placement. (**B**) Lateral view of the suture placement, noting that the suture passes deep into the tongue base. This type of closure allows the tongue base to bulge over the neolarynx postoperatively. 1, cricoid cartilage; 2, mucosa of tongue base; 3, tongue base; 4, stitch exits 2 cm anterior to hyoid bone.

A
B

◆ **Postoperative Management** In general, a patient needs the feeding tube for twice as long after a CHP as after a CHEP (about 2 months as opposed to 1). However, Naudo[311] has reported how wide the results can be, in a retrospective review of 124 patients with a mean follow-up period of 7 years. The average time until NG feeding tube removal in Naundo's series was 22 days. Normal swallowing without a gastrostomy was achieved by the first postoperative year in 91%. (Put another way, one patient in 10 could *not* overcome dependence on a feeding tube within the first year.) Note that postoperative radiotherapy is more frequent after a CHP (because unfavorable neck disease is more common in supraglottic cancer than in glottic disease). This of course may aggravate the swallowing prognosis.[311]

◆ **Complications** Fourteen patients developed pneumonia from aspiration (11.5%) in Naudo et al's series. Three required a completion total laryngectomy and three a permanent gastrostomy. The average time until the tracheostomy tube removal was 8 days. Almost everyone lost their tracheotomy tube by 1 year, and all patients but one were eventually decannulated.[311]

The main presenting symptom of local recurrence after SCPL is dyspnea. Laccourreye et al found none of 15 patients with local recurrences to be unresectable, although one patient refused any form of salvage treatment. In patients who underwent salvage total laryngectomy, there were no perioperative or postoperative deaths, no pharyngocutaneous fistulae, and no peristomal recurrences. Of the patients with local recurrences, 26.6% also experienced nodal recurrence, and 53.3% eventually developed distant metastases. Laccourreye et al's local control rate was 66.6%, and the 5-year survival rate was 33.3%. The causes of death were distant metastasis in eight patients, local recurrence in two, and intercurrent disease in one.[312]

◆ **Results** In 1987, Laccourreye et al reported their results for 113 previously untreated patients in whom they performed SCPL.[312] The actuarial survival rate at 3 years was 86.5%, after SCPL with CHEP and 71.4% after SCPL with CHP (reflecting the higher incidence of neck disease in vestibular cancer).

De Vincentiis et al reported 149 SCPLs, 98 repaired by CHP and 51 by CHEP.[313] Of these, 101 had a minimum follow-up of 3 years. The disease-related survival rate in this cohort was 94% (95/101). Overall, there were nine recurrences in the 149 patients (6.04%), two in the neck and seven locally. Six of the seven local recurrences followed a CHP—three in the hypopharynx and two in the peristomal area, and one in the arytenoid region. The lower rate of local recurrence in CHEP patients (1/51) probably reflects the restriction of this slightly more limited operation to smaller-volume exclusively glottic tumors.

The functional results of SCPL are discussed in several series,[306–313] most of which show that CHP patients face harder challenges in the postop period than do CHEP patients. All of Laccourreye's[314] SCPL patients were decannulated. Oral deglutition was eventually restored in 97.2% of those with CHEP and slightly fewer (95.5%) of those undergoing SCPL

with CHP. All 149 patients undergoing an SCPL reported by de Vincentiis and Minni[313] retained a laryngeal voice, but not all lost their tracheotomy. Of the 51 CHEP patients, one (2.0%) remained tracheostomy dependent. Following CHP, 14.3% of patients (14/98) failed to achieve decannulation. CHEP patients recovered tube-free swallowing in an average of 2 weeks (range, 9 to 90 days). CHP patients required tube feeding for an average of 4 weeks after surgery (range, 15 to 90 days). Swallowing recovery was presumably twice as lengthy in CHP patients because of the disadvantage conferred by the total loss of the suprahyoid epiglottis. In most patients, swallowing was eventually regained, as normal or minimally symptomatic. However, in 14% (21/149), special swallowing maneuvers like head posturing during meals were required, so that adequate nutrition could be sustained.

To this point in the chapter, SCPL has been discussed as if it is completely contraindicated in patients with glottic cancer but involvement down to the cricoid level. Therefore, it may come as a surprise to note that Laccourreye et al attempted an extended SCPL with tracheocricohyoidoepiglottopexy (TCHEP) as an alternative to total laryngectomy in 16 patients with this feature. All had glottic carcinoma presenting with 10 to 15 mm of anterior subglottic extent. The authors reported results for tumor-free margins, tracheostomy decannulation, oral alimentation, phonation, and disease-free interval, as well as a 3-year survival of 68% and a local control rate of 86.7%, respectively, projecting that the TCHEP procedure may well be a viable alternative to total laryngectomy for highly selected patients.[314] Two years later, Laccourreye and colleagues updated this series to 21 patients with glottic carcinoma presenting anterior infraglottic extension (over 15 years). The 5-year actuarial survival was 74.7%. Eighteen achieved local tumor control; 11.1% experienced nodal recurrence; 22.4% developed distant metastasis; and the metachronous second primary tumor estimate was 15%. Overall, the authors reported a 95.2% (20/21) local control rate and a 90.5% (19/21) laryngeal preservation rate.[315] For the technique of the procedure, the duration of the tracheotomy and NG feeding tubes, and the hospital stay, as well as a description of the postoperative complications and management, see their 1996 report.[315]

De Vincentiis et al published results for SCPL with CHP and CHEP involving 149 patients treated between January 1984 and December 1995.[313] This included 98 CHP patients and 51 with a CHEP. Nine recurrences appeared in the 149 patients. Eight recurrences occurred after CHP: three in the hypopharynx, four in the peristomal area, and one in the arytenoid area. Only one appeared after a CHEP. The average NG tube duration was 28 days (range 15 to 90) in the CHP patients, and 15 days (range 9 to 90) in the CHEP patients. Twenty-one patients were obliged to assume a particular posture during meals to facilitate swallowing.

Transoral Laser Microresection for Intermediate Laryngeal Cancer

Transoral Laser Supracricoid Laryngectomy

◆ **Results** In July 2003, the author (BWP) and his colleagues published a review of 39 patients with squamous carcinoma involving the AC of the larynx, 20 with subglottic spread, 25 with prior treatments for cure.[316] All 39 were managed with TLM. Within this series were 22 patients with pT2b (intermediate), pT3, or pT4 (advanced) disease whose laser excisions amounted to a transoral laser SCPL. None qualified as very advanced. Two had N2b neck metastases. At second-look laryngoscopies, two had small residual foci amenable to second-stage laser resection. One patient developed a prelaryngeal soft tissue recurrence and, after wide local excision and radiotherapy, retained his larynx. Two patients (both previously irradiated) developed delayed recurrences requiring total laryngectomy. Four of the five retreated patients remained alive without disease—one patient died of other causes. In the overall series, voice after TLM remained no worse in 19 patients and became one level worse (on a scale of 0 to 5) for 16 patients. Eleven patients received temporary tracheotomies, some for airway, some for exposure. Twelve patients left the hospital on a same-day basis, and the average hospital stay was 3.3 days.

This experience leads us to believe that TLM has a role to play in intermediate laryngeal cancer. It seems as good as open resection at achieving local control of the primary cancer, thus better than radiotherapy alone. This cannot be stated with certainty, however, because no two studies contain identical cohorts of patients, by stage or by patient factors, for comparison, and most surgical and laser series include patients who were also irradiated (because of the neck findings), which may inflate the reported local results.

Laser microresection also provides the patient with undeniable tangible benefits beyond excellent local control and a very serviceable voice. For example, it probably provides the least chance of overtreatment, and the most reliable staging information. The surgical specimen may provide evidence for or against the addition of postresectional radiotherapy. Laser microresection takes the fewest days to complete treatment of the primary cancer, and, compared with an open operation, offers the better chance of avoiding a temporary tracheotomy. In the event of failure, all treatment options remain possible, including further transoral laser resection. In the event of a second primary, all treatment modalities remain available, including laser microresection. Later, the voice may be amenable to further enhancement.

Steiner's 1993 report on the results of curative laser microsurgery in 81 patients with laryngeal carcinoma includes 38 cases with intermediate glottic cancer.[30] Thirty patients had supraglottic cancer (most of them "early"), and 23 patients had what we would clearly have considered advanced disease (17 pT3 cases, and six staged pT4). Twenty-three (28%) of Steiner's patients received neck dissections (19 of which were conservative), and 29 patients (35%) received postoperative radiotherapy. Overall, this is a more challenging group of patients than a pure cohort of intermediate cases. There were 18 local recurrences (22%) in the entire 81. Six patients required a total laryngectomy. The overall 5-year survival rate (Kaplan-Meier) was 59%.

In 1996, Steiner reported on the results of TLM ± neck dissection ± radiotherapy for 54 patients with early and intermediate supraglottic cancer.[276] Forty-two were staged T2.

There were seven local recurrences (13%). Two came to laryngectomy. The 5-year overall Kaplan-Meier survival rate was 67%.

Delphian or Cricothyroid Lymph Node Involvement

Cancer infiltrating the muscle attachments of the anterior glottic/subglottic region has extralaryngeal access through the cricothyroid triangle. The angle of the thyroid cartilage will be intact. The first node encountered is the Delphian (cricothyroid) node.

The frequency of neck metastasis or death from cancer or both is unusually high in patients with a positive Delphian node. The discovery of cancer in a Delphian node in a patient with intermediate cancer or above should always prompt strong consideration of either or both postop radiotherapy and a paratracheal node resection. In one whole organ serial section study, eight of 92 laryngectomy specimens showed Delphian lymph node involvement.[317] Four of the eight died of disease, *three with stomal recurrence*. None had received postoperative radiation therapy. None had undergone surgical management of the paratracheal lymph nodes. Olsen reviewed the medical records of 20 patients with laryngeal carcinoma and histologically proven Delphian node metastasis seen over a 25-year period (1960 to 1985).[318] In 12 of these patients (all T1–T3 glottic cancer with a clinically negative neck), the positive Delphian node was discovered at partial or total laryngectomy. Six of the 20 went on to develop ipsilateral neck metastases. Eleven of the 20 patients eventually died from their laryngeal cancer.

Early Pyriform Cancer Related to Intermediate Laryngeal Cancer

Pyriform cancer begins adjacent to the laryngeal introitus (the supraglottis) and within the embrace of the thyroid cartilage. It is never discovered at a stage analogous to "very early," or even "early," because it is never suitable for such a limited formal excision as a simple "cure by biopsy" or of a straightforward supraglottic laryngectomy. The earliest pyriform cancer we could include in a clinical classification would be one characterized by Ogura's classic criteria for conservation surgery:

- Both vocal folds are mobile.
- Pyriform apex is free.
- No cartilage invasion.

This would make it limited enough to be, at least in Ogura's scheme, a candidate for partial laryngopharyngectomy (PLP).

PLP was an expansion of supraglottic laryngectomy. The supraglottic bloc was extended laterally to include the pyriform. This escalated the expected dysphagia. Postoperative swallowing difficulties reached a level we would now associate with supracricoid laryngectomy. To keep the terminology consistent with larynx cancer descriptors, we should call this "intermediate" pyriform cancer. Everyone would have to agree that in clinical practice, "very early" and "early" species do not exist for pyriform cancer. Or we could call this "early," and recognize only two other grades—"intermediate" and "advanced," analogous to "advanced" and "very advanced" on the laryngeal scale. This would require taxonomists to understand that there were only three pyriform types, named with respect to each other. They did not appear until the third or intermediate level when compared with larynx cancer. The fact the correlations do not start until the *intermediate* laryngeal type reflects that the fact that the best pyriform cancer has the functional prognosis of an intermediate laryngeal one. A total laryngectomy is more than the patient needs. The open conservation operation is challenging. A permanent tracheotomy would not be expected of surgery. A lung-powered voice is expected. The neck and the restoration of swallowing are the most prominent challenges.

Supracricoid Partial Laryngopharyngectomy (SCPP)

◆ **Preoperative Considerations**   The goal of a supracricoid SCPLP is to produce physiological phonation, respiration, and swallowing while achieving the same local control rate for small pyriform cancers as one would expect of pharyngolaryngectomy. Candidates have carcinoma of the lateral laryngeal margin and supracricoid upper part of the pyriform sinus with normal vocal cord mobility. Contraindications include fixation of the true vocal cord and invasion of the apex of the pyriform sinus, the retrocricoid region, or the posterior pharyngeal wall.

◆ **Surgical Techniques**   The resection will encompass the supracricoid hemilarynx and ipsilateral pyriform sinus.

Aspiration may require secondary surgery. Rather than having to convert a patient to a total laryngectomy with tracheoesophageal puncture, near-total laryngectomy should be considered. Laccourreye et al reported one case in which they used near-total laryngectomy to treat severe aspiration after supracricoid hemilaryngopharyngectomy (SCHLP).[319] They found that near-total laryngectomy provided a reasonable option with acceptable functional results.

◆ **Results**   SCPLP appears to be a safe method of voice preservation in selected cases of pyriform sinus carcinomas. From 1964 to 1985, SCHLP was performed at Laccourreye's institution for 34 selected pyriform sinus carcinomas staged as T2. All cancers involved the anterior part of the pyriform sinus, the lateral wall, the medial wall, and the whole AE fold. [T2 in the hypopharynx meant more than one subsite, or an adjacent site, or 2 to 4 cm, *without* fixation of the hemilarynx. T3 hypopharynx cancers (> 4 cm or fixation of the hemilarynx) were considered to be too invasive; thus SCHLP was contraindicated.]

Patients were monitored for at least 6 years or until death. No patients were lost to follow-up. The 5-year cause-specific survival was 55.8%. The 5-year actuarial local recurrence rate was 3.4%. The main cause of death was a second primary tumor, something all too familiar with pyriform disease.[320]

Transoral Laser Microsurgery for Early Pyriform Cancer

◆ **Preoperative Considerations**   Despite more radical surgery, higher doses of radiotherapy, and the addition of chemotherapy, the poor prognosis of pyriform cancer (25% 5-year survival) continues. TLM is eminently feasible for the early cases. If the rate of local control is similar to that of more aggressive approaches, as it seems to be, TLM offers at least a way to reduce the morbidity of treatment and improve, in the survivors, a reasonable quality of life.

◆ **Surgical Techniques**   Laser surgery for pyriform cancer proceeds in the same way as is described elsewhere in this chapter for laryngeal cancer. Study the outlines of the cancer with all the endoscopic tools available, including the angled telescopes. Resect the tumor a block at a time, superior to inferior. The mucosal edges are always laser incised under direct microscopic vision. The deep margins are always validated by the frozen section pathologist. Maintain orientation. Clip the superior laryngeal artery to prevent the major immediate complication—hemorrhage in the pharynx in the absence of a tracheotomy. The neck does not *have* to be treated at the same time as the primary cancer. This issue is discussed elsewhere in this chapter.

◆ **Results**   Steiner[276] reported the results of primary laser microsurgery in 103 patients with hypopharyngeal cancer, 94 with pyriform sinus carcinoma, treated between 1981 and 1993. Eighteen patients had pT1 disease, 63 were staged pT2, 14 pT3, and 8 pT4. Sixty percent had cancer in the neck. Ten percent of the patients were treated with laser microsurgery only. Twenty-nine percent had a neck dissection as well. Thirteen percent had laser microsurgery and postoperative radiotherapy. Forty-eight percent had surgery for the primary tumor and the neck and postoperative radiotherapy.

With a median follow-up of 44 months, 93 patients were locally controlled. Six patients had salvage therapy, one by laser microsurgery and five by laser surgery and postoperative radiotherapy. Two patients had open salvage surgery—one partial pharyngectomy with laryngeal preservation and one with total laryngectomy. Two patients refused total laryngectomy and were treated palliatively. Eighteen patients (17%) died of their tumor, 13 (13%) of second primaries, and 16 patients (15%) of intercurrent disease. The overall 5-year Kaplan-Meier survival rate was 70% for stage I and II disease and 52.5% for stage III and IV.

◆ Treatment of Advanced Laryngeal Cancer (Species IV)

Advanced laryngeal cancers are lateralized lesions that exhibit fixation. Fixation is a critical observation for treatment selection and a vital determinant in prognosis. Fixation implies muscle invasion or penetration into the laryngeal framework. Muscle invasion brings access to the regional lymphatics. Framework invasion foreshadows extralaryngeal extension.

The astute clinician distinguishes between impaired mobility and unequivocal fixation. However, certain pitfalls abound. Mobility is a moot point in fixed structures like the AC or the cricoid arch. Bulk alone can impair mobility in a narrow laryngeal lumen. The arytenoid often moves when the anterior portion of a membranous cord is in fact fixed. And transmitted motion from pharyngeal activity or paradoxical movement of a paralyzed cord (adducting on inspiration due to the inflow of air) can mislead the occasional examiner. The TNM system acknowledges the importance of fixation and also attempts to capture the degree. Unfortunately, the retrospective chart reviewer may find this worthwhile distinction less evident—especially if the cancer was biopsied before it was classified and recorded.

Hemilaryngeal fixation signals a higher treatment morbidity, a worse prognosis, and much more functional disability in the survivors. Olofsson and Van Nostrand[251] have shown that cancers invasive enough to fix a vocal cord often extend to the thyroid and cricoid cartilages. Hemilaryngectomies (except for that described originally as an extended hemilaryngectomy,[8] and now known as near-total laryngectomy) leave the cricoid behind, violate the PES, and also leave the pyriform and AE mucosa behind. Therefore, except for selected anecdotal cases, to offer hemilaryngectomy to patients with a fixed cord is to practice surgical brinksmanship. Supracricoid resections for this group are also problematic, in both selection and performance. Most cases cannot undergo SCPL due to the potential inferior extent of the disease, the risk of aspiration from loss of the cricoarytenoid unit, and the difficulty of managing the patient through the complicated phases of rehabilitation after extending the operation for margins.

Radiation alone does poorly in "advanced" laryngeal cancer. It is offered as a possibility to patients who adamantly object to a stoma, however. Most radiotherapy-based treatment programs expect progression to salvage surgery (RRSS) in over half of their patients. This can be seen as "larynx preservation" in the successful half, however, on the assumption that all would have lost their larynx if the treatment first offered was surgery. As we noted previously, some programs use chemoresponsiveness to select for radiosensitivity before committing advanced cancer patients to radiotherapy. Others use chemotherapy in an adjuvant role, in the hopes of improving survival.

Among the advanced cases, some are more aggressive than most. Later, they will be separately discussed, as *very* advanced. Subglottic or postcricoid cancers are examples. Too many of these in an article on "advanced" cases can quickly skew treatment results in a decidedly negative direction.

Postcricoid cancer and extensive pyriform cancer point up another feature of the advanced laryngeal cancers. It becomes difficult to exclude the hypopharyngeal cancers. Pyriform cancer clearly originates within the confines of the thyroid cartilage, and postcricoid disease soon infiltrates the laryngeal muscles that lie on the back of the larynx, on and outside the cricoid. From the patient's perspective, these two extrinsic malignancies threaten the same indignities as intrinsic or "true" laryngeal cancer, total laryngectomy, and a stoma.

Finally, advanced cancers often pose a problem in staging. As they spread, they obscure their TNM site of origin. A medial pyriform cancer, a ventricular cancer, and an aryepiglottic-supraglottic cancer all destroy similar tissues in their advanced stages. Is a transglottic cancer to be listed as glottic or supraglottic? As laryngeal cancer becomes advanced, the TNM designation becomes less reliable.

Radiotherapy

◆ **Radical Radiotherapy and Surgical Salvage for Advanced Laryngeal Cancer** Radical radiotherapy and surgery for salvage (RRSS) is a controversial treatment for locally intermediate and locally advanced squamous cell carcinoma (SCC) of the larynx. DeSanto argued that RRSS cannot match the rates of locoregional control and survival reported for primary surgery in this setting.[64] Others criticize the semantic construction. Radiation failure is not *failure*—it is the first leg of a two-part treatment in which responders are simply spared the second treatment (surgery), thereby saving their larynx. MacKenzie et al described 61 "surgery-eligible patients" treated with RRSS for T2/T3/T4 SCC of the larynx. The operation deemed suitable had surgery been offered was laryngectomy and neck dissection. They justified the selection of total laryngectomy by empanelling several surgeon-judges to review the records for indications. They do not describe whether the same judges ever offered supracricoid laryngectomy, near-total laryngectomy, or TLM to patients with T2/T3/T4 cancer during the period under study (1980 to 1990).[321]

For a 3-year follow-up, the first treatment, radiotherapy, failed to control the primary in 32 of the 61 cases (12 of 20 glottic, 20 of 41 supraglottic). Three years was a median, so some cases must have been tabulated *before* 3 years had elapsed. Three years is usually considered the minimum period of observation to confirm local cure. Many editors insist on 5, and most senior head and neck surgeons have seen patients considered cured at 5 years only to have local disease reappear at 6 or 7. Thirteen of the 29 evaluable relapsing patients were not able to be salvaged with surgery. Advocates conclude RRSS offers a good chance of "laryngeal conservation" without compromising locoregional control or survival. Skeptics argue this is a high local failure rate, and the quality-of-life metric should be how all patients speak, swallow, and breathe, not whether they retain an irradiated (possibly symptomatic) laryngopharynx. Half the patients required two treatments to achieve a total laryngectomy, possibly more with longer follow-up. The main disability the other half or third have eluded is a permanent stoma. But is RRSS the only way they could have done so? Or would surgeons with extensive experience of laser and conservation operations have achieved the same selection through initial surgical treatment, while achieving better rehabilitation in the totally laryngectomized patients avoiding radiotherapy?

Over half of "advanced" cancer patients treated with radiotherapy require salvage later by surgery.

◆ **Chemoradiation and Surgical Salvage for Advanced Laryngeal Cancer** Organ preservation strategies have already been discussed elsewhere in this chapter, but they still deserve mention and a perspective. Chemotherapy for laryngeal cancer is not forbidden, but it has potential for harm, and in advanced disease in particular, it remains investigational as this chapter is prepared.

Open Surgery for Advanced Laryngeal Cancer

Near-Total Laryngectomy

When near-total laryngectomy was described in the 1980s, it had not been fully characterized as to outcome. This was rectified in 1998 with the publication of an extensive series from the Mayo Clinic.[324] With this information, and the reported experiences of several other surgical teams, the salient points about near-total laryngectomy have been clarified. Near-total laryngectomy is for *lateralized* infiltrative laryngeal cancer, in which the primary locus is the PGS. Glottic, supraglottic, or pyriform cancers may be candidates, but extensive subglottic or postcricoid disease is not well enough lateralized. Patients appreciate the sustained prosthesis-free biological (fistula) voice they achieve, and its quality, but acquisition of a permanent tracheotomy reduces their distinction over a total laryngectomy. Radiotherapy is quite tolerable *after* near-total laryngectomy (more so than after many lesser partial laryngectomies). But near-total laryngectomy *after* radiotherapy is treacherous. The variation known as near-total laryngopharyngectomy is valuable in dealing with pyriform cancer, but a pharyngeal flap is unavailable to augment the speaking fistula, so the patient will depend on what can be saved from the larynx.

◆ **Preoperative Considerations** The preoperative workup for a near-total laryngectomy includes a chest x-ray, blood count, urinalysis, chemistry profile, VDRL, tuberculin test, fungal serology, and preanesthetic medical evaluation. We have not found preoperative laryngograms or CT scans to add enough information consistently to justify their expense. A presurgical consultation with the speech pathologist is invaluable. Surgery should be delayed if necessary for alcoholic detoxification, platelet function recovery after heavy aspirin use, or a pulmonary preparation. Blood is cross-matched, with one unit retained for the neck dissection. Antibiotics are initiated preoperatively.

◆ **Surgical Technique**
Near-Total Laryngectomy Resection At the beginning of the procedure, the larynx is carefully examined to confirm the extent of the cancer. It is essential to make sure the ventricle on the "good side" is free because this will be the point of entry into the lumen. The typical glottic case will deeply ulcerate the true cord and involve the arytenoid posteriorly, the AC and opposite cord anteriorly, the false cord superiorly, and the cricoid ring inferiorly. After the biopsy, a feeding tube is placed in the nose and directed into the esophagus. With the head comfortably extended, a tracheotomy is performed below the thyroid isthmus, and the anesthesia is continued through this location.

By extending the incision across the sternomastoid and up to the mastoid process, flaps are elevated in the prevenous subplatysmal plane. The associated neck dissection removes all fat and lymph nodes from the neck on the involved side, along with the sternomastoid, digastric, and omohyoid muscles; the submandibular gland; the internal jugular vein; the sensory cervical nerves; and the enveloping fascia. The carotid arterial system and the accessory, vagus, hypoglossal, phrenic, and marginal mandibular nerves are carefully preserved.

On the tumor side, the procedure for a near-total laryngectomy is identical to that for a total laryngectomy (**Fig. 4.85**). The pedicle, comprising the superior laryngeal nerve and the superior thyroid vascular supply, is divided. The greater horn of the hyoid is skeletonized. The suprahyoid muscles attached to the greater horn and body of the hyoid are released. The strap muscles are cut low on the tumor side, exposing the thyroid. The lobe is elevated to expose the inferior neurovascular pedicle for resection, and the recurrent laryngeal nerve is divided. The larynx is rotated aside and skeletonized along the posterior border of the tumor-side thyroid cartilage and the cricoid, from the upper trachea to the hyoid.

The distinctive steps of a near-total laryngectomy are now taken on the nontumor side (**Fig. 4.86**). The fascia near the medial edge of the sternohyoid muscle is incised and elevated to expose muscle. The medial edge of the muscle is retracted until the thyrohyoid membrane is visible above and the cricothyroid below. The prelaryngeal soft tissues, including the Delphian nodes, must stay with the specimen. The sternohyoid and medial half of the thyrohyoid muscles are cut free from the hyoid bone on the good side and reflected to the oblique line of the thyroid ala. The thyroid gland is divided at the junction of its isthmus, which goes, and the "good side" lobe, which stays. The "good" cricothyroid muscle is elevated from the cricoid ring with a scalpel, and the leash of blood vessels connecting the cricothyroid arcade and the laryngeal interior, which passes through the cricothyroid triangle, is cauterized.

The larynx is entered on the nontumor side by means of the following steps (**Fig. 4.87**).

A segment of hyoid bone is removed with a rongeur at the junction of the body and the greater horn. An offside wedge of thyroid ala is removed. (Remember that this is on the nontumor side, and the ventricle is known to be clear.) The ventricle is opened at the upper border of the thyroarytenoid muscle (**Fig. 4.88**). The assistant spreads the ventriculotomy with hooks, and the operator visualizes the undersurface of the ventricular band. A heavy scissors is directed upward with one blade in the ventricle and the other outside the larynx (**Fig. 4.89**). The blades close to divide the ventricular band and false cord. This division is continued superiorly until the epiglottis can be clearly identified and retrieved. The scissors transection is continued across the vallecula, with the body of the hyoid and the entire PES kept with the specimen (**Fig. 4.90**).

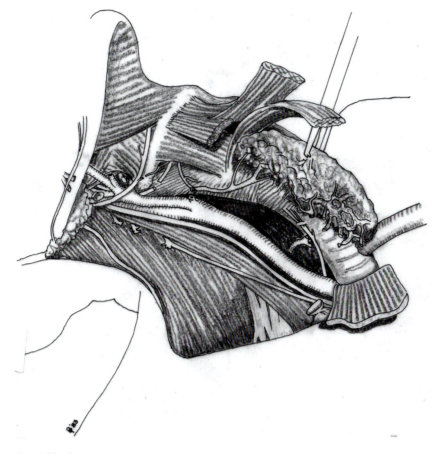

Fig. 4.85 See text.

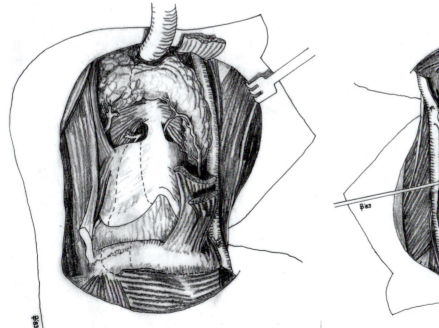

Fig. 4.86 See text.

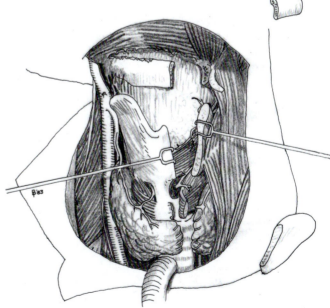

Fig. 4.87 See text.

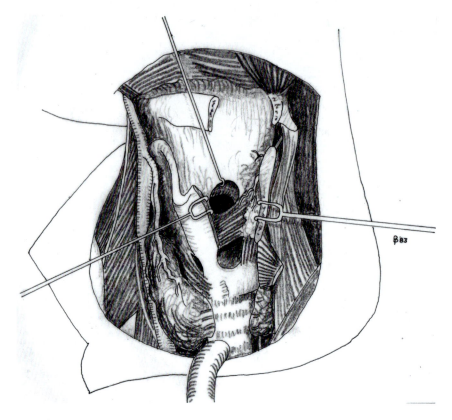

Fig. 4.88 See text.

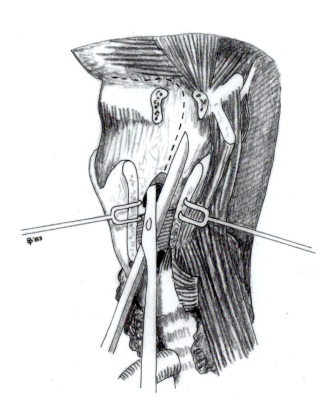

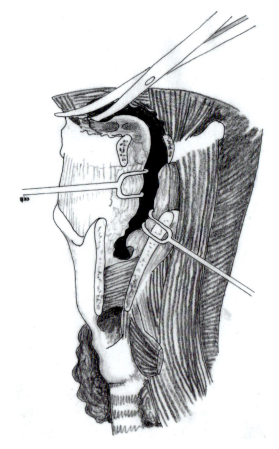

Fig. 4.89 See text.

Fig. 4.90 See text.

A muscle relaxant is given. With an Allis clamp on the epiglottis and a double hook on the cut edge of the false cord, the laryngotomy is opened to allow direct visualization of the tumor, which is principally situated on the opposite side (**Fig. 4.91**). The scissors is then directed downward to straddle the better vocal cord at the optimal division between tumor and normal tissue. The cord is divided and subglottic visualization is gradually improved (**Fig. 4.92**). The exact site of the cord cut is determined by the lesion. In the extreme case it approaches the vocal process of the arytenoid; in others it is closer to the AC. As the cut descends, it angles to fit the tumor, crosses the anterior cricoid arch, and reaches the first tracheal ring. If necessary, a portion of the trachea on the tumor side is included in the specimen.

Hooks are used to separate the anterior cricotomy, and good visualization of the subglottic lumen, the tumor, and the posterior cricoid plate is obtained (**Fig. 4.93**). The cricoid is split posteriorly in approximately the midline with a no. 15 blade. As soon as this cut passes through the anterior lamina of the cricoid plate, the cricoid fractures in the midline through its cortical portions under the stress of the traction (**Fig. 4.94**). Now the entire larynx is open like a book. The tumor-bearing portion is elevated to allow the final release across the pyriform fossa to be performed under direct vision (**Fig. 4.95**).

While the specimen margins are being studied in the surgical pathology laboratory (**Fig. 4.96**), the anterior portion of the remaining cricoid arch is resected from the patient (**Fig. 4.97A**). The resection is submucosal. A finger in the pyriform sinus is useful to elevate and stabilize the cartilage for this maneuver. All of the remaining glottic and subglottic soft tissues are preserved during this resection, which does not include the entire cricoid remnant but just enough to allow the mucosa to be tubed. Injury to the recurrent laryngeal

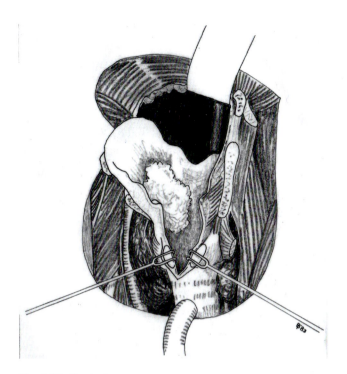

Fig. 4.92 See text.

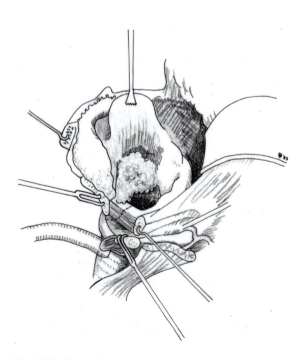

Fig. 4.91 See text.

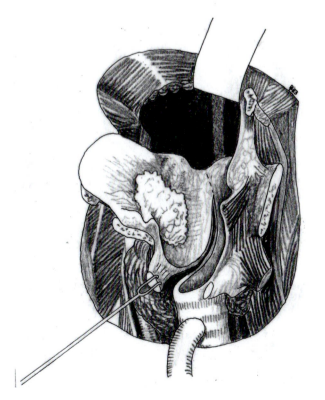

Fig. 4.93 See text.

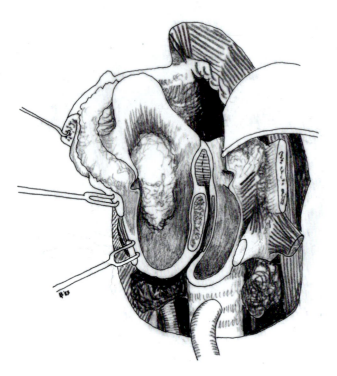

Fig. 4.94 See text.

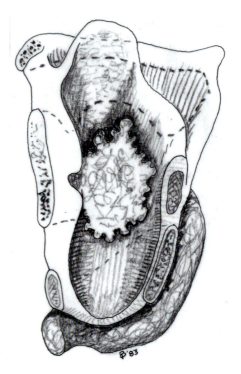

Fig. 4.96 See text.

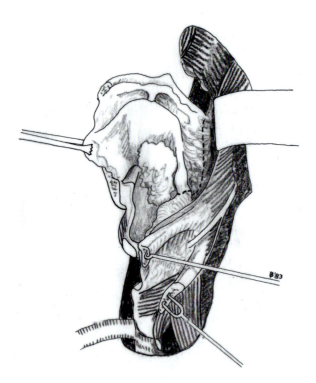

Fig. 4.95 See text.

nerve still supplying this small musculomucosal complex is avoided by preserving the cartilage deep to the inferior thyroid cornu. Some additional cricoid plate is resected submucosally from the midline margin posteriorly, and the posterior strip of thyroid cartilage (both cornua and the oblique line and posterior border) is preserved on the "good" side.

Reconstruction of a Composite (Larynx–Pharynx) Voice Shunt
The operator is now faced with a pharyngotomy, connected to the trachea by a strip of endolaryngeal mucosa. The mucosa joins the pharynx over the remaining arytenoid. By resecting the cricoid, sufficient flaccidity has been achieved that this endolaryngeal remnant can be tubed. It is often not wide enough to encircle a no. 14 French catheter (the measuring device used to assure an adequate shunt lumen). Therefore, a narrow strip of "lateral" pharyngeal wall (posterior pharyngeal wall if the entire pyriform sinus is gone) is transposed down to augment the endolaryngeal remnant (**Fig. 4.97B**). Its mucosal surface automatically faces the shunt lumen. The base of this flap should be level with the remaining arytenoid, and its medial margin is sewn to the posterior midline margin of the laryngeal strip. The entire complex is then rolled into a tube to make the vocal shunt. Starting at the tracheal end, the mucosa of the shunt is approximated with 3–0 chromic catgut. The no. 14 French catheter used to gauge the lumen is removed; no stenting or supportive device is left in place that might damage the mucosa.

The pharyngeal opening is closed in a T with 2–0 chromic catgut, similar to closure in a total laryngectomy (**Fig. 4.98**). The cricothyroid muscle is incorporated into the shunt wall. The strap muscles from the "good" side are retrieved and sewn across the upper portion of the closure, where they

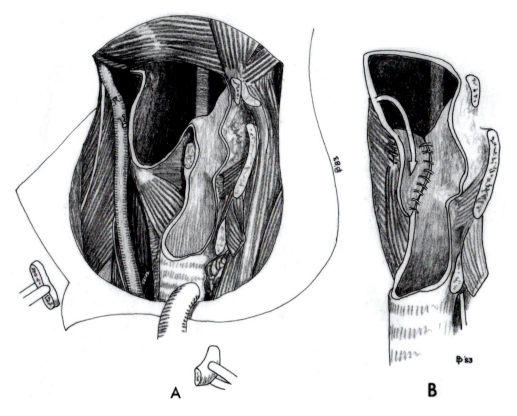

Fig. 4.97 See text.

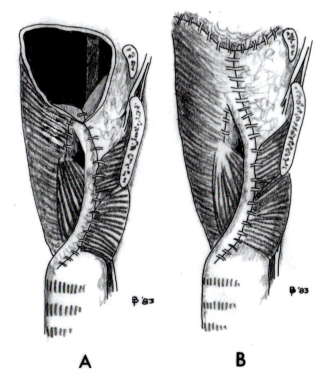

Fig. 4.98 See text.

reach the suprahyoid muscular remnants (**Fig. 4.99**). These two additional measures are aimed at reducing the possibility of aspiration, the first by adding to the sphincteric capacity of the shunt; the second by restoring some dynamic elevation. The wound is thoroughly irrigated, two Hemovac drains (Zimmer, Inc., Warsaw, IN) are led out through stab wounds to suction, and the apron flap is closed (**Fig. 4.100**). The skin at the stoma is sewn to the tracheal wall margin, and a metal tracheotomy tube is installed.

◆ **Postoperative Management** For the first postoperative week the patient is managed as for a total laryngectomy. Problems with the tracheal stoma need to be addressed first. An anterior wall stoma presents more delays due to granulation than are to be expected with the end-on stoma of a total laryngectomy. This is compounded by the patient's need to valve. The secret of stomal healing is meticulous regional hygiene (i.e., frequent tube changes, clean dressings, and use of local peroxide and/or povidone-iodine) until the skin-mucosal junction is stable.

After many months, the stoma loses its tendency to contract. The tracheotomy tube may be removed (unless the patient prefers to continue using it for the advantages it may have over his or her own stoma when valving). In the absence of a tracheotomy tube, the stoma may be fitted with a Blom-Singer tracheostoma valve[42] (Blom-Singer InHealth Technologies, 1110 Mark Avenue, Carpentaria, CA 93013) (not to be confused with the Blom-Singer tracheoesophageal

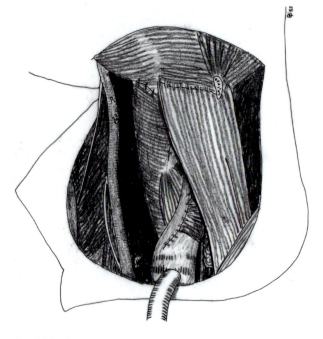

Fig. 4.99 See text.

voice prosthesis). This frees patients of the need to use their hand during speech; the valve closes at the stoma automatically on phonation.

A mechanical instrument is useful for communication in the initial postoperative period. Valving the stoma too early, in a premature effort to initiate voice, only serves to delay healing at the stomal site. Attempts to use the shunt are usually not made before the second week. The patient starts by simply occluding the stoma and exhaling when he or she is engaged in changing the tracheotomy tube. At this time the pressures are usually high, and only a small squeak of air will come up. Sometime around 8 weeks postoperatively, if healing has progressed satisfactorily, use of this shunt for a voice may commence. A speech pathologist will prove invaluable in dealing with the patient's early frustrations (and subsequent successes) in acquiring shunt speech. Technical errors that have to do with valving, articulation, speaking rate, and proficiency should not be overlooked after this procedure because they are readily identified and corrected with the help of the rehabilitation team.

◆ **Results** Lima et al reported 28 patients with T3/T4 squamous cell carcinoma of the larynx treated with near-total laryngectomy and lateral neck dissection from 1990

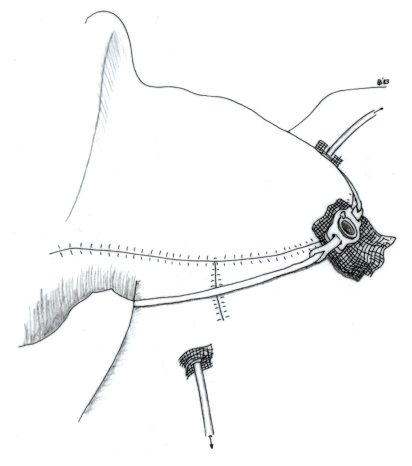

Fig. 4.100 See text.

to 1994. Twenty-six patients achieved voice preservation. Three patients died of their disease, but none had local recurrence.[322]

Laccourreye et al obtained good results with near-total laryngectomy.[323] They presented preliminary speech and voice parameters achieved by the third postoperative month in a series of 10 patients consecutively managed with near-total laryngectomy during the year 1995 and followed from 6 to 13 months. Nine patients achieved successful rehabilitation of speech and voice. One patient refused to use a functional shunt. Postoperative swallowing impairment was not encountered. None of the patients recurred locally or died of surgically related complications. The authors suggested that near-total laryngectomy should be discussed in patients conventionally managed with total laryngectomy or pharyngolaryngectomy and tracheoesophageal puncture with voice prosthesis insertion.

The authors reviewed the clinical records of 225 patients undergoing primary or salvage near-total laryngectomy for laryngeal cancer or near-total laryngopharyngectomy (NTLP) for pyriform cancer; achievement of lung-powered shunt speech; and incidence of aspiration. The 5-year local control of the primary cancer local was similar to that expected with total laryngectomy or laryngopharyngectomy. Conversational voice was achieved in 85% of patients surviving beyond 1 year. Some patients required additional surgery for voice—usually endoscopic dilation. Aspiration was absent if primary healing was achieved. It was troublesome in patients who suffered wound breakdowns, if the shunt was directly affected. Nine percent of near-total laryngectomy or NTLP patients required secondary procedures to control aspiration, but usually control could be established without sacrificing the patient's shunt speech.[324]

◆ Treatment of Very Advanced Laryngeal Cancer (Species V)

Preoperative Considerations

Total Laryngectomy

A total laryngectomy is indicated when fixation of the vocal cord with cancer is complicated by invasion of the interarytenoid space, the subglottic circumference, the postcricoid region, or both arytenoids. In unirradiated patients, extensive posterior bilateral or circumferential involvement, or both, is not too common. For tumors to reach these proportions in the airway, the symptoms must have been woefully neglected. In such cases, a total laryngectomy will often be performed solely on the basis of cord fixation. The fact that near-total laryngectomies have been conducted successfully on a few radiation failures should not obscure the more frequent need for a total laryngectomy in this situation.

Because the larynx is to be removed in its entirety, little attention is usually paid to the anatomical planning for total laryngectomy. A knowledge of the direct extralaryngeal routes of spread of laryngeal cancer is important, however.[44] Radio-recurrent cancer can spread from the AC to the Del-

phian node anteriorly, and thence into the overlying fascia and even the skin of the neck. The skin over the thyroid angle ought to be included with the specimen when its mobility is questionable. Cordal cancer may spread into the PGS, then out between the cricoid and thyroid cartilages into the lobe of the thyroid gland. It is prudent, therefore, in removing the thyroid lobe (and isthmus) with the specimen, to maintain its apposition to the larynx. Cancer of the ventricle and supraglottic region can spread directly into the neck through the thyrohyoid membrane, and laterally in the vicinity of the superior laryngeal nerve. Pain and a slight fullness in this area are ominous clinical warnings. Ventricular cancer backs up against the floor of the pyriform fossa. The implications for the hypopharyngeal resection line are obvious, especially when one considers the possibilities for submucosal spread downward into the narrower parts of the gullet. Subglottic cancer spreads circumferentially and downward to involve the trachea. It also threatens the paratracheal lymph nodes bilaterally. The surgeon must section the trachea at the appropriate level and include the surrounding paratracheal nodes in these cases.

Over half the deaths following laryngectomy are attributable to failure to control disease in the neck.[43] This fact places a heavy responsibility on the surgeon (and the patient) whenever the neck is violated to perform a laryngectomy without using the same opportunity to remove the nodes. The principal indications for lateral neck dissection in fixed cord cancers are spread to adjacent areas with rich lymphatics (e.g., the supraglottic larynx), the presence of a neck mass, and a poorly differentiated endophytic primary. A thick neck and an unreliable patient are factors that will delay prompt recognition of cervical metastasis, so these may be relative indications.

Prior to a laryngectomy it is vitally important to counsel the patient and the family on the expectations of a tracheotomy, an NG feeding tube, an intravenous line, and wound suction in the early postoperative period. Good handbooks are available to familiarize everyone with the details of stomal management and the potential for vocal rehabilitation through esophageal speech. The basic concepts and the proof of hope can be detailed in a preoperative consultation with the speech pathologist. The medical preparations for surgery are identical to those mentioned under the near-total procedure.

In a patient with stridor, the airway is established by performing the tracheotomy under local anesthesia, then inducing the anesthetic. Patients without stridor can be intubated. When quick-section diagnosis is flawlessly reliable, one may conduct the laryngoscopy and confirmatory biopsy and proceed on the basis of the frozen-section report. The dividends are time saved in the hospital, the avoidance of a second anesthetic, and a minimal period of anxiety. Carrillo et al studied 90 cases with T3 transglottic squamous cell carcinoma requiring a total laryngectomy.[325] Thirty-two patients had preoperative tracheotomies, whereas 58 did not. Only 20% of those with preoperative tracheotomies remained alive at 5 years, versus 80% of those not subjected to a preoperative tracheotomy. The authors recommended an emergency total laryngectomy in patients with obstructing lesions or a subglottic extension of 3 cm.

◆ **Surgical Technique**

Laryngectomy Ten steps are needed to accomplish an orderly and rapid total laryngectomy:

1. Establish an airway.
2. Make the incision and raise the flaps.
3. Ligate the superior neurovascular pedicles.
4. Cut the strap muscles.
5. Mobilize what thyroid you need.
6. Free the hyoid margins.
7. Transect the trachea and remove the larynx (from below upward).
8. Close the pharynx.
9. Create the stoma.
10. Close the neck and dress the wounds.

A U-shaped incision may be planned to include the permanent tracheostoma site. Alternatively, the transverse limb of the U may cross the larynx at the cricoid level so the tracheotomy site can be subsequently centered in an infinity-shaped skin excision in the middle of the lower flap. Radical neck dissection is performed discontinuously, and the accessory nerve is preserved only when the exigencies of the metastatic disease permit. Considerable judgment must be exercised in this regard, and an over-radical approach is recommended in cases where doubt exists. The significantly higher failure rates seen when an overly conservative neck dissection is done to preserve the accessory nerve make it clear that such conservatism is to be decried.

The deep cervical fascia near the hyoid and along the sternomastoid muscle is opened to visualize the carotid triangles. This is a good opportunity to palpate for nodes in cases in which a neck dissection has not been done. The superior vascular pedicles are identified by blunt dissection and divided. The superior laryngeal nerves, which can be identified by separating the hyoid and thyroid cornua with hooks, are also divided.

The sternohyoid and sternothyroid muscles are cut low over the thyroid with a knife, avoiding the gland itself. The lower segments are reflected downward to reveal the lower poles of the gland and the paratracheal fat.

The thyroid lobe on the involved side is elevated with its paratracheal fat and nodes, together with the inferior thyroid artery, exposing the posterior border of the thyroid cartilage. This border is skeletonized by dividing the inferior constrictor all along the cartilages (cricoid as well as thyroid).

The hyoid is retracted inferiorly with a Kocher forceps and the suprahyoid muscles are released. Several large veins can be cauterized as they are exposed. The lesser horns and the greater horns are freed so the entire hyoid will exit with the specimen. The thyroid gland is divided lateral to the isthmus on the uninvolved side, and the lobe to be preserved is elevated laterally until the inferior laryngeal artery and recurrent nerve are exposed at the inferior thyroid cornu. Care is taken to preserve the only remaining blood supply to the thyroid by avoiding injury to the inferior thyroid artery.

The trachea is severed on a bevel. The entry incision is usually between the third and fourth rings, but it bevels upward to approach the inferior edge of the cricoid posteriorly. By pulling the larynx strongly forward and completing the beveled airway transection at the lower edge of the posterior cricoid plate, the release of the larynx is initiated. It is usually possible by blunt dissection to elevate up under the cricoid, thus preserving the postcricoid mucosa of the hypopharynx. With strong traction toward the ceiling, the whole postcricoid area is skeletonized up to the arytenoids, and the apices of both pyriform fossae come into view. The larynx is pulled to the involved side, the superior thyroid cornua are freed, and the pyriform mucosa is cut into with a knife. The rest of the pyriform fossa is opened and the retroarytenoid mucosa is transected with scissors. Continuing the traction upward inverts the larynx, and the epiglottis flips into view. This is grasped with an Allis clamp, and one then cuts across the vallecula. Now the larynx is free to fold outward, like a book, hinged on the ipsilateral pyriform fossa. The laryngectomy is completed by dividing this final pharyngeal attachment with scissors.

Careful attention must be paid to closing the pharyngotomy to avoid a fistula. Chromic catgut corner tags help maintain orientation. The object is to close the pharyngotomy transversely or in a T, with a running 2–0 chromic catgut. Vertical closures cause a hypopharyngeal web. A second layer of interrupted sutures through the muscular layer helps support the mucosal closure. The wound is heavily irrigated, and immaculate hemostasis is secured. Drains are placed so their tips shun the suture line. An airtight wound is created by closing the subcutaneous tissues with catgut and reapproximating the skin with nylon sutures.

The postoperative course will be greatly simplified if the stoma is created properly. An infinity shape is cut from the skin of the lower flap to create a continuously smooth-edged opening with minimal loss of skin. The lower lip is sewn to the anterior tracheal wall with heavy chromic catgut. The sutures are "simple" with respect to the trachea and grasp at least one ring. They are "mattress" with respect to the skin, and they draw the skin toward the cut edge of the trachea so that no bare cartilage is left exposed. The endotracheal tube (which is crossing through the neck wound at this point) is removed and passed through the stomal opening in the skin, into the trachea. This allows sufficient access to complete the skin closure to the tracheal sides and posterior wall.

Primary Tracheoesophageal Puncture The voice loss suffered by a laryngectomy is a psychic blow that often exceeds the trauma of surgery. This has spurred surgeons to develop surgical procedures and mechanical contrivances to produce a vocal tone. After laryngectomy, of course, the articulators of speech (tongue, lips, and palate primarily) remain. If a communication is established between the airway and the foodway, the patient will speak. Air from the lungs provides 400 cc of breath support as opposed to the 90 cc by the esophagus. Air in the esophagus, as esophageal speakers show, sets the pharyngoesophageal soft tissues (the "PE segment") into vibration and establishes an acceptable vocal tone. The problems are to maintain the opening free of stenosis, to have the patient valve it on swallowing to prevent aspiration, and to arrange for exhaled air to be impeded from exiting the stoma when the patient wants it to pass into the esophagus for speech.

Cricopharyngeal Myotomy Occasionally the tracheo-esophageal puncture (TEP) procedure is unsuccessful in producing significant voicing, and the prognosis for speech development is determined to be poor on the preoperative insufflation (Taub) test.[326,327] Singer et al reported on their 3-year experience with 16 speech failures in 119 patients in whom a TEP had been attempted.[328] Fourteen patients consented to further investigation concerning the cause of their failure. Cine contrast fluoroscopy with air insufflation through a no. 14 French catheter placed in the pharyngoesophageal segment showed pharyngoesophageal spasm as the main reason for poor voice production. A parapharyngeal nerve block with lidocaine from C2 to C5 was done transcervically and the insufflation test was repeated. All patients achieved adequate voicing once the pharyngeal muscle spasm was relieved by the block. Subsequent pharyngeal myotomy in these patients resulted in successful speech in all 14 patients.

The surgical technique for secondary myotomy proceeds as follows: Under general anesthesia, a Hurst bougie is placed in the hypopharynx and cervical esophagus to act as a guide. A horizontal incision is made in a skin crease, preferably through the scar from the previous laryngectomy. Skin flaps are developed superiorly and inferiorly to expose the pharynx from the level of the oropharynx to the cervical esophagus. The carotid sheath is identified and retracted laterally. The bougie can be palpated through the pharyngeal wall. The pharynx is usually encased in a layer of fibrous tissue, the residuum of the previous dissection. Dissect the pharynx free from the paraspinal muscles, via the prevertebral fascia, and split the fibrous layer posteriorly throughout the length of the pharynx. The pharynx is turned and the sphincters are cut in the posterior midline from as high as possible down into the cervical esophagus. The muscles are cut completely through so that the submucosa bulges through the incision. If accidental penetration of the mucosa occurs, the perforation is closed with 3–0 or 4–0 absorbable suture. The wound is closed in layers and drained.

◆ **Postoperative Management** Patients are nursed postoperatively, with the head of the bed elevated. Adequate mist and suctioning are provided to maintain a clear tracheostomy tube. Feeding through the NG tube is begun on the second postoperative day, with the patient starting very slowly to avoid the risk of vomiting against the pharyngeal closure. By gradually increasing the strength and the volume, a full tube feeding formula is reached by the fifth postoperative day. The dressing is removed the day after surgery; drains are usually left for ~72 hours. The staples and NG tube can usually be removed on the twelfth day. The patient should be relatively free of pain, afebrile, and able to swallow saliva.

Prior to discharge most laryngectomy patients should have their hemoglobin, electrolytes, and calcium evaluated. They should be fully capable of looking after their tracheostomies alone or with the help of their family. A home vaporizer or suction, or both, should be supplied if necessary. Specific arrangements for speech therapy are clarified before dismissal.

With proper hygiene, stomal healing is usually complete by 4 months. Once the wound has healed, the patient is gradually weaned off the tube, omitting it for 1 hour 1 day, and escalating to 2 hours and so on, so long as there is no difficulty with reinsertion. Gradually and safely the patient demonstrates whether the stomal caliber is stable, but breaks the escalation for a week or so if contraction remains. Once the tube can be omitted for 24 hours, yet replaced smoothly at the end of this period, the stoma no longer requires its support. If satisfactory esophageal speech is not well under way by this time, the puncture-prosthesis method of vocal rehabilitation is advised.

◆ **Complications** Fistula rates are quite low with laryngectomy except for patients who were previously irradiated or in whom a deltopectoral flap reconstruction is required. Fortunately, when fistulas do develop they are usually small and close spontaneously. A fistula is heralded by an unexplained low-grade fever. The neck wound develops a reddened area, and a small part of the incision either swells or dehisces. Dressing with gauze soaked in dilute acetic acid or povidone-iodine usually results in slow resolution of the problem.

The onset of planned postoperative radiation need not be delayed because of a fistula unless the carotid artery is exposed. There is some indication in the literature that, to be useful, postoperative radiation should be given within 4 to 6 weeks following surgery. The best insurance against both a fistula and ineffective radiation is a complete and adequate resection at the time of the operation.

Significant endocrine hypofunction occurs following the treatment of laryngopharyngeal carcinoma, more so with radiotherapy and combined therapy than with surgery alone. Hypothyroidism is well known, but the incidence of partial and hypocalcemic hypoparathyroidism is also surprisingly high—63 to 88% in Thorp et al's selected material.[329]

Secondary (Delayed) Tracheoesophageal Puncture

The speaking fistula of a near-total laryngectomy can only be constructed *during* a primary excision. What about voice *after* a total laryngectomy? In 1972, Asai had resurrected the possibility that an air-powered voice could be restored after total laryngectomy by reconstructing a fistulous connection between the trachea and the esophagus with a flap.[330] Just because a cancer destroyed the internal airway and required a tracheotomy, the voice was not automatically doomed. All it needed was air power from the lungs—in the absence of a glottic sound generator, the mucosa in the esophagus would vibrate. An esophageal voice supported by the 350 cc of air one could expel from the lungs was clearly superior to one powered by the 80 cc one could gulp into the esophagus. A long list of attempts to apply Asai's insights to more patients, with less onerous interventions, soon followed but no technique to produce a "post-total" reconstruction that was consistently free of aspiration took hold. Fistulae for speech became entry points for swallowed fluids to contaminate the airway. Fistulae free from aspiration were too frequently plagued by stenosis. Eventually, Blom et al provided the most practical approach. They kept a simple direct fistula open (stenosis free) with an indwelling silicone tube, like a myringotomy vent-tube in concept.[10] The tube was modified to incorporate a one-way valve at its tip. Thus the problem of aspiration was overcome. An esophageal voice, powered by the lungs, was made widely possible by the technique of tracheoesophageal puncture and prosthesis. At the time of this writing, this concept has become the basis of virtually all post-total surgical voice reconstruction.

◆ **Preoperative Considerations**   The history of vocal rehabilitation surgery is long and interesting. It begins with Gussenbauer's[331] attempt to rehabilitate a laryngectomy of Billroth's[331] with a reed-containing device around which the tracheopharyngocutaneous wound could granulate. Many ingenious contrivances were subsequently constructed, but the natural materials available at the turn of the century (metal, ivory, leather, etc.) were hard to adapt to the healing wound and the salivary conditions in which they were expected to function.

Every subsequent generation of surgeons rediscovered the concept of a vocal shunt. Guttman in 1935 reported a spontaneous case that occurred in an individual following a suicide attempt.[332] Attempts to reproduce the physiology were made in 1958 by Conley et al,[333] and in 1965 by Asai and others.[330] But the skin tubes used to connect the two visceral tracts were not very dependable, and by 1979, Woods and Pearson[334] had demonstrated that cutaneous shunts would never supersede esophageal speech in terms of their frequency of success. In more recent times mucosal techniques developed by Calcaterra and Jafek[335] and by Staffieri[336] with modifications by Komorn[337] and Griffiths[338] and others rekindled enthusiasm for fistula techniques by showing that some degree of success was possible without a second stage and without dependence on large skin flaps. The tendency toward aspiration continued to thwart these developments; however, in addition, when a fistula was open enough to permit speech, it leaked, and when modifications were employed to tighten the fistula, it stenosed.

By the late 1970s, Sisson et al[339,340] and Leipzig[341] had shown that, once the larynx had been totally sacrificed by a laryngectomy, rebuilding a biological connection between the airway and the foodway was an unpredictable venture. Attention shifted to a prosthetic solution again, and advantage was taken of materials and concepts that had not been available to Gussenbauer.

Blom and Singer[342] and Panje[343] solved the problem of stenosis by obturating the tracheoesophageal fistula with silicone rubber tubes. The problem of aspiration was overcome by fitting the tube with a one-way valve. When sufficient attention is paid to the details of postoperative management and instruction, these methods now supersede esophageal speech in terms of the frequency of communicative success. The question of whether they should be deferred until after an attempt at esophageal speech has failed remains debatable. Esophageal speech uses the same vibrator (the PE segment), is free of any operative risk, and avoids the use of the hands, a prosthesis, or the stoma valve.

Patient requirements for successful puncture rehabilitation are sufficient coordination to plug the stoma with a finger, and the willingness and ability to clean and reapply the prosthesis on a daily basis. Prior radiotherapy, repeated surgery, or previous surgical complications do not constitute contraindications.

A Taub test[326] should be performed prior to a secondary tracheoesophageal fistula procedure. A red rubber catheter is placed through the nose into the upper esophagus and connected to an office air jet. While the operator insufflates air, the patient attempts to phonate. This suggests the spasticity of the cricopharyngeal region under airflow and the ease with which sound might be generated. Failure of this test suggests the need for repetition under fluoroscopic control, with the addition of contrast media. If the pharyngoesophageal segment is open at rest, but spastic contraction is seen in response to the insufflation of air, an associated cricopharyngeal myotomy will be required if a tracheoesophageal puncture is to succeed.

◆ **Surgical Techniques**   The initial puncture can be performed under local or general anesthesia. We have found Singer's[342] technique to be reliable; under general anesthesia an esophagoscope is introduced with the beveled end facing forward and the longer lip against the posterior pharyngeal wall. The room is darkened, the light is located at the upper end of the posterior tracheal wall, and the anterior lip is palpated through the tracheal stoma. The upper posterior tracheal wall is punctured with a smoothly precurved 14 gauge intercath needle, and the catheter in its lumen is passed up through the esophagoscope into the mouth. The esophagoscope is removed. At the stoma, a curved, pointed hemostat grasps the catheter, and as the catheter is pulled up at the mouth, the hemostat follows the puncture into the esophagus. A large enough opening is made (**Fig. 4.101**), with a few spreading movements, to enable a no. 14 red rubber catheter to be introduced. The no. 14 catheter is tied to the intercath and pulled up until it is visible in the mouth. The intercath is removed. This leaves the no. 14 red rubber catheter passing like a keeper through a puncture wound in the tracheoesophageal wall. The catheter may be brought out through the nose and secured to itself with a silk tie.

Alternatively, the catheter is repositioned so that it is directed down the gullet; its tip is lubricated and placed in an endotracheal tube and the endotracheal tube is advanced down the esophagus, well past the puncture. The endotracheal tube is then simply withdrawn. Gentle movements up and down on the catheter can confirm that it is properly positioned down the esophagus. The skin is carefully dried around the stoma and painted with tincture of benzoin. The catheter is taped very securely to the lower neck, and one must make sure that the length of free catheter is as short as possible. This is vital to ensure that the catheter is not dislodged from the puncture by regurgitation. If this happens inadvertently, the opening will rapidly close. The catheter stents the puncture for 2 weeks, during which time the patient may return home. When the patient returns to the

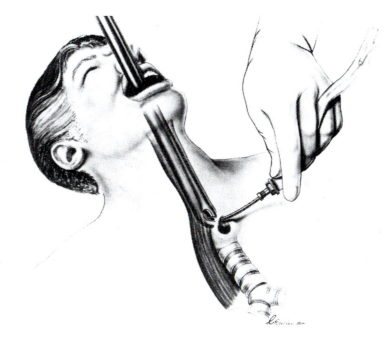

Fig. 4.101 Esophagoscope placed with the distal flange facing anteriorly. The tip is situated just below the upper lip of the tracheostoma. A 14 gauge French intracath needle is punctured through the party wall and threaded into the esophagoscope lumen. (From Johns ME, Cantrell RW. Voice restoration of the total laryngectomy patient: the Singer-Blom technique. Otolaryngol Head Neck Surg 1981;89:82.)

hospital for a fitting of the Singer-Blom prosthesis, 3 days are allowed for troubleshooting and for instruction in the care and cleaning of the device. These activities are managed in the department of speech pathology.

The prosthesis itself varies in length from 2.2 to 3.6 cm and is made of medical grade silicone rubber. The open tracheal end has two flexible tabs that are taped to the skin (**Fig. 4.102**). A double-sided tape bonds the deep side of the tab, while paper surgical tape overlaps the outside to produce extra security. The blunt-tipped esophageal end features a very thin retention flange and a razor-thin slit that permits the passage of air but not the admission of saliva. There are two openings at the tracheal end, an end-lumen for cleaning,

and a small side port that is positioned to face downward into the tracheal lumen. When the tracheostomy (and the end-lumen) is occluded, air will enter the prosthesis through this port to pass up into the esophagus.

Before fitting the prosthesis, the therapist removes the rubber catheter and establishes that voice is present through the unsupported fistula. If sound is obtained, this provides the initial elation the patient seeks and also excludes the diagnosis of pharyngoesophageal spasm if there are subsequent difficulties. The puncture is gauged for depth with a marked catheter, and the prosthesis is fitted. Several factors may interfere with its immediate success. These include inserting the prosthesis upside down, so the port faces upward; over-

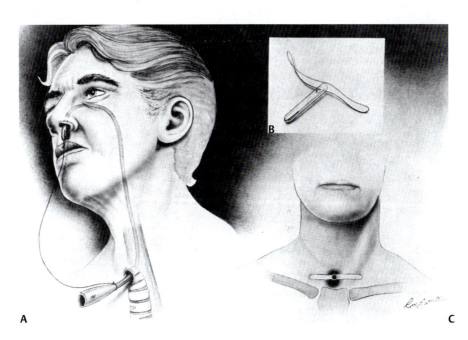

Fig. 4.102 (**A**) Red rubber catheter left in situ secured by a heavy silk ligature. (**B**) Singer-Blom prosthesis. (**C**) Prosthesis in place. (From Johns ME, Cantrell RW. Voice restoration of the total laryngectomy patient: the Singer-Blom technique. Otolaryngol Head Neck Surg 1981;89:82. Reprinted with permission.)

A

B

C

fitting, or pushing too hard on the stoma so that the valve impinges against the posterior esophageal wall; underfitting, or using too short a prosthesis, so that the tube does not traverse the whole fistula; and neglecting to check the slit valve, which may not be adequately patent.

◆ **Postoperative Management**   Once a successful fitting is obtained, the patient is instructed in off-site emergencies. The biggest danger is that during the first few months, at the time of a prosthesis change (which is conducted daily) the patient will lose the puncture. This may happen because the patient swallows when the prosthesis is out, aspirates saliva, and induces a prolonged coughing fit. Rough attempts to reinsert the prosthesis traumatize the posterior tracheal wall, and the wound closes when successful navigation is abandoned. In anticipation of this problem, the patient should carry a short length of catheter reinforced with a wooden Q-tip. This is used to probe and reopen the puncture if a temporary period elapses without the prosthesis in place.

The problem of occluding the tracheal stoma for speech has traditionally been handled manually. Recently, however, Blom and Singer[342] developed a tracheostomal vent, available commercially from the same source as the tracheoesophageal prosthesis, which relieves many patients of this restriction. The vent consists of two parts: a housing that is bonded to the skin near the stoma, and a valve that is fitted with an internal diaphragm capable of closure on exhalation. At the low pressures of normal breathing, the valve remains open. With slightly stronger exhalation, as in speech, it closes. During a cough, it can be blown out completely without unseating the housing. The patient simply needs to pull the valve from the housing and readjust the diaphragm to resume normal use.[344]

References

1. Thomas JV, Olsen KD, Neel HB III, DeSanto LW, Suman VJ. Early glottic carcinoma treated with open laryngeal procedures (see comments). Arch Otolaryngol Head Neck Surg 1994;120:264–268

2. Jako GJ. Laser surgery of the vocal cords: an experimental study with carbon dioxide lasers on dogs. Laryngoscope 1972;82:2204–2216

3. Strong MS, Jako GJ. Laser surgery in the larynx: early clinical experience with continuous CO_2 laser. Ann Otol Rhinol Laryngol 1972;81:791–798

4. Som M. Hemilaryngectomy: a modified technique for cordal carcinoma with extension posteriorly. Arch Otolaryngol 1951;54:524–533

5. Alonso J. Conservative surgery of cancer of the larynx. Trans Am Acad Ophthalmol Otolaryngol 1947;51:633–642

6. Ogura JH. Supraglottic subtotal laryngectomy and radical neck dissection for carcinoma of the epiglottis. Laryngoscope 1958;68:983–1003

7. Majer EH, Reider W. Technique de laryngectomie permetant de conserver la permeabilité respiratoire la cricohyoido-pexie. Ann Otolaryngol Chir Cervicofac 1959;76:677–681

8. Pearson BW, Woods RD II, Hartman DE. Extended hemilaryngectomy for T3 glottic carcinoma with preservation of speech and swallowing. Laryngoscope 1980;90:1950–1961

9. Singer MI, Blom ED. An endoscopic technique for restoration of voice after laryngectomy. Ann Otol Rhinol Laryngol 1980;89(6 Pt 1):529–533

10. Blom ED, Singer MI, Hamaker RC. Tracheostoma valve for postlaryngectomy voice rehabilitation. Ann Otol Rhinol Laryngol 1982;91(6 Pt 1):576–578

11. Singer MI, Blom ED. Selective myotomy for voice restoration after total laryngectomy. Arch Otolaryngol 1981;107:670–673

12. Annyas AA, Nijdam HF, Escajadillo JR, Mahieu HF, Leever H. Groningen prosthesis for voice rehabilitation after laryngectomy. Clin Otolaryngol Allied Sci 1984;9:51–54

13. Hilgers FJ, Schouwenburg P. A new low-resistance, self-retaining prosthesis (Provox) for voice rehabilitation after total laryngectomy. Laryngoscope 1990;100:1202–1207

14. Bourhis J, Pignon J. Meta-analyses in head and neck squamous cell carcinoma. What is the role of chemotherapy? Hematol Oncol Clin North Am 1999;13:769–775 vii

15. Clayman GL, Weber RS, Guillamondegui O, et al. Laryngeal preservation for advanced laryngeal and hypopharyngeal cancers. Arch Otolaryngol Head Neck Surg 1995;121:219–223

16. Eisbruch A, Thornton AF, Urba S, et al. Chemotherapy followed by accelerated fractionated radiation for larynx preservation in patients with advanced laryngeal cancer. J Clin Oncol 1996;14:2322–2330

17. Eschwege F, Bourhis J, Luboinski B, Lefebvre JL. Organ preservation in ORL oncology: myth or reality: the case for laryngeal preservation [in French]. [Review] Cancer Radiother 1998;2:437–445

18. Wolf GT, Hong W. Induction chemotherapy for organ preservation in advanced laryngeal cancer: is there a role? [Review] Head Neck 1995;17:279–283

19. Forastiere AA, Goepfert H, Maor M, et al. Concurrent chemotherapy and radiotherapy for organ preservation in advanced laryngeal cancer. N Engl J Med 2003;349:2091–2098

20. Salassa JR. A functional outcome swallowing scale for staging oropharyngeal dysphagia. Dig Dis 1999;17:230–234

21. Lazarus CL, Logemann JA, Pauloski BR, et al. Swallowing disorders in head and neck cancer patients treated with radiotherapy and adjuvant chemotherapy. Laryngoscope 1996;106(9 Pt 1):1157–1166

22. Ackerstaff AH, Hilgers FJ, Aaronson NK, Balm AJ. Communication, functional disorders and lifestyle changes after total laryngectomy. Clin Otolaryngol 1994;19:295–300

23. Terrell JE, Fisher SG, Wolf GT. Long-term quality of life after treatment of laryngeal cancer. The Veterans Affairs Laryngeal Cancer Study Group. Arch Otolaryngol Head Neck Surg 1998;124:964–971

24. Stoeckli SJ, Guidicelli M, Schneider A, Huber A, Schmid S. Quality of life after treatment for early laryngeal carcinoma. Eur Arch Otorhinolaryngol 2001;258:96–99

25. Brandenburg JH. Laser cordotomy vs radiation therapy: an objective cost analysis. Ann Otol Rhinol Laryngol 2001;110:312–318

26. Cragle SP, Brandenburg J. Laser cordectomy or radiotherapy: cure rates, communication, and cost. Otolaryngol Head Neck Surg 1993;108:648–654

27. Foote RL, Buskirk SJ, Grado GL, Bonner JA. Has radiotherapy become too expensive to be considered a treatment option for early glottic cancer? Head Neck 1997;19:692–700

28. Vaughan CW, Strong M, Jako G. Laryngeal carcinoma: transoral treatment utilizing the CO_2 laser. Am J Surg 1978;136:490–493

29. Steiner W. Endoscopic therapy of early laryngeal cancer: indications and results. In: Wigand ME, Steiner W, Stell PM, eds. Functional Partial Laryngectomy. New York: Springer-Verlag; 1984:163–170

30. Steiner W. Results of curative laser microsurgery of laryngeal carcinomas. Am J Otolaryngol 1993;14:116–121

31. Rudert HH. Transoral CO_2-laser surgery in advanced supraglottic cancer. In: Smee R, Bridger GP, eds. Laryngeal Cancer. Amsterdam: Elsevier Science BV; 1994:457–461

32. Motta G, Esposito E, Cassiano B, Motta S. T1–T2-T3 glottic tumors: fifteen years experience with CO_2 laser. Acta Otolaryngol Suppl 1997;527:155–159

33. Iro H, Waldfahrer F, Altendorf-Hofmann A, Weidenbecher M, Sauer R, Steiner W. Transoral laser surgery of supraglottic cancer: follow-up of 141 patients. Arch Otolaryngol Head Neck Surg 1998;124:1245–1250

34. Ambrosch P, Kron M, Steiner W. Carbon dioxide laser microsurgery for early supraglottic carcinoma. Ann Otol Rhinol Laryngol 1998;107:680–688

35. Peretti G, Nicolai P, Piazza C, et al. Oncological results of endoscopic resections of Tis and T1 glottic carcinomas by carbon dioxide laser. Ann Otol Rhinol Laryngol 2001;110:820–826

36. Hoffman H, Karnell L. Laryngeal cancer. In: Steele G, et al, eds. National Cancer Data Base: Annual Review of Patient Care. Atlanta: American Cancer Society; 1995:84–99

37. Lydiatt WM, Shah J, Lydiatt K. Conservation surgery for recurrent carcinoma of the glottic larynx. Am J Surg 1996;172:662–664

38. Harwood AR, Hawkins NV, Keane T, et al. Radiotherapy of early glottic cancer. Laryngoscope 1980;90:465–470

39. Fein DA, Mendenhall WM, Parsons JT, Million RR. T1–T2 squamous cell carcinoma of the glottic larynx treated with radiotherapy: a multivariate analysis of variables potentially influencing local control. Int J Radiat Oncol Biol Phys 1993;25:605–611

40. Hawkins NV. The treatment of glottic carcinoma: an analysis of 800 cases. Laryngoscope 1975;85:1485–1493

41. Stutsman AC, McGavran M. Ultraconservative management of superficially invasive epidermoid carcinoma of the true vocal cord. Ann Otol Rhinol Laryngol 1971;80:507–512

42. Lillie JC, DeSanto L. Transoral surgery of early cordal carcinoma. Trans Am Acad Ophthalmol Otolaryngol 1973;77:ORL92–ORL96

43. Bailey BJ. Glottic reconstruction after hemilaryngectomy: bipedicle muscle flap laryngoplasty. Laryngoscope 1975;85:960–977

44. Kambic V. Epiglottoplasty—new technique for laryngeal reconstruction. Radiologia Ivgoslavika 1977;(Suppl 2):33–43

45. Vaughan CW. Transoral laryngeal surgery using the CO_2 laser: laboratory experiments and clinical experience. Laryngoscope 1978;88(9 Pt 1):1399–1420

46. Davis RK, Jako GJ, Hyams VJ, Shapshay SM. The anatomic limitations of CO_2 laser cordectomy. Laryngoscope 1982;92(9 Pt 1):980–984

47. Shapshay SM. Newer methods of cancer treatment: laser therapy for the cancer patient. In: DeVita VT Jr, Hellman S, Rosenberg SA, eds. Cancer Principles and Practice of Oncology. 2nd ed. Philadelphia: Lippincott; 1985

48. Blakeslee D, Vaughan CW, Shapshay SM, Simpson GT, Strong MS. Excisional biopsy in the selective management of T1 glottic cancer: a three-year follow-up study. Laryngoscope 1984;94:488–494

49. Steiner W. Transoral microsurgical CO_2-laser resection of laryngeal carcinoma. In: Wigand ME, Steiner W, Stell PM, eds. Functional Partial Laryngectomy. Berlin: Springer-Verlag; 1984:121–125

50. Peretti G, Nicolai P, Redaelli De Zinis LO, et al. Endoscopic CO_2 laser excision for tis, T1, and T2 glottic carcinomas: cure rate and prognostic factors. Otolaryngol Head Neck Surg 2000;123(1 Pt 1):124–131

51. Werner JA, Dunne AA, Folz BJ, Lippert BM. Transoral laser microsurgery in carcinomas of the oral cavity, pharynx, and larynx. Cancer Control 2002;9:379–386

52. Shapshay SM, Hybels RL, Bohigian RK. Laser excision of early vocal cord carcinoma: indications, limitations, and precautions. Ann Otol Rhinol Laryngol 1990;99:46–50

53. Zeitels SM, Vaughan CW, Domanowski GF. Endoscopic management of early supraglottic cancer. Ann Otol Rhinol Laryngol 1990;99:951–956

54. Zeitels SM. Infrapetiole exploration of the supraglottis for exposure of the anterior glottal commissure. J Voice 1998;12:117–122

55. McGuirt WF, Koufman J. Endoscopic laser surgery: an alternative in laryngeal cancer treatment. Arch Otolaryngol Head Neck Surg 1987;113:501–505

56. Bradley PJ. Treatment of the patient with upper airway obstruction caused by cancer of the larynx. Otolaryngol Head Neck Surg 1999;120:737–741

57. Steiner W, Ambrosch P, Martin A, Liebmann F, Kron M. Results of transoral laser microsurgery of laryngeal cancer in 3rd European Congress of the European Federation of Oto-rhino-laryngological Societies (EU-FOS). Budapest: Bologna Monduzzi Editore A.p.A.; 1996

58. Rudert HH, Werner JA, Hoft S. Transoral carbon dioxide laser resection of supraglottic carcinoma. Ann Otol Rhinol Laryngol 1999;108:819–827

59. Eckel HE. Local recurrences following transoral laser surgery for early glottic carcinoma: frequency, management, and outcome. Ann Otol Rhinol Laryngol 2001;110:7–15

60. Ferlito A, Harrison DF, Bailey BJ, DeSanto LW. Are clinical classifications for laryngeal cancer satisfactory? Ann Otol Rhinol Laryngol 1995;104(9 Pt 1):741–747

61. Bryce DP, Rider WD. Pre-operative irradiation in the treatment of advanced laryngeal carcinoma. Laryngoscope 1971;81:1481–1490

62. Harwood AR, Bryce DP, Rider WD. Management of T3 glottic cancer. Arch Otolaryngol 1980;106:697–699

63. DeSanto LW, Lillie J, Devine K. Surgical salvage after radiation for laryngeal cancer. Laryngoscope 1976;86:649–657

64. DeSanto LW. T3 glottic cancer: options and consequences of the options. Laryngoscope 1984;94:1311–1315

65. Al-Sarraf M, Kinrie J, Jacobs J, et al. New way of giving chemotherapy as part of multi-disciplinary treatment for patients with head and neck cancers: preliminary report. Proc Am Assoc Cancer Res 1982;23:134

66. Hong WK, Popkin JD, Shapshay SM. Preoperative adjuvant induction chemotherapy in head and neck cancer. Cancer Treat Res 1984;22:287–300

67. Jacobs JR, Pajak TF, Kinzie J, et al. Induction chemotherapy in advanced head and neck cancer. A Radiation Therapy Oncology Group Study. Arch Otolaryngol Head Neck Surg 1987;113:193–197

68. Pfister DG, Strong E, Harrison L, et al. Larynx preservation with combined chemotherapy and radiation therapy in advanced but resectable head and neck cancer. J Clin Oncol 1991;9:850–859

69. Induction chemotherapy plus radiation compared with surgery plus radiation in patients with advanced laryngeal cancer. The Department of Veterans Affairs Laryngeal Cancer Study Group. N Engl J Med 1991;324:1685–1690

70. Wolf GT, Urba S, Hazuka M. Induction chemotherapy for organ preservation in advanced squamous cell carcinoma of the oral cavity and oropharynx. [Review] Recent Results Cancer Res 1994;134:133–143

71. Urba SG, Forastiere AA, Wolf GT, Esclamado RM, McLaughlin PW, Thornton AF. Intensive induction chemotherapy and radiation for organ preservation in patients with advanced resectable head and neck carcinoma. J Clin Oncol 1994;12:946–953

72. Bradford CR, Zhu S, Wolf GT, et al. Overexpression of p53 predicts organ preservation using induction chemotherapy and radiation in patients with advanced laryngeal cancer. Department of Veterans Affairs Laryngeal Cancer Study Group. Otolaryngol Head Neck Surg 1995;113:408–412

73. Kies M, Vokes E. Chemoradiation in the management of advanced laryngeal cancer. In: Robbins K, Murry T, eds. Head and Neck Cancer: Organ Preservation, Function, and Rehabilitation. San Diego: Singular Publishing Group; 1998:45–49

74. Mantz CA, Vokes EE, Kies MS, et al. Sequential induction chemotherapy and concomitant chemoradiotherapy in the management of locoregionally advanced laryngeal cancer. Ann Oncol 2001;12:343–347

75. Spaulding MB, Fischer SG, Wolf GT. Tumor response, toxicity, and survival after neoadjuvant organ-preserving chemotherapy for advanced laryngeal carcinoma. The Department of Veterans Affairs Cooperative Laryngeal Cancer Study Group. J Clin Oncol 1994;12:1592–1599

76. Forastiere AA. Larynx preservation trials: a critical appraisal. Semin Radiat Oncol 1998;8:254–261

77. Rodriguez-Cuevas S, Labastida S, Gonzalez D, Briseño N, Cortes H. Partial laryngectomy as salvage surgery for radiation failures in T1–T2 laryngeal cancer. Head Neck 1998;20:630–633

78. Suen JY, Wetmore SJ, Wetzel WJ, Craig RD. Blastomycosis of the larynx. Ann Otol Rhinol Laryngol 1980;89(6 Pt 1):563–566

79. Kheir SM, Flint A, Moss JA. Primary aspergillosis of the larynx simulating carcinoma. Hum Pathol 1983;14:184–186

80. Yencha MW, Linfesty R, Blackmon A. Laryngeal tuberculosis. Am J Otolaryngol 2000;21:122–126

81. Victoria LV, Hoffman HT, Robinson RA. Granular cell tumour of the larynx. J Laryngol Otol 1998;112:373–376

82. Issing WJ, Struck R, Naumann A. Positive impact of retinyl palmitate in leukoplakia of the larynx. Eur Arch Otorhinolaryngol Suppl 1997;254(Suppl 1):S105–S109

83. McCaffrey TV, Witte M, Ferguson M. Verrucous carcinoma of the larynx. Ann Otol Rhinol Laryngol 1998;107(5 Pt 1):391–395

84. Damm M, Eckel HE, Schneider D, Arnold G. CO_2 laser surgery for verrucous carcinoma of the larynx. Lasers Surg Med 1997;21:117–123

85. Cattaruzza MS, Maisonneuve P, Boyle P. Epidemiology of laryngeal cancer. Eur J Cancer B Oral Oncol 1996;32B:293–305

86. Kokoska MS, Piccirillo JF, Haughey BH. Gender differences in cancer of the larynx. Ann Otol Rhinol Laryngol 1995;104:419–424

87. Burch JD, Howe GR, Miller AB, Semenciw R. Tobacco, alcohol, asbestos, and nickel in the etiology of cancer of the larynx: a case-control study. J Natl Cancer Inst 1981;67:1219–1224

88. Olsen J, Sabroe S. Occupational causes of laryngeal cancer. J Epidemiol Community Health 1984;38:117–121

89. Shettigara PT, Morgan RW. Asbestos, smoking, and laryngeal carcinoma. Arch Environ Health 1975;30:517–519

90. Wortley P, Vaughan TL, Davis S, Morgan MS, Thomas DB. A case-control study of occupational risk factors for laryngeal cancer. Br J Ind Med 1992;49:837–844

91. Maier H, Tisch M. Epidemiology of laryngeal cancer: results of the Heidelberg case-control study. Acta Otolaryngol Suppl 1997;527:160–164

92. Mineta H, Ogino T, Amano HM, et al. Human papilloma virus (HPV) type 16 and 18 detected in head and neck squamous cell carcinoma. Anticancer Res 1998;18(6B):4765–4768

93. Garcia-Milian R, Hernández H, Panadé L, et al. Detection and typing of human papillomavirus DNA in benign and malignant tumours of laryngeal epithelium. Acta Otolaryngol 1998;118:754–758

94. Rehberg E, Kleinsasser O. Malignant transformation in non-irradiated juvenile laryngeal papillomatosis. Eur Arch Otorhinolaryngol 1999;256:450–454

95. Freije JE, Beatty TW, Campbell BH, Woodson BT, Schultz CJ, Toohill RJ. Carcinoma of the larynx in patients with gastroesophageal reflux. Am J Otolaryngol 1996;17:386–390

96. Copper MP, Smit CF, Stanojcic LD, Devriese PP, Schouwenburg PF, Mathus-Vliegen LM. High incidence of laryngopharyngeal reflux in patients with head and neck cancer. Laryngoscope 2000;110:1007–1011

97. Zagraniski RT, Kelsey JL, Walter SD. Occupational risk factors for laryngeal carcinoma: Connecticut, 1975–1980. Am J Epidemiol 1986;124:67–76

98. Kupisz K, Chibowski D, Klatka J, Klonowski S, Stepulak A. Tumor angiogenesis in patients with laryngeal cancer. Eur Arch Otorhinolaryngol 1999;256:303–305

99. Wain SL, Kier R, Vollmer RT, Bossen EH. Basaloid-squamous carcinoma of the tongue, hypopharynx, and larynx: report of 10 cases. Hum Pathol 1986;17:1158–1166

100. Barnes L, Ferlito A, Altavilla G, MacMillan C, Rinaldo A, Doglioni C. Basaloid squamous cell carcinoma of the head and neck: clinicopathological features and differential diagnosis. Ann Otol Rhinol Laryngol 1996;105:75–82

101. Banks ER, Frierson HF Jr, Mills SE, George E, Zarbo RJ, Swanson PE. Basaloid squamous cell carcinoma of the head and neck: a clinicopathologic and immunohistochemical study of 40 cases. Am J Surg Pathol 1992;16:939–946

102. Kleinsasser OK, Glanz H. Sarcomalike patterns in laryngeal carcinoma (pseudosarcoma, carcinosarcoma, spindle-cell-carcinoma, pleomorphic carcinoma) (author's transl). Laryngol Rhinol Otol (Stuttg) 1978;57:225–234

103. Vollrath M, Osborn M, Altmannsberger M. Immunohistological demonstration of the intermediate filaments in a laryngeal carcinosarcoma: considerations on its histogenesis. Laryngol Rhinol Otol (Stuttg) 1987;66:307–310

104. Balercia G, Bhan AK, Dickersin GR. Sarcomatoid carcinoma: an ultrastructural study with light microscopic and immunohistochemical correlation of 10 cases from various anatomic sites. Ultrastruct Pathol 1995;19:249–263

105. Batsakis JG, Suarez P. Sarcomatoid carcinomas of the upper aerodigestive tracts. Adv Anat Pathol 2000;7:282–293

106. Alguacil-Garcia A, Alonso A, Pettigrew NM. Sarcomatoid carcinoma (so-called pseudosarcoma) of the larynx simulating malignant giant cell tumor of soft parts. A case report. Am J Clin Pathol 1984;82:340–343

107. Madrigal FM, Godoy LM, Daboin KP, Casiraghi O, Garcia AM, Luna MA. Laryngeal osteosarcoma: a clinicopathologic analysis of four cases and comparison with a carcinosarcoma. Ann Diagn Pathol 2002;6:1–9

108. Klijanienko J, Vielh P, Duvillard P, Luboinski B. True carcinosarcoma of the larynx. J Laryngol Otol 1992;106:58–60

109. Goldman RL, Weidner N. Pure squamous cell carcinoma of the larynx with cervical nodal metastasis showing rhabdomyosarcomatous differentiation: clinical, pathologic, and immunohistochemical study of a unique example of divergent differentiation. Am J Surg Pathol 1993;17:415–421

110. Ballo MT, Garden AS, El-Naggar AK, et al. Radiation therapy for early stage (T1–T2) sarcomatoid carcinoma of true vocal cords: outcomes and patterns of failure. Laryngoscope 1998;108:760–763

111. Pesce C, Tobia-Gallelli F, Toncini C. APUD cells of the larynx. Acta Otolaryngol 1984;98:158–162

112. Johnson GD, Abt AB, Mahataphongse VP, Conner GH. Small cell undifferentiated carcinoma of the larynx. Ann Otol Rhinol Laryngol 1979;88(Pt 1):774–778

113. Gnepp DR, Ferlito A, Hyams V. Primary anaplastic small cell (oat cell) carcinoma of the larynx. Review of the literature and report of 18 cases. Cancer 1983;51:1731–1745

114. Soga J, Osaka M, Yakuwa Y. Laryngeal endocrinomas (carcinoids and relevant neoplasms): analysis of 278 reported cases. J Exp Clin Cancer Res 2002;21:5–13

115. Wenig BM, Hyams VJ, Heffner DK. Moderately differentiated neuroendocrine carcinoma of the larynx: a clinicopathologic study of 54 cases. Cancer 1988;62:2658–2676

116. Benisch BM, Tawfik B, Breitenbach EE. Primary oat cell carcinoma of the larynx: an ultrastructural study. Cancer 1975;36:145–148

117. Weidauer H, Blobel GA, Nemetschek-Gansler H, Gould VE, Mall G. Neuroendocrine larynx cancer of the small cell (oat cell) type: morphologic and immunohistochemical findings and their significance for therapy. Laryngol Rhinol Otol (Stuttg) 1985;64:121–127

118. Bishop JW, Osamura RRY, Tsutsumi Y. Multiple hormone production in an oat cell carcinoma of the larynx. Acta Pathol Jpn 1985;35:915–923

119. Porto DP, Wick MR, Ewing SL, Adams GL. Neuroendocrine carcinoma of the larynx. Am J Otolaryngol 1987;8:97–104

120. el-Naggar AK, Batsakis JG, Vassilopoulou-Sellin R, Ordonez NG, Luna MA. Medullary (thyroid) carcinoma-like carcinoids of the larynx. J Laryngol Otol 1991;105:683–686

121. Ferlito A, Barnes L, Rinaldo A, Gnepp DR, Milroy CM. A review of neuroendocrine neoplasms of the larynx: update on diagnosis and treatment. J Laryngol Otol 1998;112:827–834

122. Dictor M, Tennvall J, Akerman M. Moderately differentiated neuroendocrine carcinoma (atypical carcinoid) of the supraglottic larynx: a report of two cases including immunohistochemistry and aspiration cytology. Arch Pathol Lab Med 1992;116:253–257

123. Logue JP, Banerjee SS, Slevin NJ, Vasanthan S. Neuroendocrine carcinomas of the larynx. J Laryngol Otol 1991;105:1031–1035

124. Olofsson J, van Nostrand A. Anaplastic small cell carcinoma of larynx. Ann Otol Rhinol Laryngol 1972;81:284–287

125. Medina JE, Moran M, Goepfert H. Oat cell carcinoma of the larynx and Eaton-Lambert syndrome. Arch Otolaryngol 1984;110:123–126

126. Aguilar EA III, Robbins KT, Stephens J, Dimery IW, Batsakis JG. Primary oat cell carcinoma of the larynx. Am J Clin Oncol 1987;10:26–32

127. Gnepp DR. Small cell neuroendocrine carcinoma of the larynx: a critical review of the literature. ORL J Otorhinolaryngol Relat Spec 1991;53:210–219

128. Vrabec DP, Bartels L. Small cell anaplastic carcinoma of the larynx: review of the literature and report of a case. Laryngoscope 1980;90:1720–1726

129. Lawson W, Zak FG. The glomus bodies ("paraganglia") of the human larynx. Laryngoscope 1974;84:98–111

130. Prasad ML, Patel SG, Huvos AG, Shah JP, Busam KJ. Primary mucosal melanoma of the head and neck: a proposal for microstaging localized, stage I (lymph node-negative) tumors. Cancer 2004;100:1657–1664

131. Nandapalan V, Roland NJ, Helliwell TR, Williams EM, Hamilton JW, Jones AS. Mucosal melanoma of the head and neck. Clin Otolaryngol Allied Sci 1998;23:107–116

132. Browne JD. Management of nonepidermoid cancer of the larynx. [Review] Otolaryngol Clin North Am 1997;30:215–229

133. Mahlstedt K, Ussmuller J, Donath K. Malignant sialogenic tumours of the larynx. J Laryngol Otol 2002;116:119–122

134. Thompson LD, Gannon FH. Chondrosarcoma of the larynx: a clinicopathologic study of 111 cases with a review of the literature. Am J Surg Pathol 2002;26:836–851

135. Lippert BM, Claassen H, Bäumken J, Jänig U, Werner JA. Chondrosarcoma of the Larynx [in German]. Laryngorhinootologie 1997;76:28–35

136. Lewis JE, Olsen KD, Inwards CY. Cartilaginous tumors of the larynx: clinicopathologic review of 47 cases. Ann Otol Rhinol Laryngol 1997;106:94–100

137. Mochloulis G, Irving RM, Grant HR, Miller RF. Laryngeal Kaposi's sarcoma in patients with AIDS. J Laryngol Otol 1996;110:1034–1037

138. Schiff NF, Annino DJ, Woo P, Shapshay SM. Kaposi's sarcoma of the larynx. Ann Otol Rhinol Laryngol 1997;106(7 Pt 1):563–567

139. Friedman M, Venkatesan TK, Caldarelli DD. Intralesional vinblastine for treating AIDS-associated Kaposi's sarcoma of the oropharynx and larynx. Ann Otol Rhinol Laryngol 1996;105:272–274

140. Dittrich C. Current status of interferon therapy. Wien Med Wochenschr 1986;136(7–8):163–172

141. Tami TA, Ferlito A, Rinaldo A, Lee KC, Singh B. Laryngeal pathology in the acquired immunodeficiency syndrome: diagnostic and therapeutic dilemmas. Ann Otol Rhinol Laryngol 1999;108:214–220

142. Freeland AP, Van Nostrand A, Jahn A. Metastases to the larynx. J Otolaryngol 1979;8:448–456

143. Nicolai P, Puxeddu R, Cappiello J, et al. Metastatic neoplasms to the larynx: report of three cases. Laryngoscope 1996;106:851–855

144. McCaffrey TV, Lipton RJ. Thyroid carcinoma invading the upper aerodigestive system. Laryngoscope 1990;100:824–830

145. Lipton RJ, McCaffrey TV, van Heerden JA. Surgical treatment of invasion of the upper aerodigestive tract by well-differentiated thyroid carcinoma. Am J Surg 1987;154:363–367

146. McCaffrey TV, Bergstralh EJ, Hay ID. Locally invasive papillary thyroid carcinoma: 1940–1990. Head Neck 1994;16:165–172

147. Czaja JM, McCaffrey TV. The surgical management of laryngotracheal invasion by well-differentiated papillary thyroid carcinoma. Arch Otolaryngol Head Neck Surg 1997;123:484–490

148. Broyles FN. The anterior commissure tendon. Ann Otol Rhinol Laryngol 1943;52:342–345

149. Rucci L, Gammarota L, Gallo O. Carcinoma of the anterior commissure of the larynx, II: Proposal of a new staging system. Ann Otol Rhinol Laryngol 1996;105:391–396

150. Hirano M. Morphological structure of the vocal cord as a vibrator and its variations. Folia Phoniatr (Basel) 1974;26:89–94

151. Tucker GF Jr, Smith HR Jr. A histological demonstration of the development of laryngeal connective tissue compartments. Trans Am Acad Ophthalmol Otolaryngol 1962;66:308–318

152. Reidenbach MM. Borders and topographic relationships of the paraglottic space. Eur Arch Otorhinolaryngol 1997;254:193–195

153. Reidenbach MM. The periepiglottic space: topographic relations and histological organization. J Anat 1996;188(Pt 1):173–182

154. Reidenbach MM. The paraglottic space and transglottic cancer: anatomical considerations. Clin Anat 1996;9:244–251

155. Gilbert RW, Cullen RJ, van Nostrand AW, Bryce DP, Harwood AR. Prognostic significance of thyroid gland involvement in laryngeal carcinoma. Arch Otolaryngol Head Neck Surg 1986;112:856–859

156. Pearson BW. Laryngeal microcirculation and pathways of cancer spread. Laryngoscope 1975;85:700–713

157. Reidenbach MM. Subglottic region: normal topography and possible clinical implications. Clin Anat 1998;11:9–21

158. Steiner W, Ambrosch P. Larynx: anatomical definitions: superior and inferior boundaries of the glottis. In: Hermanek P, Henson DE, Hutter RVP, Sobin LH, editors. TNM Supplement 1993, a Commentary on Uniform Use. New York: Springer-Verlag International Union Against Cancer [Union Internationale Contre le Cancer]; 1993:27

159. Brasnu D, Laccourreye H, Dulmet E, Jaubert F. Mobility of the vocal cord and the arytenoid in cancer of the larynx and the hypopharynx: anatomo-clinical study. Ann Otolaryngol Chir Cervicofac 1988;105:435–441

160. Reidenbach MM. Aryepiglottic fold: normal topography and clinical implications. Clin Anat 1998;11:223–235

161. Dursun G, Keser R, Aktürk T, Akìner MN, Demireller A, Sak SD. The significance of pre-epiglottic space invasion in supraglottic laryngeal carcinomas. Eur Arch Otorhinolaryngol 1997;254(Suppl 1):S110–S112

162. Weinstein GS, Laccourreye O, Brasnu D, Tucker J, Montone K. Reconsidering a paradigm: the spread of supraglottic carcinoma to the glottis. Laryngoscope 1995;105:1129–1133

163. Kirchner JA. Glottic-supraglottic barrier: fact or fantasy? Ann Otol Rhinol Laryngol 1997;106:700–704

164. Cabelguenne A, Blons H, de Waziers I, et al. p53 alterations predict tumor response to neoadjuvant chemotherapy in head and neck squamous cell carcinoma: a prospective series. J Clin Oncol 2000;18:1465–1473

165. Ries L, Eisner MP, Kosary CL, et al. SEER Cancer Statistics Review, 1973–1999, ed. LAG Ries, MP Eisner, CL Kosary, et al. Bethesda, MD: Cancer Statistics Branch of the National Cancer Institute; 2002

166. American Joint Committee on Cancer. AJCC Cancer Staging Handbook from the AJCC Cancer Staging Manual, Sixth Edition, ed. FL Greene, DL Page, ID Fleming, et al. New York: Springer-Verlag; 2002:469

167. Hermans R, Van den Bogaert W, Rijnders A, Doornaert P, Baert AL. Predicting the local outcome of glottic squamous cell carcinoma after definitive radiation therapy: value of computed tomography-determined tumour parameters. Radiother Oncol 1999;50:39–46

168. Freeman DE, Mancuso AA, Parsons JT, Mendenhall WM, Million RR. Irradiation alone for supraglottic larynx carcinoma: can CT findings predict treatment results? Int J Radiat Oncol Biol Phys 1990;19:485–490

169. Leroux-Robert J. La chirurgie conservatrice par laryngofissure ou laryngectomie partielle dans les cancers du larynx (Resultats de 150 cas personnels avec recul de plus 5 ans). Ann Otolaryngol Chir Cervicofac 1957;74:40–74

170. Schade G, Kothe C, Leuwer R. Sonography of the larynx: an alternative to laryngoscopy? HNO 2003;51:585–590

171. Righini C, Mouret P, Wu D, Blanchet C, Reyt E. Is hepatic ultrasonography necessary in the initial check-up of patients with squamous cell carcinoma of the upper respiratory and digestive tract? Ann Otolaryngol Chir Cervicofac 2001;118:359–364

172. Kau RJ, Alexiou C, Stimmer H, Arnold W. Diagnostic procedures for detection of lymph node metastases in cancer of the larynx. ORL J Otorhinolaryngol Relat Spec 2000;62:199–203

173. Duflo S, Chrestian M, Guelfucci B, Champsaur P, Moulin G, Zanaret M. Comparison of magnetic resonance imaging with histopathological correlation in laryngeal carcinomas. Ann Otolaryngol Chir Cervicofac 2002;119:131–137

174. Sievers KW. Rational imaging strategies in laryngeal diseases. Radiologe 1998;38:77–82

175. Yousem DM, Tufano RP. Laryngeal imaging. Magn Reson Imaging Clin N Am 2002;10:451–465

176. Castelijns JA, Becker M, Hermans R. Impact of cartilage invasion on treatment and prognosis of laryngeal cancer. [Review] Eur Radiol 1996;6:156–169

177. Walshe P, Hamilton S, McShane D, McConn Walsh R, Walsh MA, Timon C. The potential of virtual laryngoscopy in the assessment of vocal cord lesions. Clin Otolaryngol 2002;27:98–100

178. Castelijns JA, Hermans R, van den Brekel MW, Mukherji SK. Imaging of laryngeal cancer. Semin Ultrasound CT MR 1998;19:492–504

179. Murakami R, Baba Y, Furusawa M, et al. Early glottic squamous cell carcinoma: predictive value of MR imaging for the rate of 5-year local control with radiation therapy. Acta Radiol 2000;41:38–44

180. Becker M, Moulin G, Kurt AM, et al. Atypical squamous cell carcinoma of the larynx and hypopharynx: radiologic features and pathologic correlation. Eur Radiol 1998;8:1541–1551

181. Greess H, Lell M, Römer W, Bautz W. Indications and diagnostic sensitivity of CT and MRI in the otorhinolaryngology field. HNO 2002;50:611–625

182. Berkiten G, Topaloğlu I, Babuna C, Türköz K. Comparison of magnetic resonance imaging findings with postoperative histopathologic results in laryngeal cancers. Kulak Burun Bogaz Ihtis Derg 2002;9:203–207

183. Declercq A, Van den Hauwe L, Van Marck E, Van de Heyning PH, Spanoghe M, De Schepper AM. Patterns of framework invasion in patients with laryngeal cancer: correlation of in vitro magnetic resonance imaging and pathological findings. Acta Otolaryngol 1998;118:892–895

184. Becker M. Neoplastic invasion of laryngeal cartilage: radiologic diagnosis and therapeutic implications. Eur J Radiol 2000;33:216–229

185. Atula T, Markkola A, Leivo I, Mäkitie A. Cartilage invasion of laryngeal cancer detected by magnetic resonance imaging. Eur Arch Otorhinolaryngol 2001;258:272–275

186. Carriero A, Scarabino T, Vallone A, Cammisa M, Salvolini U, Bonomo L. MRI T-staging of laryngeal tumours: role of contrast medium. Neuroradiology 2000;42:66–71

187. Giovanni A, Guelfucci B, Nazarian B, Marciano S, Moulin G, Zanaret M. X-ray imaging in assessing the extent of laryngeal cancer. Rev Laryngol Otol Rhinol (Bord) 1999;120:155–159

188. Hermans R, Op de Beeck K, Delaere PR, Marchal G. Computed tomography and magnetic resonance imaging of laryngeal tumours. Acta Otorhinolaryngol Belg 1999;53:79–86

189. Yuan YG, Han DM, Fan EZ, Li Y, Yan F, Xian JF. The evaluation of cervical lymph node metastasis of laryngeal cancer using magnetic resonance

imaging (MRI). Lin Chuang Er Bi Yan Hou Ke Za Zhi 2000;14:449–451

190. Fried MP, Hsu L, Jolesz FA. Interactive magnetic resonance imaging-guided biopsy in the head and neck: initial patient experience. Laryngoscope 1998;108(4 Pt 1):488–493

191. Steiner W, Aurbach G, Ambrosch P. Minimally invasive therapy in otorhinolaryngology and head and neck surgery. Minimally Invasive Therapy 1991;1:57–70

192. Mendenhall WM, Parsons JT, Stringer SP, Cassisi NJ, Million RR. T1–T2 vocal cord carcinoma: a basis for comparing the results of radiotherapy and surgery. Head Neck Surg 1988;10:373–377

193. Haenggeli CA, Dulguerov P, Slosman D, et al. Value of positron emission tomography with 18-fluorodeoxyglucose (FDG-PET) in early detection of residual tumor in oro-pharyngeal-laryngeal carcinoma. Schweiz Med Wochenschr Suppl 2000;116:8S–11S

194. Courtois A, Foehrenbach H, Maszelin P, et al. Positron emission tomography in head and neck oncology: five cases. Ann Otolaryngol Chir Cervicofac 2001;118:254–260

195. Brouwer J, Bodar EJ, De Bree R, et al. Detecting recurrent laryngeal carcinoma after radiotherapy: room for improvement. Eur Arch Otorhinolaryngol 2004;261:417–422

196. De Boer JR, Pruim J, Burlage F, et al. Therapy evaluation of laryngeal carcinomas by tyrosine-pet. Head Neck 2003;25:634–644

197. Dietz A, Rudat V, Harms W, Jungehülsing M, Dollner R, Henze M. Diagnosis with (18)F-FDG PET scan after larynx preservation by primary radiochemotherapy. HNO 2004;52:38–44

198. Nowak B, Di Martino E, Jänicke S, et al. Diagnostic evaluation of malignant head and neck cancer by F-18-FDG PET compared to CT/MRI. Nucl Med (Stuttg) 1999;38:312–318

199. Slevin NJ, Collins CD, Hastings DL, et al. The diagnostic value of positron emission tomography (PET) with radiolabelled fluorodeoxyglucose (18F-FDG) in head and neck cancer. J Laryngol Otol 1999;113:548–554

200. Terhaard CH, Bongers V, van Rijk PP, Hordijk GJ. F-18-fluoro-deoxyglucose positron-emission tomography scanning in detection of local recurrence after radiotherapy for laryngeal/pharyngeal cancer. Head Neck 2001;23:933–941

201. Bongers V, Hobbelink MG, van Rijk PP, Hordijk GJ. Cost-effectiveness of dual-head 18F-fluorodeoxyglucose PET for the detection of recurrent laryngeal cancer. Cancer Biother Radiopharm 2002;17:303–306

202. Kim HJ, Boyd J, Dunphy F, Lowe V. F-18 FDG PET scan after radiotherapy for early-stage larynx cancer. Clin Nucl Med 1998;23:750–752

203. Zeitels SM. Universal modular glottiscope system: the evolution of a century of design and technique for direct laryngoscopy. Ann Otol Rhinol Laryngol Suppl 1999;179:2–24

204. Arens C, Eistert B, Glanz H, Waas W. Endolaryngeal high-frequency ultrasound. Eur Arch Otorhinolaryngol 1998;255:250–255

205. Arens C, Glanz H. Endoscopic high-frequency ultrasound of the larynx. Eur Arch Otorhinolaryngol 1999;256:316–322

206. Zargi M, Smid L, Fajdiga I, et al. Laser induced fluorescence in diagnostics of laryngeal cancer. Acta Otolaryngol Suppl 1997;527:125–127

207. Arens C, Malzahn K, Dias O, Andrea M, Glanz H. Endoscopic imaging techniques in the diagnosis of laryngeal carcinoma and its precursor lesions. Laryngorhinootologie 1999;78:685–691

208. Wardrop PJ, Sim S, McLaren K. Contact endoscopy of the larynx: a quantitative study. J Laryngol Otol 2000;114:437–440

209. Andrea M, Dias O, Santos A. Contact endoscopy during microlaryngeal surgery: a new technique for endoscopic examination of the larynx. Ann Otol Rhinol Laryngol 1995;104:333–339

210. Reibel JF, Jahrsdoerfer RA, Johns MM, Cantrell RW. Histoplasmosis of the larynx. Otolaryngol Head Neck Surg 1982;90:740–743

211. Osorio LE, Castillo CM, Ochoa MT. Mucosal leishmaniasis due to Leishmania (Viannia) panamensis in Colombia: clinical characteristics. Am J Trop Med Hyg 1998;59:49–52

212. Filntisis GA, Moon RE, Kraft KL, Farmer JC, Scher RL, Piantadosi CA. Laryngeal radionecrosis and hyperbaric oxygen therapy: report of 18 cases and review of the literature. Ann Otol Rhinol Laryngol 2000;109:554–562

213. Hao SP, Chen HC, Wei FC, Chen CY, Yeh AR, Su JL. Systematic management of osteoradionecrosis in the head and neck. Laryngoscope 1999;109:1324–1328

214. McGuirt WF, Greven KM, Keyes JW Jr, Williams DW III, Watson N. Laryngeal radionecrosis versus recurrent cancer: a clinical approach. Ann Otol Rhinol Laryngol 1998;107:293–296

215. Delap TG, Lavy JA, Alusi G, Quiney RE. Tuberculosis presenting as a laryngeal tumour. J Infect 1997;34:139–141

216. Kaur S, Malik SK, Kumar B, Singh MP, Chakravarty RN. Respiratory system involvement in leprosy. Int J Lepr 1979;47:18–25

217. Waxman J, Bose WJ. Laryngeal manifestations of Wegener's granulomatosis: case reports and review of the literature. J Rheumatol 1986;13:408–411

218. Rasmussen N. Management of the ear, nose, and throat manifestations of Wegener granulomatosis: an otorhinolaryngologist's perspective. Curr Opin Rheumatol 2001;13:3–111

219. McDonald TJ, DeRemee RA, Harrison EG Jr, Facer GW, Devine KD. The protean clinical features of polymorphic reticulosis (lethal midline granuloma). Laryngoscope 1976;86:936–945

220. Payne J, Koopmann CF Jr. Laryngeal carcinoma—or is it laryngeal blastomycosis. Laryngoscope 1984;94(5 Pt 1):608–611

221. Hanson JM, Spector G, El-Mofty SK. Laryngeal blastomycosis: a commonly missed diagnosis: report of two cases and review of the literature. Ann Otol Rhinol Laryngol 2000;109:281–286

222. Lambert PR, Ward P, Berci G. Pseudosarcoma of the larynx: a comprehensive analysis. Arch Otolaryngol 1980;106:700–708

223. Orvidas LJ, Olsen KD, Lewis JE, Suman VJ. Verrucous carcinoma of the larynx: a review of 53 patients. Head Neck 1998;20:197–203

224. Baugh RF, Wolf GT, Beals TF, Krause CJ, Forastiere A. Small cell carcinoma of the larynx: results of therapy. Laryngoscope 1986;96:1283–1290

225. Woodruff JM, Senie R. Atypical carcinoid tumor of the larynx: a critical review of the literature. ORL J Otorhinolaryngol Relat Spec 1991;53:194–209

226. Shonai T, Hareyama M, Sakata K, et al. Mucoepidermoid carcinoma of the larynx: a case which responded completely to radiotherapy and a review of the literature. Jpn J Clin Oncol 1998;28:339–342

227. Whicker JH, Neel HB III, Weiland LH, Devine KD. Adenocarcinoma of the larynx. Ann Otol Rhinol Laryngol 1974;83:487–490

228. Marioni G, Bottin R, Staffieri A, Altavilla G. Spindle-cell tumours of the larynx: diagnostic pitfalls: a case report and review of the literature. Acta Otolaryngol 2003;123:86–90

229. Amin HH, Petruzzelli GJ, Husain AN, Nickoloff BJ. Primary malignant melanoma of the larynx. Arch Pathol Lab Med 2001;125:271–273

230. McCaffrey JC. Evaluation and treatment of aerodigestive tract invasion by well-differentiated thyroid carcinoma. Cancer Control 2000;7:246–252

231. Lee J. Resection margins of carcinoma of the oral cavity, oropharynx, hypopharynx and larynx: a clinical study. In: . Iowa City: Department of Otolaryngology—Head and Neck Surgery, University of Iowa; 1973

232. Di Nicola V, Resta L, Rotundo L, Fiorella ML, Fiorella R. Evaluation of resection margins as a prognostic factor in the surgical treatment of laryngeal carcinoma. (Original Italian) Il valore prognostico della valutazione dei margini di resezione nel trattamento chirurgico del carcinoma laringeo. Acta Otorhinolaryngol Ital 1999;19:325–341

233. Franklin S, Pho T, Abreo FW, et al. Detection of the proto-oncogene EIF4E in larynx and hypopharynx cancers. Arch Otolaryngol Head Neck Surg 1999;125:177–182

234. Bradford CR, Zhu S, Poore J, et al. p53 mutation as a prognostic marker in advanced laryngeal carcinoma. Department of Veterans Affairs Laryngeal Cancer Cooperative Study Group. Arch Otolaryngol Head Neck Surg 1997;123:605–609

235. Narayana A, Vaughan AT, Gunaratne S, Kathuria S, Walter SA, Reddy SP. Is p53 an independent prognostic factor in patients with laryngeal carcinoma? Cancer 1998;82:286–291

236. Golusinski W, Olofsson J, Szmeja Z, Biczysko W, Krygier-Stojałowska A, Kulczyński B. A comprehensive analysis of selected diagnostic methods with respect to their usefulness in evaluating the biology of neoplastic cells in patients with laryngeal cancer. Eur Arch Otorhinolaryngol 1999;256:306–311

237. Krecicki T, Jeleń M, Zalesska-Krecicka M, Szkudlarek T. Ki-67 immunostaining and prognosis in laryngeal cancer. Clin Otolaryngol Allied Sci 1998;23:539–542

238. Magnano M, Cavalot AL, Gervasio CF, et al. Surgery or radiotherapy for early stage carcinomas of the glottic larynx. Tumori 1999;85:188–193

239. Zeitels S, Vaughan CW, Domanowski GF, Fuleihan NS, Simpson GT II. Laser epiglottectomy: endoscopic technique and indications. Otolaryngol Head Neck Surg 1990;103:237–243

240. DiNardo LJ, Kaylie D, Isaacson J. Current treatment practices for early laryngeal carcinoma. Otolaryngol Head Neck Surg 1999;120:30–37

241. Maheshwar AA, Gaffney C. Radiotherapy for T1 glottic carcinoma: impact of anterior commissure involvement. J Laryngol Otol 2001;115:298–301

242. Hirota S, Soejima T, Obayashi K, et al. Radiotherapy of T1 and T2 glottic cancer: analysis of anterior commissure involvement. Radiat Med 1996;14:297–302

243. Burke LS, Greven KM, McGuirt WT, Case D, Hoen HM, Raben M. Definitive radiotherapy for early glottic carcinoma: prognostic factors and implications for treatment. Int J Radiat Oncol Biol Phys 1997;38:1001–1006

244. Spector JG, Sessions DG, Chao KS, et al. Stage 1 (T1 N0 M0) squamous cell carcinoma of the laryngeal glottis: therapeutic results and voice preservation. Head Neck 1999;21:707–717

245. Spector JG, Sessions DG, Chao KS, Hanson JM, Simpson JR, Perez CA. Management of stage II (T2N0M0) glottic carcinoma by radiotherapy and conservation surgery. Head Neck 1999;21:116–123

246. Hamoir M, Ledeghen S, Rombaux P, et al. Conservation surgery for laryngeal and hypopharyngeal cancer. Acta Otorhinolaryngol Belg 1999;53:207–213

247. Schwaab G, Mamelle G, Lartigau E, Parise O Jr, Wibault P, Luboinski B. Surgical salvage treatment of T1/T2 glottic carcinoma after failure of radiotherapy. Am J Surg 1994;168:474–475

248. Persky MS, Lagmay VM, Cooper J, Constantinides M, O'Leary R. Curative radiotherapy for anterior commissure laryngeal carcinoma. Ann Otol Rhinol Laryngol 2000;109(February):156–159

249. Ton-Van J, Lefebvre JL, Stern JC, Buisset E, Coche-Dequeant B, Vankemmel B. Comparison of surgery and radiotherapy in T1 and T2 glottic carcinomas. Am J Surg 1991;162:337–340

250. Gilbert RW, Lundgren JA, van Nostrand AW, Keane TJ. T3N0M0 glottic carcinoma: a pathologic analysis of 41 patients treated surgically following radiotherapy. Clin Otolaryngol Allied Sci 1988;3:467–479

251. Olofsson J, Van Nostrand AW. Growth and spread of laryngeal and hypopharyngeal carcinoma with reflections on the effect of preoperative irradiation. Acta Otolaryngol Suppl 1973;308:1–84

252. Ward PH, Calcaterra TC, Kagan AR. The enigma of post irradiation oedema and recurrent residual carcinoma of the larynx. Laryngoscope 1975;85:522–529

253. Lawson S, Som M. Second primary cancer after irradiation of laryngeal cancer. Ann Otol Rhinol Laryngol 1975;84:771–775

254. Watters GW, Patel S, Rhys-Evans P. Partial laryngectomy for recurrent laryngeal carcinoma. Clin Otolaryngol Allied Sci 2000;25:146–152

255. Kies MS, Gordon LI, Hauck WW, et al. Analysis of complete responders after initial treatment with chemotherapy in head and neck cancer. Otolaryngol Head Neck Surg 1985;93:199–205

256. Forastiere AA. Induction and adjuvant chemotherapy for head and neck cancer: future perspectives. Acta Otorhinolaryngol Belg 1999;53:277–280

257. Pignon JP, Bourhis J, Domenge C, Designé L. Chemotherapy added to locoregional treatment for head and neck squamous-cell carcinoma: three meta-analyses of updated individual data. MACH-NC Collaborative Group. Meta-Analysis of Chemotherapy on Head and Neck Cancer. Lancet 2000;355:949–955

258. Laccourreye O, Brasnu D, Bassot V, Ménard M, Khayat D, Laccourreye H. Cisplatin-fluorouracil exclusive chemotherapy for T1–T3N0 glottic squamous cell carcinoma complete clinical responders: five-year results. J Clin Oncol 1996;14:2331–2336

259. Laccourreye H. "Limited" cancers of the glottic stage of the larynx and exclusive chemotherapy: 15 years of experience. (French). Bull Acad Natl Med 1997;181:641–648, discussion 648–649

260. Laccourreye O, Diaz EM Jr, Bassot V, Muscatello L, Garcia D, Brasnu D. A multimodal strategy for the treatment of patients with T2 invasive squamous cell carcinoma of the glottis. Cancer 1999;85:40–46

261. Har-El G, Paniello RC, Abemayor E, Rice DH, Rassekh C. Partial laryngectomy with imbrication laryngoplasty for glottic carcinoma. Arch Otolaryngol Head Neck Surg 2003;129:66–71

262. Krajina Z, Kosokovic F, Vecerina S. Laryngeal reconstruction with sternohyoid fascia in partial laryngectomy. J Laryngol Otol 1979;93:1181–1189

263. Krajina Z. The Zagreb method of partial laryngectomy: a retrospective study 1970–1986. Acta Med Croatica 1999;53:179–183

264. Sheen TS, Ko J, Chang Y. Partial vertical laryngectomy in the treatment of early glottic cancer. Ann Otol Rhinol Laryngol 1998;107:593–597

265. Laccourreye O, Gutierrez-Fonseca R, Garcia D, et al. Local recurrence after vertical partial laryngectomy: a conservative modality of treatment for patients with stage I–II squamous cell carcinoma of the glottis. Cancer 1999;85:2549–2556

266. Kambic V, Radsel Z, Smid L. Laryngeal reconstruction with epiglottis after vertical hemilaryngectomy. J Laryngol Otol 1976;90:467–473

267. Sedlacek K. Application of the epiglottis as a pedunculated lobe in reconstructive surgery of the larynx. Otolaryngol Pol 1966;20:81–85

268. Sedlacek K. Reconstructive anterior and lateral laryngectomy with the use of the epiglottis for the pedicle graft. Cesk Otolaryngol 1965;14:328–334

269. Tucker HM, Wood BG, Levine H, Katz R. Glottic reconstruction after near-total laryngectomy. Laryngoscope 1979;89:609–618

270. Eckel HE, Jungehülsing M, Thumfart W. Indications, technic and results following Sedlacek-Kambic-Tucker reconstructive partial resection of the larynx [in German]. [Review] HNO 1997;45:915–922

271. Lelievre G, Laccourreye O, Strunski V, Juvanon JM, Bedbeder P, Peynegre R. Critical study and role of partial vertical reconstructive laryngectomies with epiglottoplasty by the Tucker method: apropos of 18 cases [in French]. Ann Otolaryngol Chir Cervicofac 1987;104:323–328

272. Tu G, Tang P, He Y. The use of hyoid osteomuscular flap in extended partial laryngectomy. Zhonghua Er Bi Yan Hou Ke Za Zhi 1996;31:39–42

273. Pearson B. Minimally-invasive transoral resection of head and neck cancers. Jacksonville Medicine 1998;49:68–71

274. Moreau PR. Treatment of laryngeal carcinomas by laser endoscopic microsurgery. Laryngoscope 2000;110:1000–1006

275. Eckel HE, Schneider C, Jungehülsing M, Damm M, Schröder U, Vössing M. Potential role of transoral laser surgery for larynx carcinoma. Lasers Surg Med 1998;23:79–86

276. Steiner W, Ambrosch P. Laser microsurgery for cancer of the larynx. Minim Invasive Ther Allied Technol 1996;5:159–164

277. Sittel C, Eckel HE, Eschenburg C, Vössing M, Pototschnig C, Zorowka P. Voice quality after partial laser laryngectomy [in German]. Laryngorhinootologie 1998;77:219–225

278. Rosier JF, Grégoire V, Counoy H, et al. Comparison of external radiotherapy, laser microsurgery and partial laryngectomy for the treatment of T1N0M0 glottic carcinomas: a retrospective evaluation. Radiother Oncol 1998;48:175–183

279. Wagenfeld DJ, Harwood AR, Bryce DP, van Nostrand AW, de Boer G. Second primary respiratory tract malignant neoplasms in supraglottic carcinoma. Arch Otolaryngol 1981;107:135–137

280. Lee NK, Goepfert H, Wendt C. Supraglottic laryngectomy for intermediate-stage cancer: U.T. M.D. Anderson Cancer Center experience with combined therapy. Laryngoscope 1990;100:831–836

281. Pinilla M, González FM, Górriz C, et al. Oncologic surgery of the larynx after failure of radiotherapy [in Spanish]. Acta Otorrinolaringol Esp 1998;49:633–636

282. Laramore GE. Treatment of nodes in the clinically N0 neck. In: L. GE, ed. Radiation Therapy of Head and Neck Cancer. New York: Springer-Verlag; 1989

283. Steiniger JR, Parnes S, Gardner G. Morbidity of combined therapy for the treatment of supraglottic carcinoma: supraglottic laryngectomy and radiotherapy. Ann Otol Rhinol Laryngol 1997;106:151–158

284. Mendenhall WM, Parsons JT, Mancuso AA, Stringer SP, Cassisi NJ. Radiotherapy for squamous cell carcinoma of the supraglottic larynx: an alternative to surgery. Head Neck 1996;18:24–35

285. Leonard JR, Litton WB. Selection of the patient for conservation surgery of the larynx. Laryngoscope 1971;81:232–252

286. Weinstein G, Laccourreye O, Brasnu D, et al. The role of computed tomography and magnetic resonance imaging in planning for conservation laryngeal surgery. In: Yousem D, ed. Neuroimaging Clinics of North America. Philadelphia: WB Saunders; 1996:497–504

287. Maroldi R, Battaglia G, Maculotti P, Farina D, Milesi F, Chiesa A. Computerized tomography in the surgical planning of supraglottic carcinoma: analysis of cost-effectiveness in 69 patients [in Italian]. Radiol Med (Torino) 1996;91:590–595

288. Ogura J, Biller H. Conservation surgery in cancer of the head and neck. Otolaryngol Clin North Am 1969;2:641–665

289. Ogura JH, Sessions D, Spector G. Conservation surgery for epidermoid carcinoma of the supraglottic larynx. Laryngoscope 1975;85:1808–1815

290. Weems DH, Mendenhall WM, Parsons JT, Cassisi NJ, Million RR. Squamous cell carcinoma of the supraglottic larynx treated with surgery and/or radiation therapy. Int J Radiat Oncol Biol Phys 1987;13:1483–1487

291. Moe K, Wolf GT, Fisher SG, Hong WK. Regional metastases in patients with advanced laryngeal cancer. Department of Veterans Affairs Laryngeal Cancer Study Group. Arch Otolaryngol Head Neck Surg 1996;122:644–648

292. Brasilino de Carvalho M. Quantitative analysis of the extent of extracapsular invasion and its prognostic significance: a prospective study of 170 cases of carcinoma of the larynx and hypopharynx. Head Neck 1998;20:16–21

293. Lutz CK, Johnson JT, Wagner RL, Myers EN. Supraglottic carcinoma: patterns of recurrence. Ann Otol Rhinol Laryngol 1990;99:12–17

294. Myers EN, Alvi A. Management of carcinoma of the supraglottic larynx: evolution, current concepts, and future trends. [Review] Laryngoscope 1996;106(5 Pt 1):559–567

295. Mendenhall WM, Parsons JT, Stringer SP, Cassisi NJ. Radiotherapy for carcinoma of the supraglottis. [Review] Otolaryngol Clin North Am 1997;30:145–161

296. Parsons JT, Mendenhall WM, Stringer SP, Cassisi NJ. T4 laryngeal carcinoma: radiotherapy alone with surgery reserved for salvage. Int J Radiat Oncol Biol Phys 1998;40:549–552

297. Laccourreye O, Weinstein G, Naudo P, Cauchois R, Laccourreye H, Brasnu D. Supracricoid partial laryngectomy after failed laryngeal radiation therapy. Laryngoscope 1996;106:495–498

298. Laccourreye O, Brasnu D, Merite-Drancy A, et al. Cricohyoidopexy in selected infrahyoid epiglottic carcinomas presenting with pathological preepiglottic space invasion. Arch Otolaryngol Head Neck Surg 1993;119:881–886

299. Laccourreye H, Laccourreye O, Weinstein G, Menard M, Brasnu D. Supracricoid laryngectomy with cricohyoidopexy: a partial laryngeal procedure for selected supraglottic and transglottic carcinomas. Laryngoscope 1990;100:735–741

300. Weinstein GS, Laccourreye O. Supracricoid laryngectomy with cricohyoidoepiglottopexy. Otolaryngol Head Neck Surg 1994;111:684–685

301. Piquet JJ, Desaulty A, Hoffman Y, Decroix G. La chirurgie sub-totale et reconstructive dans le traitement des cancers de larynx. Ann Otolaryngol Chir Cervicofac 1974;91:311–320

302. Labayle J, Bismuth R. Total laryngectomy with reconstitution. Ann Otolaryngol Chir Cervicofac 1971;88:219–228

303. Brasnu D, Menard M, Fabre A, Janot F, Laccourreye H. Partial supracricoid laryngectomies: techniques, indications and results [in French]. J Otolaryngol 1988;17:173–178

304. Laccourreye H, Menard M, Fabre A, Brasnu D, Janot F. Supracricoid laryngectomy with cricohyoidoepiglottopexy: a partial laryngeal procedure for glottic carcinoma. Ann Otol Rhinol Laryngol 1990;99(6 Pt 1):421–426

305. Laccourreye O, Muscatello L, Laccourreye L, Naudo P, Brasnu D, Weinstein G. Supracricoid partial laryngectomy with cricohyoidoepiglottopexy for "early" glottic carcinoma classified as T1–T2N0 invading the anterior commissure. Am J Otolaryngol 1997;18:385–390

306. Naudo P, Laccourreye O, Weinstein G, Jouffre V, Laccourreye H, Brasnu D. Complications and functional outcome after supracricoid partial laryngectomy with cricohyoidoepiglottopexy. Otolaryngol Head Neck Surg 1998;118:124–129

307. Laccourreye O, Brasnu D, Laccourreye L, Weinstein G. Ruptured pexis after supracricoid partial laryngectomy. Ann Otol Rhinol Laryngol 1997;106:159–162

308. Chevalier D, Laccourreye O, Brasnu D, Laccourreye H, Piquet JJ. Cricohyoidoepiglottopexy for glottic carcinoma with fixation or impaired motion of the true vocal cord: 5-year oncologic results with 112 patients. Ann Otol Rhinol Laryngol 1997;106:364–369

309. Hassmann E, Skotnicka B. Feasibility of supracricoid laryngectomy based on pathological examination. Eur Arch Otorhinolaryngol 1998;255:68–73

310. Laccourreye O, Cauchois R, Menard M, Brasnu D, Laccourreye H. Deglutition and partial supracricoid laryngectomies [in French]. Ann Otolaryngol Chir Cervicofac 1992;109:73–75

311. Naudo P, Laccourreye O, Weinstein G, Hans S, Laccourreye H, Brasnu D. Functional outcome and prognosis factors after supracricoid partial laryngectomy with cricohyoidopexy. Ann Otol Rhinol Laryngol 1997;106:291–296

312. Laccourreye H, Ménard M, Fabre A, Brasnu D, Janot F. Partial supracricoid laryngectomy: technics, indications and results [in French]. Ann Otolaryngol Chir Cervicofac 1987;104:163–173

313. de Vincentiis M, Minni A, Gallo A, Di Nardo A. Supracricoid partial laryngectomies: oncologic and functional results. Head Neck 1998;20:504–509

314. Laccourreye O, Ross J, Brasnu D, Chabardes E, Kelly JH, Laccourreye H. Extended supracricoid partial laryngectomy with tracheocricohyoidoepiglottopexy. Acta Otolaryngol 1994;114:669–674

315. Laccourreye O, Brasnu D, Jouffre V, Couloigner V, Naudo P, Laccourreye H. Supra-cricoid partial laryngectomy extended to the anterior arch of the cricoid with tracheo-crico-hyoido-epiglottopexy: oncologic and functional results [in French]. Ann Otolaryngol Chir Cervicofac 1996;113:15–19

316. Pearson BW, Salassa J. Transoral laser microresection for cancer of the larynx involving the anterior commissure. Laryngoscope 2003;113:1104–1112

317. Thaler ER, Montone K, Tucker J, Weinstein GS. Delphian lymph node in laryngeal carcinoma: a whole organ study. Laryngoscope 1997;107:332–334

318. Olsen KD, DeSanto LW, Pearson BW. Positive Delphian lymph node: clinical significance in laryngeal cancer. Laryngoscope 1987;97:1033–1037

319. Laccourreye O, Laccourreye L, Crevier-Buchman L, Brasnu D, Weinstein GS. Supracricoid hemilaryngopharyngectomy conversion to Pearson's near-total laryngectomy: a case report. Head Neck 1997;19:232–234

320. Laccourreye O, Mérite-Drancy A, Brasnu D, et al. Supracricoid hemilaryngopharyngectomy in selected pyriform sinus carcinoma staged as T2. Laryngoscope 1993;103:1373–1379

321. MacKenzie RG, Franssen E, Balogh JM, Gilbert RW, Birt D, Davidson J. Comparing treatment outcomes of radiotherapy and surgery in locally advanced carcinoma of the larynx: a comparison limited to patients eligible for surgery. [Review] Int J Radiat Oncol Biol Phys 2000;47:65–71

322. Lima RA, Freitas EQ, Kligerman J, et al. Near-total laryngectomy for treatment of advanced laryngeal cancer. Am J Surg 1997;174:490–491

323. Laccourreye O, Crevier-Buchman L, Hacquart N, Naudo P, Muscatello L, Brasnu D. Laryngectomies and pharyngo-laryngectomies with tracheo-laryngo-pharyngeal shunt of Pearson type: technique, indications and preliminary results [in French]. [Review] Ann Otolaryngol Chir Cervicofac 1996;113:261–268

324. Pearson BW, DeSanto LW, Olsen KD, Salassa JR. The results of near-total laryngectomy. Ann Otol Rhinol Laryngol 1998;107(10 Pt 1):820–825

325. Carrillo JF, Frías-Mendívil M, Lopez-Graniel C, Beitia AI, Ochoa-Carrillo FJ. The impact of preoperative tracheotomy on T3 transglottic carcinomas of the larynx. Eur Arch Otorhinolaryngol 1999;256:78–82

326. Taub S, Bergner L. Air bypass voice prosthesis for vocal rehabilitation of laryngectomees. Am J Surg 1973;125:748–756

327. Blom ED, Singer M, Hamaker R. An improved esophageal insufflation test. Arch Otolaryngol 1985;111:211–212

328. Singer MI, Hamaker RC, Blom ED. Revision procedure for the tracheoesophageal puncture. Laryngoscope 1989;99(7 Pt 1):761–763

329. Thorp MA, Levitt NS, Mortimore S, Isaacs S. Parathyroid and thyroid function five years after treatment of laryngeal and hypopharyngeal carcinoma. Clin Otolaryngol Allied Sci 1999;24:104–108

330. Asai R. Laryngoplasty after total laryngectomy. Arch Otolaryngol 1972;95:114–119

331. Gussenbauer C. Uber die Erste durch Th. Billroth am Menschen ausgefuhrte Kehlkopf-Extirpation und die Anwendung eines Kunstlichen Kehlkopfes. Arch Klin Chirurg 1874;17:343–356

332. Guttman M. Tracheo-hypopharyngeal fistulization. Trans Am Laryngol Rhinol Otol Soc 1935;41:219–226

333. Conley JJ, DeAmesti F, Pierce J. A new surgical technique for the vocal rehabilitation of the laryngectomized patient. Ann Otol Rhinol Laryngol 1958;67:655–664

334. Woods RD II, Pearson B. Alaryngeal speech and development of an internal tracheopharyngeal fistula. Otolaryngol Head Neck Surg 1980;88:64–73

335. Calcaterra TC, Jafek B. Tracheo-esophageal shunt for speech rehabilitation after total laryngectomy. Arch Otolaryngol 1971;94:124–128

336. Staffieri M. Laryngectomie totale avec reconstruction De La Glotte Phonatoire. Rev Laryngol 1974;95:63–83

337. Komorn R. Vocal rehabilitation after total laryngectomized patient with a tracheoesophageal shunt. Ann Otolaryngol Chir Cervicofac 1974;83:445–451

338. Griffiths CM. Neoglottic reconstruction after total laryngectomy. Arch Otolaryngol 1980;106:77–79

339. Sisson GA, McConnel FM, Logemann JA, Yeh S Jr. Voice rehabilitation after laryngectomy. Arch Otolaryngol 1975;101:178–181

340. Sisson GA, Goldman M. Pseudoglottis procedure: update and secondary reconstruction techniques. Laryngoscope 1980;90(7 Pt 1):1120–1129

341. Leipzig B. Neoglottic reconstruction following total laryngectomy: a reappraisal. Ann Otol Rhinol Laryngol 1980;89:534–537

342. Blom ED, Singer MI. Tracheoesophageal puncture prostheses. Arch Otolaryngol 1985;111:208–209

343. Panje WR. Prosthetic vocal rehabilitation following laryngectomy. Ann Otol Rhinol Laryngol 1981;90(2 Pt 1):116–120

344. Hilgers F, Ackerstaff A, van As C. Tracheoesophageal puncture: prosthetic voice management. Curr Opin Otolaryngol 1999;7:112–118

5

Cancer of the Nose and Paranasal Sinuses

Paul J. Donald

Paranasal sinus carcinoma has traditionally carried a poor prognosis. The principal reasons for this are the dearth of clinical signs and symptoms until the lesion has obtained considerable size, and the proximity of the sinuses to the brain. In addition, palpable cervical lymph node metastases, although uncommon, are occasionally accompanied by non-palpable retropharyngeal lymph node metastases.

◆ Anatomy

The intricate interrelated anatomy of the nasal fossae and paranasal sinuses must be thoroughly understood to appreciate the pathophysiology of the tumors contained therein. Further, the relationship of these sinuses to the floor of the cranial cavity is integral to the conceptualization of en bloc resection of these malignancies. Increased knowledge of these anatomical principles resulted in the evolution of craniofacial surgery, a procedure that has markedly improved the prognosis in paranasal sinus cancer.

Whereas the relationship of the maxillary sinus to the lateral wall of the nose, the orbital floor, the alveolar ridge, and the hard palate is commonly understood, appreciation of the proximity of the lateral and lateroposterior wall to the inferior aspect of the infratemporal fossa is less often considered (**Fig. 5.1**). The buccal fat pad as well as the anterior and posterior superior alveolar neurovascular bundles approximates the periosteum at this point. Slightly more lateral are the temporalis and pterygoid muscles. As the narrow posterior sinus wall is approached, the internal maxillary artery is encountered as it enters the pterygomaxillary space through the teardrop aperture of the pterygomaxillary fissure. The artery ascends to this point from its course deep to the mandibular neck, often insinuating itself between the two heads of the lateral pterygoid muscle. The troublesome bleeding so commonly encountered in maxillectomy is often due to a severance of this vessel as well as disruption of the pterygoid venous plexus that invests and drains the pterygoid musculature.

The posterior wall of the maxillary sinus forms the anterior wall of the pterygomaxillary space in its superior half, and the site of articulation of the ascending process of the palatine bone and the pterygoid plates in its inferior half. The maxillary tuberosity extends below the plates for 5 to 7 mm, allowing a point of surgical entry into the sinus in less radical operations in which the pterygoid plates are spared. The maxillary sinus roof medially forms the floor of the ethmoid labyrinth. Tumors of either region, namely the maxillary sinus and the infratemporal fossa, commonly extend into the other.

The thin osseous laminae that compose the medial walls of the orbits permit early penetration of ethmoidal carcinoma into the orbit. The roof of the ethmoid sinus, the fovea ethmoidalis, is only slightly thicker than the lamina papyracea and may make up a significant portion of the medial aspect of the anterior cranial floor (**Fig. 5.2**). The cribriform plates, which form the bony connection between the ethmoid blocks of the right and left sides, also connect both foveae. Olfactory filaments that are extensions of the subarachnoid space penetrate the cribriform plates, creating an easy access route for tumor spreading from the ethmoid sinus directly into the subdural compartment. According to Lang[1] there are 26 to 71 (with an average of 43) foramina in the cribriform plate of each side (**Fig. 5.3**). The number of ethmoid cells is highly variable, ranging from four to 17, with an average of nine.[2] As an anteroposterior progression is made, the cells become larger. The posterior cells may even encircle the optic foramina, thus increasing the vulnerability of the eye to the spread of carcinoma. The most posterior ethmoid cells abut the anterior aspect of the sphenoid sinus. The posterior aspect of the ethmoid labyrinth is much wider than the anterior.

The sphenoid sinus is the most surgically inaccessible of the paranasal sinuses. It ranges in size from a mere dimple in the basisphenoid (conchal pneumatization) to extensive pneumatization of the sphenoidal lesser wing. Tumors originating in or invading the sphenoid sinus present a serious

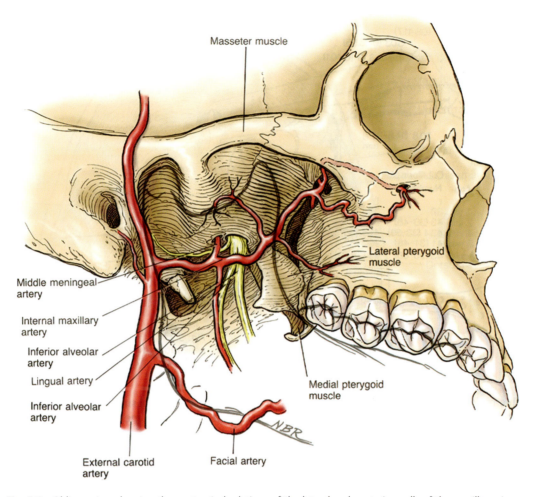

Fig. 5.1 Oblique view showing the anatomical relations of the lateral and posterior walls of the maxillary sinus to the infratemporal fossa and skull base structures.

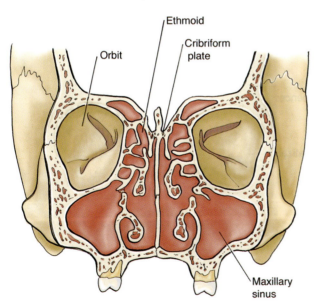

Fig. 5.2 Coronal section of ethmoid sinuses. The cribriform plates and fovea make a considerable contribution to the anterior cranial fossa floor.

therapeutic dilemma because of the plethora of vital anatomical structures approximating its walls. The internal carotid artery lies directly on the bone of the lateral wall posteriorly, often producing an appreciable bulge into the sinus cavity (**Fig. 5.4**). This portion of the artery lies within the cavernous sinus. The posterior roof of the sphenoid sinus is the sella turcica, which produces another, more pronounced bulge that protrudes inferiorly into the sinus lumen. Just anterior to the pituitary gland is the optic chiasm, on the cranial side of the sphenoid sinus anteriorly. From the chiasm the optic nerves pass anteriorly and slightly inferiorly to gain the optic canals. In this course the optic nerves are intimately related to the posterosuperior aspect of the lateral wall of the sphenoid sinus (**Fig. 5.4**).

The bone that extends anteriorly from the optic chiasm to the cribriform area is called the planum sphenoidale (**Fig. 5.5**). It is made up of the sphenoid sinus roof as well as the fovea ethmoidalis. This is often a critical area of excision in craniofacial resection and a crucial area of identification from below by the head and neck surgeon. The intimate re-

Resection using the craniofacial technique is the most commonly employed treatment for esthesioneuroblastoma. Occasionally the lesion clears the nasal vault and ethmoidal fovea sufficiently to permit successful transfacial excision through a lateral rhinotomy, sparing the patient a craniotomy (**Fig. 5.9**). A combination of surgery and postoperative irradiation is recommended.

The 5-year survival rate is reported to be 57 to 88% for stage A disease, 58 to 60% for stage B disease, and 0 to 50% for stage C.[24] In the author's personal series of 15 esthesioneuroblastomas, eight have been followed for 5 or more years. All, with one exception, were treated with a craniofacial excision. Two patients had a so-called impact tumor composed of both esthesioneuroblastoma elements and areas of squamous cell carcinoma. Seven out of 11 are alive and disease free, for a survival rate of 63.6%. We have, however, seen a patient who lived with persistent tumor for 20 years (**Fig. 5.10**).

◆ Diagnosis

One of the primary reasons for the poor prognosis in paranasal sinus cancer is its lack of early symptoms. The few symptoms that do occur (i.e., purulent drainage, nasal obstruction, and epistaxis) (**Fig. 5.11**) are so commonly encountered in benign diseases that carcinoma of the sinonasal tract may not be suspected. Late signs of proptosis, chemosis (**Fig. 5.12**), lateral displacement of the eye (**Fig. 5.11**), facial swelling (**Fig. 5.13**), or frank erosion through the skin (**Fig. 5.14**) signify a poor prognosis. Maxillary sinus lesions may erode inferiorly into the palate (**Fig. 5.15**) or alveolar ridge, producing loose teeth, a denture that quickly loses its fit, a swelling, or an ulcer.

Vigilance on the part of the physician in detecting and pursuing the cause of nasal bleeding of undetermined origin, the reasons for unilateral nasal obstruction of recent onset, or the source of purulent drainage that is refractory to antibiotic therapy is necessary to make an early diagnosis. Although intranasal examination may reveal the tumor in some cases (**Fig. 5.16**), in others the lesion may remain obscure within the sinus cavities and be detectable only by radiographic exam. The average delay from onset of symptoms to final diagnosis is 6 months.[25] The patient in **Fig. 5.17** had symptoms of purulent rhinorrhea, epistaxis, and nasal obstruction that had progressed over a period of 2 years until the diagnosis of sinonasal undifferentiated carcinoma was made.

As a screening device, standard paranasal sinus computed tomographic (CT) scan is very helpful given that 80% of patients with maxillary sinus tumors have evidence of bone erosion.[9] However, as a means of judging tumor extent the standard examination is extremely limited. One of the biggest problems in managing paranasal sinus cancers is the determination of tumor extent. Robin and Powell[26] analyzed 282 cases of paranasal sinus malignancy and found an error in estimate of tumor extension in one third of the cases. A serious source of diagnostic error in our own experience is the difficulty in interpretation of a density in a sinus cavity on the CT scan. A tumor plugging a sinus ostium can result in the accumulation of secretions that are often distinguishable on the scan from tumor.

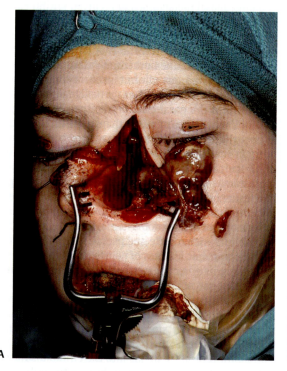
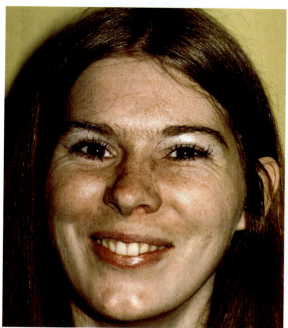

Fig. 5.9 **(A)** Young woman with an esthesioneuroblastoma on the superior meatus of the nose. Craniofacial resection was not necessary. **(B)** Photograph following full course of planned postoperative irradiation.

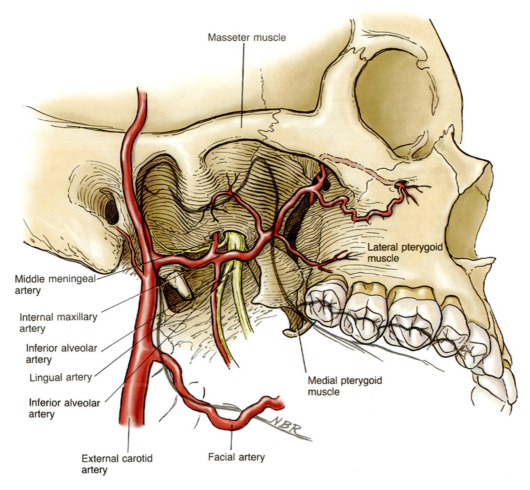

Fig. 5.1 Oblique view showing the anatomical relations of the lateral and posterior walls of the maxillary sinus to the infratemporal fossa and skull base structures.

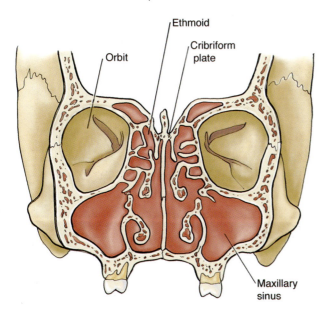

Fig. 5.2 Coronal section of ethmoid sinuses. The cribriform plates and fovea make a considerable contribution to the anterior cranial fossa floor.

therapeutic dilemma because of the plethora of vital anatomical structures approximating its walls. The internal carotid artery lies directly on the bone of the lateral wall posteriorly, often producing an appreciable bulge into the sinus cavity (**Fig. 5.4**). This portion of the artery lies within the cavernous sinus. The posterior roof of the sphenoid sinus is the sella turcica, which produces another, more pronounced bulge that protrudes inferiorly into the sinus lumen. Just anterior to the pituitary gland is the optic chiasm, on the cranial side of the sphenoid sinus anteriorly. From the chiasm the optic nerves pass anteriorly and slightly inferiorly to gain the optic canals. In this course the optic nerves are intimately related to the posterosuperior aspect of the lateral wall of the sphenoid sinus (**Fig. 5.4**).

The bone that extends anteriorly from the optic chiasm to the cribriform area is called the planum sphenoidale (**Fig. 5.5**). It is made up of the sphenoid sinus roof as well as the fovea ethmoidalis. This is often a critical area of excision in craniofacial resection and a crucial area of identification from below by the head and neck surgeon. The intimate re-

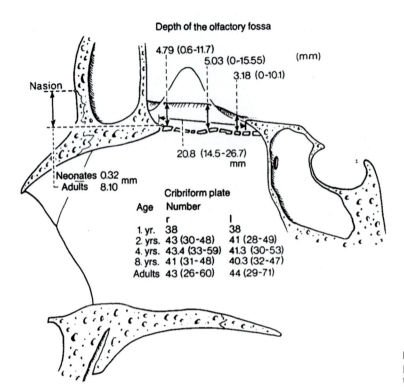

Depth of the olfactory fossa

4.79 (0.6-11.7)

5.03 (0-15.55)   (mm)

3.18 (0-10.1)

Nasion

20.8 (14.5-26.7) mm

Neonates 0.32 mm
Adults   8.10

Cribriform plate

Age	Number	
	r	l
1. yr.	38	38
2. yrs.	43 (30-48)	41 (28-49)
4. yrs.	43.4 (33-59)	41.3 (30-53)
8. yrs.	41 (31-48)	40.3 (32-47)
Adults	43 (26-60)	44 (29-71)

Fig. 5.3 Diagram illustrating the numbers of foramina penetrating the cribriform plate. (From Donald PJ. Surgery of the Skull Base. Philadelphia: Lippincott-Raven; 1998:55.)

lationship of this region to the optic chiasm and optic foramina makes the close cooperation of neurosurgeon and head and neck surgeon absolutely essential for the safe conduct of surgery in this area. Crucial decisions regarding the patient's sight and the safety of the internal carotid arteries arise when tumors encroach upon this vital area.

The frontal sinus is related inferiorly to the anterior ethmoidal cells so closely that one of the theories of origin of the frontal sinus is that it is simply a superior extension of the ethmoid labyrinth into the frontal bone.[3] Tumors originating in the anterior ethmoid cells have a tendency to invade su-

periorly to the frontal sinus via the frontonasal duct; because the latter is actually merely a foramen in 23.7% of individuals,[1] it provides even a shorter journey for the tumor. The thin bone of the posterior wall provides a weak barrier to the penetration of malignancy to the frontal dura and underlying brain.

The superior sagittal sinus takes origin in the frontal vein as it exits the foramen cecum and ascends on the anterior wall of the anterior fossa (**Fig. 5.6**), on the spine of the posterior frontal sinus wall. Fortunately this large venous sinus can safely be tied below the coronal suture without any un-

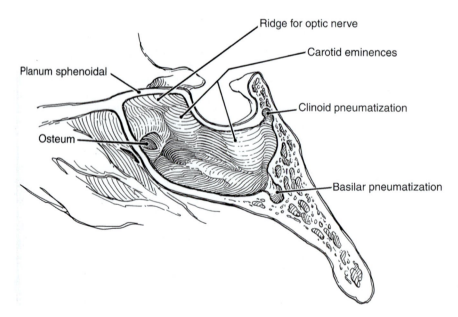

Ridge for optic nerve

Carotid eminences

Planum sphenoidal

Clinoid pneumatization

Osteum

Basilar pneumatization

Fig. 5.4 Coronal view of the sphenoidal sinus illustrating the close relationships of the internal carotid artery and the cavernous sinus.

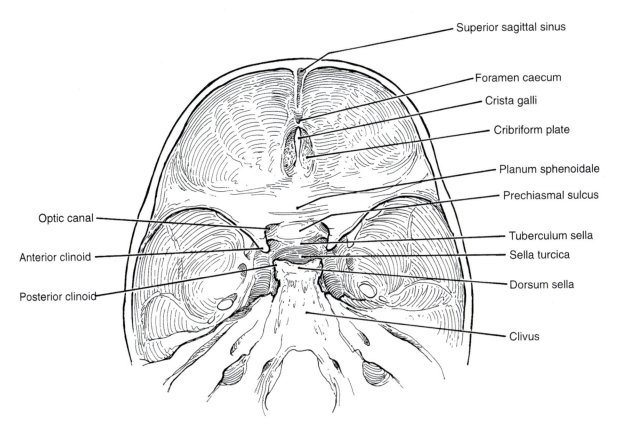

Superior sagittal sinus

Foramen caecum

Crista galli

Cribriform plate

Planum sphenoidale

Prechiasmal sulcus

Optic canal

Anterior clinoid

Posterior clinoid

Tuberculum sella

Sella turcica

Dorsum sella

Clivus

Fig. 5.5 Anterior cranial fossa and body of sphenoid. Note: Planum sphenoidale.

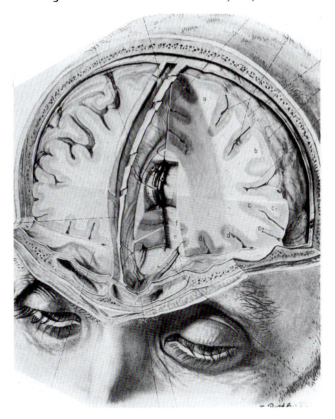

Fig. 5.6 Relationship of superior sagittal sinus to posterior frontal sinus wall.

toward effects.[4] In older patients the dura of this region tends to be thin, brittle, and adherent to the frontal bone. Because the superior sagittal sinus runs within the dura of the frontal lobe, it may be necessary to resect both sinus and dura at this level to achieve a satisfactory resection margin.

Lymphatic Drainage

The lymphatics of the nasal skin and anterior third of the nasal cavity drain into the submandibular nodes,[5] whereas those of the maxillary and ethmoidal sinuses drain in a manner similar to the posterior two thirds of the nasal cavities. Approximately 50% of these vessels coalesce in the peritubal lymphatic plexus adjacent to the eustachian tube and then pass to the lateral pharyngeal and high retropharyngeal lymph nodes, or, alternatively, directly to nodes of the superior deep cervical chain. The remaining 50% bypass the peritubal network and go directly to these latter cervical nodes.[5,6] The wisdom of combining irradiation and surgery to eradicate microscopic tumor foci in this region is readily apparent.

Although one would assume that the mucosal lymphatic drainage of the sphenoidal and frontal sinuses would follow that of the nasal mucosa adjacent to it, namely to the peritubal lymphatics or directly to the nodes of the jugulodigastric area, the precise anatomy of the lymphatic system in this area remains obscure.

◆ Pathology

Because paranasal sinus tumors are so rare, making up only between 0.2 and 0.5% of all body tumors,[6–8] and ~3% of all head and neck tumors, any significant degree of experience in their management is unfortunately limited to a few surgeons in large regional centers. Maxillary sinus cancers are the most common, representing about two thirds to three fourths of paranasal sinus tumors in most series, with malignancies of the ethmoid bloc making up most of the rest. Frontal and sphenoidal sinus malignancies are very rare.[6,9] **Table 5.1** lists a large series of cases compiled by Batsakis,[10] showing the distribution of paranasal sinus and nasal fossa carcinomas.

Table 5.1 Orbital Preservation

	Malignancy		
	Well Diff	**Poorly Diff**	**Sq. Cell Ca.**
1. Orbital Bone	P	P	P
2. Periorbita	P	±P	P
3. Orbital Fat	P	E	E
4. Muscle	E	E	E

*P = Preservation
 E = Exenteration

Squamous cell carcinoma and its variants, *transitional cell carcinoma* and *lymphoepithelioma*, make up 50 to 80% of all sinus tumors.[6,10,11] As a general rule the more anteriorly located tumors (e.g., those in the anterior aspect of the maxillary antra and the nasal cavities) tend to be better differentiated histologically, whereas those in the posterior regions are more anaplastic.[6] *Inverting papilloma*, a locally aggressive but generally nonmetastasizing tumor, has the potential for frank malignant degeneration.[6] In a large meta-analysis of 1390 patients reported by 22 separate sources of patients with inverting papilloma by Barnes et al[39] the average rate of carcinoma in an inverting papilloma was 14%, with a range of 2 to 27% among the series. The malignancies were synchronous in 61% and metachronous in 39%. The association between inverting papilloma and the human papilloma virus (HPV) has been long suspected but only until recently has been established in some cases. The commonest forms are HPV 6 and 11, occasionally 16 and 18, and rarely 57. In a further meta-analysis by Barnes et al[39] of 341 cases of inverting papilloma 50% were positive for HPV. The HPV types that seem to most carcinogenic are 16 and 18 and to a lesser degree 6 and 11.

Malignant degeneration is characterized mainly by the appearance of atypical cells or a marked increase in the number of mitotic figures. Often these changes occur as one or multiple foci in a tumor that otherwise is characteristic for inverting papilloma. The orderly cellular maturation pattern of squamous epithelium with considerable acanthosis and endophytic growth typifies this lesion. The erosion of bone, seen in inverting papilloma, is said to be caused by pressure rather than infiltration.[12] Squamous cell cancer, on the other hand, is characterized by direct invasion of bone by chords and islands of tumor cells. Late diagnosis is so common that bone destruction is present in 70 to 80% of cases.[9] There is a subset of inverting papillomata characterized by an extremely aggressive behavior with frequent local recurrence, but it remains histologically bland (**Fig. 5.7**). A much more radical approach needs to be taken in these cases because they will deeply invade bone and can even invade the overlying skin.

There is an additional, fortunately rare, form of malignancy whose histology is indistinguishable from the usual inverting papilloma, called a Schneiderian carcinoma, which is characterized by frequent local recurrences despite what appear to be resections with adequate margins. The origin in this tumor appears to be from the fungiform type of Schneiderian papilloma. One such patient in the author's experience finally died of intracranial involvement despite aggressive skull base surgery, radiation, and chemotherapy (**Fig. 5.8**).

Adenocarcinoma is seen in 10 to 14% of cases. According to Batsakis[13] even histologically benign lesions behave in an aggressive manner. Cohen and Batsakis[14] found that even oncocytomas of the maxillary sinus act clinically in an uncharacteristically malignant way. Adenocarcinomas arise in the minor salivary glands of the sinonasal tract. Most of them are adenoid cystic in type and develop in the maxillary sinus.[6,13] They express their usual behavior of local infiltration and extension along nerve sheaths, with the proximity of the cranial nerves of the sinuses to the skull base allowing early extension of these neoplasms toward the brain. Of the remaining adenocarcinomas, Batsakis et al[15,16] have identified and described three distinct growth patterns: papillary, sessile, and alveolar-mucoid. These lesions favor the ethmoid sinuses and superior nasal vault as their site of origin. Those of the nasal cavity have a more favorable prognosis than ones involving the sinuses. Of the three types, the papillary variety, whose cells resemble those of the respiratory epithelium, has the best prognosis. The sessile variety features a more anaplastic cell and is widely based. The alveolar-mucoid tumors arise presumably from the seromucinous gland below the lamina propria of the epithelium.

Adenocarcinomas are extremely aggressive locally and tend to metastasize by blood rather than lymphatics. Unlike the more commonly occurring adenoid cystic carcinoma, metastases from the other varieties are less frequent, and prolific direct spread is their principal malignant feature. However, Rafla[17] reported distant metastases in eight of 15 patients. Local recurrence following resection is common, and the tumors are relatively radioinsensitive. The prognosis is poor, with 5-year survival rates on the order of 20%.[15]

Melanoma makes up only 1% of the total number of nasal and paranasal sinus malignancies, but this site is second in frequency to only the oral cavity for mucosal melanoma of

Fig. 5.7 (**A**) Patient with aggressive inverting papilloma eroding into the anterior cranial fossa. (**B**) Coronal C.T. showing tumor.

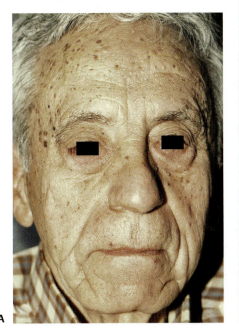

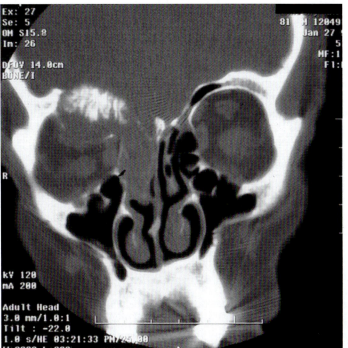

the head and neck. The multicentric nature and satellitosis of these tumors render them difficult to resect. Melanomas of the nasal cavity have a better prognosis, (31.5% with 5-year survival) than those arising in the sinuses.[18] Unfortunately, due to the protean nature of this disease, the 5-year survival

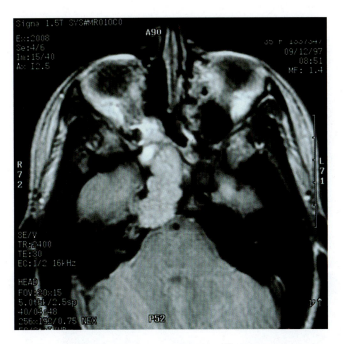

Fig. 5.8 Axial magnetic resonance imaging of a young woman who died of recurrent fungiform papilloma despite aggressive surgery, radiation, and chemotherapy. Radiograph depicts widespread intracranial disease.

is not as meaningful as the 10-year or 15-year survival rate in terms of overall cure. One patient in our experience with a melanoma of the nasal floor and septum recurred locally 12 years postoperatively and died of her tumor. This is in contrast to another patient who had a wide field resection of an intranasal melanoma and recurred within ~2 weeks of having his sutures removed.

Radiation response is poor and should be reserved for those cases that are unresectable or for attempted control of local recurrences. Chemotherapy, immunotherapy, and interferon have had sporadic but inconsistent successes.

Esthesioneuroblastoma is a rare malignancy that may arise anywhere in the nasal olfactory epithelium. It originates in cells of the neural crest rather than in the esthesioneuroblast as once thought.[19,20] This lesion may appear in the vault of the nose, in the superior meatus, or on the superior turbinate. In all the cases reviewed by Obert et al,[21] the esthesioneuroblastomas occurred high in the nose. In our experience, one lesion originated on the middle turbinate and extended into the maxillary sinus. The histological picture is characteristic of that of a neuroblastoma, featuring neurocytes and neuroblasts with rosette and pseudorosette formation. Electron-microscopic features of neurites and secretory granules containing biogenic amines help to differentiate this tumor from other sarcomas and anaplastic carcinomas.[22] The biological behavior of this tumor belies its seemingly benign histology. Local recurrences and regional and distant metastatic disease are not uncommon, with cervical lymph nodes and the lungs being the most frequent sites of metastases.[23] The tumor typically extends into the ethmoid sinuses, orbit, maxillary sinus, and superiorly through the cribriform plate and fovea ethmoidalis.

Resection using the craniofacial technique is the most commonly employed treatment for esthesioneuroblastoma. Occasionally the lesion clears the nasal vault and ethmoidal fovea sufficiently to permit successful transfacial excision through a lateral rhinotomy, sparing the patient a craniotomy (**Fig. 5.9**). A combination of surgery and postoperative irradiation is recommended.

The 5-year survival rate is reported to be 57 to 88% for stage A disease, 58 to 60% for stage B disease, and 0 to 50% for stage C.[24] In the author's personal series of 15 esthesioneuroblastomas, eight have been followed for 5 or more years. All, with one exception, were treated with a craniofacial excision. Two patients had a so-called impact tumor composed of both esthesioneuroblastoma elements and areas of squamous cell carcinoma. Seven out of 11 are alive and disease free, for a survival rate of 63.6%. We have, however, seen a patient who lived with persistent tumor for 20 years (**Fig. 5.10**).

◆ Diagnosis

One of the primary reasons for the poor prognosis in paranasal sinus cancer is its lack of early symptoms. The few symptoms that do occur (i.e., purulent drainage, nasal obstruction, and epistaxis) (**Fig. 5.11**) are so commonly encountered in benign diseases that carcinoma of the sinonasal tract may not be suspected. Late signs of proptosis, chemosis (**Fig. 5.12**), lateral displacement of the eye (**Fig. 5.11**), facial swelling (**Fig. 5.13**), or frank erosion through the skin (**Fig. 5.14**) signify a poor prognosis. Maxillary sinus lesions may erode inferiorly into the palate (**Fig. 5.15**) or alveolar ridge, producing loose teeth, a denture that quickly loses its fit, a swelling, or an ulcer.

Vigilance on the part of the physician in detecting and pursuing the cause of nasal bleeding of undetermined origin, the reasons for unilateral nasal obstruction of recent onset, or the source of purulent drainage that is refractory to antibiotic therapy is necessary to make an early diagnosis. Although intranasal examination may reveal the tumor in some cases (**Fig. 5.16**), in others the lesion may remain obscure within the sinus cavities and be detectable only by radiographic exam. The average delay from onset of symptoms to final diagnosis is 6 months.[25] The patient in **Fig. 5.17** had symptoms of purulent rhinorrhea, epistaxis, and nasal obstruction that had progressed over a period of 2 years until the diagnosis of sinonasal undifferentiated carcinoma was made.

As a screening device, standard paranasal sinus computed tomographic (CT) scan is very helpful given that 80% of patients with maxillary sinus tumors have evidence of bone erosion.[9] However, as a means of judging tumor extent the standard examination is extremely limited. One of the biggest problems in managing paranasal sinus cancers is the determination of tumor extent. Robin and Powell[26] analyzed 282 cases of paranasal sinus malignancy and found an error in estimate of tumor extension in one third of the cases. A serious source of diagnostic error in our own experience is the difficulty in interpretation of a density in a sinus cavity on the CT scan. A tumor plugging a sinus ostium can result in the accumulation of secretions that are often distinguishable on the scan from tumor.

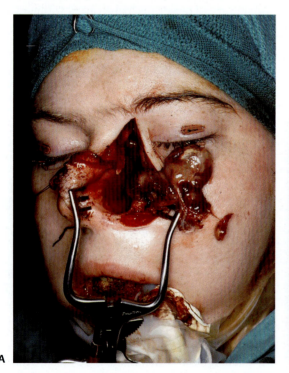

A

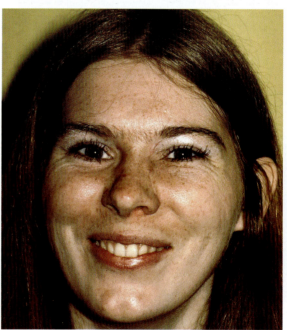

B

Fig. 5.9 **(A)** Young woman with an esthesioneuroblastoma on the superior meatus of the nose. Craniofacial resection was not necessary. **(B)** Photograph following full course of planned postoperative irradiation.

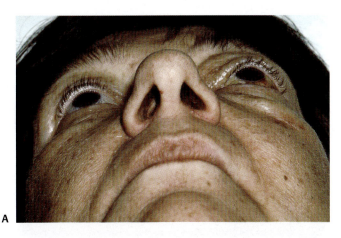

A

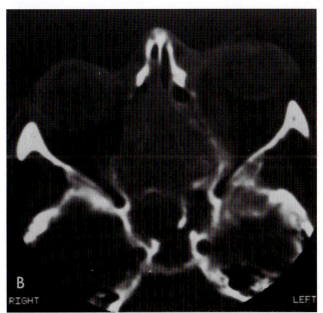

B

RIGHT   LEFT

B

Fig. 5.10 (**A**) Sixty-year-old woman with an esthesioneuroblastoma of the ethmoid sinuses for 20 years. Note displacement of left globe. (**B**) Computed tomographic (CT) scan showing horizontal section through both orbits. Large tumor fills the superior nasal cavities and ethmoid sinuses. The left orbit is full of tumor and the right orbital apex is involved but to a lesser degree. (**C**) CT scan in coronal section showing intracranial extension.

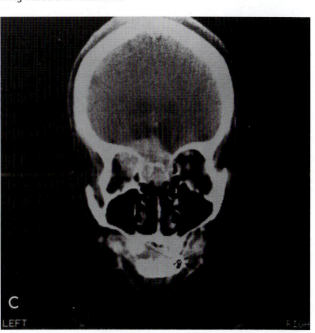

C

LEFT   RIGHT

C

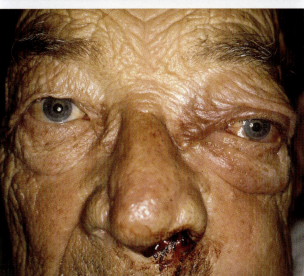

Fig. 5.11 Advanced carcinoma of the ethmoid sinus in an elderly man presenting with epistaxis, nasal swelling, and orbital displacement.

The radiographic findings suggesting a diagnosis of malignancy are (1) sinus opacification, (2) a soft tissue mass, (3) sclerosis of bony walls, and (4) erosion or destruction of bony walls.[27] None of these findings alone are diagnostic, a soft tissue mass with bone destruction being the most suggestive combination of signs. Fine-cut CT scanning in the axial, sagittal, and, especially, coronal planes using soft tissue technique and bone windows supplemented by magnetic resonance imaging (MRI) with gadolinium contrast and, when indicated, fat suppression imaging, will give a fairly accurate demonstration of tumor extent. The MRI will be able in most instances to differentiate between fluid in the sinuses secondary to sinus obstruction by tumor and the neoplasm itself. Occasionally, the distinction will be difficult if the secretions are of long standing and have become inspissated.

Critical areas of bone erosion will help in surgical planning. Tumor penetration of the anterior wall of the maxillary sinus will provide access to the subcutaneous fat, which produces characteristic signal changes that can be picked up on the MRI (**Fig. 5.18**). Further invasion of the lymphatics

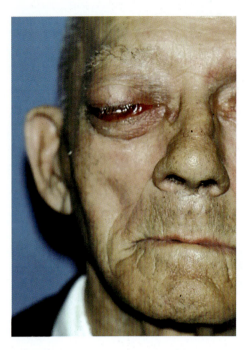

Fig. 5.12 Carcinoma of the ethmoid sinus in an 82-year-old man who presented with chemosis and proptosis. The cause of these ocular symptoms remained undiagnosed for months until finally routine sinus x-rays were obtained.

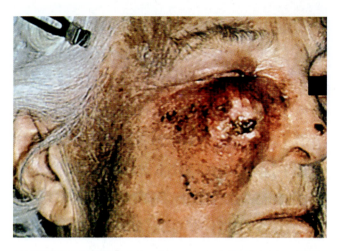

Fig. 5.14 An elderly woman with a large maxillary carcinoma that remained undiagnosed until it ulcerated through the skin.

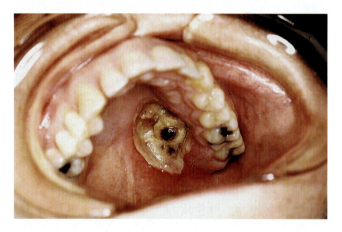

Fig. 5.15 A maxillary sinus carcinoma ulcerating through the palate.

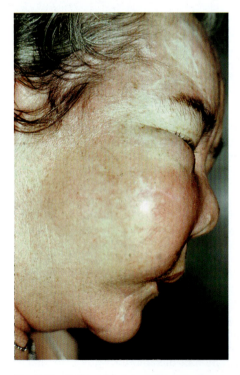

Fig. 5.13 Profound facial swelling in a woman of late middle age. A carcinoma of the maxillary sinus had breached the anterior sinus wall and infiltrated the overlying soft tissue.

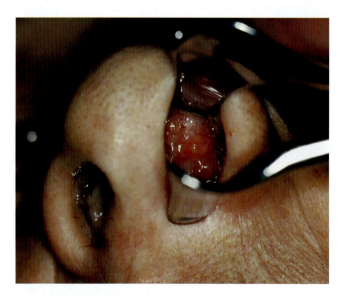

Fig. 5.16 Elderly woman with a large maxillary sinus carcinoma obstructing the nasal airway.

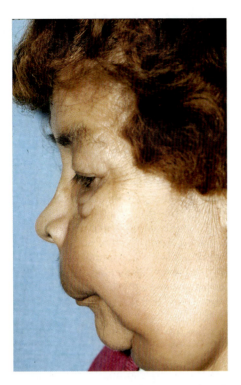

Fig. 5.17 Patient with massive squamous cell carcinoma of the maxillary sinus eroding through the anterior maxillary sinus wall into the adjacent soft tissues of the cheek.

of the cheek skin will produce thickening that indicates the likelihood of the requirement for full-thickness cheek excision. Septal invasion and opacification of the opposite nasal cavity indicate that the tumor may be invading the lateral nasal wall and even the sinuses of the opposite side. Posterior wall invasion of the maxillary sinus may indicate that the infratemporal fossa is invaded, but this is even more strongly indicated by pterygoid plate erosion. MRI will add more information by detailing the soft tissue extent of tumor (**Fig. 5.19**). The absence of the normal fat planes around the pterygoid muscles, and an alteration in their normal configuration, are strong signs of tumor invasion. However, a caveat must be extended when one is attempting to establish the possibility of recurrent tumor in the infratemporal fossa in the patient who has had prior surgery and irradiation (**Fig. 5.20**). False positives are not uncommon. The use of the positron emission tomographic (PET) scan or PET CT may help in establishing occurrence and provide a gross idea of tumor extent, but the fine-cut CT scan and MRI are the best means of delineating the degree of tumor spread.

Bone erosion of the orbital floor on the CT scan suggests intraorbital invasion. MRI gives additional information regarding the degree of intraorbital extension and whether the periorbital fat or extraocular muscles are invaded. Extension of maxilloethmoidal tumors into the intracranial fossa is suggested by bone erosion of the anterior fossa floor. The MRI once more adds information concerning the possibility of dural involvement and invasion of the cerebral hemi-

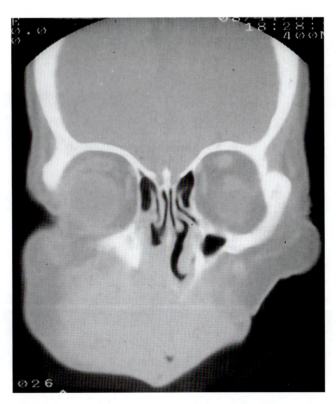

Fig. 5.18 Magnetic resonance imaging showing penetration of the anterior maxillary wall and invasion of the soft tissues.

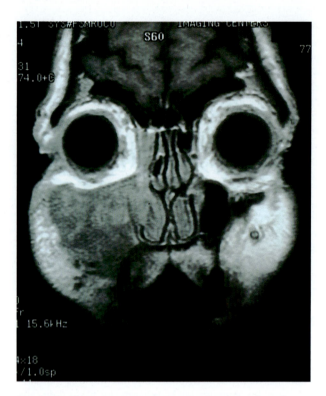

Fig. 5.19 Magnetic resonance imaging illustrating the soft tissue extent of tumor in a patient with a maxillary sinus carcinoma invading the pterygoid plates with extension into the infratemporal fossa.

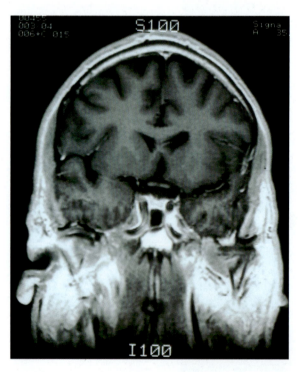

Fig. 5.20 Coronal view magnetic resonance imaging of a patient with infratemporal fossa extension of squamous cell carcinoma into the cavernous sinus following radiation therapy. Persistence of disease is difficult to discern from postradiation fibrosis.

sphere. Absence of the normal cerebrospinal fluid shadow between the dura and brain is highly suggestive of tumor invasion of dura. The absence of this shadow combined with an alteration in the normal configuration of the brain at that site, especially when accompanied by a halo of radiolucency indicating edema at the periphery, is an almost certain sign of brain invasion (**Fig. 5.21**). Enlargement of a cranial nerve branch or increased enhancement on MRI suggests perineural spread of tumor (**Fig. 5.22**). Unfortunately, the absence of this sign does not necessarily indicate that the nerve is tumor free. The maxillary sinus has the infraorbital nerve traversing through its roof, providing easy access to tumor, especially in view of the fact that dehiscences in the neural canal are not uncommon at this site. When tumor gains the infratemporal fossa the mandibular branch of the trigeminal nerve may become invaded. Erosion of the bone of the foramen rotundum or ovale is a late sign of perineural involvement and almost always portends intracranial spread. If the gasserian ganglion is enlarged and lights up with gadolinium contrast (**Fig. 5.23**) then a middle fossa/infratemporal fossa approach will be needed (see chapter 9).

In tumors involving the sphenoidal sinus, erosion of the lateral wall gives direct access to the cavernous sinus. Small degrees of cavernous sinus dural invasion can be resected and repaired through the transfacial approach, but more extensive invasion involving the proximity of the internal carotid artery will need a middle fossa/infratemporal fossa approach. The coronal projection of the CT scan will suggest bony wall erosion, and the MRI may show the degree of involvement of the cavernous sinus and internal carotid.

Despite the use of the most modern diagnostic techniques, often the establishment of the extent of tumor can be determined only at the time of resection. If resectability can

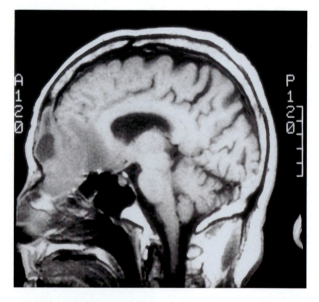

Fig. 5.21 Sagittal magnetic resonance imaging showing a halo around the intracerebral invasion of a sinus malignancy. This represents a zone of edema and necrosis that precedes the tumor as it invades the frontal lobes of the brain. (From Donald PJ. Surgery of the Skull Base. Philadelphia: Lippincott-Raven; 1998:64)

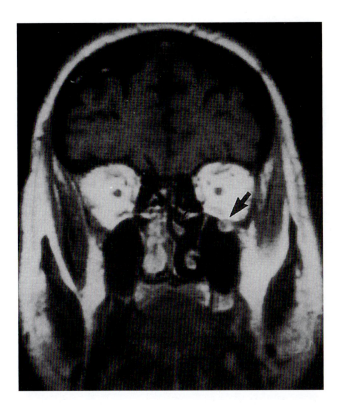

Fig. 5.22 Coronal view computed tomographic scan showing gadolinium enhancement of the second division of the trigeminal nerve by perineural spread of squamous cell carcinoma. (From Donald PJ, Gluckman JL, Rice DH, eds. The Sinuses. New York: Raven; 1995:453)

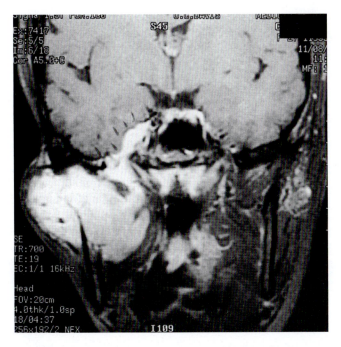

Fig. 5.23 Coronal view magnetic resonance imaging showing enhancement of the gasserian ganglion secondary to perineural spread of the malignant schwannoma. (From Donald PJ. Surgery of the Skull Base. Philadelphia. Lippincott-Raven; 1998:291)

be established only at the time of surgery, the patient must be so apprised. As the surgery proceeds, great care is taken to perform mainly a debulking procedure without compromising any major function or producing any major cosmetic defect. If the lesion is deemed unresectable, as much gross tumor is removed as possible, and postoperative irradiation is done once healing has taken place.

◆ Treatment

Nasal Vestibule Lesions

Lesions of the vestibular region of the nose (**Fig. 5.24**) are sneaky and treacherous. Whereas even squamous cell cancers of the nasal dorsum are not regarded with much apprehension, because local resection and the application of a skin graft are usually sufficient to eradicate the disease and reconstruct the defect, the vestibular area of the nose is distinctly different. Extension of a seemingly innocuous tumor on the nasal sill or columella into the premaxilla and for a considerable distance along the nasal floor is a common finding. Resection of a generous margin of tissue in the region of the nasal tip, nasal floor, premaxilla, and upper lip is important. If the alveolar bone is to be spared (**Fig. 5.25**), the patient must be warned about the likelihood of losing the vitality of the upper central teeth.

A skin incision is made outlining the tumor by at least 2 cm (**Fig. 5.26**). This invariably results in the loss of the nasal columella, one or both alae, and the superior central part of the upper lip. Intranasally a much wider resection of up to 4 cm from the visible edge of the tumor is done along the septum, nasal floor, and even the anterior maxilla. A lateral rhinotomy (**Fig. 5.27**) may be required for improved exposure. The premaxilla is excised (**Fig. 5.28**) using a power saw or a cutting needle. Bleeding from the incisive artery is controlled with bone wax or cautery. The upper lip is approximated or

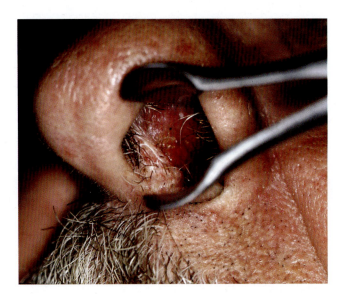

Fig. 5.24 Squamous cell carcinoma of the nasal vestibule.

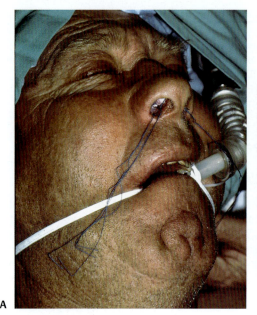

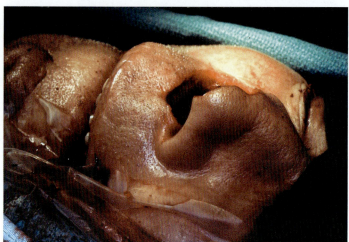

Fig. 5.25 (**A**) A small, innocuous-appearing nasal vestibular lesion. (**B**) Resection required through a lateral rhinotomy to achieve adequate tumor-free margins.

A

B

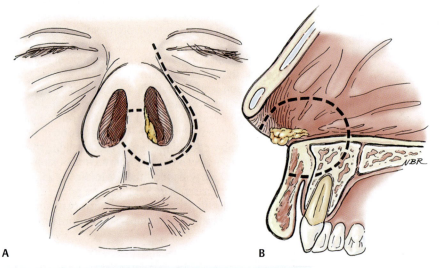

A

B

Fig. 5.26 Resection of nasal vestibular cancer. (**A**) Outline of area of resection, frontal view. (**B**) Parasagittal view outlining resection of premaxilla, columella, and septum.

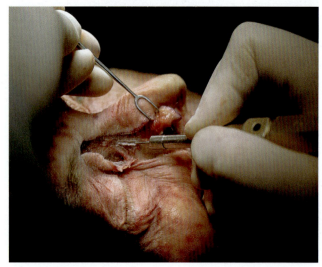

Fig. 5.27 Lateral rhinotomy.

reconstructed by the Karapandzic, Abbe flap, or Gillies technique and the raw area covered with a split-thickness skin graft. The postoperative cosmetic appearance is usually quite acceptable (**Fig. 5.29**), and further reconstruction should be delayed for at least a year because of the danger of local recurrence. At that time, a nasolabial flap with a previously implanted cartilage graft for structural support of the nasal ala is used for reconstruction (**Fig. 5.30**). The conchal cartilage of the ear provides an excellent source for a composite graft (**Fig. 5.31**). It beautifully mimics the nasal alar curve, and the cosmetic impact on the donor site is minimal.

If the defect is larger, and especially if it involves all or part of the nasal lobule, reconstruction of the tip as a unit is best done utilizing a midline forehead flap (**Fig. 5.32**). Tip support is essential for good aesthetic restoration, and grafts of cartilage or bone are necessary to shore up the framework. When reconstructing the nose, it is also vital to remember to provide an internal as well as an external lining. The internal lining can be contributed by the skin of a composite graft or

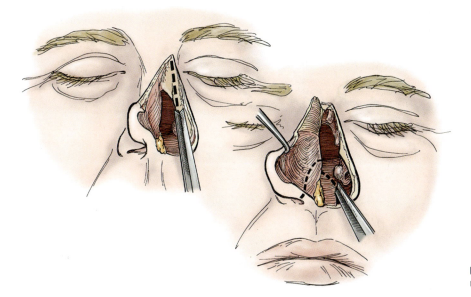

Fig. 5.28 Osteotome used to resect the nasal floor portion of the premaxilla.

it can be contributed by the nose itself. Millard has developed an ingenious method of reconstructing the support of the nasal tip. If a sufficient portion of the nasal septum remains, an L-shaped chondromucosal flap is constructed that when advanced will provide tip support. The flap is pedicled superiorly on the mucoperichondrium, the cartilage cut subperichondrially under this pedicle, and the strut swung forward on this hinge (**Fig. 5.33**). Septal mucosa is advanced to cover all raw cartilage, and all otherwise exposed areas are

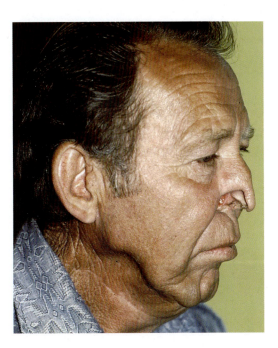

Fig. 5.29 Postoperative appearance following resection of nasal vestibular carcinoma. Delay in reconstruction of 1 year is necessary to detect early recurrences.

lined with split-thickness skin. At the next stage, deficient nasal lining is replaced by utilizing the skin of the dorsum, which is cut, elevated to the rim, and turned under. A midline forehead flap pedicled on either the supratrochlear or supraorbital arteries or both is turned to cover the raw area and to refashion the nasal alae, columella, and lobule.

In the delayed case, the skin of the nasal dorsum is used to provide the inner lining as just described (**Fig. 5.34**). The midline forehead flap is used for the external coverage and formation of the nasal tip (**Figs. 5.32** and **Fig. 5.33**). It may be created as a regular cutaneous or as an island flap. If the latter is used, a subcutaneous tunnel may be made in the residual nasal skin through which the flap may be introduced. Alternatively, the skin bridge can be split, the flap rotated into place, and continuity restored over the pedicle (**Fig. 5.32**). The advantage of the island flap is the elimination of a second stage. The disadvantages are bulkiness in the glabella–nasion region and the risk of pedicle compression by subsequent edema of the skin bridge. The midline flap is rotated into the defect and the columella and tip areas reconstructed. The forehead defect is approximated in the midline. If there is much tension in the closure, large stay sutures can be placed well to the outside of the suture line. These remain for 2 to 3 weeks.

Anterior Facial Lesions

A few facial lesions acquire such a size or extent that they are beyond curative resection (**Fig. 5.35**). However, some that may initially appear to be hopeless can be rescued with a heroic procedure (**Fig. 5.36**). So many cutaneous carcinomas of either basal or squamous cell type are readily curable by limited resection, and reconstruction is simply achieved with application of a skin graft or the rotation of a small flap into the defect. Occasionally, a pernicious lesion that persistently recurs despite repeated limited local excisions frustrates such efforts. At this point "whittling away" of the tumor

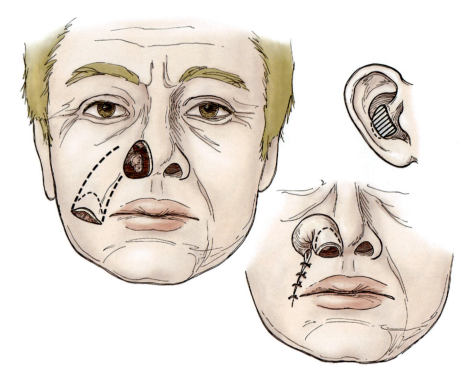

Fig. 5.30 Staged nasal alar reconstruction using a nasal labial flap and conchal composite graft.

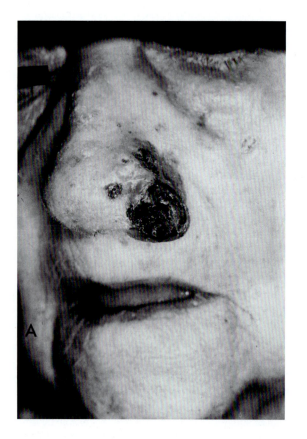

Fig. 5.31 (**A**) Lesion. (**B**) Composite cartilage graft used to reconstruct the nasal ala.

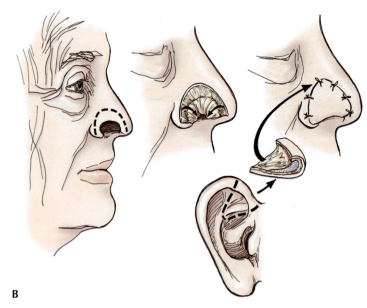

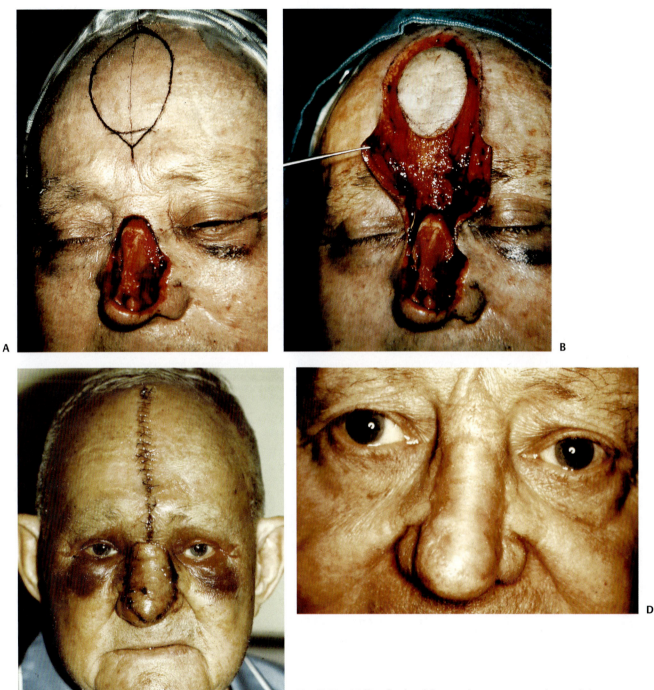

Fig. 5.32 Midline forehead flap used to reconstruct the nasal dorsum.
(**A**) Flap outlined. (**B**) Island flap pediculed on the supraorbital and
supratrochlear arteries, elevated and ready to transpose into defect.
(**C**) Flap turned and sutured into position. (**D**) Six weeks postoperatively.

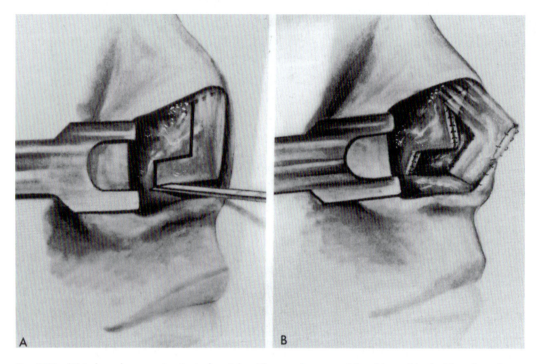

Fig. 5.33 (**A**) L-shaped composite strut of septal cartilage and mucoperichondrium of both sides of nasal septum. (**B**) Flap is pedicled on the mucoperiosteum of the nasal dorsum and adjacent septum. Cartilage is fractured to the dorsal extent of the septum, and the flap is swung anteriorly. (From Millard R. Anesthetic reconstructive rhinoplasty. Clin Plast Surg 1981;8:169)

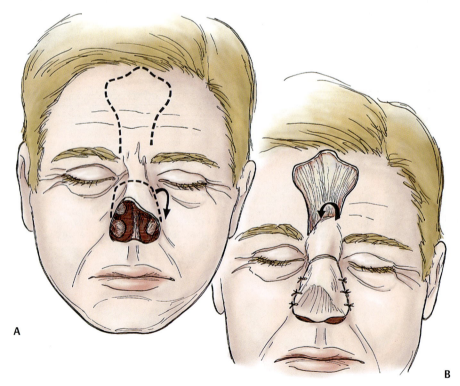

A

B

Fig. 5.34 (**A**) Midline forehead flap used to reconstruct the nasal dorsum. Turn-down flap on nasal tip is outlined and ready to dissect to nasal rim, where it is pedicled and used to provide the inner nasal lining. Midline forehead flap is outlined and may be delayed. Inner ling is provided by a turn-down flap of skin of the nasal dorsum. Midline forehead flap is rotated under the subcutaneous tunnel after a portion of the flap has been deepithelialized. (**B**) Flap rotated into place.

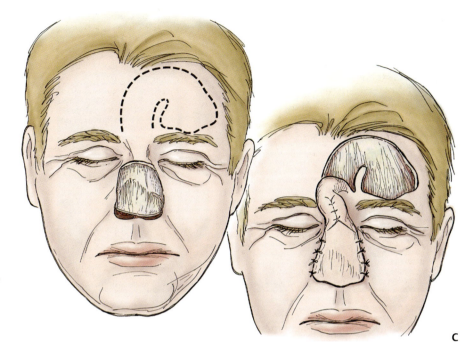

Fig. 5.34 (*continued*) (**C**) Alternatively the flap is rotated extracutaneously, with the pedicle then divided and returned to the forehead at a later stage. When a longer pedicle is required, an "up-down" design may be utilized.

C

must cease and a definitive resection with wide margins be done. The tumor specimen in such a case will reveal deep infiltration into the skeletal elements of the nose and even into the adjacent maxillary sinuses.

The patient in **Fig. 5.36** exemplifies such a case. Following numerous attempts at local excision the tumor had deeply infiltrated the soft tissues of the anterior part of the face and the cartilaginous portion of the nasal dorsum and had breached the anterior walls of the maxillary sinuses. The cutaneous resection margin is outlined in **Fig. 5.37**. A wide skin margin must be taken to avoid cutting across tumor that may have infiltrated laterally into the dermis, previous scar

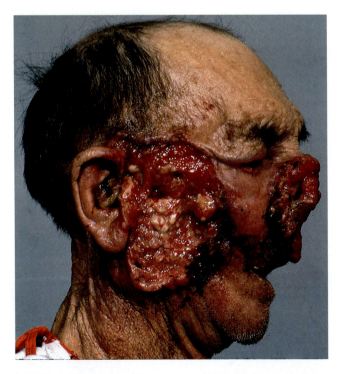

Fig. 5.35 Elderly man with extensive multifocal squamous cell carcinoma of the face.

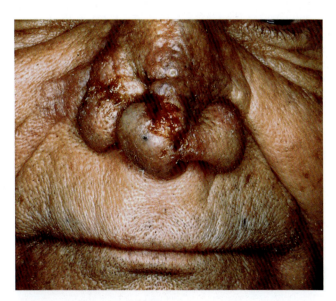

Fig. 5.36 Midline nasal squamous cell cancer that had been repeatedly treated by small conservative excisions and radiation therapy. Tumor extended throughout the skin of the entire nose as well as its framework. In addition, spread to the cheek skin and underlying tissue was also palpable.

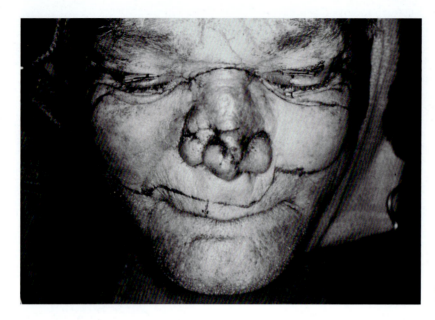

Fig. 5.37 Margins of resection for patient in Fig. 5.36 are outlined.

tissue, or muscle planes, a phenomenon that is very often seen in these cases.[4] Spread along embryological cleavage lines is another common trend in these aggressive cancers. Through-and-through excision is done into both nasal cavities and maxillary antra (Fig. 5.38). Also included is a portion of premaxilla, because of tumor infiltration into the nasal sill and vestibule.

Coverage of such a defect presents a significant reconstructive challenge. An extensive rebuilding effort using flaps should be resisted, since the burying of a local recurrence under a large flap may result in the tumor becoming unresectable by the time it is detected (Fig. 5.39). In the patient shown in Fig. 5.36, coverage was achieved by local advancement of the facial soft tissue utilizing two large Kuhnt-Szymanowski flaps (Fig. 5.40), which permitted closure of the defect and clear visualization of the resection margins on follow-up. The unsightly area of the amputated nose can be covered by a prosthesis until a 12- to 18-month follow-up

ensures the absence of local recurrence. At that time, the patient may even decide to retain the prosthesis rather than undergo the rigors of a nasal reconstruction.

Another site that produces substantial difficulties in management is the nasal–jugal area. This region of skin between the caruncle of the eye and the dorsum of the nose just lateral to the nasion occasionally harbors malignancies, usually of the basal cell variety (Fig. 5.41), that acquire a particularly pernicious character. They have a tendency to extend deeply and laterally from the cutaneous surface into the underlying ethmoid and even the maxillary sinuses, thereby jeopardizing the eye. The morpheaform type of basal cell tumor is common in this area, and local recurrences following conservative local resections are the rule (Fig. 5.42). Many surgeons are lulled into a sense of complacency usually engendered by their favorable experience with this lesion in other sites. However, with such tumors in this dangerous site, even rather aggressive excisions may prove unsuccessful

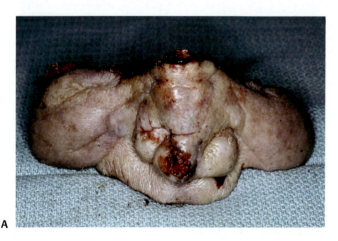

A

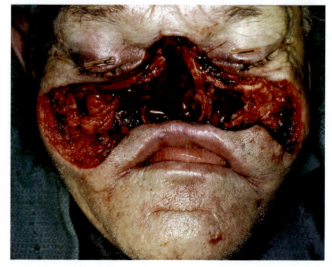

B

Fig. 5.38 A total rhinectomy and bilateral anterior maxillectomies were necessary, as was excision of overlying facial skin. (A) Specimen. (B) Defect.

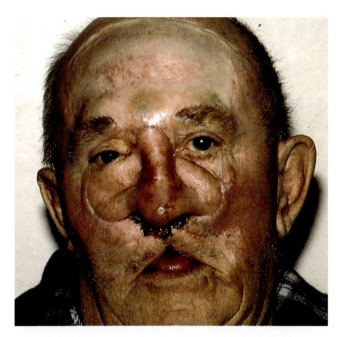

Fig. 5.39 Immediate reconstruction of a similar defect in this patient, in whom a bipedicled forehead flap obscured a local recurrence that had become inoperable prior to its detection.

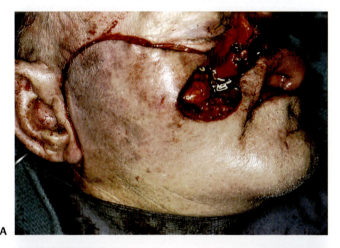

A

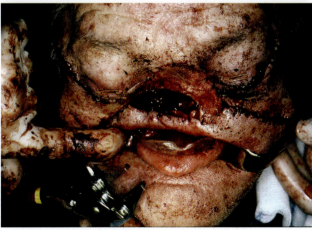

B

Fig. 5.40 Bilateral Kuhnt-Szymanowski flaps were used to obtain closure in the patient in **Fig. 5.38**. (**A**) Flap outlined. (**B**) Defect closed.

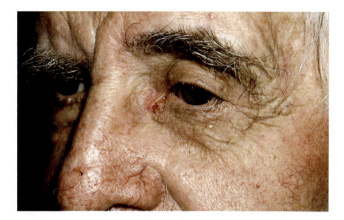

Fig. 5.41 Small, innocuous-appearing basal cell carcinoma of the inner canthal skin of the eye. This is an extremely dangerous position for basal cell carcinoma.

(**Fig. 5.43**). Mohs fresh tissue technique (see chapter 7) has one of its most pertinent applications in these cases. It is not uncommon for the recurrent and larger lesions to require an orbital exenteration and even a craniofacial procedure.

Several cutaneous malignancies acquire through some unknown mechanism the ability to spread along the perineural spaces. Malignant melanoma, basal cell, and squamous cell carcinoma all may acquire this propensity. These patients usually have a skin cancer that has been present for some time, often removed on several occasions. The first sign of perineural spread is numbness. The tumor spreads from the peripheral branches of the nerve to the main trunk. In the midfacial region this is to the infraorbital nerve, and with time the tumor spreads, often with histologically normal-appearing skip areas back through the foramen rotundum to the gasserian ganglion.

Effective treatment entails resection of the primary tumor with wide margins with a connecting area of subcutaneous tissue to the infraorbital foramen. The presence of tumor at this site means removal of the infraorbital nerve to the ptery-

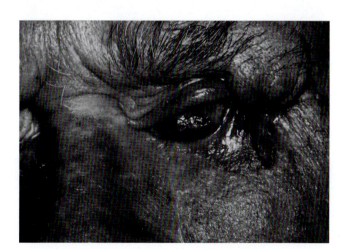

Fig. 5.42 Past conservative resection of the medial canthal basal cell carcinoma shown in the preceding figure. The tumor eventually claimed this patient's eye.

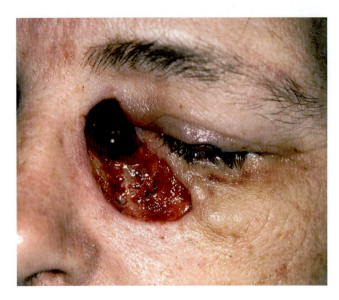

Fig. 5.43 Basal cell carcinoma of the inner canthus managed by an aggressive skin excision, exenteration of the ethmoid sinus, and resection of part of the bony wall of the nose. Despite this resection, most tumor margins were positive. Curative excision required orbital exenteration and a craniofacial procedure.

gomaxillary space. An area of anterior maxillary sinus wall in the vicinity of the foramen needs excision. The bone along the course of the nerve in the sinus roof, which of course, is the orbital floor, is also removed. The periorbita is sampled along the course of the nerve to determine involvement. If the nerve is positive in the pterygomaxillary space then the nerve is dissected to the foramen rotundum, the bone around the foramen is drilled away, and the nerve trunk is severed at the level of the dura. If the frozen section of the nerve is negative for tumor at this site then the operation is complete. If the nerve is still positive then a middle fossa/infratemporal

fossa approach must be done to dissect the ganglion from the Meckel cave and complete the excision. Chapter 9 covers this topic in greater depth.

Craniofacial Resection

The standard maxillectomy and external ethmoidectomy procedures are not covered in this chapter because they are well described in several surgical atlases and texts. Although the maxillary portion of these operations can usually be accomplished en bloc, the ethmoidal part is more of a piecemeal affair. A significantly wide margin of healthy tissue is often difficult to attain, and the bony nature of the specimen makes frozen sections unobtainable. Considerable judgment is required to establish a good cancer ablative procedure at this site. The goal in resection of any head and neck cancer is to strive for an en bloc removal with histological negative margins. It is not always possible to achieve such a resection in one single block. This is especially pertinent in many skull base resections when the sheer bulk of the tumor obtunds the view of the margins and an unnecessarily large removal of normal tissue must be done to achieve complete tumor extirpation. This obviously occurs in any traditional en bloc removal when positive margins are obtained and a repeat excision is done at those margins to remove the entire tumor. The violation of the en bloc rule is commonplace in parotid salivary gland resection for cancer as when preservation of the facial nerve is attempted. In skull base surgery initially a debulking procedure removes the tumor that obstructs the view of the margins. Second the main specimen containing most of the tumor is excised with most of the periphery of the specimen histologically negative. This is the first layer of the resection. The second layer is removed and the margins checked with frozen sections. Subsequent resection layers are excised until all margins are negative. This is similar to the Mohs technique so successfully used in dermatology, and the technique has evolved. It is not a piecemeal resection

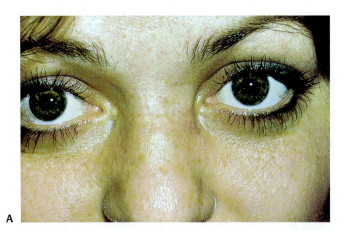
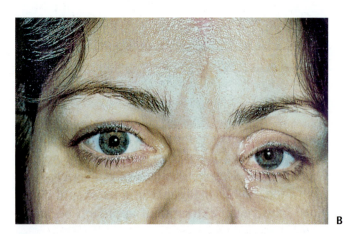

A   B

Fig. 5.44 (**A**) A 21-year-old woman with a well-differentiated fibrosarcoma of the anterior ethmoid sinuses invading the soft tissue adjacent to the glove and medial canthal skin. The tumor invaded the periorbita and a small amount of periorbital fat. The medial one third of the lids was removed as well as the lacrimal system. A window of periorbita and adjacent fat was removed down to the medial rectus muscle. Tumor-free margins were obtained. The medial canthus was reconstructed and the nasal-orbital skin resection replaced with a midline forehead flap. Lacrimal drainage was accomplished by the insertion of a Jones tube. (**B**) Patient 15 years postoperative and tumor free. She has mild restriction at the terminal parts of lateral and medial gaze but has no diplopia on straight-ahead gaze. Despite multiple attempts at reconstruction of a lacrimal drainage system she still has occasional epiphora. (From Donald PJ. Surgery of the Skull Base. Philadelphia: Lippincott-Raven; 1998:168)

but an orderly approach layer by layer to achieve total tumor extirpation with negative margins. "Gross tumor removal" is not the goal of this exercise. Craniofacial resection facilitates the establishment of superior and lateral tissue margins and has significantly broadened the perspective in ethmoidal and maxilloethmoidal cancer surgery. Surgical resection has traditionally been the method of choice in the management of paranasal sinus cancer. Irradiation therapy is usually reserved for adjunctive therapy or palliation in patients with hopeless unresectable disease or in those who are too debilitated by intercurrent disease to operate upon. For tumors of the maxilla located below the Ohngren line, maxillectomy is the standard approach and is often curative. Simple maxillectomy is much less successful with tumors above this line because of their proximity to the orbit and pterygomaxillary space. A much more radical procedure is required, often involving orbital resection.

The performance of orbital resection has undergone considerable debate over the years. Even the notion that the prognosis is so bad when paranasal sinus tumors have become so advanced that the removal of the eye is not worth it, has been posited. Prior to the advent of skull base surgery, resection of advanced sinus tumors that invaded the orbit was poor. Currently, 5-year tumor-free survival rates for anterior skull base malignancy range from 50 to 65%. With this, an evolution of thought has occurred regarding ocular resection. In the past many surgeons believed that invasion of the periorbita and even the orbital bone was an indication for orbital exenteration. The seminal work of Perry et al[28] showed that the eye could be preserved in many cases of advanced maxilloethmoidal malignancy. We made our first attempt at this in 1986 in a case of fibrosarcoma of the ethmoid sinuses that invaded the periorbita and periorbital fat of the eye. The

involved tissues with negative margins were removed down to the medial rectus muscle. The patient remains tumor-free to this day (**Fig. 5.44A,B**). Over the years we have developed a treatment algorithm depicted in **Table 5.1**. Unfortunately, many advanced sinus tumors that have grown large enough to require skull base resection have more often invaded the orbital apex than the area of the globe (**Fig. 5.45A,B**).

Although small ethmoidal tumors can be adequately excised transfacially, usually these tumors, because of their occult nature, are not detected until they are quite large. Adequate excision in these instances must include the floor of the anterior cranial fossa, the medial and superior orbital walls, and often the orbital contents.

To enhance the survival rate, follow-up radiotherapy is employed. The histopathologic establishment of integrity of the surgical margins in these cases is exceptionally difficult because of the modified en bloc nature of portions of the resection and the presence of cure at the margins. The addition of radiotherapy greatly enhances the opportunity for complete tumor ablation.

Craniofacial resection is used for cancers whose geographic center may be either maxillary or ethmoidal in origin. If the lesion originated in the ethmoid sinus, occasionally a portion of the maxilla can be spared. A primarily maxillary tumor may not have as much cranial spread, thus reducing the amount of anterior fossa floor needing resection. Occasionally maxillary encroachment by an ethmoid tumor is minimal, permitting salvage of the dental arch of the affected side. However, in. many instances, a maxilloethmoidectomy and orbital exenteration are required. When there is cutaneous involvement, a wide margin of skin must be excised, compounding the reconstructive problem.

If oncologically possible, because of its vital role in the aesthetics of the face, an attempt should be made to preserve

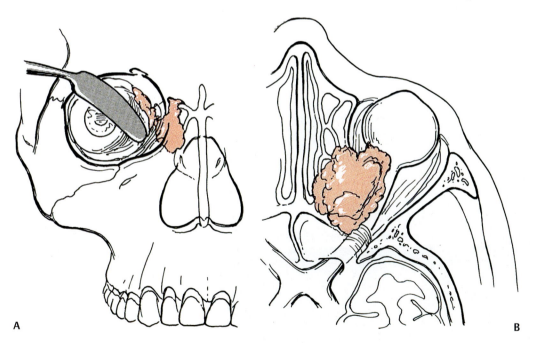

Fig. 5.45 (**A,B**) Illustration of the commonest scenario in advanced ethmoidal carcinoma. Invasion of the orbital apex. (**A**) Frontal view. (**B**) Cross sectional view. (From Donald PJ. Surgery of the Skull Base. Philadelphia: Lippincott-Raven; 1998:289)

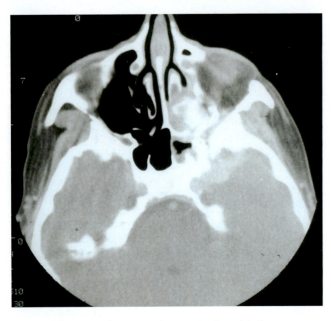

Fig. 5.46 Computed tomographic scan in the axial plane illustrating a chondrosarcoma of the ethmoid sinuses extending across the orbital apex into the anterior aspect of middle cranial fossa displacing the anterior horn of the temporal lobe of the brain.

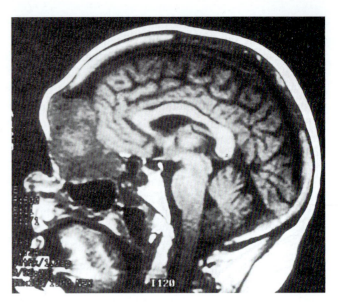

Fig. 5.47 Sagittal view magnetic resonance imaging showing squamous cell carcinoma of the frontal sinus extending into the cranial fossa. (From Donald PJ. Surgery of the Skull Base. Philadelphia: Lippincott-Raven; 1998:184)

some aspect of the malar eminence. This can be done when there is only a small amount of bone invasion on the sinus side of the malar eminence. The bone is hollowed out with the cutting bur. A frozen section of marrow curetting at this site can establish a negative margin.

The greatest advance in the management of paranasal sinus malignancy has been the advent of skull base surgery. Following Ketcham's[40] initial report in 1964, small series of patients were reported on a sporadic basis. It was not until the 1980s that organized skull base teams became established, and reports of cases in significant numbers were published. A clear survival advantage over subtotal removal and follow-up irradiation stimulated widespread interest in cranial base resection techniques.

Skull base surgery should be a well-coordinated cooperative venture between the head and neck surgeon and the neurological surgeon. These combined intracranial/extracranial resections exploit the knowledge of these two disciplines, enabling a safe and usually complete resection of malignancies that were once considered inoperable and incurable. The team approach is essential. One of the principal reasons sinus tumors that invaded the intracranial cavity were thought to be inoperable was that they crossed the arbitrary anatomical barriers established by specialty tradition. Now that skull base surgery is more commonplace there arises the concern that individuals in a single specialty will attempt these operations without the assistance of their partner in the sister-discipline.

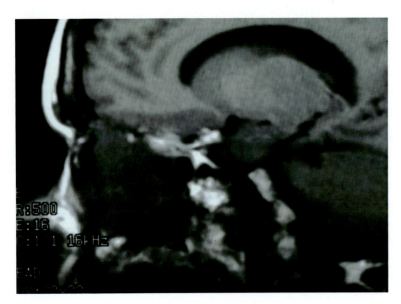

Fig. 5.48 Sagittal-cut magnetic resonance imaging scan showing sphenoethmoidal carcinoma invading through the planum sphenoidale and into the frontal lobe of the brain.

It is the coordination of the expertise of both surgical specialties that is essential to produce the best results.

Pathophysiology

Although each individual cell type of malignancy has its own idiosyncratic behavior, these tumors as a whole have some growth and spread characteristics in common. Most malignant tumors of the paranasal sinuses are of epithelial origin (**Table 5.1**). Squamous cell cancer, adenocarcinoma, acinic cell, and adenoid cystic carcinomas are most common. Esthesioneuroblastoma, although of olfactory epithelial origin, characteristically invades the adjacent ethmoid sinuses. Mucosal melanoma, probably the deadliest of all sinonasal tumors, is fortunately very uncommon. Sarcomas may take origin in the bone of the sinuses or in the bony and cartilaginous septum. Fibrosarcoma, chondrosarcoma, and osteogenic sarcoma are the most usual tumors of this type, although uncommon as a whole. Intracranial tumors and those of the supporting skeleton of the skull base may even present as neoplasms in the nose or sinuses. Chordomas and chondrosarcomas of the sphenoid or ethmoid bone, meningioma (although not usually malignant), and craniopharyngioma make up most of the tumors at this site. Plasmacytomas, lymphomas, and metastatic tumors from primary sites below the clavicles are occasionally seen.

Method of Spread

Sinus malignancies make their way into the intracranial compartment by way of direct bone erosion, penetration of cranial base foramina, perivascular and perineural spread, and, exceedingly rarely, by metastasis. Although referred to on occasion in literature of other medical specialties, brain metastasis from head and neck cancer, other then that of the thyroid, is very rare. This is more so the situation in the paranasal sinus malignancy.

Direct erosion of bone can occur anywhere along the interface of the sinus cavities and the supporting bone of the cranial floor. The fovea ethmoidalis is the thinnest bone of the anterior skull base and is a common site of erosion from carcinomas of the ethmoid sinuses. Malignancies primary to the maxillary sinuses may invade the orbit and the globe itself. They then extend superiorly through the orbital roof into the anterior cranial fossa. A common site of orbital invasion is in the posterior aspect near the apex. From there the tumor may erode the posterior or posterolateral wall into the middle cranial fossa (**Fig. 5.46**). Frontal sinus tumors, although rare, erode the posterior wall to enter this anterior fossa and invade the dura over the anterior pole of the frontal lobe and the inferior reaches of the superior sagittal sinus (**Fig. 5.47**). The sphenoidal sinus is usually involved with tumor by virtue of extension rather than per premum. Tumors in this site may invade superiorly through the planum sphenoidale to the anterior fossa dura (**Fig. 5.48**), laterally to that of the cavernous sinus in the middle cranial fossa (**Fig. 5.49**) or posteriorly, through the clivus, into the posterior cranial fossa (**Fig. 5.50A,B**).

The foramina of the skull base that provide access for vascular and neural structures also provide a portal of entry for direct tumor extension. Notable among these are the small neurovascular foramina that emit the fila olfactoria. There

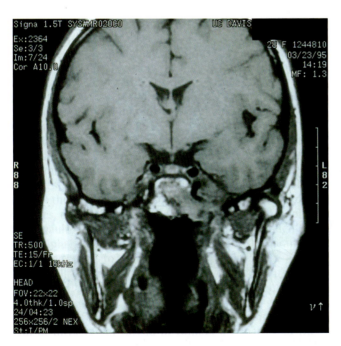

Fig. 5.49 Coronal magnetic resonance imaging showing extension of sphenoethmoidal carcinoma into the cavernous sinus and middle cranial fossa.

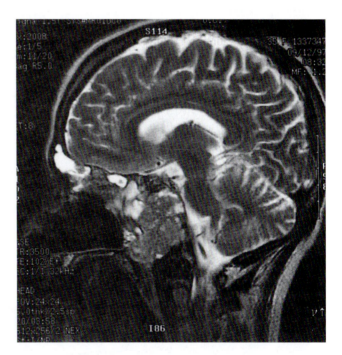

Fig. 5.50 Sagittal magnetic resonance image showing direct spread of tumor originating in the posterior ethmoid and sphenoid sinuses through the posterior sphenoid wall into the posterior cranial fossa. This is especially important in patients with postsellar pneumatization. Axial magnetic resonance image showing proximity of tumor to the basilar artery and pontine dura. (From Donald PJ. Surgery of the Skull Base. Philadelphia: Lippincott-Raven; 1998:64)

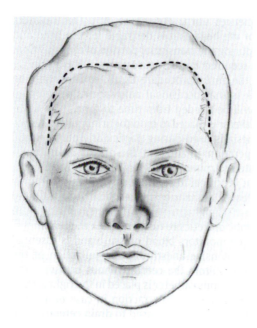

Fig. 5.60 Bitemporal coronal incision commonly employed in craniofacial surgery to provide access to anterior cranial fossa. Care is taken to avoid damage to the superficial temporal artery on the side opposite the lesion, in case the scalp flap is used in reconstruction. The pericranium is preserved as well because it also may be employed in adding support to the cranial floor.

invaded by cancer. In these instances the tumor is debulked with the hope that subsequent chemotherapy and irradiation therapy may at least produce a significant period of palliation. On the other hand, if the preoperative assessment raises a question merely of the proximity of tumor to the cranial floor, or there is no concern of inoperability of the intracranial component, then the transfacial approach is done first.

If the craniotomy is done first, a bitemporal coronal incision is made ~2 cm behind the hairline (**Fig. 5.60**). Care is taken to preserve the pericranium (**Fig. 5.61**) because it will

be used later in the reconstruction of the cranial floor. Rainey clips are placed for hemostasis, and the flap is turned inferiorly. Two bur holes are placed with a craniotome through the frontal bone on either side of the superior sagittal sinus to dissect the sinus off the frontal spine on the intracranial side of the frontal sinus posterior wall. One or two additional bur holes are placed low on the supraorbital rim or rims marking the lateral aspects of the craniotomy flap (**Fig. 5.62**). A skull flap is removed that is large enough to permit exposure of the anterior fossa floor back to the planum sphenoidale. It is important to construct the bone flap as close to the superior wall of the orbit as possible to reduce brain retraction in exposing the dura of the anterior fossa floor. Once some experience is gained with this procedure, a smaller cranial flap is sufficient for adequate resection. Cheeseman[30] for instance, recommended bone removal just larger than a bur hole. However, we have found such limited access is too difficult to work through and impossible when there is extensive intracranial involvement. Schramm[31] uses a frontal sinusotomy approach in patients with minimal intracranial extension. An osteoplastic flap of the anterior frontal sinus wall is created pedicled on the periosteum of the brow. The frontal sinus cavity is exposed, and tumor invading the frontal sinus floor (**Fig. 5.63**) and or the posterior wall is visualized. A cranialization[32] of the sinus is done by removing the entire posterior wall of the sinus. The frontal dura is elevated and the involved dura resected. If the size of the tumor and extent of dural involvement were underestimated by the preoperative studies then a larger frontal bone flap can be removed to enhance exposure.

The approach by Raveh et al may be used, which combines the craniotomy and the facial approach with one bone flap[33] (**Fig. 5.64**). The approach can be expanded by adding a facial degloving and by adding a larger craniotomy. This provides direct access to the central skull base with minimal brain retraction. The drawbacks are the necessity to detach both medial canthal tendons, the resection of the superior aspect of the nasal septum, and the difficulty in visualizing the plane above the cribriform plate, especially in the superior part of the sphenoid sinus. The cribriform plate needs to be fractured and then retracted or resected. The tumors arising in the ethmoid sinuses that invade the intracranial

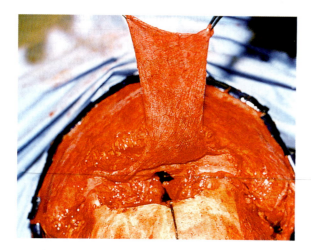

Fig. 5.61 Pericranial flap. (From Donald PJ. Surgery of the Skull Base. Philadelphia: Lippincott-Raven; 1998:184)

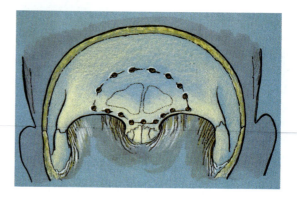

Fig. 5.62 The flap must be sufficient to allow for exposure of the anterior fossa floor all the way to the planum sphenoidale.

It is the coordination of the expertise of both surgical specialties that is essential to produce the best results.

Pathophysiology

Although each individual cell type of malignancy has its own idiosyncratic behavior, these tumors as a whole have some growth and spread characteristics in common. Most malignant tumors of the paranasal sinuses are of epithelial origin (**Table 5.1**). Squamous cell cancer, adenocarcinoma, acinic cell, and adenoid cystic carcinomas are most common. Esthesioneuroblastoma, although of olfactory epithelial origin, characteristically invades the adjacent ethmoid sinuses. Mucosal melanoma, probably the deadliest of all sinonasal tumors, is fortunately very uncommon. Sarcomas may take origin in the bone of the sinuses or in the bony and cartilaginous septum. Fibrosarcoma, chondrosarcoma, and osteogenic sarcoma are the most usual tumors of this type, although uncommon as a whole. Intracranial tumors and those of the supporting skeleton of the skull base may even present as neoplasms in the nose or sinuses. Chordomas and chondrosarcomas of the sphenoid or ethmoid bone, meningioma (although not usually malignant), and craniopharyngioma make up most of the tumors at this site. Plasmacytomas, lymphomas, and metastatic tumors from primary sites below the clavicles are occasionally seen.

Method of Spread

Sinus malignancies make their way into the intracranial compartment by way of direct bone erosion, penetration of cranial base foramina, perivascular and perineural spread, and, exceedingly rarely, by metastasis. Although referred to on occasion in literature of other medical specialties, brain metastasis from head and neck cancer, other then that of the thyroid, is very rare. This is more so the situation in the paranasal sinus malignancy.

Direct erosion of bone can occur anywhere along the interface of the sinus cavities and the supporting bone of the cranial floor. The fovea ethmoidalis is the thinnest bone of the anterior skull base and is a common site of erosion from carcinomas of the ethmoid sinuses. Malignancies primary to the maxillary sinuses may invade the orbit and the globe itself. They then extend superiorly through the orbital roof into the anterior cranial fossa. A common site of orbital invasion is in the posterior aspect near the apex. From there the tumor may erode the posterior or posterolateral wall into the middle cranial fossa (**Fig. 5.46**). Frontal sinus tumors, although rare, erode the posterior wall to enter this anterior fossa and invade the dura over the anterior pole of the frontal lobe and the inferior reaches of the superior sagittal sinus (**Fig. 5.47**). The sphenoidal sinus is usually involved with tumor by virtue of extension rather than per premum. Tumors in this site may invade superiorly through the planum sphenoidale to the anterior fossa dura (**Fig. 5.48**), laterally to that of the cavernous sinus in the middle cranial fossa (**Fig. 5.49**) or posteriorly, through the clivus, into the posterior cranial fossa (**Fig. 5.50A,B**).

The foramina of the skull base that provide access for vascular and neural structures also provide a portal of entry for direct tumor extension. Notable among these are the small neurovascular foramina that emit the fila olfactoria. There

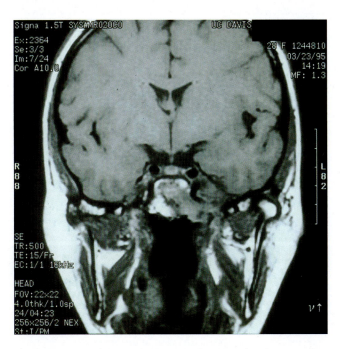

Fig. 5.49 Coronal magnetic resonance imaging showing extension of sphenoethmoidal carcinoma into the cavernous sinus and middle cranial fossa.

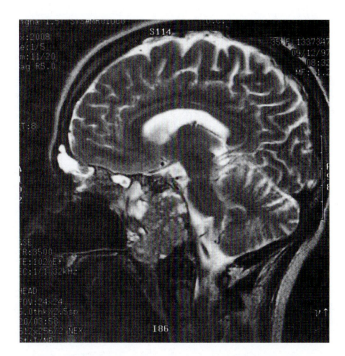

Fig. 5.50 Sagittal magnetic resonance image showing direct spread of tumor originating in the posterior ethmoid and sphenoid sinuses through the posterior sphenoid wall into the posterior cranial fossa. This is especially important in patients with postsellar pneumatization. Axial magnetic resonance image showing proximity of tumor to the basilar artery and pontine dura. (From Donald PJ. Surgery of the Skull Base. Philadelphia: Lippincott-Raven; 1998:64)

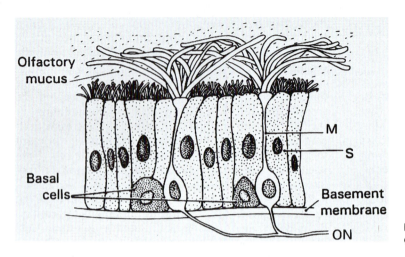

Fig. 5.51 Diagram of the olfactory epithelium. ON = optic nerve, M = mitral body layer, S = suppporting cells.

are ~43 foramina per side in the cribriform plate that emit these first-order neurons whose cell bodies are contained and that synapse in the olfactory bulbs. Each olfactory filament is sheathed in dura. Therefore tumors that erode through the cribriform plate, by definition, invade dura. In the case of esthesioneuroblastoma, because the tumor begins in the supporting cells (**Fig. 5.51**) of the olfactory epithelium, virtually all of them have invaded dura. The rare exception to this may be the unusual case in which the tumor arises in the infrequently and occurring islands of olfactory epithelium in the supreme meatus of the nose. In our series of esthesioneuroblastomas we have seen only one such case (**Fig. 5.8**).

There are three foramina in the posterior orbit, which allow direct tumor spread: the superior orbital fissure, the optic foramen, and the foramen rotundum (**Fig. 5.52**). All three lead into the middle cranial fossa. The superior fissure leads into the cavernous sinus, the optic foramen, and the foramen rotundum into the middle cranial fossa. The optic canal exits at the superior border of the cavernous sinus, but the optic nerve is outside the dura of the sinus as it exits the foramen and enters the middle fossa. At a variable point in the canal the periosteum becomes continuous with the middle fossa dura, and the nerve is subdural as it enters the intracranial space, then meets its fellow nerve of the opposite side to become the optic chiasm.

The foramen rotundum admits the maxillary division of the trigeminal nerve that enters the gasserian ganglion in the Meckel cave, which in turn is situated in the trigeminal impression on the middle fossa floor (**Fig. 5.53**). A direct extension of the cavernous sinus often encloses this nerve trunk. The cavernous sinus dura marks the medial boundary of the Meckel cave. Sinus tumors can extend along the intra-

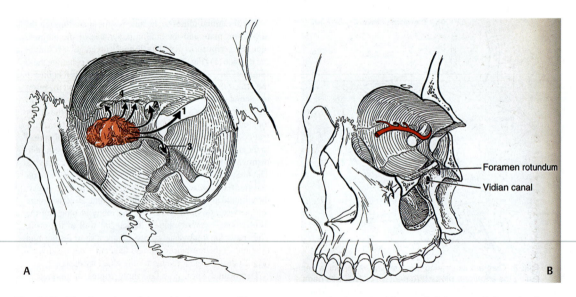

Fig. 5.52 The foramina of the orbital apex provide an easy avenue for intracranial spread. (**A**) View of the orbital apex showing routes of tumor spread. 1, superior orbital fissure; 2, optic foramen; 3, inferior orbital fissure; 4, vascular foramina for the ethmoid vessels. (**B**) Sagittal cutaway view of the orbital apex with orbital floor and portion of posterior wall of the maxillary sinus removed. (From Donald PJ. Surgery of the Skull Base. Philadelphia: Lippincott-Raven; 1998:56)

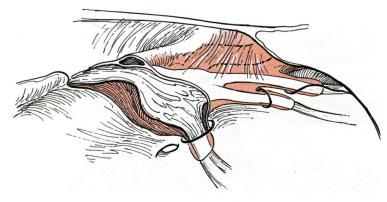

Fig. 5.53 Diagram of the Meckel cave showing dural investment of the gasserian ganglion and branches of the trigeminal nerve. (From Donald PJ. Surgery of the Skull Base. Philadelphia: Lippincott-Raven; 1998:57)

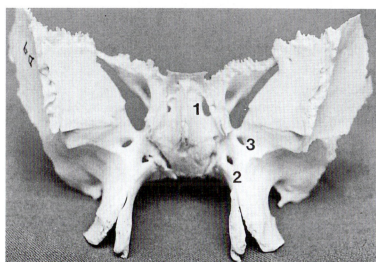

Fig. 5.54 Anterior face of the sphenoid bone. 1, sphenoid ostium; 2, vidian canal; 3, foramen rotundum. (From Donald PJ. Surgery of the Skull Base. Philadelphia: Lippincott-Raven; 1998:27)

cranial aspect of the middle fossa deep in the infratemporal fossa. From there they can spread through the foramen ovale and from there to the Meckel cave.

Tumors involving the sphenoidal sinus can spread through the pterygoid (vidian) canal to the middle fossa floor and the internal carotid artery. The positions of the optic canal, foramen rotundum, and vidian canal occupy a triangular point of access to the anteroinferior part of the middle fossa near the cavernous sinus (**Fig. 5.54**).

Vascular spread of tumors can also proceed through skull base foramina. Regarding tumors the most notable foramen is the foramen lacerum. Although not intimately related to the sinuses, it is closest to the sphenoidal sinus. Tumors originating in the sinus or having spread from the ethmoid block, turbinates, or nasal septum can spread along the nasopharyngeal vault, penetrate the mucosa, and erode through the cartilage plug that fills the inferior aspect of the foramen, thus gaining access to the cavernous sinus (**Fig. 5.55**).

Rarely will a sinus tumor be so extensive as to creep across the undersurface of the sphenoid bone and penetrate the jugular foramen.

Perineural spread, already alluded to, is a common mechanism of intracranial spread of tumors originating in the sinuses. The method of spread was once thought to be via the perineural lymphatics; however, these structures do not exist to any extent. The mode of spread appears to be via

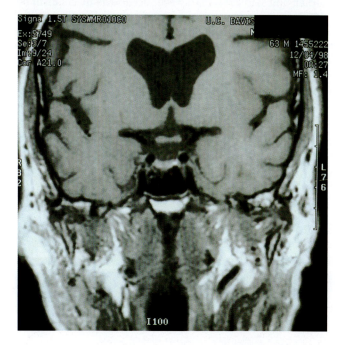

Fig. 5.55 Magnetic resonance imaging in the coronal plane showing a squamous cell carcinoma of the sphenoethmoid area invading the foramen lacerum, extending into the carotid canal and encasing the internal carotid artery as it made its course into the cavernous sinus.

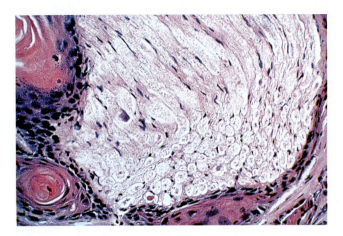

Fig. 5.56 Histological section showing spread of tumor in the perineural space of cranial nerve V (H&E, ×100). (From Donald PJ. Surgery of the Skull Base. Philadelphia: Lippincott-Raven; 1998:57)

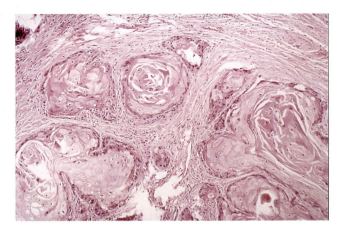

Fig. 5.57 Intraneuronal spread of squamous cell carcinoma in the optic nerve (H&E, ×100). (From Donald PJ, Gluckman JL, Rice DH, eds. The Sinuses. New York: Raven; 1995:73)

the perineural spaces of the nerve trunks or branches[29] (**Fig. 5.56**). Rarely is there penetration into actual nerve substance (**Fig. 5.57**), and for some curious reason, the tumor, once intracranial, appears to stay confined mostly to the nerve and only occasionally invades the overlying dura. Another interesting phenomenon is that in the extracranial course, neurotropic tumors tend to have skip areas. This is especially characteristic of adenoid cystic carcinoma, where one focus of perineural tumor may be separated by as much as 2 cm from another tumor deposit. This is rarely seen once the nerve becomes intracranial. The tumor seems packed together, and skip areas hardly ever occur. The mechanism by which perineural invasion takes place is as yet obscure. Some tumors that have extensive perineural spread such as neuroblastomas have high concentrations of polysialated neuronal cell adhesion molecules (NCAMs). This class of proteins is ubiquitous throughout embryogenesis, but rapidly disappears shortly after birth. Some NCAMs, however, persist, and they are found mainly in the brain. These compounds are

seen in relatively high concentrations in multiple myeloma and some lymphomas. In our series they were particularly prominent in primary carcinomas of the salivary gland, especially those with distant metastasis. In our first series of patients, no clear difference was seen in concentrations of polysialated NCAMs in tumors with perineural spread compared with those without. Because of some potential flaws in this study, especially the freshness of the tissue under study and the quality of the markers used, the study continues.

There are certain other characteristics that head and neck cancers express once intracranial invasion has taken place. The dura forms a rather solid barrier to the spread of these malignancies. Perhaps the dense collagenous structure of this tissue impedes the movement of the cancerous tissue within it. The tumor tends to become rather densely concentrated and has often a pushing rather than an infiltrative margin of advance (**Fig. 5.58**). The underlying brain is rarely invaded. In our series of cases of dural invasion only 20 patients have spread to the brain. Even when the tumor does spread to underlying brain, meningeal carcinomatosis is rarely seen. Our 5-year tumor free survival rate for these 20 patients is 27.6%.

◆ **Preparation** Preparing the patient for surgery requires the coordinated efforts of the head and neck surgeon, neurosurgeon, and maxillofacial prosthodontist. The planning and timing of each surgeon's step in the procedure is anticipated and agreed upon ahead of time. Each participant should plan to be present for most of his or her partner's contribution to the procedure because the most difficult aspect of the operation is to establish clear surgical margins. Both surgical participants contribute to and jointly decide on the determination of these margins, which are especially crucial in the region of the fovea ethmoidalis and planum sphenoidale. The patient needs to understand the gravity of the procedure and that it is "brain surgery," with its possible aftereffects as well as the attendant problem of the usually inevitable facial deformity.

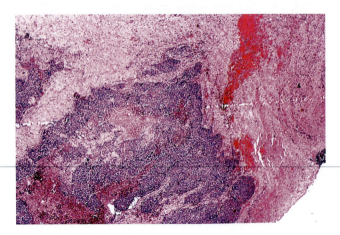

Fig. 5.58 Compact nature of tumor in dura (H&E, ×40). (From Donald PJ. Surgery of the Skull Base. Philadelphia. Lippincott-Raven; 1998:62)

Although in some instances the eye can be saved, the loss of the eye, especially if little preoperative disturbance in vision has been experienced, is an exceptionally traumatic psychological prospect for most patients. Even the eye already blinded by disease is precious, and thus orbital exenteration is a highly charged emotional consideration. Nevertheless, surgeons must not allow their judgment to be swayed into compromising a chance of cure in these circumstances. The surgeon, not the patient, must dictate surgical margins. On the other hand, some patients with a longstanding aggravating problem find the afflicted eye an anathema and actually request its excision (**Fig. 5.42**).

Compared with loss of the eye, defects in the lower part of the face are relatively less traumatic, and the functional improvement and psychological boost a patient gets from the use of an "immediate" dental obturator is remarkable. Planning the extent of palatal, alveolar ridge, and soft tissue resection in advance with the prosthodontist allows sufficient time for a functional palatal prosthesis to be made. The dentition that is to remain is carefully checked so that any restorative work necessary can be completed preoperatively. Once the resection has been done and the closure completed, the obturator is fitted into the defect. The prosthesis forms a platform on which a bolster can be placed to support the skin graft lining the cavity (**Fig. 5.59**).

◆ **Procedure** General anesthesia is induced and maintained through either an oral endotracheal tube or a tracheostomy tube. Over the past 15 years we did tracheostomies on virtually all the patients who were to have an anterior approach skull base resection. The tracheostomy eliminates the nuisance posed by the tube in the mouth, may contribute to a cleaner operative field, and is excellent prophylaxis to the development of tension pneumocephalus. The head may be supported on a headrest such as the Mayfield

(Integra Lifesciences Corp., Plainsboro, NJ). This restricts the mobility of the head that is desirable for the head and neck surgeon during the transfacial portion of the resection, but it may be required by the neurosurgeon. It is perfectly feasible to do the entire procedure using the headrest. The only drawback is that occasional adjustments to improve visualization will be needed from time to time.

A urinary catheter is placed to monitor urinary flow. Hypotensive anesthesia is used during particularly hemorrhagic parts of the operation. In addition, the patient is kept relatively dehydrated to minimize cerebral volume. Monitoring of urine output is critical to continuously assess renal function and, indirectly, vascular perfusion. Finally, the catheter is needed to drain the large volumes of urine resulting from the use of osmotic diuretics to further shrink the brain.

An arterial line monitors blood pressure and is essential when using hypotensive anesthesia. Cannulization of the subclavian vein monitors the central venous pressure. The tip of the central venous catheter is placed in the right atrium to provide a ready means of extraction in case of air embolism. A lumbar drain is often used to drain cerebrospinal fluid, thus facilitating the intracranial dissection. Temporary tarsorrhaphy sutures are placed to prevent corneal exposure. Occasionally, the operation will be one that is to establish operability. If the MRI suggests that both cavernous sinuses and both intracavernous carotids may be invaded by tumor, then the operation may be a procedure to ensure surgical feasibility. The definitive procedure will be done at a second stage 1 to 2 weeks later. This initial staging operation will provide adequate exposure to view and biopsy the cavernous sinus and pericarotid tissue, but especially if the eye is present, will not permit a complete resection of the cavernous sinus or the carotid. For further information on staging and resection of these structures see chapter 9. Sometimes the use of the sinus endoscope may provide valuable information in the establishment of tumor extension. Currently patients are considered inoperable if they have distant metastasis, the optic chiasm is invaded by tumor, both carotids or both cavernous sinuses are involved, or the brainstem or other vital areas of the brain are invaded that the neurosurgical member of the team considers inviolable.

Before the definitive operation is done, a surgical confirmation of actual tumor respectability is undertaken if this is in question. This is an essential step to avoid the tragedy of being committed to a major impairment of the patient's subsequent function by doing a massive procedure only to find at the end of the operation that the tumor is surgically unencompassable. Making this determination necessitates piecemeal removal of gross tumor, entirely violating the principle of en bloc resection. It unfortunately is the only means of determining tumor extent. The violation of the en bloc principal was initially a concern because of the potential problem of seeding of tumor in the surgical wound. The issue of seeding of tumor in the operative bed has not been seen in our patients.

If there is any question about the possible inoperability of the total amount of intracranial tumor, then the craniotomy must be done first and the undersurface of the cerebrum checked to see if unresectable areas of the brain have been

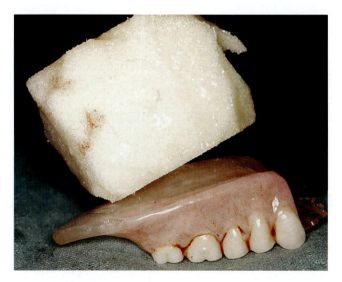

Fig. 5.59 Preoperative maxillary prosthesis that restores the dental arch and can support a bolster to stent the skin grafts within the maxillectomy cavity.

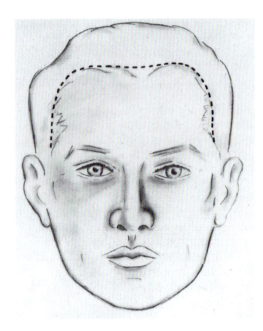

Fig. 5.60 Bitemporal coronal incision commonly employed in craniofacial surgery to provide access to anterior cranial fossa. Care is taken to avoid damage to the superficial temporal artery on the side opposite the lesion, in case the scalp flap is used in reconstruction. The pericranium is preserved as well because it also may be employed in adding support to the cranial floor.

invaded by cancer. In these instances the tumor is debulked with the hope that subsequent chemotherapy and irradiation therapy may at least produce a significant period of palliation. On the other hand, if the preoperative assessment raises a question merely of the proximity of tumor to the cranial floor, or there is no concern of inoperability of the intracranial component, then the transfacial approach is done first.

If the craniotomy is done first, a bitemporal coronal incision is made ~2 cm behind the hairline (**Fig. 5.60**). Care is taken to preserve the pericranium (**Fig. 5.61**) because it will

be used later in the reconstruction of the cranial floor. Rainey clips are placed for hemostasis, and the flap is turned inferiorly. Two bur holes are placed with a craniotome through the frontal bone on either side of the superior sagittal sinus to dissect the sinus off the frontal spine on the intracranial side of the frontal sinus posterior wall. One or two additional bur holes are placed low on the supraorbital rim or rims marking the lateral aspects of the craniotomy flap (**Fig. 5.62**). A skull flap is removed that is large enough to permit exposure of the anterior fossa floor back to the planum sphenoidale. It is important to construct the bone flap as close to the superior wall of the orbit as possible to reduce brain retraction in exposing the dura of the anterior fossa floor. Once some experience is gained with this procedure, a smaller cranial flap is sufficient for adequate resection. Cheeseman[30] for instance, recommended bone removal just larger than a bur hole. However, we have found such limited access is too difficult to work through and impossible when there is extensive intracranial involvement. Schramm[31] uses a frontal sinusotomy approach in patients with minimal intracranial extension. An osteoplastic flap of the anterior frontal sinus wall is created pedicled on the periosteum of the brow. The frontal sinus cavity is exposed, and tumor invading the frontal sinus floor (**Fig. 5.63**) and or the posterior wall is visualized. A cranialization[32] of the sinus is done by removing the entire posterior wall of the sinus. The frontal dura is elevated and the involved dura resected. If the size of the tumor and extent of dural involvement were underestimated by the preoperative studies then a larger frontal bone flap can be removed to enhance exposure.

The approach by Raveh et al may be used, which combines the craniotomy and the facial approach with one bone flap[33] (**Fig. 5.64**). The approach can be expanded by adding a facial degloving and by adding a larger craniotomy. This provides direct access to the central skull base with minimal brain retraction. The drawbacks are the necessity to detach both medial canthal tendons, the resection of the superior aspect of the nasal septum, and the difficulty in visualizing the plane above the cribriform plate, especially in the superior part of the sphenoid sinus. The cribriform plate needs to be fractured and then retracted or resected. The tumors arising in the ethmoid sinuses that invade the intracranial

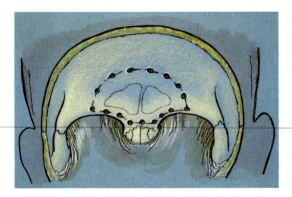

Fig. 5.61 Pericranial flap. (From Donald PJ. Surgery of the Skull Base. Philadelphia: Lippincott-Raven; 1998:184)

Fig. 5.62 The flap must be sufficient to allow for exposure of the anterior fossa floor all the way to the planum sphenoidale.

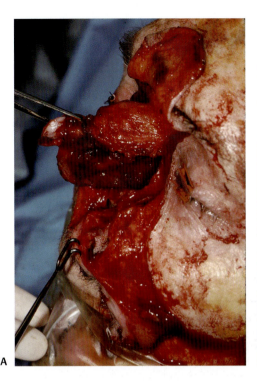
A

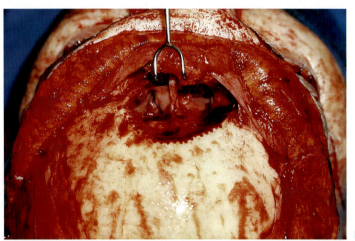
B

Fig. 5.63 Squamous cell carcinoma invading the frontal sinus involving the anterior ethmoid sinuses and the nasal bones. (**A**) Transfacial approach showing tumor in anterior ethmoid sinuses, septum, and nasal bones. (**B**) Low anterior craniotomy showing extension of tumor through frontal sinus floor.

space commonly involve the cribriform plate so its excision is necessary in any event.

The dura can either be retracted after careful dissection or incised at the craniotomy site. The dura of the anterior pole of the frontal lobe is brittle in the elderly and prone to injury during craniotomy. In addition, the area of the cribriform plate is perforated by dural extensions surrounding the olfactory filaments and is often torn during extradural dissection. We have used both approaches, but when the CT and MRI scans suggest intracranial invasion,[6] the intradural approach makes exposure of the tumor much easier. In addition, intracerebral extension is far more easily assessed and dealt with when this latter exposure is used.

The frontal lobes are gently retracted and the tumor extent determined (**Fig. 5.65**). A margin of 3 to 5 mm is taken around the tumor and checked with frozen section. The dense connective tissue compromising the dura mater offers a stout barrier to the spread of tumor. Even the arachnoid layer with

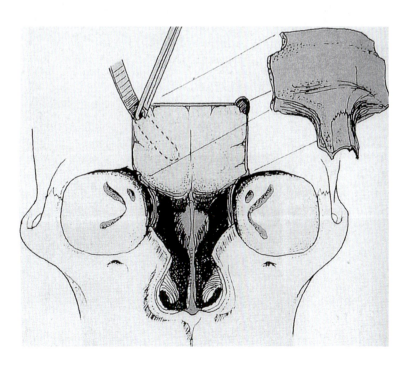

Fig. 5.64 Bone flap for extended anterior subcranial approach. Allows direct view of the anterior skull base with minimal or no brain retraction. (From Donald PJ. Surgery of the Skull Base. Philadelphia: Lippincott-Raven; 1998:242)

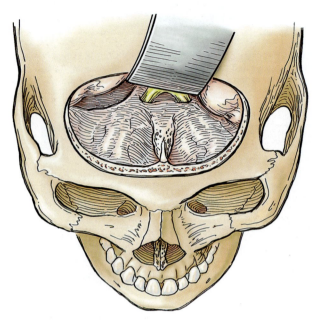

Fig. 5.65 Exposure of the entire floor of the anterior cranial fossa is possible up to the lesser wing of the sphenoid by this approach.

its thin filamentous makeup offers significant resistance to tumor spreads, especially to the brain. The patient whose MRI is seen in **Fig. 5.16** had extensive arachnoid involvement by the malignancy, which displaced the brain and compressed the third ventricle but did not invade the cerebral tissue per se. Involvement of the superior sagittal sinus can be safely resected up to the level of the coronal suture.

A biopsy of the frontal lobe adjacent to the areas of dural penetration must be done to determine whether there is intracerebral invasion. A generous cuff of frontal lobe must be resected surrounding any site of such involvement. Most patients tolerate this quite well.

The area encompassing the extent of tumor into the anterior fossa is clearly exposed and outlined, and margins of uninvolved dura surrounding the neoplasm are established.

In those cases in which the craniotomy was done first the transfacial part now begins. The transfacial exposure is usually done first. The extent of incision on the face varies with the amount of tumor spread. An ethmoidectomy incision in continuity with a lateral rhinotomy may be sufficient if the tumor is limited to the ethmoid block with no orbital and minimal maxillary invasion (**Fig. 5.66**). The incision begins just in the inferior hairs of the medial aspect of the brow. Care is taken to angle the knife so that it parallels the hair follicles. The incision proceeds inferiorly in a gentle curve that traverses a point midway between the midline of the nose, near the nasion, and the medial canthus of the eye. The lateral rhinotomy portion of the incision extends in the

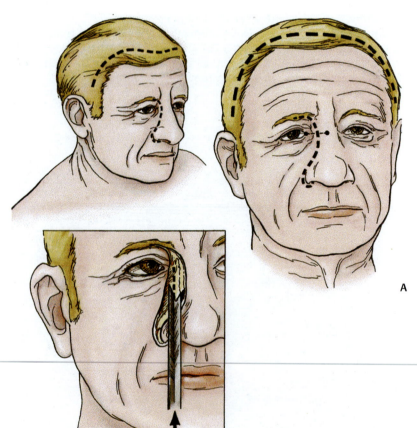

Fig. 5.66 (A) Lateral rhinotomy incision coupled with an ethmoidectomy incision provides excellent exposure for limited access to the ethmoid bloc, orbit, and upper maxilla. (B) Lateral osteotomy portion of rhinotomy.

natural facial cleavage line between the lateral nose and the anterior cheek skin. It courses around the nasal ala and into the vestibule of the nose. The soft tissue part of the incision is carried both intra- and extranasally up to the edge of the pyriform rim. Soft tissue elevation is carried over the maxillary face encircling and at the same time protecting the infraorbital nerve. No soft tissue elevation is done over the nasal dorsum except a small tunnel at the level of the nasion. A bone-cutting needle such as the Midas Rex B5 (Medtronic, Inc., Minneapolis, MN) is used to make the lateral osteotomy in the ascending process of the maxilla. This is carried up to the level of the nasion where it is turned horizontally and extended to the nasal septum. The scalpel blade is slipped in this narrow osteotomy cut to completely incise the nasal mucosa. A broad, flat osteotome is placed in the nose under the incised nasal bone, and a lateral twist will produce a greenstick fracture at the level of the septum.

The lateral rhinotomy gives a limited view of the field. An extended anterior wall maxillary ostectomy will provide a much superior exposure, especially when a medial maxillectomy is added to it. The outline of the ostectomy is portrayed in **Fig. 5.67**. Encirclement of a narrow collar of bone surrounding the infraorbital nerve is done to protect the nerve from damage unless the nerve has been invaded by tumor. The most difficult of the bony incisions is the vertical cut made with the Midas Rex B5 (Medtronic) just inside the nasal cavity in the medial wall of the maxilla. Prior to the actual bony incisions it is wise to drill the holes and contour the miniplates and microplates that will be placed to secure the bone flap back into position at the end of the resection. The bony fragment is removed and stored at the back table in

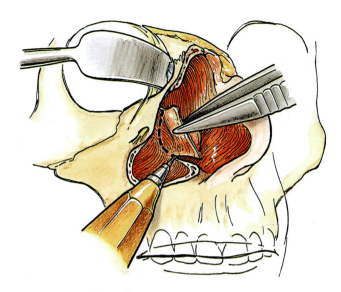

Fig. 5.68 Medial maxillectomy. (From Donald PJ. Surgery of the Skull Base. Philadelphia: Lippincott-Raven; 1998:172)

saline-soaked gauze. Any part of this bone invaded by tumor must of course be resected. The next stage is to resect the medial maxillary wall. A bone cut is made horizontally flush with the floor of the nose that extends from the ostectomy cut to the most posterior extent of the medial maxillary wall near the nasopharynx. A right-angled scissors is placed in the most posterior extent of this incision and is directed superiorly toward the ethmoid sinuses (**Fig. 5.68**).

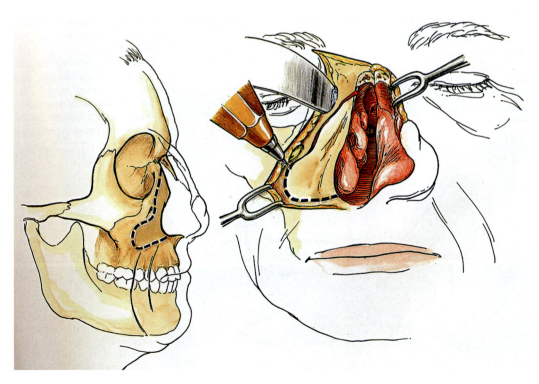

Fig. 5.67 Anterior maxillary ostectomy.

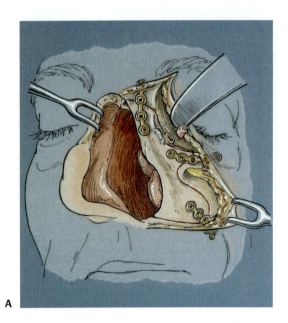

A

Fig. 5.69 Anterior wall bony segment returned with plates. (**A**) Diagram. (**B**) In patient after completion of craniofacial resection.

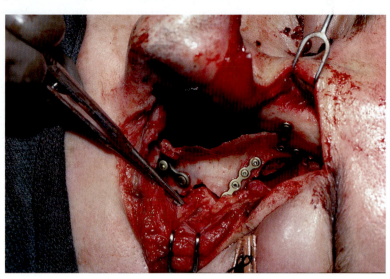

B

Excision of the lacrimal bone and lamina papyracea with biting forceps exposes the anterior ethmoidal extent of the tumor. The ethmoidectomy is completed, all the time debulking the tumor. The medial maxillary wall is now removed. Piecemeal tumor removal is often required to visualize the superior limits of the tumor. Another factor limiting visualization is bleeding. This is usually controlled by hypotensive anesthesia and the use of an intranasal pack of 1-inch ribbon gauze soaked in 0.5% lidocaine and 1:200,000 epinephrine. If possible, the nasal septum is preserved because it will be of great value in reconstruction of the anterior fossa floor.

Once the superior margins of the tumor have been delineated, the neurosurgeon deflects the coronal scalp flap and retracts the brain. The neurosurgeon can then guide the head

and neck surgeon who is tapping out the bony margins of the tumor from below. From above, the neurosurgeon protects the brain and other vital structures with a malleable Teflon-coated retractor. The two surgeons working in concert can then clearly and safely establish the limits of resection. Once the bloc is free, it is delivered through the facial wound.

Reconstruction entails the establishment of a watertight dural seal. Resected dura is replaced with a fascial graft. Temporalis fascia is preferred to fascia lata and is readily available through the coronal incision. Any rents in the dura, such as biopsy sites, can usually be repaired by careful suturing.

The maxillary ostectomy flap is replaced and secured with the previously contoured miniplates and microplates (**Fig. 5.69A,B**). Support for the cranial floor is best provided by a

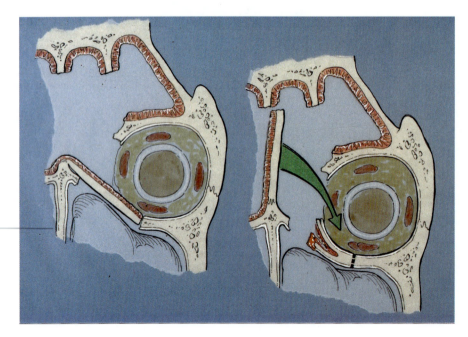

Fig. 5.70 The nasal septum is denuded of mucosa on one surface and then cut from its attachments to the nasal crest and the nasal dorsum. It is greenstick-fractured at the nasal vault, and the flap is swung superiorly to reconstruct the cranial floor. The flap is held in position with packing.

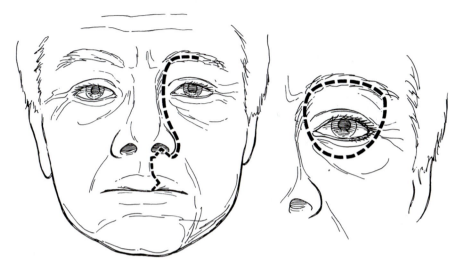

Fig. 5.71 Weber-Fergusson incision. Note darts in nasal sill and surrounding sucking tubercle of upper lip. (From Donald PJ, Gluckman JL, Rice DH, eds. The Sinuses. New York: Raven; 1995:468)

nasal septal chondralosseous–mucosal flap. The mucosa is denuded from the tumor side of the septum, and the septal flap is detached from the surrounding attachments and fractured across the nasal vault. A greenstick fracture will allow hinging of the flap on a mucoperiosteal pedicle. The flap is swung superiorly and packed into position (**Fig. 5.70**). In the remaining cases either the septum or the opposite cribriform plate and fovea ethmoidalis requires resection to clear the tumor. This flap has been feasible in only three cases in our series. The lumbar drain is maintained to control intracerebral pressure. The drain can usually be removed by the third postoperative day.

Postoperative antibiotics are a controversial subject in any area of surgery. We have elected to give a short course of a broad-spectrum antibiotic on the day prior to surgery, intraoperatively, and 3 to 5 days postoperatively. Postoperative infection has not been a problem. Most series quote a less than 4% incidence of meningitis.[34]

Craniofacial Resection with Maxillectomy

Many patients requiring craniofacial surgery for paranasal sinus cancer have extensive neoplasms. Orbital exenteration and maxillectomy with an ethmoid-sphenoidectomy are usually necessary. The face of the sphenoid is completely removed, and the frontal sinus may require exenteration.

The cranial portion of the operation remains the same as previously described; however, extension of tumor through the orbital roof and the frontal sinus should be anticipated. Marked restriction of ocular motility and visual impairment are danger signs indicating orbital apex involvement. Tumor extending this far requires resection of portions of the lesser wing of the sphenoid bone and a part of the middle fossa floor. The cavernous sinus and the intercavernous and intrapetrous portions of the internal carotid artery present special problems. The CT scan and MRI are invaluable in the preoperative evaluation of this potential problem. Often the degree of tumor involvement is more extensive in these cases, with tumor extending across the nasal septum and involving both cribriform plates.

The maxillectomy is done through the standard Weber-Fergusson incision (**Fig. 5.71**). A triangular dart in the lip helps to prevent notching of the vermilion border later on. A second dart into the floor of the nose preserves the nasal sill. If there is skin involvement, a generous cutaneous margin of 3 to 4 cm is taken to ensure complete tumor encompassment (**Fig. 5.72**). If any doubt at all exists concerning tumor fixation to skin, the area must be resected (**Fig. 5.73**) because the dissemination of cutaneous tumor via skin lymphatics occurs with astounding rapidity, with subcutaneous tumor spreading wide of the primary.

The maxillectomy is performed in the usual way. The exception is that the posterior bony cut is made such that a small triangular piece of bone that is the posterior wall is

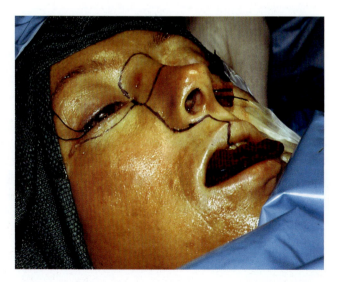

Fig. 5.72 Because of skin involvement, a wide cutaneous margin was necessary in this case.

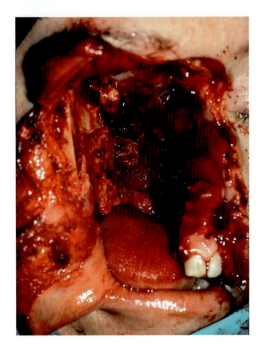

Fig. 5.73 Although skin involvement was suspected, there was no fixation to tumor. Biopsy of the overlying skin showed tumor invasion, and a generous excision was required. Operative appearance of tumor from the maxilla and ethmoid bloc invading the nasal cavity and the overlying skin.

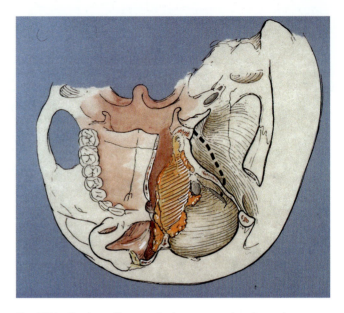

Fig. 5.74 Total maxillectomy is done, preserving the malar eminence of the zygoma when possible and leaving a residual triangle of the posterior maxillary wall.

left behind (**Fig. 5.74**). An attempt is made to preserve the malar eminence. If minimal tumor exists within the zygomatic recess of the maxilla then the residual tumor may be removed with a cutting bur, followed by curetting of the cancellous bone taken for a margin and the preservation of the malar eminence. If tumor penetrates the posterior wall then the first bloc that has been excised is considered as the

"first layer." A cutting bur is used to remove the posterior wall; then if tumor extends beyond, removal of the pterygoid plates is done (**Fig. 5.75**). As the plates are removed the muscles retract. Small encroachments of tumor on the immediate areas of the muscle can be widely resected, but significant invasion will need complete removal up to and often including the muscular insertions. This may require a separate cervical incision and partial mandibulectomy from the glenoid fossa to the area just beyond the angle. While dissecting in the region of the pterygoids, brisk bleeding is commonplace from the branches of the maxillary artery, es-

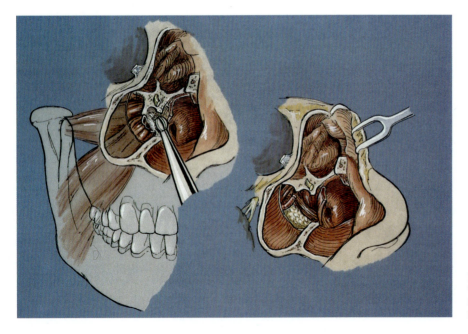

Fig. 5.75 Residual tumor in the maxillary wall extending into the pterygomaxillary space pterygoid plates and body of the sphenoid excised with cutting bur.

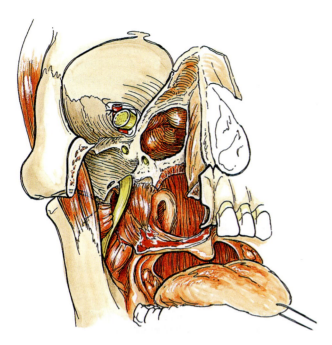

Fig. 5.76 The pterygoid plates are removed, the pterygoid muscles retracted, and the palatal muscles exposed. (From Donald PJ. *Surgery of the Skull Base.* Philadelphia: Lippincott-Raven; 1998:300)

pecially in the pterygomaxillary space. Access to invasion of the clivus, eustachian tube, palatal muscles, and basisphenoid and sphenoidal sinus is provided (**Fig. 5.76**).

The amount of alveolar ridge and nasal floor to be resected is determined by the extent of tumor. Extension of disease across the septum and into the opposing sinus requires a wide maxillary excision, but unfortunately this severely compromises prosthetic rehabilitation (**Fig. 5.77**) (see chapter 15). An attempt is made to save as much alveolar ridge and as many teeth as is feasible within the limits of adequate cancer resection. Bearing in mind the same constraints, as much soft palate as possible is preserved. This helps enormously in the rehabilitation of speech and swallowing.

The ethmoid bloc is resected as already described. Lesions in the posterior region of the maxilla and ethmoid labyrinth present a special problem because the optic chiasm lies adjacent to the planum sphenoidale. Gentle retraction by the neurosurgeon exposes the region, and careful removal of affected bone can be done without disturbing the optic nerves. The roof and even the lateral wall of this side of the orbit may require removal. If the eye cannot be preserved then it is resected, dissecting around the periorbita and cross-clamping at the orbital apex. The apex is often invaded by tumor and the margin of resection at the annulus of Zinn will contain tumor. Once the eye has been removed from the field the cutting bur is used to remove some of the bone of the optic

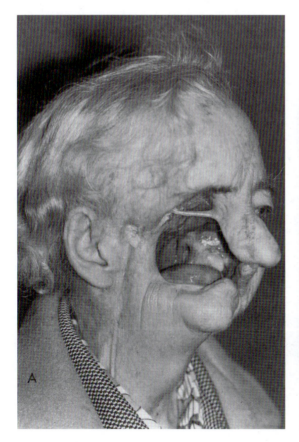
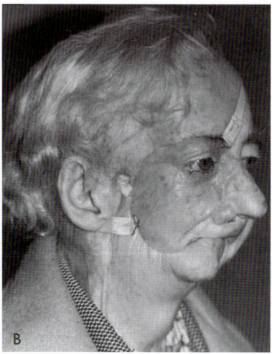

Fig. 5.77 (**A**) Aggressive verrucous carcinoma crossing the septum into the opposing maxillary sinus, requiring repeated resections. (**B**) Prosthetic rehabilitation is an improvement, but the result is still less than perfect.

foramen an the "second layer" containing the optic nerve, ophthalmic artery, and ophthalmic veins as well as the residual muscle and the annulus (**Fig. 5.78A,B**). If tumor is still present along the optic nerve it can be resected back to the optic chiasm.

With the eye removed there is an increased access to the skull base, and in some cases a subcranial craniotomy can be performed to resect dural infiltration by the cancer. It is possible to do some resections of the anterior aspects of the cavernous sinus as long as the internal carotid artery is not involved (**Fig. 5.79**). This avoids a formal craniotomy and essentially eliminates any brain retraction.

Reconstruction of the area involves use of both flaps and free grafts. Covering the resected area with a skin flap provides an excellent durable surface, good support for the intracranial contents, and also partially obliterates the cavity. The single deterring factor to using a flap is the masking of any local recurrence, which then does not become obvious until it has reached a large and most often unresectable size. The exception to this rule may be the radial forearm free flap, which is relatively thin. Although more durable than a split-thickness skin graft the major benefit of this flap is that it provides an excellent vascular supply to the area. In a patient who has had prior irradiation to the area of resection this is a distinct advantage (**Fig. 5.80**).

Some form of cranial support is essential. The septal flap used in the more limited ethmoid resection is usually not available in this more extensive operation. A pericranial flap created at the time of craniotomy provides bulk, resilience, excellent blood supply, and close proximity for this portion of the reconstruction (**Fig. 5.81**). The pericranial flap pro-

vides all the necessary support, even in individuals who have had a large portion of the anterior fossa floor resected. Bone grafts, titanium mesh, and other grafts or alloplasts are unnecessary. The dura is sutured and patched with temporalis fascia and the pericranial flap turned into position. A split-thickness skin graft is placed against the pericranial flap, and the remaining maxillectomy cavity. A graft of good quality is necessary against the raw cheek. Failure to resurface this area results in severe retraction of the cheek flap. The skin is held in place by a sponge bolster and packing, which in turn is held in place by a prosthetic obturator.

The packing material is removed 7 to 10 days postoperatively. Careful cleansing of the cavity and frequent observations are made until the cavity is reepithelialized.

Frontal Sinus Carcinoma

Frontal sinus carcinoma is most often mistaken for a mucocele. Because bone erosion occurs in both entities, this finding cannot serve as the important differential feature that is so relevant with lesions in the other paranasal sinuses. Robinson[35] reports that in a 4-year period, three of 12 patients presenting with a frontal sinus mucopyocele had an underlying carcinoma. Chronic infection commonly produces frontal sinus opacification and bony sclerosis. Unfortunately, findings of sclerosis have also been cited by several authors[34–36] in cases of cancer, thus eliminating another important differentiating sign.

An excellent article by Brownson and Ogura[37] reviewing 102 cases in the literature revealed pain and swelling to be the most common of the presenting symptoms of frontal si-

Fig. 5.78 (**A**) Right-angled clamp placed around soft tissues of the orbital apex, which are transected with right-angled scissors. (**B**) Second echelon of orbital apex tissue resected to establish resection margin. (From Donald PJ. Surgery of the Skull Base. Philadelphia. Lippincott-Raven; 1998:177)

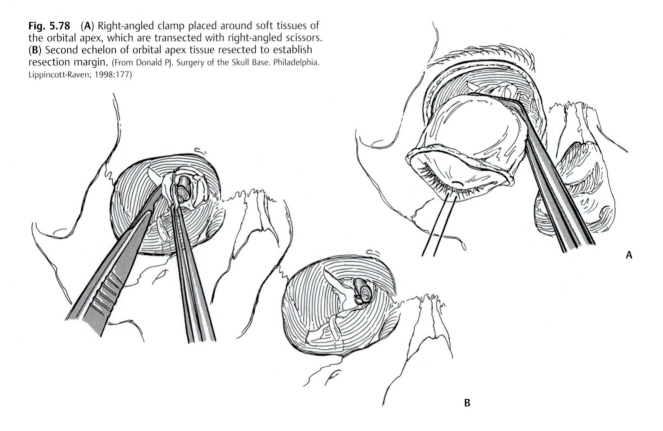

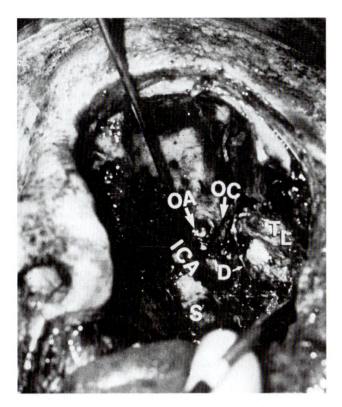

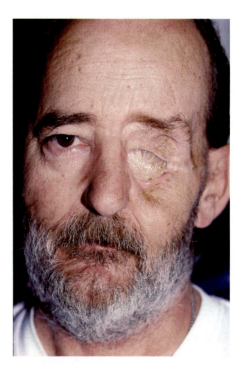

Fig. 5.79 Following tumor resection. S, sphenoid sinus; ICA, internal carotid artery; OA, orbital apex; OC, optic canal; D, temporal lobe dura; TL, temporal lobe brain. (From Donald PJ. Surgery of the Skull Base. Philadelphia: Lippincott-Raven; 1998:301)

Fig. 5.80 Man with extensive adenoid cystic carcinoma of the ethmoid sinuses. Following slough of the pericranial flap the necrotic brain was removed and a radial forearm free flap placed. Flap seen through orbital socket.

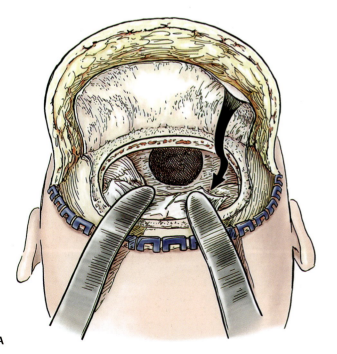

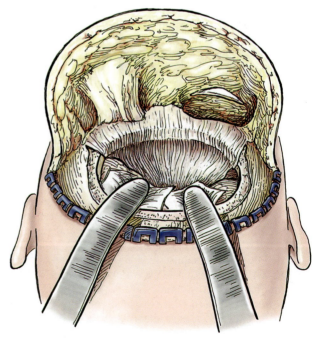

A

B

Fig. 5.81 (**A**) Pericranial flap is elevated at the time the scalp incision is made. (**B**) Flap is brought through the craniotomy defect, folded, and tucked to lie along the defect in the floor of the anterior cranial fossa.

nus carcinoma. Radiographic evidence of bone erosion on plane films was seen in 48% of patients. Most demonstrated anterior wall involvement, with only 17% showing posterior wall erosion. However, on exploration 75% of the patients in the entire group were found to have erosion of the back wall. Intracranial extension was found in 19%.

Although metastases were found in only 12% of cases, survival rates were miserable. This is probably due to the lack of experience of any one individual with this lesion. Because of the frequency of posterior wall penetration, a combined craniofacial excision should be employed. Both walls of the sinus, the dura, the adjacent superior sagittal sinus, and the frontal lobe, if necessary, should be removed. Removal of the adjacent ethmoid sinuses and orbital contents depends on the degree of involvement. If tumor has extended into the overlying skin, wide excision followed by coverage with a scalp flap must be done.

Reconstruction of the bony defect should be delayed 1 to 2 years to permit early discovery of local recurrences should they develop.

Sphenoid Sinus Carcinoma

Sphenoid sinus carcinoma is fortunately exceedingly rare. One of the largest, published series contains only seven patients.[38] Deep-seated head pain and ocular palsies are the most common presenting symptoms. The abducens nerve is most frequently affected because of its proximity to the lateral sphenoid sinus wall during its traverse through the cavernous sinus. The frequency of sixth nerve palsy in these patients illustrates the problem of extension of tumor beyond the confines of the sinus prior to diagnosis, rendering the tumor in most cases done in the past, inoperable and incurable.

Most tumors residing in the sphenoid are extensions from either the ethmoid labyrinth or the nasopharynx. Care must be taken in these instances not to assign an inoperable status to these patients prior to exploration. Obturation of the sphenoid sinus ostium will cause mucous accumulation and opacify the sinus on CT scan. T1 and T2 MRI imagery can usually make the distinction between tumor and fluid. Explora-

Case Reports

Case 1 (Fig. 5.82–5.87, pp. 255–256)

Mrs. R.A. was a 34-year-old woman who presented with a 3-year history of nasal obstruction and occasional nasal discharge. On physical examination she had a diffuse swelling over the right cheek, and her right nasal cavity was completely obstructed by a pink, fleshy, firm mass. A CT scan showed a mass in the right nasal cavity that extended into the right maxillary sinus, the ethmoid, and the frontal sinuses (**Fig. 5.82**). The lamina papyracea and the floor of the anterior cranial fossa were eroded. Tumor extended into the orbit, and MRI confirmed the presence of tumor in the sinuses and the invasion of the right globe. The tumor invading the anterior cranial fossa extended into the gyrus rectus of the frontal lobe (**Fig. 5.83**). Biopsy of the mass revealed a poorly differentiated fibrosarcoma.

She was taken to the operating room where a lateral rhinotomy and Denker resection of the maxilla was done (**Fig. 5.84**). Tumor was debulked from the maxilla, and only the medial maxillary wall and orbital floor were invaded by tumor. The orbit was exenterated, the ethmoid portion was debulked, and all of the ethmoid sinuses on that side were then removed, with the exception of the tumor extending through the eroded fovea ethmoidalis and the orbital roof (**Fig. 5.85**). The subcranial specimen was thus removed. A frontal craniotomy was done (**Fig. 5.86**) and the dura dissected to the point of obvious tumor involvement. The invaded dura was circumscribed and the portion of gyrus rectus with tumor extension was removed with a 3- to 5-mm margin of healthy brain.

The dura was closed with a flap of falx cerebri and a temporalis fascia graft. A pericranial flap was laid across the defect, a skin graft placed over the flap and onto the raw cheek surface and into the maxillary cavity. No adjunctive irradiation therapy was given.

The patient is alive and well without disease 15 years postoperatively (**Fig. 5.87**).

Discussion

Long-standing symptoms of nasal obstruction and rhinorrhea are not uncommonly dismissed by the family physician as innocuous symptoms, and these neoplasms of the paranasal sinuses often go unnoticed for many years. The findings of dural and especially brain invasion by malignancy originating in the head and neck have long been thought to be signs of inoperability and incurability.

In our series of over 185 operations for skull base tumors, the survival for those without dural involvement is better than those with the dura invaded by tumor, by a margin of ~19%. Those with brain involvement (25 cases) have a 27.61%, 5-year tumor-free survival rate.

Case 2 (Fig. 5.88–5.96, pp. 256–259)

Mrs. I.S. was a 65-year-old woman who presented with ulceration in the upper eyelid and ocular displacement in the inferior and lateral direction (**Fig. 5.88**). She complained of an 8-week history of diplopia and the appearance of a red turgid swelling over the right eye for 5 weeks. She had no past history of sinus disease.

On physical exam in addition to the above findings she had a mass in the right nasal cavity emanating from the middle meatus. A MRI revealed a large mass in the frontal sinus invading the orbit and the ethmoid sinuses with bone erosion and considerable extension into the anterior cranial fossa (**Fig. 5.89A**). MRI showed the invasion of the eye and the frontal lobe dura with questionable involvement of the brain (**Fig. 5.89B**). Biopsy showed squamous cell carcinoma.

A lateral rhinotomy incision in continuity with a wide field resection of the periocular skin and proposed orbital exenteration was done (**Fig. 5.90**). The lateral rhinotomy revealed some invasion of the superior maxilla, the eye, and the anterior ethmoid sinuses. An anterior craniotomy through a coronal scalp incision revealed widespread invasion of the frontal bone (**Fig. 5.91**), and when the cranial bone flap was removed, extensive invasion of the dura. Remarkably, the brain was uninvolved by malignancy, but much of the anterior aspect of the frontal dura, the falx, the inferior part of superior sagittal sinus, and a considerable amount of the anterior fossa floor dura required excision. A large graft of lyophilized cadaver dura was necessary to cover this defect (**Fig. 5.92**). The large pericranial flap, having lost one of its pedicles because of tumor infiltration, was pedicled on the vessels of the opposite side (**Fig. 5.93**). The cavity was lined with split-thickness skin grafts. The patient then underwent a full course of irradiation therapy.

The patient is now 16 years alive and without tumor recurrence (**Fig. 5.94**).

Discussion

It is remarkable what a strong barrier of resistance to tumor penetration is provided by the dura. The massive involvement of the anterior fossa dura in this case held the tumor at bay without invasion of the underlying brain. In the early postoperative period the patient lost much of the skin graft covering the pericranial flap (**Fig. 5.95**). Meticulous wound care allowed the dead skin to slough and the remaining epithelial islands as well as the adjacent mucosal remnants to resurface the raw area (**Fig. 5.96**). The pericranial flap was sufficient to support the brain and provide a sufficiently vascularized bed for reepithelialization.

Case 3 (Fig. 5.97 and 5.98, p. 259)

Mr. E.P. was a 58-year-old man with a 3-year history of nasal obstruction, purulent nasal drainage from the right side of his nose, and intermittent blood staining of the drainage. Over the 7 months prior to his admission he had the gradual onset of progressive forgetfulness, disorientation, and behavior characteristic of dementia. MRI revealed a massive intracranial tumor that produced marked deformation of the right frontal lobe and third ventricle (**Fig. 5.97**). There was a small extracranial component in the ethmoidal sinuses that represented ~10% of the total tumor volume. Biopsy of the mass in the nose revealed the diagnosis of sinonasal-undifferentiated carcinoma.

A low craniotomy including an orbital bar was done (**Fig. 5.98**). Extensive invasion of the frontal lobe dura was seen that at some sites invaded the underlying arachnoid. At the points where brain was invaded it was removed with a 5 mm margin of grossly healthy tissue. Adequacy of removal was monitored by frozen section. Tumor was dissected from the optic chiasm, the diaphragma sella, the interhemispheric fissure, and the hypothalamus. The subcranial portion was removed with little difficulty through a lateral rhinotomy.

The patient has made a full recovery, has had postoperative irradiation, and is 7 years postoperative with no signs of disease.

Discussion

The importance of the skull base team is exemplified by this case. The subcranial part of this tumor was small relative to the massive intracranial extension. The neurosurgical member of the team concluded that this patient was clearly operable. This case also illustrates how the dura and the arachnoid prevented the major potion of the tumor from invading the brain. The low anterior craniotomy provides excellent access to the anterior cranial fossa while minimizing brain retraction. Postoperative irradiation therapy is an essential component of the treatment.

Case 4 (Fig. 5.99–5.101, pp. 260–261)

Mr. E.W. was a 53-year-old postman who presented with a 10-month history of nasal stuffiness and purulent discharge that eventually progressed to complete nasal obstruction and anosmia. On examination an obvious tumor was present in the right nasal cavity. Repeated courses of antibiotics and saline nasal irrigations were without effect. CT scanning revealed a tumor in the ethmoidal sinuses with invasion of the superior part of the maxilla, the anterior cranial fossa, and the orbit as well as the optic nerve. Intranasal biopsy revealed adenoid cystic carcinoma.

A lateral rhinotomy, complete ethmoidectomy, and orbital exenteration were done leaving residual tumor on the orbital roof and fovea ethmoidalis to be removed under careful control via an anterior craniotomy (**Fig. 5.99**). Complete removal was then resected through the anterior fossa exposure. Perineural spread of tumor was seen on the optic nerve and was resected back to the level of the optic chiasm where a negative margin was obtained (**Fig. 5.100**). A pericranial flap was placed and the subcranial defect lined with split-thickness skin grafts. The patient then had a full course of irradiation therapy.

The patient is alive and free of disease 21 years postoperatively (**Fig. 5.101**).

Discussion

Perineural spread is a common method of tumor extension in adenoid cystic carcinoma. Fortunately, a negative margin was possible at the optic chiasm just short of the optic nerve of the opposite side. The patient has retained normal vision in the remaining eye and has remained tumor free to date.

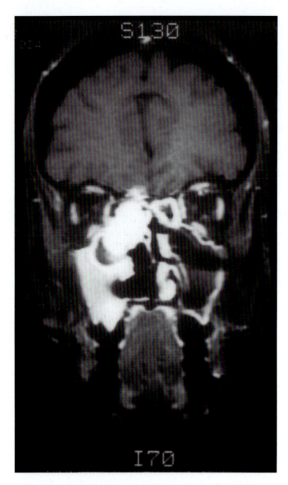

Fig. 5.82 *Case 1* Coronal section magnetic resonance imaging scan showing invasion of the lamina papyracea, ethmoid sinuses, and anterior fossa floor.

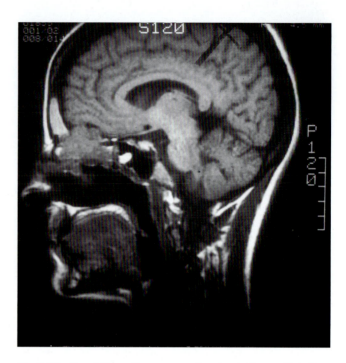

Fig. 5.83 *Case 1* Magnetic resonance imaging in the sagittal plane illustrating invasion of dura and encroachment on the frontal lobe of the brain.

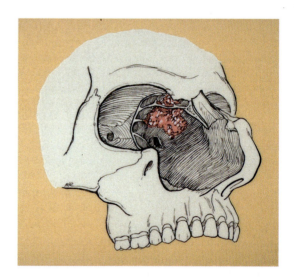

Fig. 5.84 *Case 1* Lateral rhinotomy and Denker procedure done.

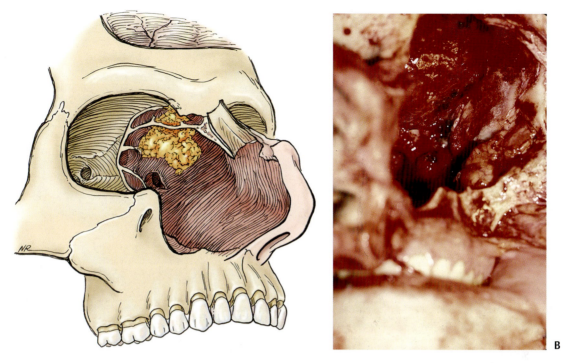

A

B

Fig. 5.85 *Case 1* All subcranial tumor is removed and the patient is ready for craniotomy. (**A**) Diagram showing residual tumor. (**B**) Residual tumor on anterior skull base.

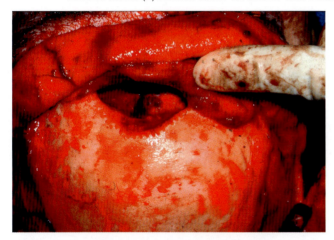

Fig. 5.86 *Case 1* Craniotomy done and tumor exposed.

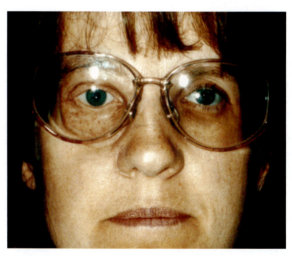

Fig. 5.87 *Case 1* Patient alive and well without disease at 10 years postoperatively.

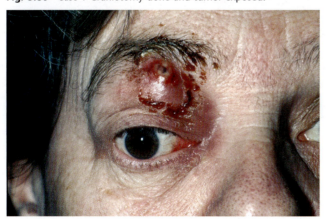

Fig. 5.88 *Case 2* Frontal sinus squamous cell carcinoma invading the upper eyelid.

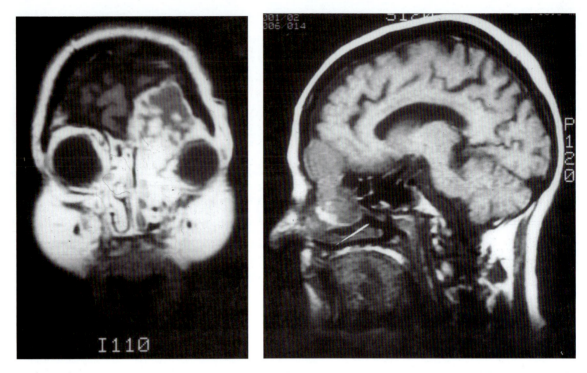

Fig. 5.89 *Case 2* Coronal-cut computed tomographic scan illustrating extensive bone erosion of the frontal calvarium and orbit with soft tissue extending into the orbit.

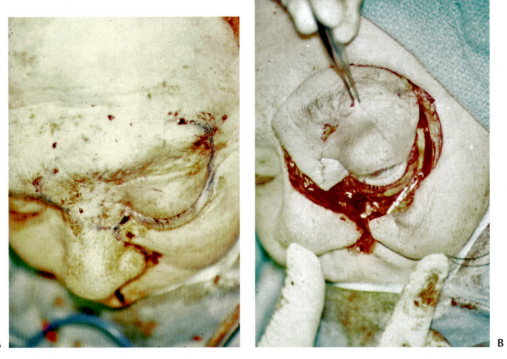

Fig. 5.90 *Case 2* Facial incision made. (**A**) Incision outlined. (**B**) Rhinotomy and periorbital incisions made.

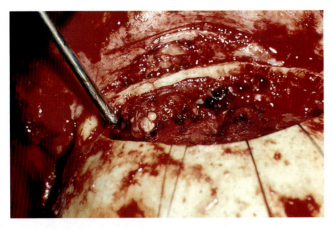

Fig. 5.91 *Case 2* Extensive tumor of the frontal and ethmoid sinuses extending into the anterior cranial fossa through the frontal calvarium.

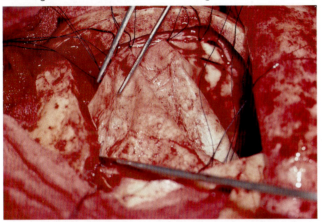

Fig. 5.92 *Case 2* Larger lyophilized dural graft required to replace extensive dural resection.

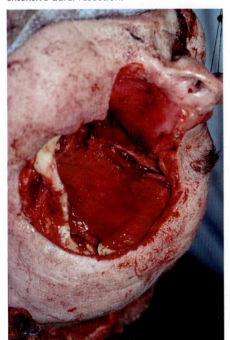

Fig. 5.93 *Case 2* Unipedicled pericranial flap in place.

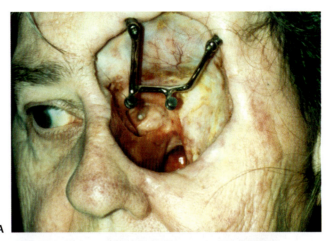

A

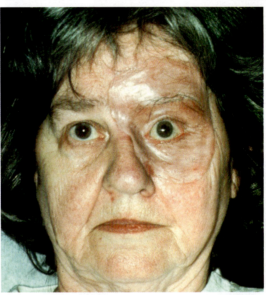

B

Fig. 5.94 *Case 2* Patient 2 years following surgery. She is now 10 years postoperative and free of disease. (**A**) Patient with operative site healed, Branemark implants and connecting framework in place, ready for attachment of prosthesis. (**B**) Prosthesis in place.

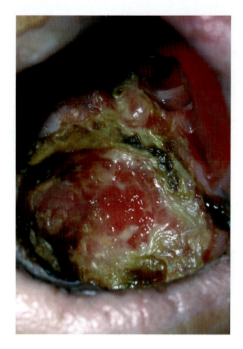

Fig. 5.95 *Case 2* Partial slough of split-thickness skin graft lining exenteration cavity.

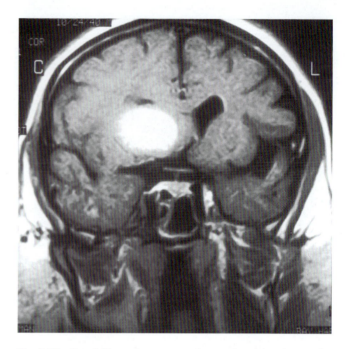

Fig. 5.97 *Case 3* Magnetic resonance images in axial and coronal planes. Sinonasal undifferentiated carcinoma with large intracranial component showing deformation of the third ventricle.

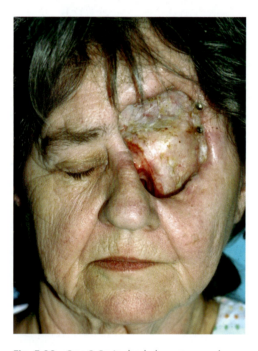

Fig. 5.96 *Case 2* Cavity healed spontaneously.

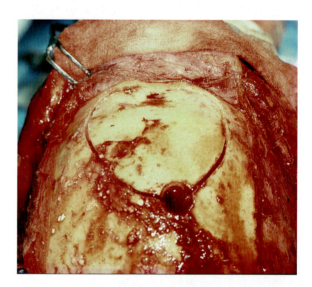

Fig. 5.98 *Case 3* Illustration of a low anterior craniotomy with removal of the superior orbital bandeau to give wide field access to the anterior cranial fossa while minimizing brain retraction.

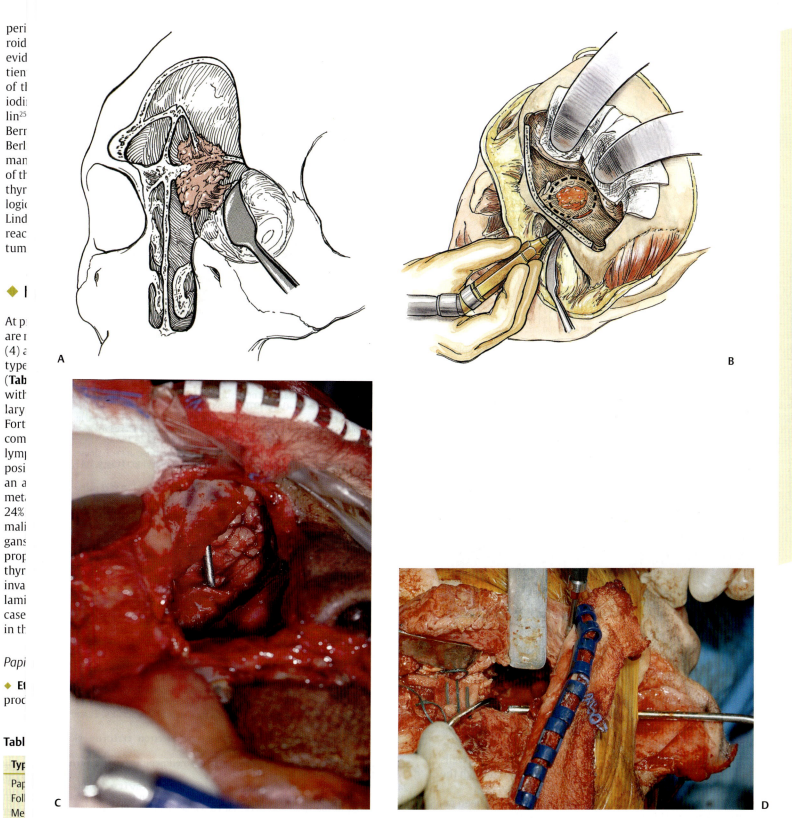

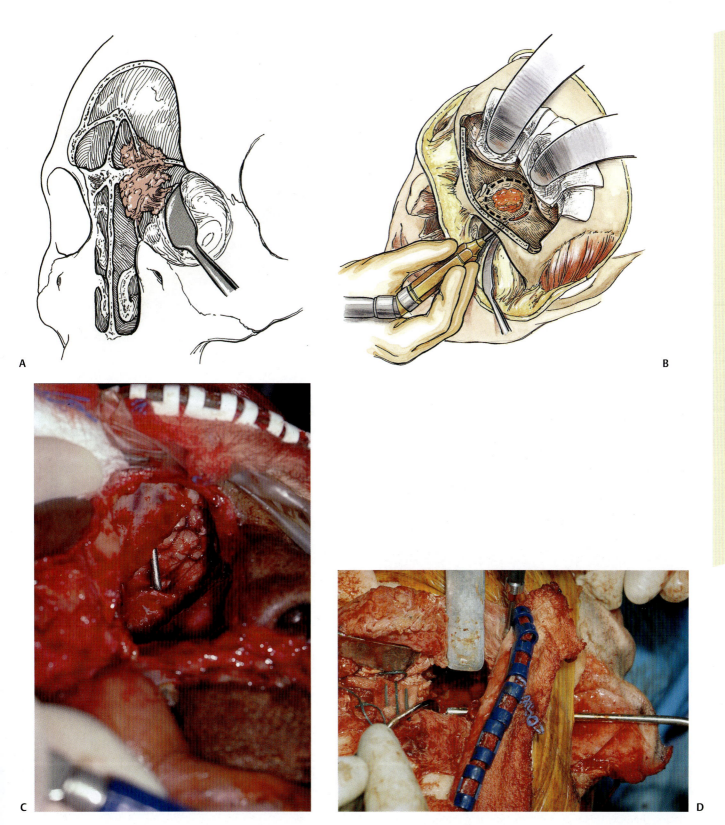

A

B

C

D

Fig. 5.99 *Case 4* Adenoid cystic carcinoma of the ethmoid sinuses with orbital invasion and intracranial presentation. (**A**) Diagram showing tumor extent. (**B**) Diagram showing subcranial resection with intracranial control. (**C**) Defect in anterior fossa seen from below. (**D**) Defect following resection seen from above.

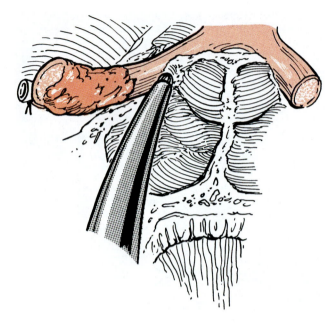

Fig. 5.100 Diagram showing tumor resection at the orbital apex and dissection back to the optic chiasm.

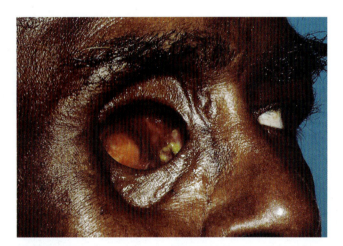

Fig. 5.101 *Case 4* Patient 7 years postoperative, currently 22 years without disease.

tion and delineation of tumor extent must be done, often as a staged procedure and commonly done endoscopically.

The floor of the sinus and sphenoid rostrum are the areas least frequently involved with tumor. Cancers commonly penetrate the sella turcica or extend through the lateral walls and roof of the sinus. Occasionally they protrude through the sinus ostium and present in the nose or nasopharynx.

Treatment of these malignancies has traditionally been radiation therapy. This region is remarkable in that it can withstand the rigors of more than one full course of irradiation. Only rarely is a patient cured; in sphenoid sinus carcinoma, radiotherapy is usually only palliative, with the patient succumbing to the disease 6 to 24 months later. Recent advances in craniofacial surgery may make many of these patients amenable to resection. A combined infratemporal fossa/middle fossa approach and a transfacial exposure will permit a clivectomy, cavernous sinus resection, and sphenoidectomy (see chapter 9).

References

1. Lang J. Clinical Anatomy of the Nose, Nasal Cavity and Paranasal Sinuses. New York: Thieme; 1989:121
2. Van Alyea OE. Nasal Sinuses. 2nd ed. Baltimore: Williams & Wilkins; 1951
3. Schaeffer JP. The Embryology, Development and Anatomy of the Nose, Paranasal Sinuses, Nasolacrimal Passageways and Olfactory Organ in Man. Philadelphia: Blakiston; 1920
4. Donald PJ. Frontal Sinus and Nasofrontal Ethmoidal Complex Fractures. Self Instructional Package #80400. Alexandria, VA: American Academy of Otolaryngology; 1980:12
5. Goss CM. Gray's Anatomy of the Human Body. 29th ed. Philadelphia: Lea & Febiger; 1975:741
6. Sisson GA, Becket SP. Cancer of the Nasal Cavity and Paranasal Sinuses. In: Suen JY, Myers EN, eds. Cancer of the Head and Neck. New York: Churchill Livingstone; 1981:242–279
7. Birt BD, Briant TD. The management of malignant tumors of the maxillary sinuses. Otolaryngol Clin North Am 1976;9:249–254
8. Jesse RH, Butler JJ, Healey JE Jr, et al. Paranasal sinuses and nasal cavity. In: MacComb WS, Fletcher GH, eds. Cancer of the Head and Neck. Baltimore: Williams & Wilkins; 1967:329–356
9. Conley J. Concepts in head and neck surgery. In: The Paranasal Sinuses. New York: Grune & Stratton; 1970:54–68
10. Batsakis JG. Cancer of the nasal cavity and the paranasal sinuses. In: Batsakis JG, ed. Tumors of the Head and Neck—Clinical and Pathological Considerations. Baltimore: Williams & Wilkins; 1974:112–122
11. Chandler JR, de la Cruz A, Pickard RE. Tumors of the nose and sinuses and their surgical treatment. In: English, GM, ed. Otolaryngology. Vol 3. Hagerstown, MD: Harper & Row; 1978:1–17
12. Vrabec DP. The inverted Schneiderian papilloma: a clinical and pathological study. Laryngoscope 1975;85:186–220
13. Batsakis JG. Neoplasms of the minor and "lesser" major salivary glands. In: Tumors of the Head and Neck—Clinical and Pathological Considerations. Baltimore: Williams & Wilkins; 1974:Chap. 2
14. Cohen MA, Batsakis JG. Oncocytic tumors (oncocytoma) of minor salivary glands. Arch Otolaryngol 1968;88:71–73
15. Batsakis JG. Mucous gland tumors of the nose and paranasal sinuses. Ann Otol Rhinol Laryngol 1970;79:557–562
16. Batsakis JG, Holtz F, Sueper RH. Adenocarcinoma of the nasal and paranasal cavities. Arch Otolaryngol 1963;77:625–633
17. Rafla S. Mucous gland tumors of paranasal sinuses. Cancer 1969;24:683–691
18. Manolidis S, Donald PJ. Malignant mucosal melanoma of the head and neck. Cancer 1997;80:1373–1386
19. Cantrell RW, Ghorayeb BY, Fitz-Hugh GS. Esthesioneuroblastoma: diagnosis and treatment. Ann Otol Rhinol Laryngol 1977;86:760–765
20. Mendeloff J. The olfactory neuroepithelial tumors. Cancer 1957;10:944–956
21. Obert GJ, Devine KD, McDonald JR. Olfactory neuroblastomas. Cancer 1960;13:205–215
22. Kahn LB. Esthesioneuroblastoma: a light and electron microscopic study. Hum Pathol 1974;5:364–371
23. Skolnik EM, Massari FS, Tenta LT. Olfactory neuroepithelioma. Arch Otolaryngol 1966;84:644–653
24. Ordoez BP, Huvos AG. Nonsquamous lesions of nasal cavity, paranasal sinuses, and nasopharynx. In: Gnepp DR, ed. Diagnostic Surgical Pathology of the Head and Neck. 1st ed. Philadelphia: WB Saunders; 2000:79–139
25. Harrison DF. The management of malignant tumors of the nasal sinuses. Otolaryngol Clin North Am 1971;4:159–177
26. Robin PE, Powell DJ. Diagnostic errors in cancers of the nasal cavity and paranasal sinuses. Arch Otolaryngol 1981;107:138–140
27. Dodd GD, Jing B-S. Radiology of the Nose, Paranasal Sinuses and Nasopharynx. Baltimore: Williams & Wilkins; 1977:215–276

28. Perry C, Levine PA, William BR, Cantrell RW. Preservation of the eye in paranasal sinus cancer. Arch Otolaryngol Head Neck Surg 1988; 114:632–634

29. Jackson K, Donald PJ, Gandoor-Edwards R. Pathophysiology of skull base malignancies. In: Donald PJ, ed. Surgery of the Skull Base. Philadelphia: Lippincott-Raven; 1998:51–72

30. Cheeseman AD. Non-healing granulomata and tumors of the nose and sinuses. In: Kerr A, MacKay IS, Bull TR, eds. Scott Brown's Otolaryngology. London: Butterworth-Heinemann Ltd, 5th rev. ed. Vol 4. 5th ed. 1987:308–311

31. Schramm VL. Anterior craniofacial resection. In: Jackson CG, ed. Surgery of Skull Base Tumors. New York: Churchill Livingstone; 1991:67–83

32. Donald PJ. Frontal Sinus Fractures. In: Donald PJ, Gluckman JL, Rice DH ed. The Sinuses. New York: Raven Press; 1995:369–399

33. Raveh J, Laedrach K, Iizuka T, Leibenger F. Subcranial extended approach for skull base tumors: surgical procedure and reconstruction. In: Donald PJ, ed. Surgery of the Skull Base. Philadelphia: Lippincott-Raven; 1998:239–261

34. Donald PJ. Complications. In: Donald PJ, ed. Surgery of the Skull Base. Philadelphia: Lippincott-Raven; 1998:585–597

35. Robinson JM. Frontal sinus cancer manifested as a frontal mucocele. Arch Otolaryngol 1975;101:718–721

36. Brunner H. Primary tumors of the frontal bone. Arch Otolaryngol 1953;57:158–172

37. Brownson RJ, Ogura JH. Primary carcinoma of the frontal sinus. Laryngoscope 1971;81:71–89

38. Van Wart CA, Dedo HH, McCoy EG. Carcinoma of the sphenoid sinus. Ann Otol Rhinol Laryngol 1973;82:318–322

39. Barnes L, Brandwein M, Som P. Diseases of the nasal cavity and paranasal sinuses and nasopharynx. Surgical Pathology of the Head and Neck. Barnes L, ed. 2nd ed. Vol 1. New York: Informa Healthcare; 2001; 10:439–556

40. Ketcham AS, Wilkins RH, Van Buren JM, Smith RR. A combined intracranial facial approach to the paranasal sinuses. Am J Surg 1963; 106:698–703

41. Ireland PE, Bryce DP: Carcinoma of the accessory nasal sinuses. Ann Otol Rhinol Laryngol 1966;75:698

42. Osborn DA, Winston P: Carcinoma of the paranasal sinuses. J Laryngol 1961;75:187

43. Frazell EL, Lewis JS: Cancer of the nasal cavity and accessory sinuses: a report of the management of 416 patients. Cancer 1963;16;1293

44. Tabah EJ: Cancer of the paranasal sinuses: a study of the results of various methods of treatment in fifty-four patients. Am J Surg 1962;104:741.

45. Conley J: Concepts in head and neck surgery. Georg Thime Verlag, Stuttgart, 1970;57

46. Lederman M: Cancer of the upper jaw and nasal chambers. Proc R Soc Med 1969;62:55

47. Lewis JS, Castro EB: Cancer of the nasal cavity and paranasal sinuses. J Laryngol 1972;86:255

48. Larsson LG, Martensson G: Carcinoma of the paranasal sinuses and the nasal cavities. Acta Radiol 1954;42:149

49. Boone ML, Harle TS, Higholt HW, Fletcher GH: Malignant disease of the paranasal sinuses and nasal cavity. Am J Roentgenol 1968;86:255

6

Cancer of the Thyroid and Parathyroids

Paul J. Donald

Nowhere in the considerations of head and neck cancer is there more controversy than over the management of thyroid malignancy. Part of the problem is the uncommonness of the disorder, depriving individual surgeons with the wealth of data in their own experience necessary for accurate decision making. In a public health survey conducted from 1969 to 1971, only 37 new cases of thyroid carcinoma per million population were reported each year.[1] According to the Armed Forces Institute of Pathology (AFIP) fascicle on thyroid tumors, the attack rate for most countries averages two to three cases per 100,000 population.[2] Another factor contributing to the therapeutic enigma is the protean behavior of these tumors. Autopsy studies reveal the incidence of occult thyroid malignancy to vary from 0.08 to 5.7% in individuals who were not suffering from any known history of thyroid disorder.[3,4] On the other hand, patients have been reported who suddenly developed and quickly succumbed to widespread papillary carcinoma, a disease that usually enjoys a benign reputation.[5–11]

◆ Incidence

Despite the relatively low incidence of thyroid cancer as already noted, it does seem to have increased in frequency over the years. Carroll et al[12] showed a twofold increase in the incidence of thyroid carcinoma from 1941 to 1962 in New York State. In an extensive review of the literature, Mazzaferri et al[13] allude to the increased incidence of the disease over roughly the same time period. Although part of this may be due to an improvement in diagnostic accuracy, the increased frequency has been mainly ascribed to the irradiation of the thymus so commonly done in the 1940s. This well-publicized relationship between cervical and mediastinal irradiation and thyroid malignancy is one of the best-promulgated pieces of public health information in modern experience. The findings of Favus et al,[14] who discovered a palpable thyroid mass in 16.5% of individuals with histories

of cervical or mediastinal irradiation, are frightening. In addition, they found an abnormal ^{131}I scan in 10.5% of those with a palpably normal gland. Of those who subsequently underwent thyroidectomy, 33% had carcinoma.

In an analysis of 576 cases of papillary carcinoma, Mazzaferri et al[13] found a female-to-male ratio of 16:1. More recent studies quoted in the AFIP fascicle state the ratio in the United States to be in the range of 2:1 to 3:1.[2] They found the peak age incidence to be in the third decade of life, with a rather constant female-to-male ratio throughout each age group. According to Sommers,[15] most children and adolescents with thyroid carcinoma have undergone prior irradiation. Becker et al[16] state that 50% of children with solitary thyroid nodules have cancer. Further evidence implicating radiation exposure in the genesis of thyroid cancer comes from the experience in the Chernobyl nuclear accident. An increase in the incidence of thyroid carcinoma was markedly apparent after only 4 years had passed following the accident where large amounts of I-131 and other short-lived radio-iodides were released into the atmosphere. The tumors were predominantly papillary carcinomas, and the majority were highly aggressive.[17–19] An exhaustive epidemiological review by Clark et al[20] revealed an extremely consistent female predilection for thyroid malignancy, with females generally outnumbering the males by a ratio of 2:1.

It is important to note here that a much higher frequency of overall thyroid disease is seen in females as compared with males, with Clark et al[20] reporting a ratio of 5:1. Moreover, the incidence of thyroid nodules is significantly higher in women than in men, and carcinoma is reputed to occur in 4 to 12% of patients with nodular disease.[21,22] The implication of other thyroid diseases in the genesis of carcinoma is undecided. Meissner and Adler[23] found five cases of carcinoma in 226 glands that were excised primarily for Graves disease. Olen and Klinck[24] found 53 cancers in 2000 excised hyperfunctioning glands. Of Mazzaferri et al's 576 patients with papillary carcinoma, 17 had Graves disease, and two others had hyperfunctioning nodules.[13] There is some experimental evidence in animals of malignant change in thyroid glands that have been made hyperplastic.[22] There is also evidence that endemic adenomatous goiter predisposes patients to thyroid tumors. Unfortunately, in many of the areas of the world where iodine-poor diets are not treated with iodine prophylaxis, good statistics are not available. Wegelin[25] showed a higher incidence of malignancy at autopsy in Berne (1.04%), where endemic goiter was common, than in Berlin (0.09%), where it was not. In the modern literature, many studies conflict and fail to show conclusive evidence of this association. Although a common association between thyroiditis and thyroid cancer has been observed, the etiologic significance of this remains obscure. Hirabayashi and Lindsay[26] propose that it represents the usual inflammatory reaction observed around most tumors, or the response to a tumor-elaborated antigen.

◆ Pathology

At present, four basic histological forms of thyroid carcinoma are recognized: (1) papillary, (2) follicular, (3) medullary, and (4) anaplastic or undifferentiated. The distribution of tumor types is reflected in Mazzaferri et al's[13] review of 714 cases (**Table 6.1**). The predominance of papillary carcinoma agrees with most other series of an incidence of ~65 to 90%. Papillary makes up almost all of the thyroid cancers in children.[2,17] Fortunately the more benign varieties are by far the most common. The thyroid can be the site of rare tumors such as lymphoma, teratoma, or sarcoma, and it may also be a depository of secondary carcinoma. In Mazzaferri et al's series, an additional three cases of lymphoma were found. Of 62 metastasizing tumors described by Silverberg and Vidone,[27] 24% had secondaries in the thyroid. Shimaoka et al[28] listed malignancies of the breast, lung, and kidney as common organs of origin. Malignant melanoma, because of its similar propensity to spread by blood, also frequently spreads to the thyroid.[29] The tendency of laryngeal carcinoma to directly invade the thyroid gland by direct penetration of the thyroid lamina is well known. In our experience we have had one case of squamous cell carcinoma that had its primary origin in the thyroid gland.

Papillary Carcinoma

◆ **Etiology** The most significant etiological factor in the production of papillary carcinoma is exposure to irradiation.

Table 6.1 Analysis of 714 Thyroid Cancers

Type	No.	Percentage
Papillary	585	81.9
Follicular	114	16.0
Medullary	9	1.3
Anaplastic	6	0.8

Source: Mazzaferri EL, Young RL, Oertel JE, et al. Papillary thyroid carcinoma: the impact of therapy in 576 patients. Medicine 1977;56:171. Reprinted with permission.

Usually there is a gap of 20 years between the exposure and manifestation of the tumor. In the Chernobyl experience, children under the age of 12 months had a much more rapid development of the tumor than older children or adults.[17] There is a reported association between certain genetic syndromes and papillary carcinoma, notably Gardener syndrome and Cowden syndrome.[30] The papillary carcinoma associated with Cowden syndrome has unusual cellular morphologies consisting of a cribriform pattern and solid spindle cell configurations. Rearrangements of the *ret* and *trk* oncogenes have also been implicated as mechanisms of the production of papillary carcinoma.[31]

◆ **Gross Appearance** Small tumors may appear as nothing more than a scar that is fibrotic or calcific in nature. Larger ones are generally well encapsulated, but the very large lesions usually show some evidence of invasion beyond the capsule. These larger varieties commonly have colloid-filled cysts that may be up to 4 cm in diameter (**Fig. 6.1**). The colloid material is usually thin, brown, and watery in consistency. Numerous papillae project into the cyst's lumina,[9] giving the epithelial surface the appearance of a shag rug. Calcification and even ossification may occur in the more heavily fibrosed areas of the tumor.

◆ **Microscopic Features** The tumors have both solid and cystic areas, the latter varying widely in size. The epithelium lining of the cysts is composed of a single layer of cuboidal amphophilic cells of rather uniform size. They project into the cyst lumina on a vascularized stalk in the form of many villus-like fronds (Fig. 6.2). The cells themselves have infrequent mitotic figures and no evidence of nuclear hyperchromatism or pleomorphism, the hallmarks of malignancy in other tissues.

The more dense areas have foci of fibrosis and calcific deposits. Calcified, laminated spherules called psammoma bodies (**Fig. 6.3**) are usually present. Nests of cells, some of which show evidence of squamous metaplasia complete with keratin pearl formation, may be seen. Some cells have nuclei that have a "ground-glass" appearance and appear devoid of nuclear material. This tissue as well as the nucleoli, are compressed against the inner surface of the nuclear membrane in the process of fixation. These so-called Orphan Annie cells are characteristic of papillary carcinoma. In some regions the cells form actual follicles. About 10% of papillary carcinomas are of the so-called tall cell variety. The tumor should be made up of over 30% tall cells to qualify as such. In these tumors usually 90% of the tumor cell population are tall cells. The cells are twice as tall as they are wide, and they have a distinctive pink, granular cytoplasm. These tumors are generally more aggressive and occur most commonly in the elderly.

Lymphatic invasion is common. In the AFIP series[2] of 226 papillary carcinomas, lymphatic invasion was seen in 75% of cases. Blood vessel invasion was much less common, being present in only 10%.

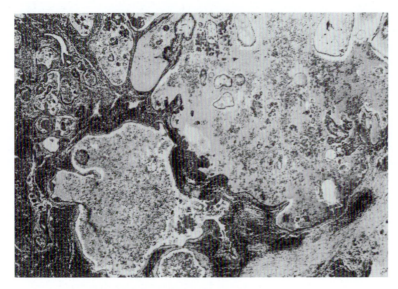

Fig. 6.1 Photomicrograph of large cyst in a papillary carcinoma of the thyroid (H&E, ×48). (From Meissner WA, Warren S. Tumors of the thyroid gland. Fascicle 4, Atlas of Tumor Pathology. 2nd ed. Washington, DC: Armed Forces Institute of Pathology; 1969:73. Reprinted with permission.)

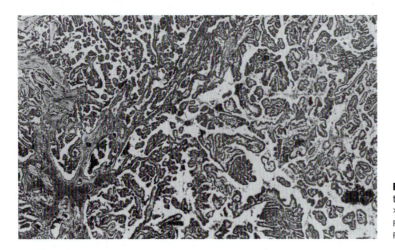

Fig. 6.2 Photomicrograph of a papillary carcinoma of the thyroid showing the many villous-like fronds of tumor (H&E, ×50). (From Meissner WA, Warren S. Tumors of the thyroid gland. Fascicle 4, Atlas of Tumor Pathology. 2nd ed. Washington, DC: Armed Forces Institute of Pathology; 1969:72. Reprinted with permission.)

The presence of multiple foci of tumor in any one gland is extremely common, having been noted in as many as 89 to 90% of cases in some series.[26] This may represent multiple spontaneous foci of disease or intraglandular metastasis. This finding has strongly dissuaded many surgeons from performing only lobectomy for papillary disease.

The differentiation of benign papillary adenoma from papillary carcinoma is made on the basis of invasiveness because the morphological characteristics of the cells are virtually indistinguishable. The presence in carcinoma of capsular and extracapsular invasion and the permeation of adjacent lymphatics or blood vessels are the prime histological differentiating features. Benign papillary adenomas are fortunately rare and are highly unlikely to be a precursor to malignancy. Psammoma bodies, although not a feature distinguishing a benign from a malignant tumor, are characteristic of papillary cancer and are exceedingly rare in normal thyroid tissue.[32,33]

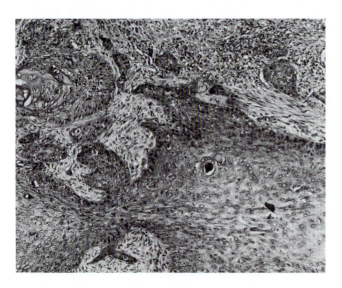

Fig. 6.3 Photomicrograph of papillary carcinoma of the thyroid, showing a psammoma body (H&E, ×100).

◆ **Pathophysiology** Papillary carcinoma is the most common and the most benign-behaving malignancy of the thy-

roid gland. Although early metastases to cervical lymph nodes are common, the progress of the disease is slow, with 5- to 10-year survival rates in the 90 to 95% range.[29] Even with distant metastases the progression is protracted.

One of the most common presentations of papillary adenocarcinoma is a lump in the neck. The misnomer "lateral aberrant thyroid" was applied in the past to papillary carcinoma metastatic to a lateral cervical lymph node, which was thought to arise as a mass of ectopic tissue. There are rare instances when small foci of normal-appearing thyroid follicles appear in a lymph node or even outside the nodal capsule.[34–36] However, for practical purposes, these should be considered as possible metastases, and a thorough investigation as well as careful continued observation should be made on such patients.

Normal thyroid tissue can be found anywhere along the track of migration of the thyroid gland in its embryological development. Because of the one-time proximity of the developing heart to the embryonic thyroid, portions of the gland may be found in the chest, mediastinum, aortic arch, and even the heart itself.[2] Normal thyroid tissue can be found occasionally in adjacent strap muscles and must not be misconstrued as cancer. Thyroglossal duct remnants are generally epithelium, normal thyroid tissue, or cyst. However, more than 30 cases of carcinoma have been reported originating in a thyroglossal duct remnant.[37]

The course of papillary cancer is slow, especially in children and young adults. The tumor is often present for a long time and reaches a considerable size before invading adjacent tissues. It is not uncommon to see large papillary tumors in patients who have no hoarseness, dysphagia, or vocal cord paralysis. In Mazzaferri et al's series,[13] contiguous structures were involved in only 4.7% of patients. However, patients over the age of 40 have a worse prognosis. In a series by Sedgwick and Bookwalter,[38] 270 cases were followed for a minimum of 10 years. The mortality rate for patients younger than 40 was 8% and for those older than 40 was 30%. Over 80% of the patients who died were over the age of 40 when first treated. An aggressive variant of papillary carcinoma is occasionally seen that does not follow the usual benign course that is commonly a feature of this disease. Both papillary and follicular varieties may assume this aggressive course. In the author's experience there have been patients with invasion of the larynx and trachea, including a young woman who had metastasis to 70 lymph nodes in the neck and mediastinum.

As mentioned, lymph node involvement is very common. In a series of 393 patients by Frazell and Foote,[39] 50% had cervical adenopathy and 11% had bilateral disease. In Mazzaferri et al's group there was cervical or mediastinal involvement in 46%.[13] The AFIP[2] study showed lymph node involvement in 76% of patients. Lymph node disease does not necessarily mean that blood vessel invasion has also taken place, and there are also cases in which distant metastases are present and cervical involvement is limited entirely to the gland.

The tall cell variant of papillary carcinoma is more aggressive with not only the lymph nodes involved with metastatic cancer but those of the mediastinum as well. The tumors are usually large when seen, and direct extension to adjacent structures is common. The prognosis is worse than the usual papillary carcinoma of the thyroid.

Follicular Carcinoma

◆ **Etiology** The second most common thyroid malignancy is follicular carcinoma. Some controversy surrounds the relationship of chronic dietary iodine deficiency and follicular carcinoma. In geographic areas in which the dietary source of iodine is deficient, follicular cancers make up 30 to 40% of all thyroid malignancies compared with 5 to 15% in iodine-rich areas.[40] Mutations of the *ras* gene have been found more commonly in both benign follicular adenomas and carcinomas in these iodine-poor areas.[41] There is much skepticism concerning the relationship of follicular cancer and multinodular goiter.

◆ **Gross Appearance** Follicular carcinoma tends to be of firmer consistency than the papillary variety, grayish-pink, gritty when cut, and tends to be solid all the way through. Often a central scar is present that may be calcified. Any cavitation is usually the result of infarction and subsequent liquefaction, but this is uncommon. Tumor tissue may invade surrounding structures and permeate lymphatics. The propensity of these tumors for blood vessel invasion is far greater than in papillary carcinoma and may even be obvious on gross examination.

◆ **Microscopic Features** The microscopic picture of follicular carcinoma is highly variable. Follicles containing colloid may be seen, and the overall picture closely resembles that of an adenoma (**Fig. 6.4**). The only clue to malignancy is capsular invasion or the invasion of a blood vessel or lymphatic channel. The great variation in follicle size among these tumors has fostered several subclassifications based upon this parameter, and indeed there appears to be some correlation between follicle size and prognosis. Small size or no follicle formation at all is associated with aggressiveness, invasiveness, and a poor prognosis.

Generally, there is little variation in cell size in any one tumor, and few or no mitotic figures are seen. Occasionally, the histological picture is one of packed follicular cells with no colloid formation and significant cellular pleomorphism. A cellular picture of mixed morphology is not uncommon. In an examination of 80 differentiated tumors by Russell et al,[29] a consistent follicular pattern was found in only 2.5%. A mixed papillary and follicular picture and even some areas of undifferentiated tumor are frequently seen. Some authorities feel that any tumor showing a mixed picture should be described as such, whereas others state that the tumor should be named according to its most predominant component. The behavior of these tumors generally corresponds to that of the most predominant cell type.

◆ **Pathophysiology** The slowly progressive character of papillary carcinoma is somewhat characteristic of the follicular form as well. However, because of the propensity of

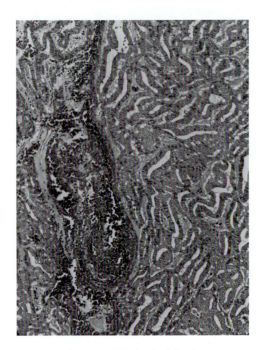

Fig. 6.4 Photomicrograph of a follicular carcinoma of the thyroid, showing vascular invasion (H&E, ×100).

follicular tumors for blood vessel invasion, bloodborne metastases are much more common. Follicular cancer is much more common in females and often appears to originate in an adenomatous goiter. A prolonged history of thyroid adenoma preceding the development of tumor is not uncommon. Most benign adenomas, however, remain as such. How and why a particular adenoma undergoes malignant transformation remains a total mystery.

Lymph node metastases are less common in follicular cancer than in the papillary variety. Although bloodborne secondaries are common, they may remain dormant for a considerable time before becoming symptomatic. In fact, histological confirmation of blood vessel invasion does not necessarily mean that there are distant metastases. In 34 cases of follicular cancer followed by Warren,[42] all of whom had histological evidence of vascular invasion, only 2% died of subsequent metastasis. The Hürthle cell variant of follicular carcinoma is distinguished by its characteristic oncocytic cells. Although oncocytic adenomas do exist some controversy surrounds their distinction from its malignant counterpart, with some authorities stating that all Hürthle cell tumors are malignant. The current thought is that the same criteria distinguishing a follicular adenoma from a carcinoma, namely capsular invasion or vascular spread, separate the oncocytic adenoma from oncocytic carcinoma. Lymph node metastasis are more frequent than in follicular carcinoma and the 5-year tumor-free survival rate is 50 to 60%.[43] Shaha et al[44] found the Hürthle cell variety of follicular carcinoma in 59 out of 228 patients (26%) in their series and found that it was one of the factors for an adverse prognosis in their series. They classified their patients into low, medium, and high risk. **Table 6.2** illustrates the prognosis at 10 and 20 years. Patients in the high-risk group were older than

Table 6.2 Ten- and 20-Year Survival Rate versus Risk Category in Follicular Carcinoma of the Thyroid

Risk Category	10-Year (%)	20-Year (%)
Low	98	97
Intermediate	88	87
High	56	49

Source: Shaha AR, Loree TR, Shah S. Prognostic factors and risk group analysis in follicular carcinoma of the thyroid. Surgery 1995;18:1131. Reprinted with permission.

45 years of age and had tumors greater than 4 cm in diameter, Hürthle cell histology, and distant metastasis. Gender and lymph nodal invasion had no prognostic significance.

Overall 10-year survival rates range from 34 to 68%.[45–47] In a series of 100 cases in which the cancer was limited to the thyroid gland itself, Beahrs and Pasternak[48] reported a 10-year survival rate of 90%. Meissner[23] and Warren[42] state that with extensive invasion the 5-year survival rate is around 50%. They further quote a collective series of the American Cancer Society that gives an overall 5-year survival rate of 64.7%.

Medullary Carcinoma

◆ **Etiology** Among thyroid cancers, the medullary variety is distinguished by several systemic peculiarities. The tumor has a strong familial tendency[49] and is associated with several other tumor states and endocrinopathies. Medullary carcinoma makes up ~5 to 10% of all thyroid malignancies. The tumor is a malignancy of the calcitonin-producing C cells. The tumors may occur spontaneously as a part of a genetic syndrome. The multiple endocrine neoplasia (MEN) syndromes of the type 2 variety are autosomal dominant syndromes that are responsible for the development of 75% of cases of medullary carcinoma. MEN2A is characterized by medullary carcinoma of the thyroid, pheochromocytoma, and parathyroid chief cell hyperplasia or adenoma. MEN2B is composed of medullary carcinoma, pheochromocytoma, multiple ocular and gastrointestinal ganglioneuromatosis, and skeletal abnormalities. A final familial disorder is seen that is manifest only by medullary carcinoma.[43]

In contrast to the sporadically appearing tumors the MEN type2 tumors tend to present in childhood or under the age of 20. These tumors are also usually bilateral compared with the unilaterality characteristic of the sporadic tumors.

Familial tumors are associated with a mutation of the ret gene, whereas some of the sporadic tumors tend to be associated with abnormalities at codon 918.[50] Boultwood et al[51] reviewed a series of 21 patients with medullary carcinoma searching for the levels of the *N-myc* and *C-myc* oncogenes. They found six of the patients had the *N-myc* gene and one had the *C-myc* gene, but none in C cells tested in normal patients without medullary cancer.

◆ **Gross Appearance** Medullary carcinoma is a hard, dense, solid tumor of gray-white coloration occasionally marked by hemorrhages. It varies in size from 1.5 to 10 cm. Unlike the differentiated malignancies, it is not generally well encapsulated and is locally infiltrative. One of its characteristic features is gross angioinvasion.

◆ **Microscopic Features** The tumor is composed of clusters or trabeculae of cells interspersed by a dense fibrotic stroma containing amyloid (**Fig. 6.5**). The cells are round or polyhedral but can be spindle shaped or assume the appearance of a follicular cell. The cytoplasm is eosinophilic and granular, and the nuclei are hyperchromatic. Some parenchymal cells are binucleate, and occasionally giant cells may be seen in reaction to the amyloid deposits. Mitoses may be present but are infrequent. There are no colloid-containing follicles, although some of the cells may assume a follicular pattern. The cellular arrangement may be a more palisaded trabecular configuration and may even resemble a carcinoid tumor.

The amyloid found in the hyaline stroma takes up most of the characterizing stains. Its ultrastructure reveals a composition of glycoproteins and acid mucopolysaccharides peculiar to primary and secondary amyloid deposits in other disease states. The material is commonly found in the metastases as well; however, medullary carcinoma does not result in generalized amyloidosis.

Calcium deposits are also found in the stroma, some of them resembling the psammoma bodies found in papillary carcinoma. Some plasma cells and lymphocytes are also seen. Blood vessel and lymphatic invasion is very common.

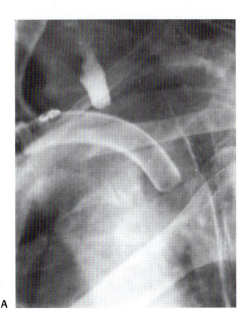

Fig. 6.5 Photomicrograph showing chords of irregular cuboidal cells with hyperchromatic nuclei in a fibrous stoma characteristic of medullary carcinoma of the thyroid. Tumor is interspersed with deposits of an amorphous material that will take up a stain specific for amyloid (H&E ×100).

◆ **Pathophysiology** This tumor is commonly seen in patients beyond the fourth decade of life. It is usually unifocal, with the remaining thyroid gland showing little reaction to it. As with the differentiated types, the course of medullary carcinoma is slow. Metastases to lymph nodes and the bloodstream are common. Over half the cases demonstrate cervical metastases on first presentation.

The tumors are also highly locally invasive, extending into the trachea and larynx. The pharynx and cervical esophagus may be constricted by retropharyngeal encroachment of tumor (**Fig. 6.6**). Death occurs as a result of distant blood metastases, lymph node involvement, and local extension. Beahrs and Pasternak[48] reported an 85% 10-year survival among 36 patients whose disease was confined to the thyroid gland on initial presentation. The survival rate dropped precipitously to 42% among 41 additional patients who presented with lymph node involvement. In Freeman and Lindsay's series of 33 patients, 39% died of their disease.[52] Hazard et al[53] reported a 30% mortality rate, and Williams et al[54] a rate of 33%, with most of the patients in both series being followed for at least 10 years.

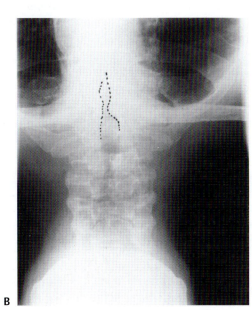

Fig. 6.6 (**A**) Barium swallow of an elderly patient with a longstanding medullary carcinoma of the thyroid. Note the tumor producing extensive pressure on the esophagus. (**B**) Soft tissue x-ray shows marked narrowing of trachea.

Thyroid adenomas and hyperplasia are more commonly seen with medullary carcinoma than with any other cell type. The production of thyrocalcitonin linking the cell of origin in medullary cancer to the parafollicular or C cell has already been alluded to. These patients may even present with the clinical picture of hyperparathyroidism. However, many patients with medullary thyroid cancer, even with the genetic syndrome, do not have hyperparathyroidism.

Medullary tumors have been known to elaborate an adrenocortical hormone in sufficiently high amounts to produce Cushing disease. Prostaglandins, serotonin, and histaminase have all been identified as secretory products of these neoplasms. The most consistent laboratory test for following patients with these tumors is the monitoring of thyrocalcitonin levels. Tumor production of this hormone can be stimulated by artificially inducing hypercalcemia by calcium infusions. Pentagastrin can stimulate calcitonin secretion as well, although not in all cases. Wells et al[55] used the pentagastrin stimulation test in several families with a genetic trait for medullary carcinoma. They operated upon four children who had elevated calcitonin levels on pentagastrin stimulation but palpably normal thyroid glands. They found the gland in each case to be riddled by multiple foci of medullary carcinoma.

Undifferentiated Carcinoma

◆ **Etiology** The incidence of undifferentiated carcinoma varies from one to 15%.[2,12] The average age of presentation is 60 to 65 years of age. It has an increased incidence in regions where endemic goiter is common. A preexisting enlarged or nodular gland is almost always present. It is a highly aggressive neoplasm with a poor prognosis.

◆ **Gross Appearance** The tumor is a typical cancer: firm, generally solid throughout, whitish in color, and without the usual cystic or hemorrhagic areas seen in the less malignant types. Local invasion into the opposite lobe and into adjacent structures is the rule.

◆ **Microscopic Features** The predominant histological type is either small cell or large cell. Differentiation between the two types is important in that the small cell type has a somewhat better prognosis. The small cell variety has two forms: compact and diffuse. The compact (**Fig. 6.7**) shows a plethora of small cells packed together in tight clusters with an intervening stroma similar to that found in medullary carcinoma. Mitotic figures are frequent, but pleomorphism is minimal. In both this and the large cell variety, occasional follicles may be seen. The diffuse type has the small cells loosely arranged without any clear organization. The appearance is very similar to a lymphoma. Blood vessel invasion in both types is exceedingly common.

The large cell type is composed of a wide variety of large, bizarre cells (**Fig. 6.8**). Marked pleomorphism, frequent mitoses (some of which are abnormal), and hyperchromatism of the nuclei are prominent features. The cells may resemble those of the strap cells of a rhabdomyosarcoma. Giant cell

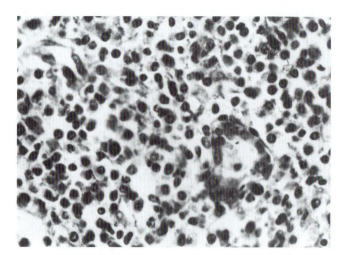

Fig. 6.7 Photomicrograph of a small cell variety of undifferentiated carcinoma of the thyroid. The monotonous cellular pattern is reminiscent of a lymphoma (H&E, ×1500). (From Meissner WA, Warren S. Tumors of the thyroid gland. Fascicle 4, Atlas of Tumor Pathology. 2nd ed. Washington, DC: Armed Forces Institute of Pathology; 1969:105. Reprinted with permission.)

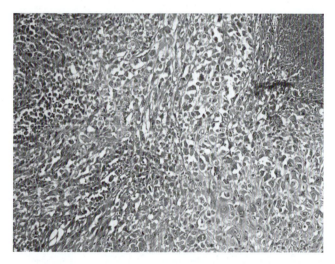

Fig. 6.8 Photomicrograph of a large cell type of undifferentiated carcinoma of the thyroid (H&E, ×100).

formation is also seen. The predominant large cell may be more spindle shaped and have a morphology strikingly similar to that of a fibrosarcoma (**Fig. 6.9**).

A mixed picture of small and large cells is not too uncommon, and foci of undifferentiated tumor in a papillary-follicular setting are also seen. It is possible that the undifferentiated variety may be a further degenerative step in the gradual progression of malignancy in a neoplasm that may even have originated as an adenoma.

◆ **Pathophysiology** Rapid lymph- and bloodborne metastasis and early progressive local invasion are the hallmarks

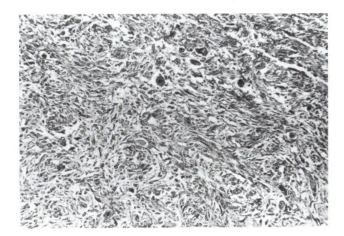

Fig. 6.9 Photomicrograph of a large cell type of undifferentiated carcinoma of the thyroid wherein the predominant morphology is a spindle-shaped cell (H&E, ×100). (From Meissner WA, Warren S. Tumors of the thyroid gland. Fascicle 4, Atlas of Tumor Pathology. 2nd ed. Washington, DC: Armed Forces Institute of Pathology; 1969:107. Reprinted with permission.)

Table 6.3 Factors Favoring Malignancy or Benignity of Solitary Thyroid Nodule

Factors	Benign	Malignant
History		
Age	20–40	<20; >40
Sex	Female	Male
Previous irradiation	No	Yes
Dysphagia	No	Yes
Hoarseness	No	Yes
Airway obstruction	No	Yes
Physical examination		
Mass consistency	Firm; cystic	Stony-hard
Extra thyroid mass	No	Yes
Vocal cord paralysis	No	Yes
Fixation	No	Yes
Pain and tenderness	Yes	No
Hyperthyroidism	Yes	No
Investigation		
^{131}I scan	Hot or warm	Cold
Ultrasound	Cyst	No cyst

of this extremely aggressive cancer. In a large series of 160 patients reported by Woolner et al,[56] 50% died within 5 months, and most by 3 years. Only four of the original 160 patients were alive after 5 years. In a review of 84 cases by Aldinger et al,[57] the mean survival time following diagnosis was 6.2 months and the 5-year survival rate was 7.1%.

At a symposium on the management of thyroid cancer at the annual meeting of the American Academy of Otolaryngology in 1980,[58] there was universal pessimism expressed by the panelists regarding the fate of victims of this disease. Early, aggressive surgery coupled with external irradiation may be the only possible means of salvaging any afflicted patients. Unfortunately, even the most radical local attack on these tumors is usually doomed to failure because of distant metastases.

◆ The Solitary Nodule

Management of the solitary thyroid nodule is a conundrum whose precise solution has evaded medical practitioners for decades. An overwhelming number of erudite dissertations, flow sheets, and algorithms have been put forth in attempts to clarify this dilemma. Opinions have varied over the years from the philosophy of test, wait, and watch to recommendations for surgical excision of most or all of these nodules. From a general statistical standpoint, there are certain clinical and investigative factors that tend to sway the opinion toward either watchful waiting or surgical excision. However, each individual patient independent of the balancing of these factors can harbor a malignancy in the thyroid gland.

Table 6.3 shows the various clinical and investigative factors that favor either malignancy or benignity. Although such information can serve as an aid in decision making, it will become clear from the following discussion that what, for example, appears to be a perfectly benign lump in a fe-

male patient in a favorable age group, with an encouraging-looking scan, can indeed be malignant.

Diagnostic Factors

◆ **Age** A mass in the thyroid gland of a child must be assumed to be malignant. Although these patients most often present with cervical adenopathy and even distant metastases, the course of the disease is usually markedly protracted. Patients often survive for 20 years or longer after the diagnosis is made before succumbing to the disease.

A relatively equal distribution of case incidence is present from the second to the fourth decade. In patients over the age of 60, the incidence of carcinoma in a nodule is much higher and tends to be of the more malignant variety.[59] Cutler and Mustacchi[60] observed that, although the incidence of papillary carcinoma changes little with increasing age, the other histological varieties occur more frequently in the older age groups. This is especially relevant in that thyroid masses are relatively common in the elderly.

◆ **Sex** Thyroid nodules are much more common in females. Although they outnumber males in the incidence of malignant masses, the frequency of benign lumps is much higher in women than in men. The inference, therefore, is that a thyroid nodule in a male is much more likely to be cancerous than one in a woman.

◆ **Prior Irradiation** The widespread irradiation of infants for the prophylaxis of sudden infant death syndrome due to "status thymus lymphaticus" is well-known history. The use of ionizing irradiation for the treatment of acne was also popular years ago. A thyroid nodule in an individual with such a history carries with it some ominous statistics, with as many as one third of these patients harboring thyroid carcinoma.

Numerous studies have indicated that as many as 80% of all patients with thyroid carcinoma may have had prior irradiation.[61] A large study by Raventos and Winship[62] of 528 patients revealed an average latent period of 10.9 years between exposure to irradiation and subsequent diagnosis of disease. The data from the Chernobyl experience have already been mentioned.

Such statistics make it clear that a history of prior cervical irradiation in a patient with a thyroid mass is one of the strongest indications for excisional biopsy.

Symptoms

Symptoms related to a thyroid mass may develop either from compression caused by the mass or from its invasion of other structures. Adenomatous goiters and individual adenomas may reach substantial size (**Fig. 6.10**) and by pressure alone cause dysphagia, dyspnea, and stridor. Retrosternal adenomas are especially infamous for this because of their con-

finement in the upper thoracic cavity. However, most benign processes do not cause such symptoms, and complaints of dysphagia, hoarseness, or airway obstruction strongly suggest malignancy.

Hoarseness is usually secondary to invasion of one or both recurrent laryngeal nerves. It is, however, remarkable how much involvement can be tolerated without actual paralysis.

Signs

Although Graves disease is seen occasionally with carcinoma, a thyroid nodule in a hyperthyroid patient is usually a toxic nodular goiter. In a study of 150 cases of thyroid cancer, Fitzgerald[63] could not find one tumor that would concentrate radioiodine more than a normal gland. As already mentioned, however, Meissner and Adler[23] found five carcinomas in glands from 226 patients who had Graves disease.

Pain and tenderness are most often seen in viral thyroiditis and the early stages of Hashimoto thyroiditis. The presence of circulating antithyroid antibodies is not helpful in ruling out carcinoma. Malignancy may coexist with both of these states.

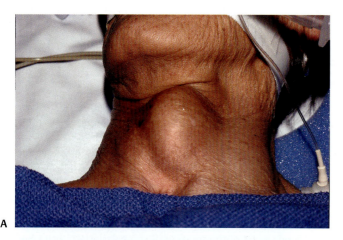

A

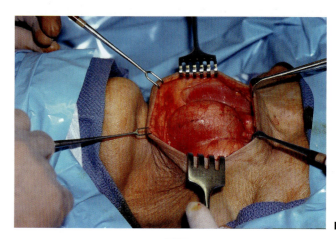

B

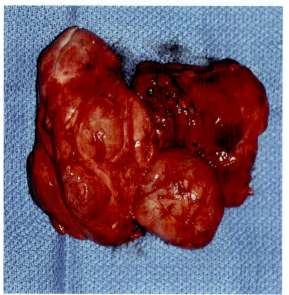

C

Fig. 6.10 (**A**) Elderly man with symptoms of dysphagia, stridor, and airway distress and a large adenomatous goiter. (**B**) Large adenoma at time of surgical removal. (**C**) Pathological specimen.

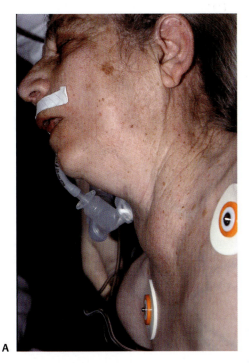

A

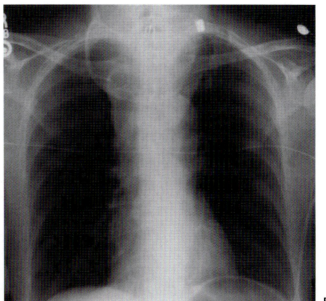

B

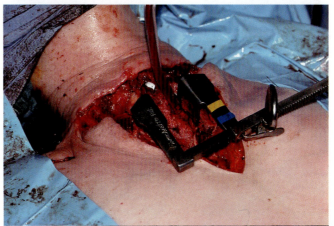

C

Fig. 6.11 (**A**) Elderly woman who presented with a 6-month history of a fairly rapidly enlarging neck mass that was stony hard. She had severe dysphagia, severe dyspnea, and stridor requiring emergency tracheostomy. (**B**) Chest x-ray following emergency tracheostomy, showing mediastinal widening secondary to tumor. (**C**) Intraoperative photograph of mediastinotomy illustrating a relatively avascular, hard, stony tumor. Signs and symptoms were strongly suggestive of undifferentiated carcinoma of the thyroid. Diagnosis was desmoid tumor of the neck and mediastinum.

The actual consistency of the mass is often difficult to discern because of the overlying soft tissue. A stony-hard mass definitely suggests carcinoma, as does fixation to, or infiltration of, surrounding structures (**Fig. 6.11**). On the other hand, a fluctuant cyst or softish mass is much more suggestive of a benign process (**Fig. 6.12**).

Vocal cord paralysis or a palpable mass elsewhere in the neck strongly indicates malignant disease, and the presence of a thyroid mass together with vocal cord paralysis is almost always an indication for surgery. A benign process almost never causes paralysis. One must bear in mind, however, the possibility of idiopathic paralysis coexisting with a benign adenoma. Conversely, the absence of paralysis in the presence of even a large tumor does not rule out carcinoma.

A palpable mass elsewhere in the neck raises alarm because of the high probability of metastasis. However, an incident in the author's experience might serve as a warning against overzealous treatment in some of these cases. A middle-aged

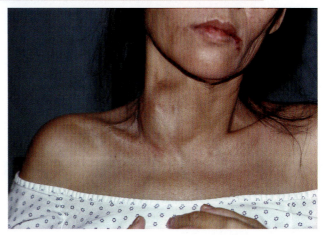

Fig. 6.12 A middle-aged Laotian woman with a large cystic mass in the neck. The scar marks the site of previous incisions and drainage; one was done in her native village with a hot umbrella spoke. In the wall of the cyst was a thyroid carcinoma.

woman with a hard thyroid mass and a 2 cm firm neck node was explored with a plan of node biopsy and lobectomy, to be followed by definitive surgical therapy based upon the pathological findings at frozen section. The neck node revealed microscopic foci of amorphous material resembling amyloid and dense fibrous tissue but no definitely identifiable cells of thyroid origin. The pathologist suggested a diagnosis of medullary carcinoma. Thyroid lobectomy produced a frozen section diagnosis that was equivocal. The neck was closed with plans for reexploration when a definitive diagnosis of cancer was established. Paraffin sections with Congo red stains subsequently established the amorphous deposits as hyaline in a lymph node, representing end-stage chronic inflammation, and the thyroid tumor was a follicular adenoma with densely packed cells.

Laboratory Investigations

◆ **131I Scan** One of the most useful differentiating tests for diagnosing a thyroid mass is the ^{131}I scan. By analyzing the pattern of the gamma emissions emanating from the radioactive iodide trapped by the gland, nodules can be portrayed. They are classified according to ^{131}I uptake as "hot" or "cold." The hot, hyperfunctioning nodule is generally considered to be benign, although a few isolated instances of malignancy have been found in hot nodules.[64–66] A hot nodule, moreover, may screen and obscure a cold area adjacent to it. Carcinomas generally tend to be autonomous, and their radioactive iodine uptake is not influenced by the administration of exogenous thyroid. The lack of depression of ^{131}I following administration of triiodothyronine and the failure of the thyrotropin-releasing hormone test both demonstrate this autonomy.

Normal or irregular functioning is not an uncommon finding in differentiated carcinomas. In Fitzgerald's autoradiography experiment on 150 cancers, 40 of the tumors were shown to contain organified iodine. The use of ^{131}I as a means of therapy for papillary and follicular carcinoma, as well as its combination with TSH stimulation to elevate its uptake by the tumor, illustrates the frequency of function and coexistent malignancy in a nodule.

The cold nodule may be a cyst, a tumor of other than thyroid origin, or a carcinoma. Approximately 10 to 20% of cold nodules are determined to be carcinomatous. **Table 6.4** compares the various radioisotope uptake findings in benign and malignant nodules. It is somewhat disheartening to see the

similarity of isotope findings between the two groups. However, a solitary solid cold nodule should be generally considered to be carcinoma until proved otherwise.

◆ **Ultrasonography** The differentiation of a solid from a cystic cold nodule can be made with 90% accuracy with the B mode ultrasound scanner. Although cyst formation is a feature of both papillary and follicular lesions, these cysts are small. Furthermore, the probability of the residual solid tissue in a predominantly cystic lesion being carcinomatous is slight, For example, if the entire lesion measures less than 3 cm in size, the chance of it being malignant is only 2%.[58]

Fine-Needle Aspiration Cytology

Thyroid carcinoma is often difficult to diagnose histologically. The principle problem is the differentiation of benign papillary and follicular adenomas from their malignant counterparts. As is obvious from the discussion earlier in the chapter, the major differentiating histological features are not based on cellular morphology; rather, a diagnosis of malignancy is made on the basis of capsular, blood vessel, or lymphatic invasion. This information is difficult to extract from material procured by needle biopsy. Furthermore, the stromal component of medullary carcinoma strongly resembles the fibrosis of some of the inflammatory disorders. Small-cell anaplastic carcinoma closely resembles lymphoma, and large-cell anaplastic tumors may resemble sarcoma.

Some pathologists have acquired considerable skill in the interpretation of fine-needle aspiration (FNA) cytology. Because of the relative rarity of thyroid cancer, it is difficult for most pathologists to acquire the degree of experience required unless they undergo special training. This is especially true when the FNA shows "normal follicular cells."

Open biopsy remains the surest method of establishing the diagnosis of the suspicious thyroid nodule.

◆ Surgical Management

The cornerstone of treatment of thyroid carcinoma is surgery. Papillary carcinoma is not only the most common malignancy but also the most controversial in terms of surgical management. Opinions vary from lobectomy through lobectomy-isthmusectomy to total thyroidectomy. Because of the frequency of bilateral involvement with these tumors, total thyroidectomy with parathyroid preservation is probably the safest procedure. If total thyroidectomy devascularizes the parathyroid glands, then one gland is removed, carefully diced, and implanted in the antecubital fossa of the arm. However, any tumor involvement of these glands militates against their preservation. Similarly, in the author's opinion, direct infiltration of the recurrent laryngeal nerves demands that they be sacrificed.

The management of the cervical lymph nodes in differentiated thyroid cancer remains somewhat controversial. In the absence of manifest nodal disease the lymph nodes of the central compartment of the neck adjacent to the thyroid gland and in the upper mediastinum should be removed

Table 6.4 Findings in Radioactive [131]I Scans in Two Major Groups*

	Normal Nodule (%)	Hot Nodule (%)	Cool Nodule (%)	Cold Nodule (%)	Multiple Nodule (%)
Colloid Nodule	23.07	3.6	12.07	58	3.6
Carcinoma	22.0	3.7	11.0	63.0	0.0

Source: Data from Hoffman GL, Thompson NW, Heffron C. The solitary thyroid nodule. Arch Surg 1972;105(2):379–385.

along with the affected thyroid. Metastases are more commonly seen in papillary than in follicular tumors. If lateral neck secondaries are present then the nodal chain in the vicinity of the involved node is taken in addition. In some individuals extensive neck disease is seen with nodes attached to the internal jugular vein and sternocleidomastoid muscle. A radical or modified radical neck dissection will be required in these atypical cases.

In medullary carcinoma metastatic disease is common. A radical or modified radical neck dissection is usually performed. Similarly, in undifferentiated carcinoma, especially of the large cell type, a modified or radical neck dissection is done.

Residual disease and distant metastases can be effectively managed for a considerable time by the administration of [131]I. In Mazzaferri et al's series, in which 116 patients were treated, ^{131}I in total doses ranging from 50 to 800 mCi was given.[13] The dose was less than 200 mCi in 87% of the patients and less than 300 mCi in 90%. Following surgical and medical therapy, 44.8% of these patients had no demonstrable ^{131}I uptake. However, in 70 individuals, representing 12.2% of the entire group of 504 patients who were judged to be free of disease at the cessation of their initial therapy, the disease recurred. The recurrences were treated by revision therapy, and half of the patients in this group were given ^{131}I in addition. Four of the eight patients with distant disease eventually died. During their prolonged period of observation, 19 patients died. Of these, seven who had persistent tumor died of other causes and five died as a direct result of the carcinoma. Given these statistics, a more conservative approach to surgical management with adjunctive ^{131}I administration would appear to be an effective therapeutic combination.

Follicular carcinoma requires slightly more aggressive management because of its increased invasive potential. Lymph nodal metastasis in follicular carcinoma, in my experience, is relatively uncommon. However, Tollefson et al[68] reported an overall 49% incidence of neck secondaries in follicular carcinoma, 28% of which were manifest and 21% were occult.

On the other hand, Pomorski and Bortos[69] reviewed their experience with 975 patients with thyroid carcinoma, and lymph node metastasis was the first sign of cancer in only 1.6% of their cases of follicular carcinoma. The efficacy of conservation neck dissection in the management of follicular carcinoma is yet to be proved.[70] An important deterrent factor to the conservation procedure is the incidence of recurrent neck disease following thyroidectomy *without* neck dissection, with Black et al[71] noting a 22% recurrence rate in necks thus treated. Witte et al,[72] in their meta-analysis from 35 studies taken from a review of 2186 articles in the literature on the subject, found that the presence of neck metastasis was a negative influence at a rate of 7.62/4.0 compared with papillary at a rate of 3.25/2.97 for 5- and 10-year survival. In Shaha's series[44] neck metastasis had no overall influence on survival. Adjunctive ^{131}I therapy is still effective because of the propensity of most follicular tumors to trap and organify the isotope. Most tumors can be safely excised without having to remove adjacent laryngeal or tracheal skeletal elements. Only when there is direct invasion of these

structures need there be any resection, and then it should be of a limited nature.

Medullary carcinoma is highly invasive locally and often accompanied by cervical lymphadenopathy. In a study of 40 such cancers by Gordon et al,[73] 67% of those who had a radical neck dissection survived 5 years. However, a 43% survival rate was seen in those whose necks were not dissected. Occult adenopathy was present in 70% of the latter group; ^{131}I is almost never taken up by the tumor and is of little value in the management of this disease. Despite the optimism of some,[73] external beam irradiation has marginal efficacy in medullary cancer.

Undifferentiated carcinoma has a dismal prognosis. The only possibility for cure may be with an aggressive combination of surgery and external beam irradiation. Millburn and Ameen[74] report cure rates of between 25 and 35% in totally unresectable disease with external irradiation alone, but few therapists share their enthusiasm. The experience of Crile and Hawk,[75] who had only one survivor among 24 patients treated by surgery or surgery and radiotherapy, is more the rule.

Problems arise regarding radicalism of surgery and determination of prognosis when areas of poor differentiation and frank anaplasia occur within an otherwise well-differentiated follicular or papillary carcinoma. Generally, if disease is confined to the gland and the areas of poor differentiation are small, the characteristic highly aggressive behavior pathognomonic of anaplastic or poorly differentiated malignancy is not seen. The distinction between different histological types of poorly differentiated carcinoma and anaplastic carcinoma appear to be important in that the prognosis for anaplastic cancer is extremely poor, whereas that for the poorly differentiated types is better. The pathological concept of insular carcinoma[76] characterized by islands of round and oval cells surrounded by a capsule of fibrous connective tissue is interesting. They are usually seen in older patients, most commonly female, and are often larger than 5 cm in diameter. The tumor comprises up to 4% of thyroid cancers in central Italy and is even more common in Paraguay,[76–78] but it is extremely rare in the United States. The prognosis is generally poor; for example, in Carcangui et al's[79] series of 25 patients, 14 were dead of disease, and seven were alive with persistent disease at last follow-up. Both anaplastic tumors have been classified as squamoid, spindle cell, and giant cell.[80] The squamoid type have the appearance of a nonkeratinizing squamous cell carcinoma, the spindle cell variety a sarcomatous appearance, and the giant cell type is composed of highly pleomorphic cells with multinucleated giant cells.

Thyroidectomy

Because the standard procedure is well described in other texts,[81–83] only points of importance in the resection will be stressed. Once the diagnosis of cancer is made, total extracapsular thyroidectomy is always performed because of the frequency of bilateral disease. A neck dissection of level 6 (the so-called central compartment of lymph nodes in the juxtathyroid area) is always done in differentiated carcinoma even when there is no palpable adenopathy.

With the patient's neck hyperextended due to the midline shoulder bolster, the nodes of the upper mediastinum are easily dissectible in the lower neck. In these tumors, any other palpable lymph nodes are removed with a small surrounding area of connective tissue. Any structures that are invaded by tumor, such as the sternomastoid muscle or internal jugular vein, should be removed. A "node plucking" or limited neck dissection is usually done; modified radical and radical neck dissections are rarely necessary.

In medullary and poorly differentiated carcinoma of the thyroid a modified radical or radical neck dissection is usually done because of the high incidence of manifest and occult disease. In anaplastic tumors a more conservative neck dissection may be done because of the poor prognosis. However, it is far better for the patient to succumb to distant metastasis than to die of local disease coming through the neck.

Incision

A "collar-type" incision is made in a crease line in the neck at the level of the inferior border of the cricoid cartilage (**Fig. 6.13**), ~2.5 to 3 cm above the sternal notch. The skin incision extends about midway across the width of the sternocleidomastoid muscle on each side. The incision is carried through the platysma, exposing the superficial layer of deep cervical fascia investing the strap muscles. If a neck dissection is to be done, the "collar" incision is continued to a point 2 cm anterior to the trapezius muscle, where it is joined by a vertical incision made from the mastoid tip to the clavicle, forming a type of "half-H" incision.

Flaps are developed through this avascular plane superiorly to the level of the hyoid bone and inferiorly to the level of the sternum. The incision is propped open with self-retaining retractors.

◆ **Strap Muscles**   The fascia over the midline is incised to reveal the thyroid perichondrium, that of the cricoid, and the isthmus of the thyroid. The strap muscles are thus separated in the midline and dissected laterally. If the tumor is stuck to the strap muscles, they are excised en bloc with the tumor. However, if the neoplasm is restricted to the gland, the straps are retracted laterally. If the tumor is exceptionally large and strap muscle retraction is inadequate for exposure then the strap muscles are detached from the hyoid bone. Incision of the straps at their insertion into the hyoid, followed by dissection inferiorly, will preserve the blood and nerve supplies that enter the muscles inferiorly (**Fig. 6.14**). This facilitates dissection of the tumor and is probably the safest and most expedient method of exposure in very large tumors. The thyroid lobe on the tumor side is thus exposed.

◆ **Recurrent Laryngeal Nerve**   In the catalogue of head and neck procedures, thyroidectomy is one of the easier to perform. The principal factor that makes it difficult is the proximity of the recurrent laryngeal nerve. There is little doubt that careful dissection of the nerve and direct visualization are the surest means of its preservation.

Although it is classically described as occupying the triangle formed by the trachea and esophagus medially, the carotid

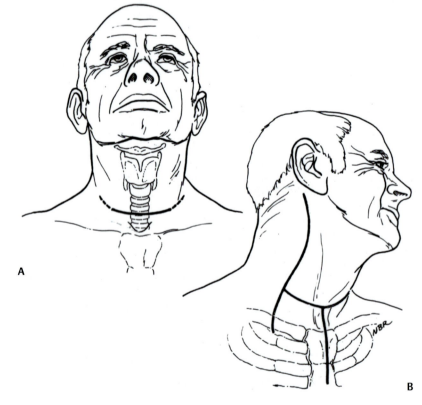

A

B

Fig. 6.13 (**A**) Standard thyroidectomy "collar-type" incision. (**B**) Skin incision extending from the collar incision to accommodate the sternal split necessary to dissect thyroid tumor from the mediastinum.

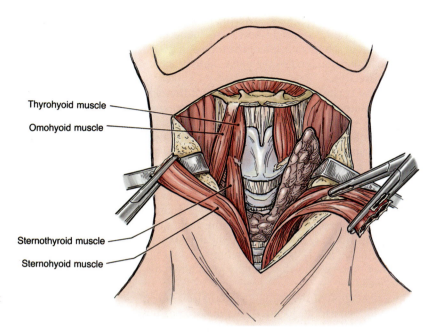

Thyrohyoid muscle

Omohyoid muscle

Sternothyroid muscle

Sternohyoid muscle

Fig. 6.14 The strap muscles on the side of the tumor are cut from the hyoid bone, with care taken to preserve the nerve and blood supply that is located inferiorly. Interference with either may cause disfiguring atrophy and fibrosis.

laterally, and the lobe of the thyroid superiorly, the course of the nerve may be highly variable. **Figure 6.15** shows the location of both recurrent nerves in their extraglandular and retroglandular courses. On the left side, the nerve usually emerges from its origin on the vagus to pass under the arch of the aorta and ascend in the tracheoesophageal groove. Behind the thyroid gland, it penetrates the inferior constrictor muscle and then dips posteriorly behind the cricothyroid articulation. The nerve commonly divides into anterior and posterior branches. In some cases, only the posterior branch assumes a course posterior to the joint. In rare instances, the nerve may divide prior to penetrating the inferior constrictor, creating the possibility of a pure abductor paralysis if only one branch is injured.

On the right side, the nerve passes under the subclavian artery and, like its left-sided counterpart, seeks the tracheoesophageal groove, ascends, and pierces the inferior constrictor to reach the larynx. It tends to be more lateral to

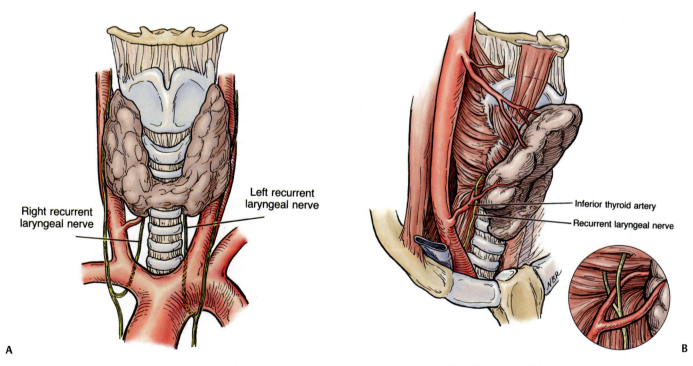

Right recurrent laryngeal nerve

Left recurrent laryngeal nerve

Inferior thyroid artery

Recurrent laryngeal nerve

A

B

Fig. 6.15 Relationship of the recurrent laryngeal nerves in (**A**) the extraglandular course and (**B**) the intraglandular course.

the tracheoesophageal groove than the left. In an anatomical study by Hunt,[84] the right nerve was found in a lateral relationship to the groove 33% of the time and the left 22%. This lateral position renders the nerve more prone to injury during dissection.

The nerve is closely related to the inferior thyroid artery, and some authors have described this common anatomical association as a guide to its safe dissection.[85,86] However, the profusion of anatomical variations (**Fig. 6.16**) should dissuade the surgeon from using this relationship as a reliable guideline. Loré et al[87] actually warn against using this landmark and advocate beginning the dissection at the thoracic inlet, identifying the nerve either in the groove or lateral to it, and then following it up to the gland. They advise ligating the inferior thyroid artery adjacent to the gland rather than out laterally. Not only does this avoid the danger of traumatizing the nerve if it is entangled in branches of the artery, but it may preserve the blood supply to parathyroids in the area as well.

Once dissection of the thyroid from the adjacent trachea and larynx begins, the recurrent nerve becomes obscured by a substantial sheet of fibrous tissue binding the posterior surface of the gland to the esophagus and hypopharynx. This ligament (**Fig. 6.17**), first described by Berry,[88] lies directly over the nerve.[89] The safest way to protect the nerve is to dissect it as one would the facial nerve in parotidectomy. A Mixter clamp is slipped over the epineurium of the nerve, gently elevated and parted, and the intervening connective tissue free of the nerve is cut with scissors (**Fig. 6.17**).

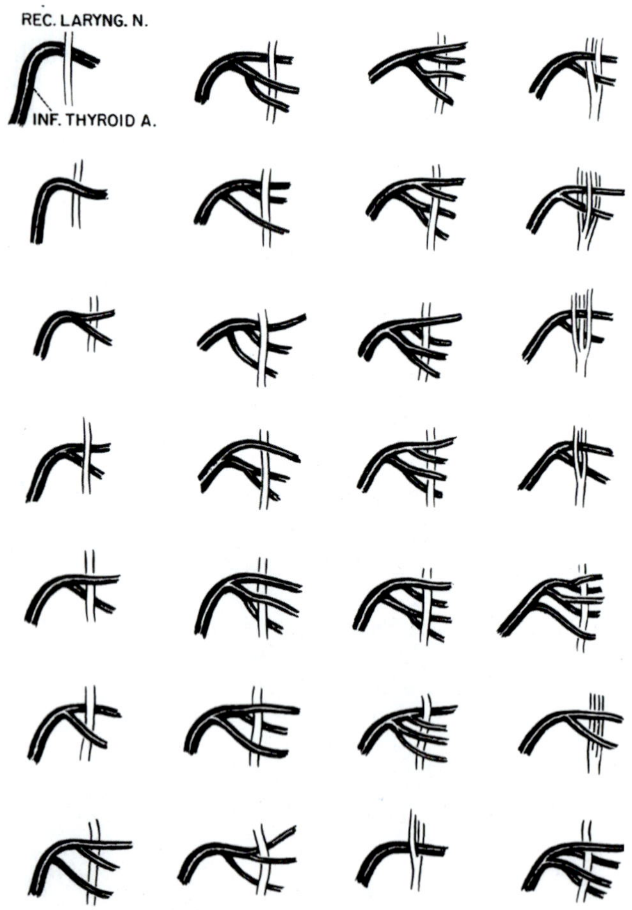

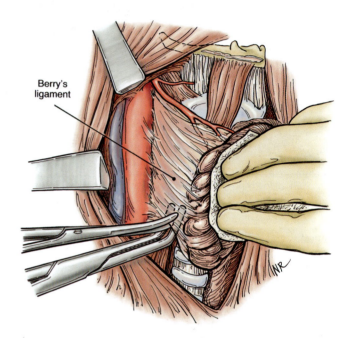

Fig. 6.17 Dissection of the Berry ligament, with preservation of the recurrent laryngeal nerve.

Fig. 6.16 Anatomical variations of the course of the recurrent laryngeal nerve in relationship to the inferior thyroid artery. (From Sedgwick CE, Bookwalter JR. Thyroid tumors. In: Sedgwick CE, ed. Surgery of the Thyroid Gland. Philadelphia: WB Saunders; 1974;207. Reprinted with permission.)

The superior laryngeal nerve, especially the external laryngeal branch to the cricothyroid muscle, is in jeopardy during the dissection of the superior pole of the thyroid. Although the consequences of injury are not as severe as with damage to the recurrent nerve, interference with pitch modulation if the external laryngeal nerve is cut, hemilaryngeal anesthesia if the inferior branch of the superior laryngeal nerve is cut, or both, represent significant complications. The superior laryngeal nerve is high in relation to the thyroid gland proper (**Fig. 6.18**) and should be out of danger in most cases. However, the anterior suspensory ligament of the gland may be mistaken for a glandular attenuation, and indeed such an attenuation or thyroid lingula may reach and even wrap around this nerve. The superior thyroid artery and vein should be ligated close to the glandular tissue of the upper pole. If a lingula is present, the superior laryngeal nerve is isolated and the external laryngeal nerve dissected free from the vessel and gland. Usually, careful isolation of the vessels in the ligament close to the gland with identification of the external nerve until the area of the cricothyroid muscle is past will keep these neural structures safe.

In the body of the gland, careful attention should be paid to the position of the carotid sheath. If the tumor is large, the internal jugular vein may be adherent to it. Inadvertent

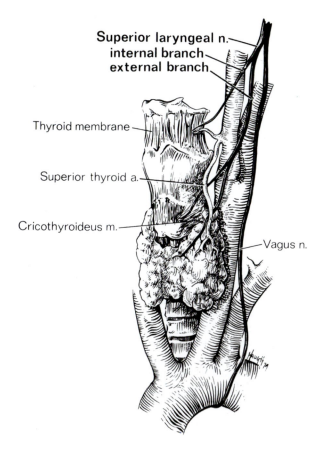

Fig. 6.18 Relationship of the superior laryngeal nerve to the superior pole of the thyroid gland. (From Caldarelli DD, Holinger LD. Complications and sequelae of thyroid surgery. Otolaryngol Clin North Am 1980;13:93. Reprinted with permission.)

incision of the vein can be prevented if, following dissection of the inferior and superior poles, the middle thyroid vein is identified and ligated.

◆ **Parathyroid Glands** A careful search for the parathyroid glands is an important step in total thyroidectomy. Hypoparathyroidism is one of the most difficult of medical management problems. However, in malignant disease, especially medullary or undifferentiated cancer, preservation of these vital glands may be impossible because of tumor invasion by direct extension. Fortunately, in a high percentage of individuals the parathyroids are in an extrathyroid location. It has been estimated that in most people two thirds of the glands are in the neck, with most of the remainder located in the upper mediastinum. Although the usual number of glands is four, 33% of individuals have more (usually five or six).[90] The location of the two superior glands is fairly constant, usually on the posteromedial surface of the superior pole. Although they are often positioned close to the superior thyroid artery, the inferior usually supplies them. Dissection in the region of the inferior border of the cricoid to the cricothyroid articulation and up the inferior cornua of the thyroid cartilage will usually reveal the superior para-

thyroids. The inferior glands are usually found near the inferior pole of the thyroid but are commonly extraglandular in location. A frequent location is the crossing of the inferior thyroid artery by the recurrent laryngeal nerve, but the gland is usually a little more superficial in location than the nerve. The inferior parathyroids may even be extraglandular, entrapped in a fold of thyroid parenchyma. These glands are also found in the tracheoesophageal area anywhere from the inferior thyroid pole to the pericardium.

If parathyroid preservation can be achieved but the blood supply is in jeopardy, the gland can be prepared and implanted in the sternocleidomastoid muscle or the antecubital fossa as described by Tenta and Keyes.[91] The gland is diced into 2 × 2 × 2 mm pieces, with control under the dissecting microscope if desired. A transverse crease incision is made in the antecubital fossa. Parallel furrows are cut in the flexor and pronator muscles in the forearm, and the diced parathyroid tissue is implanted. Parathyroid function can be monitored by taking serial calcium levels.

◆ **Mediastinal Resection** Resection of the thyroid gland for cancer requires removal of all adjacent lymph node and loose connective tissue. The lymphatic tissue is directly adjacent to the thyroid and drains laterally to the internal jugular chain as well as to the nodes of the pharyngoesophagus and mediastinum. Most of this tissue, even that of the upper mediastinum, can be readily dissected from a cervical approach. **Figure 6.19** shows a 56-year-old man with a large papillary carcinoma of the thyroid with bilateral cervical metastases. The tumor pushed the right common carotid artery aside and hugged the brachiocephalic trunk. Complete

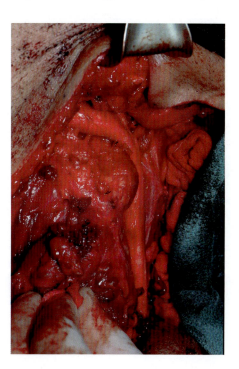

Fig. 6.19 Large carcinoma of the thyroid in a 50-year-old man. Tumor displaced the right common carotid artery in the root of the neck.

resection was possible through a transcervical approach. No palpable adenopathy was apparent in the mediastinum, which was also negative on CT scanning.

The tumor occasionally descends into the mediastinum, and adequate resection is possible only with a transsternal approach (**Fig. 6.20**). Unlike resections for squamous cell carcinomas of the upper aerodigestive tract, the transsternal approach for thyroid cancer does not require removal of bone. Although mediastinotomy might appear to be radical treatment for a disease with an often somewhat benign course, it must be remembered that thyroid cancer kills.[92] Moreover, those who die often do so as a direct result of extensive local disease.[93]

The skin incision is in the midline, bisecting the collar incision and descending over the upper third of the sternum (**Fig. 6.13b**). Soft tissue is incised down to the sternal periosteum. The tough fibrous tissue band that stretches over the rostral surface of the manubrium and extends onto its deep surface forms a protective sheet for the underlying structures during the sternal osteotomy. Careful finger dissection between the manubrium and this fascia will permit insertion of a ribbon retractor to protect the underlying soft tissue. A periosteal elevator is used to clear a track for the sternal split as outlined in **Fig. 6.21**. A single angled cut with a power saw into the second interspace may be sufficient; however, a second relaxation osteotomy into the first interspace facilitates retraction and enhances the exposure. The heavy protective retromanubrial fascia can now be cut and the sternotomy propped open with a self-retaining retractor such as a pediatric Finochietto.

The contents of the upper anterior mediastinum are now well visualized (**Fig. 6.22**). Care must be exercised to avoid the pleural reflections that form the lateral boundaries of the space. The principal features obvious at this juncture are direct extension of tumor, the thymus, and lymphatic and loose connective tissue. The somewhat amorphous thymus gland is dissected free of the vascular twigs that supply and drain it, with care taken to ensure hemostasis. As recommended by Loré,[82] dissections should proceed from right to left, over the superior vena cava and the left innominate vein (**Fig. 6.23**). The left innominate vein crosses the mediastinal space, and if tumor extensions or involved lymphatics course deep to the innominate, it may be ligated (**Fig. 6.24**). This also facilitates dissection around the aorta. Care must be taken to avoid damaging the recurrent laryngeal nerve at this level as it courses around the ligamentum arteriosum. Tumor may invade the trachea, the larynx, or the cervical esophagus. This is more commonly seen in the older patient. These structures must be removed and appropriate reconstruction done. The entire dissection can be done in continuity with the cervical block, and the tissue is now all removed.

After implantation of the parathyroid tissue, the sternum is closed with braided nonabsorbable suture or wire and threaded through drill holes (**Fig. 6.25**). A soft drain is placed in the mediastinum, and the wound is closed.

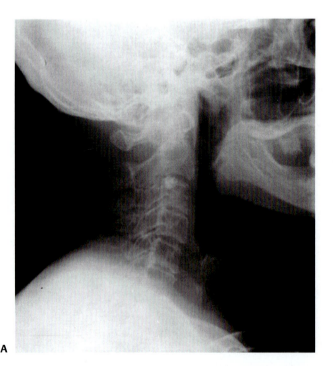

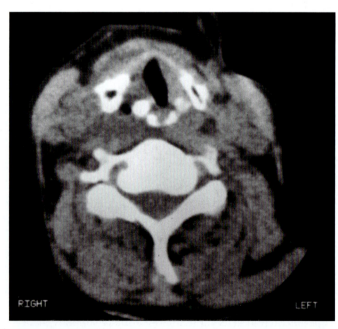

A   B

Fig. 6.20 *Case 2* Large undifferentiated carcinoma of the thyroid gland in an elderly woman, causing erosion of the larynx and severe airway obstruction. (**A**) Lateral soft tissue x-ray showing invasion of the larynx and trachea. (**B**) Computed tomographic scan showing erosion of the thyroid cartilage and soft tissue swelling into the laryngeal lumen.

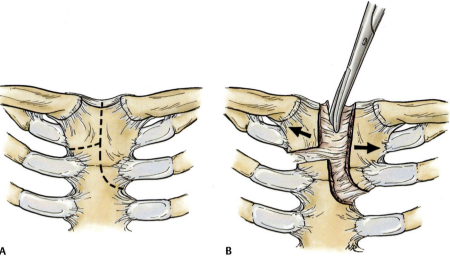

A

B

Fig. 6.21 (**A**) Sternal split outlined. (**B**) Thick protective periosteum on the deep surface of the manubrium being incised.

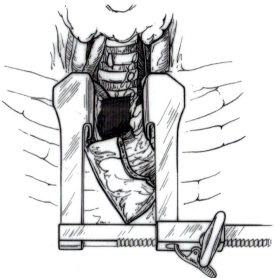

Fig. 6.22 The pediatric sternal retractor is inserted and the mediastinal contents are exposed. Note how the left innominate vein obscures a complete view of the mediastinal structures.

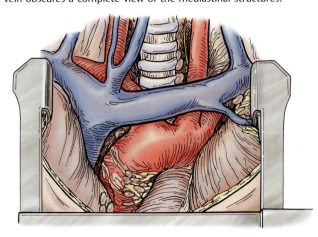

Fig. 6.23 Mediastinal exposure to the level of the aorta. The left innominate vein is exposed from the superior vena cava to the takeoff of the left jugular vein. Illustration reveals more exposure than is usually apparent.

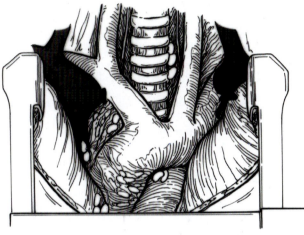

Fig. 6.24 The left innominate vein is carefully ligated with silk stick-ties and incised; the rest of the anterior mediastinum is now exposed.

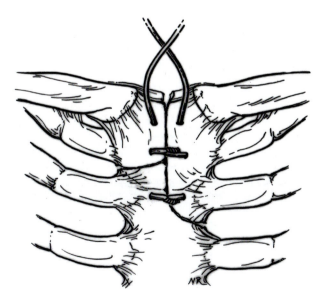

Fig. 6.25 Sternotomy closed with braided wire.

Case 1 (Figs. 6.26–6.30, pp. 281–282)

Fig. 6.26 shows a ^{131}I scan of the thyroid of a 25-year-old man who 6 years before had a neck node determined by biopsy to be follicular carcinoma. His practitioner took no further diagnostic or therapeutic steps. On presentation the patient had multiple nodules in his right neck, including one in the right submandibular triangle. His trachea was markedly deviated to the left, and the thyroid gland itself was huge. **Figure 6.27** is a CT scan showing mediastinal extension of tumor. Because tumor invaded the sternocleidomastoid muscle and the wall of the internal jugular vein, a radical neck dissection was done with sparing of the spinal accessory nerve (**Fig. 6.28**). An upper median sternotomy enabled the excision of a large projection of tumor (**Fig. 6.29**). The thymus and adjacent lymph nodes were removed (**Fig. 6.30**).

The patient was discharged on the seventh postoperative day. Follow-up treatment with ^{131}I was done, and the patient is well 8 years after treatment.

Case 2 (Figs. 6.20, 6.30, and 6.31, p. 282)

The elderly woman depicted radiographically in **Fig. 6.20** had an undifferentiated thyroid cancer that was locally very aggressive but was without symptoms, signs, or laboratory evidence of metastatic disease at the time of presentation. Extrinsic pressure on the esophageal lumen and erosion of the larynx rendered the patient severely dysphagic and caused considerable airway obstruction. Through a median sternotomy (**Fig. 6.30** and **Fig. 6.31**) complete extirpation of tumor was possible. A total laryngectomy was necessary, but lack of esophageal extension allowed sparing of the food conduit. She was discharged 3.5 weeks postoperatively, but succumbed to pulmonary metastases 1 year later. Although a rather radical procedure was done, it provided excellent palliation, allowing her full ambulation and normal swallowing until shortly before her death.

Case 3 (Figs. 6.32–6.34, p. 282)

A 63-year-old woman presented with a 7-month history of feeling a sense of choking that was most marked when brushing her teeth at first, but then became progressive. She experienced no hoarseness but complained of some hemoptysis and dysphagia, and then airway obstruction that was slowly progressive. She noted a mass in her neck 6 months prior that was gradually enlarging. One month prior she had a laser excision of an endotracheal mass that on biopsy revealed papillary thyroid carcinoma.

On examination she had obvious hoarseness and biphasic stridor with airway distress on minimal activity. There was no vocal cord paralysis and she had normal phonation. She had an 8 cm mass attached to her trachea on the right side. A CT scan revealed a thyroid mass eroding into the proximal trachea and occluding 65% of her airway (**Fig. 6.32**). Endoscopic biopsy revealed papillary carcinoma of the thyroid.

A total thyroidectomy and regional node dissection of level VI was done, along with a resection of the lateral and anterior wall of the trachea, which included a portion of three rings (**Fig. 6.33**). The tracheal defect was reconstructed with a composite graft of nasal septal cartilage and attached mucoperichondrium (**Fig. 6.34**). Her tracheostomy was discontinued after 1 week, and she has a completely unobstructed airway. She is over 21 years postoperative with no evidence of recurrence.

Case 4 (Figs. 6.35–6.37, p. 283)

A 61-year-old male presented with a history of a gradual increase in his collar size over a period of 12 months. He developed odynophagia centered low in the neck about 6 weeks prior to his hospital admission followed by hoarseness and dysphagia. On examination he had a mass in his thyroid gland measuring ~6 cm in diameter. He had a left vocal cord paralysis. CT scan revealed a large thyroid malignancy invading the larynx, trachea, and upper esophagus. Open biopsy was interpreted as a probable squamous cell carcinoma of the thyroid. The more likely diagnosis is large cell–type undifferentiated carcinoma of the thyroid.

Because of the extensive invasion of all adjacent structures a laryngotrachectomy and cervical esophagectomy with a regional as well as mediastinal nodal dissection was required (**Fig. 6.35** and **Fig. 6.36**). A permanent tracheostomy was established low in the neck and a gastric pull-up was done to restore the integrity of the upper digestive tract (**Fig. 6.37**). On pathological examination only two mediastinal nodes had metastatic cancer and there was no nodal involvement in the neck.

His postoperative course was complicated by a pleural effusion, which cleared after 10 days, and hypocalcemia secondary to hypoparathyroidism. He was discharged on postoperative day 23.

At his last visit he was 16 years postsurgery, disease free, swallowing without difficulty, and communicating well with an electrolarynx.

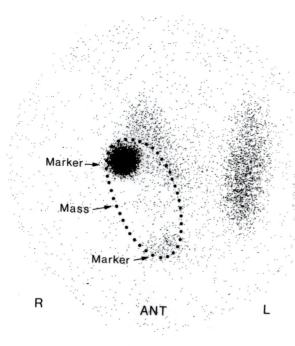

Fig. 6.26 *Case 1* ¹³¹I scan of a 25-year-old man with a large follicular carcinoma in the right lobe of the thyroid gland. Encircled area represents the tumor.

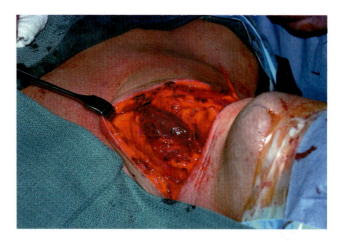

Fig. 6.28 *Case 1* Large follicular carcinoma of patient in **Fig. 6.26** and **Fig. 6.27**.

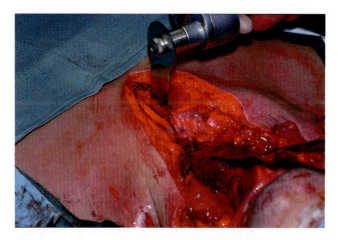

Fig. 6.29 *Case 1* Median sternotomy done with oscillating saw. Note the large flat malleable retractor inserted between the underlying thick manubrial periosteum and the bone, protecting the underlying vessels from the saw blade. (See also chapter 3, Fig. 3.36.)

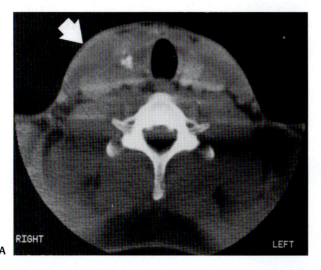

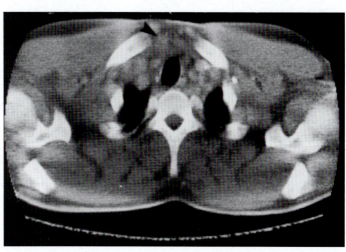

Fig. 6.27 *Case 1* (**A**) Computed tomographic (CT) scan showing large cervical metastasis (*arrow*) from thyroid carcinoma shown in **Fig. 6.26**. (**B**) CT scan of upper mediastinum showing thyroid tumor extension into its superior aspect.

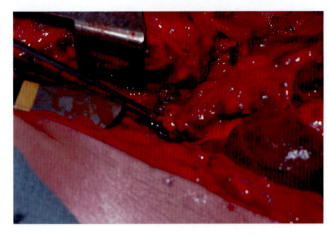

Fig. 6.30 *Case 1* Mediastinal extension of a large thyroid tumor.

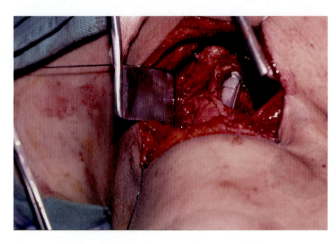

Fig. 6.33 *Case 3* Thyroidectomy and regional nodal dissection completed. Partial tracheotomy defect seen (*arrow*).

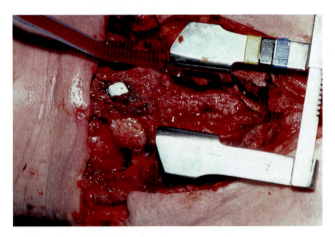

Fig. 6.31 *Case 2* Operative photograph of woman whose tumor is depicted radiographically in **Fig. 6.20**. Sternal split has been done, giving excellent access to tumor extension in the mediastinum.

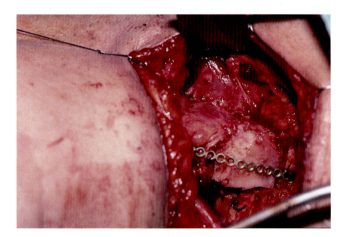

Fig. 6.34 *Case 3* Tracheal wall reconstructed with a free composite graft of nasal septal cartilage and mucoperiosteum.

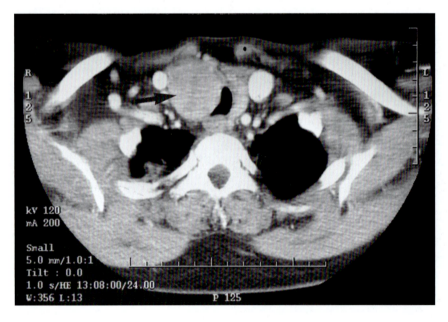

Fig. 6.32 *Case 3* Computed tomographic scan in the axial plane showing thyroid malignancy (*arrow*) eroding through the tracheal wall and occupying 65% of the tracheal lumen.

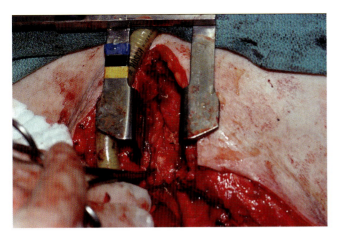

Fig. 6.35 *Case 4* Tumor exposed with a wide collar incision with a "T" extension onto the manubrium and a midsternal split. A Finochietto retractor is used to retract the sternum.

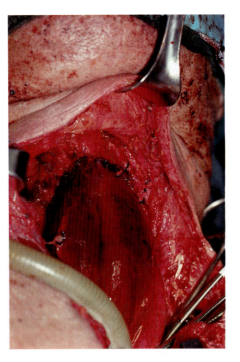

Fig. 6.37 *Case 4* Gastric pull-up completed.

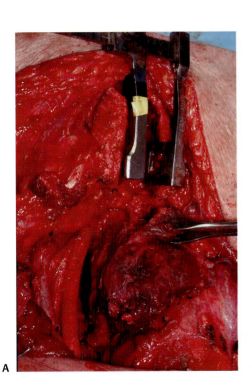

A

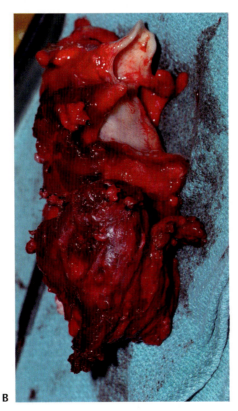

B

Fig. 6.36 *Case 4* (**A**) Large tumor in situ prior to removal. (**B**) Specimen containing larynx, trachea, esophagus, thyroid gland, and cervical as well as mediastinal lymphatics.

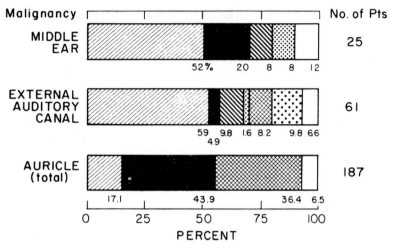

HISTOLOGIC DISTRIBUTION OF MALIGNANCIES
OF THE MIDDLE EAR, EXTERNAL AUDITORY CANAL
AND AURICLE

273 PATIENTS
PACK MEDICAL FOUNDATION......1945-1972

Fig. 7.1 Distribution of 273 patients with malignancies of the ear and temporal bone according to histological diagnosis. (From Conley J, Schuller DE. Malignancies of the ear. Laryngoscope 1976;86:1147)

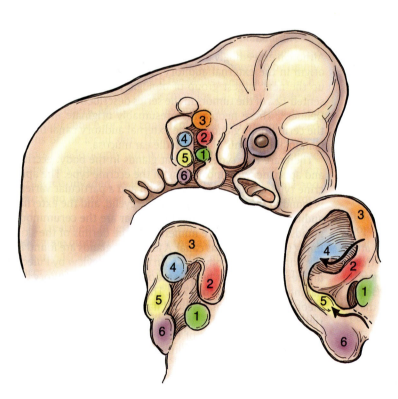

Fig. 7.2 Basal cell tumors of the auricle tend to spread along the fusion lines of the first and second and first and sixth embryological hillocks.

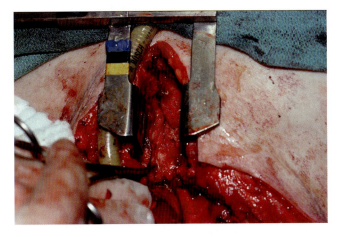

Fig. 6.35 *Case 4* Tumor exposed with a wide collar incision with a "T" extension onto the manubrium and a midsternal split. A Finochietto retractor is used to retract the sternum.

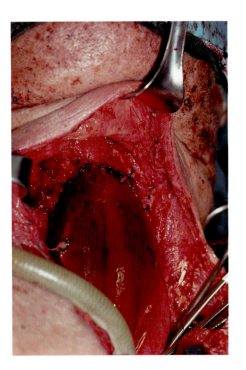

Fig. 6.37 *Case 4* Gastric pull-up completed.

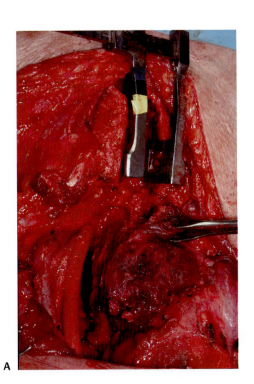

A

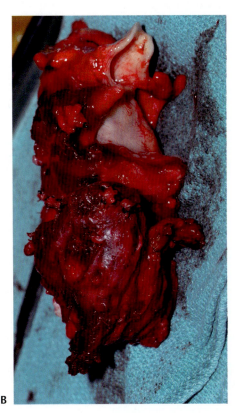

B

Fig. 6.36 *Case 4* (**A**) Large tumor in situ prior to removal. (**B**) Specimen containing larynx, trachea, esophagus, thyroid gland, and cervical as well as mediastinal lymphatics.

References

1. National Cancer Institute. Information for physicians on irradiation-related thyroid cancer. CA Cancer J Clin 1976;26:150–159

2. Rosai J, Carcangiu ML, Delellias RA. Atlas of Tumor Pathology: Tumors of the Thyroid Gland. 3rd Series, Fascicle 5. Washington, DC: AFIP; 1992:65

3. Lacher AB, Stucker FJ, Kirokawa RH. Management of the thyroid nodule. Otolaryngol Clin North Am 1980;13:59–67

4. Sampson RJ, Woolner LB, Rahn RC, et al. Occult thyroid carcinoma in Olmstead County, Minnesota: prevalence at autopsy compared with that in Hiroshima and Nagasaki, Japan. Cancer 1974;34:2072–2076

5. Crocker DW. Thyroid carcinoma. Surgery 1973;73:671–676

6. Djalilian M, Beahrs OH, Devine KD, et al. Intraluminal involvement of the larynx and trachea by thyroid cancer. Am J Surg 1974;128:500–504

7. Geissinger WT, Horsley JS III, Parker FP, et al. Carcinoma of the thyroid. Ann Surg 1974;179:734–739

8. Ibanez ML, Russell WO, Saavedra JA, et al. Thyroid carcinoma—biological behavior and mortality. Cancer 1966;19:1039–1052

9. Shelley WB, Beerman H, Enterline HT. Metastatic thyroid carcinoma. JAMA 1973;226:173–174

10. Silverberg SG, Huller RVP, Foote FW Jr. Fatal carcinoma of the thyroid: histology, metastases, and causes of death. Cancer 1970;25:792–802

11. Sutton JP, McSevain B, Diveley WL. Carcinoma of the thyroid. Ann Surg 1968;167:839–846

12. Carroll RE, Haddon W Jr, Handy VH, et al. Thyroid cancer: cohort analysis of increasing incidence in New York State, 1941–1962. J Natl Cancer Inst 1964;33:277–283

13. Mazzaferri EL, Young RL, Oertel JE, et al. Papillary thyroid carcinoma: the impact of therapy in 576 patients. Medicine 1977;56:171–196

14. Favus MJ, Schneider AB, Stachura ME, et al. Thyroid cancer occurring as a late consequence of head-and-neck irradiation: evaluation of 1056 patients. N Engl J Med 1976;294:1019–1025

15. Sommers SC. Thyroid gland. In: Anderson WAD, ed. Pathology. Vol 2. 6th ed. St. Louis: CV Mosby; 1971:1431

16. Becker SP, Skolnik EM, O'Neill JV. The nodular thyroid. Otolaryngol Clin North Am 1980;13:53–58

17. LiVolsi VA. Pathology of the thyroid gland. In: Barnes L, ed. Surgical Pathology of the Head and Neck. 2nd ed. Vol 3. New York: Marcel Dekker; 2001:1673–1718

18. Becker DV, Robbins J, Beebe GW, et al. Childhood thyroid cancer following the Chernobyl accident: a status report. Endocrinol Metab Clin North Am 1996;25:197–211

19. Nikiforov Y, Gnepp NR, Fagin JA. Thyroid lesions in children and adolescents after the Chernobyl accident. J Clin Endocrinol Metab 1996;81:9–14

20. Clark LR, Cole VW, Fuller LM, et al. Thyroid. In: Fletcher GH, McComb WS, eds. Cancer of the Head and Neck. Baltimore: Williams & Wilkins; 1967:293

21. Cole WH, Slaughter DP, Rossiter LJ. Potential dangers of nontoxic nodular goiter. JAMA 1945;127:883–888

22. Veith FJ, Brooks JR, Grigsby WP, et al. The nodular thyroid gland and cancer: a practical approach to the problem. N Engl J Med 1964;270:431–436

23. Meissner WA, Adler A. Papillary carcinoma of the thyroid: a study of the pathology of 225 cases. Arch Pathol 1958;66:518–525

24. Olen E, Klinck GH. Hyperthyroidism and thyroid cancer. Arch Pathol 1966;81:531–535

25. Wegelin C. Malignant disease of the thyroid gland and its relation to goiter in man and animals. Cancer Rev 1928;3:297–313

26. Hirabayashi RN, Lindsay S. The relation of thyroid carcinoma and chronic thyroiditis. Surg Gynecol Obstet 1965;121:243–252

27. Silverberg SG, Vidone RA. Metastatic tumors in the thyroid. Pac Med Surg 1966;74:175–180

28. Shimaoka K, Takeuchi S, Pickren IW. Carcinoma of the thyroid associated with other primary malignant tumors. Cancer 1967;20:1000–1005

29. Russell WO, Ibanez ML, Clark RL, et al. Thyroid carcinoma: classification, intraglandular dissemination and clinicopathological study based upon whole organ sections of 80 glands. Cancer 1963;16:1425–1460

30. Harach HR, Williams GT, Williams ED. Familial adenomatous polyposis (Gardener's syndrome) and thyroid carcinoma: a distinct type of follicular cell neoplasm. Histopathology 1994;25:549–561

31. Burman KD, Ringel MD, Wartofsky L. Unusual types of thyroid neoplasms. Endocrinol Metab Clin North Am 1996;25:49–68

32. Batsakis JG, Nishigama RH, Rich CR. Microlithiasis (calcospherites) and carcinoma of the thyroid gland. Arch Pathol 1960;69:493–498

33. Klinck GH, Winship T. Psammoma bodies and thyroid cancer. Cancer 1959;12:656–662

34. Block MA, Wylie JH, Patton RB, et al. Does benign thyroid tissue occur in the lateral part of the neck? Am J Surg 1966;112:476–481

35. Nicastri AD, Foote FW Jr, Frazell EL. Benign thyroid inclusions in cervical lymph nodes. JAMA 1965;194:1–45

36. Roth LM. Inclusions of non-neoplastic thyroid tissue within cervical lymph nodes. Cancer 1965;18:105–111

37. Toomey JM. Cysts and tumors of the pharynx. In: Paparella MM, Shumrick DA, eds. Otolaryngology. Vol 3. 2nd ed. Philadelphia: WB Saunders; 1980:2323

38. Sedgwick CE, Bookwalter JR. Thyroid tumors. In: Sedgwick CE, ed. Surgery of the Thyroid Gland. Major Problems in Clinical Surgery, Vol 15. Philadelphia: WB Saunders; 1974:133

39. Frazell EL, Foote FW Jr. Papillary cancer of the thyroid: a review of 25 years of experience. Cancer 1958;11:895–922

40. Farid NR, Sou M, Shi Y. Genetics of follicular cancer. Endocrinol Metab Clin North Am 1995;24:865–883

41. Rosai J, Carcangiu ML, Delellias RA. Atlas of Tumor Pathology: Tumors of the Thyroid Gland. 3rd Series, Fascicle 5. Washington, DC: AFIP; 1992:49

42. Warren S. The significance of invasion of blood vessels in adenomas of the thyroid gland. Arch Pathol (Chic) 1931;11:255–257

43. DeLellis RA, Guiter G, Weinstein BJ. Pathology of the Thyroid and Parathyroid Glands in Diagnostic Pathology of the Head and Neck. Gnepp DR ed. Philadelphia: WB Saunders; 2001:476

44. Shaha AR, Loree TR, Shah S. Prognostic factors and risk group analysis in follicular carcinoma of the thyroid. Surgery 1995;118:1131–1136

45. Buckwalter JA, Thomas CG Jr. Selection of surgical treatment for well differentiated thyroid carcinomas. Ann Surg 1972;176:565–578

46. Sutton JP, McSwain B, Diveley WL. Carcinoma of the thyroid. Ann Surg 1968;167:839–846

47. Hirabayashi RN, Lindsay S. Carcinoma of the thyroid gland: a statistical study of 390 patients. J Clin Endocrinol Metab 1961;21:1596–1610

48. Beahrs OH, Pasternak BM. Cancer of the thyroid gland. Curr Probl Surg 1969;3:1–38

49. Block MA, Horn RC, Miller JM, et al. Familial medullary cancer of the thyroid. Ann Surg 1967;166:403–4126

50. DeLellis RA. Multiple endocrine neoplasia syndromes revisited: clinical morphological and molecular features. Lab Invest 1995;72:494–505

51. Boultwood J, Wyllie FS, Williams ED, Winford-Thomas D. N-myc expression in neoplasia of human thyroid C-cells. Cancer Res 1988;48:4073–4077

52. Freeman D, Lindsay S. Medullary carcinoma of the thyroid. Arch Pathol 1965;80:575–582

53. Hazard JB, Hawk WA, Crile G Jr. Medullary (solid) carcinoma: a clinicopathological entity. J Clin Endocrinol 1959;19:152–161

54. Williams ED, Brown CL, Doniach L. Pathological and clinical findings in a series of 67 cases of medullary carcinoma of the thyroid. J Clin Pathol 1966;19:103–113

55. Wells SA Jr, Ontjes DA, Cooper CW, et al. The early diagnosis of medullary carcinoma of the thyroid gland in patients with multiple endocrine neoplasia type II. Ann Surg 1975;182:362–370

56. Woolner LB, Beahrs OH, Black BM, et al, eds. Thyroid Neoplasia: Proceedings of the Second Imperial Cancer Research Fund Symposium, London, April 1967. London/New York: Academic Press; 1968

57. Aldinger KA, Samaan NA, Ibanez M, et al. Anaplastic carcinoma of the thyroid. Cancer 1978;41:2267–2275

58. Loré JM, Marchetta F, Conley JJ. Thyroid cancer update. Meeting of the American Academy of Otolaryngology—Head and Neck Surgery, September 1982, New Orleans

59. Hoffmann GL, Thompson NW, Heffron C. The solitary thyroid nodule. Arch Surg 1972;105:379–385

60. Cutler SJ, Mustacchi P. Some observations on the incidence of thyroid cancer in the United States. N Engl J Med 1956;255:889–893

61. Winship T, Rosvall RV. A study of thyroid cancer in children. Am J Surg 1961;102:747–752

62. Raventos A, Winship T. The latent period for thyroid cancer following irradiation. Radiology 1964;83:501–506

63. Fitzgerald PJ. I[131] concentration and thyroid morphology in the thyroid. In: Upton (New York) Biology Department. The Thyroid. Brookhaven National Laboratory Symposia in Biology, Number 7. Brookhaven, NY: Brookhaven National Laboratory; 1954:220

64. Becker FO, Economou PG, Schwartz TB. The occurrence of carcinoma in "hot" thyroid nodules: report of 2 cases. Ann Intern Med 1963;58:877–882

65. Dische S. The radioisotope scan applied to the detection of carcinoma in thyroid swellings. Cancer 1964;17:473–479

66. Meadows PM. Scintillation scanning in the management of the clinically single thyroid nodule. JAMA 1961;177:229–234

67. Bain J, Walfish PG. The assessment of thyroid function and structure. Otolaryngol Clin North Am 1978;11:419–443

68. Tollefson HR, Shah JP, Huvos AG. Follicular carcinoma of the thyroid. Am J Surg 1973;126:523–528

69. Pomorski L, Bartos M. Metastasis as the first sign of thyroid cancer. Neoplasma 1999;46:309–312

70. Sisson GA, Feldman DE. The management of thyroid carcinoma metastatic to the neck and mediastinum. Otolaryngol Clin North Am 1980;13:119–126

71. Black BM, Yadeau RE, Wollner LB. Surgical treatment of thyroidal carcinomas: a study of 885 cases observed in a 30-year period. Arch Surg 1964;88:610–618

72. Witte J, Schlotmann U, Simon D, Dotzenrath C, Ohmann C, Goretzki PE. Significance of lymph node metastasis of differentiated thyroid carcinomas and C-cell carcinomas for prognosis: a metaanalysis. Zentralbl Chir 1997;122:259–265

73. Gordon PR, Huvos AG, Strong EW. Medullary carcinoma of the thyroid gland. Cancer 1973;31:915–924

74. Millburn L, Ameen D. The place of ionizing radiation in the treatment of thyroid carcinoma. Otolaryngol Clin North Am 1980;13:109–113

75. Crile G Jr, Hawk WA. Carcinomas of the thyroid. In: Anderson R, Hoopes JE, eds. Symposium on Malignancies of Head and Neck. St. Louis: CV Mosby; 1975:153

76. Carcangiu ML, Zampi G, Rosai J. Poorly differentiated ("insular") thyroid carcinoma: a reinterpretation of Langhans' "wuchernde Struma." Am J Pathol 1984;8:847–860

77. Nishiyama RH. Pathology of Thyroid Tumors. In: Comprehensive Management of Head and Neck Tumors. Vol 2. 2nd ed. Thawley SE, Panje WR, Batsakis JG, Lingberg RD, eds. 1999:1710–1721

78. Rosai J, Carcangui J, DeLellis RA. Tumors of the Thyroid Gland. In: Rosai J, Carcangui J, DeLellis RA eds. Atlas of Tumor Pathology: Tumors of the Thyroid Gland. 3rd ed. Washington: Armed Forces Institute of Pathology, fascicle 5. 1992:123–128

79. Carcangiu ML, Gerard-Marchand R, Heimann R, Williams ED. Poorly differentiated ("insular") carcinoma: a reinterpretation of Langhans' "Wuchernde struma. Am J Surg Pathol 1984;8:655–668

80. Rosai J, Carcangui J, DeLellis RA. Tumors of the Thyroid Gland. In: Rosai J, Carcangui J, DeLellis RA eds. Atlas of Tumor Pathology: Tumors of the Thyroid Gland. 3rd ed. Washington: Armed Forces Institute of Pathology, fascicle 5. 1992:135–159

81. Freund HR. Principles of Head and Neck Surgery. 2nd ed. New York: Appleton-Century-Crofts; 1979:322

82. Loré JM Jr. An Atlas of Head and Neck Surgery. Vol 2. 2nd ed. Philadelphia: WB Saunders; 1973:620

83. Sedgwick CE, ed. Surgery of the Thyroid Gland. Philadelphia: WB Saunders; 1974:170

84. Hunt PS. A reappraisal of the surgical anatomy of the thyroid and parathyroid glands. Br J Surg 1968;55:63–665

85. Beahrs OH. Complications of surgery of the head and neck. Surg Clin North Am 1977;57:823–829

86. Sedgwick CE. Surgical techniques. In: Sedgwick CE, ed. Surgery of the Thyroid Gland. Philadelphia: WB Saunders; 1974:133

87. Loré JM Jr, Duck JK, Elias S. Preservation of the laryngeal nerves during total thyroid lobectomy. Ann Otol Rhinol Laryngol 1977;86:777–788

88. Berry J. Suspensory ligaments of the thyroid gland. Proc Anat Soc Gr Brit Ireland 1887:4

89. Loré JM Jr. Surgery of the thyroid gland. Otolaryngol Clin North Am 1980;13:69–837367009

90. Goss CM, ed. Gray's Anatomy. 23rd ed. Philadelphia: Lea & Febiger; 1973:1345

91. Tenta LT, Keyes GR. Transcervical parathyroidectomy with microsurgical autotransplantation and the viscerovertebral angle. Otolaryngol Clin North Am 1980;13:169–179

92. Beierwaltes WH. The treatment of thyroid carcinoma with radioactive iodine. Semin Nucl Med 1978;8:79–94

93. Silliphant WM, Klinik GH, Levitin MS. Thyroid carcinoma and death. Cancer 1964;17:513–525

7

Cancer of the Ear and Temporal Bone

Paul J. Donald

Malignant tumors of the ear range from small lesions that can be adequately handled by desiccation and curettage to lesions involving the temporal bone proper that require a full temporal bone resection, the most formidable operative procedure that challenges the head and neck surgeon. Unfortunately, inadequate treatment of what initially seems to be an innocuous "skin tumor" of the pinna too often leads to the need for this dangerous extensive resection. In the last decade or two, there has been considerable reevaluation of what was previously considered to be optimal therapy for lesions of both the auricle and the temporal bone. Standard resection techniques for removal of basal cell and squamous cell cancers primary to the auricle have been shown to be highly ineffective in comparison with the Mohs chemosurgery technique.[1,2] Over the years the dermatological technique developed by Frederic Mohs[3–5] has become widely accepted as the method of choice for the control of small and medium-sized lesions of the facial skin. The technique breaks down when tumors invade deeply into bone and cartilage. The technique is especially applicable to lesions of the auricle, even when cartilage is invaded, as long as it is limited to the pinna and there is no invasion of the cartilage of the external auditory canal.

The treatment of lesions involving the temporal bone has undergone quite a transition in the last 2 to 3 decades. Until the early 1950s, the standard treatment for temporal bone cancer was irradiation therapy, radical mastoidectomy, or occasionally a combination of both. Cure rates were dismal, and a pessimism that in some quarters persists today pervaded any consideration of management. Thanks to the pioneering work of Campbell et al[6] and Parsons and Lewis,[7] however, the combined extracranial-intracranial approach to the temporal bone is now standard and, together with advances in anesthesia and intensive care management, has greatly enhanced patient survival.

◆ Pathology

Basal and Squamous Cell Carcinomas

By far the most common malignant neoplasms of the peri-auricular area, pinna, external auditory canal, and middle ear are basal cell and squamous cell cancers (**Table 7.1**). In Bumstead et al's series of 71 auricular malignancies, 40 were basal cell, and 29 were squamous cell cancers.[1] In the authors' review of the literature describing 780 malignancies of this site, 746 were either basal or squamous cell tumors, with 40% being basal cell and 55% squamous cell, there is an almost even distribution. On the other hand, in Conley's[8] series of 100 cancers of the external auditory canal, middle ear, and mastoid, 67% were squamous cell and less than 10% were basal cell tumors.[7] Of 100 patients followed for 5 years, Lewis[9] reported 86% with squamous cell and only 8% with basal cell carcinoma.

Later, Lewis,[9] in describing 150 of his own cases, found that 60% of these tumors originated in the auricle, 28% in the external auditory canal, and 12% in the middle ear and mastoid. To emphasize that he had a skewed distribution of cases he quotes Broders, who, drawing from a more general patient population and less of a tertiary referral setting, reported that 84% of his auricular and temporal bone tumors originated in the auricle. In Conley and Schuller's series,[10] 69% of the tumors originated in the pinna, 22% in the external auditory canal, and 9% in the middle ear and mastoid (**Fig. 7.1**).

The basal cell tumors vary considerably in their malignant potential. The morphea-type lesions are most resistant to therapy, one of the major problems being the difficulty in achieving tumor-free margins in the surgical specimen. Recurrent lesions are similarly difficult to adequately resect. These basal cell tumors of the auricle are so often diagnosed in the early stages that they are often regarded casually. Desiccation and curet-

Table 7.1 Incidence and Type of Ear Malignancies

Epithelial tumors		
Squamous cell carcinoma		
External auditory canal	24	
Auricle	17	
Total	**41 (45)**	
Neuroepithelial tumors		
Paraganglioma	14	
Melanocytic nevus	2	
Malignant melanoma	1	
Total	**17 (18)**	
Glandular tumors		
Adenoma	4	
Pleomorphic adenoma (mixed tumor)	2	
Adenoid cystic carcinoma	2	
Low-grade adenocarcinoma	2	
High-grade adenocarcinoma	3	
Total	**13 (14)**	
Basal cell carcinoma		
Auricle	3	
External and auditory canal	1	
Total	**4 (4)**	
Mesenchymal tumors		
Benign		
Osteoma	5	
Chondroma	1	
Lipoma	1	
Hemangioma	1	
Total	**8 (9)**	
Malignant		
Rhabdomyosarcoma	6	
Total	**6 (7)**	
Other tumors		
Meningioma	3	
Total	**3 (3)**	
TOTAL	**92 (100)**	

Source: Data from Chen KTR, Dehner LP. Primary tumors of the external and middle ear. Arch Otolaryngol 1978;104:247.

tage, shave excision, and other ultraconservative methods are so often successful that many physicians can hardly believe that what was formerly an innocuous-appearing little "skin cancer" has now become an invasive life-threatening malignancy. Once basal cell cancers assume a more aggressive demeanor, they freely invade bone and adjacent periauricular soft tissue.

Squamous cell tumors, like basal cell lesions, are usually seen in a background of solar skin damage. The surrounding pinna commonly demonstrates multiple scaling and roughened and pigmented areas in a thin atrophic skin. Squamous cancers are most commonly seen in the helix and postau-

ricular area.[10] The lesion itself is usually ulcerated and indurated with a peripheral area of erythema. In a series by Chen and Dehner[11] (**Fig. 7.1**) of 92 malignancies of the ear, the 17 squamous cell cancers of the pinna had associated periauricular lymphadenopathy when the primary lesion was ulcerated and erythematous. The lymph node was cancerous, however, in only one instance. Histologically there is a dense chronic inflammatory response. When auricular cartilage invasion occurs, cervical lymph node metastases are much more common.[11]

Both squamous cell and basal cell cancers show a propensity to spread along the perichondrium of the auricle. Bailin et al[12] showed that pre- and postauricular cancers tend to spread toward the ear itself. They also discovered that helical tumors spread both above and below along the helix, then proceed anteriorly to the antihelix as well as posteriorly to the retroauricular area. Antihelical lesions, on the other hand, show a more concentric pattern of spread. Ceilley et al[13] have shown that these tumors tend to follow embryological fusion lines, especially extending along the lines of fusion of the first and second, and first and sixth auricular hillocks (**Fig. 7.2**). In more recent times the area of greatest vulnerability to spread has been expanded to the so-called H zone.[15] The significance of this is discussed in more detail in chapter 12. The notion of the importance of embryological fusion line spread is supported in the author's experience.

Squamous cell cancers made up approximately half of the middle ear and external auditory canal malignancies in the series by Conley and Schuller.[10]

Glandular Neoplasms

Although exceedingly uncommon, malignancies of glandular origin in the external auditory canal and middle ear make up the next largest group of otologic cancers. They represented 12% of the tumors in the series described by Chen and Dehner.[11] These neoplasms presumably originate in either the ceruminous glands of the external auditory canal or the glandular elements of the middle ear mucosa.

There are two types of sweat glands in the body: eccrine and apocrine, with most being of the eccrine type. The apocrine type are relatively uncommon and a particular variety is found in the mammary gland, the eyelid, and the external auditory canal. Those in the middle ear are the ceruminous glands.[16] They are more numerous in the dermis of the skin lining the cartilaginous canal. A few scant glands are found in the skin lining the bony canal. An excellent review by Pulec[14] divides the glandular neoplasms of the external auditory canal into four types (**Table 7.2**). The only addition to this list, pleomorphic adenoma, which I have never seen in my experience, was suggested by Barnes.[16]

Glandular neoplasms of the external auditory canal are rare tumors and are often lumped under the common appellation "ceruminoma." The adenoma is the benign variant whose cells resemble the double-layered epithelial configuration of normal ceruminous glands with an inner colum-

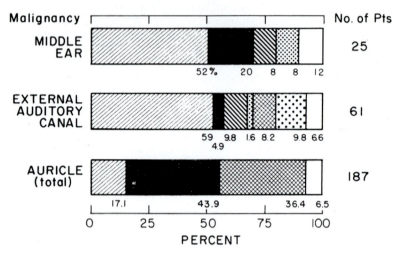

HISTOLOGIC DISTRIBUTION OF MALIGNANCIES OF THE MIDDLE EAR, EXTERNAL AUDITORY CANAL AND AURICLE

273 PATIENTS
PACK MEDICAL FOUNDATION......1945-1972

Malignancy		No. of Pts
MIDDLE EAR	52% 20 8 8 12	25
EXTERNAL AUDITORY CANAL	59 4.9 9.8 1.6 8.2 9.8 6.6	61
AURICLE (total)	17.1 43.9 36.4 6.5	187

PERCENT 0 25 50 75 100

Legend:
- ▨ Squamous Cell Ca
- ■ Malignant Melanoma
- ▩ Basal Cell Ca
- ▧ Adenocarcinoma
- ⬚ Adenoid–Cystic Ca
- ⬚ Paraganglioma
- ☐ All Others

Fig. 7.1 Distribution of 273 patients with malignancies of the ear and temporal bone according to histological diagnosis. (From Conley J, Schuller DE. Malignancies of the ear. Laryngoscope 1976;86:1147)

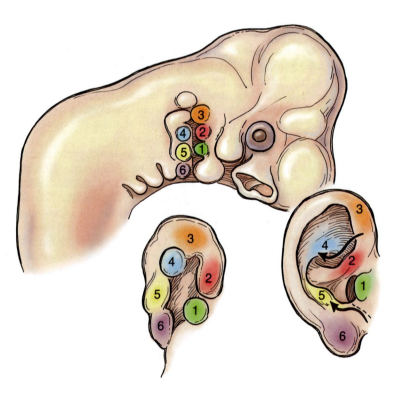

Fig. 7.2 Basal cell tumors of the auricle tend to spread along the fusion lines of the first and second and first and sixth embryological hillocks.

Table 7.2 Histological Analysis of 37 Tumors of Glandular Origin

Cell Type	No. of Cases
Adenoma	6
Mucoepidermoid carcinoma	2
Adenoid cystic carcinoma	24
Adenocarcinoma	5

Source: Data from Pulec JL. Glandular tumors of the external auditory canal. Laryngoscope 1977;87:1601.

nar eosinophilic layer and an outer myoepithelial layer. The adenoid cystic cancer is unfortunately the most common malignancy of these glands, but overall is distinctly rare. By 1977, only 58 cases[15] had been reported in the world literature, the old-fashioned cylindromatous type with a "Swiss cheese" histological pattern being the most common. The tumor has the same malevolent disposition characteristic of its behavior in other body sites. Lymphatic and blood vessel spread to regional and distant sites is common. Frequently there is perineural and perivascular spread, and local recurrence following conservative resection is the rule. The conchal cartilage appears to offer some resistance to invasion, and this tumor seems to creep alongside the cartilage rather than penetrate it. The malignancy is highly radioresistant. Spread through the fissures of Santorini in the cartilaginous external canal to the adjacent parotid gland is common.

Adenocarcinoma of ceruminous gland origin is highly variable in its degree of cellular differentiation. It may be so well differentiated as to completely mimic the adjacent ceruminous glands; only its characteristic of local invasiveness distinguishes it from normal cerumen glands or a benign adenoma.[17] These tumors are very aggressive, with rapid local invasiveness being characteristic. Metastatic disease is uncommon, and patients usually succumb to cerebral extension. Adenocarcinoma of the middle ear, however, has its origin in the glandular epithelium lining the cavity rather than in the cerumen glands.

Mucoepidermoid tumor of the external auditory canal is the most rare, with only two cases reported in the literature. The local invasiveness of this tumor as manifested in the salivary glands is seen in the external canal. Histologically the tumor mimics the salivary lesion, although the canal tumors do not originate in salivary glandular tissue.

Melanotic Lesions

The bulk of malignant melanomas of the ear are found on the pinna; external auditory canal and middle ear lesions are decidedly rare (see chapter 10). In the series by Conley and Schuller,[10] 9.1% of the melanotic lesions had metastatic nodes in the neck and 4.6% had distant metastases at the time of initial examination. Nonmelanotic lesions were present in 8.1% of the cases. Most lesions in the group were less than 1 cm in size.

Glomus Body Tumors

The glomus body tumor is usually benign, although it will run a course eventuating in death if not adequately treated. These tumors arise in the parenchymal cells of the glomus bodies of the skull base, particularly of the internal jugular vein. Although the latter structure is the most common site of origin, these tumors may also arise from similar bodies on the internal carotid artery, the vagus nerve, and the tympanic plexus.[18] These organs function as chemoreceptors. Their cells are of neural crest origin and are nonchromaffin staining and nonepinephrine secreting in type. They are epithelioid in appearance and cluster around the numerous blood vessels that richly populate the tumor. Glomus tumors slowly enlarge and gradually erode the surrounding bone, which is usually that adjacent to the jugular foramen.

Arteriography reveals a characteristic flush that is caused by the rich blood supply (**Fig. 7.3**). Retrograde jugular venography commonly demonstrates a lack of filling of the jugular bulb (**Fig. 7.4A**). These two signs are pathognomonic of the disease. Further evaluation by computed tomographic (CT) scanning and magnetic resonance imaging (MRI) of the temporal bone helps to delineate the extent of the neoplasm (**Fig. 7.4B**).

Malignancy is uncommon, being found in only ~10% of cases.[19] Local persistence after inadequate excision should not be construed as a sign of malignancy, but local recurrence after complete excision or the presence of metastases does signify malignancy. It is important to remember that

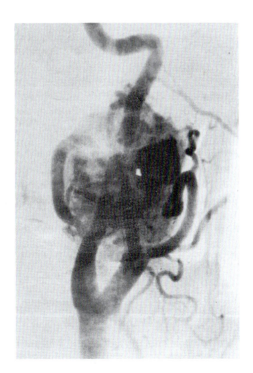

Fig. 7.3 Arteriogram showing marked blush of a large glomus jugulare tumor.

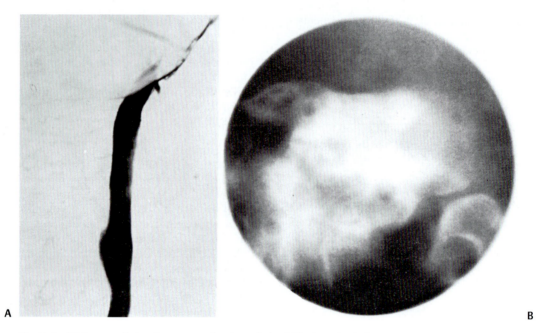

Fig. 7.4 (**A**) Retrograde jugular venography shows lack of fill of jugular bulb. (**B**) Polytomograph showing enlargement of jugular foramen.

the usual histological criteria of a malignant tumor cannot be applied to these lesions. Even the most blatantly metastasizing ones may show a uniform population of cells with infrequent mitoses, and without pleomorphism or dysplasia.

Carcinoid Tumor

According to Barnes,[16] middle ear adenoma and carcinoid tumor are part of the same pathological spectrum. They have similar presentations and a spectrum of histological appearance, with the adenomatous type demonstrating more endothelial cells and the carcinoid more neuroendocrine cells. The same symptoms of carcinoid elsewhere in the body may present when the tumor arises in the middle ear; facial flushing, palpitations, asthma, and diarrhea. In addition the symptoms of earache, otorrhea, and diminished hearing characteristic of other middle ear tumors are seen. They are very rare and hardly mentioned in standard texts on head and neck neoplasia or pathology. I have seen only one in my experience.

Sarcomas

These malignancies are rare in the ear and temporal bone. Rhabdomyosarcoma is basically a disease of childhood and mainly occurs in the first year of life. It begins in the middle ear and mastoid and spreads to both middle and posterior cranial fossae via the internal acoustic canal, usually along the fallopian canal.[19,20] Local recurrences are the rule, and distant metastatic disease (especially to the lung) is common.[20] Unfortunately, the early, somewhat quiescent period in which the patient presents with only hearing loss may

be the only time the tumor may remain within resectable bounds. In Myer et al's review[19] all patients succumbed to the disease. Lewis[21] states that the most effective treatment is combined radiotherapy and triple agent chemotherapy (see chapter 11 and chapter 15).

In a series of 211 sarcomas reported on by Naufal[22] in an extensive review spanning 100 years of the literature, the most common sarcoma was an undifferentiated variety composed of cells of either a spindle, round, or anaplastic configuration. The histological distribution of the remainder is summarized in **Table 7.3**. Little additional information has been added to the literature since Naufal's exhaustive study. The rarity of the tumor renders a well-established course of

Table 7.3 Histological Analysis of 211 Cases of Primary Sarcoma of the Temporal Bone

Cell Type	No. of Cases
Undifferentiated	89
Rhabdomyosarcoma	64
Fibrosarcoma	17
Osteogenic Sarcoma	12
Ewing Sarcoma	7
Hemangiosarcoma	8
Myxosarcoma	5
Chondrosarcoma	1
Liposarcoma	1
Meningiosarcoma	1

Source: Data from Naufal PE. Primary sarcomas of the temporal bone. Arch Otolaryngol 1973;98:44.

treatment a matter of extrapolation from the treatment of head and neck sarcomas at other sites.

Osteogenic sarcoma may originate in a previous exostosis in a patient with multiple exostoses of the external auditory canal. Chondrosarcoma or chondromyxosarcoma may arise from cartilaginous rests within the petrous bone.

Most patients with sarcomas involving the temporal bone are not initially seen until the disease is massive, with the normal anatomical structure already replaced by tumor. Management at this stage is difficult. If the disease is resectable the basic rhabdomyosarcoma protocol of complete excision followed by radiation and chemotherapy will give the best survival results. Even if the margins are histologically positive but there has been a gross total removal of the malignancy the survival results are better than treatment limited to primary chemotherapy and radiation. Chemotherapy, especially in combination with irradiation therapy, is usually the treatment of choice. Small lesions encompassable by temporal bone resection are rarely seen.

◆ Surgical Management

Mohs Chemosurgery

To compare the relative efficacy of standard resection technique in the excision of basal cell carcinoma of the pinna with the Mohs technique a prospective study of 71 basal and squamous cell cancers of the pinna has been done; a comparison of projected resection using standard margins to the actual tumor-free margins was done using Mohs technique.[23] The standard resection margins used were as follows: 8 mm for basal cell cancers less than 3 cm in diameter; 10 mm for squamous cell cancers less than 3 cm; and 15 mm for any lesion larger than 3 cm and all recurrent lesions. Once the proposed resection was mapped out, the area was measured and then the lesion was excised using Mohs chemosurgery. Employing the histopathologic control of the margins characteristic of conventional surgical, inadequate excision would have occurred in 24% of the lesions (**Table 7.4**).

For the Mohs technique the inadequate excision rate was 4% overall based on this rate of local recurrence. As would be expected, lesions that were larger than 1 cm or were recurrent in nature, or both, showed an increasingly higher incidence of positive margins with the theoretical surgery. Lesions smaller than 1 cm would have had a 13% recurrence

Table 7.4 Results of Hypothetical Conventional Excision

Lesion	Size (cm)	Inadequate Excision (%)
Primary	< 1	13
Recurrent	> 1	28
All	< 1	13
	> 1	33
All	All	24

Source: Bumstead RM, Ceilley RL. Auricular malignant neoplasms. Arch Otol 1982;108:226, Table 1.

rate, and those that were recurrent and larger than 1 cm in diameter, a 33% recurrence rate. On the other hand, if the proposed conventional surgery would have actually successfully removed the tumor, the amount of tissue that would have been unnecessarily excised was estimated to be 180% larger on the average in primary lesions and 347% larger in recurrent cancers (**Table 7.5**).

Table 7.5 Comparison of Defect Area of Mohs Technique with Conventional Excision*

Lesion	Size (cm)	% Excess Area Excised† Average Range
Primary (average, 180; range, 28–589)	< 1	333 35–589
	> 1	78 28–125
Recurrent (average, 347; range, 28–1051)	< 1	412 79–851
	> 1	317 28–1051

Source: Bumstead RM, Ceilley RL. Auricular malignant neoplasms. Arch Otol 1982;108:226, Table 2.

*Only lesions successfully excised by conventional excision were included.

†Excess area excised is percentage of the area of noninvolved tissue excised by conventional excision in relation to the area of the tissue involved with tumor (area of Mohs defect), which is equal to the area of noninvolved tissue excised divided by the area of Mohs defect.

In the judgment of those doing the study, the high-risk lesions included all tumors larger than 1 cm in diameter, all morpheaform basal cell carcinomas, and all recurrent neoplasms. The morpheaform basal cell lesion was particularly pernicious because of the high unpredictability of its extent and its propensity to recur within the scar of the initial excision.

Use of the Mohs technique was justified in all the cases studied on the basis of the 4% local recurrence rate with a follow-up of 3.5 years or longer. All recurrences were nests of cells in discontinuity with the initial primary lesion that developed within the scar of the initial resection. This cure rate compares favorably to the projected 24% theoretical recurrence rate in these lesions had they been resected by conventional surgical techniques. Recurrence rates with resections quoted in the literature are around 16%.[24–26] This contrasts with a 47 to 50% recurrence rate when a third and often recommended modality, radiotherapy, is used.[26,27] This classic study definitively establishes the role of the Mohs technique in the management of these tumors. The elaboration of the fresh frozen technique of micrographic analysis of the specimen by Tromovitch and Stegman[28] rather than the zinc chloride fixation originally described by Mohs has made the technique easier on the patient and quicker for the surgeon (refer to chapter 12).

The following case report illustrates the use of the fresh frozen Mohs technique in the removal of a basal cell carcinoma of the auricular concha.

Case Report

Case 1 (Fig. 7.5–7.10, pp. 292–294)

A 45-year-old male had been treated over the years for actinic-induced basal cell carcinomas of the facial skin. He presented with a short history of a lesion of the concha with multiple small areas of breakdown (**Fig. 7.5**). Incisional biopsy revealed basal cell carcinoma. Because of the absence of any clear delineating margin surrounding the tumor, Mohs fresh frozen technique was elected.

In the first resection all visible tumor was excised with a very narrow margin. These margins were marked with India ink and separated into orderly fragments (**Fig. 7.6**). Close cooperation between surgeon and pathologist is essential at this stage. Care is taken to examine both lateral and deep margins by taking cuts close but parallel to the actual margin of resection. Those areas that were positive for cancer had a further resection done. These were again carefully marked, correctly oriented (**Fig. 7.7**), and sectioned. A tumor-free margin was established on the third series of resections (**Fig. 7.8**). The wound was then covered with a split-thickness skin graft held in place with a tie-over bolster and a mastoid dressing (**Fig. 7.9**). In 2 weeks, the operative site was healed, and the patient has an excellent cosmetic result by virtue of the narrow excision allowed by this technique (**Fig. 7.10**). The patient is tumor free at this site now for 20 years.

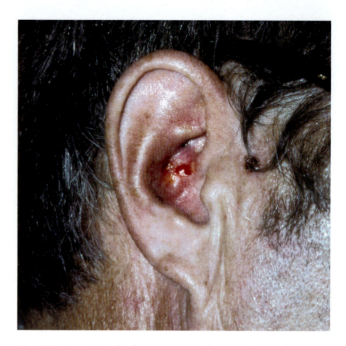

Fig. 7.5 *Case 1* Basal cell carcinoma of the auricular concha with indistinct borders.

Temporal Bone Resections

One of the most frighteningly difficult operations for the head and neck surgeon is temporal bone resection. In the early years of this procedure the operative mortality rate was 10%. Thanks to modern anesthesia, sophisticated monitoring equipment, innovations in surgical instrumentation, and the

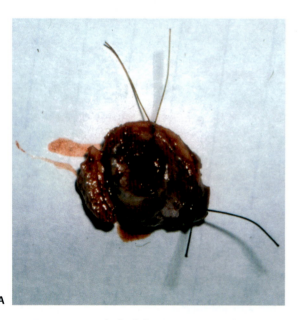

A

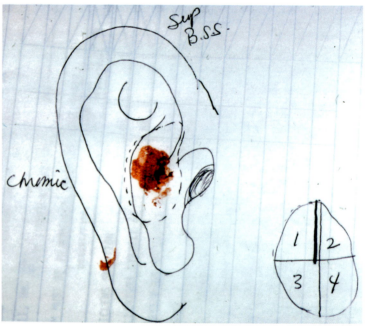

B

Fig. 7.6 *Case 1* Mohs fresh frozen resection technique. (**A**) Initial specimen mounted. (**B**) Initial specimen with margins marked out. It is vital to transpose margin numbers to the operative site when taking next specimens.

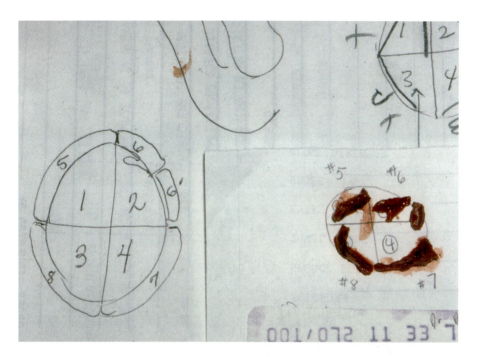

Fig. 7.7 *Case 1* Second resection done in areas with positive margins.

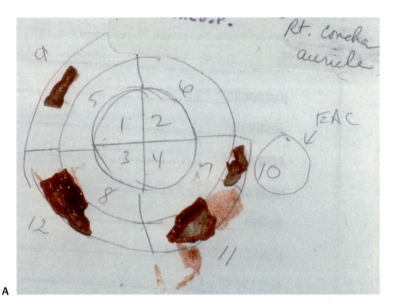

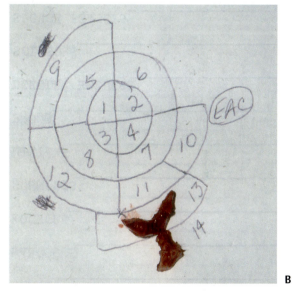

A
B

Fig. 7.8 *Case 1* (**A**) Third resection established negative margins in all but two sites. (**B**) Fourth specimen yields final negative margin.

wisdom acquired from the experience of several courageous surgeons in the past, this catastrophic figure has become considerably lower. I have not had such a fatality in over 30 years of doing this procedure. However, temporal bone resection remains a substantial surgical challenge.

Because of the sensitive location of the temporal bone, under the cerebrum and anterior to the cerebellum, surrounded, as Lewis[22] describes, by an interconnecting series of blood-filled "lakes" (**Fig. 7.11**), a precise anatomical understanding is essential to this operation. Separation of the bone from these blood-containing channels and judicious protection of the cerebral contents will ensure the safe removal of tempo-

ral bone cancers, with an adequate margin yielding a reasonable prognosis for an eventual tumor-free course.

The procedures are divided into lateral temporal bone resection, total temporal bone resection, total temporal bone resection with petrous apicectomy (**Fig. 7.12**), transcervical-transmastoid resection for removal of glomus jugulare and neurogenic tumors of the skull base, and, finally, temporal bone resection with intracranial extension. In this latter category are those tumors that have extended beyond the confines of the temporal bone and have intracranial extension with dural or brain involvement. Considerable judgment and experience are necessary not only to do this operation

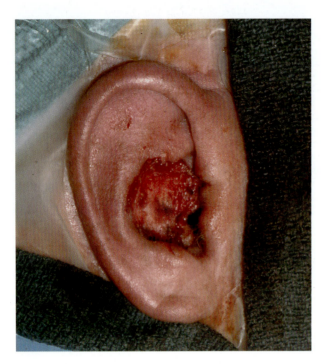

Fig. 7.9 *Case 1* Wound prior to coverage with a split-thickness skin graft with a tie-over bolster.

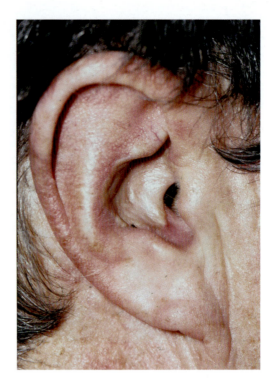

Fig. 7.10 *Case 1* Postoperative result.

as a team with a neurosurgeon but also to make the judgment as to who is a good surgical candidate. One of the main problems with the management of intracranial spread is the threat posed by the vein of Labbé. If this vessel needs sacrifice because of dural involvement there is a very high risk of death that is obviously a contraindication to surgery.

Lateral Temporal Bone Resection

This procedure is indicated for cancers in the external auditory canal that do not transgress the tympanic annulus. Lewis[19] uses a margin of 5 mm lateral to the tympanic membrane as his limit to lateral resection. Many of these tumors

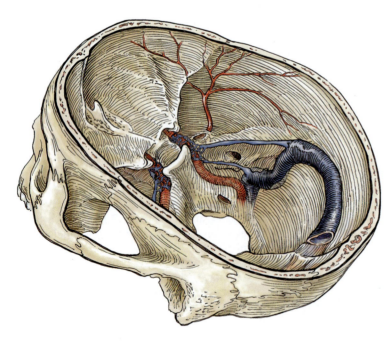

Fig. 7.11 Intracranial view depicting the temporal bone encircled by blood-filled "lakes," represented by the internal carotid artery, internal jugular vein, sigmoid sinus, inferior and superior petrosal sinuses, cavernous sinus, and middle meningeal artery.

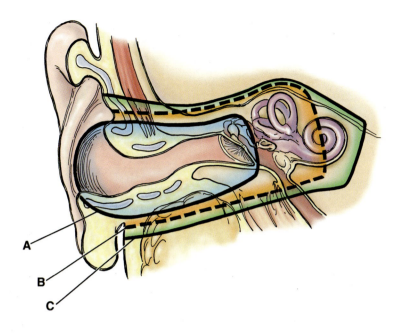

Fig. 7.12 Coronal schematic representation of extent of resection for A, lateral, B, subtotal, and C, total temporal bone resections.

begin in the skin over the conchal cartilage and extend into the external canal. Several patients have had repeated limited resections of the pinna (**Fig. 7.13A,B**) and even total auriculectomy (**Fig. 7.14**), only to later require temporal bone resection because of surgery that was too conservative.

External canal malignancies either have manifest palpable disease in the parotid gland or have highly probable microscopic extension. The fissures of Santorini in the cartilaginous portion of the canal provide free access for the passage of lymphatic disease directly into the glandular tissue that abuts it. A parotidectomy is mandatory in all cases. The facial nerve trunk and its branches are carefully dissected,

sacrificing only those stuck or close to tumor. If either the zygomatic, buccal, or mandibular branches are removed, they are replaced by interposing greater auricular or sural nerve grafts.

Lesions of the conchal skin may penetrate the postauricular skin and be affixed to the periosteum of the mastoid cortex. If there is radiographic evidence of bone erosion, especially close to the middle ear space, total rather than lateral temporal bone resection may be necessary. As long as just the lateral cortex of the mastoid air cell system is involved, a lateral resection will suffice (**Fig. 7.15**). External auditory canal invasion may proceed anterosuperiorly into the zygo-

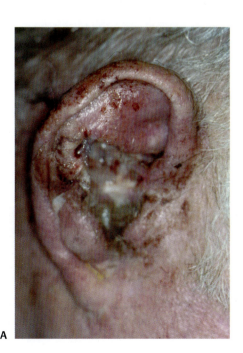

A

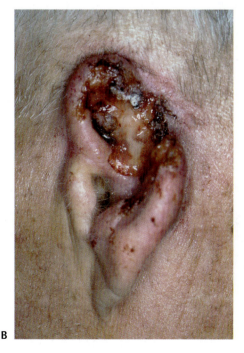

B

Fig. 7.13 (**A**) Numerous hyphercations and curettage followed by limited resections of this squamous cell carcinoma of the pinna were ineffective. (**B**) Numerous limited resections plus irradiation therapy were insufficient to rid this patient of basal cell carcinoma of the pinna.

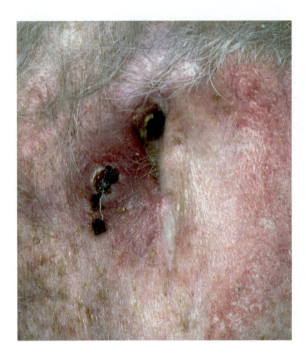

Fig. 7.14 Total auriculectomy was done but with an inadequate margin that resulted in a recurrence of squamous cell carcinoma of the premastoid soft tissue.

matic root (**Fig. 7.16**). In these instances, zygomatic resection with excision of the contents of the infratemporal fossa and even underlying skull may be necessary. With both posterior and anterior extension of tumor, often a large skin excision is necessary as well.

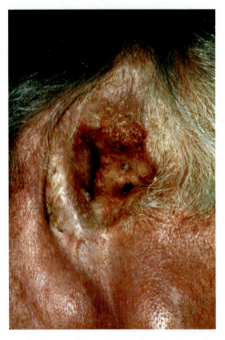

Fig. 7.15 Defect following lateral temporal bone resection as illustrated in **Fig. 7.12A**. Split-thickness skin graft used to line defect to facilitate early detection of recurrences.

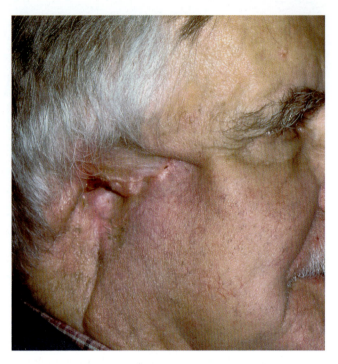

Fig. 7.16 Defect following lateral temporal bone resection that included the zygomatic arch, infratemporal fossa, underlying cranium, and dura. Because of intracranial intervention the defect was lined with a scalp flap.

The patient is positioned on the table as for a mastoidectomy. The amount of postauricular skin resected is proportional to the degree of cutaneous involvement, usually taking a 2 to 3 cm margin. The face of the involved side is covered by a transparent "adherent" drape to permit visualization of the facial muscles. The region of the squamosal aspect of the temporal bone is sufficiently exposed to accommodate the exigencies of anterosuperior extension.

The excision is again dependent upon the soft tissue extent of the cancer. If the helical rim can be preserved, especially in conjunction with the concha, then it is included in a superiorly based flap. The basic surgical approach combines a mastoidectomy and parotidectomy type incision (**Fig. 7.17**). The auricular remnant, if any, is reflected superiorly. If a radical neck dissection is employed, a lazy S incision is dropped from the inferior limb of the modified Blair incision behind the carotid artery. If an extension posteriorly into the occipital scalp is required to enter the posterior fossa, it can be extended in a gentle looping arc superoposteriorly. If an anterior craniotomy or anterior access to the infratemporal fossa is mandated, an irregular loop into the anterior temporal scalp is made. The cancer itself is circumscribed by an incision that allows the neoplasm and its cutaneous margin to stay with the temporal bone. The auricular remnant can then be reflected superiorly (**Fig. 7.18**).

The lymph nodes adjacent to the ear are palpated for evidence of metastatic disease. A frozen section is taken of any suspicious lymph nodes. If any are positive, a radical neck dissection is done. However, parotidectomy should precede the neck dissection. This sequence allows the parotid dis-

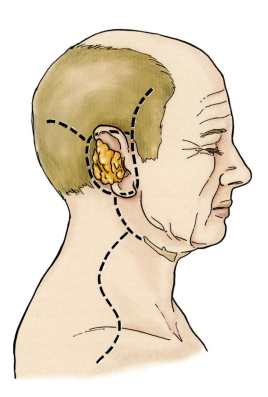

Fig. 7.17 Incision for temporal bone resection, with extension outlined (*dashed lines*) for exposure of the anterior reaches of the middle cranial fossa, the posterior fossa, and inferiorly if a radical neck dissection is required. In the complete resection the superior limbs usually need to be higher and more extensive than in the lateral operation.

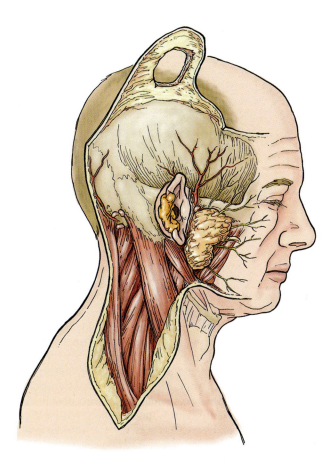

Fig. 7.18 Lateral temporal bone resection. The flaps are retracted, and the cutaneous involvement with tumor and an adequate margin of healthy tissue remain with the temporal bone.

section to proceed unhindered by the troublesome bleeding that results when the internal jugular vein is tied as part of the radical neck dissection. If during the parotidectomy facial nerve branches are sacrificed, the ends are tagged with silk sutures or clips for nerve grafting later in the operation.

The external auditory canal is injected with Xylocaine and 1/100,00 epinephrine. The incision in the canal skin is made with an otologic knife within a few mm of the tympanic annulus. If the tumor is found to encroach on the tympanic membrane then it will require excision, and essentially no incision in the canal skin will be done.

The next step is a complete mastoidectomy. The mastoid portion of the fallopian canal is skeletonized carefully throughout its length, to the stylomastoid foramen. This step is facilitated by meticulously outlining the digastric ridge. The mastoid tip is amputated, and the facial recess is developed and carried inferiorly as far as possible within the bounds of safety imposed by the facial nerve. If the canal skin is involved with tumor up to the annulus or onto the tympanic membrane then the deep margin of resection at this point will be the nerve, and the resection skives directly over its lateral aspect. If at any point it becomes obvious that tumor has extended into the mastoid air cell system proper, or if in viewing through the facial recess it is seen to have invaded the middle ear, the lateral resection is abandoned and the operation expanded to a full temporal bone excision. As

the lateral procedure continues, an atticotomy is done, with care taken to preserve the ossicular chain when possible. Drilling the lateral attic bone to a thin plate and then excising it with a stapes curette greatly aids in ossicular preservation. As the atticotomy proceeds, obvious tumor extension into the zygomatic root may be found (**Fig. 7.19**), in which case continued removal of the root and even the arch to the lateral orbital rim may be required (see **Fig. 7.17**). If anything beyond a minimal amount of zygomatic extension is present, it is probably wise at this point to do a mandibular condylectomy. The condylectomy may be done either at this juncture or, if anticipated earlier, following the parotidectomy.

The mandibular condylectomy is performed as follows. The microscope is pushed to the side and an exposure of the temporomandibular joint is done. Keeping the temporal branch of the facial nerve as well as the main trunk in view, the fascia and periosteum over the zygoma are incised with a scalpel in an inverted L configuration. The horizontal portion of this incision should be only ~3 to 4 mm long, to avoid damage to the temporal branch. Further dissection forward is done with a Joseph or similar elevator. The joint capsule is incised with the cautery and the joint cavity entered. The meniscus is separated from its superior attachment. The cutting bone needle is used to cut across the condylar neck. Care

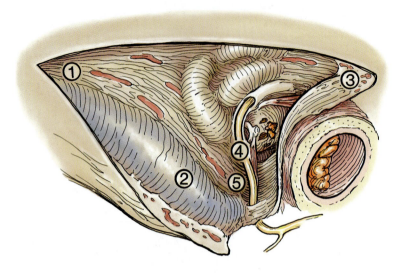

Fig. 7.19 Lateral temporal bone resection: Mastoidectomy completed, the facial nerve skeletonized, and the facial recess opened. The atticotomy is proceeding. 1, sinodural angle sharply outlined; 2, sigmoid plate skeletonized; 3, atticotomy; 4, facial nerve skeletonized and facial recess opened, revealing no tumor beyond tympanic membrane; 5, cerebellar plate skeletonized.

is taken as the medial cortical surface is reached. The deep periosteum is not transgressed if at all possible, to avoid injury to the internal maxillary artery, which usually lies just deep to the mandibular neck. The condyle is grasped with bone-holding forceps, and the insertion of the lateral pterygoid muscle and the remaining attachments of the sphenomandibular and temporomandibular ligaments are cut close to the bone (**Fig. 7.20**). With a bone needle, a fissure is created in the glenoid fossa that will enable the anterior aspect of the external auditory canal wall to be incised just lateral to the tympanic annulus (**Fig. 7.21**). It is not uncommon to expose the middle fossa dura during this maneuver. If this occurs, a careful check is made to ensure that no damage has occurred to the middle meningeal artery. If there is extensive tumor involvement in the zygomatic root, it is necessary to remove not only the zygoma up to the lateral orbital rim but the temporalis muscle and occasionally the skull deep to the infratemporal fossa as well. In the patient shown in **Fig. 7.16**, basal cell carcinoma not only had penetrated the temporal and sphenoidal squama but had also involved the underlying dura (**Fig. 7.22**).

The last step in the resection is now at hand. The inferior aspect of the resection is delineated with an osteotome. An imaginary line is drawn between the most inferior aspect of the facial recess and its natural extension inferiorly, just lateral to the facial canal and the fissure previously created in the glenoid fossa with the bur. If the tympanic annulus and tympanic membrane can be preserved, which is often the case, then the posterior cut in the bony external canal is just lateral to the annulus and not through the facial recess. The excision then will be essentially of the external auditory canal only. This will take the osteotome across the tympanic bone just lateral to the tympanic annulus (**Fig. 7.23**). The technique is to tap the osteotome until it is well seated, and then with an alternating tapping and gentle lateral torquing motion drive the instrument in an anterosuperior direction. Usually the bone will fracture just lateral to the annulus. If the break is placed too far laterally, the remaining bone can be removed with the bur. Occasionally, the fracture will be too medially located. If so, a careful check is made to ensure

the integrity of the facial nerve. The medial course of the osteotome will carry it to the hypotympanum. In this instance, a fascia graft must be placed under the tympanic membrane and beneath the skin graft used to line the cavity.

The specimen is removed and the cavity inspected. Because of the complexity of the specimen and the difficulty the pathologist has in establishing margins, it is vital at this point to check the specimen and relate it to the defect, ensuring the integrity of the resection margins.

The cavity should be lined with split-thickness skin (see **Fig. 7.15**). This enables the physician to accurately follow the patient and pick up any early locally recurrent tumor. It is very tempting to fill the cavity with a flap for the sake of aesthetics; however, patient safety should never be sacrificed for this cosmetically laudable but oncologically unsound practice. The exception to this is the patient with a considerable amount of exposed dura or in whom the dura or underlying brain have been resected, especially if the patient has had irradiation therapy in the past (see **Fig. 7.16**). A bipedicled or unipedicled flap is used because of its proximity and hair-bearing qualities. For large defects, a deltopectoral or pectoralis major musculocutaneous flap or free flap (**Fig. 7.24**) may be used.

Prior to closure, interposition of a facial nerve cable graft is done to replace any of the three critical facial nerve branches that may have been sacrificed. A greater auricular or sural nerve graft is performed under microscopic control. Approximately four to six 10–0 nylon sutures are used in the anastomosis.

The skin graft is bolstered with sponge or mechanics waste. A modified mastoid dressing is applied and changed only when the bandage is soaked. Unless the wound becomes purulent, the bolster is left in place unchanged for 10 days.

Total Temporal Bone Resection

The complete resection can be done entirely by the head and neck surgeon. However, a margin of expertise and safety is added by including a neurological surgeon in the operative team. This is because, although management of the dura and

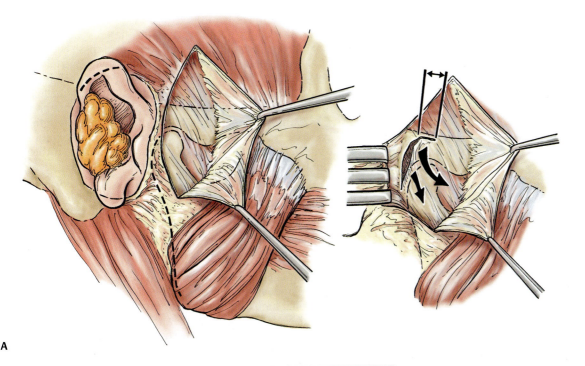

A

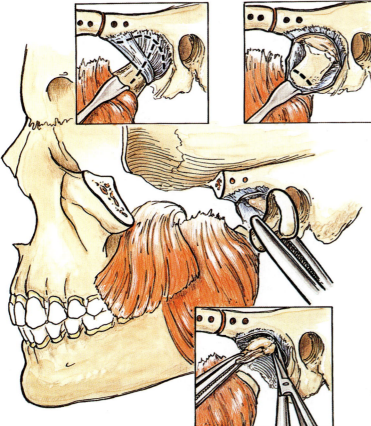

B

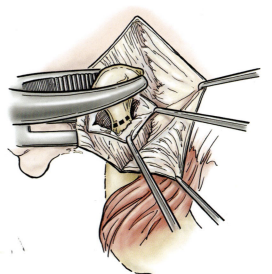

C

Fig. 7.20 Lateral temporal bone resection: Condylectomy. (**A**) A short (3 to 4 mm) incision in fascia over the zygomatic root is extended by blunt dissection with the Joseph elevator. (**B**) The joint capsule is incised and the joint entered. The dissection is facilitated by downward traction exerted on the angle of the mandible. (**C**) A subperiosteal excision of the condyle helps avoid injury to the internal maxillary artery.

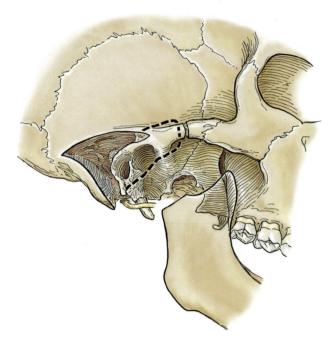

Fig. 7.21 Lateral temporal bone resection. A cutting bur incises the zygomatic arch and creates a fissure in the glenoid fossa to create a fracture line to enable excision of the bony external auditory canal.

dural sinuses is easy and routine for the neurosurgeon, it often adds unnecessary anxiety to the work of the head and neck surgeon who is "going it alone." The only drawback to having the neurosurgeon along is the potential difficulty of

dissuading him or her from using a static or semifixed headrest. The mobility necessary to do the mastoid portion of the operation is severely impeded by the use of these headrests.

A stepwise plan that is devised preoperatively and followed religiously *during* the procedure is exceedingly helpful. Because the operation is so complex and done so infrequently, the dictum of "doing the operation the night before on paper" is nowhere more important than in complete temporal bone resection. Following an orderly plan will avoid the time-wasting folly of jumping from place to place throughout the large operative field during the procedure.

The operation is divided into 11 steps: (1) incision, (2) parotidectomy, (3) neck dissection (if indicated), (4) mastoidectomy, (5) condylectomy, (6) anteroinferior exposure, (7) temporal craniotomy, (8) bony cuts, (9) cavity ablation, (10) hypoglossal to facial nerve graft, (11) closure. These are discussed in sequence in the following paragraphs.

1. *Incision.* The incision is similar to that for lateral temporal bone resection except that both anterior and posterior cranial limbs are carried more superiorly (**Fig. 7.17**). This is necessary to perform the small temporal craniotomy required for the medial bone cut. If the auricle is uninvolved, an incision encircling the extreme lateral aspect of the external auditory canal and the cavum concha will leave the involved part with the specimen. The auricular remnant is left attached in the superiorly based flap. The superficial temporal artery can be preserved if possible, but even with both it and the occipital artery cut, the flap will usually survive because of the wealth of collateral supply over the vertex. Rainey clips used on the incised scalp help to achieve hemostasis. Dissection of the flaps is done widely enough to expose the parotid gland, the temporal squama,

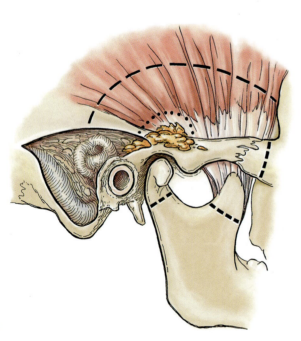

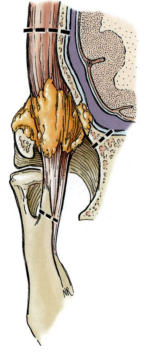

Fig. 7.22 Lateral temporal bone resection. (**A**) Extension of tumor into the zygomatic root requires excision of the arch up to the lateral orbital rim. The temporalis muscle is excised as well in the patient shown in **Fig. 7.15**. (**B**) The underlying skull and dura require resection as well.

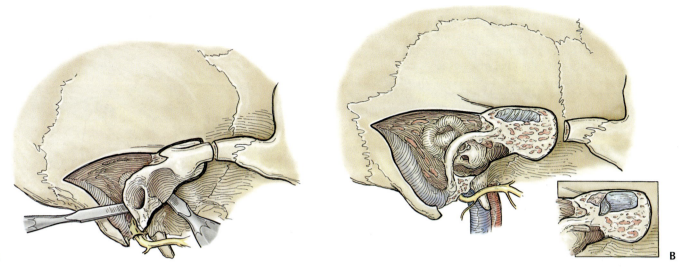

Fig. 7.23 Lateral temporal bone resection. (**A**) The osteotome is placed anteriorly in the fissure cut in the glenoid fossa, just medial to the tympanic bone, and posteriorly through the facial recess. A gentle tapping action with the hammer followed by a twisting of the osteotome usually results in a fracture in the desired plane. (**B**) Resection completed with margin deep to the tympanic annulus. Facial nerve is intact. (*Inset*) Inadvertent exposure of middle fossa dura is not uncommon and is covered with a skin graft.

the temporomandibular joint, and the mastoid tip with its attached muscles.

2. *Parotidectomy.* The parotid gland, including both superficial and deep lobes, should be resected in all cases. The facial nerve is dissected and any tumor involvement excised with a wide margin. The main trunk or branches are clearly tagged for the hypoglossal to facial crossover anastomosis later on. Even if cervical adenopathy is present, the parotid should be done first, because of the problems of increased hemorrhage brought about by internal jugular vein ligation.

The facial nerve branches are very gently retracted with a nerve hook as the deep lobe is separated from the nerve. This lobe can extend a long way along the undersurface of the mandibular ramus. It is often difficult to separate the

last remnants of deep lobe that abut the undersurface of the temporal bone deep to the facial nerve as it exits the stylomastoid foramen.

3. *Neck dissection.* Either before or after the parotidectomy, exploration of the lymphatics of the upper neck is done in search of possible metastatic disease. The preauricular, subauricular, and postauricular nodal areas are examined. Suspicious nodes are submitted for frozen section analysis; if they are found positive for cancer, a radical neck dissection is performed. If the postauricular nodes are positive for tumor, then the occipital nodes and usually a strip of underlying trapezius muscle are resected.

At this stage, control of the internal carotid artery and— if a neck dissection is not done—the internal jugular vein is secured. Vascular loops are passed around the internal

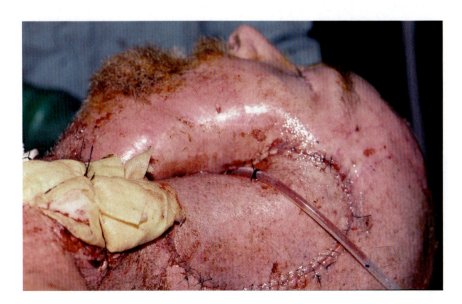

Fig. 7.24 Reconstruction of total temporal bone resection with pectoralis musculocutaneous flap.

jugular vein and external and internal carotid arteries (**Fig. 7.25**). If a major vessel within the temporal bone is inadvertently breached during resection, instant pressure is exerted by tightening the loops, to prevent the rapid exsanguination that would otherwise ensue.

In cases in which the neck is not dissected, the origin of the sternocleidomastoid muscle is then severed from the mastoid tip. The posterior belly of the digastric muscle is

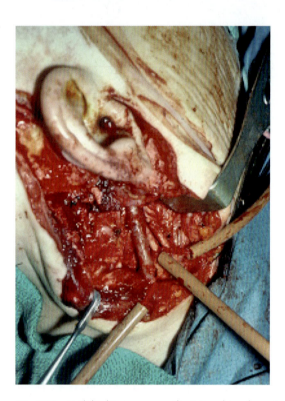

Fig. 7.25 Umbilical tapes secure the internal jugular vein and the internal carotid artery in case of inadvertent massive hemorrhage.

removed from the digastric groove and dissected anteriorly. Just medial to this muscle is the groove for the occipital artery. This artery is isolated and ligated (**Fig. 7.26**).

The styloid process is now isolated deep to the artery and anteriorly. The inferior margin of resection is medial to the process against which lies the lateral lip of the jugular foramen. The stylopharyngeus and styloglossus muscles are dissected from the styloid to facilitate the correct placement of the osteotome.

4. *Mastoidectomy.* In the original descriptions of temporal bone resection a saw chisels and gouges were used for this dissection. The operational concept of the procedure was an en bloc resection. Currently the surgeon uses the bur to perform a modified mastoidectomy that will establish a tumor-free plane to enable the final en bloc tumor removal with osteotomes. Even if tumor is actually encountered during the mastoidectomy portion of the resection, complete tumor removal can be effected using the drill. Tumor-free margins need to be insured, which may mean periodically sampling dura and cancellous bone for frozen-

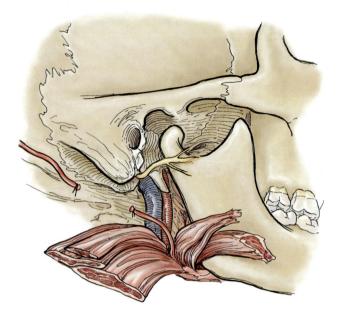

Fig. 7.26 Total temporal bone resection. The mastoid tip is exposed by incision and transposition of the sternomastoid muscle. The digastric muscle is prized from its sulcus, and the occipital artery lying deep to it is tied. The vaginal process over the styloid process together with the styloid process itself is exposed by dissecting the styloid muscles from it.

section evidence of disease. A complete mastoidectomy is done with excision of the tip and careful skeletonization of the sigmoid sinus. The cerebellar plate is skeletonized deep to it. An osteotome driven through this thin lamina will establish the posterolateral resection margin. The tegmen mastoideum and the sinodural angle are definitively outlined. The latter is a vital spot because it is near the junction of the superior petrosal and lateral venous sinuses.

An atticotomy is done extending to the zygomatic root. Extent of disease may now be more precisely defined because a full view of the epitympanum and mesotympanum can be obtained. A facial recess aperture may be required to facilitate the latter (**Fig. 7.27**).

5. *Condylectomy.* If not done at the time of parotidectomy, this step is now performed. A triangular cuff of soft tissue is raised over the proximal zygomatic arch to expose the temporomandibular joint while at the same time protecting the facial nerve (**Fig. 7.20**). The joint capsule is incised and the joint entered. An incision in the periosteum of the mandibular neck permits an intraperiosteal dissection of the condyle. The neck is cut across with the bone needle. Staying within the periosteum avoids injury to the internal maxillary artery. While grasping the condyle with bone-holding forceps, the surgeon cuts away the remaining soft tissue connections.

This exposes the glenoid fossa, through which a connection between the craniotomy and the anteroinferior bone cut will be made in the final stages of the resection.

6. *Anteroinferior exposure.* The zygomatic arch is transected just anterior to the articular eminence with a cutting bur or a bone needle. The glenoid fossa is cut inferiorly. The

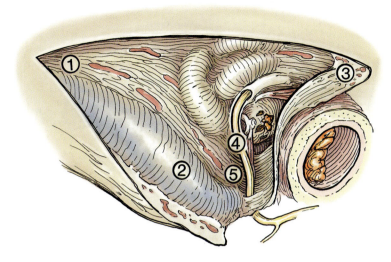

Fig. 7.27 Total temporal bone resection. The mastoidectomy is completed, including 1, a clearly defined sinodural angle; 2, a well-skeletonized sigmoid plate; 3, an atticotomy extending into the zygomatic root; 4, a skeletonized facial nerve and open facial recess; and 5, a well-delineated retrofacial space.

cut in the glenoid fossa is only 2 or 3 mm deep because of the proximity of the internal carotid artery, which is at a variable depth from the surface (**Fig. 7.28**). The artery, because of its thin media, is particularly vulnerable to injury in its intratemporal course. As the superior aspect of this incision is made, care is taken to avoid cutting across the middle meningeal artery.

The resection line proceeds along the glenoid fossa toward the styloid process. If the styloid muscles had not been completely stripped from the process earlier, this step is now done. In this anteroinferior aspect of the resection it is important to keep in mind that the deep limit of this bony cut is the internal carotid artery as it enters the skull via the carotid canal, and the internal jugular vein as it exits the jugular foramen. The carotid canal is more

anteriorly and deeply placed, located just deep to the most anterior extent of the tympanic process of the temporal bone. The jugular fossa is just behind it in a slightly lateral direction toward the more posterior part of the tympanic bone and the styloid process. The purpose of the fissure cut in the bone just lateral to these vessels is to provide a groove to safely seat the osteotome.

7. *Temporal Craniotomy.* The temporal craniotomy is most expeditiously outlined according to the method described by Montgomery.[28] A cutting bur is used to outline a small bony incision in the temporal squama. The incision should extend in a smooth arc from the sinodural angle to a point 4 cm above the external auditory canal, and then arch forward to the cut in the zygomatic arch (**Fig. 7.29**). Before extending the cut to the dura, the intracranial fluid volume is diminished by extracting cerebrospinal fluid either from a previously placed lumbar drain, through a lumbar puncture, or by use of an osmotic diuretic such as mannitol.

Next the inner table of skull is carefully cut through and the bone flap carefully dissected from the underlying dura. This is usually fairly easy to do, except in the elderly, in whom the dura is brittle and adherent to the skull. This part of the procedure may be done by either the neurosurgeon or the head and neck surgeon. I prefer to cut the bone flap myself and leave the rest to the neurosurgeons. The purpose of this operative step is to control the superior petrosal sinus and the middle meningeal artery, detect and resect any dural invasion or temporal lobe extension if possible, and establish the medial margin of resection. As the temporal lobe dura is elevated from the floor of the middle fossa and retracted with a Teflon-coated retractor, the superior petrosal sinus is prized from its fissure in the posterosuperior extremity of the temporal bone (**Fig. 7.29**). This elevation proceeds toward the cavernous sinus and Meckel cave, judiciously staying lateral to them.

Exposure of the middle fossa floor to the portion of temporal bone medial to the arcuate eminence is done with the dural elevator.

All aspects of the circumference of the temporal bone are now outlined, and final bony cuts may now be made. Up to

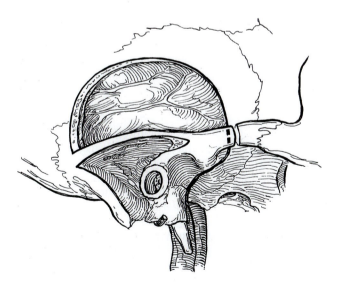

Fig. 7.28 Total temporal bone resection. The glenoid fossa is cut across medially and often transects the eustachian tube and proceeds into the middle cranial fossa. This latter extension may be delayed until the completion of the craniotomy. The inferior aspect of the fissure is carried down to the level of the medial aspect of the styloid process.

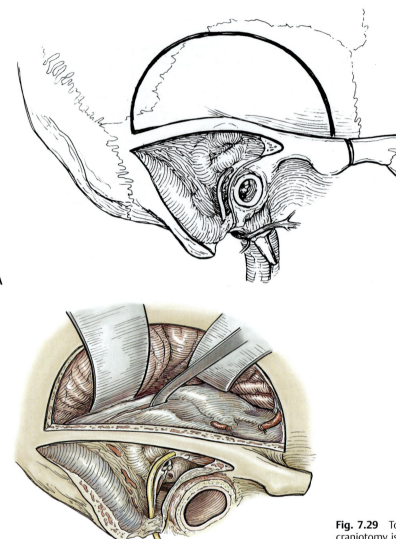

A

B

Fig. 7.29 Total temporal bone resection. (**A**) The temporal craniotomy is outlined with the cutting bur. (**B**) The temporal lobe is elevated and the superior petrosal sinus elevated from its sulcus.

this point all the bony exposure has been the result of the use of the combination cutting bur and the Midas Rex cutting needle (Medtronic, Inc., Minneapolis, MN). Most of the remaining steps will be done with osteotomes.

8. *Final bony cuts.* This critical part of the resection is where most surgical disasters occur. The problem is that the internal cuts that will sever the temporal bone from the skull run adjacent to the course of the internal carotid artery and the jugular bulb. Injury to the latter structure is no great problem because bleeding can be controlled from below by the vascular loop and from above through tamponade of the sigmoid or lateral sinuses. However, hemorrhage from a rent in the internal carotid can be life threatening given that bleeding can be only partially controlled in the neck. Moreover, occlusion of the vessel may result in stroke and even death. Preoperative assessment with an internal carotid balloon test occlusion and single photon emission computed tomography (SPECT) scan will establish the necessity of carotid grafting or the safety of internal carotid artery sacrifice (see chapter 9).

Osteotome cuts are initiated at the following sites:
1. Posteriorly through the back surface of the bone at its most medial aspect, through the most medial limit of cerebellar plate skeletonization
2. From cut #1 a superolaterally directed bony incision is made to the sinodural angle. A cut through the tegmen mastoideum connects this to the craniotomy and is carried medially.
3. Inferiorly just medial to the styloid process and directly lateral to the jugular bulb. This cut is directed superiorly and slightly medially.
4. Anteroinferiorly through the fissure in the glenoid fossa
5. The "coup de grâce": superiorly through the floor of the middle fossa just medial to the arcuate eminence (**Fig. 7.30**)

These bony incisions are made with an osteotome. The instrument is guided toward the theoretical center of the temporal bone near the internal acoustic meatus by being angled slightly medially. A gentle tapping with the mallet is followed by a slight twisting of the osteotome.

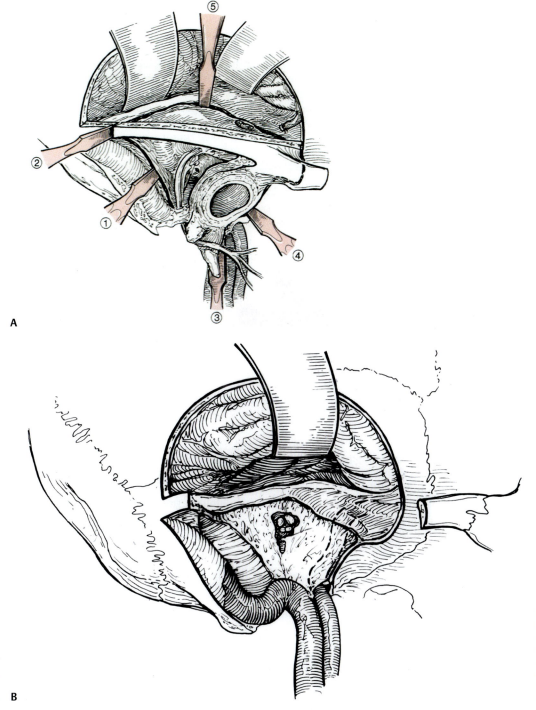

A

B

Fig. 7.30 Total temporal bone resection. (**A**) The five osteotome cuts necessary to finally excise the bone are outlined. (The numbers correspond to those in the text.) (**B**) Defect following excision.

This results in a more controlled type of incision. The cut made medial to the arcuate eminence has to penetrate the otic capsule and thus requires a more brisk blow with the hammer.

Anteroinferiorly the cutting and twisting motion of the osteotome usually results in the bone splitting along the plane of the initial ascending portion of the internal carotid artery. The bone is most commonly transected through either the cochlea or the internal auditory canal.

9. *Cavity ablation*. If the bone transection is quite medial in the internal auditory canal, a cerebrospinal fluid leak may result. A fat graft taken from the subcutaneous area of the abdomen and placed at the site of the leak is usually an effective plug.

Temporalis muscle flaps may be used to ablate the cavity. However, the cavity should not be so effaced that possible tumor recurrences might be obscured in their early stages.

303

The most important aspect of closure is the careful replacement of any resected dura with fascia together with the securing of a watertight closure of any rents. Occasionally, because of the extensive resection of temporal lobe dura and even temporal lobe of the brain, the area is covered by a pectoralis musculocutaneous flap or a rectus abdominis free flap (**Fig. 7.24**).

10. *Hypoglossal to facial nerve.* Full temporal bone resection always necessitates transection of the facial nerve. Although some thought may be given to cable grafting the nerve, this connection must extend from the proximal internal acoustic canal to the transected main trunk near the resected parotid bed. This is a difficult maneuver, and I have elected in most cases to do a hypoglossal to facial nerve crossover anastomosis.

The hypoglossal nerve is cut as far down in the neck as possible so the anastomosis will be tension free. The approximation is made under microscopic control using 10–0 nylon sutures. About 10 sutures are placed through the epineurium of these nerves (**Fig. 7.31**).

11. *Closure.* When a portion of the auricle remains, the flap is returned, and the gap created by the conchal and external canal skin excision is bridged with a split-thickness skin graft. The graft is inverted into the cavity and packed with iodoform or antibiotic-impregnated gauze packing. The graft is sutured to the auricular cut edges, and the remaining wound in the neck and scalp is closed with interrupted sutures.

The neck is drained and a large pressure dressing applied or suction drains are used. Excision of the entire auricle occasionally presents a problem in closure. Because most patients who are afflicted with temporal bone carcinoma are elderly, an elevation of the facial skin similar to that of a facelift will enhance flap advancement. When this is not enough, a relaxation incision can be done and a bipedicled scalp flap advanced into the wound. The donor site on the skull is skin grafted and the wound closed and drained.

Transcervical-Transmastoid Resection

Management of acoustic neuroma is beyond the scope of this book. However, some vasoformative and neurogenic tumors originate within the temporal bone and extend into the neck, or have a cervical origin and spread superiorly, usually through the neural or vascular foramina of the bone.

Nonchromaffin staining paragangliomas arise most commonly on the jugular vein (glomus jugulare), at the carotid bifurcation (carotid body tumor), or on the vagus nerve (glomus vagale). The large tumors that present simultaneously in the neck and ear require a combined transcervical and transtemporal approach. If the tumor extends to the posterior or middle fossa, this approach may need to be augmented by a transcranial exposure.

Most procedures described for the removal of these tumors require either mobilization and transposition of the facial nerve or its transection and later reconstruction. A transoccipital, retrofacial approach described initially by Gardner et al[29] and then by Mischke and Balkany[30] provides an excellent exposure between the occiput and the transverse process of C1 without mobilization of the facial nerve and often with preservation of hearing. A small occipital craniotomy in continuity with the mastoid defect provides the necessary exposure of the posterior fossa contents so that the continuity of the tumor can be adequately visualized and the neoplasm easily removed.

The head is placed in the lateral position and flexed acutely forward. The usual postauricular incision for mastoidectomy is made ~2 cm posterior to the postauricular crease and extended into the neck, similar to the inferior limb of the modified Blair parotidectomy incision. A superiorly placed limb arching posteriorly over the occiput gives excellent access for an occipital craniotomy (**Fig. 7.32**). The incision is placed through skin and mastoid periosteum and the auricle dissected anteriorly.

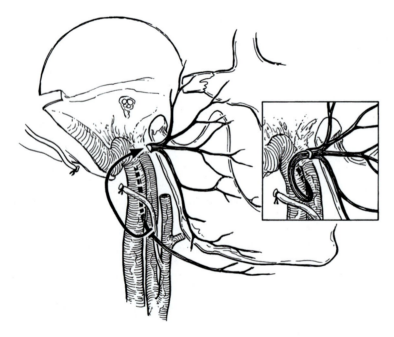

Fig. 7.31 Total temporal bone resection. Hypoglossal nerve to facial nerve crossover anastomosis.

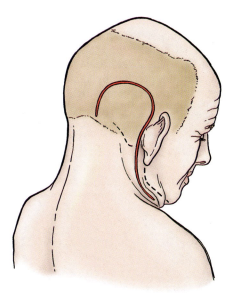

Fig. 7.32 Patient's head is flexed acutely forward, and a postauricular incision is directed posterosuperiorly over the occipital scalp and anteroinferiorly toward the hyoid bone.

The inferior limb of the incision exposes the contents of the upper neck. The sternocleidomastoid, lateral trapezius, and posterior belly of the digastric muscle are dissected from the mastoid tip and occipital bone. In addition, some of the laterally placed deep cervical muscles inserting on the occiput are dissected from the calvarium; specifically the splenius capitis, longissimus capitis, and even the obliquus capitis superior. This opens a space up between the undersurface of the temporal bone and the transverse process of C1 (**Fig. 7.33**).

A complete mastoidectomy is performed, with emphasis on careful skeletonization of the sigmoid sinus and the facial canal. The mastoid tip is completely removed with a Lem-

pert rongeur, and at least 180 degrees of the sigmoid sinus is skeletonized. It becomes readily apparent that as the inferior aspect of the sigmoid approaches the region of the facial canal it begins to sharply deviate medially, moving deeply into the substance of the temporal bone. As the facial nerve is skeletonized, it is important to preserve a surrounding thin shell of bone to protect it during the subsequent resection. The stylomastoid foramen is also skeletonized, and the part of the nerve that exits the foramen is exposed for a short distance. The subsequent dissection is performed deep to the nerve both in its mastoid and upper cervical parts.

At this point attention is turned to the neck. The internal jugular vein and internal carotid artery are identified below the cervical extent of tumor. An umbilical tape is placed around each in case of sudden hemorrhage. Preoperative embolization of any feeding vessels as well as nitroprusside-induced hypotension during the part of the operation in which the tumor is being dissected helps immensely in reducing blood loss. As dissection proceeds, meticulous care must be exercised to preserve the vagus, hypoglossal, and spinal accessory nerves as well as the sympathetic plexus. Unfortunately, in the case of large tumors, impairment of these nerves may already have occurred preoperatively as a result of tumor encroachment in the jugular foramen.

Dissection of the tumor at the carotid bifurcation may produce wide fluctuations in pulse rate. Deposition of lidocaine in this region is advised prior to tumor manipulation. The space between the proximal internal and external carotids and the skull base is very narrow. This is the parapharyngeal space. Strong lateral traction on the angle of the mandible with a large bone hook opens it up. This is often sufficient; but if not, a transverse osteotomy of the mandibular ramus provides excellent exposure. The osteotomy is done between the insertions of the lateral and medial pterygoid muscles. If the transection is high enough, transection of the inferior alveolar neurovascular bundle may be avoided. A stair-step osteotomy is done to facilitate approximation later (**Fig. 7.34**).

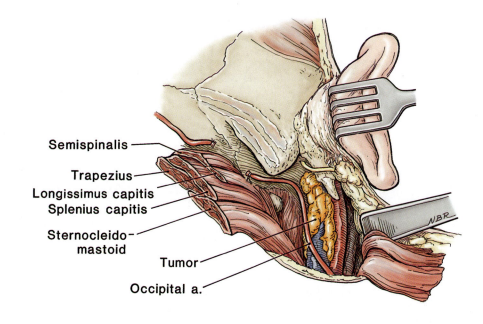

Fig. 7.33 Incision of the sternocleidomastoid, trapezius, posterior belly of digastric, splenius capitis, and longissimus capitis opens up a space between the mastoid tip and C1.

Semispinalis

Trapezius

Longissimus capitis

Splenius capitis

Sternocleido-mastoid

Tumor

Occipital a.

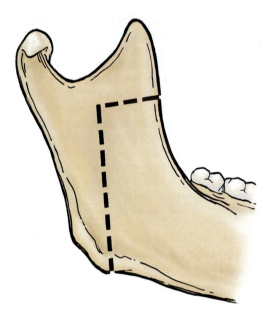

Fig. 7.34 A stair-step osteotomy is done in the mandibular ramus and the bone reflected to improve visualization of the skull base.

Sectioning of the stylomandibular ligament as it inserts on the medial aspect of the mandibular angle facilitates retraction of the fragments and enhances the exposure of the great vessels all along their course to the skull base. The internal jugular vein is ligated just below the tumor and the vessel transected (**Fig. 7.35**).

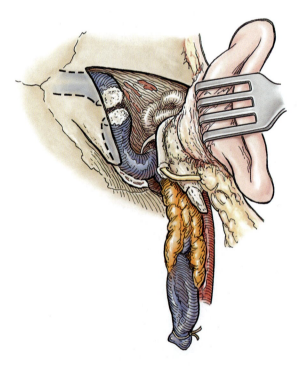

Fig. 7.35 The internal jugular vein is tied below the skull base, and the sigmoid sinus is controlled with a hemostatic absorbable cotton plug.

The tumor is now approached from both above and below the jugular foramen. Returning to the ear, the sigmoid sinus is dissected deep to the facial nerve until the point where it becomes the jugular bulb. The jugular bulb and attached tumor are exposed as much as possible by finally removing a portion of the posterolateral rim of the jugular foramen (**Fig. 7.36**).

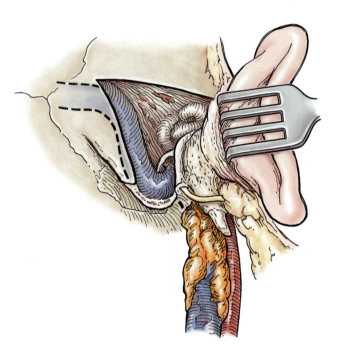

Fig. 7.36 The final portion of the tumor is exposed by removing bone lateral to the sigmoid sinus and the lateral lip of the jugular foramen.

Bleeding from the lateral venous sinus is controlled either by circumferential ligation or by venorrhaphy and stuffing the lumen with hemostatic gauze. The sigmoid sinus is transected and with contained tumor is dissected toward the foramen. Near the jugular bulb the inferior petrosal sinus is identified, transected, and plugged with surgical gauze (**Fig. 7.37**). This site is the most troublesome area for bleeding during the procedure.

The infratemporal portion of the tumor is delivered into the neck and the specimen removed. In the case of intracranial extension, which is usually into the posterior fossa, an occipital craniotomy is done in continuity with the mastoid defect. Dura is reflected and tumor removed (**Fig. 7.38**). The mandible is plated, a suction drain placed, and the wound closed.

Temporal Bone Resection with Petrous Apicectomy

At the completion of a "total temporal bone resection" usually not all of the temporal bone has been excised. The petrous tip and the bone immediately lateral to the internal acoustic canal as well as some of the bone housing the labyrinth often still remains. At times small amounts of residual tumor may

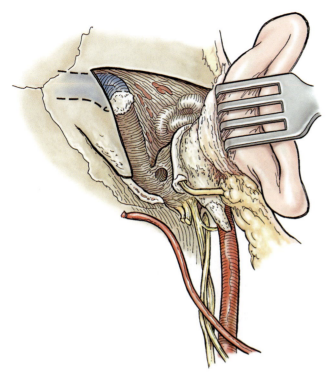

Fig. 7.37 Bleeding from the inferior petrosal sinus is controlled with a hemostatic cotton plug.

anteriorly toward the cavernous sinus. Management of this structure and adjacent areas is covered in chapter 9. As progression from the cochlear portion of the temporal bone is made the diminishing triangular aspect of the petrous bone is appreciated (**Fig. 7.39**). A relatively small venous sinus exists at the suture line between the temporal bone tip and the sphenoidal contribution to the clivus, which sometimes bleeds profusely (**Fig. 7.40**).

be seen within the remaining bone. Further osteotome cuts to obtain a more medial margin are extremely dangerous. A cutting bur is used to remove them with a healthy margin of petrous bone or even beyond the suture with adjacent clival sphenoid bone. Tumor may extend more medially and

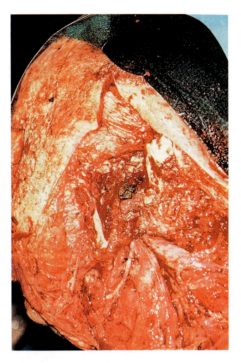

Fig. 7.39 Complete temporal bone resection showing petrous apex.

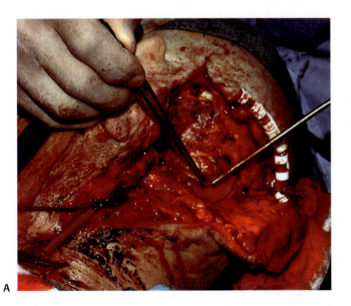

A

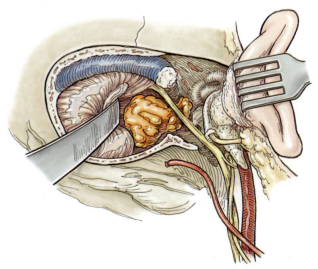

B

Fig. 7.38 (**A**) Massive glossopharyngeal schwannoma, with tissue forceps shown grasping cerebellar dura. Arrow indicated tumor in the mastoid extending into the posterior cranial fossa. (**B**) Drawing of lesion in (**A**). Extensions into the posterior fossa are exposed by occipital craniotomy and reflection of cerebellar dura.

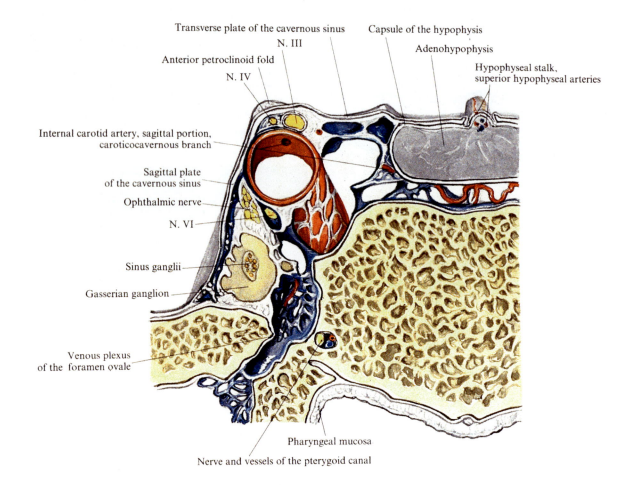

Transverse plate of the cavernous sinus
N. III
Anterior petroclinoid fold
N. IV
Capsule of the hypophysis
Adenohypophysis
Hypophyseal stalk, superior hypophyseal arteries
Internal carotid artery, sagittal portion, caroticocavernous branch
Sagittal plate of the cavernous sinus
Ophthalmic nerve
N. VI
Sinus ganglii
Gasserian ganglion
Venous plexus of the foramen ovale
Pharyngeal mucosa
Nerve and vessels of the pterygoid canal

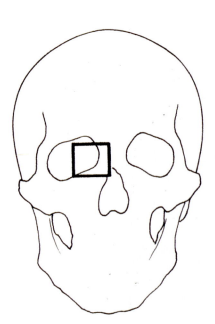

Fig. 7.40 Illustration of carotid artery in cavernous sinus near the foramen lacerum. Note substantial venous structure in the suture line between the petrous tip and the sphenoidal contribution to the clivus.

References

1. Bumstead RM, Ceilley RI, Panje WR, et al. Auricular malignant neoplasms: when is chemotherapy (Mohs technique) necessary? Arch Otolaryngol 1981;107:721–724

2. Bumstead RM, Ceilley RI. Auricular malignant neoplasms. Arch Otolaryngol 1982;108:225–231

3. Mohs FE. Mohs micrographic surgery: a historical perspective. Dermatol Clin 1989;7:609–612

4. Mohs FE. Microscopically controlled surgery for skin cancer: past, present and future. J Dermatol Surg Oncol 1978;4:41–53

5. Mohs FE. Chemosurgery: Microscopically Controlled Surgery for Skull Cancer. Springfield, IL: Charles C Thomas; 1978

6. Campbell E, Volk BM, Burkland CW. Total resection of the temporal bone for malignancy of the middle ear. Ann Surg 1951;134:397–404

7. Parsons H, Lewis JS. Subtotal resection of the temporal bone for cancer of the ear. Cancer 1954;7:995–1001

8. Conley J. Concepts in Head and Neck Surgery. New York: Grune & Stratton; 1970:69

9. Lewis JS. Temporal bone resection. Arch Otolaryngol 1975;101:23–25

10. Conley J, Schuller DE. Malignancies of the ear. Laryngoscope 1976; 86:1147–1163

11. Chen KTK, Dehner LP. Primary tumors of the external and middle ear. Arch Otolaryngol 1978;104:247–252

12. Bailin PL, Levine HL, Wood BG, et al. Cutaneous carcinoma of the auricular and periauricular region. Arch Otolaryngol 1980;106:692–696

13. Ceilley RI, Bumstead RM, Smith WH. Malignancies on the external ear: methods of ablation and reconstruction of defects. J Dermatol Surg Oncol 1979;5:762–767

14. Pulec JL. Glandular tumors of the external auditory canal. Laryngoscope 1977;87:1601–1612

15. Lambert DR, Siegel RJ. Skin cancer: a review with consideration of treatment options including Moh's micrographic surgery. Ohio Med 1990;86:745–747

16. Barnes L, Peel R. Diseases of the external auditory canal, middle ear, and temporal bone. In: Barnes L, ed. Surgical Pathology of the Head and Neck. Vol 1. 2nd ed. New York: Marcel Dekker; 2001:557–559

17. Wetli CV, Pardo V, Millard M, et al. Tumors of ceruminous glands. Cancer 1972;29:1169–1178

18. Schuknecht HE. Neoplastic growth. In: Pathology of the Ear. Schuknecht HF, ed. Cambridge, MA: Harvard University Press; 1974:420

19. Myers EN, Stool S, Weltschew MA. Rhabdomyosarcoma of the middle ear. Ann Otol Rhinol Laryngol 1968;77:949–958

20. Karatay S. Rhabdomyosarcoma of the middle ear. Arch Otolaryngol 1949;50:330–334

21. Lewis JS. Tumors of the external ear and temporal bone in otolaryngology. In: English GM, ed. Otolaryngology. Vol 2. Hagerstown, MD: Harper & Row; 1979:chapter 26

22. Naufal PM. Primary sarcomas of the temporal bone. Arch Otolaryngol 1973;98:44–50

23. Mohs FE. Chemosurgery for skin cancer: fixed tissues and fresh tissue techniques. Arch Dermatol 1976;112:211–215

24. Fredericks S. External ear malignancy. Br J Plast Surg 1956;9:136–160

25. Pless J. Carcinoma of the external ear. Scand J Plast Reconstr Surg 1976;10:147–151

26. Blake GB, Wilson JSP. Malignant tumors of the ear and their treatment. Br J Plast Surg 1974;27:67–76

27. Tromovitch TA, Stegman SJ. Microscopically controlled excision of skin tumors: (Mohs) fresh technique. Arch Dermatol 1974;110:231–232

28. Montgomery WW. Surgery of the Upper Respiratory Tract. Vol 1. Philadelphia: Lea & Febiger; 1971:471

29. Gardner G, Cocke EW Jr, Robertson JT, et al. Combined approach surgery for removal of glomus jugular tumors. Laryngoscope 1977;87:665–688

30. Mischke RE, Balkany TJ. Skull base approach to glomus jugulare. Laryngoscope 1980;90:89–94

8

Cancer of the Salivary Glands

Paul J. Donald

Tumors of the salivary glands are unique among head and neck tumors in that their cell type may be of epithelial or glandular origin or a mixture of both. Each specific gland appears to have a peculiar predisposition to develop a particular variety of tumor with a greater frequency than its neighbor does. This is true both of the quality of benignity versus malignancy and of the specific cell type. The salivary glands are classified as major or minor and are principally ringed in a roughly U-shaped pattern around the oral cavity. The parotid, submandibular, and sublingual are the major glands, whereas the small submucosal glands of the oral cavity make up the minor glands. Other minor salivary glands are found throughout the upper air and food passageway, but these appear to be firmly resistant to the development of neoplasms. The oral cavity is the site of 95% of the tumors of minor salivary gland origin.[1]

◆ Anatomy

A thorough knowledge of the anatomy of these glands aids in the anticipation of the pathophysiology of malignancies that may arise therein.

The paired parotid glands are wrapped around the vertical rami of the mandible. The superficial lobe is lateral to the ramus and overlies the masseter muscle, whereas the deep lobe lies against the periosteum of the bone's medial surface and the medial pterygoid muscle (**Fig. 8.1**). The deep lobe resides between the medial pterygoid muscle medially and the styloid process laterally; the so-called stylomandibular tunnel (**Fig. 8.2**). The axial computed tomographic (CT) scan can clearly differentiate a deep lobe tumor from neoplasm of the carotid sheath by the former tumor's location in the stylomandibular tunnel and the latter's location posterior to the styloid process (**Fig. 8.3**). The facial nerve splits the gland into these two lobes. Although there is still some debate concerning the existence of an anatomical separation between them, dissection during surgery on the gland consistently re-

veals a facial plane at the level of the nerve (**Fig. 8.4**). The tail of the gland lies over the mastoid tip and may be of considerable size (**Fig. 8.5**). The gland abuts the anterior aspect of the external auditory canal and occasionally the undersurface of the temporal bone. It may extend superiorly to overlie the temporomandibular joint and the root of the zygomatic arch. The close relationship of the parotid to the mandible and external auditory canal requires their frequent inclusion in the resection of large tumors afflicting the gland. The deep lobe of the gland is intimately related to the external carotid artery. It may, especially if involved with a malignant tumor, involve both the internal jugular vein laterally and the internal carotid artery medially (**Fig. 8.6**). A third small accessory lobe is often found along the course of the Stensen duct. In one series of 96 consecutive cadaver dissections, an accessory lobe was found in 21 instances.[2]

As the parotid wraps around the mandible, the submandibular gland similarly wraps around the posterior edge of the mylohyoid muscle (**Fig. 8.1**). The amount of gland on the superior surface of the mylohyoid is highly variable. The superior portion of the gland is covered by oral mucosa, whereas the inframylohyoid part is wedged between the anterior belly of the digastric and the mylohyoid muscle. As the patient ages, the mylohyoid muscle relaxes and the gland becomes more of an upper cervical structure than a paramandibular one. This allows the gland to be more easily palpated by both physician and patient, occasionally frightening these patients into thinking they may have cancer. The ramus mandibularis of the facial nerve frequently courses across the gland superficial to the investing fascia. The hypoglossal and lingual nerves have a close relationship to the submandibular gland; the hypoglossal in the neck and the lingual to Wharton's duct in the floor of the mouth.

The sublingual gland is about one half the size of the submandibular gland, lying in the middle third of the floor of the mouth and related to the mylohyoid inferoposteriorly and to the inferior longitudinal portion of the hyoglossus medially. It may partially overlap the submandibular gland and at

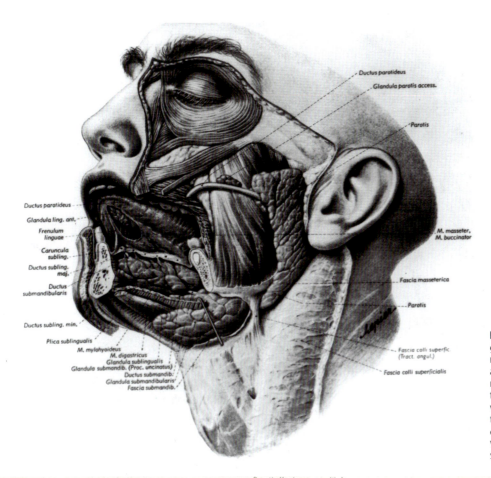

A

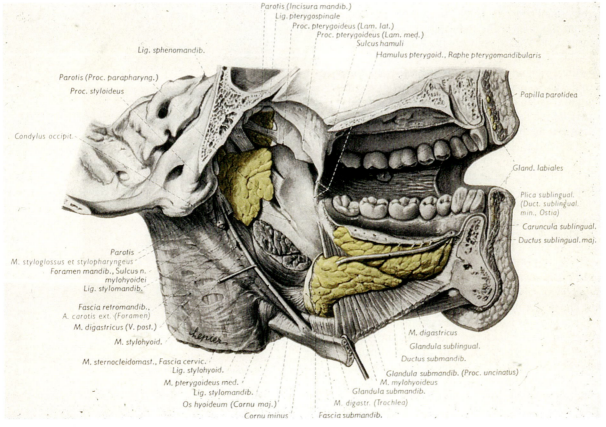

B

Fig. 8.1 The major salivary glands and their anatomical relations. (**A**) Lateral view with a portion of the body of the mandible removed to expose the sublingual gland. (**B**) Medial view of the salivary glands of the left side. (From Pernkopf E. Atlas of Topographical and Applied Anatomy. Vol 1: Head and Neck. Philadelphia: WB Saunders; 1980.)

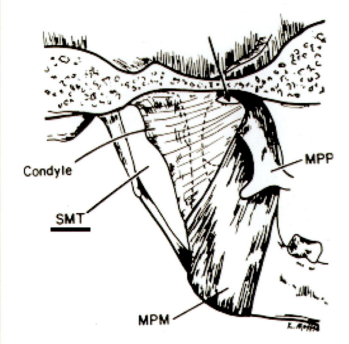

Fig. 8.2 The stylomandibular tunnel (SMT). MPM, ??; MPP, ??.

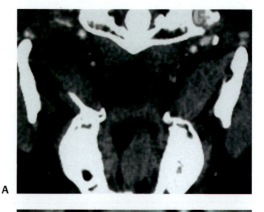

A

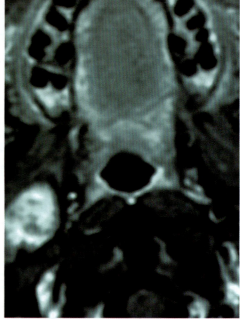

B

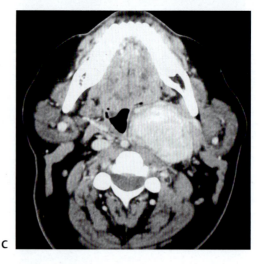

C

Fig. 8.3 (**A**) Axial view computed tomographic scan showing an apparent deep lobe parotid gland tumor in parapharyngeal space with small extension through the stylomandibular tunnel. (**B**) Axial view magnetic resonance imaging scan T1-weighted image showing parapharyngeal space tumor. (**C**) Parapharyngeal space tumor-vagal paraganglioma. Note location posteriorly to the carotid artery.

times appears almost in continuity with it. The gland abuts the lingual plate of the parasymphyseal aspect of the mandible. Anteromedially the gland is related to the genioglossus. The lingual nerve courses between this muscle and the gland. Numerous small short ducts lead from the gland and open directly into the floor of the mouth along the sublingual fold adjacent to the Wharton duct of the submandibular gland.[3,4]

The minor salivary glands are scattered throughout the oral mucosa and vary somewhat in form and function with their site of origin. The labial and buccal glands are situated in the submucosa of the lips and cheek. They may be extensive enough to penetrate through the fibers of the orbicularis oris and buccinator muscles. Although they are classically described as mixed serous and mucus-secreting glands similar in histological structure to the submandibular and sublingual glands, recent ultrastructural studies reveal evidence of mucous elements only. The glossopalatine glands extend along the palatoglossal fold. The palatine glands are richly distributed throughout the soft palate, making up half of its bulk. Both are of the pure mucous variety. The lingual minor salivary glands are anteriorly and posteriorly located. The anterior glands (Nuhn glands, or the glands of Blandin) are located in the undersurface of the tip of the tongue and are mixed in type. The posterior glands are of two types. Those of the mucous variety are lateral to the circumvallate papillae and related to the lingual tonsil. The more numerous serous glands (von Ebner glands) are entwined by lingual muscle in the posterior third of the tongue, lying under the circumvallate papillae and emptying into their troughs. They are also related to the foliate papillae on the posterolateral tongue surface.

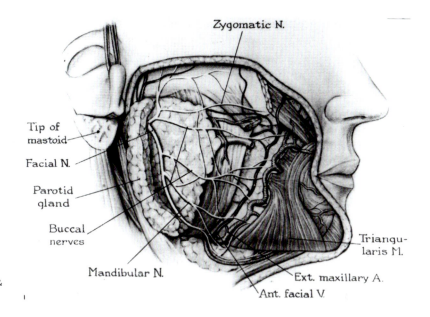

Fig. 8.4 The facial nerve branches separate the parotid gland at its superficial and deep lobes. (From Conley J. Salivary Glands and the Facial Nerve. New York: Grune & Stratton; 1975.)

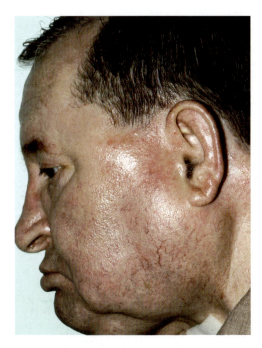

Fig. 8.5 Parotid gland hypertrophy showing enlargement of the glandular tail over the mastoid process.

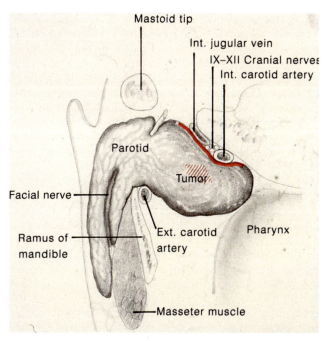

Fig. 8.6 Relationship of the deep lobe of the parotid gland to the external carotid artery. There is encroachment on the internal jugular vein and the internal carotid artery when the deep lobe of the gland is involved with tumor. (From Rankow RM, Polayes IM. Diseases of the Salivary Glands. Philadelphia: WB Saunders; 1976.)

◆ Pathology

In an attempt to sort out the most appropriate treatment of salivary gland cancer, one of the greatest dilemmas is to unravel the complexity of nomenclature that surrounds this protean group of tumors. A variety of classifications have emerged over the years, but considerable order was restored by the excellent work of Foote and Frazell in 1953).[5] Since then several investigators have contributed to the understanding of these lesions.[6–8] Kleinsasser, through an extensive investigation of the light- and electron-microscopic appearance of a large number of tumors, which he then correlated

with operative findings and personal clinical follow-up of the patients involved, has developed a most meaningful classification.[9] More recently Barnes[15] has produced a more complete classification of parotid tumors in a very understandable format (**Table 8.1**).

Pleomorphic Adenoma and Carcinoma

Pleomorphic adenoma is considered by most authorities to be a benign lesion with only a rare malignant variant. Benign

313

Table 8.1 Frequency of Malignant Mixed Tumors*

Authors	No. of Salivary Gland Tumors	No. of Malignant Mixed Tumors	Percentage of Malignant Mixed Tumors
Foote & Frazell	877	57	7
Eneroth	802	16	2
Morgan & Mackenzie	151	14	9.3
Moberger & Eneroth	2211	34	1.8
Skolnik et al	116	2	1.7
Brown et al	286	12	4.2
Mustard & Anderson	287	16	5.5
Wheelock et al	209	15	5.3
Freeman et al	545	5	0.9
Chaudhry et al	1414	29	2.0

*Except for the data from the study by Chaudhry et al, all other information is from a series dealing with the major salivary glands (predominantly the parotid gland).

mixed tumors, as they are also called, occur in the parotid gland 84% of the time[10] and represent 60 to 65% of all parotid tumors.[11] The malignant variant makes up only 2 to 5% of all mixed tumors (**Table 8.1**), and these are limited almost exclusively to the parotid gland. This neoplasm in its benign form has an unusual pathophysiological characteristic that distinguishes it from most other benign tumors. Without wide excision it has a marked propensity for local recurrence. This was initially thought to be due to the phenomenon of satellitosis or multicentricity. Using histological serial sectioning, Eneroth[12] established that the peculiar character of multiple tumor bosselations or outgrowths on the tumor's surface is responsible for the frequent recurrences following "lumpectomy" of benign mixed tumors.

Hubner et al established that pleomorphic adenomas originate from two stem cells of the ectodermal layer: the ductal epithelial cell and the myoepithelial cell.[13] They conceptualize that the malignant mixed tumor is a "new" cancer that arises within the substance of usually a longstanding benign pleomorphic adenoma. Its cell type is often mixed epidermoid and adenomatous. A focus of anarchistic cancer cells is seen to have developed in an otherwise perfectly unremarkable, benign-appearing pleomorphic adenoma. It is not thought of as a "degenerative process" because the lesion begins unifocally, without signs of such malignant transformation appearing elsewhere within the tumor. In support of this notion is the frequent finding of malignant degeneration being seen most commonly in those tumors that are of long standing.

The histological picture of pleomorphic adenoma is characteristic (**Fig. 8.7**). Cell lines of both epithelial and mesenchymal origin must be present to make the diagnosis. The appearance of stellate mesenchymal cells, islands of cartilage with chondrocytes, mucinous deposits, and structures resembling glandular acini provoked the name of "mixed tumor." Occasionally, a more spindle-shaped cell may predominate, in which case the lesion is called a monomorphic adenoma. The malignant variant is characterized by a par-

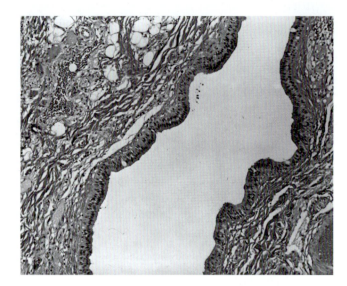

Fig. 8.7 Photomicrograph of patient with pleomorphic adenoma. Note large epithelium-lined cyst. Some chondroid and myxoid material is dispensed in loosely arranged connective tissue. (H&E, ×100)

tial or complete replacement of the usual cellular makeup of pleomorphic adenoma by a "malignification" of one or more of its cellular components (**Fig. 8.8**).

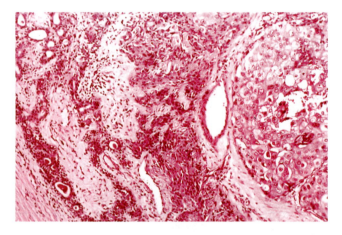

Fig. 8.8 Photomicrograph of patient with malignant mixed tumor. (H&E, ×90)

A painless hard lump that is often irregular in outline is the usual clinical presentation of pleomorphic adenoma. The tumor may attain considerable size and is occasionally cystic (**Fig. 8.9**). Malignant mixed tumors may be indistinguishable from the benign variety but may present with the common stigmata of malignancy: pain, fixation, and facial nerve paralysis.

Adenocarcinoma

Most neoplasms of benign or malignant type originate in the cells of the ductal elements of the gland. Adenocarcinomas by definition ought to include all those lesions that take their

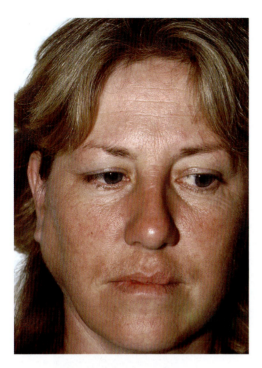

Fig. 8.9 Young woman with moderately sized pleomorphic adenoma containing a large cystic area.

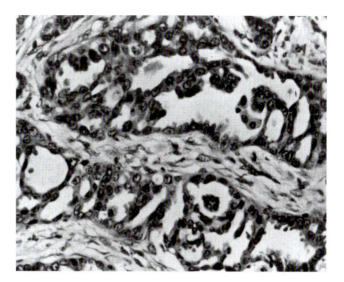

Fig. 8.10 Photomicrograph of a patient with adenocarcinoma of the parotid gland. Note similarity to gastrointestinal malignancy. (×250) (From Thackray AC, Lucas RB. Tumors in the major salivary glands. Fascicle 10. Atlas of Tumor Pathology. 2nd ed. Washington, DC: Armed Forces Institute of Pathology; 1974:101.)

origin in the glandular elements of the parenchyma. Strictly speaking, these cancers would be primarily from the serous or mucous acinar cells. Complicating the picture are those malignancies that are obviously glandular but for which no definitive stem cell can be identified, as well as others in the class of mucoepidermoid cancers that form mucin-secreting acini. Finally, many authorities, beginning with Foote and Frazell,[5] have included adenoid cystic carcinoma under the heading of adenocarcinoma.

Kleinsasser[9] used the term *adenocarcinoma* to comprise those lesions that could not be clearly identified as either acinic cell, adenoid cystic, mucoepidermoid, or mixed cancers. As Batsakis[14] has clearly outlined, many of the salivary adenocarcinomas are papillary or cystic, or both, in type, and closely resemble adenocarcinomas of the gastrointestinal tract (**Fig. 8.10**). However, many are rather undifferentiated, albeit glandular in type. Their biological behavior is variable, ranging from highly malignant to relatively benign depending on histological invasiveness rather than on any particular cellular structure. Barnes,[15] in his exhaustive text on pathology of the head and neck, describes four different varieties of adenocarcinoma: polymorphous low-grade adenocarcinoma, basal cell adenocarcinoma, adenosquamous carcinoma, and cystadenocarcinoma (sometimes called papillary adenocarcinoma). Polymorphous low-grade adenocarcinoma is predominantly a malignancy of the minor salivary glands of the oral cavity. Only 20% of them occur in the parotid salivary gland. They have a characteristic histology with a very bland appearance of columnar and cuboidal cells, no mitotic figures, and no necrosis. Their clinical behavior is highly variable, ranging from no recurrence after simple enucleation to widespread

recurrence after wide-field resection. Basal cell adenocarcinoma is the malignant equivalent of basal cell adenoma. It is a low-grade malignancy with rare to no incidence of regional or distant metastasis. Adenosquamous carcinoma has the histological characteristics of both adenocarcinoma and squamous cell carcinomas. It is highly malignant with a nodal metastatic rate of over 80% and a 5-year tumor-free survival rate of only 25%. Cystadenocarcinoma is so-called because of its pathognomonic histological appearance of large cysts. The lining epithelia are often thrown into papillary projections. Unlike the polymorphous low-grade adenocarcinoma with which it is often confused, cystadenocarcinoma is characterized by frequent metastasis and a poor prognosis.

Adenocarcinomas probably make up ~20% or less of the malignancies in the salivary glands and are found in both the major and the minor glands. The highly invasive type are extremely malignant and are characterized by frequent regional and distant metastases.[16] They present as hard, firm, mixed masses. They are rapid growing and frequently invade the mandible and temporal bone (**Fig. 8.11**). They may ulcerate through the overlying skin of these structures or that of the external auditory canal; invasion of the adjacent masseter muscle may produce trismus.

Acinic Cell Cancer

Acini of the salivary glands are serous, mucous, or mixed seromucinous in type. Tumors of the acinic type are almost exclusively serous (**Fig. 8.12**).[17,18] This has been proved not only by light microscopy (by which the zymogen granules of the tumor are seen to be identical to those of the normal serous acinar cell) but by ultrastructural and histochemical analysis as well. These acinic tumors are found almost exclusively in the superficial lobe and tail of the parotid gland and make up 2% of all tumors and 17 to 19% of all malignancies there. They

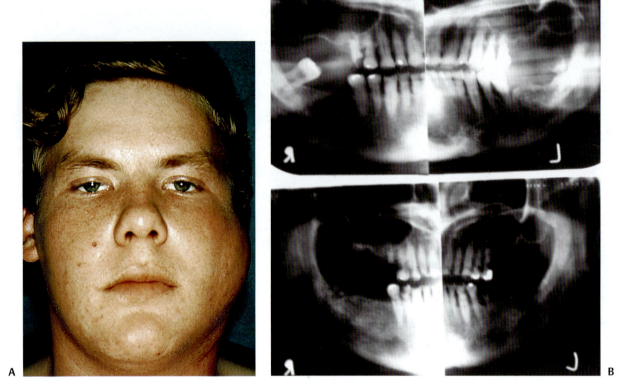

Fig. 8.11 (**A**) A 19-year-old male with a large adenocarcinoma of the parotid gland. (**B**) Orthopantomograph showing extensive erosion of the left mandibular ramus from tumor in (**A**). The patient died 1 year after radical resection of distant metastasis.

are rarely found in the submandibular and sublingual glands. Only seven acinous tumors of intraoral minor salivary gland origin have been identified.[19]

Histologically the tumors appear benign. It is impossible to differentiate those that will undertake a malignant course from the benign lesions. Fortunately, the benign variety is the most frequently encountered type; however, it is important to bear in mind that the pathologist cannot make a judgment concerning the malignancy or benignity of the tumor's

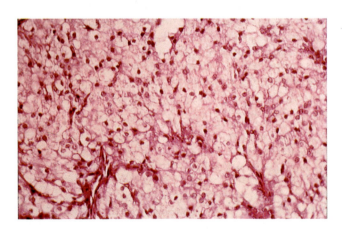

Fig. 8.12 Photomicrograph of acinic cell tumor of the minor salivary glands of the buccal mucosa. (H&E, ×100)

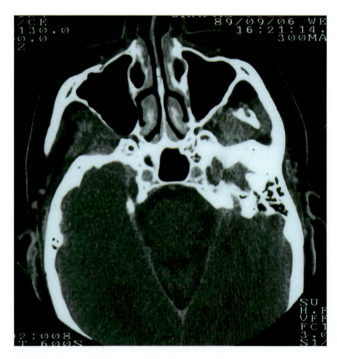

Fig. 8.13 Computed tomographic scan in coronal plane of patient with recurrent acinic cell carcinoma of the parotid resected by superficial lobe parotidectomy 12 years earlier.

eventual course on the basis of histology. Only the biological activity exhibited in each individual case can determine this. Two cellular variants of the serous cell exist—the granular and the clear cell. The clear cell type is very uncommon and its ultrastructural appearance suggests that it originates from ductal epithelial rather than acinar cells.

Acinic cell tumors are slow growing, and local recurrences are seen many years after primary excision (**Fig. 8.13**). Eneroth et al[20] quote a 90% 5-year survival and a 50% 25-year survival rate for patients with acinic cell cancer of the parotid gland. The patient whose CT scan is seen in **Fig. 8.13** exemplifies the findings of Eneroth. The patient had a recurrent acinic cell carcinoma 15 years after the primary resection in which we obtained negative margins. The recurrence was very extensive, invading the lateral pharynx from just above the pyriform sinus to the nasopharynx. Invading the infratemporal fossa, it extended up the foramen ovale, along V3 intracranially, and medially into the clivus. An extensive skull base resection included a lateral pharyngectomy from the aryepiglottic fold to the vault of the nasopharynx. The lateral clivus, infratemporal fossa, eustachian tube, floor of the middle cranial fossa and Meckel cave were also excised (**Fig. 8.14**). Reconstruction was done with a pectoralis major musculocutaneous flap (**Fig. 8.15**). She survived for 9 more years without local recurrence but eventually died of pulmonary metastasis.

A compendium of cases involving 296 patients revealed a local recurrence rate of 27%, a metastatic rate of 10.8%, and a mortality rate of 14%.[14]

Adenoid Cystic Cancer

Adenoid cystic carcinoma is an enigmatic tumor with an unpredictable course. It is locally invasive with a peculiar propensity to invade nerve sheaths (**Fig. 8.16**). This invasiveness can extend in discontinuity a considerable distance from the primary lesion. A not uncommon finding is that of nests of tumor cells along an involved nerve an unexpectedly long way from the main lesion, sometimes even as far as the cranial foramina. Metastases are both lymphatic and bloodborne. A tragic but more than occasional scenario in the treatment of these tumors is to have achieved local control only to be thwarted by a pulmonary nodule presenting 5 or 10 years after the initial resection. Because such a course is seen so often, an air of pessimism tends to pervade any consideration of management of these tumors.

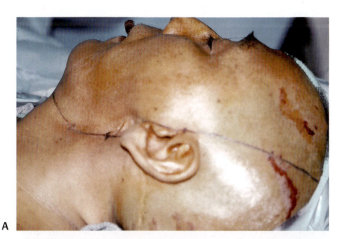

A

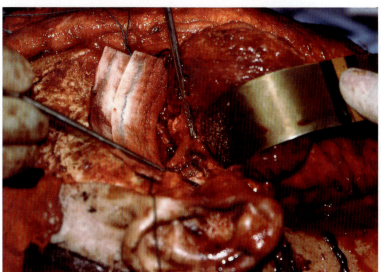

B

Fig. 8.14 Infratemporal fossa approach. (**A**) Incision marked out. (**B**) Infratemporal fossa exposed. Arrow shows tumor coursing along V3.

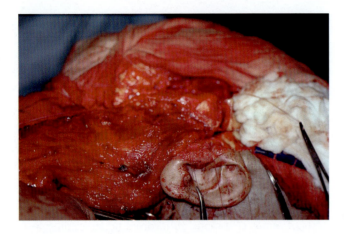

Fig. 8.15 Reconstruction of defect with pectoralis major musculocutaneous flap. Muscle with applied skin graft faces the pharyngeal excision. Pectoralis muscle fills the infratemporal fossa and extends along the floor of the resected middle fossa floor.

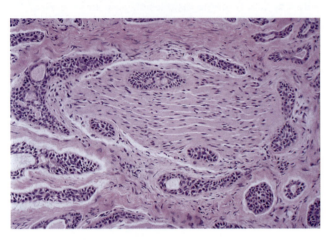

Fig. 8.16 Perineural invasion of adenoidcystic carcinoma.

The cell of origin is thought to be derived from the epithelium of the intercalated ducts. These basaloid cells often form a cribrose or lacy pattern and have a tendency to form glandular or cystlike structures. However, the cystic spaces may be missing and, because of its stromal component, made up of an eosinophilic hyaline or mucinous element, the tumor is occasionally confused with mucoepidermoid tumors or pleomorphic adenoma. The other two histological patterns are the solid and so-called tubular configurations. The solid type consists of a monotonous sheet of cells. The tubular configurations are represented by numerous small rounded structures; the result of cutting across closely packed thin tubules of cells (**Fig. 8.17**).[21]

Perzin et al[22] have shown an interesting correlation between survival and the predominant histological type of the tumor. Tumors with a 30% or greater solid pattern have the worst prognosis, whereas those with a predominantly tubular pattern have the best, with intermediate survival rates seen with tumors of the cribrose variety.

In an extensive review of the literature by Batsakis,[14] the parotid gland was found to be the site of origin of only 17.3% of all adenoid cystic tumors of head and neck origin. The submandibular and sublingual glands are much more common sites, and adenoid cystic tumors are the most prevalent type found in the minor salivary glands. In Conley's series,

58% of all adenoid cystic cancers were in these glands.[23] Conley's review of his experience with 134 adenoid cystic carcinomas graphically illustrates the metastatic potential of these tumors.[24] Pulmonary metastases occurred in 41% of his patients, 22% had secondaries in the brain, 16% in lymph nodes, 13% in bone, and 4% in other body organs. A fascinating aspect of these tumors is the ability of the patient to live for prolonged periods of time, even 5 years or longer, often asymptomatically, with obvious metastatic disease (**Fig. 8.18**). In Conley's series,[23] 42% of the patients had at least one local recurrence, and most had more.

There were several patients in Conley's series[24] who had repeated local recurrences that were controlled by repeated resection. Their survival ranged from 11 to 30 years. However, in my more limited experience, local recurrence in most instances heralded a demise from the disease within 1 to 2 years.

Adenoid cystic carcinoma is commonly painful and locally tender. The lesion may be present for a long time before the patient seeks medical attention. In the parotid gland, the lesion commonly causes a facial paralysis, which may be the presenting symptom in the absence of a palpable mass.[22] Because the tumor is the most important malignancy of the minor salivary glands, pain, ulceration, bleeding, and a local mass are symptoms in these sites. Nasal, paranasal sinus, and nasopharyngeal tumors present with airway obstruction and epistaxis; those of the soft palate and pharynx with dysphagia and ulceration.

Mucoepidermoid Tumor

Mucoepidermoid tumor is a highly variable neoplasm whose most innocuous form has been classified by some as "benign." The lesions form 6 to 9% of all primary salivary gland tumors. About 60% of them occur in the parotid gland.[14,16] With some exceptions there appears to be a fairly close correlation between the cellular composition of the tumor and its biological behavior. There are six morphological types of cells found in these tumors: "maternal cells," intermediate, epidermoid, clear, columnar, and mucous (**Table 8.2**). A predominance of intermediate and epidermoid cells (especially pleomorphic forms of the latter) signifies malignancy (**Fig. 8.19**). These more invasive tumors are characterized by relatively rapid

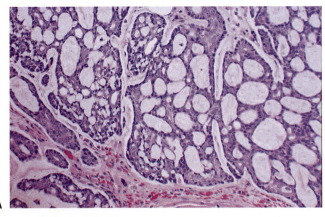

A

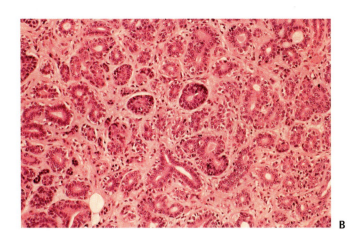

B

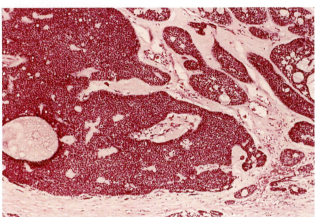

C

Fig. 8.17 Three histological configurations assumed by adenoid cystic carcinoma. (**A**) Cribrose variety. Note large cystic spaces filled with mucoid material and lined by cells only one or two layers thick (×100). (**B**) Tubular variety. A small ductlike or tubular pattern is seen in this adenoid cystic tumor invading the bone of the hard palate (×150). (**C**) Solid configuration. This type is the most malignant in behavior (×60). (From Thackray AC, Lucas RB. Tumors of the major salivary glands. Fascicle 10. Atlas of Tumor Pathology. 2nd ed. Washington, DC: Armed Forces Institute of Pathology; 1974:74.)

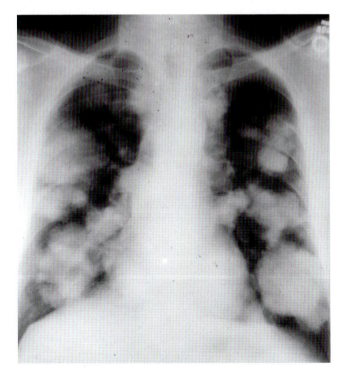

Fig. 8.18 Chest x-ray of a patient with extensive metastatic adenoid cystic carcinoma to the lung. The patient had no lower respiratory tract symptoms at the time this x-ray was taken.

Table 8.2 Cellular Characteristics of Mucoepidermoid Tumors

Cell Type	Description	Type of Cytoplasm	Characteristic
Maternal	Small; round or oval	Scant basophilic	Progenitor of other cell types
Intermediate	Oval; larger than maternal	Pale eosinophilic; scant	Characteristic of malignancy
Epidermoid	Squamous cell appearance; may form keratin	Eosinophilic	Characteristic of malignancy
Clear	Variable size; central nucleus	Water-clear	Characteristic of benignity
Columnar	Similar to secretory cells of ducts	Granular to foamy	None diagnostic
Mucous	Large, swollen, balloon-shaped; small eccentric nucleus	Foamy or reticular	Characteristic of benignity

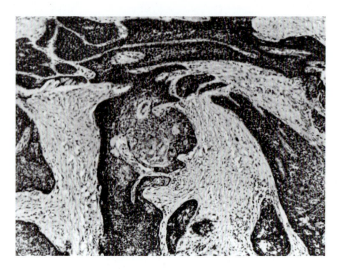

Fig. 8.19 Photomicrograph of a malignant mucoepidermoid tumor (×60). (From Thackray AC, Lucas RB. Tumors of the major salivary glands. Fascicle 10. Atlas of Tumor Pathology. 2nd ed. Washington, DC: Armed Forces Institute of Pathology; 1974:74.)

growth, local invasion of skin and facial nerve, and regional as well as distant metastases. The more benign forms display glandular structures with formation of mucin, well-differentiated epidermoid cells, and a dearth of intermediate cells (**Fig. 8.20**). The problem is that, despite a completely benign histological appearance, an occasional low-grade mucoepidermoid tumor will metastasize. These lesions thus are all potentially malignant and must be treated accordingly. If local recurrences or metastases do occur, they do so within 5 years.[25] Another favorable factor is that the bulk of the tumors are of the more benign variety.[23]

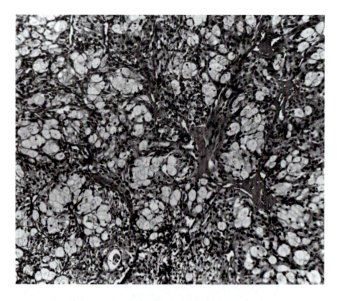

Fig. 8.20 Photomicrograph of a low-grade mucoepidermoid tumor. Note the number of mucous cells with scant squamous or intermediate cells. (×75) (From Thackray AC, Lucas RB: Tumors of the major salivary glands. Fascicle 10, Atlas of tumor Pathology, 2nd ed. Washington, DC, Armed Forces Institute of Pathology, 1974: 74.)

These neoplasms present most commonly as a firm, painless, slow-growing mass in the superficial lobe of the parotid. Facial nerve involvement, cutaneous fixation, and pain are common in only the most malignant types. The more benign are indistinguishable clinically from a benign mixed tumor. The lesion has a pseudocapsule, and the cut surface may be solid or cystic. The cysts, which are variable in size, contain clear but usually viscid material.

Squamous Cell Carcinoma

Squamous cell carcinoma is an uncommon malignancy of the salivary glands, being mainly limited to the parotid and the submaxillary. This tumor makes up 0.1 to 3.4% of all parotid neoplasms and 12% of those in the submaxillary gland.[14] It is often difficult to determine whether a squamous cell cancer is primary in the parotid or is a metastatic lymph node from a primary in the skin or elsewhere in the upper aerodigestive tract. The skin primaries that produce the metastases are usually 2 cm or greater in diameter. Metastatic squamous cancer in a partial lymph node is far more common than the primary neoplasm in the gland itself, especially in Caucasians who live in the "sunbelt" areas of the world.

Clinically, these malignancies are usually very obvious. They are rock hard and are often fixed to the underlying structures or overlying skin, even eroding through the latter, producing an ugly suppurating ulcer (**Fig. 8.21**). The lesion is painful, tender, and rapid growing. Facial nerve paralysis is found in ~30% of patients. Neck metastases are present ~25% of the time.

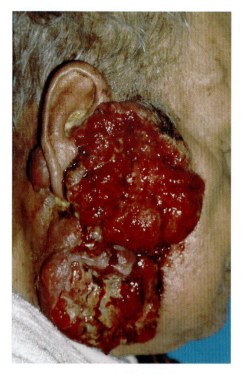

Fig. 8.21 Extensive squamous cell carcinoma of the parotid gland that has eroded through the skin.

Histologically the tumors are composed of keratin-producing cells with intercellular bridges. There is no mucin production. If the cancer is the result of metastasis to the lymph node from a cutaneous lesion, some residuum of the node may be seen. However, these metastases are often substantial prior to resection, and the lymphatic architecture may be entirely replaced by tumor.

◆ Diagnosis

Unfortunately, the clinical differentiation between benign and malignant lesions may be determined only when the signs of malignancy become evident. Pain, ulceration, facial nerve paralysis, fixation to surrounding structures, and metastases are the hallmarks of cancer, although notable exceptions to this rule occur. Many salivary gland cancers, for instance, are painless and do not produce paralysis, while on the other hand, it is not uncommon to find a benign pleomorphic adenoma arising in the minor salivary glands of the palate that ulcerates (**Fig. 8.22**). Recurrent pleomorphic adenomas are commonly fixed to deep structures and even the adjacent skin, despite their benign histology. Facial nerve paralysis is almost a sure sign of malignancy, but there are rare exceptions even to this rule (**Fig. 8.23**).

The use of contrast sialography has become obsolete. CT and magnetic resonance imaging (MRI) scanning and fine-needle aspiration (FNA) cytology have become the most useful tests. MRI will delineate extension of tumor into surrounding soft tissue (**Fig. 8.24**), and the CT scan will identify erosion of bone in the mandible, zygoma, or temporal bone. Obviously, any extraglandular extension is highly suggestive of malignancy. The CT scan may also differentiate intraglandular from extraglandular pathology. Lesions of the mandibular condyle or zygoma (**Fig. 8.25**) present as a hard mass

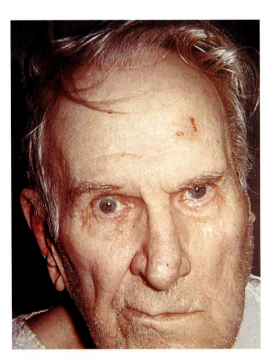

Fig. 8.23 Elderly man with a swelling of the parotid gland and a facial palsy, raising a high index of suspicion for malignancy of the gland. The patient in actuality had an abscess.

in the parotid bed but are extraglandular. On axial view CT scanning arteriovenous malformations may present as parotid masses (**Fig. 8.24**). The differentiation from a parotid tumor may be very difficult even on MRI. Lesions in the deep lobe of the gland will be seen to extend through the stylomandibular tunnel, whereas carotid sheath primaries, such as Schwannomas, will be seen to be outside the tunnel. Dumbbell-shaped tumors will be seen to occupy a position in both the superficial and the deep lobes (**Fig. 8.26**). MRI will suggest invasion of the carotid arteries and internal jugular vein extension of tumor up the facial nerve or into the third division of the trigeminal nerve. Whereas vascular involvement may be suggested by displacement of the vessels, irregularity of the vascular lumena, flow voids, or vascular encirclement by tumor are more definitive signs of direct vascular invasion by tumor. Microscopic invasion of nerves is seldom picked up on CT scan or MRI. Gross thickening of a nerve or erosion of the bone of a skull base foramen is usually indicative of perineural or direct neural invasion. Extension of advanced lesions through the floor of the middle cranial fossa are best seen in the coronal projections. The CT scan will show bone erosion (**Fig. 8.27**) and the MRI will suggest dural, cavernous sinus, or brain involvement (**Fig. 8.28**).

FNA cytology, although well established in lymph node and thyroid pathologies, is more controversial in the analysis of salivary gland tumors. FNA as developed by Eneroth[26] and others is the definitive diagnostic test in Sweden and other European countries. However, Conley[27] has seriously questioned the validity of this approach, and with considerable justification. Considering the difficulty in establishing a definitive diagnosis even on the basis of the large tissue

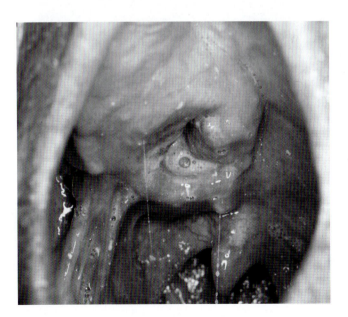

Fig. 8.22 Large pleomorphic adenoma of the hard palate with ulceration.

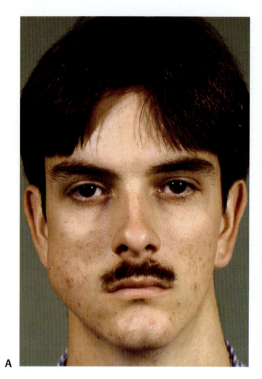

A

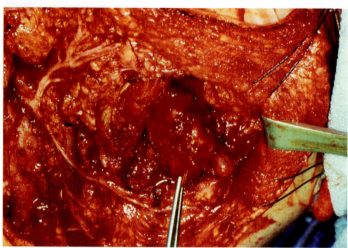

B

Fig. 8.24 (**A**) Vascular malformation deep to superficial lobe parotid. (**B**) Tumor removal.

volume produced by resection, it is hard to conceive of making this diagnosis from the minute specimen produced by needle biopsy. The wisdom of predicating therapy on the basis of this small portion of tumor from a limited area is therefore open to question. FNA biopsy requires special training

and substantial experience on the part of the pathologist. False negatives and false positives are not uncommon. The most difficult distinction is differentiating pleomorphic adenoma from adenoid cystic and mucoepidermoid carcinoma. However, a strong suspicion of malignancy on FNA coupled

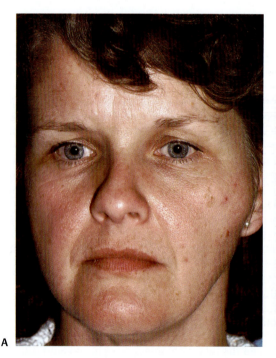

A

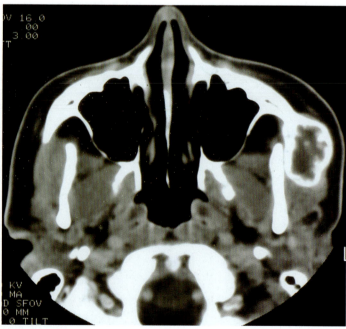

B

Fig. 8.25 (**A**) Middle-aged woman presenting with a mass "in parotid gland." (**B**) Computed tomographic scan in axial plane shows mass in zygoma deep to the superior aspect of the parotid. Mass was a fibromyxoma.

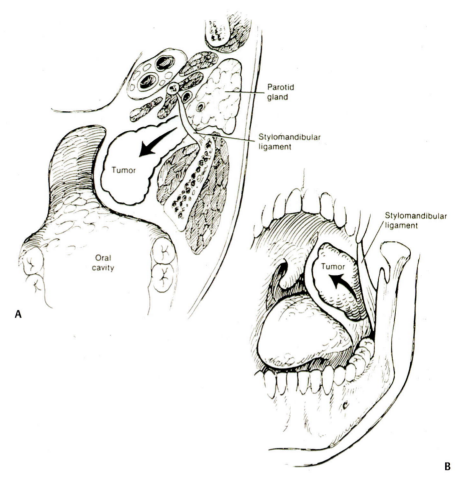

Fig. 8.26 (**A**) Coronal view. (**B**) "Cut away" coronal view. Dumbbell tumor of the parotid extending from the superficial to the deep lobe.

with suggestive symptoms of carcinoma and evidence of extraglandular spread on CT and MRI can prepare the patient and the surgeon for the strong possibility of a more radical operation.

Tumors of the minor salivary glands are amenable to incisional biopsy, as they present in the oral cavity, pharynx, or nasal cavities. Lesions of the major glands, however, do not lend themselves to this diagnostic exercise, and excisional

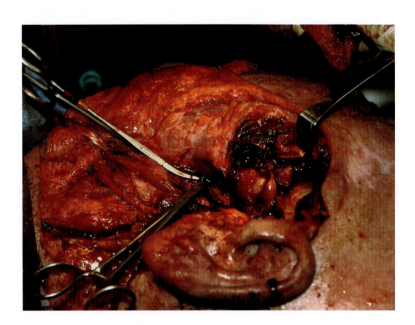

Fig. 8.27 Bone erosion of the middle fossa secondary to carcinoma of the parotid.

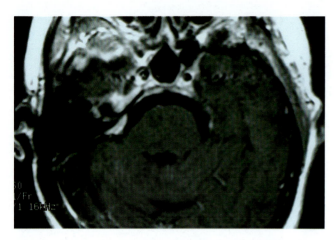

Fig. 8.28 T1-weighted magnetic resonance imaging with gadolinium contrast in the axial plane showing middle fossa, cavernous sinus, and posterior fossa dural enhancement of direct extension of a mucoepidermoid carcinoma of the parotid.

biopsy is the method of choice. This is particularly true with regard to parotid gland tumors.

Parotidectomy with facial nerve preservation has become the definitive procedure for excisional biopsy of a parotid neoplasm. The recurrence rate of benign tumors is exceptionally small following this procedure, especially when compared with recurrence rates seen with the fortunately discarded procedure of "lumpectomy," or worse, incisional biopsy. The unfortunate results of these latter procedures are still with us and provide a considerable therapeutic challenge. If after superficial parotidectomy, a definitive diagnosis of malignancy cannot be categorically stated by the pathologist after review of the frozen section histology, then a more radical procedure must be deferred until the permanent sections can be examined. It is always wise to warn the patient preoperatively of the possible need for a second staged operation.

◆ Surgical Considerations

Recurrent Pleomorphic Adenoma

Once a pleomorphic adenoma recurs, it acquires a tenacious hold on adjacent tissue. It assumes an almost malignant demeanor with numerous extensions and tumor excrescences in seeming discontinuity. In the truly benign form, however, metastases never occur. The surgical problem is that of encompassing local tumor extension, which can be accomplished only by a radical attack on the tumor. Even with an aggressive excision, if tumor-free margins are not obtained, the lesion will recur (**Fig. 8.29**).

One of the most difficult facts to accept is that occasionally portions of the facial nerve will need to be excised to achieve an adequate resection. Work and Hecht[11] established this as a basic principle in these cases as long ago as 1976. A fruitless attempt to dissect through a mass of fibrous tissue and tumor to preserve the nerve will produce not only further recurrence but neural injury as well.

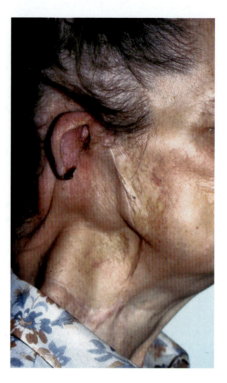

Fig. 8.29 Middle-aged woman following 14 attempts at resecting a pleomorphic adenoma. The original operation was an incisional biopsy. Radical neck dissection, mandibulectomy, and temporal bone excision were fraught with recurrence. The patient died of brain stem invasion.

The patient in **Fig. 8.29** presented with a history spanning 20 years of 14 prior attempts at eliminating a pleomorphic adenoma. The tumor had been initially diagnosed by incisional biopsy and then locally excised. The surgeon when faced with repeated recurrence had, in a desperate attempt at removing the lesion, even resorted to a radical neck dissection. In light of the benign form of this tumor, this was unnecessary, as nodal metastases never occur. However, the tumor may locally invade muscle, bone, and skin. Resection of this recurrent lesion required partial mandibulectomy, mastoid tip excision, and removal of the posterior belly of the digastric muscle, part of the trapezius, splenius capitis, and masseter muscles, the main trunk of the facial nerve, and substantial neck skin.

A modified Blair incision[28] (**Fig. 8.30**) yields excellent access to the gland. It was modified in this instance to include a large portion of postauricular and superior neck skin to circumscribe the area of cutaneous involvement (**Fig. 8.31**). Skin flaps are developed to expose the tumor and the peripheral branches of the facial nerve. In the previously operated patient, much fibrosis between the facial skin and the underlying tissue is encountered, and frequent use of the facial nerve stimulator helps to localize the various branches. Although I avoid the use of the facial nerve monitor in most parotidectomies it is invaluable in the performance of revision surgery in recurrent pleomorphic adenoma. Also in such cases, the elevation of the facial flap over the parotid bed and the site of tumor recurrence is extremely tedious,

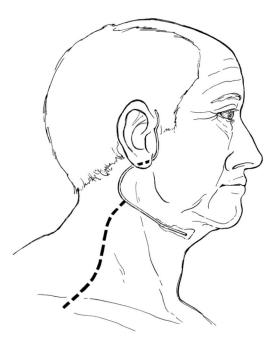

Fig. 8.30 Modified Blair incision. Dotted line represents extension if radical neck dissection is required.

in marked contrast to the easy, quick dissection that is the norm in the previously unoperated case. Pleomorphic adenomas tend to push the various branches of the facial nerve in front of them. In the recurrent cases, however, the tumor has more of a tendency to envelop the nerves. In addition, fibrosis secondary to past surgical intervention also envelops and further binds the branches into the bed.

Once the flaps are elevated, the main trunk of the facial nerve is located. The key to all parotid gland surgery is the isolation of this nerve, and for a detailed account of this step, the beautifully exact description of facial nerve localization by McCabe and Work[28] is unsurpassed in the literature. The most consistent landmark is the tragal "pointer" on the cartilaginous external auditory canal. The trunk of the nerve is usually found approximately 1 cm deep to it (**Fig. 8.32**). In the case of the patient in **Fig. 8.31B**, the nerve could not be identified because of tumor envelopment. A simple mastoidectomy with skeletonization of the fallopian canal was done. Parchment-thin layers of the bone of the canal were chipped away, unroofing the nerve, and tumor was seen invading the stylomastoid foramen. The nerve was sectioned about half the distance up the mastoid portion of the facial canal. The nerve stump and tumor excrescences were dissected from the canal into the upper neck. Attempts to isolate the upper and lower main divisions were thwarted by the presence of tumor and fibrosis. The distal branches of the nerve were then identified, tagged, and severed.

Posteriorly and superiorly an incision was made outside of tumor involvement and carried through the underlying trapezius and splenius capitis muscles to the skull. Because the deeper muscles were not involved, the dissection stopped at this level. Sweeping the dissection inferiorly, the digastric and stylohyoid muscles were excised, with care taken to ligate the occipital artery, which sits in its own groove deep to the digastric muscle. The mastoid tip was excised at this point and the bloc carried forward (**Fig. 8.33**).

Recurrent pleomorphic adenomas are usually attached to the masseter muscle, and a generous portion surrounding the tumor is resected. The deep margin anteriorly may be either the ramus of the mandible or the medial pterygoid muscle. If there is bone involvement, however, the ramus must be

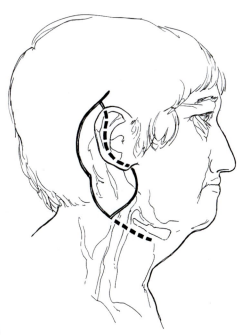

A

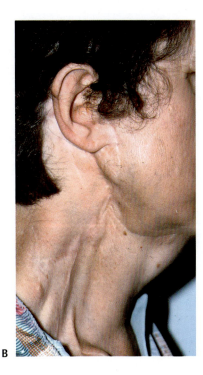

B

Fig. 8.31 (**A**) Extension of Blair incision necessary to encompass tumor invasion of skin in patient depicted in **Fig. 8.31B**. (**B**) Appearance of patient postoperatively. After years of follow-up, no recurrences were seen.

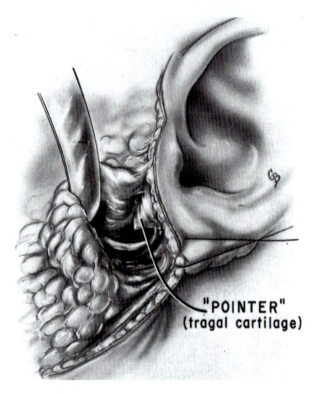

Fig. 8.32 Dissection of the facial nerve showing relationship to the tragal pointer. (From McCabe BF, Work PW. Parotidectomy with special preference in the facial nerve. In: English GM, ed. Otolaryngology. Vol 4. Hagerstown, MD: Harper & Row; 1967:43.)

sacrificed (**Fig. 8.34**). If the tumor wraps around its medial surface or if the deep lobe remnant is infiltrated, not only the mandibular ramus but the pterygoid muscles as well are taken (**Fig. 8.35**). Bleeding from the internal maxillary artery on the medial surface of the mandibular neck, as well as from the pterygoid venous plexus, can be somewhat troublesome. Stick ties of 3–0 vascular silk may be necessary to ensure hemostasis in the pterygoid plexus. Sometimes bleeding is so persistent that only a pack of hemostatic cotton or gauze such as Surgicel (Ethicon, Inc., Somerville, NJ) or fibrin products will stop it. Tumor invasion of the pterygoid musculature renders complete excision difficult. The internal carotid artery presents in the bed as further deep progression is made along the skull base. Superior invasion of the external auditory canal may require lateral temporal bone resection (see chapter 7). The bloc is removed and suspicious margins checked by frozen section.

The head is turned and excision of the greater auricular nerve is done from the opposing side. In revision cases, the ipsilateral nerve has invariably been sacrificed previously. The nerve graft is approximated to the facial trunk in the fallopian canal. Although it is not essential to have a suture at this site, if one or two sutures can be placed, this is done. The distal branches are sutured to the other end of the graft with 8–0 or 10–0 nylon under microscopic control (**Fig. 8.36**). Closure of the wound is by skin grafting or a local rotation flap (**Fig. 8.37**). Thick regional skin flaps or musculocutaneous flaps are initially avoided to prevent obscuring possible early local recurrences. If resection margins are found to be positive on per-

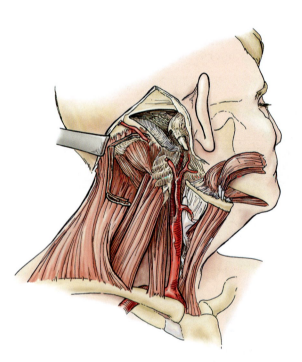

Fig. 8.33 Resection of the upper aspects of the trapezius and splenius capitis muscles as well as of the digastric and stylohyoid is required to achieve a tumor-free margin on the superior and deep aspects. The sternomastoid muscle was resected in a prior operation. The mastoid tip is amputated. The facial nerve is resected within the fallopian canal.

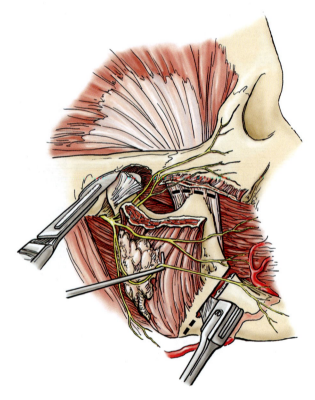

Fig. 8.34 Resection of persistent recurrent pleomorphic adenoma with adherence to the mandible. Lateral view showing cuts in temporal-mandibular joint and at angle of mandible.

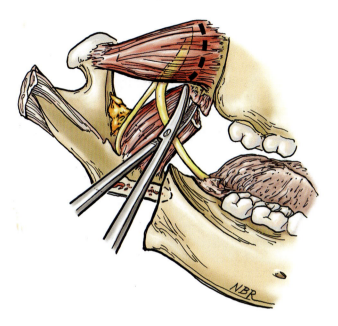

Fig. 8.35 Resection of the medial and lateral pterygoid muscles when deep lobe of parotid involved medial view.

manent pathological section, immediate revision is advised in the hope of getting ahead of the disease. This has been necessary on several occasions in my experience and was successful in ablating the tumor in each instance. Radiation therapy is not an effective means of dealing with residual tumor.[6]

Although a study by Buchman et al[29] showed a 24% local recurrence rate in where pleomorphic adenomas that had positive margins or tumor spill when treated with postoperative irradiation therapy. This is little better than the historical local recurrence rate of 30 to 35%.

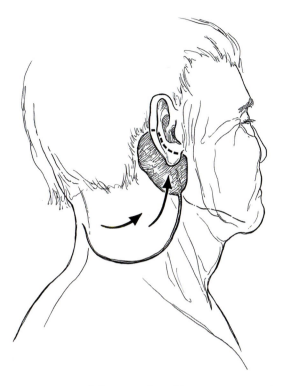

Fig. 8.37 Wound closure is affected by using a rotation flap from the nape of the neck.

Mucoepidermoid Tumor

The treatment of this lesion is problematic. If the surgeon could be assured that all histologically benign tumors would pursue a benign course, they could be safely excised with a narrow margin. However, the protean nature of mucoepider-

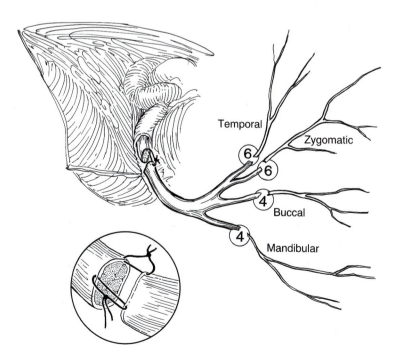

Fig. 8.36 A greater auricular nerve graft is placed, with the thickest end of the graft within the fallopian canal secured to the main trunk by one or two sutures when possible. The distal arborization of the graft is sutured to at least the three most functionally important facial nerve branches; the zygomatic, buccal, and mandibular.

moid tumors is such that resection with adequate margins is mandatory. The issue of the facial nerve is a tricky one. Direct tumor invasion by tumor of a branch or of the main trunk of the nerve necessitates its sacrifice. In the cases of a very well differentiated tumor, some tempering of this harsh dictum may be in order because local recurrences are very uncommon, and their reexcision is not necessarily associated with a poor prognosis.[23] A negative frozen section of the nerve sheath generally ensures no later local recurrence.

The more histologically malignant types have a marked tendency to metastasize with rates quoted as high as 66%.[5,22] On the other hand, the low-grade tumors rarely spread. Distant metastases are again a feature of the more poorly differentiated tumors and are much more common in patients with cervical adenopathy,[5,23,25]

The overall 5-year survival rate of patients with mucoepidermoid tumor is between 80 and 90%.[17,23,25] Those with the most highly differentiated tumors have a rate close to 100%. However, the more malignant, poorly differentiated mucoepidermoid carcinomas have a much different clinical course and eventual prognosis. In Conley's series of 278 patients with cancer of the parotid gland, 27% had mucoepidermoid tumors, and of these only 30 were of the poorly differentiated type.[23] Of those with this poor differentiation who were initially treated by Conley, the 5-year survival rate was 56%. These patients all had radical excisions as the primary attack. The ones who presented with recurrent disease and had their initial management elsewhere did not do nearly as well. The surgical technique for the more malignant forms of mucoepidermoid tumor is the same as that for squamous cell cancer (see next section).

Squamous Cell Cancer

The best treatment of squamous cell carcinoma is radical excision. Postoperative irradiation should be added if significant spread beyond the gland has occurred or when there are neck metastases. Even though the prognosis of poorly differentiated mucoepidermoid carcinoma is better than that of squamous cell, the surgical management should be just as aggressive.

One of the few violations of the en bloc technique of cancer removal in head and neck surgery is the isolation of the facial nerve in parotid gland tumor resection. As dissection of the main trunk and its branches proceeds, constant vigilance is required in keeping track of the tumor margins. Branches of the nerve are preserved whenever possible, the most important functionally being the zygomatic or eye branch. Once branches of the facial nerve have been found to be invaded, the piecemeal excision in that part of the gland is halted and a complete en bloc resection of the gland and any involved overlying skin and deep muscle are done.

In planning the excision, any skin fixation or penetration must be skirted by a wide margin of at least 4 cm because skin recurrences are common when narrower margins are employed. Conley's principle of the first attack being by far the most successful is epitomized in salivary gland cancer surgery. Anticipation of the possible adjacent structures that will require resection also helps in planning the excision. Provision must be made for exposing the mastoid tip if a portion of the temporal bone requires resection. Extending the

incision into the scalp allows excellent exposure of the temporomandibular joint and zygomatic roots. If a radical neck dissection is required, a lazy S excision can be dropped from the inferior limb of the modified Blair incision (**Fig. 8.30**). The neck dissection is done only in the presence of manifest cervical metastases because these occur in only 25% of patients. However, if the parotid lesion is itself secondary to a tumor elsewhere in the upper aerodigestive tract, a neck dissection is indicated.

Tumor stuck to the cartilaginous portion of the external auditory canal requires removal of the portion of the canal and a generous margin of conchal cartilage. Often some bony canal must be removed as well. When the neoplasm is fixed to the osseous external canal, a lateral temporal bone resection must be done (**Fig. 8.38B**) (see chapter 7).

In squamous cell cancer of the parotid gland, frequently the tumor has extended beyond the deep margin of the superficial lobe. This area is often neglected by many surgeons who pay more attention to the aesthetic implications of the proximity of the tumor to the facial nerve and skin. The masseter muscle lies in the parotid bed and should always be included in resections of malignancies of the superficial lobe when tumor is fixed or close to the muscle. Deep lobe involvement automatically dictates inclusion of portions of the medial and even lateral pterygoid muscles in the resection. Fixation of tumor to the paraspinal muscles requires removal of these muscles, including possibly the transverse process of C2 and even part of the lateral mass of C1. Careful attention must be paid to the vertebral artery as it passes through the foramen transversarium of C2 and around the posterior aspect of the lateral mass of the C1. If anticipation of vertebral arterial involvement is made then it is wise to get a preoperative Balloon Test Occlusion (BTO) and cerebral Single photon emission computed tomography (SPECT) scan. Almost always one vertebral artery can be sacrificed. Any compromise of the internal carotid, however, could lead to a disastrous stroke if the vertebral is taken. If invasion of the occipital condyle has occurred then removal with the cutting bur using the far lateral approach to the upper cervical spine and brain stem described by George and Laurian,[30,31] Sen and Catalano,[32] and Spetzler and Graham[33] should enable encompassment of the tumor. The position of the hypoglossal nerve as it passes through the anterior one third of the condyle should be remembered and the nerve avoided if not invaded by tumor. Approximately one half of the condyle can be removed without a concern of spinal destabilization or the need for rigid spinal fixation. Tumor invasion of the internal carotid, except in a few rare cases (see chapter 9), is a dire prognostic sign. "Mopping up" with postoperative irradiation in these cases does little to improve survival, although it may prolong temporary local control. Gross residual disease, even though scant in amount, almost invariably dooms the patient to death from the cancer. Internal carotid involvement requires excision and grafting with either a saphenous vein graft or a synthetic Gore-Tex polytetrafluoroethylene graft (W.L. Gore and Associates, Inc., Flagstaff, AZ). The vein graft is preferred because of delayed clotting off of Gore-Tex grafts that is not uncommonly seen.

Both superficial and deep lobe involvement usually necessitates partial mandibulectomy. Whereas in resections involv-

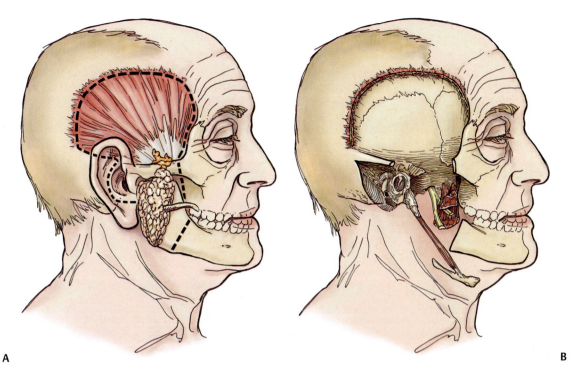

Fig. 8.38 (**A**) When a malignancy approximates the zygomatic arch or temporalis muscle, resection includes the temporalis, the arch, neck, and condyle of the mandible, and usually the ramus. (**B**) Often a lateral temporal bone resection is necessary because of the proximity of the tumor to the external auditory gland.

ing the oropharynx the mandibular condyle is usually preserved, here the condyle must be included in the resection of the mandibular ramus (**Fig. 8.24**). Vigilance for the internal maxillary artery during this phase will prevent the problem of troublesome bleeding. If tumor extends beyond the mandibular ramus, it may be necessary to remove the glenoid fossa itself and the posterior aspect of the zygomatic arch. Temporalis muscle excision and removal of the contents of the infratemporal fossa (**Fig. 8.38**) may also be required to achieve a safe margin (**Fig. 8.39**). The resection of bone in this region (with the exception of the condyle) is most easily achieved with a cutting bur. Care must be taken to get well beyond the tumor, even if it means exposing middle fossa dura. Extensions of tumor through the middle fossa floor or through the foramen ovale along V3 into the Meckel cave are resected using the middle fossa/infratemporal fossa technique (see chapter 9).

Those branches of the facial nerve sacrificed during resection are replaced with nerve grafts. When the main trunk is taken, the sural or the greater auricular nerve can be used as a cable graft. The branching network of the greater auricular may be employed to graft in various severed branches of the facial nerve. If sufficient graft arborization is not available, the graft can be split longitudinally. The nerve is sutured with 10–0 monofilament nylon, using 8 to 10 sutures in the trunk, 6 to 8 in a main division, and 4 to 6 in a named branch. The operating microscope, especially if fitted with a zoom lens, greatly facilitates this part of the surgery.

Lost skin is replaced by a flap. A myocutaneous flap improves the cosmetic appearance by virtue of the bulk supplied by the muscular portion. The only problem with these

flaps is that they will obscure any local recurrence. The trapezius or pectoralis flaps are the most commonly used. For facial defects no greater than 6 to 7 cm in diameter a cervicopectoral rotation flap can be used (**Fig. 8.40**). The advantages of skin of similar color, texture, and thickness are an

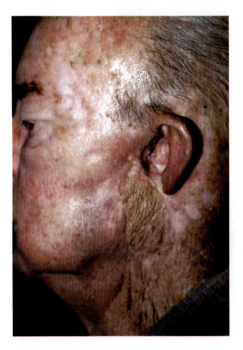

Fig. 8.39 Patient following the resection illustrated in **Fig. 8.38**.

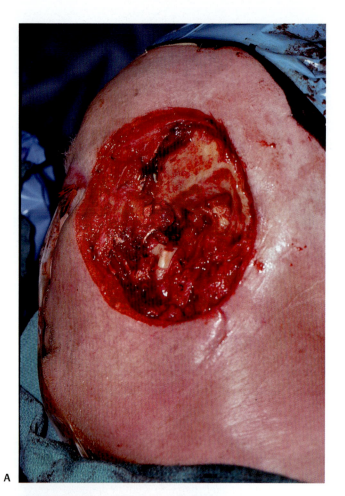

A

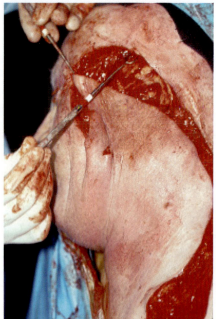

B

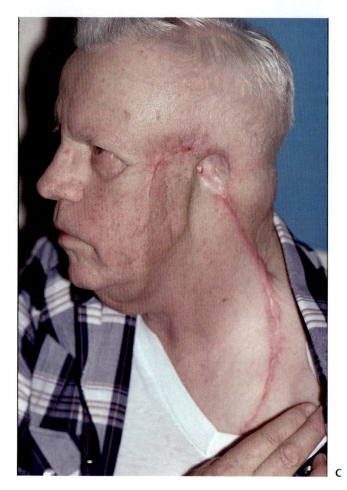

C

Fig. 8.40 Cervicopectoral rotation flap used to cover skin defect after radical parotidectomy with overlying skin excision. (**A**) Defect after resection. (**B**) Flap elevated. (**C**) Twelve months postop.

immense aesthetic advantage. However, lining the surgical defect with a split-thickness skin graft, although unsightly, is the safest method for early detection of local recurrences. In some instances a split-thickness skin graft will not provide sufficient cover for the upper cervical spine, the internal carotid artery, exposed mandible, and denuded temporal and sphenoid bone. In addition, patients who have had prior radiation are unsuitable for skin grafting. The rectus abdominis free flap provides excellent cover and can at a later stage be debulked, providing good cosmetic result.

Adenoid Cystic Carcinoma

A philosophy of therapy directed at these pernicious, aggressive, and unpredictable tumors must bring to bear a host of considerations relative to the patient's age and general state of health, the presence of regional or distant metastases, and the local extent of tumor. The basic foundation of effective long-term local control is aggressive surgical resection.[21,34,35] Although distant metastases are not uncommon, the sooner the entire primary tumor is removed, the less vulnerable the patient will be to the risk of metastasis. The local "recurrence" of cancer is in reality local persistence. As long as tumor persists at the primary site, there is an increasing likelihood that the patient may have tumor emboli that are continually breaking away from the lesion to lodge elsewhere in the body. This is especially important to remember in the management of adenoid cystic cancer, in which locally persistent disease often remains occult for prolonged periods of time before finally becoming manifest. During these extended periods when tumor is present but obscured at the primary site, the patient is at continuous risk for metastases. Thus the importance of complete surgical removal cannot be overemphasized. In a series of 58 patients with adenoid cystic carcinoma reported by Smith et al,[35] with one exception, all of those patients clinically free of disease 10 years or longer had negative surgical margins. No patient with a negative margin had metastatic disease. On the other hand, when surgical margins were inadequate, 79% developed metastatic disease, and only 8.8% of these patients were alive and clinically free of disease at 10 years. In Conley and Dingman's series of 40 patients followed longer than 10 years, 11 (27.5%) were alive and tumor free.[24] An analysis relative to margins was not made, but Conley and Dingman's impression of an association between aggressive surgery and increased longevity has guided our management philosophy.

In a young person, an aggressive operation is done that includes total parotidectomy, resection of all involved or adjacent facial nerve branches, mastoidectomy, excision of the infratemporal fossa and the masseter muscle, and occasionally mandibulectomy, which is done only if the mandible is directly invaded. If the soft tissues of the temporomandibular joint are infiltrated the condyle, mandibular neck, and adjacent soft tissue are excised. A 2 mm thickness of glenoid fossa is removed at the medial end of the temporal bone resection to ensure a complete encompassing of the tumor.

Both the deep and superficial lobes of the gland are removed. Facial nerve branches that are anywhere near the tumor are excised. If no perineural invasion is evident and no facial paralysis was present preoperatively, all branches outside a 2 to 3 cm perimeter are spared. When neural invasion is evident, the safest procedure is to excise the nerve as far as the region of the stylomastoid foramen into the fallopian canal. A cable graft is interposed, or if this is not feasible, a hypoglossal to facial crossover anastomosis is done. Mastoidectomy and resection of the external auditory canal, including both its cartilaginous and bony portions, must be performed in most cases because of the proximity of the gland to these structures. The need for masseter and temporalis muscle as well as mandibular and zygomatic arch resection is determined on an individual basis, depending on tumor proximity. If the external auditory canal needs resection, the mandibular condyle is removed. Access to the glenoid fossa and hence the bony wall is thus affected. Often the root of the zygomatic bone is excised as well. A substantial resection margin must be maintained in all planes. The issue of radical neck dissection is a difficult one to resolve. Because lymph node metastases occur infrequently,[24,31] the absence of clinically involved nodes militates against radical neck dissection. However, a neck dissection should be done when any suspicion of nodal disease is encountered.

The older or infirm patient, and all patients with distant metastases, should be treated by a lesser procedure. Because of the slowly progressive nature of the disease and its sensitivity, albeit limited, to irradiation therapy, local control can be maintained for a reasonable time. Extensive resections resulting in profound aesthetic and functional compromise should be limited to the younger patients.

The extreme arduousness of these decisions makes management of adenoid cystic carcinoma difficult. Evaluation of each case on an individual basis is absolutely essential to determining the best possible treatment plan. The prognosis for survival is better when the disease is in the major salivary glands, especially the parotid, than in the minor glands. Conley's disease-free survival rate was 75% at 5 years, 30% at 10 years, and 20% at 15 years for all sites.[24]

Adenocarcinomas and Acinic Cell Tumor

Resection for these tumors is similar to that for squamous cell and poorly differentiated mucoepidermoid carcinoma. The limits of excision are dictated by tumor extent. Lymph node metastases are uncommon, and therefore neck dissection is rarely performed. Mandibular and lateral temporal bone resections are usually necessary, and often even the zygomatic arch and the muscles deep in the parotid bed have to be removed. Deep lobe involvement may extend under the skull base, almost to the nasopharynx. In some cases, tumor may extend beyond these confines into the middle fossa (**Fig. 8.41**). At this point, a combined neurosurgical head and neck procedure through an infratemporal fossa/middle fossa approach may completely expose the tumor in its intracranial and extracranial extents. Details of this procedure are given in chapter 9.

Submandibular and Sublingual Gland Tumors

Whereas most parotid neoplasms are benign, the submandibular and sublingual gland tumors are more often

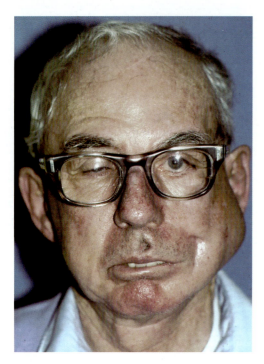

Fig. 8.41 Patient with a large deep lobe parotid gland malignancy extending under the skull base, presenting with findings of compromise of the maxillary division of the trigeminal nerve. Tumor had eroded through the floor of the middle cranial fossa.

malignant. In Conley's series[23] 47% of submandibular gland tumors and 90% of sublingual glands were carcinomatous. Neoplasms of the sublingual glands are unusual. Although some mucoepidermoid, squamous cell, and acinic cell tumors are seen, most are adenoid cystic carcinoma. The same philosophy of radical excision applied to this tumor in the parotid gland is followed when it arises in the submaxillary and sublingual glands. The excision includes partial glossectomy and resection of the floor of the mouth. The adjacent mandible is resected if invaded by tumor, and lymph nodal dissection is reserved for those individuals with palpable nodal metastasis. The lingual and hypoglossal nerves as well as the ramus mandibularis of the facial nerve will need to be resected because of the propensity of adenoid cystic carcinoma to invade the nerve sheath. Excision of these nerves as close to their origin as possible is important to ensure completeness of tumor removal.

If there is numbness of the lip, denoting inferior alveolar nerve involvement, much wider resection must be done. The tumor in these instances must be considered to have extended into the marrow cavity along the sheath of the nerve. To get above possible tumor, the mandibulectomy incision must be through the neck above the coronoid notch. The anterior incision is curved through the parasymphyseal area well in front of the mental foramen. The inferior alveolar nerve should be cut as closely as possible to its emergence from the submandibular division of the trigeminal nerve near the foramen ovale. Similarly, the lingual, buccal, and hypoglossal nerves should be excised if they show clinical evidence of tumor involvement. Cranial nerve invasion is a poor prognostic sign.

Sublingual primaries involve the undersurface of the tongue. The patient in **Fig. 8.42** had the tongue sectioned horizontally through much of its width, with preservation of its upper half and attendant blood supply from the lingual arteries (**Fig.**

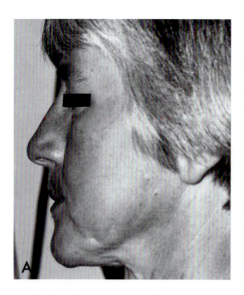

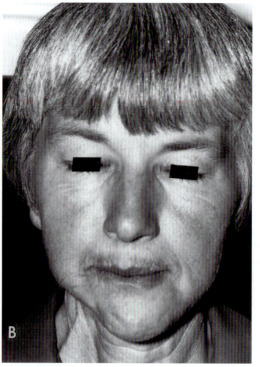

Fig. 8.42 Appearance of patient following anterior mandibulectomy, including the arch, required for excision of a sublingual gland adenoid cystic carcinoma. The arch was reconstructed with a contoured rib graft. (**A**) Side view. (**B**) Frontal view.

8.43). The primary reconstruction of the defect created from the tongue to the buccal and labial mucosa may leave the patient "tongue-tied" and require a sulcoplasty later on. If there is further invasion of tumor requiring more extensive resection, reconstruction with a nasolabial flap, split-thickness skin graft, or radial-foreman free flap may be necessary.

For low-grade malignant tumors of these glands, a more conservative resection that includes adjacent muscles and mandibular periosteum is appropriate. If tumor proximity to mandible presents any doubts as to its preservation, an excision employing a lingual splitting procedure can be done.

Minor Salivary Gland Tumors

Considering that there are 400 to 500 minor salivary glands in the oral cavity alone, it is remarkable that the incidence of neoplasm is only one fifth that of the major glands.[36] In Conley's series[23] of 200 minor salivary gland tumors, 65% were malignant. Adenoid cystic carcinoma accounts for the biggest percentage of tumor types, comprising 35 to 50% of all malignancies.[23,37,38] Mucoepidermoid, malignant mixed, adenocarcinoma (mainly of the poorly differentiated type), and finally the rare acinic cell tumors make up the remaining varieties in descending order of frequency.

The palate is a common site for the benign mixed tumor (**Fig. 8.44**), which often attains significant size before the sufferer seeks help. Careful histological examination is important to ensure that the lesion is neither a malignant mixed tumor nor an adenoid cystic carcinoma. Unlike squamous cell tumors of the same site, intraoral tumors of minor gland origin, either benign or malignant, are usually nonulcerating.

Extraoral sites may be involved but less commonly so. However, in Conley and Dingman's[24] series of 78 adenoid cystic carcinomas, 19 of the lesions involving the minor salivary glands were located in the nose or paranasal sinuses. This site is extremely unfortunate both because of the long delay to diagnosis that is characteristic of sinus malignancy and because of the affinity of the tumor for adjacent nerves that are so close to the cranial foramen from which they emerge.

The trachea, larynx, and even the bronchi can harbor adenoid cystic tumor. The responsiveness of small squamous cell cancers of the larynx to irradiation therapy should not delude one into thinking that this modality is equally applicable to adenoid cystic cancers in this site. Conservation laryngeal surgery and irradiation are *not* adequate for cure. Rather, the same wide-field resection principles used for treating this tumor in the major salivary glands should be applied to the laryngeal lesion as well (**Fig. 8.45**).

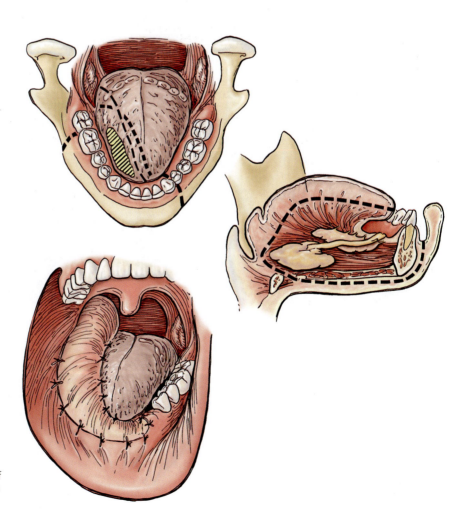

Fig. 8.43 Resection of the inferior aspect of the tongue and the anterior mandibular arch required for patient in **Fig. 8.42**.

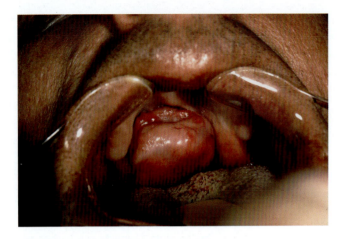

Fig. 8.44 Benign mixed tumor of the palate.

Salivary gland lesions of the oral cavity are resected according to the same criteria imposed by the various tumor types in the major salivary glands. Mucoepidermoid tumors of the minor salivary glands tend to be of low malignancy, and conservatism in resection is generally justifiable (**Fig.**

8.46). However, limited resection of mucoepidermoid tumors of minor glands is not always successful, and these patients suffer disastrous results. Careful attention must be paid to the histological grade of the tumor, and histologically negative margins must be ensured at the time of resection. In the poorly differentiated varieties this inevitably requires the excision of bone.[39]

Adenoid cystic tumors are resected with a wide margin, which for buccal mucosal or lip tumors often requires through-and-through excision and replacement with a flap. Adenocarcinomas require a similar approach. **Figure 8.47** illustrates a patient with an acinic cell tumor of the labial mucosa that, because of its proximity to skin, required resection from the skin to the mucosa in the labial sulcus as well as removal of the underlying bone of the anterior wall of the maxillary sinus. The malignant potential of the acinic cell tumor is very hard to predict on the basis of histological appearance. Therefore, it is better to be overcautious to assure a sufficiently radical excision. The fact that for adenoid cystic cancer the local recurrence rate was 50% in Conley's series, compared with 30 to 47% for the other tumor types,[23] emphasizes this point. Repeated resection is often needed, and even histopathological evidence of clear surgical margins is no guarantee of success.

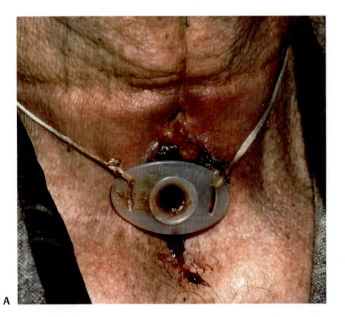

A

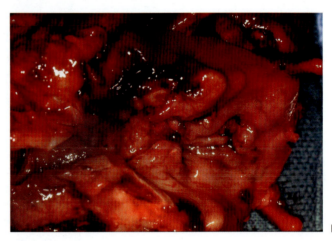

B

Fig. 8.45 (**A**) In this patient, an adenoid cystic carcinoma of the vocal cord was initially treated by hemilaryngectomy and postoperative irradiation. (**B**) There was massive local recurrence in the larynx and tracheotomy site.

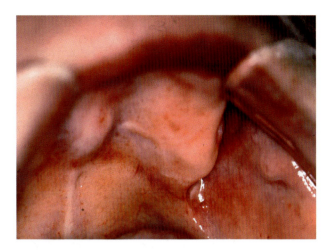

Fig. 8.46 Minor defect in the hard palate seen 7 years following local excision for a low-grade mucoepidermoid carcinoma.

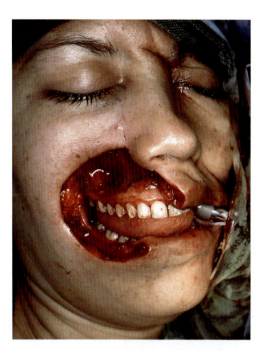

Fig. 8.47 Defect following excision of an acinic cell carcinoma of the right upper buccal and labial mucosa.

Case Reports

Case 1 (Figs. 8.48 and 8.49, page 338)

Mr. A.Y. was a 56-year-old male who presented with a 4-month history of a mass in the right parotid gland area. The mass had recently undergone an accelerated enlargement and was occasionally painful. There was no facial weakness and no numbness. On physical examination there was a 5 cm by 2.5 cm firm mass in the body of the right parotid gland (**Fig. 8.48**) fixed to the underling structures.

The facial nerve was dissected, and an open biopsy revealed a sebaceous carcinoma of the parotid gland. A portion of the facial nerve was imbedded in tumor, so a portion of the main trunk and proximal branches at the pes ansirinus had to be included in the specimen. A total parotidectomy, overlying skin excision, lateral temporal bone resection, and radical neck dissection were done. A cable graft taken from the greater auricular nerve was used to reestablish the continuity of the facial nerve. A gold weight was placed in the upper eyelid to ensure closure until facial nerve reinnervations occurred. He underwent a full course of irradiation to the parotid bed and neck. The patient is alive and well without disease 15 years later (**Fig. 8.49**).

Case 2

Mr. B.L. was a 41-year-old man who developed a pigmented lesion in the frontotemporal scalp of undetermined duration. The lesion was scaly on the surface, without ulceration or bleeding, and he noticed no cervical adenopathy. About 6 months prior to presentation he noticed a subcutaneous mass developing in the region of the ipsilateral parotid salivary gland. There was no facial nerve paralysis and no facial numbness. The skin lesion measured ~5 mm in diameter and the periparotid mass was ~3 cm in diameter and there were no palpable masses in the neck. A local otolaryngologist resected the pigmented lesion as well as the parotid gland at the same sitting. The skin lesion was 2 mm in thickness and was described as a compound nevus without malignant change, but the mass in the parotid was a metastatic melanoma. Because the margins of resection were close the patient was referred to University of California Davis Medical Center (UCDMC) for revision surgery. Three weeks later the patient underwent a radical parotidectomy, lateral temporal bone resection, and radical neck dissection. No postoperative radiotherapy was administered. The lateral temporal bone resection was done at about the level of the tympanic annulus sparing the tympanic membrane. He is now 15 years since surgery with no evidence of recurrence.

This is an example of a metastasis of a "sun-belt" tumor to the parotid gland. Such tumors, more commonly originating in squamous cell carcinoma of the skin, are the commonest parotid malignancies seen in our institution. This patient is a typical example of the type of resection that I think is most appropriate for advanced malignancies of the parotid.

Case 3 (Figs. 8.50 and 8.51, page 339)

Mr. G.M. was a 57-year-old male who presented with a rapidly growing mass in his left parotid gland that was first noticed 12 months before. It was massive in size (**Fig. 8.50**) and classified as T4bN2bM0. He had widespread invasion of the skin, a complete facial nerve paralysis, numbness over V3, invasion of the temporalis and masseter muscles as well as the zygoma and mandible, and metastases in the neck. Fine-needle biopsy showed poorly differentiated mucoepidermoid carcinoma.

He had an incontinuity resection of the parotid gland, seventh nerve, temporalis and masseter muscles, zygoma and mandible, and a radical neck dissection. He also had a lateral temporal bone resection (**Fig. 8.51**). The wound was closed with a cervicopectoral rotation flap. He had a positive margin on permanent section of the facial nerve so was taken back to surgery and had a re-resection of the nerve. Postoperative radiation therapy was done in a timely fashion. Although the patient remained locally free of tumor he died of pulmonary metastases 12 months later.

Radical resection and postoperative irradiation therapy controlled the disease locally, but the patient succumbed to distant metastatic disease.

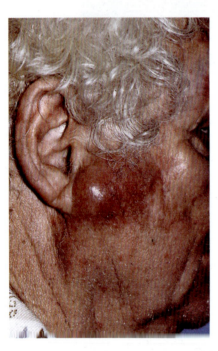

Fig. 8.48 *Case 1* Sebaceous carcinoma of the parotid.

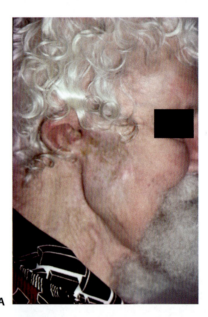

Fig. 8.49 *Case 1* Sebaceous carcinoma of the parotid. (**A**) 3.5 years after radical surgical excision and postoperative irradiation. (**B**) Patient is now 20 years since recurrence.

A

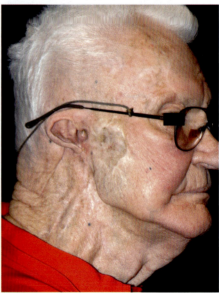

B

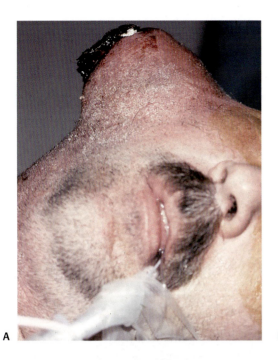

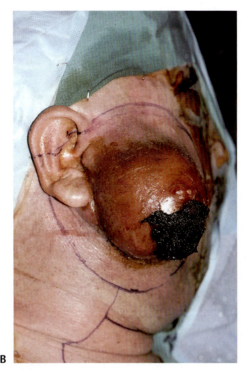

Fig. 8.50 *Case 3* Adenocarcinoma of the parotid. (**A**) Frontal view. (**B**) Lateral view.

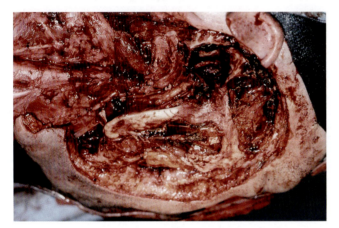

Fig. 8.51 *Case 3* Resection bed after radical removal.

References

1. Conley J. Concepts in Head and Neck Surgery. New York: Grune & Stratton; 1970:255–260
2. McFarland J. Adenoma of the salivary gland with report of a possible case. Am J Med Sci 1927;174:362–378
3. Polayes IM, Rankow RM. Cysts, masses and tumors of the accessory parotid gland. Plast Reconstr Surg 1979;64:17–23
4. Rankow RM, Polayes IM. Diseases of the Salivary Glands. Philadelphia; WB Saunders; 1976:162–163
5. Foote FW, Frazell EL. Tumors of the major salivary glands. Cancer 1953;6:1065–1113
6. Conley J. Salivary Glands and the Facial Nerve. New York: Grune & Stratton; 1975:151
7. Eneroth CM. Histological and clinical aspects of parotid tumors. Acta Otolaryngol Suppl 1964;188:1–99
8. Evansweather RW, Cruickshank AH. Epithelial Tumors of the Salivary Glands. Philadelphia: WB Saunders; 1970
9. Kleinsasser O. Behavior and adequate treatment of epithelial tumors of the parotid gland. In: Conley J, ed. Salivary Glands and the Facial Nerve. New York: Grune & Stratton; 1975:15–33
10. Rauch S, Seifert G, Gorlin RJ. Disease of the salivary glands: tumors. In: Gorlin RJ, Goldman HM, eds. Thomas' Oral Pathology. 6th ed. St. Louis: CV Mosby; 1970:1013
11. Work WP, Hecht DW. Tumors and cysts of major salivary glands. In: Shumrick DA, Paparella MM, eds. Otolaryngology. 2nd ed. Vol 3. Philadelphia: WB Saunders; 1980:2244
12. Eneroth CM. Mixed tumors of major salivary glands: prognostic role of capsular structure. Ann Otol Rhinol Laryngol 1965;74:944–953
13. Hubner G, Klein HJ, Kleinsasser O, et al. The role of the myoepithelial cells in the development of salivary gland tumors. Cancer 1971;27:1255–1261
14. Batsakis JG. Tumors of the major salivary glands. In: Tumors of the Head and Neck–Clinical and Pathological Considerations. Baltimore: Williams & Wilkins; 1974:1–37
15. Peel RL. Diseases of the salivary glands. In: Barnes L, ed. Surgical Pathology of the Head and Neck. Vol 1. 2nd ed. New York: Marcel Dekker; 2001:633–757
16. Blanck C, Eneroth CM, Jakobsson PA. Mucus-producing adenopapillary (nonepidermoid) carcinoma of the parotid gland. Cancer 1971;28:676–685
17. Rankow RM, Polayes IM. Diseases of the Salivary Glands. Philadelphia: WB Saunders; 1976:119–123
18. Seifert G. Mundspeicheldrusen Tonsillen und Rachen. In: Doerr-Seifert-Vehlinger: Spezielle Pathol. Anatomie Bd 1. Berlin: Springer; 1966
19. Wertheimer FW, Georgen GJ. Intraoral acinic cell adenocarcinoma. Oral Surg Oral Med Oral Pathol 1971;32:923–926
20. Eneroth CM, Jakobsson PA, Blanck C. Acinic cell carcinoma of the parotid gland. Cancer 1966;19:1761–1772
21. Thackray AC, Lucas RB. Tumors in the major salivary glands. In: Atlas of Tumor Pathology. 2nd ed. Fascicle 10. Washington, DC: Armed Forces Institute of Pathology; 1974
22. Perzin KH, Gullane P, Clairmont AC. Adenoid cystic carcinomas arising in salivary glands. Cancer 1978;42:265–282
23. Conley J. Salivary Glands and the Facial Nerve. New York: Grune & Stratton; 1975:153–154
24. Conley J, Dingman DL. Adenoid cystic carcinoma in the head and neck (cylindroma). Arch Otolaryngol 1974;100:81–90

25. Jakobsson PA, Blanck C, Eneroth CM. Mucoepidermold carcinoma of the parotid gland. Cancer 1968;22:111–124

26. Zajicek J, Eneroth CM. Cytological diagnosis of salivary gland carcinomata from aspiration biopsy smears. Acta Otolaryngol Suppl 1969;263:183–185

27. Conley J. Salivary Glands and the Facial Nerve. New York: Grune & Stratton; 1975:81

28. McCabe BF, Work PW. Parotidectomy with special preference in the facial nerve. In: English GM, ed. Otolaryngology. Vol 4. Hagerstown, MD: Harper & Row; 1967:39

29. Buchman C, Stringer SP, Mendenhall WM, Parson JT, Jordan JR, Cassisi NJ. Effect of tumor spill and inadequate resection on tumor recurrence. Laryngoscope 1994;104:1231–1234

30. George B, Laurian C. The Vertebral Artery: Pathology and Surgery. New York: Springer-Verlag; 1987

31. George B, Laurian C. Surgical approach to the whole length of the vertebral artery with special reference to the third portion. Acta Neurochir (Wien) 1980;51:259–272

32. Sen C, Catalano PJ. Extreme lateral transcondylar approach to the craniocervical junction. In: Donald PJ, ed. Skull Base Surgery. New York: Lippincott Raven; 1998:25:491–506

33. Spetzler RRF, Graham TW. The far lateral approach to the inferior clivus and the upper cervical region: technical note. BNI Q 1990;6:35–38

34. Conley J. Salivary Glands and the Facial Nerve. New York: Grune & Stratton; 1975:183

35. Smith LC, Lane N, Rankow RM. Cylindroma (adenoid cystic carcinoma): a report of fifty-eight cases. Am J Surg 1965;110:519–526

36. Rankow RM, Polayes IM. Disease of the Salivary Glands. Philadelphia: WB Saunders; 1976:38–5l

37. DelBalso AM. Malignant disease of the minor oral salivary glands. Otolaryngol Clin North Am 1979;12:135–140

38. Rafla-Demetrious S. Mucous and Salivary Gland Tumours. Springfield, IL: Charles C Thomas; 1970

39. Smitheringale A, Hoyek AM, Chapnik JS, et al. Mucoepidermoid carcinoma of the palate. J Otolaryngol 1981;10:261–266

9

Cancer of the Infratemporal Fossa and Skull Base

Paul J. Donald

Possibly the most challenging area in head and neck surgery is the region of the skull base. It was only a short time ago that neoplasms, especially malignancies, close or adherent to the undersurface of the cranium were considered inoperable. Once the barrier had been breached and tumor had spread intracranially, the patient's prognosis became entirely hopeless. This pessimistic situation has radically changed in recent years, however, thanks to the concurrence of three major developments: the advent of microvascular surgery, the emergence of the era of combined craniofacial surgery, and the advances in modern anesthesia in the areas of pharmacological manipulation and monitoring.

In 1972, McLean and Buncke[1] first transplanted omentum to the cranium using a microvascular anastomosis. During the past decade, the work of such pioneers as O'Brien, Acland, Taylor, and Harii established the techniques of free flap transplantation as a viable clinical tool. The application of these principles to the revascularization of compromised cerebral circulation was one of the major breakthroughs in expanding the scope and safety of skull base surgery.[2] One of the principal stumbling blocks in this area has always been the inviolability of the internal carotid artery. If this vessel was compromised, the viability of the ipsilateral cerebral hemisphere became severely jeopardized. Despite the assurance of numerous investigative procedures indicating collateral supply, this viability could not be guaranteed. The development of the superficial temporal-to-middle cerebral artery vascular anastomosis provided hope of making internal carotid artery sacrifice possible.[3] However, the low flow often seen through this anastomosis may be insufficient to provide adequate supply to the hemisphere deprived of its internal carotid supply. Currently the internal carotid artery is always replaced when feasible, even when a patient passes his or her balloon test occlusion (BTO) study and single photon emission computed tomography (SPECT) scan.

In recent years, much has been made of the so-called team approach, in which paramedical and medical personnel coordinate their efforts in the management of patients.

The impetus for this has largely come from the paramedical disciplines. It is curious that this most laudable concept had somewhat slow acceptance among some of the surgical disciplines when it concerned cooperation between certain surgical specialties. Cooperation between head and neck surgeons, especially otorhinolaryngologists, and neurological surgeons was initially halting. The neurosurgeons' reluctance to cooperate was based not so much on a lack of trust in their counterparts' ability to handle the cervicofacial end of the surgery, but on a deep concern that the carefully guarded, sterile cranial cavity would be exposed to the profusion of microorganisms inhabiting the environs of the upper aerodigestive tract. The work of Paul Tessier clearly demonstrated that a substantial surgical communication could be temporarily created between the cranial cavity and the upper aerodigestive system without undue hazard to the patient. The experiences of Ketcham et al[3,4] and Sisson et al[5] in the resection of extensive paranasal sinus tumors proved that combined craniofacial surgery can be done safely and with a low infection rate.

The cooperation between the neurological surgeon and the head and neck surgeon should be "a natural" because their respective skills are complementary with regard to the skull base region. The areas that hold a morbid fear for the head and neck surgeon—the contents of the cranial cavity—are regions of easy familiarity for the neurosurgeon. Those areas beneath the skull base and deep in the face that for the neurosurgeon are an anatomical and physiological mystery are common ground for head and neck surgeons.

The advances of modern anesthesia are largely responsible for the safety of the technical manipulations of the surgical team. Air embolism is a constant threat, especially if the patient is operated upon in the sitting position. In general, most of the procedures done by the author are done with the patient in the supine position. However, despite this, air embolism via the dural venous sinuses or the large veins in the neck, although less frequently a problem, is still a constant threat. Considerable evidence has been accumulated to show that the Doppler ultrasound can monitor the emergence of an air embolus much more precisely than any other monitoring system.[6] Its sensitivity compared with other methods is illustrated in **Table 9.1**. In the dog, a volume of air as scant as 0.12 to 0.25 mL can be detected. The characteristic murmur of an air embolus heard over the precordium is not heard until at least 15 to 30 mL of air is present.[7]

Table 9.1 Detectable Levels of Emboli in Dogs

Method	Embolus Volume per Body Weight (mL/kg)
Doppler	0.01–0.02
	0.10
Decreased end-tidal CO₂	0.25–0.50
	0.50–1.00
Elevated pulmonary artery pressure	0.25–0.50
Decreased blood pressure	4.00–8.00
Electrocardiography	4.00–8.00

Source: Hybels R. Venous air embolism in head and neck surgery. Laryngoscope 1980;90:950. Reprinted with permission.

The profusion of blood vessels in the region of the skull base, as well as in the equivalent area intracranially, creates a problem of significant blood loss. Controlled hypotension using nitroprusside or similar agents reduces hemorrhage markedly. A mean circulating blood pressure of 60 to 70 mm Hg adequately perfuses vital organs while markedly facilitating dissection, thus reducing both blood loss and operating time. Central venous and arterial pressure monitoring devices are essential in the safe application of this technique. A continuous digital readout displaying these parameters, as well as pulse and respiratory rates, greatly facilitates observation of the patient's intraoperative course.

Monitoring of intracranial pressure with a catheter in the third ventricle permits an indirect assessment of intracranial volume. A clear understanding of the relationship between intracranial volume and intracranial pressure is vital. Diminution of intracranial volume is an essential step in promoting optimal conditions for the neurosurgical part of the operation. Several measurements are involved in determining this critical factor. As cerebral blood flow increases, so does the cerebral volume (**Fig. 9.1**). A mean circulating blood pressure of between 60 and 100 mm Hg has little effect on blood flow to the brain. However, once 100 mm Hg is exceeded, cerebral blood flow and, concomitantly, intracranial volume increase. Cerebral vascular tone is exquisitely sensitive to concentrations of carbon dioxide partial pressure (PCO_2). An elevation of PCO_2 of 1 mm Hg will increase the cerebral blood flow by 2%. Although intracranial blood flow, and hence intracranial volume, is highly sensitive to PCO_2, there is no change in cerebral blood flow when the pressure of arterial oxygen (PaO_2) is between 40 and 300 mm Hg. Therefore it is essential to maintain a low PCO_2 during the intracranial part of the procedure. The insertion of a Dean tube, a catheter inserted into the endotracheal tube and connected to a CO_2 analyzer, records end tidal CO_2, providing a continuous precise moni-

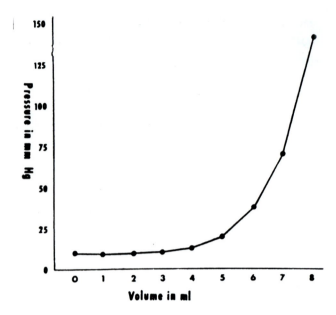

Fig. 9.1 A pressure-volume curve relating rises of intracranial pressure to increases in intracerebral volume. Pressure is in millimeters of Hg and volume is in cubic cm. This curve was extrapolated from an experiment relating intracranial volume and pressure using an inflatable balloon in the cranium of a Rhesus monkey. (From Youmans JR. Neurological Surgery. Vol 2. 2nd ed. Philadelphia: WB Saunders; 1982:854. Reprinted with permission.)

toring of this vital parameter. Care must be taken to maintain the airway pressure on the respirator below 25 cm H_2O. Pressures in excess of this will raise intracranial pressure.

Anesthetic agents may have an effect on cerebral blood flow as well. Inducting agents such as Althesin (GlaxoSmith Kline, Brentford, UK) and thiopental bring about a decrease in cerebral flow, and hence a fall in intracranial pressure. On the other hand, halothane causes an increase in pressure. Although methoxyflurane appears to be the agent of choice at some institutions,[8] the best anesthetic for minimizing cerebral flow is a combination of nitrous oxide and narcotics (**Table 9.2**).

Successful craniofacial surgery depends not only on the smooth coordination of the surgical team but on expert nursing care as well. Diligent postoperative observation and rapid intervention in the event of an alteration in the patient's status is vital in the care of these patients. Following a technically successful procedure, the loss of life or the development of permanent morbid sequelae as a result of inadequate, inattentive postoperative care is an execrable tragedy. A therapeutic dilemma that occasionally follows extensive craniofacial procedures is the problem of poor systemic perfusion in a hypotensive patient in whom restoration of an adequate blood pressure with intravascular volume augmentation will result in an intolerable increase in cerebral volume. Early intervention by an experienced skilled medical team for the delicate management of volume replacement and pharmacological regulation of systemic pressure is the only hope of saving the patient from the ravages of profound cerebral edema. Monitoring of the patient's hemodynamics, blood gases, and cerebrospinal fluid (CSF) pressure must be a continuous and compulsively exercised pursuit.

Table 9.2 Physiological Factors and Drugs Affecting Cerebral Blood Flow

Factors during Anesthesia Causing an Increase in Intracranial Pressure
Straining during induction
Increased blood flow
Increased intrathoracic or intraabdominal pressure
Agents
Halothane
Methoxyflurane
Trichloroethylene
Enflurane
Ketamine

Factors during Anesthesia Causing a Decrease in Intracranial Pressure
Hyperventilation
Osmotic diuretics
Nitroprusside
Atropine
Agents
Innovar
Nitrous oxide
Barbiturates

◆ Anatomy

Skull base anatomy is complex, requiring the head and neck surgeon who endeavors to perform surgical procedures here to have a meticulous three-dimensional conception of the topography and contents of the region. Moreover, it is mandatory to comprehend the structures that lie on the opposing cranial surfaces of the plates and buttresses on which one is working. Much like acquiring an appreciation of the anatomy of the temporal bone during dissections prior to performing ear surgery, the central anatomy must be studied "from the outside in." Preparation for surgery is done in the dissecting laboratory or the autopsy room where, with the aid of anatomical texts, a spatial conception of this region can be formulated. Surgery in the skull base area is very demanding but is not outside the scope of any well-trained head and neck surgeon who is willing to do a little homework and acquire the necessary team members.

Nasopharyngeal carcinoma has been generally considered and still remains essentially a nonsurgical disease. The mucosa of this region suffers the disadvantage of being adherent and adjacent to several vital structures. It is tightly affixed to the bone of the clivus, precluding a clean plane of dissection, as is usually found throughout the rest of the pharynx. In addition, the internal carotid artery in the lateral recesses is separated from the nasopharynx by a mere plug of cartilage in the inferior aspect of the foramen lacerum, and the brain stem is located on the deep surface of the clivus (**Fig. 9.2**). However, despite these complicating factors, recent surgical advances have permitted nasopharyngeal resections in highly selected cases.

Soon after the eustachian tube enters the region of the nasopharynx, the upper portion of the superior constrictor muscle forms a sort of sling under the tube. The superior constrictor muscle of the nasopharynx has its origin on the pharyngeal tubercles of the basiocciput and inserts into the inferior aspect of the medial pterygoid plate and hamulus as well as the pterygomandibular raphe. The tubercles are the origin of both the pharyngobasilar and the buccopharyngeal fascial sheaths that encase the superior constrictor muscle in its anterior and posterior aspects, respectively (**Fig. 9.3**). The remainder of the clivus is covered by a thick layer of mucosa that overlies a very heavy layer of periosteum. The lateral walls of the nasopharynx are made up mainly of the structures in the foramen of Morgagni—the gap that extends between the clivus and the superior border of the superior constrictor. The eustachian tube and its pharyngeal elaboration, the torus tubarius, along with the tensor and levator muscles of the palate, are the principal structures occupying this gap (**Fig. 9.4**). They are leashed together by the pharyngobasilar fascia. At the anterior aspect of the lateral extent of the nasopharyngeal roof, just medial to the region of the pterygoid plates, is the foramen lacerum. The inferior portion of the foramen is obliterated by a cartilage plug, but the superior part harbors the internal carotid artery as it sweeps out of the petrous apex into the cavernous sinus. The proximity of the internal carotid artery and cavernous sinus, and the presence of the brain stem on the intracranial side of the clivus, had until recently precluded the use of surgery for lesions in the nasopharynx. Over the last 2 decades surgical procedures on the clivus such as those developed by Fang and Ong,[9] Crockard,[10] and Donald and Bernstein[11] have been developed to resect nasopharyngeal neoplasms. The transpalatal approach by Fee and colleagues,[12,13] which gives limited but adequate access for small tumors, has been complemented by the procedures of Cocke and Robertson,[14] Wei and colleagues,[15,16] and Janecka et al,[17] who approach the nasopharynx from the midface, and those of Sekhar and Schramm,[18] Fisch,[19] and Yasergil,[59] who gain the exposure of this region from the lateral aspect. These procedures have enabled surgeons to achieve complete resection of even squamous cell carcinoma at this site.

Sphenoid Sinus

The sphenoid sinus resides in a unique area in the head, occupying its anatomical center. Lying above it, suspended from the region of the hypothalamus, in the sella turcica, is the grand orchestrator of bodily hormonal function, the pituitary gland (**Fig. 9.5**). It is related laterally to the cavernous sinus and its contents.

Posterior to the sphenoid sinus is the posterior extent of the basisphenoid and its articulation with the basiocciput; these latter two bones are commonly called collectively the clivus. The anterior surface of the sinus contains its ostium, emptying into the sphenoethmoidal recess in the posterior vault of the nasal chamber. The sphenopalatine artery runs under the sinus ostium and may be a source of troublesome bleeding if not adequately coagulated prior to severance. In cases of marked pneumatization, the thick floor of the sinus may form a small part of the anterior roof of the nasopharynx. The inferior aspect of the anterior sinus wall forms the

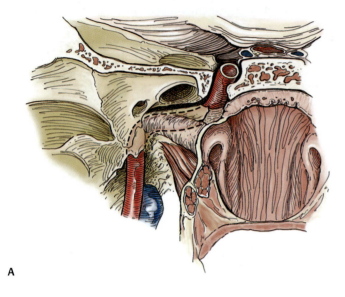

A

Fig. 9.2 (**A**) Coronal section through the nasopharynx and overlying brain at the level of the foramen lacerum. (**B**) Parasagittal cut through the nasopharynx and clivus through the petrous apex. (Fig. 9.2B from Pernkoff E. Atlas of Topographical and Applied Human Anatomy. Vol 1. Philadelphia: WB Saunders; 1963. Reprinted with permission.)

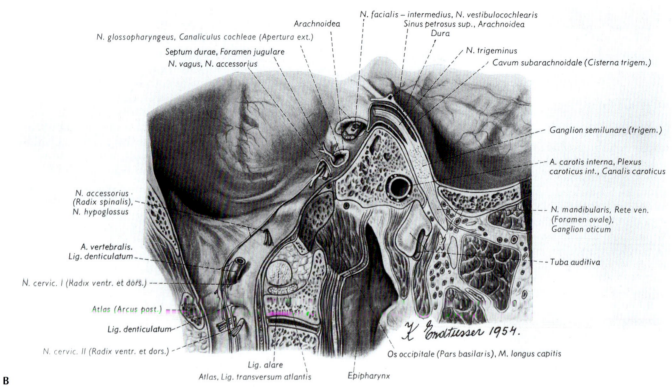

B

sphenoid rostrum, which is at the posteriormost extremity of the roof of the nasal cavity.

The sphenoid sinus may be highly variable in its extent (**Fig. 9.6**). It is described in relation to the sella turcica, which is a vital consideration in the transsphenoidal approach to the pituitary. Pneumatization may consist merely of a dimple on the anterior surface of the basiocciput. Presellar and especially postsellar pneumatization will permit a satisfactory approach to the gland. Although the optic nerve is usually related to the sphenoid sinus high on its lateral wall (see chapter 5, Fig. 5.3), in certain individuals the sinus actually wraps around

the optic nerve (**Fig. 9.7**). Before extensive surgery in this area, a careful study of the computed tomographic (CT) scan of the sinuses and skull base in the coronal view is mandatory to establish the nature of this anatomical relationship.

Cavernous Sinus and Clivus

The cavernous sinus lies directly against the bone making up the lateral wall of the sphenoid sinus (**Fig. 9.8**). The dura that forms each sinus is derived from the sphenoidal periosteum. Each cavernous sinus extends from the orbital apex anteri-

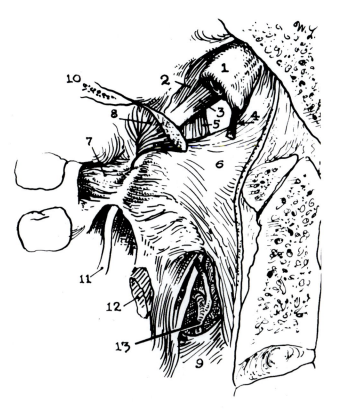

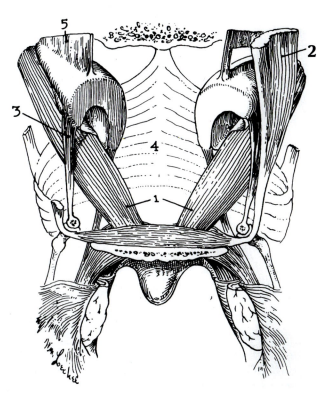

Fig. 9.3 Lateral view of the nasopharynx and oropharynx to show superior constrictor of the pharynx (6), which is shown attaching to the hamulus and pterygomandibular raphe and continuing on as the buccinator (7). The levator muscle (3) and the tubal cartilage (1) are shown passing through the sinus of Morgagni. The tensor muscle (2) is shown descending and passing around the hamulus (8). 5, medial pterygoid muscle; 4, salpingopharyngeal muscle; 10, hard palate; 9, middle constrictor muscle; 11, lingual nerve; 12, palatoglossus; 13, facial artery. (From Proctor B. Anatomy of the eustachian tube. Arch Otolaryngol 97:6, 1973. Reprinted with permission.)

Fig. 9.4 Schema showing the position of the levator muscle (1) with respect to the eustachian tube, superior tubal ligament (5), and two components of the tensor veli palatine muscle—one that tenses the palate (2) and another that pulls the hook of the eustachian cartilage downward (3). The superior pharyngeal constrictor muscle (4) is also shown.

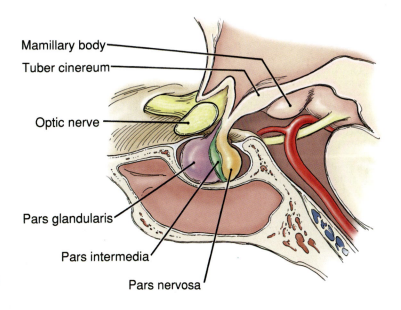

Mamillary body
Tuber cinereum
Optic nerve
Pars glandularis
Pars intermedia
Pars nervosa

Fig. 9.5 The pituitary gland, its immediate relations and physiological compartments.

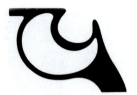
Sellar
226 (85%)

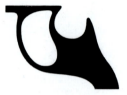
Presellar
32 (12%)

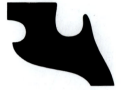
Conchal
8 (3%)

Fig. 9.6 Varieties of sphenoid sinus pneumatization. (From Hardy J, Maina G. Microsurgical anatomy in transsphenoidal hypophysectomy. J Neurol Sci 1977;21:151. Reprinted with permission.)

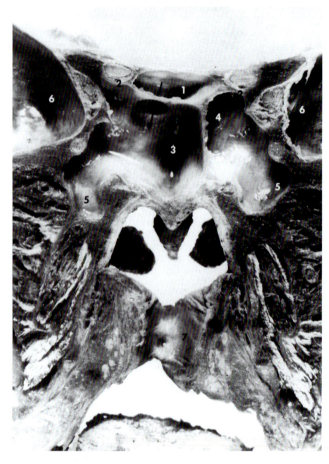

Fig. 9.7 Anatomical specimen cut in coronal section through the sphenoid sinus, illustrating the sinus surrounding ~200 degrees of the left optic nerve. Posterior facing surface. 1, superior compartment in the sphenoid sinus; arrow demonstrates foramen communication with the main body of the sinus; 2, optic nerves separated by a thin plate of bone from the sphenoid sinus, which wraps around it on the left side for 280 degrees; 3, left sphenoid sinus larger than the right; 4, right sphenoid sinus; 5, pterygoid extensions of the sphenoid sinuses; 6, greater wings of the sphenoid bone; 7, cleft palate defect. (Adapted from Ritter FN. The Paranasal Sinuses: Anatomy and Surgical Techniques. 2nd ed. St Louis: CV Mosby; 1976:83. Reprinted with permission.)

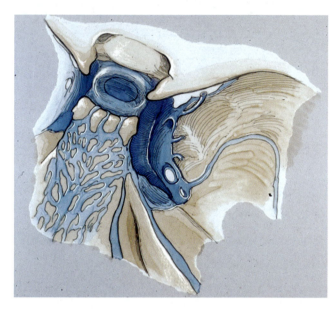

Fig. 9.8 Cavernous sinus showing connections across the midline via the circular sinus and the basilar plexus.

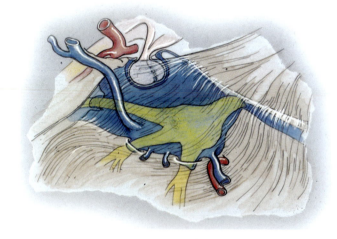

Fig. 9.9 Venous connections of the cavernous sinuses and the bridging cerebral veins leading into it: (**A**) lateral view; (**B**) top view.

344

orly to the petrous ridge posteriorly. The petrous apex terminates in the floor of the sinus. A plethora of veins drain into it, making it vulnerable to a variety of sources of infection. The cavernous sinus connects to both the superior and the inferior petrosal sinuses, as well as the sphenoparietal sinus. Further anteriorly, connections to the superior and inferior orbital veins establish a direct connection to the veins of the face. The neurovascular foramina in the floor of the cavernous sinus establish routes to the paranasal sinuses, the principal vein being the connection to the pterygoid plexus through the foramen of Vesalius. The foramen lacerum, the conduit for the internal carotid artery, is also in the sinus floor. In addition, there are several bridging veins that go from the cerebral surface to the cavernous sinus. The commonest ones are from the anterior and middle cerebral veins (**Fig. 9.9**). Each of the dural venous cavernous sinuses is connected to

its fellow on the opposite side of the sphenoid sinus by the circular sinus. The circular sinus, although it encircles the pituitary stalk, is in reality a labyrinth of blood-filled channels and spaces rather than a single venous conduit (**Fig. 9.8**).

The second connection across the midline is through the basilar plexus, which lies over the cranial surface of the clivus (**Fig. 9.9**). Running through the cavernous sinus are the optic nerve; the third, fourth, and sixth cranial nerves; the first, second, and occasionally the third branches of the trigeminal nerve; and the internal carotid artery (**Fig. 9.10**). The artery may indent the posterolateral wall of the sphenoid sinus and appear from the interior perspective of the sinus as a bulge. The third cranial nerve (the oculomotor) lies superiorly in the superior aspect of the lateral dura of the cavernous sinus encased in a double layer. The fourth cranial nerve (trochlear nerve) is much smaller than the oculomotor and lies just below it.

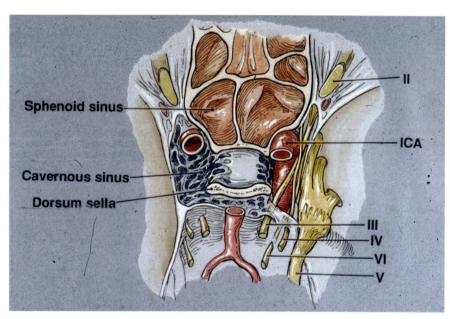

Fig. 9.10 Cavernous sinus internal carotid artery and cranial nerves. ICA, internal carotid artery.

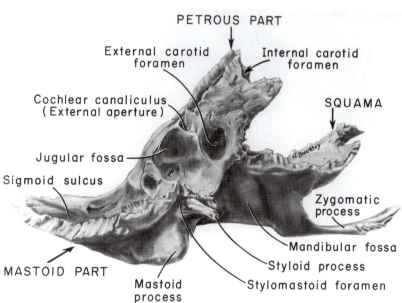

Fig. 9.11 The inferior surface of the temporal bone. (From Anson BJ, Donaldson JA. Surgical Anatomy of the Temporal Bone and Ear. 2nd ed. Philadelphia: WB Saunders; 1973:9. Reprinted with permission.)

The clivus is composed of the basisphenoid bone anteriorly and the basiocciput posteriorly. The two bones are connected by a synostosis. Much of the basisphenoid is often occupied by the sphenoid sinus.

Undersurface of the Temporal Bone

To most otorhinolaryngologists, the anatomy of the temporal bone is well understood. However, unless they are engaged in considerable inner ear surgery, most practitioners find that their comprehension of the inferior surface of the bone (**Fig. 9.11**) dims with time.

Although the temporal bone itself is shaped roughly like a triangle, with the base situated laterally and the apex at the petrous tip medially, it may be helpful to envision its undersurface as a rectangular area canted at roughly 45 degrees to the side of the skull (**Fig. 9.12**). The lateral corners are bounded by the articular eminence anteriorly and the

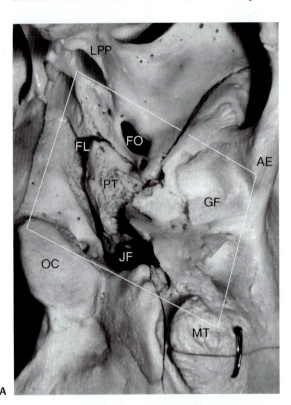

A

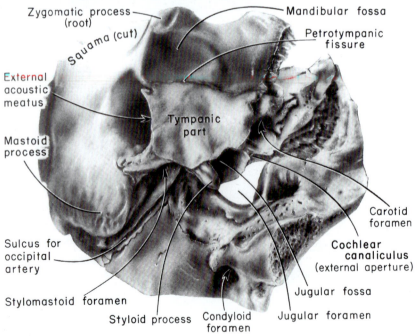

B

Fig. 9.12 **(A)** The undersurface of the skull base. This area is roughly rectangular and is canted anteromedially at 45 degrees. LPP, lateral pterygoid plate; AE, articular eminence; FL, foramen lacerum; FO, foramen ovale; PT, petrous tip; GF, glenoid fossa; JF, jugular foramen; OC, occipital condyle; MT, mastoid tip). **(B)** Anteroinferior view of temporal bones. (Fig. 9.12B from Anson BJ, Donaldson JA. Surgical Anatomy of the Temporal Bone and Ear. 2nd ed. Philadelphia: WB Saunders; 1973:11. Reprinted with permission.)

anterior lip of the occipital condyle posteriorly. Although the inferior surface of the temporal bone makes up 90% of this area of the skull base, the sphenoid anteromedially and the occiput posteromedially make small contributions.

Deep to the mastoid tip, the posterior belly of the digastric muscle takes its origin and receives its innervation directly from the main trunk of the facial nerve. A notch medial to the muscle houses the occipital artery. This artery can be responsible for considerable hemorrhage during surgery if not well controlled. As further progress anteromedially is made, the styloid process is seen with the origin of the styloid muscles and ligament. Just deep and posterior to it are the stylomastoid foramen and the emergence of the facial nerve.

Directly medial to the styloid process is the jugular foramen, and just deep and anterior to it, separated by a thin ridge of bone, the carotid canal. Posteromedial to the carotid is the occipital condyle and its articulation with C1. Posteromedial to the carotid canal and under the lip of the occipital condyle is the foramen of the hypoglossal canal, the iter of the hypoglossal nerve. The vagus, glossopharyngeal, and spinal accessory nerves exit the skull adjacent to the medial surface of the jugular vein, through the incisura between the temporal and occipital bones.

Returning more laterally to the anterolateral corner of the skull base rectangle, and proceeding from the articular eminence medially, the remaining anatomy of this complex region is revealed. Just posterior to the eminence is the condyle of the mandible in the glenoid fossa. The glenoid fossa lies directly underneath the lateral aspect of the middle cranial fossa. Its medial extent lies anteromedial to the foramina for the great vessels. A fissure cut coronally, directly through the center of the glenoid fossa plate, will expose the eustachian tube. Surgical removal of the condylar head is essential to the complete exposure of the middle fossa floor.

With the condylar head removed and sighting from lateral to medial, the undersurface of the temporal bone appears to be a steep triangle. Anteriorly, the lateral pterygoid muscular insertions retract into the infratemporal fossa, and these, as well as the temporal muscle, form the anterior wall. The posterior wall is formed by the tympanic bone and its vaginal process. At the blunted apex of the triangle, the beginning of the cartilaginous eustachian tube, the tensor palatini anteriorly and the levator palatini posteriorly are located. At the anteriormost aspect of this apex is the sphenoid spine.

Adjacent to the medial surface of the sphenoid spine is the foramen spinosum, which contains the middle meningeal artery. The sphenoid spine is also one of the points of origin for the tensor muscle of the soft palate, which courses along and takes further origin on the lateral plate of the cartilaginous portion of the eustachian tube on its way to the nasopharynx.

The Infratemporal Fossa and Pterygomaxillary Space

The infratemporal fossa is a space on the side of the head that begins superiorly at the temporal line at the inferior limit of the temporal fossa and lays deep to the zygomatic arch just in front of the "skull base rectangle." The temporal fossa houses the temporalis muscles, whereas the pterygoid muscles and the internal maxillary artery (**Fig. 9.13**) reside in the infratemporal fossa. The medial wall of the fossa is the squamosal portion of the skull superiorly and the lateral maxillary sinus wall and lateral pterygoid plate inferiorly. The fossa leads into the pterygomaxillary space through the fissure of the same name in the middle of this medial wall.

The pterygomaxillary space (**Fig. 9.14**) is directly behind the maxillary sinus, just under the medial aspect of the skull base and just above the pterygoid plates. The internal maxillary artery enters the space following its passage between the two heads of the internal pterygoid muscle. Upon reaching the space, it ramifies into its terminal branches. The maxillary nerve, gaining entrance via the foramen rotundum, traverses the space while arborizing into branches that pass together with their accompanying vessels through the various exiting foramina. The vidian canal enters the pterygomaxillary space posteriorly, carrying the amalgamation of the deep petrosal and greater superficial petrosal nerves (**Fig. 9.15**). Although tumors rarely take origin in this space, neoplasms originating in the nasopharynx, buccal space, maxillary sinus, and infratemporal fossa often find their way to this site. The foramen ovale with its contained nerve, the mandibular branch of the trigeminal, is situated slightly anterior and medial to the middle meningeal artery. The medialmost limit of the foramen approximates the beginning of the lateral pterygoid plate. Now the anteromedial apex of the skull base rectangle has been reached. An imaginary line subtended from the medial pterygoid plate to the anterior limit of the occipital condyle marks the lateral wall of the nasopharynx.

◆ Pathology

Although this book is intended to deal mainly with malignancies, some benign tumors, because of their location and biological behavior, are considered malignant by position and proclivity. This is particularly true of tumors located at the skull base. For instance, *juvenile nasopharyngeal angiofibroma*, a vasoformative tumor of vascular channels and spaces and intervening fibrous connective tissue (**Fig. 9.16**), has a predilection for prepubertal males, often is hormonally dependent, and can remain occult for some time until presenting with nasal obstruction or epistaxis (**Fig. 9.17 and Fig. 9.18**). The tumor arises in the sphenoid bone near the origin of the pterygoid plates[20] presumably from totipotential cells that differentiate into the characteristic fibroblasts and endothelially lined vascular spaces of this tumor. It slowly expands into the nasopharynx and then extends into the paranasal sinuses, infratemporal fossa, skull base, and even the anterior and middle cranial fossae. The bony erosion produced by the tumor is probably a pressure phenomenon, and large protrusions often occur through the osseous barriers in its path. The characteristic presenting symptom of profuse epistaxis may be absent or of reduced intensity, masquerading as a routine "nuisance type" nosebleed. Such tumors may assume considerable size, as in the patient shown in **Fig. 9.18**, who presented with total nasal obstruction, a mass in the cheek and palate, and proptosis. As intracranial involve-

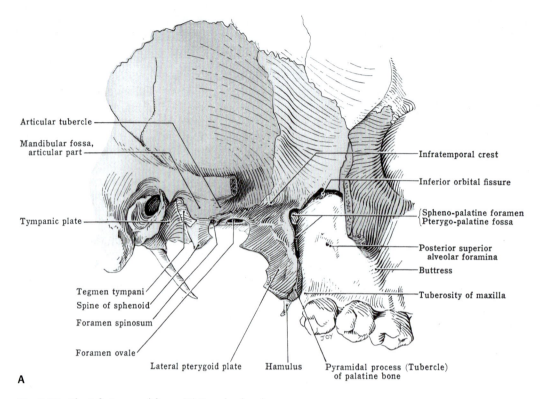

Articular tubercle

Mandibular fossa, articular part

Tympanic plate

Infratemporal crest

Inferior orbital fissure

Spheno-palatine foramen
Pterygo-palatine fossa

Posterior superior alveolar foramina

Buttress

Tuberosity of maxilla

Tegmen tympani
Spine of sphenoid
Foramen spinosum

Foramen ovale

Lateral pterygoid plate   Hamulus   Pyramidal process (Tubercle)
of palatine bone

A

Fig. 9.13   The infratemporal fossa. (**A**) Bony landmarks.

ment occurs, branches of the internal carotid artery make contributions to an already abundant blood supply.

Chordoma, a locally malignant but rarely metastasizing tumor of notochordal origin, is one of the tumors that can be best managed by partial clivectomy. It arises from cells that are remnants of the embryological notochord. The nasopharyngeal variety accounts for about one third of these tumors, which in the main take origin in the clivus at the suture line between the basisphenoid and the basiocciput. According to Binkhorst et al,[21] chordomas can also arise from the dorsum sellae, the retropharyngeal area, the apical ligament of the odontoid, and the nucleus pulposus of the cervical vertebrae. Because of their slow growth they often do not present until they have compromised cranial nerves in either the optic or the otic systems.[22,23] Histologically they are composed of trabeculations of polygonal cells containing eosinophilic granular or homogeneous cytoplasm. Cytoplasmic vacuolations are present in foci throughout the tumor and are thought to represent cellular aging.[23] This pathognomonic vacuolated cell—the so-called physaliphorous cell—is characteristic of chordoma. These grossly lobulated tumors have a tendency to erode bone and invade soft tissue structures.

Envelopment of cranial nerves and the internal carotid artery, together with aggressive invasion of the dura, renders complete resection of these lesions extremely difficult. Until recently, total excision was considered impossible, and palliative surgery and radiotherapy were often the only choices of therapy. Refinements in craniofacial surgery and the advent of transclival resection and the far lateral approach have made possible total resection in heretofore-hopeless cases.

Connective tissue tumors such as fibromas, schwannomas, lipomas, and their malignant counterparts can inhabit the skull base region. Both benign and malignant forms can erode bone and extend intracranially. Moreover, neither type can be differentiated on the basis of local behavior alone. Sarcomas of the nasopharynx or those invading the skull base from adjacent regions have a uniformly dismal prognosis because of local recurrence. On the other hand, the benign forms, if totally removed, have an excellent prognosis. Although the major problem with sarcomas is local recurrence, occasionally regional lymphatic, but especially distant bloodborne, metastases pose a significant problem.

The erosion of bone is not the only route of spread. The neural and vascular foramina of the middle fossa floor also provide portals of tumor intrusion. Often these tumors remain occult until compromise of the nerves traversing these foramina produces symptoms suggesting their presence. Schwannomas of the nerves of the jugular foramen, when high in the neck, may be mistaken for neoplasms in the tail of the parotid. Magnetic resonance imaging (MRI) and CT scans of the upper neck will make the differentiation.[24]

Malignant connective tissue tumors are rare. Leiomyosarcoma, fibrosarcoma, liposarcoma, myxoma, malignant histiocytoma, rhabdomyosarcoma, and malignant schwannomas have all been reported and commonly occur in the recesses near the skull base (**Fig. 9.19**). Malignancies of blood vessel origin, such as hemangiopericytoma and malignant glomus jugulare tumor, are also seen. *Hemangiopericytomas*, originating in the pericytes of Zimmerman, have a dismal prognosis when intracranial spread occurs because local inva-

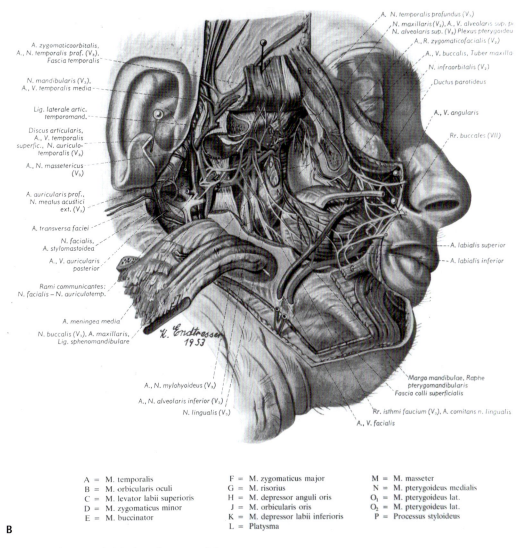

A = M. temporalis
B = M. orbicularis oculi
C = M. levator labii superioris
D = M. zygomaticus minor
E = M. buccinator

F = M. zygomaticus major
G = M. risorius
H = M. depressor anguli oris
J = M. orbicularis oris
K = M. depressor labii inferioris
L = Platysma

M = M. masseter
N = M. pterygoideus medialis
O_1 = M. pterygoideus lat.
O_2 = M. pterygoideus lat.
P = Processus styloideus

B

Fig. 9.13 (*continued*) (**B**) The infratemporal fossa contents. (Fig. 9.13A from Grant JCB. Grant's Atlas of Anatomy. 6th ed. Baltimore: Williams & Wilkins; 1972. Fig. 9.13B reprinted with permission from Pernkoff E. Atlas of Topographical and Applied Human Anatomy. Vol. I. Philadelphia: WB Saunders; 1963. Reprinted with permission.)

sion to this extent usually means that there are concomitant distant metastases. The orbit and nasopharynx are the most common sites of origin in the head and neck.[25] The skin and muscle account for the majority of tissues primarily involved, and ~25% of all such lesions occur in the head and neck.

Hemangiopericytoma is a rapidly growing, locally aggressive tumor with a high local recurrence rate. Regional lymph node metastases are uncommon. The histological diagnosis is sometimes difficult. The tumor cells are located between the flattened endothelial cells of the numerous capillaries of the tumor and the investing reticulin layer.[26] Reticulin stains are often necessary to clarify this relationship. Curiously, there is some electron-microscopic evidence indicating a similar origin of hemangiopericytoma and subungual glomus tumors.[27] Malignancy is difficult to determine histologically. Mitotic figures and anaplasia are features common to both benign and malignant varieties and are inaccurate predictors of bio-

logical activity. Disturbance of the relationship between the tumor cells and the reticulin layer has been reputed to be a sign of malignancy.[28]

Leiomyosarcoma is very uncommon and is rarely seen in the head and neck. Most of these tumors arise in the subcutis, probably from the erector pili muscles, but occasionally lesions will develop from the wall of the internal jugular vein. *Rhabdomyosarcoma* is most commonly seen in the orbit in children, with the next most frequent site being the nasopharynx.

It is not the purpose of this chapter to present an exhaustive treatise on soft tissue tumors because this confusing group of neoplasms is expertly dealt with by several other recognized authorities.[29–31] However, some attention should be given to the *fibrous neoplasms* because they are a confusing melange of tumors and proliferations. Not all types are common problems in the region of the skull base, but an un-

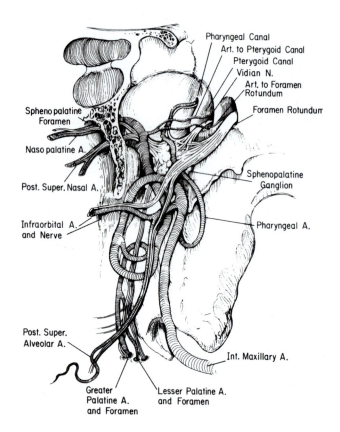

Fig. 9.14 The pterygomaxillary space. (From Morgenstein RM. Surgery of the pterygopalatine fossa. In: English GM, ed. Otolaryngology. Hagerstown, MD: Harper & Row; 1976:3. Reprinted with permission.)

derstanding of the natural history of these tumors as a group is necessary to have a clear picture of them as a pathological entity.

In describing tumors of connective tissue cell origin, Conley eloquently states, "Although these specific tissue entities lend themselves to an arbitrary academic classification, their dynamism for capricious primitive cellular development, functionalism, and partial mutation seems to create critical obstacles to their accurate microscopic classification."[32] Batsakis[29] roughly classifies fibrous lesions as benign, malignant, or indeterminate. Of the last group he explains, "Classifications of this group of tumors (proliferations and neoplasms) have often been rambling monstrosities with terms such as fasciitis, nodular fasciitis, infiltrative fasciitis, pseudosarcomatous fibromatosis, aggressive fibromatosis, cellular keloid, differentiated or Grade 1 fibrosarcoma, and non-metastasizing fibrosarcoma, either lumped together or sharply defined by ill-defined and often intangible criteria." The differentiation of *fibroma* from *fibrosarcoma* on a histological basis is often extremely difficult because the usual criteria of mitotic activity, cellular pleomorphism, nuclear hyperchromatism, and extracapsular invasion cannot be reliably used to make this distinction. The presence of metastases, of course, definitively designates the lesion as malignant, but this is an uncommon occurrence in fibrosarcoma. Very often the differentiation has to be made on the basis of biological activity. The pathological diagnosis then emerges from a composite of clues derived from historic, radiographic, and histological data. Very often the surgeon who is managing the case must make the definitive diagnosis, being the only person cognizant of the aggressiveness of the specific tumor under treatment.

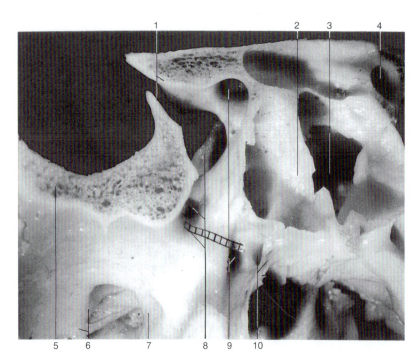

Fig. 9.15 Pterygopalatine fossa with posterior foramina and surrounding area in frontal section seen from in front. 1, superior orbital fissure; 2, oblique septum of the sphenoidal sinus; 3, left sphenoidal sinus; 4, left optic canal; 5, floor of the middle cranial fossa; 6, sphenoidal lamina; 7, lateral plate of the pterygoid process; 8, dorsum sellai and foramen rotundum: millimeter strip; 9, optic canal and anterior aperture of the pterygoid canal; 10, palatovaginal canal and palatine (sphenoidal process).

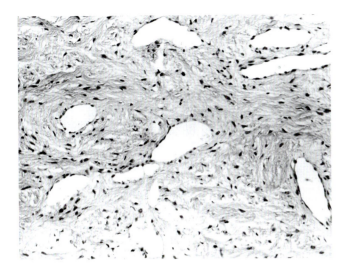

Fig. 9.16 Photomicrograph of juvenile angiofibroma showing numerous vascular spaces in a fibrous tissue stroma (H&E, ×220). (From Donald PJ. Sarcomatous degeneration in a nasopharyngeal angiofibroma. Otolaryngol Head Neck Surg 1979;87:42. Reprinted with permission.)

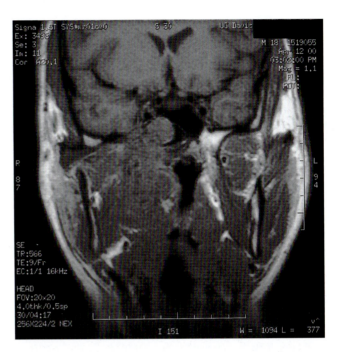

Fig. 9.17 Coronal magnetic resonance imaging scan of 17-year-old male with a large nasopharyngeal angiofibroma beginning near the superior aspect of the sphenoid bone near the origin of the pterygoid plates. Note tumor extending into the infratemporal fossa and the middle cranial fossa.

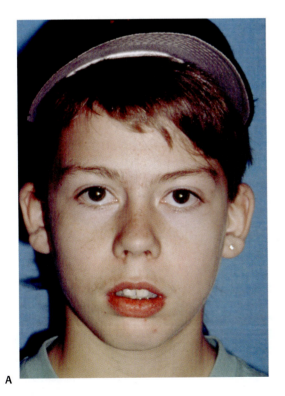

A

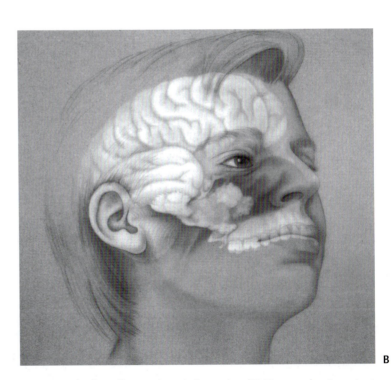

B

Fig. 9.18 (**A**) A 14-year-old male presenting with epistaxis, mild proptosis, cheek swelling, and nasal obstruction. (**B**) Diagram showing extent of tumor; note extension into the cavernous sinus.

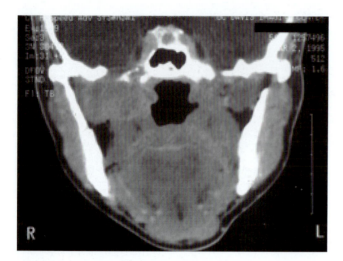

Fig. 9.19 Computed tomographic scan showing a leiomyosarcoma invading the third branch of the trigeminal nerve and extending through the foramen ovale. (Courtesy of Susan Stanton.)

Figure 9.20 portrays even more graphically the confusion that exists over the classification of fibrous tumors, although it does in some way provide a framework to work by. *Fibromas* are difficult to diagnose and are quite uncommon. Many of the tumors formerly bearing this appellation were in fact histiocytomas. Most of these tumors occur in skin and are rarely seen in the region of the skull base. One patient in our experience had a desmoid tumor of the infratemporal fossa that invaded the middle cranial fossa floor and extended into the middle fossa and cavernous sinus. He presented with a frozen globe and impairment of all branches of the trigeminal nerve on the affected side. Despite two aggressive attempts at resection including the entire cavernous sinus and the temporal lobe dura; dissection of the internal carotid artery; removal of the sphenoid sinus and the clivus; and resection of the infratemporal fossa, nasopharynx, and oropharynx, negative margins could not be obtained.

Postoperative irradiation was given, with little effect on the residual tumor. The patient was a prisoner and extended follow-up was impossible. This case illustrates the problem of classification of these fibrous neoplasms whose behavior is clearly malignant.

Fibrosarcoma was formerly one of the most commonly diagnosed soft tissue malignancies, often in error. The patient whose MRI is seen in **Fig. 9.22** had the appearance of a slowly growing mass in the left neck that suddenly over a period of 3 days became rapidly larger. The patient had severe pain over the mass, paralysis of the left side of the tongue, and a complete left vocal cord paralysis. Surgical exploration revealed a fish-flesh-appearing, hard mass encasing the common and internal carotid arteries and all the lower cranial nerves in the neck. Diagnosis was made variously as an "aggressive fibrotic process consistent with nodular fasciitis" and fibrosarcoma by several consultants from different institutions. The patient had a rapid and complete resolution of the mass with a course of steroid medication. At 5 years follow-up there is no mass and the cranial palsies have resolved.

In recent times, fibrosarcomas have been determined to make up ~0.5 to 5.5% of all soft tissue malignancies.[33] The degree of histological differentiation usually determines the biological activity. The well-differentiated tumor rarely metastasizes and tends to be less locally aggressive. Regional and distant metastases, as well as aggressive local spread, characterize the poorly differentiated. The well-differentiated variety demonstrates an admixture of fibers and cells. The cells are fairly uniform, mitoses are infrequent, and nuclear hyperchromatism is occasionally seen. Varying degrees of cellular anaplasia designate the malignancy of the undifferentiated forms. The metastatic rate in the latter is around 20 to 25%[19,20] and is usually hematogenous.

A much more common tumor in the skull base area is the *schwannoma*. Electron-microscopic and histochemical evidence definitely points to the Schwann cell as the origin of both schwannomas (also called neurilemomas) and neurofibromas.[34] Clinically and grossly, the two have characteristic differences. One of the most important, from the surgical

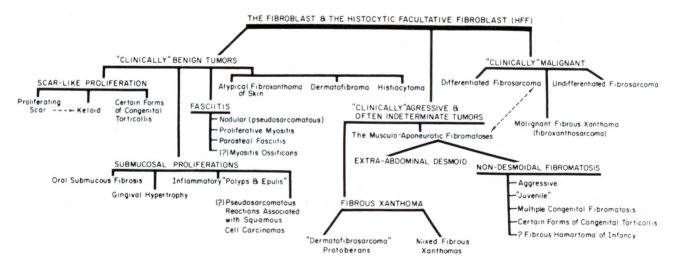

Fig. 9.20 Schematic attempts to classify fibrous tumors and fibroproliferative diseases of the head and neck. (From Batsakis JG. Tumors of the Head and Neck: Clinical and Pathological Considerations. Baltimore: Williams & Wilkins; 1974:180. Reprinted with permission.)

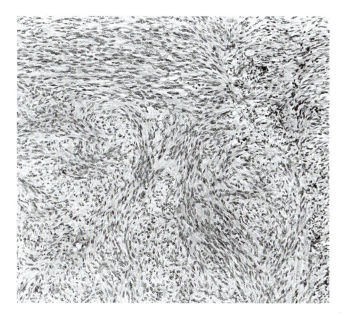

Fig. 9.21 Photomicrograph of a schwannoma (×130).

standpoint, is that the neurofibroma has neural elements that traverse the tumor, whereas the schwannoma, although attached to a nerve, has no actual nerve fibers traversing it. *Neurofibromas* are characteristic of von Recklinghausen disease and carry a significant potential for malignant degeneration. Histologically, the Antoni A and B configuration and the presence of Verocay bodies are characteristic (**Fig. 9.21**). Although the configuration of a central cytoplasmic mass encircled by palisaded nuclei that together constitute the Verocay body is occasionally seen in neurofibromas, the usual

picture is of an unencapsulated tumor composed of fibers and spindle cells insinuated within the nerve substance. The fibrous component is commonly randomly distributed, and the cellular nuclei take on a serpiginous configuration.

Batsakis[29] prefers to designate malignancies of nerve cell sheath origin as neurogenous sarcomas. *Malignant schwannoma* would appear to be a misnomer because clear evidence of malignant degeneration in a schwannoma is wanting. The appearance of some cellular pleomorphism—an occasional mitotic figure or multinucleated cells—must be recognized as a regressive step and not as a sign of malignancy.

Neurofibromas appear to be the principal source of malignancy among neural tumors of the head and neck. Histologically, the differentiation of neurogenous sarcoma from fibrosarcoma is almost impossible. The origin of the tumor in a nerve is the prime distinguishing feature. These malignancies frequently metastasize and have rapid local spread. Only wide radical local excision provides any hope of salvage.

Sarcomas are rare in the nasopharynx, and *squamous cell carcinoma* is by far the most common malignancy seen, usually of a poorly differentiated cellular type or as a lymphoepithelioma (WHO III). For some time controversy over the precise categorization of lymphoepithelioma and transitional cell cancer raged. The electron-microscopic findings of keratin granules and desmosomes[35,36] have definitively classified these tumors as variants of epidermoid carcinoma. Their biological behavior is similar to that of poorly differentiated squamous cell cancers, and, like them, they are more radiosensitive than their more differentiated relatives. Both lymphoepithelioma and transitional cell cancer may be grossly exophytic, ulcerative, or infiltrative. The occult infiltrative type is the most common (**Fig. 9.23**).

Following the palatine tonsil the nasopharynx is the most common site of lymphoma. It is frequently accompanied by cervical lymphadenopathy.

Nasopharyngeal malignancies in general are uncommon, making up only 0.25% or so of all cancers. In the population at large this is an overall incidence of only ~0.0005%.[37] A notable exception is the high incidence of nasopharyngeal can-

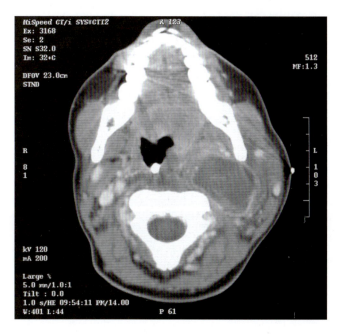

Fig. 9.22 MRI of patient with nodular fasciitis of the neck.

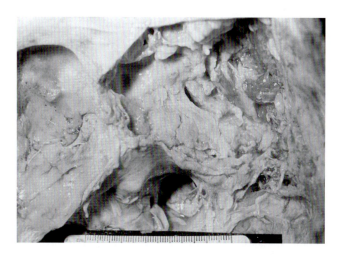

Fig. 9.23 Autopsy specimen showing massive intracranial extent of an infiltrating nasopharyngeal carcinoma arising in the fossa of Rosenmüller.

cer in China, where it is responsible for ~15% of all deaths due to malignant disease.[35] This is not true for Chinese born in other countries. Although this incidence of nasopharyngeal malignancy is still high, it diminishes among each successive generation of Chinese born outside their native country. The role of the Epstein-Barr virus in the etiology of this disease is of considerable interest. A common association between elevated titers of Epstein-Barr antibody commonly coexist with the disease. Further, Coates et al showed a decrease in antibody titers in those cured of their disease.[38] An association between nasopharyngeal carcinoma and the consumption of salt fish has been made.[39] This is especially strong when this consumption begins in early childhood.

The most common presenting sign in nasopharyngeal carcinoma is a lump in the neck. Conversely, one of the most common of the unknown primaries in patients who present initially with a lump in the neck is nasopharyngeal carcinoma.[40] Fletcher and Million[41] found only 16 cases out of a total of 112 (14.3%) that had no metastasis to the neck. Vilar[42] reported 21/24 (87.5%) of patients with nodal involvement, and another authority[43] quotes 90% of patients with unilateral and 50% with bilateral disease.

The lymphatic drainage system of the nasopharynx offers several different routes of metastatic spread. There are from one to three high laterally placed retropharyngeal lymph nodes that are the principal filtering stations of the lymphatic channels draining the nasopharynx. The lymph proceeds from these to the upper internal jugular nodal group or to the nodes of the posterior cervical triangle. In some instances, the high nodes are bypassed and the first manifestation of nasopharyngeal tumor is an enlarged node in the posterior triangle or, less commonly, in the upper internal jugular chain.[44] The original study done by Rouvière[45] over 40 years ago clearly delineating the lymphatic system in the head and neck has not been improved upon since.

Pathophysiology of Spread of Skull Base Tumors

The routes of spread of malignant neoplasms through the skull base into the intracranial cavity are varied. Although direct invasion by bone or cartilage erosion is a common method of spread, direct extension through the natural avenues provided by neural and vascular foramina provide easy access to the subdural spaces. Direct spread by bony erosion is commonly encountered in paranasal sinus malignancies because the bone of the fovea ethmoidalis and cribriform plate area is quite thin. Similarly tumor spread through the lateral walls of the sphenoidal sinus to the dura of the cavernous sinus is facilitated by the thinness of the bone whereas extension posteriorly through the clivus is uncommon because of its thickness except in cases of extensive postsellar pneumatization.

Perineural spread of tumor through the neural foramina of the skull base is probably the commonest method of spread. Adenoid cystic carcinoma has this property as its pathognomonic characteristic. Most malignant tumors of the head and neck can on occasion spread along nerve sheaths, but squamous cell and basal cell carcinoma and malignant melanoma are most likely to acquire this propensity. These latter tumors

when affecting the skin may spread along the branches of the trigeminal nerve through their respective foramina and into the gasserian ganglion. Spread of squamous cell cancers of the tonsil, inferior alveolar ridge, and even the lip and tongue may spread along the sheath of the inferior alveolar nerve to the mandibular division of the trigeminal nerve and through the foramen ovale to the ganglion. Tracking of tumor along the optic and olfactory nerves provides access to the anterior cranial fossa. A curious property of this method of spread in the subcranial route is the phenomenon of skip areas. There may be a gap of 1 cm or more between tumor deposits along the nerve until it gains its intracranial course. Once the nerve has traversed the foramen the tumor continues mainly in continuity almost entirely devoid of skip areas.

The spread of tumor along vascular structures through the skull base foramina is, in contrast to perineural invasion, in continuity. The vessels most commonly involved are the internal jugular vein and the internal carotid artery. Spread along the basilar artery, the mastoid emissary vein and the pterygoid venous plexus are examples of this avenue of spread.

Dural invasion occurs following intracranial spread via the neurovascular foramina and also when tumor spreads by direct extension. It is curious that in some cases, tumor that has eroded even a considerable amount of bone may abut against but not directly invade the dura. Dural invasion is not a contraindication to successful surgical tumor exenteration. In our series, after surgical excision, dural involvement made no statistical difference in the 2-year tumor-free survival and local tumor control rates.[46] Dura has the ability to contain malignant tumors for an extended period of time before they will invade brain substance. Furthermore the tumor in dura tends to be compact and has a tendency to expand into the tissue by a pushing action (**Fig. 9.24**). This enables adequate control of tumor when a surgical margin of only a few millimeters is taken.

Brain invasion is uncommon even when there is extensive involvement of dura. Unlike primary malignancies of the central nervous system, which have multiple satellites of the tumor at a distance from the primary, cancers of the upper digestive tract tend to spread by direct tumor extension and tend to remain in continuity (**Fig. 9.25**). They behave similarly to their spread in dura in this regard. Usually the

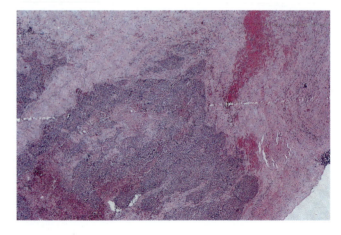

Fig. 9.24 Dural invasion by squamous cell carcinoma (H&E, ×40).

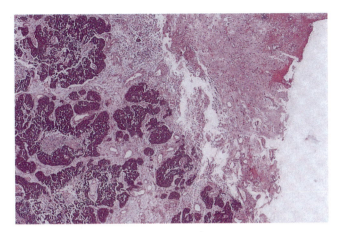

Fig. 9.25 Histological section demonstrating area of edema and necrosis (*arrows*) preceding advancing tumor front (H&E, ×100).

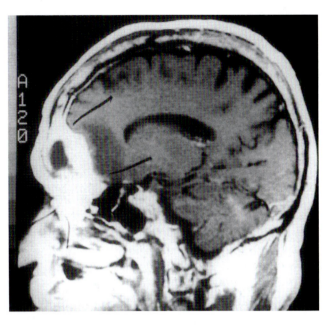

Fig. 9.26 Lateral magnetic resonance image showing area of edema and necrosis preceding tumor front (*arrows*) of poorly differentiated carcinoma.

tumor is preceded by a halo of necrosis, which is apparent on the MRI (**Fig. 9.26**). After resection for brain invasion survival rates differ little from those with dural invasion.[46] The phenomenon of meningeal carcinomatosis,[47,48] thought to be the result of spread of tumor cells in the CSF, is very uncommon in our experience, having occurred in only three of our patients.

Internal carotid artery involvement occurs by direct extension either from the neck, through the temporal bone, via the foramen lacerum or vidian canal, and finally in the cavernous sinus, either from tumor breaking through the ethmoidal or sphenoidal sinuses or from the various venous foramina entering the cavernous sinus. Metastatic carcinoma in an upper cervical lymph node from an upper aerodigestive tract primary is the usual source of tumor spread in the neck. Direct extension from a parotid gland tumor or from a deeply invasive tumor from the oropharynx or nasopharynx occasionally occurs. The cervical carotid is covered by a layer of adventitia that provides a barrier to tumor spread. The fibrous ring (**Fig. 9.27**) that encircles the carotid as it enters the undersurface of the temporal bone provides significant resistance to tumor penetration. In the carotid canal that traverses the temporal bone the carotid is protected first by a layer of stout periosteum and then a layer of loose areolar tissue that carries some of the blood supply to the wall of the artery. Finally, a layer of adventitia covers the vessel. The media of the vessel is slightly thinner than the artery in the neck (**Fig. 9.28**). The periosteum and even the loose connective tissue and adventitia provide a good barrier to tumor penetration, especially by low-grade tumors. The cavernous carotid has a thinner media and very little surrounding connective tissue to prevent tumor invasion of the artery.

The *cavernous sinuses* along with the petrous and cavernous carotid are highly controversial areas in terms of feasibility of resection. Its multiple venous connections and

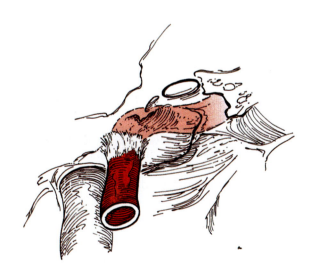

Fig. 9.27 Internal carotid artery with fibrous ring as it enters the carotid foramen. Internal jugular vein enters the jugular foramen posterolaterally.

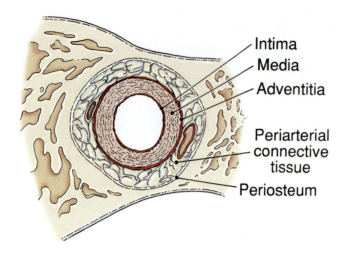

Fig. 9.28 Diagram showing histological details of the internal carotid artery in the carotid canal of the temporal bone.

its intrinsic highly vascular structure make resection of the cavernous sinus a formidable surgical challenge. Only a limited number of neurosurgeons are equipped by training or experience to tackle this challenging anatomical area. Tumors invading the sinus tend to displace the vascular channels resulting in scant bleeding at the beginning of the resection, and only when the margins of tumor are reached does hemorrhage become a problem. Tumors that extend across the midline through either the circular sinus or the basilar plexus are considered by our team to be inoperable.

◆ Surgical Procedures

Preoperative Planning

One of the most important steps in the performance of procedures in the infratemporal fossa and skull base areas is preoperative planning. A thorough history and physical examination including a comprehensive review of all past records is essential. The previous biopsies or histological sections of any past surgery must be reviewed by the skull base team pathologist. All previous radiographs are reviewed, and usually it is necessary to get more current films. MRI and CT scans are obtained with a focus on the skull base. Axial and coronal views usually give the most useful information. Gadolinium contrast and, often, fat suppression software are needed with the MRI to provide optimal information. The utility of the positron emission tomographic (PET) scan in head and neck tumors continues to evolve.

If the tumor is close to the internal carotid artery then a carotid arteriogram with a BTO and a SPECT scan is done to determine the ability of the contralateral arterial supply to supply the brain on the test side if the carotid is sacrificed.[49] If the carotid artery is sacrificed the artery is replaced with a graft, preferably the saphenous vein.

Because of the exigencies of each case, there will be considerable variation in the approach and extent of the surgery. Once a comprehensive examination and investigation have been conducted, by both the head and neck surgeon and the neurosurgeon, a presurgical conference should be scheduled. At this time the skull base surgical team will establish the sequence of operative steps, including the incisions, the temporal order of intracranial and transfacial dissections, the method of tumor delivery, and finally the stages of reconstruction and closure.

With careful planning, often the cranial and facial incisions can complement one another. Care must be taken not to compromise the cutaneous blood supply by poor flap design. In many instances, a single incision can afford a perfectly adequate exposure for both facets of the procedure. The use of curved incisions not only is more cosmetic but also enhances exposure. Determining the sequence of the steps of dissection often requires considerable deliberation. This should not take the form of a power struggle but should be a process of deciding how best the dissection should proceed.

Reconstructive efforts have as a first priority a watertight dural closure and separation of the cranial cavity from the upper aerodigestive system. Dural grafting is often required. The experience of Ketcham et al[50] of improved results with the use of temporalis fascia over fascia lata as dural replacement is borne out by my own. Dural substitutes in the form of lyophilized dura and bovine pericardium can be used as well. Dural allografts have gained popularity; however, caution must be exercised in cases that have been irradiated or in whom prior infection had occurred. Whenever possible the dural repair is covered with a flap of pericranium. Considerable time is often required to ensure precise dural integrity. This is time well spent; it is the key to the prevention of CSF leakage and subsequent meningitis. Isolation of the cranial cavity from the air- and foodstream may not be a problem. Sufficient soft tissue in the upper neck or around the skull base may exist to reinforce the dural repair. If not, the interposition of a flap or the application of a skin graft may be necessary to seal off the defect. Neurosurgeons commonly employ alloplastic materials for reestablishing cranial continuity. However, these materials should only be used when there is good vascularization of the bed. The concomitant use of a free flap adds a good measure of insurance. Adequately vascularized tissue is essential for the take of both dural and skin grafts.

A good general principle is for both surgeons to be present during most of the operation. As the partnership matures, substantial assistance can be rendered between participants. Anticipation of problems can be better predicted and more efficient dispatch of the operative process can be effected. Sudden unexpected hemorrhage may be best handled by the complementary team member; when both are present, the success of this cooperative venture will be maximized.

Lateral Approach to the Skull Base

The undersurface of the skull base, specifically the inferior surface of the temporal bone, which is in fact the floor of the middle cranial fossa, is best exposed through the lateral infratemporal fossa approach. Visualization is enhanced not only by mandibular condylectomy, but by osteotomy and mobilization of the zygoma.[51] The parotid gland is mobilized and the facial nerve is not dissected unless the tumor takes origin

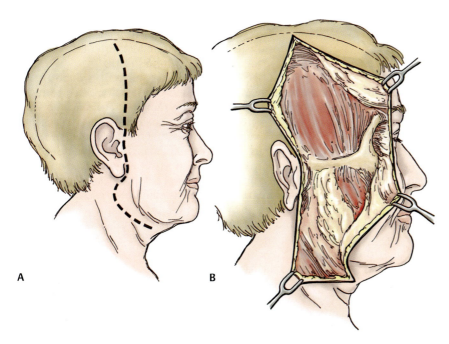

A   B

Fig. 9.29 (**A**) Standard preauricular infratemporal fossa–middle cranial fossa incision and flap elevation. (**B**) Flap elevated in patient. Note the use of the Taney clips on the scalp for hemostasis.

in the gland or the gland is invaded by tumor extension. Retraction of the gland rarely results in facial nerve weakness and does not hamper the exposure.

Fisch developed the zygomatic osteotomy approach[52] for enhancing the exposure of large acoustic neuromas and glomus jugulare tumors with extensive intracranial and upper cervical involvement. His primary motivation was to eradicate extensive otologic disease. We have found this approach useful also for deep-seated lesions such as extensive deep lobe parotid tumors and extensive schwannomas originating from the nerves of the jugular foramen, as well as tumors that reach to or extend from the nasopharynx, sphenoid sinus, and even the pituitary fossa. Sekhar and Schramm[18] modified Fisch's approach to enable the resection of the intracranial extension of subcranial neoplasms,

especially those that are malignant. Our team uses a very similar approach to that of Sekhar and Schramm with minor variations.

The incision is an adaptation of the modified Blair incision for parotidectomy (**Fig. 9.29A**). The incision extends from the vertex almost to the hyoid bone (**Fig. 9.29B**). This is used for those tumors that are more anteriorly located such as deep lobe parotid tumors, carcinomas with perineural spread along the branches of the trigeminal nerve, and recurrent nasopharyngeal carcinomas. A postauricular C-shaped incision as described by Fisch and Mattox[51] is used in those patients with more posteriorly located tumors such as clivus chordomas, temporal bone carcinomas, and glomus jugulare tumors with intracranial extension (**Fig. 9.30**). As the skin flap is dissected forward, the frontal branch of the facial

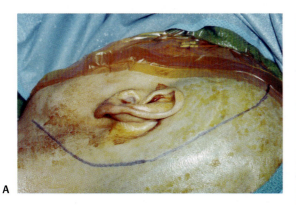

A

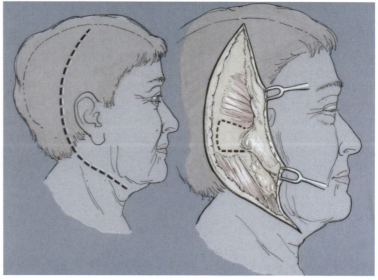

B

Fig. 9.30 Postauricular C-shaped incision for access to more posteriorly located lesions. A line drawing of posterior incision.

nerve is preserved by incising and then elevating a semicircular flap of deep temporalis fascia (**Fig. 9.31**). The external auditory canal is transected and the auricle retracted posteriorly, if the latter is to be retained. A decision now needs to be made regarding preservation of the middle ear space. If the eustachian tube is to be transected to dissect the internal carotid artery, then serious consideration should be given to eliminating the middle ear space and ablating the external auditory canal on the basis of patient age, the disease process, and whether the patient has been irradiated in the past. In young patients with juvenile nasopharyngeal angiofibromas invading the middle cranial fossa and the cavernous sinus the middle ear is preserved and a ventilating tube inserted. In an older patient who has been previously irradiated, the likelihood of postoperative infection and the danger of exposing the middle fossa dura to the outside air and a chronically infected ear put the patient at constant risk of meningitis. The hazard is even greater if the internal carotid artery is exposed, especially if it has been grafted. In the majority of cases the middle ear is ablated.

When ablating the middle ear space the method of Fisch and Mattox[51] is used (**Fig. 9.32**) because this effectively removes most of the middle ear mucosa and closes the external ear canal in two layers. The cervical extension of the incision is used not only for access to the parotid tail but also as a means of exposing the great vessels from the carotid bifurcation to the skull base. The internal jugular vein and the internal and external carotid arteries are identified and en-

circled with a vascular loop (**Fig. 9.33**). If a radical neck dissection is required, a lazy S extension is made at right angles to the cervical aspect of the incision inferiorly. As always, the junction is made behind the carotid sheath.

If a radical neck dissection is required, it is done after a parotidectomy, when the latter is necessary. Often both the superficial and deep lobes are removed. The facial nerve is carefully dissected in the manner described by McCabe and Work[52] (see chapter 6). In resecting the deep lobe, the nerve is gently retracted with a nerve hook. During the rest of the dissection, the continuity of the nerve is preserved up to the point where further retraction puts it in danger of severe neurapraxia or avulsion. At this point, severance just beyond the point of main branching is done so that when continuity is restored (near the termination of the operation), subsequent reinnervation will result in differential function. Most usually the parotid gland does not need removal and the gland and the facial nerve are preserved intact, the gland retracted inferiorly, and the nerve not dissected. The skin flap is elevated in the "face-lift" plane up to an imaginary line between the lateral orbital rim and the angle of the mandible. A radical neck dissection is done at this point, if required by the exigencies of the tumor. If not, the inferior aspect of the apex of the temporal bone is now approached in a stepwise manner from lateral to medial.

The initial exposure is gained by excising the origin of the sternocleidomastoid muscle from the mastoid tip. A slicing motion with a scalpel blade against the mastoid cortex is often quicker than the standard dissection with the mastoid elevator. Deep to this muscle is the posterior belly of the digastric. This is elevated from its fossa with a Joseph elevator (Snowden Pencer Inc., Tucker, GA), with care taken anteriorly not to traumatize the facial nerve. The occipital artery in its groove is dissected free and ligated. It is wise to control this vessel with a ligature or suture ligature at the outset because failure to do so leads to annoying hemorrhage.

As one proceeds medioanteriorly, the styloid process comes into view. The stylohyoid, stylopharyngeus, and styloglossus muscles are removed and dissected anteriorly, with the facial nerve always kept in clear view. Care is taken while dissecting the stylopharyngeus muscle not to damage the glossopharyngeal nerve. The pharyngeal anesthesia and the even minor motor disturbance that may result from damage to cranial nerve IX may render the patient dysphagic, an especially troublesome consequence in elderly patients.

Progress beyond the styloid becomes difficult because of the mandibular condyle and neck. The triangle gets tighter as the dissection proceeds more deeply. Resection of the mandibular condyle is delayed until after the next two steps in the operation.

The first phase of exposing the infratemporal fossa is the elevation and transposition of the temporalis muscle. A 2 cm wide cuff of pericranium is incised around the circumference of the temporalis muscle. The muscle is then dissected from the temporal fossa down to the level of the zygomatic arch. The object is to eventually dissect the muscle down to its insertion on the coronoid process of the mandible.

To free up the temporalis muscle it is necessary to detach the zygomatic arch. The earlier dissection of the deep layer

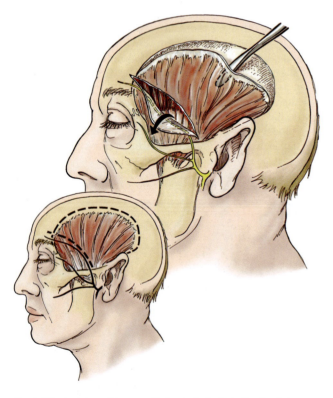

Fig. 9.31 Incision of temporalis fascia to include the frontal branch of the facial nerve, precluding it from injury. (From Donald PJ. Skull base surgery for sinus neoplasms. In: Donald PJ, Gluckman JL, Rice DH, eds. The Sinuses. New York: Raven; 1995:479. Reprinted with permission.)

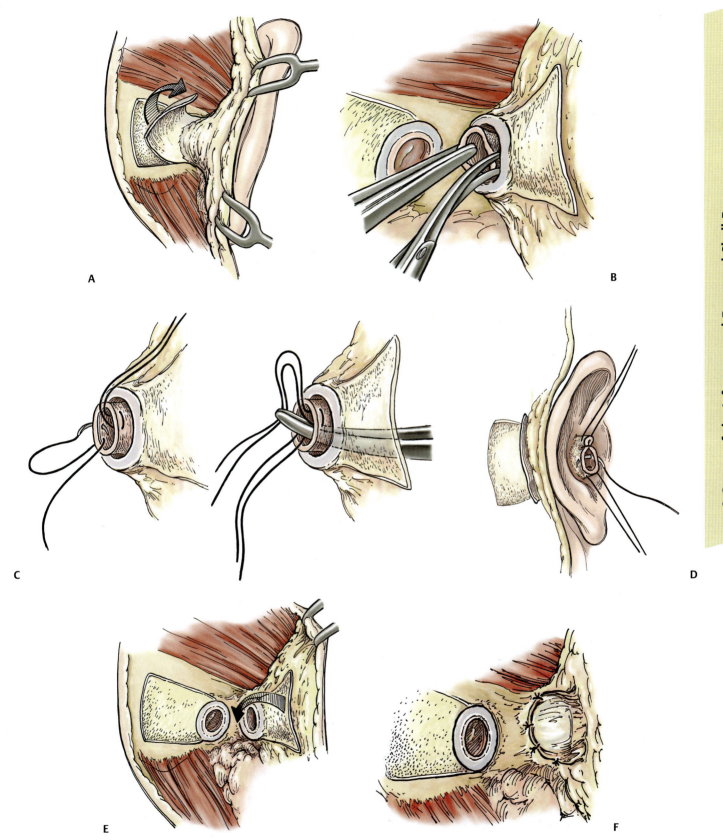

Fig. 9.32 (**A**) Periosteal-fascial flap pedicled on cartilaginous canal. (**B**) External canal skin elevated off conchal cartilage and out to level of external auditory meatus. (**C**) Suture placed through canal skin and brought out of ear with a mosquito clamp. (**D**) External auditory canal (EAC) skin closed. (**E**) Periosteal-fascial closure over EAC. (**F**) Closure complete.

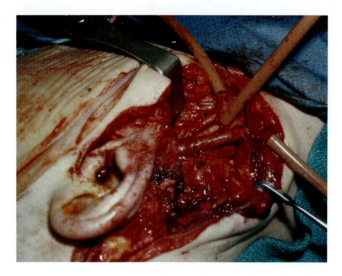

Fig. 9.33 Vascular loops placed around the internal jugular vein and the internal and external carotid arteries.

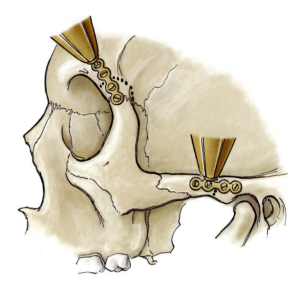

Fig. 9.35 Holes being drilled and plates applied, then removed for later osteosynthesis with the completion of the operation.

of the temporalis fascia makes exposure of the zygomatic arch much simpler and preserves the frontal branch of the facial nerve. The bony incisions in the arch are outlined as seen in **Fig. 9.34**. The posterior incision is made just in front of the articular eminence of the temporal bone and the anterior incision through the lateral orbital rim and posterior extent of the malar eminence. The fine bone-cutting needle of the Midas Rex drill (Medtronic, Inc., Minneapolis, MN) is ideal for these cuts. Prior to the cuts miniplates are bent into the appropriate shape and preregistered with drill holes (**Fig. 9.35**). Once the zygoma has been removed it is preserved in

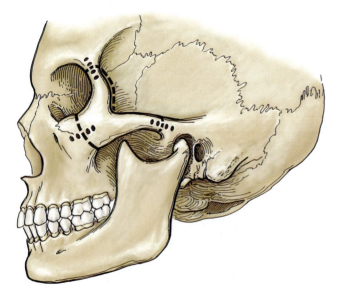

Fig. 9.34 Diagram illustrating the cuts in zygomatic ostectomy. Bone is preserved for later reconstruction. Note holes drilled for wire ligation. At least two holes are required if plate osteosynthesis is used. (From Donald PJ. Skull base surgery for sinus neoplasms. In: Donald PJ, Gluckman JL, Rice DH, eds. The Sinuses. New York: Raven; 1995:481. Reprinted with permission.)

a saline-soaked gauze sponge for later replacement. To complete the exposure of the infratemporal fossa, the condyle of the mandible is removed (**Fig. 9.36**). A T-shaped incision is made through the temporal-mandibular joint, the periosteum at the mandibular neck dissected, and a malleable retractor placed under the deep surface of the neck to protect the underlying internal maxillary artery from being cut. The internal maxillary artery gives off the deep temporal arteries, which are now the lone blood supply to the temporalis muscle. Its viability is essential if it is to be used for reconstruction of the middle fossa floor. Removal of the condyle leaves no significant postoperative functional deficit except a wandering of the jaw to one side on wide opening. Postoperative trismus is most often related to dissection of the pterygoid muscles or dissection of the temporal-mandibular joint and not removing the condyle or postoperative radiation therapy. After the condyle is removed the remaining soft tissue in the glenoid fossa is dissected free and removed so that only the bare bone of the fossa remains.

With a Deaver retractor (CS Surgical, Inc., Slidell, LA) against the temporalis insertion on the coronoid process and the leading edge of the anterior aspect of the ramus of the mandible and the other soft tissues in the infratemporal fossa a subperiosteal dissection is carried medially under the middle cranial fossa floor to the foramen spinosum and the foramen ovale. The subperiosteal dissection is continued anteriorly to the foramen ovale until the root of the pterygoid processes is exposed. Any remaining soft tissue lying on the lateral aspect of the lateral orbital wall is removed. The middle meningeal artery is clipped or tied, then divided. The dissection around the subcranial side of the foramen ovale may stir up bleeding from small extensions of the cavernous sinus. Any bleeding must be gently and carefully controlled with light bipolar cautery, thrombin-soaked Gelfoam (Pfizer Inc., New York, NY), and hemostatic gauze. Bleeding from the superior aspect of the pterygoid plexus of veins is not uncommon, and judicious

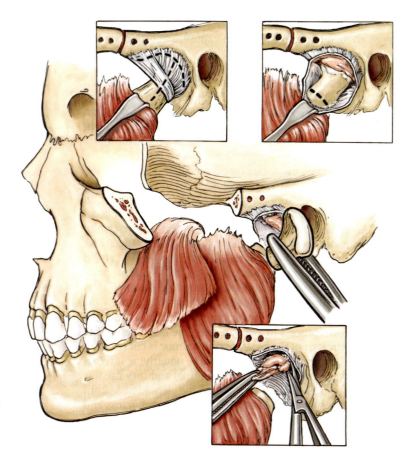

Fig. 9.36 Condylectomy: Lateral aspect of the temporomandibular joint capsule is opened and connected to a vertical incision in the periosteum of the mandibular neck. The condylar neck is transected and the condyle removed. The meniscus and attached soft tissue are removed.

use of the bipolar cautery is exercised so as to preserve the two nutrient arteries to the temporalis muscle.

The craniotomy that is now to ensue is a combined effort by the head and neck surgeon and the neurosurgeon. The goal of the craniotomy is to produce an L-shaped bone flap where the vertically oriented long limb of the "L" is made up

of a smaller portion of the greater wing of the sphenoid and the greater part the squamous part of the temporal bone and the short limb is made up of a portion of the middle fossa floor (**Fig. 9.37**). The inferior bone flap incision extends from the middle ear cleft posteriorly to the base of the pterygoid plates anteriorly. The superior potion of the flap (the vertical

Fig. 9.37 (**A**) L-shaped craniotomy. Diagram outlining cuts. (**B**) Craniotomy flap removed from patient with extensive amount of temporal lobe dura involvement.

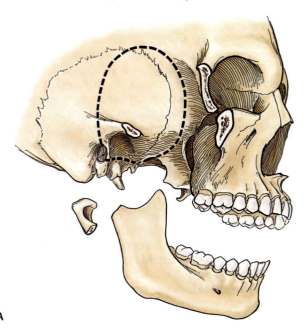

A

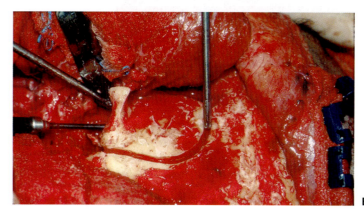

B

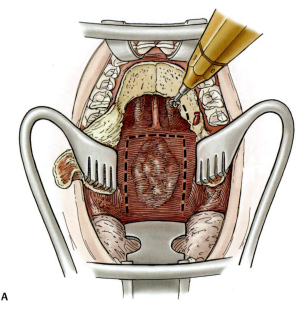

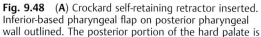

Fig. 9.48 (**A**) Crockard self-retaining retractor inserted. Inferior-based pharyngeal flap on posterior pharyngeal wall outlined. The posterior portion of the hard palate is removed with the cutting bur. (**B**) Parallel lateral incision made through the mucosa and posterior constrictor in the level of the alar fascia.

Takahashi forceps. Exposure to the level of the sphenoid sinus can be accomplished in this manner. If the oral cavity or oropharynx is too small to achieve adequate exposure, a median labial mandibuloglossotomy is done (**Fig. 9.50**). This vastly improves exposure and provides more room in which to maneuver.

The next layer that is incised is composed of the prevertebral muscles and the underlying periosteum. A midline inci-

sion is made down to bone and the soft tissue dissected from the clivus and the upper cervical vertebrae with a heavy elevator such as the Cob or that developed by the author (**Fig. 9.51A,B**). The deep-toothed Crockard retractor is now placed inside the palatal retractor to hold the muscle and periosteum to the side.

At any time during this procedure, the tumor may be encountered. A chordoma may invade or simply bulge the mu-

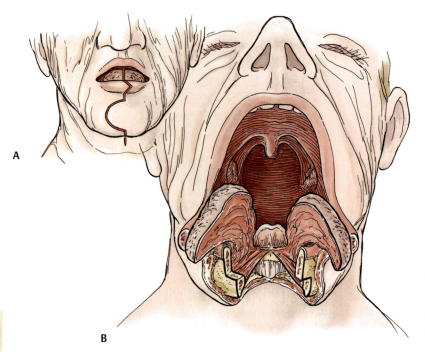

Fig. 9.49 (**A**) The pharyngeal flap has sutures with small squares of lead placed on its distal end, then stuffed into the hypopharynx to stabilize the flap during subsequent dissection. Mucosal incision in midline of posterior septum is outlined. (**B**) Bony septum removed with drill.

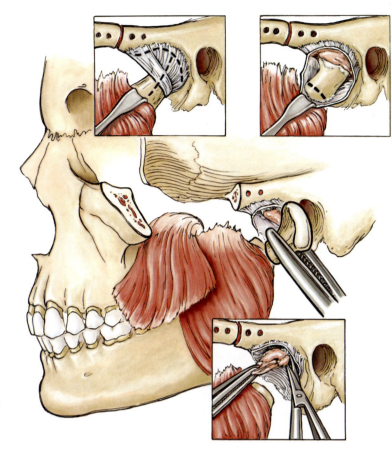

Fig. 9.36 Condylectomy: Lateral aspect of the temporomandibular joint capsule is opened and connected to a vertical incision in the periosteum of the mandibular neck. The condylar neck is transected and the condyle removed. The meniscus and attached soft tissue are removed.

use of the bipolar cautery is exercised so as to preserve the two nutrient arteries to the temporalis muscle.

The craniotomy that is now to ensue is a combined effort by the head and neck surgeon and the neurosurgeon. The goal of the craniotomy is to produce an L-shaped bone flap where the vertically oriented long limb of the "L" is made up of a smaller portion of the greater wing of the sphenoid and the greater part the squamous part of the temporal bone and the short limb is made up of a portion of the middle fossa floor (**Fig. 9.37**). The inferior bone flap incision extends from the middle ear cleft posteriorly to the base of the pterygoid plates anteriorly. The superior potion of the flap (the vertical

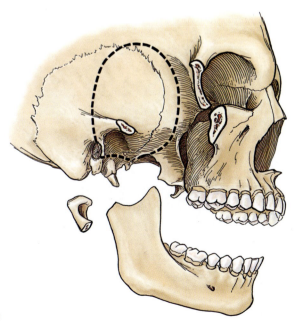

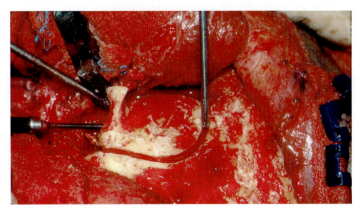

Fig. 9.37 (**A**) L-shaped craniotomy. Diagram outlining cuts. (**B**) Craniotomy flap removed from patient with extensive amount of temporal lobe dura involvement.

A

B

limb of the "L") is usually relatively small but is fashioned large enough to permit adequate exposure and resection of involved dura or brain.

Utilizing the dissecting microscope the head and neck surgeon creates an anterior-tympanomeatal flap in the external auditory canal skin going from 12 o'clock to ~7 o'clock. If the middle ear is to be ablated then the entire canal skin and tympanic membrane are removed. The flap is elevated down to the tympanic annulus and the annulus prized out of its sulcus. The protympanum, the hemicanal for the tensor tympani, and the cochleariform process are identified (**Fig. 9.38**). A small cutting bur is used to make a cut along the course of the external auditory canal at ~2 o'clock. The exposure of the protympanum and the construction of the superior canal wall cut is facilitated by making a saucer-shaped excision in the zygomatic root (the Trojanowski maneuver) (**Fig. 9.39**). The bony incision begins just outside the canal and is carried down to dura. The cut is then carried at this depth medially down the ear canal to the tympanic annulus. The annulus is cut and the bur carried through a short distance in the attic, across the hemicanal for tensor tympani well in front of the cochleariform process to avoid injuring the facial nerve. The pretympanic part of the bony eustachian tube is cut to only a depth of ~2 mm so as not to damage the underlying internal carotid artery. Inferiorly the bony external auditory canal is incised at ~5 o'clock full thickness into the glenoid fossa until the annulus is met (**Fig. 9.40**). The annulus is cut across and a 2 mm fissure cut in the floor of the hypotympanum and the inferior part of the protympanum fissured in a similar fashion to the superior cut. The cut is kept shallow in the floor of the middle ear to avoid accidentally cutting the jugular bulb. The cut through the inferior aspect of the external auditory canal and tympanic annulus is now directed along the

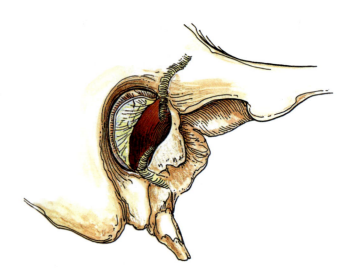

Fig. 9.38 Anterior tympanomeatal flap retracted, exposing the tympanic opening of the eustachian tube. The superior and inferior cuts into the protympanum are outlined.

glenoid fossa bone anteromedially again at a shallow depth until the sphenoid spine is reached. The middle meningeal artery is identified and clipped or ligated if not yet done so. The bone cut is now extended deeply to the level of the middle fossa dura and carried forward to the foramen ovale. The final part of the subcranial portion of the bony incision ex-

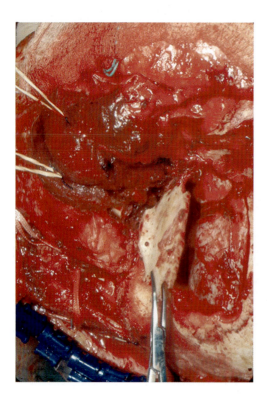

Fig. 9.39 Close-up view showing bulge in posterior eustachian tube.

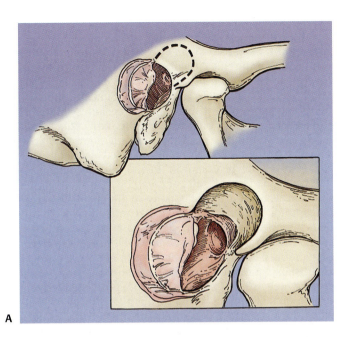

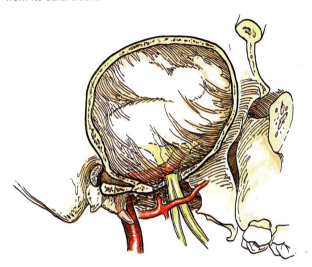

A

B

tends from the anterior lip of the foramen ovale anterolaterally through the inferior aspect of the greater sphenoid wing just above the origin of the pterygoid plates.

The neurosurgeon now makes the vertical portion of the craniotomy flap. A bur hole is usually made in the so-called key-hole at the pterion. The cut with the craniotome is made in the greater wing of the sphenoid and the squamous part of the temporal bone large enough to afford the exposure necessary to resect any involved dura or temporal lobe and exposure needed to dissect the cavernous sinus if invaded by tumor. The calvarial cuts join up with those made posteriorly in the 12 o'clock position in the external auditory canal and anteriorly at the level of the base of the pterygoid plates. The craniotomy flap thus completed is still attached by a thin bridge of bone in the middle ear. A careful dissection of the dura from superiorly to inferiorly is done while a gentle prying motion is exerted against the vertical part of the bone. The craniotomy flap fractures in a greenstick manner through the middle ear and glenoid fossa (**Fig. 40A**). It is important to construct the bone flap in this manner because the fracture through the middle ear goes through the protympanum and the bony eustachian tube in the oblique axis of the temporal bone. When the bone flap is removed a bulge in the posterior wall of the bony eustachian tube is seen. This corresponds to the position of the internal carotid artery. Occasionally this thin bony wall is dehiscent and the internal carotid can actually be seen pulsating.

The exposure of the middle cranial fossa and this removal of the middle fossa floor up to the level of the foramen ovale enormously expand the exposure of the contents of the infratemporal fossa. How the subsequent dissection proceeds is dependent on tumor extent. Limited tumor invasion up the foramen ovale or the foramen rotundum may simply require excision of the nerve trunk at the level of the gasserian ganglion in the "Meckel's Cave" with resection of the overlying dura. If tumor invades the ganglion, then this structure is

removed. If tumor tracks along the trigeminal nerve trunk, the neurosurgeon can trace the nerve along its short course on the posterior floor of the middle fossa, over the petrous ridge and along its traverse of the posterior fossa up to the level of the brain stem. Invasion of the brain stem constitutes inoperability, and the resection is terminated at this point. In only rare instances have we seen tumor extend this far. The characteristic skip areas pathognomonic of most tumors with perineural spread seen in the extracranial course of the cranial nerves when invaded by these neoplasms is rarely experienced in their intracranial course. Usually a 2 to 3 mm length of healthy nerve will provide an adequate margin of resection. Furthermore, the invasion of the dura overlying the involved nerves is usually of limited extent.

If tumor invades the eustachian tube, the tube can be removed with the cutting bur into the nasopharynx. This resection necessitates the dissection of the internal carotid artery. The entry of the artery at the fibrous ring (**Fig. 9.26**) is exposed in the upper reaches of the neck. Bone surrounding the artery is drilled up to the point at which it turns to its horizontal course posteriorly to the bony eustachian tube. A bidirectional dissection (**Fig. 9.41**) removing bone over the artery seen at the bulge in the posterior wall of the eustachian tube is directed along the horizontal part of the artery then joining that to the vertical part working superiorly from the carotid foramen. A diamond bur is used for that part of the bony canal that is next to the vessel. The artery can be exposed up to the foramen lacerum, the cartilage plug contained in the inferior part of the foramen removed, and the artery dissected up into the cavernous sinus (**Fig. 9.42**).

Cavernous sinus invasion of cancers originating in the facial skin and upper aerodigestive tract is for many surgeons a contraindication to surgical intervention. Unquestionably the prognosis of such patients is much less than other patients having skull base surgery. However, in our series the 3-year and better survival rate after cavernous sinus resection

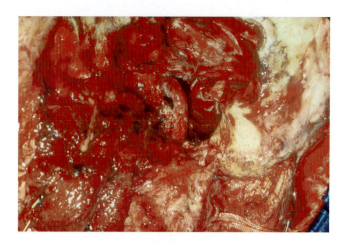

Fig. 9.41 Internal carotid artery dissected from the carotid foramen to the cavernous sinus.

for malignancy is better than 20%. Although this survival rate is only one half to one third that of the usual survival for skull base resection I believe it is worth the effort.

The cavernous sinus resection is obviously the province of the neurosurgeon. The head and neck surgeon usually does the carotid exposure in the temporal bone using the dissecting microscope. The neurosurgeon dissects the sinus, very carefully securing hemostasis by proceeding slowly using the bipolar cautery, thrombin-soaked Gelfoam, hemostatic gauze, and pressure with cottonoid. Because the cavernous sinus is a low-pressure system hemostasis can be readily achieved with pressure. The tumor tends to replace the part of the sinus that it invades and bleeding is minimal during the early phases of tumor removal. More vigorous bleeding

is not encountered until the tumor has been mostly resected, and the displaced vascular channels of the sinus are now encountered. If the resection can be confined to the anteroinferior regions of the sinus usually the third and fourth cranial nerves can be avoided because they are located superolaterally between a double layer of dura. Similarly the sixth nerve can be avoided if the tumor extension is limited to this anterior position. Unfortunately, the sixth cranial nerve is highly susceptible to damage, even with minor manipulation. The lateral rectus palsy thus produced by minor injury to the nerve often resolves over time.

Because the initial results of cavernous sinus surgery for direct invasion of malignancy were so disappointing (16.7% 5-year tumor-free survival) and local control rates were only 50%, the operation was redesigned to make the resection wider with larger margins of uninvolved tissue (**Fig. 9.42**). In addition, patients with malignancy are now often staged with an exploration of the opposite sinus to ensure the tumor has not crossed from the sinus with tumor involvement via the circular sinus or basilar venous plexus to the opposite side, which is negative or equivocal on the MRI or CT scan.

In the past 5 years the redesigned operation outlined in **Fig. 9.43** takes a wider margin of healthy tissue including the petrous apex, the entire lateral wall of the sphenoid sinus, the lateral third of the clivus, and the adjacent body of the sphenoid bone. The superior and inferior petrosal sinuses, a portion of the basilar plexus, and the carotid artery, if it is involved, are resected. The internal carotid, if sacrificed, is always grafted, even if the patient has passed the BTO and SPECT scan.

The resection of the internal carotid artery is even more controversial than the operation on the cavernous sinus. Our only long-term survivors of internal carotid sacrifice have been since the revision of the cavernous sinus operation. Prior to the new procedure we had no survivors at 5 years

Fig. 9.42 Redesigned cavernous sinus resection.

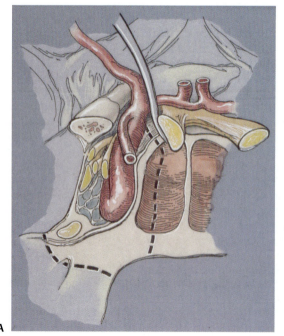

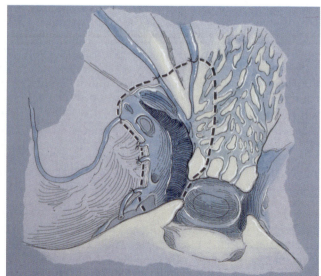

A

B

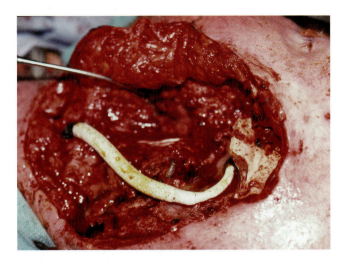

Fig. 9.43 Internal carotid artery replaced by Gore-Tex graft from petrous temporal bone at foramen lacerum to upper neck.

and only a few at 2 years postresection. On the other hand, when the tumor was dissected from the carotid canal in the petrous temporal bone, and the malignancy had not invaded the media of the artery, then 25% of patients survived 5 years. Because the carotid canal in the petrous temporal bone is lined by a sturdy periosteum and the artery has a surrounding area of areolar tissue and adventitia (**Fig. 9.27**) there is a significant barrier to tumor penetration, especially in cases of low-grade malignancy and those that tend to have a pushing margin such as adenoid cystic and acinic cell carcinoma. The preferred graft material for the carotid is saphenous vein and the second choice is Gore-Tex (W.L. Gore and Associates, Inc., Flagstaff, AZ, **Fig. 9.43**). The grafts usually extend from the neck to the take-off of the ophthalmic branch of the distal internal carotid.

Closure of the wound begins with as watertight a dural closure as possible. Commonly dura has been resected and a graft of fascia lata, temporalis fascia, lyophilized cadaver dura, or bovine pericardium is used for repair. Direct suturing is augmented with tissue glue. The floor of the middle fossa is closed by transposing the temporalis muscle across the middle fossa floor and suturing the pericranial cuff to the residual mucosa and muscle of the nasopharynx. The cranial bone flap and the zygoma are replaced (**Fig. 9.44**).

On occasion the blood supply to the temporalis muscle has been compromised or the muscle has been invaded by tumor and it is not available for reconstruction. In these instances either a myogenous flap such as the pectoralis major or the latissimus dorsi can be used or the area reconstructed with a free flap. The free flap of choice is the rectus abdominis muscle. In our series the complication rate was significantly less in patients whose middle fossa floor was reconstructed with the free flap than when the temporalis muscle is used. The calvarial flap and zygoma are replaced and fixed in place with miniplates. Suction drains are placed and the scalp and facial wound are closed.

The tracheostomy is removed once the patient is stable and the lumbar drain pulled if there is no CSF leak at the third or fourth postoperative day.

Clivectomy

The pioneering surgery in this somewhat frightening area was done initially by neurosurgeons and orthopedic surgeons in attempts to manage fracture dislocations at the atlantoaxial and atlanto-occipital joints.

A transoropharyngeal approach was employed by Southwick and Robinson[53] in 1957 to excise a bony tumor in the body of second cervical vertebra (C2). They based their technique on that of their otolaryngological colleagues, who routinely opened the retropharyngeal space for drainage of retropharyngeal abscesses, usually without incident. The absence of intercurrent infection and the rapidity of closure by secondary intention encouraged them to use this approach.

These injuries were difficult, if not impossible, to adequately reduce and fix through a posterior approach. The most logical access to this region would be through the oral cavity, but a natural reluctance existed because of the fear of contamination by oral flora. Moreover, the transoral approach was unfamiliar to these surgeons, who were used to a more direct access and extensive exposure.

Fang and Ong[9] in 1962 were the first to describe an anterior approach to the top end of the spine through the transoral transpalatal route. Four years later, De Rougemont et al[54] reported on their experience with this procedure. In the same year, Mullan et al[55] described a slightly more rostral incursion into the skull base. They executed a partial removal of a tumor in the region of the foramen magnum. Stevenson et al,[56] also in 1966, described a resection of the clivus. By using a transcervical route, they excised a chordoma that had invaded both the clivus and the upper cervical spine. In the following year, based on this procedure, Fox[57] and Wissinger et al[58] produced large enough openings in the clivus to control the hemorrhage from basilar arterial aneurysms. Both used the transcervical approach. The disadvantage of this transcervical route is that the extensiveness of the dissection required compromise of many cranial nerves. Yassargil[59] in 1969 reported his experience with two patients in whom the transoral route was used. Both patients suffered postoperative neurological deficits and eventually died. Successful control of a basilar aneurysm was done by transoral clivectomy and reported by Haselden and Brice.[60] This approach has been used by the authors and others for clivectomy and odontoidectomy in patients with basilar impression syndrome.[61-63] As resections progress superiorly beyond the body of first cervical vertebra (C1), simple soft palate retraction becomes ineffective in exposing the field. Soft palatal splitting, as well as vomerine and hard palate resection, permits extension of operative intervention up to the sphenoid sinus. The transoral/oropharyngeal route does not provide adequate exposure to manage the internal carotid artery or the cavernous sinus. If the artery is exposed and is involved with tumor then an alternative route such as the infratemporal–middle fossa exposure will be necessary to gain proximal and distal control of the vessel and hemostasis of the cavernous sinus if anything other than a small degree of the sinus is exposed.

◆ **Technique** Anesthesia is induced through an oroendotracheal tube or a tracheostomy. (The latter is preferable because

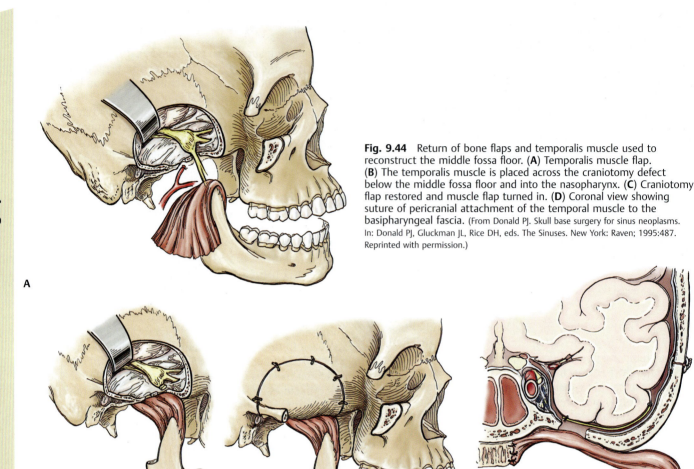

A

B

C

D

Fig. 9.44 Return of bone flaps and temporalis muscle used to reconstruct the middle fossa floor. (**A**) Temporalis muscle flap. (**B**) The temporalis muscle is placed across the craniotomy defect below the middle fossa floor and into the nasopharynx. (**C**) Craniotomy flap restored and muscle flap turned in. (**D**) Coronal view showing suture of pericranial attachment of the temporal muscle to the basipharyngeal fascia. (From Donald PJ. Skull base surgery for sinus neoplasms. In: Donald PJ, Gluckman JL, Rice DH, eds. The Sinuses. New York: Raven; 1995:487. Reprinted with permission.)

of exclusion of the delivery of anesthesia from the field and postoperative airway control.) The head is dropped into the Rose position, similar to that for tonsillectomy as long as sufficient spinal stability is ensured and there is no danger of upper cervical spinal cord compression. If the surgery is being done for clivectomy for tumor this is usually not a problem, but if any craniocervical instability is present the patient's head is secured in pins on the Mayfield headrest (Integra Lifesciences Corp., Plainsboro, NJ) and the head is not dropped back. The mouth is propped open with a mouth gag such as the Dingman or Crockard (**Fig. 9.45**). The posterior pharyngeal wall is injected with 0.5% lidocaine with 1:200,000 epinephrine. Similar injections are made in the hard and soft palates. The nose is cocainized with a 5% aqueous cocaine solution on pledgets or cotton-tipped applicators.

A linear midline incision is made in the soft palate with either a scalpel or a cutting cautery. This incision is carried directly through the nasopharyngeal mucosa up to the junction of the hard and soft palates. The tensor and levator veli palatini muscles are dissected from their insertions into the posterior surface of the hard palate with a blunt elevator. If

further exposure is required, the incision in the mucosa is extended laterally on the side requiring greatest exposure to the point where the maxillary tuberosity emerges (**Fig. 9.46**) and is then carried around the palate anteriorly, staying posterior to the foramen incisivum and carried back on the opposing side similar to the Owen incision to the opposing maxillary tuberosity. The palatal mucoperiosteal flap is elevated and pedicled on the opposing greater palatine artery. The ipsilateral neurovascular flap is elevated and pedicled on the opposing greater palatine artery. The ipsilateral neurovascular bundle should be identified at its emergence from the greater palatine foramen, isolated, and ligated (**Fig. 9.47**). With the mucosal flap retracted with self-retaining retractors, the bony palate is drilled away with a cutting bur, taking care to leave a small bony shelf such that the subsequent closure of the soft tissue will lie over bone.

An inferiorly based pharyngeal flap is constructed with its superior extent next to the vomer and the lateral limbs placed in the junction of the lateral and posterior pharyngeal walls (**Fig. 9.48**). The cut is medial to the eustachian tube tori and extends inferiorly behind the posterior tonsillar pil-

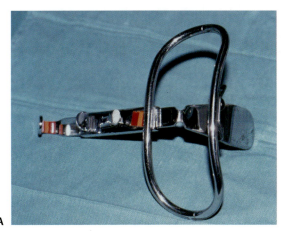

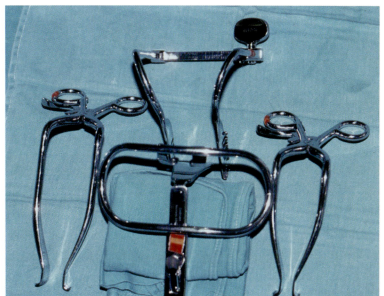

Fig. 9.45 The Crockard instrument set. (**A**) Mouth gag. (**B**) Mouth gag blades and self-retractors.

lars. The incision in the oropharynx goes to the layer of the alar fascia, which exists as a thin layer between the pharyngobasilar fascia and the prevertebral fascia. This is an easy dissection plane in the oropharynx, but it is obliterated in the nasopharynx. The plane in the posterior nasopharyngeal wall is through the origin of the superior constrictor muscle. The lateral cuts and dissection are done first and then the two vertical limbs are connected in the nasopharynx. The flap is easily dissected from its bed and proceeds from the nasopharyngeal vault to the level of the upper hypopharynx. Silk sutures with small lead weights are placed through the superior corners of the pharyngeal flap and the flap folded into the hypopharynx to keep it out of the way of the further dissection (**Fig. 9.49A**).

The posterior nasal septum is exposed, and its mucosal leaves are dissected on either side and then split along the back surface (**Fig. 9.49B**).

As much nasal septum is taken as necessary to achieve adequate exposure. The bony septum is removed in pieces as large as possible, so that they may be used later in the reconstruction of the clival defect. The septal resection is best accomplished by making a vertical cut with a small osteotome, and then fracturing the bone and removing it with Luc or

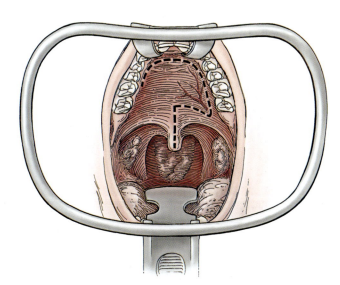

Fig. 9.46 Palatal splitting procedure to expose the undersurface of the clivus in the nasopharynx and the arch of C1 in its more posterior reaches.

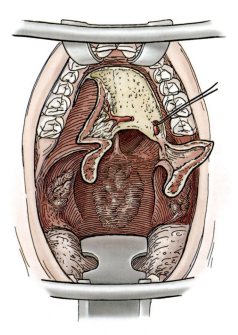

Fig. 9.47 Ligation of the greater palatine neurovascular bundle and dissection of the palatal flap to the opposing side, with care taken to stay posterior to the foramen incisivum. A dissection is used to separate the aponeurotic insertions on the posterior aspect of the bony palate on the right side.

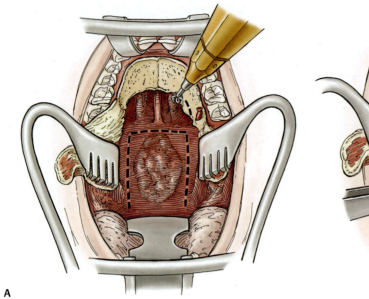

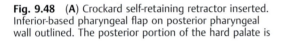

A

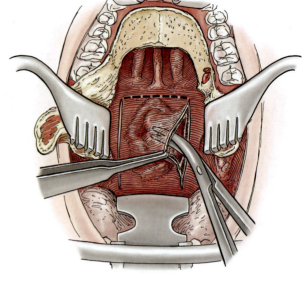

B

Fig. 9.48 (**A**) Crockard self-retaining retractor inserted. Inferior-based pharyngeal flap on posterior pharyngeal wall outlined. The posterior portion of the hard palate is removed with the cutting bur. (**B**) Parallel lateral incision made through the mucosa and posterior constrictor in the level of the alar fascia.

Takahashi forceps. Exposure to the level of the sphenoid sinus can be accomplished in this manner. If the oral cavity or oropharynx is too small to achieve adequate exposure, a median labial mandibuloglossotomy is done (**Fig. 9.50**). This vastly improves exposure and provides more room in which to maneuver.

The next layer that is incised is composed of the prevertebral muscles and the underlying periosteum. A midline incision is made down to bone and the soft tissue dissected from the clivus and the upper cervical vertebrae with a heavy elevator such as the Cob or that developed by the author (**Fig. 9.51A,B**). The deep-toothed Crockard retractor is now placed inside the palatal retractor to hold the muscle and periosteum to the side.

At any time during this procedure, the tumor may be encountered. A chordoma may invade or simply bulge the mu-

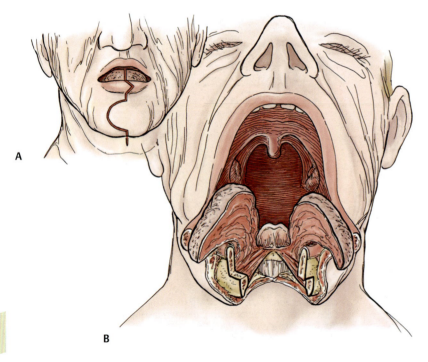

A

B

Fig. 9.49 (**A**) The pharyngeal flap has sutures with small squares of lead placed on its distal end, then stuffed into the hypopharynx to stabilize the flap during subsequent dissection. Mucosal incision in midline of posterior septum is outlined. (**B**) Bony septum removed with drill.

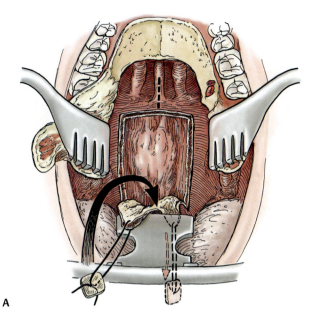

A

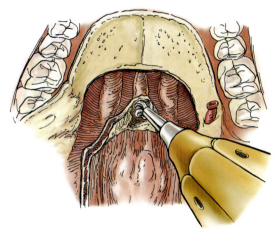

Fig. 9.50 Median labial mandibuloglossoptomy improves exposure and provides more room for surgical manipulation.

B

cosa. A squamous cell tumor in or invading the nasopharynx will be mucosal in origin and require a peripheral incision to a degree necessary to ensure a tumor-free margin. This squamous cell type of tumor, especially if it is exophytic, may obscure any attempt at underlying bony resection. The en bloc principle will then need to be violated to permit adequate exposure of the tumor bed. Tumor is then removed with bone, the latter by use of the cutting bur. The TAC attachment

of the Midas Rex drill (Medtronic, Inc., Minneapolis, MN) is ideally suited to do this resection. Its curved tube and considerable length allow bone removal with an unobstructed view (**Fig. 9.52**). The headlight in this situation is indispensable. The dissecting microscope may be needed for accurate tumor control. Bony removal proceeds until the pontine and medullary dura is encountered (**Fig. 9.53**). The basilar artery is on the opposite side and often casts a shadow on the dura

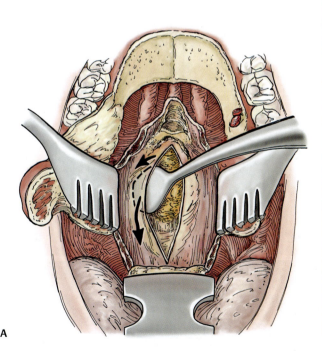

A

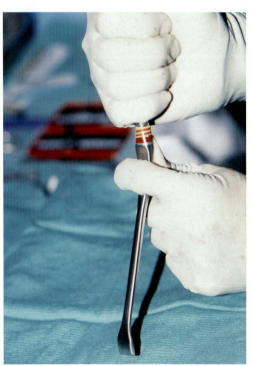

B

Fig. 9.51 (**A**) The heavy elevator is used to dissect the tough soft tissues off the clivus and cervical spine. The Crockard retractor is then reapplied to give enhanced exposure of the tumor and surrounding bone. (**B**) Donald elevator for dissecting the tough periosteum from the clivus and the cervical vertebrae.

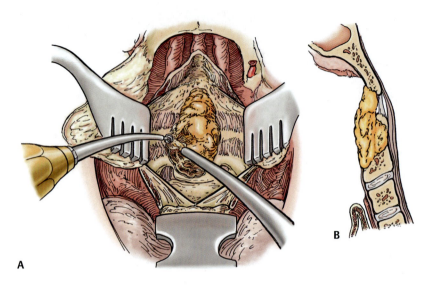

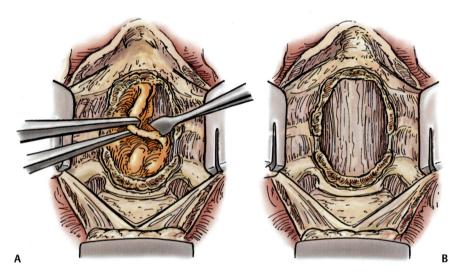

Fig. 9.52 (**A**) The curved Midas Rex TAC (Medtronic, Inc., Minneapolis, MN) attachment is used to remove bone from the clivus and cervical spinous bodies to expose the limits of tumor. (**B**) Tumor is removed completely and great care is taken to avoid injury to the dura.

Fig. 9.53 (**A**) The tumor is removed to the level of the dura. (**B**) The pontine dura is free of tumor involvement.

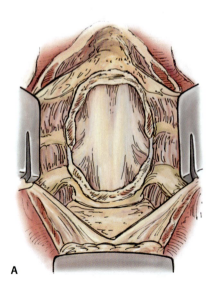

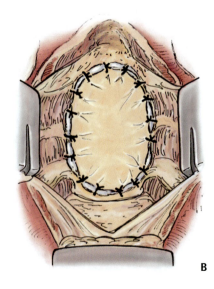

Fig. 9.54 (**A**) More advanced case than illustrated in **Fig. 9.54A** where the pontine dura is positive for tumor and must be resected. Defect following resection with the shadow of the pons shining through the arachnoid. (**B**) Pontine dura repaired with fascia graft and fibrin glue.

overlying it. If dural invasion is encountered, the neurosurgeon is required for this part of the resection (**Fig. 9.54**). The basilar arterial supply must not be interrupted. Brain stem involvement by tumor renders it unresectable.

Tumor resection is usually done piecemeal so that frequent frozen sections are mandatory. At times the transoral approach is only the first stage in the resection. This is particularly so in cases of extensive clival chordoma. The approach to the tumor at the lateral aspect of the brain stem may need the far-lateral approach.

Bilateral disease that jeopardizes the contralateral internal carotid artery renders the tumor unresectable. Under these circumstances, only attempts at reasonable palliation should be taken.

Tumor extension from the maxillary or ethmoidal sinuses may be the reason for this approach. Similarly, tumors arising in the nasopharynx, notably the angiofibroma, have a tendency to invade the paranasal sinuses. The transpalatal-transsinal excision of this and other tumors as well as management of the pterygomaxillary space are dealt with in chapter 5.

Reconstruction of the clival defect is begun by fascia lata or temporalis fascia grafting of any dural defects (**Fig. 9.54B**). The repair of dural defects and the establishment of a watertight seal are one of the greatest reconstructive challenges in neurosurgery. Any dural suturing is generously complemented by the use of fibrin glue. The bony defect is plugged with septal bony fragments and Gelfoam (**Fig. 9.55A**). The

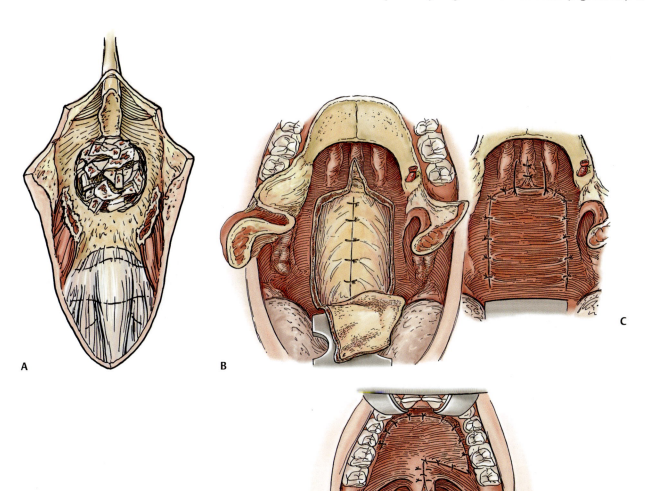

Fig. 9.55 (**A**) Clival defect filled with septal bone fragments. (**B**) Posterior paraspinous muscular closure. (**C**) Posterior pharyngeal wall and posterior septal closure. (**D**) Palatal and uvular closure.

bony removal can be repaired with hydroxyapatite bone cement if a watertight seal can be obtained with the pharyngeal mucosal closure. If the mucosa has not been sacrificed, approximation with absorbable sutures is done in one layer (**Fig. 9.55B,C**). If mucosal excision has been done, replacement with a flap is essential. The radial forearm free flap is the best choice because it is thin and has an excellent take rate. The rich blood supply, copious soft tissue, and durable cutaneous surfaces are ideal for resurfacing this area. The palate is sutured with interrupted absorbable suture (**Fig. 9.55D**). Alimentation is best administered through a piriform sinus or esophagostomy tube.

Closure of a median labial mandibuloglossoptomy is shown in **Fig. 9.56**. Lateral extensions of tumor may encroach on the cavernous sinus and the internal carotid artery as it emerges from the foramen lacerum. This is an extremely hazardous area, incursions into which are frequently fraught with serious complications. Such tumors have a hopeless prognosis unless resected, and the surgeon must carefully weigh all the factors in each case prior to venturing into this region. Tumors of this magnitude have been successfully extricated from this region by Yassargil,[59] Panje and McCabe,[64] and the author. The transoral/oropharyngeal route does not provide adequate exposure to manage the internal carotid artery or the cavernous sinus. If the artery is exposed and is involved with tumor then an alternative route such as the infratemporal–middle fossa exposure will be necessary to gain proximal and distal control of the vessel and hemostasis of the cavernous sinus if anything other than a small degree of the sinus is exposed.

Resection of "pushing tumors" such as angiofibromas, chordomas, and fibrosarcomas is more feasible than of more invasive neoplasms, such as those of epithelial origin.

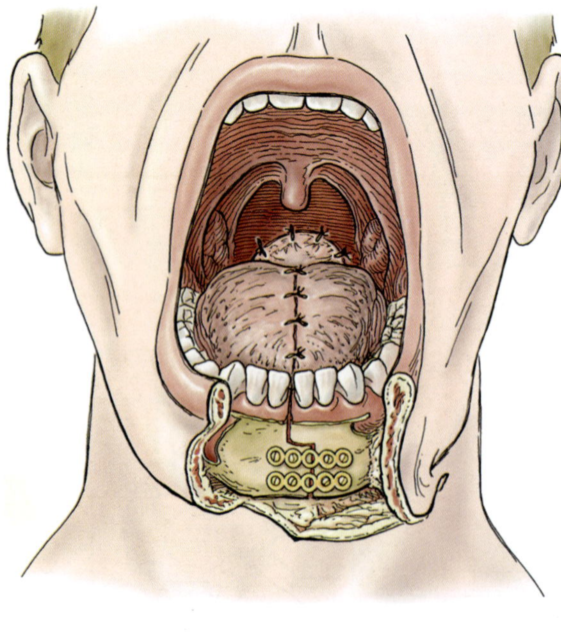

Once any chance of tumor incursion into the intracranial cavity presents itself, a temporal-parietal craniotomy must be done. This is the only way any degree of safety can be assured. **Fig. 9.57** illustrates a 20-year-old man who presented with proptosis, total nasal obstruction, and a mass that bulged his cheek, soft palate, and lateral pharyngeal wall. An arteriogram demonstrated neoplastic invasion of the middle cranial fossa and a nutrient vessel from the cavernous sinus branch of the internal carotid artery (**Fig. 9.58**). The presumptive diagnosis of juvenile nasopharyngeal angiofibroma was made. Following tumor-shrinking medication with diethylstilbestrol, a transoral/oropharyngeal resection was done through the palate. Substantial reduction in tumor volume resulted in minimal tumor in the region of the floor of the middle fossa and retraction of tumor from the orbital apex. A combined infratemporal fossa–middle cranial fossa approach was done to remove that portion of the neoplasm invading the middle cranial fossa, as well as that portion encroaching on the cavernous sinus. The rather meager blood supply from the internal carotid system was easily controlled. Complete resection of a tumor close to 800 g in weight was then done through a transpalatal–transmaxillary approach. The patient had a full, uneventful recovery and is still free of tumor 20 years later.

Additional exposure can be obtained by a lateral approach through the parotid bed. The beginning of this extension may already have been affected by virtue of the clivectomy being but the superior extension of a pharyngectomy for a cancer extending across the boundary from meso- to epipharynx.

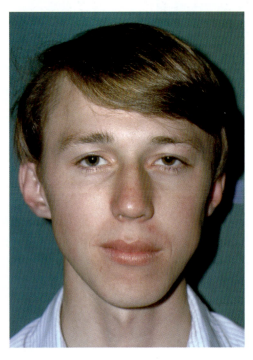

Fig. 9.57 A 20-year-old man presenting with massive nasopharyngeal angiofibroma that produced nasal obstruction, proptosis, and epistaxis. The lesion extended into the cheek, middle cranial fossa, infratemporal fossa, and pterygomaxillary space. It caused bulging of the eye, cheek and soft palate.

Fig. 9.56 Medican labiomandibuloglossoptomy incision closed.

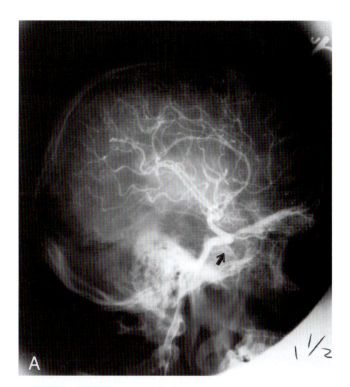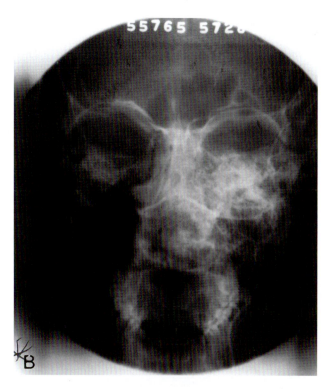

Fig. 9.58 **(A)** Arteriogram demonstrating the intracranial extent of tumor in the patient seen in **Fig. 9.56**. The arrow indicates the cavernous sinus arterial branch contribution to the tumor's blood supply. **(B)** Tumor blush in delayed phase of arteriogram, showing tumor extent. Caldwell view.

The concomitant radical neck dissection commonly done, as well as the mandibulectomy portion of the pharyngectomy, provides access. The patient's head position may have to be frequently altered to facilitate exposure, and it is important to bear in mind and prepare for it at the start of the procedure. During subsequent manipulation, exposed brain-stem dura must be carefully protected.

Antibiotic coverage is begun 24 hours preoperatively, continued intraoperatively, and terminated 48 hours postoperatively. The patient is nursed in the semi-Fowler position. Care is taken to maintain a low CSF pressure by means of fluid restriction and a lumbar subarachnoid drain. The patient is strongly discouraged from straining. The importance of sneezing through an open mouth, the use of laxatives, and the avoidance of bending over must be carefully emphasized to the patient and nursing staff in these early postoperative days.

The Far Lateral Approach

The far lateral approach is uncommonly done by head and neck surgeons, being usually employed by neurological surgeons to gain access to the upper cervical cord and lower brain stem. It is most commonly used by them to control aneurysms of the vertebral artery and to resect meningiomas afflicting the dura in this area. The approach for the head and neck surgeon provides a means to resect metastatic lymph nodes that are fixed to the transverse processes of C1 and C2, tumors of the oropharynx and nasopharynx with lateral

extension, clival and upper cervical spine chordomas, and malignancies with perineural spread that may have invaded the hypoglossal nerve up the hypoglossal canal. In our experience this approach has been used for deep lobe parotid tumors invading the craniocervical junction, tumors with perineural spread along the hypoglossal nerve, clival chordomas, and the resection of metastatic lymph nodes fixed at this site.

The approach was first developed by George and Laurian[65] as a means of exposing the vertebral artery to control aneurysms. In the mid-1970s, by doing a series of cadaver dissections, the authors devised an exposure of the upper cervical spine and occipital–cervical junction to allow mobilization of the vertebral artery and thus achieve control of aneurysms afflicting this vessel. They reported their early results in 1979.[66] In 1990 Sen and Sekhar reported their modifications to this technique to provide access for tumors.[67]

The patient is placed in the lateral decubitus position or slightly inclined with beanbags supporting the back. A Mayfield headrest provides stabilization of the head and the ability of the surgeon to stand closer to the patient. If there is spinal cord compression it is important to have the lateral position with the head in a neutral position. In most head and neck tumors compromise of the cord is not an issue so the head can be slightly flexed forward enhancing the exposure.

A generous C-shaped incision is made postauricularly or a J-shaped incision is constructed that will give an enhanced exposure of the upper lateral neck and will also facilitate a spinal fusion if necessary (**Fig. 9.59**). A vertical extension into the neck is done if a radical neck dissection will be part of the procedure.

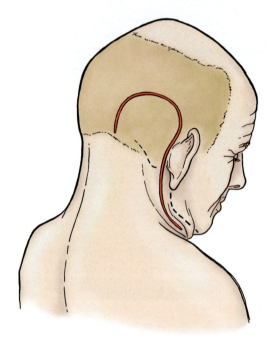

Fig. 9.59 J-shaped incision for the far lateral approach.

The soft tissue resection we do proceeds in a manner similar to that described by Sen and Sekhar.[67] Usually, the sternocleidomastoid muscle has been resected as part of the radical neck dissection. If not it is dissected free of the mastoid tip and retracted anteriorly. The muscles of the posterolateral neck are dissected in a layered fashion. The trapezius muscle is dissected free of the nuchal line and retracted inferiorly.

The splenius capitis and longissimus capitis are similarly dissected free and retracted inferiorly. The longissimus cervicis, located just lateral to the longissimus capitis, is freed up as well (**Fig. 9.60**). The deep cervical vein lies just under the splenius capitis as does a plexus of veins (**Fig. 9.61**). The transverse process of C1 with its attachment of the upper slip of the levator scapulae and the rectus capitis posterior minor is identified. These muscles are dissected free, exposing the vertebral artery (**Fig. 9.62**). The insertion of the rectus capitis posterior major from the transverse process of C2 also facilitates this exposure.

The vertebral artery is described as being in four parts. The first portion extends from its origin from the subclavian artery to its entrance into the foramen transversarium of C6. The second part traverses the vertebral foramina from C6 to C2. The third part goes from C2 around the condyle of C1 until it penetrates the dura, and, finally, the fourth, where the vertebral penetrates the dura to that point where the artery from one side joins with that of the other to form the basilar artery (**Fig. 9.63**). The third part of the artery is most germane to the head and neck surgeon. The vessel goes from the foramen in C2 through the larger foramen in C1 to slant posteromedially, coursing around the lateral mass of the atlas to enter the dura of the posterior cranial fossa (**Fig. 9.64**). In dissecting the vertebral artery it becomes apparent that it is covered in a thick sheath. This is the continuation of the periosteal sheath of the vertebral foramina. A plexus of vertebral veins travel mainly on the anterior and lateral aspects of the vertebral artery. They are especially prominent above C1.

Once the levator scapulae and inferior oblique muscles have been elevated from the transverse processes of the involved vertebrae the vertebral artery is isolated between the vertebrae. The heavy sheath surrounding the artery not always protects it during dissection but also provides a barrier to tumor penetration. The transverse processes involved with disease are removed with a rongeur or a cutting bur and the artery mobilized. If there is preoperative suspicion of arterial invasion by tumor and the vessel may need to be sacrificed, a BOT and SPECT scan are done to ensure the safety of

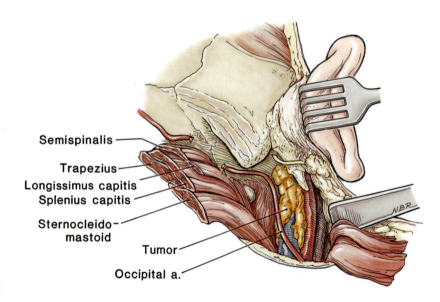

Semispinalis

Trapezius

Longissimus capitis

Splenius capitis

Sternocleido-mastoid

Tumor

Occipital a.

Fig. 9.60 Incision of the sternocleidomastoid, trapezius, posterior belly of digastric, splenius capitis, and longissimus capitis opens up a space between the mastoid tip and C1.

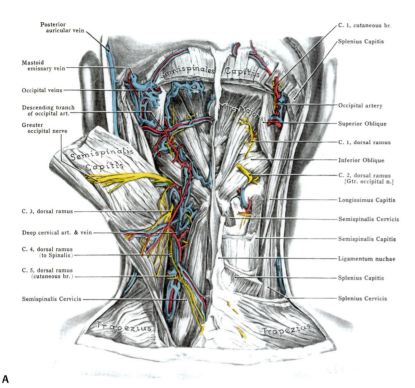

Posterior auricular vein

Mastoid emissary vein

Occipital veins

Descending branch of occipital art.

Greater occipital nerve

Semispinalis Capitis

C. 3, dorsal ramus

Deep cervical art. & vein

C. 4, dorsal ramus (to Spinalis)

C. 5, dorsal ramus (cutaneous br.)

Semispinalis Cervicis

Semispinales Capitis

Minor Major

Trapezius

Trapezius

C. 1, cutaneous br.

Splenius Capitis

Occipital artery

Superior Oblique

C. 1, dorsal ramus

Inferior Oblique

C. 2, dorsal ramus [Gtr. occipital n.]

Longissimus Capitis

Semispinalis Cervicis

Semispinalis Capitis

Ligamentum nuchae

Splenius Capitis

Splenius Cervicis

A

Fig. 9.61 (**A**) The deep cervical vein. (**B**) Occipital venous plexus.

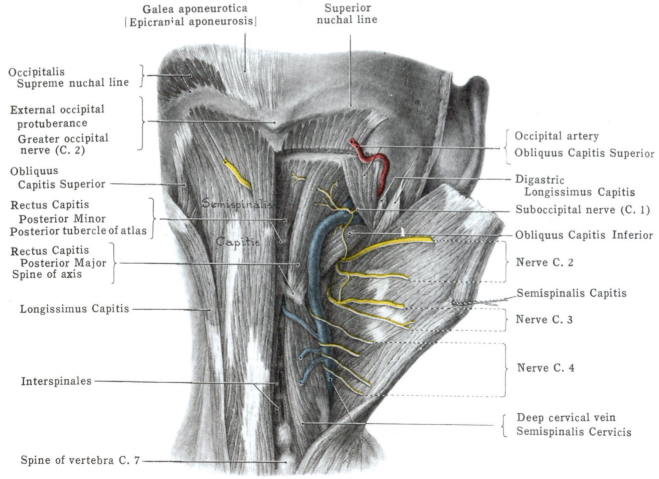

Galea aponeurotica [Epicranial aponeurosis]

Superior nuchal line

Occipitalis
Supreme nuchal line

External occipital protuberance
Greater occipital nerve (C. 2)

Obliquus Capitis Superior

Rectus Capitis Posterior Minor
Posterior tubercle of atlas

Rectus Capitis Posterior Major
Spine of axis

Longissimus Capitis

Interspinales

Spine of vertebra C. 7

Semispinalis

Capitis

Occipital artery
Obliquus Capitis Superior

Digastric
Longissimus Capitis

Suboccipital nerve (C. 1)

Obliquus Capitis Inferior

Nerve C. 2

Semispinalis Capitis

Nerve C. 3

Nerve C. 4

Deep cervical vein
Semispinalis Cervicis

B

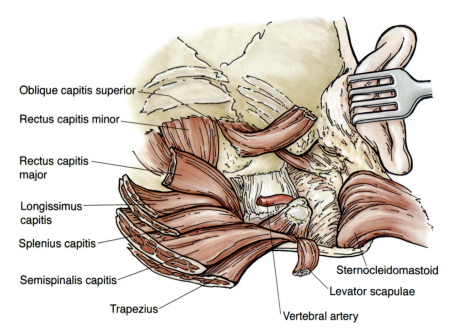

Oblique capitis superior

Rectus capitis minor

Rectus capitis major

Longissimus capitis

Splenius capitis

Semispinalis capitis

Trapezius

Sternocleidomastoid

Levator scapulae

Vertebral artery

Fig. 9.62 Dissection of the insertion of rectus capitis posterior minor and levator scapulae from the transverse process of C1 and the insertions of rectus capitis posterior major from the transverse process of C2 facilitates the exposure of the vertebral artery.

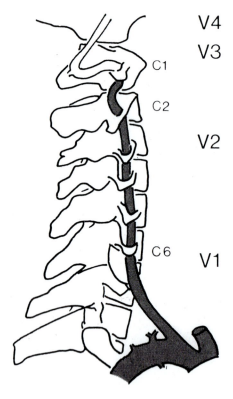

V4

V3

C1

C2

V2

C6 V1

Fig. 9.63 Anatomical division of the cervical vertebral artery. (From George B, Laurian C. The Vertebral Artery: Pathology and Surgery. New York: Springer-Verlag; 1987: Figure 1A:6. Reprinted with permission.)

sacrificing this artery. In most instances no untoward effect ensues from taking one vertebral artery.

If tumor extends up the foramen magnum or into the hypoglossal canal part or all of one lateral mass of the atlas and occipital condyle may need to be removed. The hypoglossal canal traverses the occipital condyle obliquely at a 45 degree angle from posteromedially to anterolaterally. It exits the condyle at the junction of its anterior one third and posterior two thirds ~5 mm above the craniocervical articulation and ~8 mm from the posterior edge of the occipital condyle[68] (**Fig. 9.65**). In exposing the hypoglossal nerve, if more than two thirds of the condyle require removal then the patient should undergo spinal fusion. Decisions regarding spinal instability are somewhat individual and made by the neurosurgeon.

Dissection of tumor can progress anteriorly to the jugular bulb and mastoid. This is sometimes necessary in the removal of large clival chordomas.

The wound closure is in anatomical layers and a suction drain is placed. If the dura has been resected then repaired, a suction drain may not be the best choice because it may facilitate a CSF fistula. A Penrose drain is placed instead, and a lumbar-subarachnoid drain is placed for about 3 to 5 days.

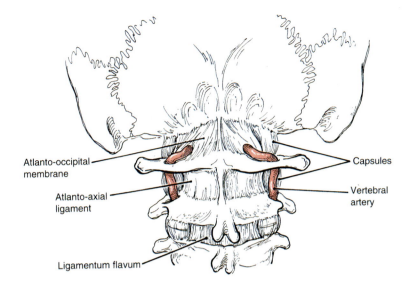

Atlanto-occipital
membrane

Atlanto-axial
ligament

Capsules

Vertebral
artery

Ligamentum flavum

Fig. 9.64 Posterior view of the craniocervical junction.

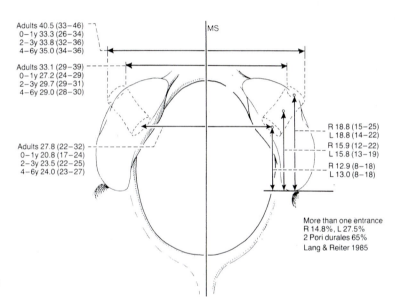

Adults 40.5 (33–46)
0–1y 33.3 (26–34)
2–3y 33.8 (32–36)
4–6y 35.0 (34–36)

Adults 33.1 (29–39)
0–1y 27.2 (24–29)
2–3y 29.7 (29–31)
4–6y 29.0 (28–30)

MS

R 18.8 (15–25)
L 18.8 (14–22)
R 15.9 (12–22)
L 15.8 (13–19)
R 12.9 (8–18)
L 13.0 (8–18)

Adults 27.8 (22–32)
0–1y 20.8 (17–24)
2–3y 23.5 (22–25)
4–6y 24.0 (23–27)

More than one entrance
R 14.8%, L 27.5%
2 Pori durales 65%
Lang & Reiter 1985

Fig. 9.65 Hypoglossal canal. Distances of its intracranial and extracranial pores and distances between the midpoints of the canal at the intracranial pore, in the middle part, and at the extracranial pore to the posterior border of the condylar process. According to Lang and Hornung. (From Lang J. Clinical Anatomy of the Posterior Cranial Fossa and its Foramina. New York: Thieme; 1991:Figure 5B:5. Reprinted with permission.)

References

1. McLean DH, Buncke HJ Jr. Autotransplant of omentum to a large scalp defect with microvascular revascularization. Plast Reconstr Surg 1972; 49:268–274

2. Yassargil MG. Reconstructive Operations on the Cerebral Blood Vessels in Microsurgery Applied to the Neurosurgery. Stuttgart: Thieme; 1969:96–114

3. Ketcham AS, Wilkins RN, Van Beuren JM, et al. A combined intracranial facial approach to the paranasal sinuses. Am J Surg 1963;106:698–703

4. Ketcham AS, Chretien PB, Schour L, et al. Surgical treatment of patients with advanced cancer of the paranasal sinuses in neoplasia of the head and neck. In: MD Anderson Hospital: Neoplasia of the Head and Neck. Chicago: Year Book Medical Publications; 1974:187

5. Sisson GA, Bytell DF, Becker SP, et al. Carcinoma of the paranasal sinuses and craniofacial resection. J Laryngol Otol 1976;90:59–68

6. Hybels RL. Venous embolism in head and neck surgery. Laryngoscope 1980;90:946–954

7. Maroon JC, Goodman JM, Hornet TG, et al. Detection of minute venous air emboli with ultrasound. Surg Gynecol Obstet 1968;127:1236–1238

8. Broderson BR, Barky N. Acoustic tumor surgery: anesthetic considerations. In: House WF, Luetje CM, eds. Acoustic Tumors. Vol 2. Baltimore: University Park Press; 1979:3

9. Fang HS, Ong GB. Direct anterior approach to the upper cervical spine. J Bone Joint Surg Am 1962;44:1588–1604

10. Crockard A. Transoral approach to intra/extradural tumors. In: Sekhar LN, Janecka IP, eds. Surgery of Cranial Base Tumors. New York: Raven; 1993:225–234

11. Donald PJ, Bernstein LB. Transpalatal excision of the odontoid process. Otolaryngology 1978;86:729–731

12. Fee WE, Gilmer PA, Goffinet DR. Surgical management of recurrent nasopharyngeal carcinoma after radiation failure at the primary site. Laryngoscope 1988;98:1220–1226

13. Fee WE Jr, Moir MS, Choi EC, Goffinet D. Nasopharyngectomy for recurrent nasopharyngeal cancer: a 2–17 year follow. Arch Otolaryngol Head Neck Surg 2002;128:280–284

14. Cocke EW Jr, Robertson JH. Anterior Fossa Approaches: Extended unilateral maxillotomy approach. In: Donald PJ, ed. Surgery of the Skull Base. Philadelphia: Lippincott-Raven; 1998:207–237.

15. Wei WI, Lam KH, Sham JS. New approach to the nasopharynx: the maxillary swing approach. Head Neck 1991;13:200–207

16. Wei WI. Salvage surgery for recurrent primary nasopharyngeal carcinoma. Crit Rev Oncol Hematol 2000;33:91–98

17. Janecka IP, Sen C, Sekhar LN, Arriaga M. Facial translocation: a new approach to the cranial base. Otolaryngol Head Neck Surg 1990;103:413–419

18. Schramm VL. Infratemporal fossa surgery. In: Sekhar LN, Schramm VL, eds. Tumors of the Cranial Base: Diagnosis and Treatment. Mount Kisco, NY: Futura; 1987:421–437

19. Fisch U. The infratemporal fossa approaches for nasopharyngeal tumors. Laryngoscope 1983;93:36–446

20. Howard DJ, Lloyd G, Lund V. Recurrence and its avoidance in juvenile nasopharyngeal angiofibroma. Laryngoscope 2001;111:1509–1511

21. Binkhorst CD, Schierbeck P, Petten GHW. Neoplasms of the notochord: report of a case of basilar chordoma and bilateral orbital involvement. Acta Otolaryngol 1957;47:10–20

22. Conley J. Concepts in Head and Neck Surgery. New York: Grune & Stratton; 1970:202

23. Batsakis JH. Soft tissue tumors of the head and neck: unusual forms. In: Batsakis JG, ed. Tumors of the Head and Neck: Clinical and Pathological Considerations. Baltimore: Williams & Wilkins; 1974:264

24. Rice DH, Manusco A, Hanafee WN. Computed tomography with simultaneous contrast sialography. West J Med 1980;133:321–322

25. Stenhouse D, Mason DK. Oral hemangiopericytoma: a case report. Br J Oral Surg 1968;6:114–117

26. Stout AP, Murray MR. Hemangiopericytoma: vascular tumor featuring Zimmerman's pericytes. Ann Surg 1942;116:26–33

27. Loke YW. Lymphoepitheliomas of the cervical lymph nodes. Br J Cancer 1965;19:482–485

28. Batsakis JG. Tumors of the Head and Neck: Clinical and Pathological Considerations. Baltimore: Williams & Wilkins; 1974:213

29. Batsakis JG. Tumors of the Head and Neck: Clinical and Pathological Considerations. Baltimore: Williams & Wilkins; 1974:178

30. Weiss SW, Goldblum JR. Enzinger and Weiss's Soft Tissue Tumors. 4th ed. St. Louis: Mosby; 2001

31. Barnes L. Surgical Pathology of the Head and Neck. Vol 2. 2nd ed. New York: Marcel Dekker; 2001

32. Conley J. Concepts in Head and Neck Surgery. New York: Grune & Stratton; 1970:199

33. Thompson DE, Forest HM, Hendrick JW, et al. Soft tissue sarcomas involving the extremities and the limb girdles. South Med J 1971;64:33–34

34. Fisher ER, Vuzevski VD. Cytogenesis of schwannoma (neurilemoma), neurofibroma, dermatofibroma, and dermatofibrosarcoma as revealed by electron microscopy. Am J Clin Pathol 1968;49:141–154

35. Laing D. Nasopharyngeal carcinoma. Otolaryngol Clin North Am 1969;2:703–725

36. Batsakis JG. Carcinomas of the nasopharynx. In: Tumors of the Head and Neck: Clinical and Pathological Considerations. Baltimore: Williams & Wilkins; 1974:123

37. Toomey JM. Cysts and tumors of the pharynx. In: Paparella MM, Shumrick DA, eds. Otolaryngology. Vol 3. 2nd ed. Philadelphia: WB Saunders; 1980:2323

38. Coates HL, Pearson GR, Nee IHB, et al. Epstein-Barr virus—associated antigens in nasopharyngeal carcinoma. Arch Otolaryngol 1978;104:427–430

39. Yu MC, Ho JH, Lai SH, Henderson BE. Cantonese-style salted fish as a cause of nasopharyngeal carcinoma: report of a case-controlled study in Hong Kong. Cancer Res 1986;46:956–961

40. Loke YW. Lymphoepitheliomas of the cervical lymph nodes. Br J Cancer 1965;19:482–485

41. Fletcher GH, Million RR. Malignant tumors of the nasopharynx. Am J Roentgenol Radium Ther Nucl Med 1965;93:44–55

42. Vilar P. Nasopharyngeal carcinoma: a report on 24 patients seen over six years. Scott Med J 1966;11:315–318

43. Raventos A, Davis LW. Cancer of the nasal cavity, paranasal sinuses, and nasopharynx: radiotherapeutic management. In: English GM, ed. Otolaryngology. Vol 3. Hagerstown, MD: Harper & Row; 1979:1–13

44. Jing BS. Tumors of the nasopharynx. Radiol Clin North Am 1970;8:323–342

45. Rouvière H. Anatomy of the Human Lymphatic System. Trans. MJ Tobias. Ann Arbor: JW Edwards; 1938

46. Donald PJ. Pathophysiology of skull base malignancies. In: Donald PJ, ed. Surgery of the Skull Base. Philadelphia: Lippincott-Raven; 1998:62

47. Donald PJ. Infratemporal fossa-middle cranial fossa approach. In: Donald PJ, ed. Surgery of the Skull Base. Philadelphia: Lippincott-Raven; 1998:335

48. Donald PJ. The significance of invasion of key intracranial structures in skull base surgery for malignancy. Presented at the Triological Society Meeting, Scottsdale, Arizona, May, 1997

49. Menzek W. Carotid artery assessment and interventional radiologic procedures before skull base surgery. In: Donald PJ, ed. Surgery of the Skull Base. Philadelphia: Lippincott-Raven; 1998:105–118

50. Ketcham AS, Chretien PB, Schour L, et al. Surgical treatment of patients with advanced cancer of the paranasal sinuses. In: M.D. Anderson Hospital: Neoplasms of the Head and Neck. Chicago: YearBook Medical Publications; 1974:187–202

51. Fisch U, Mattox D. Microsurgery of the Skull Base. New York: Thieme; 1988:22–24

52. McCabe FB, Work WP. Parotidectomy with special reference to the facial nerve. In: English GM, ed. Otolaryngology. Vol 4. Hagerstown, MD: Harper & Row; 1967:37

53. Southwick WO, Robinson RA. Surgical approaches to the vertebral bodies in the cervical and lumbar regions. J Bone Joint Surg Am 1957;39:631–644

54. De Rougemont J, Abada M, Barge M. Les possibilités de la voie d'abord antérieure dans les lésions des trois premières vertèbres cervicales. Neurochirurgie 1966;12:323–326

55. Mullan S, Naunton R, Hekmatpanah J, et al. The use of the anterior approach to ventrally placed tumors in the foramen magnum and vertebral column. J Neurosurg 1966;24:536–543

56. Stevenson GC, Stoney RJ, Perkins RK, et al. A transclival approach to the ventral surface of the brainstem for removal of clivus chordoma. J Neurosurg 1966;24:544–551

57. Fox JL. Obliteration of midline vertebral artery aneurysm via basilar craniectomy. J Neurosurg 1967;26:406–412

58. Wissinger JP, Danoff D, Wisial ES. Repair of an aneurysm of the basilar artery by a transclival approach. J Neurosurg 1967;26:417–419

59. Yassargil MC. Reconstructive operations on the cerebral blood vessels. In: Microsurgery Applied to Neurosurgery. Stuttgart: Thieme; 1969. (Also published by Academic Press, New York, 1969)

60. Haselden FG, Brice JG. Transoral clivectomy. J Maxillofac Surg 1978; 6:32–34

61. Donald PJ, Bernstein LB. Transpalatal excision of the odontoid process. Otolaryngology 1978;86:ORL-729–ORL-731

62. Menezes AH, Van Gilder JC, Graf CS, et al. Craniocervical abnormalities; a comprehensive surgical approach. J Neurosurg 1980;53:444–455

63. Apuzzo ML, Weiss MH, Heiden J. Transoral exposure of the atlantoaxial region. Neurosurgery 1978;3:201–207

64. Panje WR, McCabe BF. Transparotid approach to the infratemporal fossa and base of the skull. Presented at the Yale Symposium on Skull Base Surgery, June 1980

65. George B, Laurian C. The Vertebral Artery Pathology and Surgery. New York: Springer-Verlag; 1987

66. George B, Laurian C. Surgical possibilities in the 3rd portion of the vertebral artery (above) C2. VIth European Congress of Neurosurgery, Paris; June, 1979

67. Sen CN, Sekhar LN. An extreme lateral approach to intradural lesions of the cervical spine and foramen magnum. Neurosurgery 1990;27:197–204

68. Rhoton AL Jr. The far-lateral approach and its transcondylar, supracondylar and paracondylar extensions. Surgery 2000;47(Suppl 3): S195–S209

10

Melanoma of the Head and Neck

Paul J. Donald

Melanoma of the head and neck is a terrifying and, unfortunately, an increasingly more commonly occurring malignancy. Its propensity for rapid local spread and distant metastases often precludes adequate control. One of the deadliest of all the malignancies of the head and neck, its vicious and "capricious nature," so aptly coined by Conley,[1] is well known to all experienced head and neck oncological surgeons. The lesion, which despite adequate excision recurs many years later, the distant metastases that suddenly appear within weeks of resection, and the primary lesion that disappears once the neck metastasis becomes manifest are but a few examples of this unpredictable behavior.

The tumor arises when a melanocyte becomes autonomous in its growth pattern, rapidly replicating itself in the manner that hallmarks malignancy. The melanocyte is a cell that resides in the dermal–epidermal junction and in the matrix of hair follicles. Its dendritic processes intrude themselves between the cells of the malpighian layer of the epidermis. Melanin, a brown pigment produced in the melanocyte by the metabolism of k-tyrosine, collects in these processes in the form of granules. These are extruded into the intracellular spaces by a "pinching-off" process known as clasmatosis.[2] The granules are phagocytosed by adjacent nonpigmented cells, thereby becoming the main contributor to skin pigmentation. The concentration of melanocytes in the skin of the head and neck is double that of the trunk and extremities.

Nevi are aggregations of melanocytes that are present from birth and often do not make their appearance until puberty. According to Pack and Davis,[3] each individual has an average of 15 nevi. These benign lesions are generally classified according to the histological location of the melanocytes. The junctional nevus is found at the dermal–epidermal interface and is the most common variety to undergo malignant degeneration. The compound nevus has concentrations of melanocytes both in the junctional zone and in the dermal layer. As puberty progresses, the junctional component occasionally regresses and the intradermal portion hypertrophies, thus transforming the compound nevus to a purely intradermal

one. The intradermal nevus is usually small and like the compound nevus has a very low malignant potential. A rare form of nevus that is only rarely seen in the head and neck, but which has a frighteningly high incidence of malignant degeneration of 10%, is the giant hairy nevus. Histologically, it may be either compound or intradermal. Exquisite judgment must be exercised in the management of this lesion. It is important to remember that total prophylactic excision, which is often advised, may result in extensive scarring and deformity. Careful frequent observation is essential to detect any change indicating focal malignant degeneration.

Most malignant melanomas arise in a preexisting nevus. MacNeer and Das Gupta[4] reported a series of 557 patients in which 27% of the melanomas occurred in a nevus present since birth and 39% in a pigmented lesion that had been present for longer than 5 years. Therefore only 34% of their patients had a melanoma develop de novo. Malignant transformation can occur in any form of nevus but develops most commonly in the junctional and giant varieties. However, the chance of a pigmented lesion becoming malignant is approximately one in a million. This statistic, coupled with the fact that it would take 10,000 surgeons excising a nevus every 15 minutes for 8 hours a day ~25 years to excise all the nevi in the population,[5] has consoled many a cancerphobic patient with regard to the probable lack of necessity for excision.

◆ Epidemiology and Etiology

In the United States in 2002, there were 53,600 cases of malignant melanoma with 7400 subsequent deaths.[6] The incidence is much higher in populations exposed to high-intensity sunlight. MacDonald[7] in 1948 reported a melanoma incidence of 1.6 per 100,000 population in males and two per 100,000 population in females recorded in the Connecticut Tumor Registry. This contrasts with a 6.9 per 100,000 white population found in six counties surveyed in Texas in 1975.[8] There has been a 3% annual increase in melanoma in the white population of the United States in the past 30 years.[9]

Sex incidence in most series is equal, with a slight female predominance. Because melanomas rarely appear before puberty, theories have developed centering on the notion that they are hormone dependent. Additional evidence for this relationship was thought to be found in the once prevalent idea that pregnant women with melanoma had a poorer prognosis.[10] However, more recent work[11,12] has cast doubt on this belief, leaving obscure the implication of hormones in the disease. There is evidence to indicate a familial tendency in some melanomas.[13] In those patients who have a positive family history, Anderson[14] found a younger median age of presentation of the disease and a higher incidence of multiple pigmented tumors. He postulated that the genetic location involved multiple chromosomes and that the carrier was female.

Although Caucasians have the highest incidence of malignant melanoma, the lesion is also found in the pigmented races. African Americans commonly have nevi but have a lower frequency of melanoma than Caucasians. Curiously, however, melanoma on the sole of the foot is relatively common among black Africans. This may be explained by the fact that nevi in blacks generally tend to occur much more frequently in the less pigmented parts of the body. In addition, in the African, the sole of the foot is frequently exposed to trauma. This tends to support the still popular notion of the role of frequent irritation of a mole in the genesis of malignant melanoma. Melanoma is rare in Japanese and uncommon in Sri Lankans and Javanese. Among those of Indian-Spanish descent in Texas and in Cali, Colombia, it is as common as in the Caucasian race.[9]

The implication of sunlight as an etiologic factor has already been alluded to. The mechanism of action is unclear, but it is thought that in addition to the alteration in melanocyte metabolism resulting in malignant behavior, continued actinic exposure also causes the production of a melanoma-stimulating factor.[2] This would explain the frequent occurrence of melanoma in non-sun-exposed areas of individuals in high sunshine density geographic regions. The protection of the skin by increased melanin pigment seems indisputable. This is evidenced by the predominance of melanomas in those with blond or red hair, blue or hazel eyes, and a fair complexion.[7] The most consistent historical event predisposing Caucasians to melanoma is sun exposure with burning and blistering in childhood or adolescence. The use of protective clothing, sunscreen with SPF 15 or higher, and avoidance of the midday sun are the most effective preventatives.

Polychlorinated biphenyls, hydrazine, dimethylsulphate, DDT,[15,16] and the by-products of the steel and nonferrous[17,18] metal industries have all been implicated as etiologic agents in malignant melanoma. The epidemiological studies of Morton and Starr[19] lend further support to these findings. They showed an increased incidence of melanoma in some counties in Oregon in which there was high environmental exposure to malathion, fenthion, and DDT and little exposure to comparatively dense sunlight.

The other factors that have been associated with the production of melanoma are immunosuppression, atypical male/ dysplastic nevus syndrome, prior therapy with psoralen, the use of ultraviolet (UV) A light (200 to 320 nm), UV exposure in tanning salons, and a history of melanoma in a first-degree relative. Using a multivariate analysis Rigel[20] showed six factors that incidentally influenced the risk of contacting melanoma (**Table 10.1**). If a patient possesses one or two of these risk factors the individual has 3.5-fold increased risk of developing the disease. Three or more factors carried a 20-fold increased risk. Individuals who have had one melanoma are at a 4 to 30% risk of developing a second one compared with the 1% risk that the rest of the American population is at risk for during their lifetime.[21] Alterations in the P16 genome are also associated with melanoma development.[22]

Table 10.1 Risk Factors for Melanoma

- Family history of malignant melanoma
- Presence of blond or red hair
- A marked freckling on the upper back
- History of three or more blistering sun burns prior to age 20
- History of three or more years of an outdoor job as a teenager
- Presence of actinic keratosis

◆ Pathology

Once a melanocyte becomes autonomous, replicates rapidly, and breaks through the host's immune barrier, it may assume a variety of growth patterns and hence a highly variable clinical course. The most common case reports of spontaneous tumor regression involve melanoma patients. On the other hand, a lesion may remain relatively static for years and then suddenly enlarge and metastasize. In some cases, the primary lesion has spontaneously resolved in the presence of manifest metastasis. Furthermore, spontaneous regression of metastases has occurred coincidentally with the development of new lesions. These facts, coupled with the discovery that melanoma will often regress following inoculation with the bacillus Calmette-Guérin (BCG), strongly implicate the activity of the immune system in this disease. Further, a membrane-associated tumor-specific antigen has been identified in a large number of patients with melanoma. Antibodies to these antigens have been detected in the sera of most of the melanoma patients studied and in 20% of normal individuals.[23]

The approach to the management of malignant melanoma has been greatly facilitated in the past decade by the work of Clark.[24] By relating the morphological pattern of the disease to its natural history, he classified these lesions on the basis of gross appearance into three types: lentigo maligna melanoma (the melanotic freckle of Hutchinson), the superficial spreading type, and the nodular variety.

The lentigo maligna is a superficial, pigmented lesion found primarily in the elderly; it is two to three times more common in females. It is found on the cheek and temporal skin and has irregular borders with a smooth surface. Malignant degeneration is slow to develop and then gradually progressive, but never metastatic. Nodular thickening or ulceration in lentigo maligna melanoma denotes malignant transformation.

The superficial spreading type is smaller and more circumscribed than the lentigo maligna variety. It may demonstrate a wide spectrum of colors ranging from black through various hues of brown to the pinkish cast of amelanotic melanoma. The lesions seldom reach a size greater than 2 cm in diameter without ulcerating or bleeding. These signs denote dermal penetration. Histologically, the malignant melanocytes assume a pagetoid appearance and initially penetrate the epidermis. As the lesion progresses, dermal invasion occurs. The head and neck area is the most common site for this form of melanoma.[25]

Nodular melanoma comprises 10 to 15% of all melanomas and is the principal form of the mucosal lesion. It invades dermis immediately and frequently metastasizes. Preexisting nevi are less commonly associated with its development, and there is a positive association with actinic exposure. It is papular in type and shows no "staining" of the surrounding skin. Goldsmith[26] points out that it usually assumes various shades of blue, from blue-black through bluish-gray to blue-red. The amelanotic variety is often very difficult to diagnose and escapes detection until a high index of suspicion is aroused. The presence of melanotic spots near its base is an important diagnostic clue. Because of early dermal invasion, frequent ulceration is common in nodular lesions, even when they are still quite small. Cellular anaplasia is more marked in this type than in the others. Clark et al[24] established the diagnostic criterion that if junctional activity does not extend more than three rete pegs beyond the epidermal extent of the lesion, the lesion may be classified as nodular.

Smith[27] makes a cogent point that there are several intermediate types of melanoma that cannot be pigeonholed into one or another of these categories. For instance, a nodular ex-

crescence may develop in a superficial melanoma, have deep dermal invasion, yet spread at the junctional zone beyond three rete pegs. Thus the disease process must be recognized as a continuum with varieties that cross the boundaries of definitive classification.

Clark's histological classification,[24] based upon the depth of invasion, has greatly aided the surgeon in planning the width of excision and determining the necessity for neck dissection. **Figure 10.1** illustrates the five levels of penetration that he describes. He discovered that the incidence of metastases increases and survival rates diminish with increasing depths of tumor penetration. In most series, level I is associated with almost no metastases, and in level II they are infrequent. However, levels IV and V are associated with frequent regional and distant secondaries and a high mortality rate. Fortner et al[28] reported only one patient with lymph node metastasis among 22 patients with Clark level II penetration. Gupta[29] found no lymph node metastasis in 10 patients with this level of invasion, and Wanebo et al[30] had only one patient with secondaries in 28 such patients. But with level V involvement, these three groups of investigators found a 71, 100, and 70% incidence of metastatic disease, respectively. Curiously Gumport and Harris,[31] as well as Conley and Pack,[32] had a small number of patients with lentigo maligna melanoma who developed metastases. These idiosyncratic secondaries had a pathognomonic histological pattern characterized by a marked desmoplastic reaction similar to that of fibrosarcoma.

Breslow and Macht[33] have presented data that bring into question the accuracy of the Clark histological staging system. They quote McGovern's experience of a 48% 10-year survival rate in each of two groups of melanoma patients, one group having level II involvement and the other group, level IV. The fact that these levels of invasion had equivalent survival rates, coupled with the difficulty in determining the

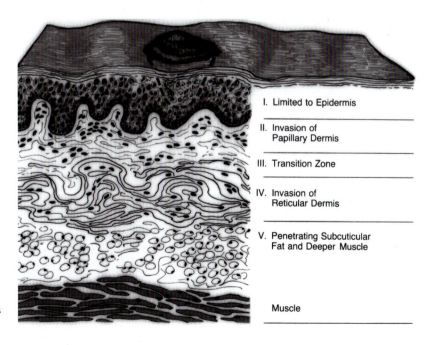

I. Limited to Epidermis

II. Invasion of Papillary Dermis

III. Transition Zone

IV. Invasion of Reticular Dermis

V. Penetrating Subcuticular Fat and Deeper Muscle

Muscle

Fig. 10.1 The five levels of invasion of malignant melanoma according to Clark. (From Clark WH Jr, Fran L, Bernardino FA et al. The histogenesis and biologic behavior of primary human malignant melanoma of the skin. Cancer Res 1969;29:705. Reprinted with permission.)

anatomical cutoff point between the two levels, encouraged Breslow and Macht to investigate an alternative method of classification. They correlated the measured depth of penetration of melanoma cells, mitotic activity, and inflammatory response to prognosis, and found that the only consistently significant factor was the measured depth of tumor extension. They had a total of 62 patients in their series whose excised tumors had penetrated less than a 0.76 mm thickness of epithelium. In a 5-year period, there has been no mortality and all the patients have remained disease free. Unfortunately, no data were presented on lymph node metastasis or local recurrence other than the statement that these situations rarely, if ever, occur with these so-called thin tumors. An earlier report by the principal author[34] described a series of 98 melanoma patients of whom 45 had lesions that were less than 0.76 mm deep, no wider than 5 mm, and less than 6.01 mm in cross-sectional area on the fixed specimen. Except in one of these patients, there was no local recurrence of tumor or development of metastasis. Unfortunately, these data were collected on cases involving the extremities, and their relevance to the head and neck can only be inferential.

In an analysis of 510 melanomas by Smith,[27] a correlation between lesion thickness in millimeters and Clark level of penetration was made (**Fig. 10.2**). **Table 10.1** correlates Clark level of stage I melanoma with 5- and 10-year survival (Bergsen-Gage), and **Table 10.2** correlates depth of penetration with survival. Stage I was defined as a primary melanoma that is not a recurrent primary and that has no metastasis. A

Table 10.2 Survival of Stage I Patients According to Clark Level of Invasion

Total No. of Patients	Males/ Females	Stage	Level	5-Year Survival	10-Year Survival
68	26/42	1	II	87.8	83.7
66	27/39	1	III	86.0	74.6
170	80/90	1	IV	56.2	40.7

Source: From Smith JL. Neoplasms of skin and malignant melanoma. In: Histopathology and Biologic Behavior of Malignant Melanoma. Chicago: Year Book Medical Publications; 1976:320. Reprinted with permission.

multivariate analysis of a large series of cutaneous melanomas of the head and neck by Medina[35] revealed a positive correlation between the four depths of tumor penetration and prognosis, although the difference between 0.76 and 1.50 was small (**Table 10.3**). Within these limitations, it is apparent that tumors fulfilling the criteria for Clark levels I, II, and III and with penetration depths of less than 0.99 mm have an excellent prognosis.

Table 10.3 Survival of Stage I Patients According to Thickness of Tumor

Total No. of Patients	Males/ Females	Stage	Thickness of Tumor (mm)	5-Year Survival	10-Year Survival
55	19/36	1	< 0.5	87.2	84.8
58	21/37	1	0.5–0.99	89.5	79.0
57	25/32	1	1.0–1.49	78.4	70.0
36	15/21	1	1.5–1.99	60.4	48.8
49	27/22	1	2.0–2.99	58.5	35.2
82	43/29	1	> 3.0	35.3	18.4

Source: From Smith JL. Neoplasms of skin and malignant melanoma. In: Histopathology and Biologic Behavior of Malignant Melanoma. Chicago: Year Book Medical Publications; 1976:321. Reprinted with permission.

Mucosal melanomas of the head and neck form a special group. They have a much poorer prognosis than cutaneous lesions of the same region but are fortunately rare, with those involving the oral mucosa making up 0.4 to 14% of all melanomas. Much less common sites of involvement include the nose, tonsils, paranasal sinuses, and larynx. Hormia and Vuori[36] reviewed 7253 cases of malignancy of the upper aerodigestive tract and found only 11 malignant melanomas. In a review of four large series of head and neck melanomas, Batsakis[25] compiled 930 cases, of which only 71 involved the mucous membranes.

Melanotic pigmentation of the mucosa is characteristic of blacks but is less common in Caucasians, except for those of Latin descent. Mucosal melanoma is exceedingly rare in blacks, has a predilection for males, and has its highest incidence in the age group of 20 to 70 years. Although primary rather than secondary lesions are reported to be by far the most common in the head and neck region, this has not been the case in the author's experience. I have found the oral and

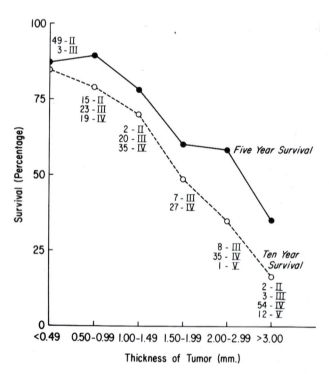

Fig. 10.2 Graph relating the survival of patients with malignant melanoma to lesion thickness and to Clark level. (From Smith JL. Neoplasms of skin and malignant melanoma. In: Histopathology and Biologic Behavior of Malignant Melanoma. Chicago: Year Book Medical Publications; 1976:321. Reprinted with permission.)

nasal septal mucosa to be a much more common site of secondary melanoma than primary.

The prognosis for mucosal melanoma is poor because of the frequency of metastases, the delay in recognition and diagnosis, the richness of lymphatic drainage, and the often-inadequate resection of the lesion.

◆ Diagnosis

The diagnosis of head and neck melanoma is suggested by any color change in a pigmented lesion. A thickening or nodularity in a Hutchinson freckle or junctional nevus usually denotes malignant degeneration. Ulceration and bleeding, a halo of inflammation, and satellitosis are even stronger indications of malignant change. In Conley and Pack's series of head and neck melanomas, 8% were amelanotic. The absence of pigment is more common in the mucosal form of the disease than in the cutaneous.[32] The frequency of occurrence of cutaneous melanomas of the head and neck in the series reviewed by Batsakis[25] is illustrated in **Fig. 10.3**.

The lesions occur most frequently in the neck, scalp, and cheek,[25,37] where the skin has the highest melanocyte density. However, lesions in these sites have the best prognosis, whereas affliction of the skin of the external ear carries the worst prognosis. In a series of 42 cases occurring in this site, Pack et al[38] describe the lesion's most frequent occurrence in the helix and antihelix.

Obviously, not all pigmented lesions are malignant melanomas. The recent introduction of epiluminescent microscopy has great promise in vivo differentiation of benign pigmented lesions from malignant melanoma.[39–41] A dermatoscope with a 10× lens is used and the lesion viewed under oil immersion. Certain subepithelial features help identify a pigmented lesion as a melanoma.

The rate of metastasis to regional lymph nodes is difficult to determine. Most series summarize the experience of a large referral center where many patients are sent who either have failed primary treatment and have a local recurrence or are already metastatic and therefore difficult to manage. Thus these lesions are automatically more aggressive and more advanced. Conley and Pack,[32] for example, observed a 48% rate of metastasis to cervical lymphatics when the patient was first seen, but in only 10% of the cases was Conley the first physician to excise the primary. In fact, in 25% of 175 cases, two or more excisions had already been done before the patient's first visit to see Conley. In contrast, the series of Storm et al[42] contained 69 patients of whom only 17 represented cases of local recurrence following therapy done elsewhere. Only 15 patients in this series (21.7%) had manifest cervical metastasis when first seen by the authors. Southwick et al[43] had 17 of 38 patients (44.7%) who presented with regional metastases, and Simons[44] had 78 of 265 (29.4%) with cervical node involvement. Both of these authors saw a large number of patients with previously treated disease.

The site of the lesion and the depth of penetration strongly influence the metastatic rate. In situ melanoma has a 0 incidence of lymph nodal metastasis and is 100% curable by local excision. As already mentioned, metastases are rarely seen in cases of lentigo maligna melanoma, and Clark level I melanoma metastases are similarly unusual. The regional metastatic rate for Clark level II is from 2 to 5%; for level III, ~20%; for level IV, 40%; and for level V, 70%.[25] In Medina's meta-analysis, lesions of less than 0.76 mm thickness had a cervical lymph nodal metastatic rate of only 2 to 3%; those between 0.76 and 1.50 thick, a 25% nodal with an additional 8% distant metastatic rate; those between 1.52 mm and 4.00 mm, 57% nodal and 15% distant rates; and those greater than 4.00 in thickness 62% nodal and 72% distant.[34] Lesions of the skin of the cheek and neck infrequently metastasize and have a good prognosis, whereas melanomas of the external ear and scalp have a higher metastatic rate and a poorer prognosis. Conley[37] quotes a 50% rate of cervical secondaries for primary tumors of the scalp, with frequent bilateral neck involvement. His pessimism regarding scalp lesions is shared by Southwick et al,[43] who had only two of nine patients survive 5 years.

Mucosal melanomas can present as flat lesions but are usually nodular. They are almost exclusively confined to the maxillary portion of the head, with the palate the most common site of origin. Lesions of the tongue and mandibular gingiva are uncommon. In the nasal cavities, the tumor may present on either the septum or turbinates and rarely may primarily involve the maxillary or ethmoid sinuses.

The oral lesions may ulcerate and bleed and may involve bone and become painful. Gingival involvement eventually

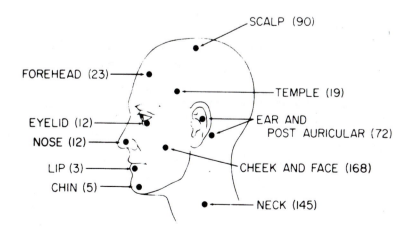

Fig. 10.3 Topographic distribution of 179 cutaneous malignant melanomas of the head and neck. (From Batsakis JG. Tumors of the Head and Neck: Clinical and Pathological Considerations. Baltimore: Williams & Wilkins; 1974:335. Reprinted with permission.)

results in loosening of the teeth. Nasal cavity melanomas cause symptoms of nasal obstruction, epistaxis, and foul nasal discharge.

Mucosal melanoma has a high incidence of regional and distant metastases with an attendant poor prognosis. The same relationships of Clark staging and Breslow penetration depth to metastatic rate and survival pertain. Unfortunately, most of these lesions are quite extensive before they are diagnosed, resulting in tragic consequences. This is borne out by the series of both Chaudhry et al[45] and Allen,[46] who cite a 4 to 6% 5-year survival rate for patients with oral melanoma. In a meta-analysis of over 1000 patients reported in the literature by Mandolidis and Donald,[47] 547 patients contained in 13 series had enough information for complete analysis. Patients with nasal mucosal melanoma had a 31% 5-year survival rate, whereas melanoma of the sinuses had a 0% 5-year survival.

The diagnosis of malignant melanoma is established primarily by the biopsy of a suspicious lesion. Electrodessication of moles and other pigmented lesions or their relegation to the trashcan after excision is to be decried. Only biopsies that skirt the lesions by at least a narrow margin of healthy tissue and extend into the subcutaneous layer are sufficient. All specimens must be submitted for histological examination. In the case of a large lesion it is often not reasonable to do a total excision because of the resultant large defect and the potential for having to do a major revisional operation if the lesion is malignant. There is no evidence available to indicate that incisional biopsy followed by definitive resection increases the local recurrence rate, increases the frequency of local and distant metastases, or diminishes survival.[25] Occasionally, the histological diagnosis on routine hemotoxylin-eosin (H&E) staining is difficult to make. Special stains, including SI00, HMB 45, and Mel 45, greatly aid in establishing the lesion definitively as a melanoma.

Because of the common development of distant metastases in the absence of cervical adenopathy, scans of potential distant metastatic sites are advisable in all level IV and V and most level III melanomas. Disseminated disease will produce a generalized change in cutaneous pigmentation and even melanuria.

◆ Treatment

The precise histological classifications of Clark and Breslow has revolutionized the surgical management of malignant melanoma. Heretofore the dictum was that all melanomas had to be resected with a 4 to 6 cm margin of surrounding healthy tissue to ensure complete excision. It has become increasingly apparent that adequate removal of lentigo maligna and Clark I melanomas can be achieved with a 1 cm resection margin. Breslow and Macht[33] found in their experience that the "thin" melanoma—one measuring less than 0.76 mm in depth—could be safely excised with a narrow resection margin. They followed 62 patients who had excision of a thin lesion in which the resection margin varied from 0.1 to 5.5 cm. A remarkable 32% of the margins were 1 cm or less. All patients were free of disease at the end of the 5-year observation period.

When the lesion penetrates the epithelial surface to the deep III, IV, or V levels, or measures greater than 0.76 mm in thickness, satellitosis, local recurrences, and regional metastases are common. These lesions require a wide margin of excision. A margin of healthy tissue at least 4 to 6 cm wide will adequately encompass the disease in most instances. Care must be taken not only to adequately skirt the lesion but to excise sufficient depth as well. The pernicious nature of melanoma dictates the most radical of excisions.

In thin melanomas of small diameter, it is often possible to close the defect by primary approximation of the wound edges. This is relatively safe because of the low incidence of local recurrence of these lesions. In wider excisions, the defect may be covered with a split-thickness skin graft, a full-thickness skin graft, or a flap. The problem with using a flap is the potential for obscuring early local recurrences. To a degree, the same problem pertains to the full-thickness graft. Although the split-thickness graft is the safest method of wound coverage, it is also the most aesthetically disagreeable. The surgeon is often faced with the dilemma of choosing between patient safety and cosmetic appearance.

Sentinel Node Biopsy

The utility of the concept of sentinel node biopsy is controversial in the head and neck region. A two-step process of detection is used to determine the location of the sentinel node. A radionuclide, usually a technetium 99 colloid, is injected into the dermis surrounding the tumor site, and a gamma camera maps out the regional lymphatics as they pick up the radioactive material to be filtered by the sentinel node. The sentinel node concentrates the isotope and shows up brightly on the lymphoscintogram. A vital dye such as patent blue violet or isosulphan blue is then injected into the tumor site, the neck opened over the previously identified nodal site, and the node or nodes stained by the dye removed and sent for frozen section analysis.[48] If the nodes are positive then a neck dissection is done. If the nodes are histologically negative then no further dissection is done. A more streamlined version of the technique was described by Van der Veen et al[49] wherein the radionuclide is injected intradermally 1 hour preoperatively, and a sterile gamma counter is used to identify the area of the sentinel node. The area of the lesion is reinjected now with lymphozurin blue. The neck is opened and the stained nodes removed. A meticulous technique and careful coordination with the nuclear medicine specialist and pathologist are essential to produce good results. It is estimated that a minimum of 25 cases is necessary to produce optimal results with this technique.

In melanoma of the extremities and trunk isolation of the sentinel node that drains the area involved with tumor is done and the node biopsied. Lack of involvement of that node with tumor has led to the practice of preclusion of a regional nodal dissection in such cases. This has been established as an oncologically safe policy in melanomas of the extremities and back,[50] saving many patients from nodal dissection without jeopardizing their overall survival. The complexity of lymphatic drainage in the head and neck with many nodes often having the potential of being a sentinel node has sig-

Table 10.4 Five-Year Follow-up Study of 224 Patients with Malignant Melanoma of the Head and Neck

	All Patients	DIED Uncontrolled Disease		Other Cause		ALIVE With Disease		Well, without Disease	
Procedure		No.	Percent	No.	Percent	No.	Percent	No.	Percent
Excision without nodal dissection	133	53	40	13	10	6	5	61	45
Excision with nodal dissection for positive nodes	37	25	68	1	3	0	0	11	29
Regional nodal dissection; no treatment to primary lesion	29	23	79	0	0	2	7	4	14
Excision with prophylactic nodal dissection	25	7	28	2	8	0	0	16	64
Total	224	108	48	16	8	8	4	92	41
Excision with late dissection for positive nodes*	28	23	82	0	0	0	0	5	18

Source: From Simons JN. Malignant melanomas of the skin of the head and neck. Am J Surg 1972;124;487. Reprinted with permission.

*Patients were in group that had undergone excision without nodal dissection.

nificantly diminished the utility of using the sentinel node concept here. The study of O'Brien[51] reinforces the dilemmas posed by the complexity of the cervicofacial lymphatics and the problem of false positives and false negatives using lymphoscintigraphy in identifying the sentinel node. Discordance between clinical findings and lymphoscintigraph was seen in 34% of patients. Other reports are more encouraging but suffer from short follow-up and lack of reporting of incidences of metastatic disease appearance in the test negative necks.

Radical Neck Dissection

◆ **Indications** In the author's opinion, the presence of palpable cervical lymphadenopathy is a definitive indication for a radical neck dissection, provided there is no evidence of distant metastases. However, the role of elective neck dissection remains highly controversial. Detection of early distant disease still remains an enormous diagnostic problem. Computed tomographic (CT) scanning of the lungs will pick up small metastatic lesions in the lungs, but metastases in other organs are a little more difficult to discern when small. Positron emission tomographic (PET) scans will only detect lesions larger than 2 cm in diameter. One of the most sensitive detectors of metastatic disease is serum LDH.

The low incidence of regional metastases in thin melanomas rules out the serious consideration of elective neck dissection for these lesions. A review of the literature by Bernstein et al[52] showed that in several large series there was good evidence of the efficacy of elective neck dissection in cases of thick melanomas. One of the major problems in analyzing the statistics on this issue is the lack of conforming data among series. Sisson and McMahan[53] have neatly summarized the major areas of discrepancy. The major problem is the small number of cases available for study, with variations in statistical method, the use of different classification systems, and the fact that patients are not always randomized to treatment groups all adding to the difficulty of drawing solid conclusions.

An analysis of the data of Simons[44] on 224 patients with head and neck melanoma shows that those who had a prophylactic neck dissection did statistically significantly better than those who had excision and a delayed therapeutic dissection once regional secondaries became manifest (**Table 10.4**). **Tables 10.5**, **10.6**, and **10.7** illustrate the efficacy of elective neck dissection in three other series of patients with head and neck melanoma. On the other hand, Sisson and McMahan[53] point to a report by Veronesi et al,[54] who analyzed a prospective, randomized study of 557 patients of whom 267 had immediate resection and regional node dissection and 286 had local excision and adenectomy only when metastases became manifest. When the patients were controlled as to sex, age, and lesion extent and site of origin there was no significant difference in survival. One of this study's major drawbacks for our purposes is that it unfortunately was done only on melanoma confined to the extremities. The patients with the highest probability to benefit from elective neck dissection are those with intermediate-thickness melanoma who have no evidence of distant metastasis.

◆ **Technique** The unpredictable and protean nature of malignant melanoma has led to considerable controversy regarding how to manage the neck. Conley's[1] classic recommendation of almost always performing a radical neck dissection including the platysma has undergone some revision.

The sentinel node biopsy has yet to withstand the test of time because there are some false-positive and false-negative results. In addition it requires close cooperation of the nu-

Table 10.5 Five-Year Definitive Cures as End Results of Treatment in 116 Determinate Cases

Therapy	Total	No.	Percent
Local excision only	42	26	62.0
Local excision and elective neck dissection	17	13	76.5
Negative nodes	8	2	25.0
Positive nodes			
Local excision and radical neck dissection with proven secondary	56	6	10.4

Source: Conley JJ, Pack GT. Melanoma of the head and neck. Surg Gynecol Obstet 1963;116:26. By permission of Surgery, Gynecology & Obstetrics.

Table 10.6 Results of Regional Node Dissections (five-year postoperative follow-up of 185 cases)

Histology	Living and Well	Recurrence	Lost to Follow-Up	Dead*	Total
Nodes microscopically negative					
Clinically negative	69 (56%)	6 (5%)	12 (10%)	37 (30%)	124
Clinically "positive"	3 (27%)	0	2 (18%)	6 (55%)	11
Nodes microscopically positive					
Clinically negative	6 (30%)	2 (10%)	1 (55%)	11 (55%)	20
Clinically "positive"	3 (10%)	0	3 (10%)	24 (80%)	30
Total					185

*Death from all causes.

Source: From Gumport SL, Harris MN. Results of regional lymph node dissection for melanoma. Ann Surg 1974;179:107, Table 2. Reprinted with permission.

clear medicine specialist, the pathologist, and the surgeon in a carefully coordinated way to make this technique work. The technique is also quite operator sensitive with those with more experience having greater success at it than a relative neophyte. If the sentinel node or nodes are positive then some form of neck dissection is required.

Table 10.7 relates melanoma thickness to incidence of nodal metastasis and survival.[35] In thin melanoma (less than 0.76 mm in thickness) no neck dissection is required. This is true also for lentigo maligna. In intermediate thickness melanoma (between 0.76 mm and 1.50 mm) some form of neck dissection is performed. In deep melanoma either with or without manifest nodal metastasis a radical neck or modified radical neck dissection is performed even though it does not seem to statistically favorably affect overall survival. It does, however, significantly impact on local tumor control.

Table 10.7 Elective Node Dissection 1954–1964, 259 Patients

Histology	No. of Patients	5-Year (%)	Cure 10-Year (%)
Negative nodes	219	83	79
Positive nodes	40 (15%)	42	42
Microscopic focus	9	67	67
One node	18	50	50
Multiple nodes	13	15	15
Total	259	76	73

Source: From Fortner JG, Woodruff J, Schottenfield D, MacLean B. Biostatistical basis of elective node dissection for malignant melanoma. Ann Surg 1977;186: 102, Table 1. Reprinted with permission.

Where no manifest lymph nodes are either palpable or are obvious on CT scanning a form of selective neck dissection is performed and if disease is detected on frozen section then a radical or modified radical neck dissection is performed predicated on the site of the primary and the proximity of the metastasis to the spinal accessory nerve. In the presence of manifest metastases a dissection that includes levels I through V is performed unless the primary is in the posterior scalp or neck skin.

In tumors involving the temporal scalp, ear, and cheek, a total parotidectomy should be done. The wealth of superficial and deep parotid lymph nodes draining these areas mandates this additional step. The posterior belly of the digastric and stylohyoid muscles should also be included in these resections.

The unknown primary is less common in melanoma than in other head and neck cancers, occurring in only ~2.5% of cases.[55] Survival following radical neck dissection in these patients is about the same as for those in whom the primary was found.

Management of Specific Sites

◆ **Scalp** The scalp is a source of a particularly aggressive form of melanoma. Most lesions in this area are nodular in type and tend to develop both satellitosis and bilateral cervical metastases. Wide-field local excision with a 4 cm margin is advisable. If the tumor is predominantly on one side, an ipsilateral neck dissection is done. However, if bilateral metastases are present, a bilateral neck dissection is required. A somewhat pessimistic view is unavoidable in cases in which there is bilateral disease. Scalp melanoma has the poorest prognosis of all cutaneous melanomas and usually requires a bilateral neck dissection.

A split-thickness skin graft is used to cover the wound. If the Clark level is IV or V, excision of the underlying periosteum and outer table of skull will be necessary to achieve an adequate margin. The bone excision is also necessary to supply a sufficient vascular bed for graft take. If some periosteum is removed and portions of the graft slough, the areas of denuded bone may be revascularized. All dead bone is removed, and multiple small penetrations through the outer table into the diploë are made with a bur (**Fig. 10.4**). A subsequent growth of granulation tissue will serve as a bed for reapplication of the skin graft.

In some instances, especially when the patient has had prior irradiation to the site or is diabetic and shows evidence of poor wound healing, a fascia-cutaneous free flap, especially from the forearm, is used for coverage.

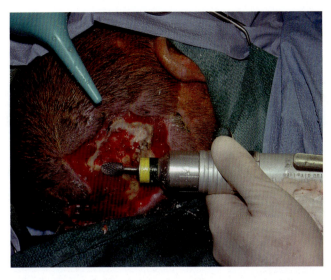

Fig. 10.4 Calvarium being prepared with multiple bur holes for a split-thickness skin graft.

◆ **Cheek** The commonest site for the most benign forms of melanoma is the midface. The lentigo maligna variety is most frequently seen on the cheek of elderly females. A neck dissection is not necessary in these cases, and a narrow margin of ~5 mm is usually sufficient to ensure adequate excision. During the resection of the primary lesion, care must be taken to avoid damage to the branches of the facial nerve. This can be achieved by keeping the dissection plane at the level of the subcutaneous fat, similar to the plane of a face-lift.

Closure can be done with the Kuhnt-Szymanowski rotation flap (**Fig. 10.5**) or, for smaller defects, the bilobed flap (**Fig. 10.6**). The unsightly scar of a split-thickness skin graft is not only ugly but also unnecessary in the thin melanoma. Great care must be taken in designing the flap when the lesion approximates the lower eyelid. If the Kuhnt-Szymanowski flap is used, the incision lateral to the lateral canthus of the eye must be swept superiorly enough to prevent the development of ectropion once the flap is rotated.

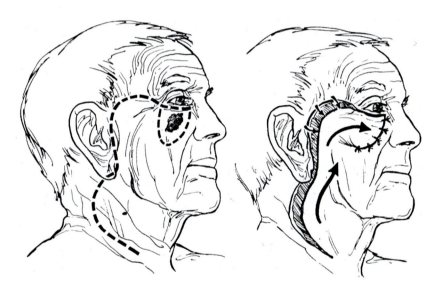

Fig. 10.5 Kuhnt-Szymanowski rotation cheek flap.

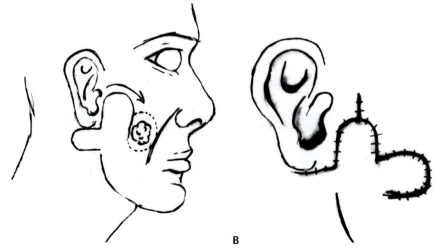

A B

Fig. 10.6 Bilobed flap. (**A**) Lesion to be excised and bilobed flap outlined. (**B**) Larger flap rotated into defect. Smaller flap used to close defect left by the first flap. Defect from smaller flap closed in a straight line.

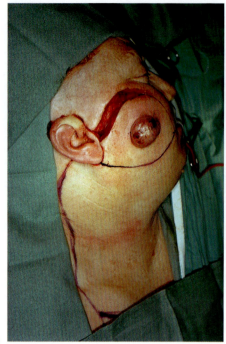
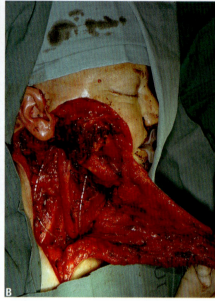
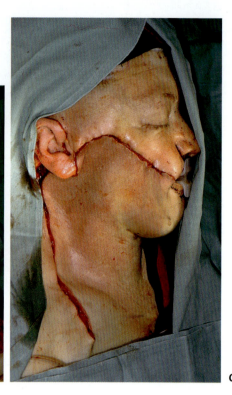

Fig. 10.7 (**A**) Nodular melanoma of the face. (**B**) Wide-field resection, parotidectomy, and radical neck dissection. (**C**) Large rotation flap used to close defect. Incision extends beneath the auricle down the posterior neck and curves onto the chest.

Nodular melanoma may also occur at this site. A wide excision must be planned along with a parotidectomy and radical neck dissection (**Fig. 10.7**). The optimal closure in terms of facilitation of follow-up is a skin graft. In a lesion such as the one in **Fig. 10.7**, the residual aesthetic deformity resulting from such a maneuver would be devastating. Wound coverage in this particular case was done using a large rotation flap. A permanent tarsorrhaphy was necessary to prevent ectropion.

The temporal region is somewhat intermediate between the cheek and the scalp proper in terms of lesion severity. **Figure 10.8** is the postoperative photograph of a patient with a Clark level II superficial spreading melanoma. He was managed by resection with a 1 cm margin and application of a split-thickness skin graft. Because thin melanomas rarely produce occult metastasis to regional nodes, neck dissection was not done.

A lesion greater than 0.76 mm in depth or deeper than Clark level II would require wide-field resection, parotidectomy, radical neck dissection, and a split-thickness skin graft for coverage.

◆ **Ear** The external ear is an uncommon site for melanoma, representing, according to Conley and Pack,[32] only 14.5% of melanotic lesions of the head and neck region. **Figure 10.9** illustrates the distribution of sites of origin in their series of 42 patients. The helix, being the most sun-exposed area, was the site with the highest incidence. One third of the patients presented with cervical lymphadenopathy, repre-

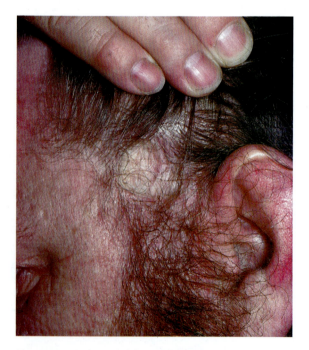

Fig. 10.8 Local excision for Clark level II melanoma of the temporal scalp utilizing a 1 cm margin. Defect covered with a split-thickness skin graft. Narrow margins are safe in "thin" melanomas.

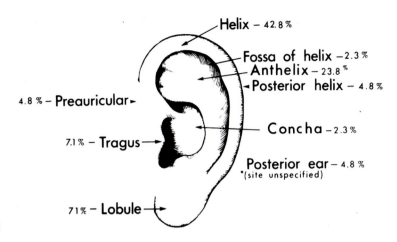

Fig. 10.9 Frequency distribution of malignant melanoma of the ear. (From Pack GT, Conley J, Orepeza R. Melanoma of the external ear. Arch Otolaryngol 1970;92:106. Reprinted with permission.)

senting the highest incidence of lymph node involvement among all head and neck melanomas, which illustrates the aggressiveness of these lesions. Because of the proximity of the external auditory canal to the parotid gland and the free access of lymphatics via the fissures of Santorini, there are excellent routes for the spread of auricular melanoma to the parotid salivary gland. Lymphatics of the auricle also drain to the lymph nodes in the occipital triangle.

The superficial lesions can be managed by wedge resection and primary approximation of the auricle. Resection of more extensive melanomas must include total auriculectomy (**Fig.**

10.10), total parotidectomy, radical neck dissection, and dissection of the occipital triangle. The incision for this resection is similar to that for temporal bone excision (see chapter 7, **Fig. 7.16**). Enough exposure can be achieved with a back cut through the parietal scalp to clearly visualize and dissect the occipital nodes. Smoothly curving incisions that interconnect at right angles permit adequate exposure and promote optimal hearing. If the lesion is stuck to the mastoid tip, a lateral temporal bone resection is advisable (see chapter 7).

One must not be lulled into a state of complacency by the seemingly innocuous appearance of a small auricular

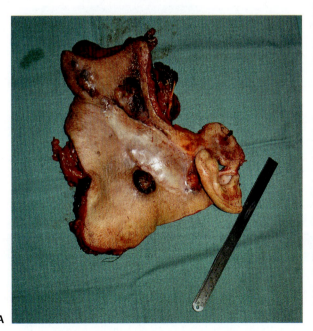

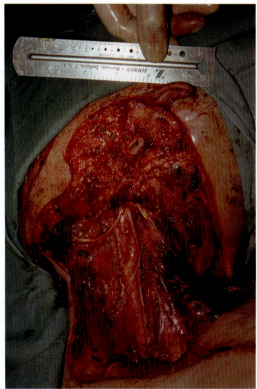

A   B

Fig. 10.10 Total auriculectomy for malignant melanoma. (**A**) Specimen following wide-field resection of nodular melanoma. (**B**) Defect following wide-field local resection and radical neck dissection.

melanoma. Most of these lesions are deeply invasive and characteristically metastasize early. The literature is replete with examples of inadequate, piecemeal, "whittling" operations in which the surgeon was always one step behind the progress of the disease. Faintheartedness in the management of this insidious lesion has devastating consequences for the patient.

Giant Hairy Nevus

Management of the giant hairy nevus is very problematic. The lesion usually presents at birth (**Fig. 10.11**). Even when the lesion is in as aesthetically unobtrusive area, as the one depicted in **Fig. 10.11**, excision will demand a reconstructive effort of considerable magnitude. Subsequent deformity of some degree is inevitable. The incidence of malignant melanoma developing in a congenital giant hairy nevus is between 15 and 42%.[56] Great care must be exercised in making a diagnosis of malignancy when biopsies are taken in the first year of life because at this stage there is a marked tendency for much cellular atypia to appear in these lesions despite an entirely benign clinical course.[56]

Excision is usually done in stages, beginning in the prepubertal years. An attempt is made to resect individual anatomical aesthetic facial units. The areas are usually resurfaced with split-thickness skin. A gap of 6 to 9 months is usual between stages. The region of the forehead together with the periorbital and cheek areas is one of the most challenging. For the lips, local flaps should be used if possible.

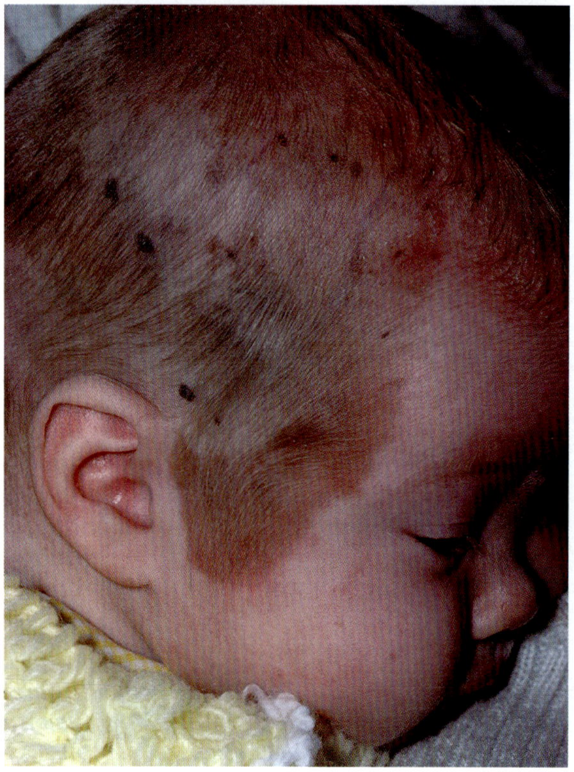

Tissue expanders are a great aid in providing cutaneous coverage in these cases.

The concern regarding the danger of incising into the substance of the lesion during the serial resection, with its possible potential for inducing malignancy, has been somewhat dispelled by the experience of Ariel.[56] He reports having had not one instance of melanoma appearing at the incision line when doing staged excisions.

There are some reports that if deep dermabrasion is done during the first year of life, most or all of the pigment can be eliminated.[57,58] Muti[59] describes a cryotherapeutic technique that unfortunately produces the same unaesthetic result as skin grafting. The problem of not being able to detect recurrent malignancies in their early stages when either dermabrasion or cryotherapy is used has yet to be resolved.

Mucosal Melanoma

Mucosal melanoma is extremely difficult to manage because of its silent nature until substantial size has been achieved and because of the relative obscurity of the sites in which it originates. A high index of suspicion must be maintained whenever a pigmented lesion in the mucosa of a Caucasian is apparent. Melanotic pigmentation in the nasal chambers is especially rare and is highly suspect (**Fig. 10.12**). The possibility of the upper aerodigestive mucosa as the site of deposition of secondary melanoma must always be entertained.

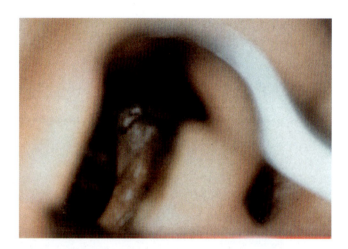

Fig. 10.12 Melanotic pigmentation in nasal cavity with malignant melanoma of nasal mucosa.

The treatment of choice is wide-field resection with, whenever possible, en bloc radical neck resection. In the region of the nasal cavities and the paranasal sinuses, en bloc dissection is impossible. However, Shah and Goldsmith[60] demonstrated no significant difference in survival between those patients in whom a neck dissection was done in continuity and those in whom it was discontinuous. The frequency of occult metastases (25% and higher) leaves little argument against prophylactic neck dissection in the clinically negative neck.

Fig. 10.11 Giant hairy nevus on scalp of newborn.

The resection must widely skirt the primary lesion. A margin double or triple that conventional for squamous cell tumor resection is required. Split-grafts or mucosal-to-skin closures are mainly impractical for the oral cavity lesions. Reconstruction with flaps is the only method whereby adequate function and acceptable cosmesis can be attained. (See also chapters 1 and 5).

The most unfortunate aspect of mucosal melanoma is the frequency of bloodborne metastases, even in the absence of lymphatic secondaries. Mucosal melanoma has the poorest prognosis of all melanomas of the head and neck. Oddly enough, although melanomas are generally relatively radioinsensitive, those involving mucosa are more responsive to gamma irradiation. However, the best opportunity for cure is early diagnosis and radical resection, including neck dissection.

The lesion of the patient in **Fig. 10.13** demonstrates the protean behavior of malignant melanoma even in a mucosal site. This melanoma had a desultory course for 40 years until it reached an accelerated growth phase and, despite two radical resections that spared only the eyes, continued to grow (**Fig. 10.14**) and finally extended intracranially (**Fig. 10.15**).

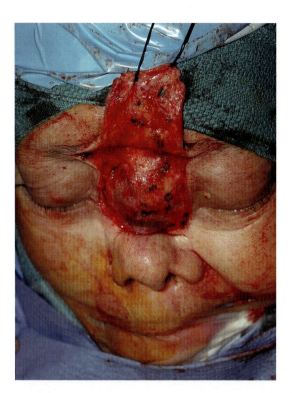

Fig. 10.14 Intraoperative view of extensive nasal mucosal melanoma that invaded both maxillary antra and ethmoid blocs.

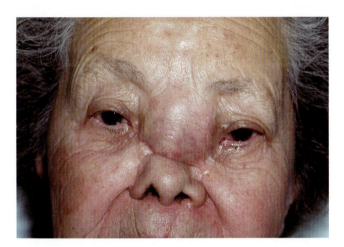

Fig. 10.13 Intranasal melanoma that was controlled with intermittent local resections for 40 years, until it reached an accelerated growth phase.

Adjunctive Therapy

There is a variable sensitivity of melanoma to irradiation therapy with mucosal melanoma being more sensitive than the cutaneous variety. In general, however, melanomas are radioresistant and offer marginal help in the treatment of malignant melanoma.

Few chemotherapeutic agents offer significant efficacy in melanoma. Dacarbazine (DTIC) is the only Food and Drug Administration (FDA)-approved drug for the treatment of metastatic melanoma. Clinical trials are proceeding with another drug that shows promise: temozolamide.

Interferon α 26 has been used with a modest improvement in some patients. Interferon gamma has not shown efficacy. Interleukins alone or in combination with lymphokine-activated killer cells have had some success but their use is fraught with multiple serious side effects, including death.

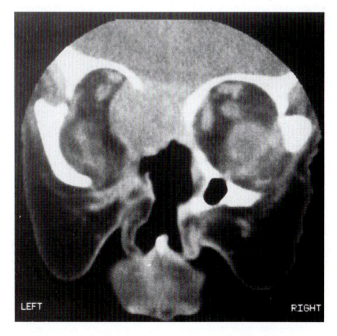

Fig. 10.15 Computed tomographic scan showing both intranasal and intracranial extent of lesion in patient from **Figs. 10.13** and **Fig. 10.14**.

Immunotherapy with vaccines has demonstrated up to 20% regression and even complete regression in some instances. One patient in our experience had a 2-year period of complete regression until she relapsed and succumbed to her disease.

Gene therapy is currently in its infancy but shows some promise either as primary treatment or as a biological sensitizer to other chemotherapeutic agents.

◆ Prognosis

Head and neck melanoma offers the best chance of survival of all the sites of melanoma. The one notable exception to this is when the lesion involves mucosa; for these cases, the 5-year survival rates are only 6 to 16%,[36] ranking second only to anorectic melanoma in bleakness.

In melanoma, 5-year survival rates are not as meaningful as 10-year rates. In fact, it is not uncommon to read reports of individuals surviving 20 to 25 years before succumbing to their disease. The overall survival rate in Conley's series of 200 patients was 35%.[37] However, it should also be noted that when local excision alone was required, the figure leapt to 62%. Local excision combined with elective neck dissection when the nodes were histologically negative yielded a 76.5% survival rate.

Catlin[61] reports a 5-year survival rate of 40.7% in his series of 179 patients, whereas Ballantyne[62] reports a 65.7% 5-year survival in a series of 405 patients. The presence of metastasis correspondingly diminishes the survival, as can be seen by referring to **Tables 10.4, 10.5, 10.6**, and **10.7**.

The superficiality of the tumor in terms of penetration is, as has been mentioned, of the utmost influence with regard to a favorable prognosis. Finally, those melanomas that have originated on sun-damaged skin also have a more favorable prognosis.

The heretofore-imponderable nature of the degree of host immunity plays a vital role. The dramatic effect of BCG administration[63] on the arrest and involution of often widespread melanoma has provided an exciting glimpse into what appears to be the hope of the future in the management of this devastating malignancy.

References

1. Conley J. Melanoma of the Head and Neck. New York: Georg Thieme Verlag, New; 1990:1
2. Ronsdahl MM, Cox IS. Biological aspects of pigment cells and malignant melanoma. In: Neoplasms of the Skin and Malignant Melanoma (Proceedings of the M.D. Anderson Hospital and Tumor Institute Symposium). Chicago: Year Book Medical Publications; 1976:251
3. Pack GT, Davis J. The pigmented mole. Postgrad Med 1960;27:370–382
4. Macneer G, Dasgupta T. Prognosis in malignant melanoma. Surgery 1964;56:512–518
5. Hugo NE. Malignant melanoma: brief review of current therapy. Mil Med 1969;134:52–56
6. Albert DM, Ryan IM, Borden EC. Metastatic ocular and cutaneous melanoma: a comparison of patient characteristics and prognosis. Arch Ophthalmol 1996;114:107–114
7. MacDonald EJ. Malignant melanoma in Connecticut. Special publication of the New York Academy of Sciences. 1948;IV:71–81
8. MacDonald EJ. Incidence and epidemiology of melanoma in Texas. In: Neoplasms of the Skin and Malignant Melanoma (Proceedings of the M.D. Anderson Hospital and Tumor Institute Symposium). Chicago: Year Book Medical Publications; 1976:279
9. Liu ZJ, Herlyn M. Melanoma. In: Bita VT, Hellman S, Rosenberg SA. eds. Cancer: Principles and Practice of Oncology. 7th ed. Philadelphia: Lippincott, Williams and Wilkins; 2005:chapter 38
10. Pack GT, Gerber DM, Scharnagle IM. End results of the treatment of malignant melanoma: a report of 1140 cases. Ann Surg 1952;136:905–911
11. White LP, Linden G, Breslow L, et al. Studies in melanoma: the effect of pregnancy on survival in human melanoma. JAMA 1961;177:235–238
12. George PA, Fortner JG, Pack CT. Melanoma with pregnancy. Cancer 1960;13:854–859
13. Miller TR, Pack GR. The familial aspect of malignant melanoma. Arch Dermatol 1962;86:35–39
14. Anderson DE. Clinical characteristics of the genetic variety of cutaneous melanoma in man. Cancer 1971;28:721–725
15. Bahn AK, Rosenwaike I, Hermann J, et al. Melanoma after exposure to PCBs [letter]. N Engl J Med 1976;295:450
16. Lawrence C. PCB and melanoma (reply to previous letter). N Engl J Med 1977;296:108
17. Albert DM, Puliafito CA. Choroidal melanoma: possible exposure to industrial toxin [letter]. N Engl J Med 1977;296:634–635
18. Houten L. Increased risk of cancer among workers in metal-related occupations [abstract]. Public Health Rep 1976;91:569
19. Morton WE, Start CF. Epidemiologic clues of the cause of melanoma. West J Med 1979;131:263–269
20. Rigel DS. Epidemiology and prognostic factors in malignant melanoma. Ann Plast Surg 1992;28:7–8
21. Rigel DS, Carucci JA. Malignant melanoma: prevention, early detection, and treatment in the 21st century. CA Cancer J Clin 2000;50:215–240
22. Greene MH. The genetics of hereditary melanoma and nevi: 1998 update. Cancer 1999; 86(11, Suppl)2464–2477
23. Currie GA. Cancer and the Immune Response. Chicago: Year Book Medical Publishers (Oulu); 1974:25
24. Clark WH Jr, Fran L, Bernardino FA, et al. The histogenesis and biologic behavior of primary human malignant melanoma of the skin. Cancer Res 1969;29:705–727
25. Batsakis JG. Tumors of the Head and Neck. Baltimore: Williams and Wilkins; 1974:332
26. Goldsmith H. Melanoma. In: Practice of Surgery. Hagerstown, MD: Harper & Row; 1978:1–26
27. Smith JL. Neoplasms of skin and malignant melanoma. In: Histopathology and Biologic Behavior of Malignant Melanoma (Proceedings of the M.D. Anderson Hospital and Tumor Institute Symposium). Chicago: Year Book Medical Publications; 1976:293
28. Fortner JG, Woodruff J, Schottenfield D, et al. Biostatistical basis of elective node dissection for melanoma. Ann Surg 1977;186:101–103
29. Gupta TK. Results of treatment of 269 patients with primary cutaneous melanoma: a five-year prospective study. Ann Surg 1977;186:201–209
30. Wanebo HJ, Woodruff J, Fortner JG. Malignant melanoma of the extremities: a clinicopathologic study using levels of invasion (microstage). Cancer 1975;35:666–6761
31. Gumport SL, Harris MN. Melanoma of the skin. In: Andrade R, Gumport SL, Popkin GL, et al, eds. Cancer of the Skin. Vol 2. Philadelphia: WB Saunders; 1976:950
32. Conley JJ, Pack CT. Melanoma of the head and neck. Surg Gynecol Obstet 1963;116:15–18
33. Breslow A, Macht SD. Evaluation of prognosis in stage I cutaneous melanoma. Plast Reconstr Surg 1978;61:342–346
34. Breslow A. Thickness, cross-sectional area and depth of invasion in the prognosis of cutaneous melanoma. Ann Surg 1970;172:902–908
35. Medina J. Malignant melanoma. In: Meyers E, Suen J, eds. Cancer of the Head and Neck. 3rd ed. Philadelphia: WB Saunders; 1996:160–183

36. Hormia M, Vuori EE. Mucosal melanoma of the head and neck. J Laryngol Otol 1969;83:349–359

37. Conley J. Concepts in Head and Neck Surgery. New York: Grune & Stratton; 1970:277

38. Pack GT, Conley J, Oropeza R. Melanoma of the external ear. Arch Otolaryngol 1970;92:106–113

39. Soyer HP, Kenet RO, Wolf IH, et al. Clinicopathalogical correlation of pigmented skin lesions using dermoscopy. Eur J Dermatol 2000;10:22–28

40. Stanganelli I, Seidenari S, Serafini M, et al. Diagnosis of skin lesions by epiluminescence microscopy: determination of accuracy improvement in a nationwide training programme for practical dermatologists. Public Health 1999;113:237–242

41. Rigel DS. Epiluminescence microscopy in clinical diagnosis of pigmented skin lesions. Lancet 1997;349:1566–1567

42. Storm FK, Eilber FR, Morton DL, et al. Malignant melanoma of the head and neck. Head Neck Surg 1978;1:123–128

43. Southwick HW, Slaughter DP, Hinkamp JF, et al. The role of radical neck dissection in malignant melanoma. Arch Surg 1962;85:63–69

44. Simons JN. Malignant melanoma of the head and neck. Am J Surg 1968;116:494–498

45. Chaudhry AP, Hampel A, Gorlin RJ. Primary malignant melanoma of the oral cavity: a review of 105 cases. Cancer 1958;11:923–928

46. Allen AC. The Skin. 2nd ed. St Louis: CV Mosby; 1967:967

47. Manolidis S, Donald PJ. Malignant mucosal melanoma of the head and neck: review of the literature and report of 14 patients. Cancer 1997;80:1373–1386

48. Morton DL, Wen DR, Cochran AJ. Management of early-stage melanoma by intraoperative mapping and selective lymphadenectomy: an alternative to routine elective lymphadenectomy or "watch and wait." Surg Oncol Clin N Am 1992;1:247–259

49. Van der Veen H, Hoekstra OS, Paul MA, et al. Gamma probe-guided sentinel lymph node biopsy to select patients for lymphadenectomy. Br J Surg 1994;81:1769–1770

50. Ali-Salaam P, Ariyan S. Lymphatic Mapping and Sentinel Lymph Node Biopsies. Clinics in Plastic Surgery 27.3. Philadelphia: WB Saunders; 2000:421–429

51. O'Brien C. Melanoma of the Head and Neck. The Eugene N. Myers International Lecture on Head and Neck Cancer. AAO-HNSF Annual Meeting. Los Angeles, California. Sept. 27, 2005

52. Bernstein L, Donald PJ, Chole RA. Prophylactic radical neck dissection in melanoma of the face and scalp. In: Snow JB, ed. Controversies in Otolaryngology. Philadelphia: WB Saunders; 1980:239

53. Sisson GA, McMahan JT. Prophylactic radical neck dissection for melanoma may not be indicated. In: Snow JB, ed. Controversies in Otolaryngology. Philadelphia: WB Saunders; 1980:245

54. Veronesi U, Adomus DC, Bandiers DC, et al. Inefficacy of immediate node dissection in stage I melanoma of the limbs. N Engl J Med 1977;297:627–630

55. Ballantyne AJ. Malignant melanoma of the head and neck region. In: Neoplasms of the Skin and Malignant Melanoma (Proceedings of the M.D. Anderson Hospital and Tumor Institute Symposium). Chicago: Year Book Medical Publications; 1976:345

56. Ariel IM. Moles and malignant melanoma of the preadolescent child. In: Malignant Melanoma. New York: Appleton-Century-Crofts; 1981:87

57. Johnson H. Permanent removal of pigmentation from giant hairy nevi by dermabrasion in early life. Br J Plast Surg 1977;30:321–323

58. Johnson H. A registry of results obtained by the abrasion of giant nevi in early infancy. Plast Reconstr Surg 1981;67:258

59. Muti E. Cryotherapy in the treatment of some facial nevi. Ann Plast Surg 1982;9:167–171

60. Shah JP, Goldsmith HS. Dissection for malignant melanoma. Cancer 1970;26:610–6145

61. Catlin D. Cutaneous melanoma of the head and neck. Am J Surg 1966;112:512–521

62. Ballantyne AJ. Malignant melanoma of the skin of the head and neck: an analysis of 405 cases. Am J Surg 1970;120:425–431

63. Eilber FR, Townsend CM Jr, Martin DL. Results of BCG adjuvant immunotherapy for melanoma of the head and neck. Am J Surg 1976;132:476–479

11

Pediatric Malignancies

Paul J. Donald

Malignancies in the pediatric age group are, fortunately, quite rare. Approximately 5% of all malignant tumors in childhood arise in the head and neck. The psychological impact of a child with cancer is devastating for parents and physician alike. One of the major difficulties in formulating a plan of attack on these tumors is the general lack of experience in the management of pediatric cancer by any one surgeon or group. In addition, unlike adult cancers, which are nearly always of epithelial origin, the vast majority of pediatric neoplasms are of mesodermal derivation, with those of epithelial origin being distinctly rare.

Malignant neoplasms are second only to accidents as a cause of mortality in children, accounting for the deaths of seven to eight per 100,000 children between the ages of 1 and 14. Head and neck malignancies make up ~27% of this group.[1,2] In the United States approximately one in 300 children will contract cancer in the first 20 years of their life.[3] By far the largest group is represented by the lymphomas, especially Hodgkin disease and lymphosarcoma.[4] Rhabdomyosarcoma is the next most common, being the most common soft tissue sarcoma and occurring with the highest frequency in the head and neck.[5,6] Fibrosarcoma, neurosarcoma, thyroid malignancy, and salivary gland cancer, in that order, are the next most frequent. The presenting symptom in 70% of all head and neck malignancies in children is a mass in the neck. **Table 11.1** illustrates the common malignant tumors

Table 11.1 Summary Data from Six Large Series of Pediatric Head and Neck Malignancies

Type	Children's Hospital Medical Center, Cincinnati (1971–1982)	Jaffe & Jaffe	Sutow	Cunningham et al	Robinson et al	Rapidis et al	Total
Hodgkin lymphoma	16	46	31	85	31	82	291 (29%)
Non-Hodgkin lymphoma	10	51	22	58	23	78	242 (24%)
Rhabdomyosarcoma	13	20	35	31	26	68	193 (19%)
Other soft-tissue sarcoma	2	15	11	8	5	31	72 (7%)
Osteogenic sarcoma	2	2	1	1			6 (0.5%)
Ewing sarcoma	1	3	4	2			10 (1%)
Salivary gland malignancy	1	2	3	6		1	13 (1%)
Thyroid malignancy	1	9	15	24	1	12	62 (6%)
Squamous call carcinoma*	5	7	7**	12	1	18	50 (5%)
Neuroblastoma	1	9	3	12	14	18	57 (6%)
Malignant melanoma		4	3				7 (1%)
Malignant teratoma		1	2	2			5 (0.5%)
Total	52	169	137	241	101	308	1008

*Includes transitional cell tumors and all nasopharyngeal carcinomas.

**Includes three basal cell carcinomas.

encountered in the head and neck in the pediatric age group. As can be seen in squamous cell carcinoma, the commonest head and neck neoplasm in adults is seen in only 5% of children with malignancies.

◆ Lymphoma

Lymphomas of the entire body present most commonly with a lump in the neck. In the M.D. Anderson series, 84% of children with Hodgkin disease had their primary presentation in the cervical nodes.[2] This is in general agreement with other series.[7,8] Much confusion has occurred over the years regarding the classification of lymphomas. Most clinicians divide these diseases into Hodgkin and non-Hodgkin lymphoma based on their cellular composition and the natural history of the disease.[9] The early classification system of non-Hodgkin lymphoma by Rappaport[10] was simple but did not relate itself well to the cellular type of origin of these neoplasms. Modern cytological techniques have revised the classification systems into two broad categories; B cell and T cell types, based upon the cell of origin. **Table 11.2** depicts the original Rappaport classification adopted in 1966.[10,11] **Table 11.3** is the Lukes-Collins classification adopted in 1992.[12,13] **Table 11.4** is the revised European-American lymphoma (REAL) system inaugurated in 1994.[14,15] None of these currently existing systems appears to be entirely satisfactory, and there is currently a revision of the REAL and a new World Health Organization (WHO) classification in progress.[14]

Table 11.2 The Rappaport Classification of the Non-Hodgkin Lymphomas (1966)

	Malignant Lymphoma
Growth Pattern	• Nodular • Diffuse (follicular)
Cell Type	• Lymphatic, well differentiated • Lymphocytic, poorly differentiated • Mixed cell (histiocytic-lymphocytic) • Histiocytic • Undifferentiated

Source: Rappaport H. Tumors of the Hematopoietic System. Washington, DC: Armed Forces Institute of Pathology; 1966.

A thorough dissertation of these complex diseases is beyond the scope of this treatise. The reader is directed to the textbook by Barnes,[14] which outlines the histopathological characteristic of each type, including the immunophenotype and genotype/karyotype of each specific tumor.

Hodgkin Disease

In children, lymphoma of the head and neck is the commonest malignancy seen, making up 40% of all cases of head and neck malignancy.[16] Non-Hodgkin lymphoma makes up roughly two thirds of all these lesions.[17] Hodgkin disease is seen four times more commonly in males than in females.[17]

Table 11.3 Lukes-Collins Revised Classification of Undefined Cell and Lymphoid Neoplasms (1992)

Undefined cell neoplasms
  Acute undefined leukemia
Lymphoid neoplasms
  T cell neoplasms
    T cell acute lymphocytic leukemia
    Adult T cell leukemia
    Small T cell neoplasms, including chronic lymphocytic leukemia T
    Convoluted T-lymphoma/lymphoblastic (thymic lymphoma)
    Immunoblastic T cell lymphoma, including peripheral T cell lymphomas
    Other T cell neoplasms, including lymphoepithelioid
      T-lymphocytic lymphoma (Lennert lymphoma),
      T-zone lymphoma
    Cerebriform T cell lymphoma (mycosis fungoides and Sezary syndrome)
    Extranodal T lymphomas
  B cell neoplasms
    B cell acute lymphocytic leukemias, including B cell precursor acute leukemia
    Prolymphocytic leukemia
    Small B cell lymphoid neoplasms, including chronic lymphocytic leukemia
    B cell neoplasms with plasmacytic differentiation, including plasmacytoid lymphocytic lymphoma and multiple myeloma
    Hairy cell leukemia (leukemic reticuloendotheliosis)
    Mantle zone lymphomas
    Marginal zone lymphomas
    Parafollicular (monocytoid) B cell lymphomas
    Follicular center cell lymphomas, including Burkitt lymphoma and non-Burkitt types
  Immunoblastic lymphoma of B cells
  Large B cell lymphomas

Source: Data from Jaffe BF. Neck masses and malignant tumors of the head and neck. In: Ferguson CF, Kendig EL Jr, eds. Disorders of the Respiratory Tract in Children. Vol 2: Pediatric Otolaryngology. Philadelphia: WB Saunders; 1972:1135.

The incidence in females appears to increase with age. Approximately 46% of cases are seen between the ages of 3 and 10 and another 30% between the ages of 10 and 14. The characteristic histological pattern is the appearance of the pathognomonic Reed-Sternberg cell, a polymorphous large cell with multiple nuclei, each with an eosinophilic nucleolus and a perinuclear halo. There are variable amounts of lymphocytes, plasma cells, and eosinophils. The sclerosing variety has thick hyaline bands containing scant amounts of collagen dividing the tumor into lobules. This latter variant makes up the majority of lymphomas in all age groups in the United States and ~38% of these diseases in children. Those with a lymphocytic infiltrate as the predominant cell type have the best prognosis.

Around 80 to 90% of Hodgkin lymphoma cases present as a lump in the upper neck. The masses are rubbery in consistency, nontender, and often matted together. Relapsing fevers,

Table 11.4 Revised European-American Lymphoma (REAL) Classification (1994)

B cell Neoplasms
1. Precursor B cell neoplasm: precursor B-lymphoblastic leukemia/lymphoma
2. Peripheral B cell neoplasms
    1. B cell chronic lymphocytic leukemia/prolymphocytic leukemia/small lymphocytic lymphoma
    2. Lymphoplasmacytoid lymphoma/immunocytoma
    3. Mantle cell lymphoma
    4. Follicle center lymphoma, follicular
       Provisional cytological grades: I (small cell), II (mixed small and large cell), III (large cell)
    5. Marginal zone B cell lymphoma
       Extranodal (Malt-type ± villous lymphocytes)
       Provisional subtype: Nodal (± monocytoid B cells)
    6. Provisional entity: splenic marginal zone lymphoma (± villous lymphocytes)
    7. Hairy cell leukemia
    8. Plasmacytoma/plasma cell myeloma
    9. Diffuse large-B cell lymphoma[a]
       Subtype: Primary mediastinal (thymic) B cell lymphoma
    10. Burkitt lymphoma
    11. Provisional entity: high-grade B cell lymphoma, Burkitt-like[a]

T cell and Putative NK-cell Neoplasms
1. Precursor T cell neoplasm: precursor T-lymphoblastic lymphoma/leukemia
2. Peripheral T cell and NK-cell neoplasms
    1. T cell chronic lymphocytic leukemia/polymphorphocytic leukemia
    2. Large granular lymphocyte leukemia (LGL)
       T cell type
       NK-cell type
    3. Mycosis fungoides/Sezary syndrome
    4. Peripheral T cell lymphomas, unspecified[a]
    5. Angioimmunoblastic T cell lymphoma (AILD)
    6. Angiocentric lymphoma
    7. Intestinal T cell lymphoma (± enteropathy associated)
    8. Adult T cell lymphoma/leukemia (ATL/L)
    9. Anaplastic large-cell lymphoma (ALCL), CD30+, T- and null-cell types
    10. Provisional entity: anaplastic large-cell lymphoma, Hodgkin-like

Hodgkin Disease
 I. Lymphocyte predominance
 II. Nodular sclerosis
 III. Mixed cellularity
 IV. Lymphocyte depletion
 V. Provisional entity: lymphocyte-rich classic HD

[a]These categories are thought likely to include more than one disease entity.

Abbreviations: HD, ??; NK, ??.

Source: Harris NL, Jaffe ES, Stein H, et al. A revised European-American classification of lymphoid neoplasms: a proposal from the International Lymphoma Study Group. Blood 1994;84:1361–1392.

occurring in the evening and late afternoon, are common. Weight loss, night sweats, and pruritus, especially, after a bath or shower, are also seen. Severe itching associated with multiple excoriations is associated with a poor prognosis.[18] The Ann Arbor classification is the most frequently used staging system (**Table 11.5**).[19] The staging is further stratified according to the presence or absence of systemic symptoms. Subtype A is assigned when the patient does not have systemic symptoms, and subtype B when these symptoms are manifest. The prognosis in subtype A is much better than in subtype B. Supraclavicular nodal involvement is commonly associated with disease below the clavicles. Right-sided supraclavicular adenopathy is most often associated with mediastinal involvement and left sided with abdominal disease. Most often the regional adenopathy is the only site of the disease.

Table 11.5 Staging in Hodgkin Disease (Ann Arbor)

Stage	Description
I	Involvement of a single lymph node region
IE	Involvement of a single extralymphatic organ
II	Involvement of two or more lymph node regions on the same side of the diaphragm
IIE	Localized involvement of extralymphatic organ or site and of one or more lymph node regions on the same side of the diaphragm
III	Involvement of lymph node regions on both sides of the diaphragm
IIIE	Involvement of lymph node regions on both sides of the diaphragm with localized involvement of extralymphatic organ or site
IIIS	As in III, with involvement of spleen
IIISE	As in III, with involvement of spleen and extralymphatic organ or site
IV	Diffuse or disseminated involvement of one or more extralymphatic organs or tissues, with or without associated lymph node enlargement

The treatment of Hodgkin disease is dependent on whether the disease is limited to the neck or has spread to the chest or below the diaphragm. Cervical disease is usually treated by radiation therapy alone and higher stages by a combination of chemotherapy and irradiation. The only role for surgery is in taking an open biopsy.

Non-Hodgkin Lymphoma

Cotton et al[3] divides childhood non-Hodgkin lymphoma into three basic types:

1. Malignant lymphoma lymphoblastic type: 30 to 50% of cases
2. Malignant lymphoma undifferentiated (Burkitt and non-Burkitt lymphoma): 40 to 50% of cases
3. Larger cell lymphomas: 15 to 20% of cases

Some authorities consider non-Hodgkin lymphoma as a spectrum of disease containing both lymphoma and acute lymphoblastic leukemia.[3] This is supported by the fact that bone marrow involvement with lymphoma is not uncommonly seen in lymphoma, and massive adenopathy is often the presenting feature of lymphoblastic leukemia. In contrast to Hodgkin disease, lymphoma is generally a systemic condition at the time of presentation. Lymphoma is usually found in the 7- to 10-year-old age group with a male to female predominance of 3:1.

Undifferentiated lymphomas have a predilection for the abdominal cavity and gastrointestinal tract as well as the Waldeyer ring. Although lymphoma most commonly presents as a lump in the neck it may be seen in extranodal locations in the head and neck.

In recent times the prognosis for children with lymphoma treated with multiple drug therapy has vastly improved. Children with early stage disease can anticipate a 90% 5-year survival and in the advanced stage a 70% survival rate. The mainstay of treatment is multiple drug chemotherapy. As many as 10 different agents may be given in some protocols to achieve a cure. For lymphoblastic lymphomas either cyclophosphamide, doxorubicin, Oncovin, prednisone (CHOP) or cyclophosphamide, Oncovin, methotrexate and prednisone (COMP) regimens have about equal efficacy. Salvage with other agents and the addition to the original protocols of such agents as anthracyclines, cytosine arabinosides, and epipodophyllotoxins add greatly to the long-term prognosis.[17]

The tonsil is the commonest site, with the disease presenting as a nontender, nonulcerating enlargement. The nasopharynx, salivary glands, lingual tonsils of the tongue, maxilla, and mandible are less commonly involved. The maxilla and maxillary sinuses are more commonly involved than the mandible.[20] Some may also arise in the skin of the face and scalp.[4]

One of the tragedies of these tumors is the risk of leukemic transformation, which may occur in as many as 50% of those with head and neck involvement.

Burkitt lymphoma, an undifferentiated lymphoma, was initially thought to be an endemic disease exclusively afflicting African children.[21] Since it was first identified, however, its worldwide distribution has become apparent.[22] In Africa Burkitt lymphoma is most often found in the head and neck, but the American variety is most usually seen in the abdomen. The tumor characteristically afflicts the mandible and maxilla, and when untreated rapidly progresses to a generalized, fatal disease. It is curious that, although cervical adenopathy is uncommon, abdominal nodes are present in 80% of cases.[23] Furthermore, the jaws are usually the only bones affected. The tumor occurs exclusively between the ages of 2 and 14, with the peak age being 5 and 6 years. In Uganda, Burkitt tumor accounts for 50% of all childhood malignancies and in Kenya 40%.[24] In children outside Africa the jaws are much less affected, and the disease itself is rare.

The lesion begins in the medullary cavity of the jaw and progresses to the alveolar bone, where the deciduous teeth become loosened and extrude. Maxillary alveolar involvement rapidly spreads into the adjacent antrum and then into the ethmoid and sphenoid sinuses and the orbit, producing proptosis.[25] Involvement of the abdominal viscera, retroperitoneal soft tissues, central nervous system, and salivary and thyroid glands rapidly follows, producing a fatal course in untreated cases.[26]

For Burkitt lymphoma cyclophosphamide was the mainstay of treatment and resulted in an initial 80% response rate. Intrathecal methotrexate is added for patients with involvement of the head and neck. For relapses, the addition of vincristine, with methotrexate or cytarabine, produces better responses. However, relapses are difficult to manage, with bone marrow transplantation probably being the only hope for a permanent cure. The prognosis in large cell lymphoma with CHOP or COMP therapy is excellent, with an 85% survival rate. The addition of irradiation therapy to these protocols does little to improve the results in any of the cell types.

◆ Rhabdomyosarcoma

This tumor is the most common nonlymphomatous malignancy of the head and neck in children. It is primarily a disease of the first decade of life.[27,28] Thirty-eight percent of all rhabdomyosarcomas occur in the head and neck.[3] Of 166 patients with rhabdomyosarcoma of the head and neck studied by Dito and Batsakis,[29] 129 (77.7%) were between the ages of 1 and 12. Five of these patients had their tumors at birth. The peak incident is age 4.[30] As Batsakis[28] eloquently points out, rhabdomyosarcomas are malignant neoplasms that recapitulate the embryological development of the myocyte. The progression of the primitive anlage, a small round cell, through the stages of a spindle cell and finally the characteristic multinucleated, straplike myocyte, complete with its typical cross-striations, is seen in the various forms of the tumor. Neoplasms, whose cell of predominance is of the more primitive variety, lack the cross-striations and in the past were often designated as other than rhabdomyosarcoma. Presently, the cellular types are classified as pleomorphic, embryonal, or alveolar, with occasionally the designation of a subclass; botryoid.

The pleomorphic variety demonstrates some relatively normal-appearing myocytes, others that appear undifferentiated although retaining their cross-striations, and a further type of a somewhat more undifferentiated variety but still with striations. The embryonal type possesses cells that are more characteristics of those of the developing muscle cell in the early embryonic period. At the 7- to 10-week stage, round and spindle-shaped cells of varying size predominate. Their dearth of cytoplasm has often led to their being confused with lymphomas. The alveolar type may be simply a variant of the embryonic tumor. It is characterized by round cells aligned in an acinar fashion, resembling a glandular structure. Although spaces between the cells occur near the lumen of the pseudogland, cytoplasmic continuity is maintained at the periphery. The botryoid subclassification is used mainly to describe the grapelike exuberant quality characteristic of some of these tumors. Botryoid tumors always originate on a mucosal surface but have no pathognomonic histological pattern. Because the appellation serves only to describe gross appearance, the utility of the term is questionable. Most botryoid rhabdomyosarcomas are of the embryonal type histologically. The commonest form in children is the embryonal type.

Next to the orbit and eyelid, the commonest site of occurrence of rhabdomyosarcoma in the pediatric age group

Table 11.6 Incidence of Rhabdomyosarcoma

Author(s)							
Site	Jaffe	Batsakis[28]	Healy	Schuller et al	Sutow and Montague	Heyn et al	Total
Orbit and eyelid	2	54	2	8	9	10	85
Ear and temporal bone	4	19	3	2	8	7	43
Cervical facial soft tissue	3	44	5	7	8	4	71
Oral cavity	2	27	—	3	1	8	41
Oropharynx	1	3	—	5	—	—	9
Nasopharynx	6	16	1	3	8	3	37
Hypopharynx	—	3	—	3	1	2	9
Nose and sinuses	1	3	1	2	3	—	10
Total							305

is the facial soft tissue. The next most frequent site is the nasopharynx (**Table 11.6**). Rhabdomyosarcoma can occur anywhere in the head and neck as a painless mass until bone erosion or neural invasion ensues. This is especially true of primaries in facial soft tissue (**Fig. 11.1**). Sarcomas in the ear often present as a polyp that causes bloody otorrhea (**Fig. 11.2**). Those in the orbit cause proptosis or appear as fungating masses. Laryngeal and hypopharyngeal lesions present

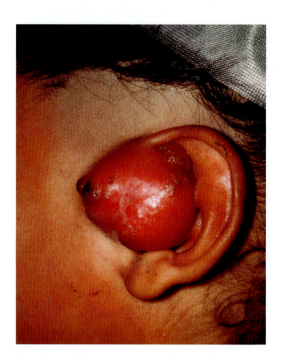

Fig. 11.2 Rhabdomyosarcoma of external auditory canal in a young girl.

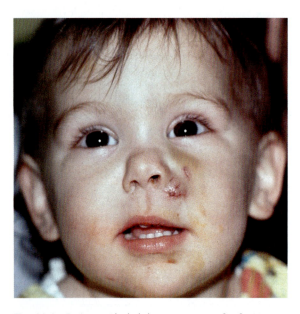

Fig. 11.1 Patient with rhabdomyosarcoma of soft tissue area adjacent to nose.

with dysphagia and hoarseness or airway compromise. Some tumors arising in the nasopharynx or nose and paranasal sinuses are so large that their site of origin is indeterminate. One such patient in our own experience presented with a massive neoplasm that filled the nasal cavities, nasopharynx, and maxillary and ethmoid sinuses, and encroached on the middle cranial fossa (**Fig. 11.3 and Fig. 11.4**). The tumors are rapidly growing, and medical attention is nearly always sought within 6 months and usually before 2 months.[26]

Metastasis to regional lymph nodes is variably reported. Lawrence et al[31] reported lymph node involvement in only three out of 96 head and neck sarcomas. Donaldson et al,[32] on the other hand, report an incidence of 26% in a group of 19 patients. In Schuller et al's series, only three of 35 cases had nodal disease.[33] All reports agree in one respect and that is that lymphatic metastases from orbital rhabdomyosarcomas are extremely rare.[31–34] This illustrates the ability of the orbit to contain the tumor within its bony confines, which is likely responsible for its good prognosis relative to other sites.

Unfortunately, the favorable prognosis of orbital rhabdomyosarcoma is not reflected by these tumors in the rest of the head and neck. The head and neck area in general has the worst prognosis of all the regions in the body.[34] With the current Intergroup Rhabdomyosarcoma Study (IRS) protocol the prognosis for pediatric patients with rhabdomyosarcoma has steadily improved. The first protocol that began in 1972 has

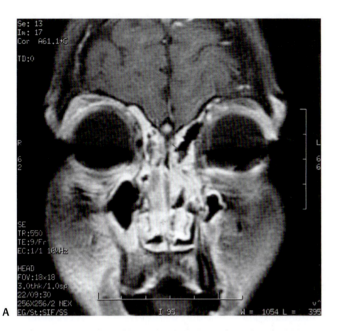

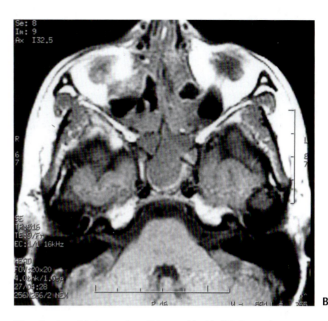

Fig. 11.3 Magnetic resonance imaging of rhabdomyosarcoma of the ethmoid and sphenoid sinuses in a 17-year-old girl. (**A**) Coronal cut showing invasion of tumor into the nasal space and orbit and proximity to the anterior cranial fossa. (**B**) Axial projection illustrating invasion into the sphenoid sinus and proximity to both orbital apices and cavernous sinuses.

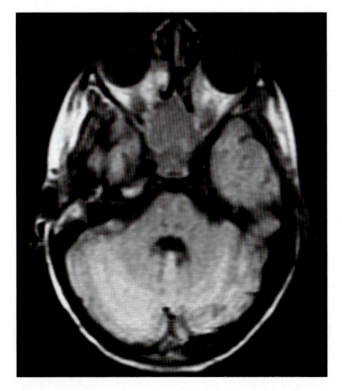

Fig. 11.4 Magnetic resonance imaging of an 8-year-old boy with a massive rhabdomyosarcoma of the ethmoid and sphenoid sinuses as well as the nasopharynx. Both orbital apices are invaded. Patient is alive and free of disease 7 years posttreatment on the Intergroup Rhabdomyosarcoma Study IV protocol.

evolved as new more effective agents have been introduced. Since 1991 IRS IV has been utilized. The prognosis of the disease seems to be related to the stage of the disease. Unlike the tumor, nodes, metastasis (TNM) system of tumor staging that we all have become accustomed to, the system used to classify rhabdomyosarcomas, devised by the IRS[35] is based on a consideration of past surgical therapy as well as extent of disease. **Table 11.7** is an abbreviation of the currently employed IRS clinical staging system.[36] A detailed analysis of this classification reveals many flaws and ambiguities. An

Table 11.7 Intergroup Rhabdomyosarcoma Study Grouping in Rhabdomyosarcoma

Stage	Description
IA	Localized disease, completely resected, confined to site of origin
IB	Localized disease, completely resected, beyond site of origin
IIA	Localized, grossly resected but positive margins
IIB	Regional disease, primary and involved lymph nodes resected
IIC	Regional disease, primary and involved lymph nodes resected with positive margins
IIIA	Local or regional disease, biopsy only
IIIB	Local or regional disease, more than 50% of primary tumor bulk resected
IV	Distant metastases found to be present at diagnosis

Source: Data from Maurer HM, et al. The Intergroup Rhabdomyosarcoma Study—I: a final report. Cancer 1988;61:209.

alternative system based on the TNM classification (**Table 11.8**) is much more helpful for end results reporting. The final designation is often based on the pathologist's findings following histological examination of the specimen.

Table 11.8 Tumor, Nodes, Metastasis (TNM) Pretreatment Staging for Rhabdomyosarcoma

Stage	Sites	T	Size	N	M
1	Orbit	T1 or T2	a or b	N0 or N1 or N2	M0
	Head and Neck (excluding parameningeal)				
	Genitourinary-nonbladder/nonprostate				
2	Bladder/prostate	T1 or T2	a	N0 or Nx	M0
	Extremity				
	Cranial parameningeal				
	Other				
3	Bladder/prostate	T1 or T2	a	N1	
	Extremity		b	N0 or N1	M0
	Cranial parameningeal			Nx	
	Other				
4	All	T1 or T2	a or b	N0 or N1	M1

T4: confined to anatomical site of origin
    a: less than 5 cm in diameter
    b: greater than 5 cm in diameter
T2: extension and/or fixation to surrounding tissue
    a: less than 5 cm in diameter
    b: greater than 5 cm in diameter
N0: regional lymph nodes not clinically involved
N1: regional lymph nodes clinically involved by tumor
Nx: clinical status of regional lymph nodes unknown
M0: no distant metastases
M1: metastases present

Treatment

As has been mentioned, since 1972, treatment of rhabdomyosarcoma in children has undergone considerable evolution. Formerly, these lesions were managed with either surgery or radiation therapy. Cotton et al[3] provide a concise historical review of this method of management. Johnson[37] quotes a study done in 1965, which reviewed the preceding 5 years' experience with surgical management of 64 cases of rhabdomyosarcoma of all sites. There were 24 sites in which complete tumor extirpation had been performed, with only five of the patients surviving 5 years. These were the only survivors in the entire group of 64; yielding a meager 7.8% overall survival rate. Johnson further reviewed several series of cases in which either irradiation or surgery alone was the method of treatment. The overall survival rate in his group was ~12%.

Complete excision of the neoplasms is often exceptionally difficult not only because of the invasive nature of the cancer but also because of the inherent reluctance on the part of the patient's parents, the pediatrician, and the surgeon to perform mutilating surgery on a child. The difficulty in completely encompassing these tumors surgically is reflected in Donaldson's experience, in which only three of 19 resections resulted in a total excision with tumor-free margins.[32]

The evolution of triple therapy, combining surgery with irradiation and chemotherapy, has produced a heartening improvement in prolonged survival rates in these children.[38] In Donaldson's series of 16 incomplete excisions out of 19 resections, 74% of the children were alive without evidence of disease at 2 years.[32] With aggressive triple therapy Ghavimi et al[39] reported a 67% actuarial 3-year survival rate in six patients with head and neck lesions. For all sites throughout the body they had a 100% 3-year survival rate for the 200 patients who had group I and group II disease. Wilbur et al[40] reported a series of 11 selected cases of inoperable nasopharyngeal and oropharyngeal tumors that were treated with radiation therapy and chemotherapy alone. At the time of treatment none had proved distant metastatic disease. Cervical nodes were involved in four patients. A regimen of 5000 to 6500 rads of Co60 irradiation was given to most patients. A combination of vincristine, actinomycin D, and cyclophosphamide was given during the radiotherapy in a maintenance schedule as outlined in **Table 11.9**. After 2 years, the chemotherapy was discontinued. Of the 11 children, nine were alive and free of disease at 28 to 62 months from the onset of therapy, with a median disease-free survival time of 41 months.

Table 11.9 Vincristine, Dactinomycin, and Cyclophosphamide Combination Chemotherapy for Rhabdomyosarcoma

Drug	Dosage
Vincristine	2 mg/m^2 IV weekly × 12 weeks (max. 2 mg)
Actinomycin D	0.075 mg/kg/course IV over 5–8 days (max. 0.5 mg/kg/day) every 3 months × five courses
Cyclophosphamide	2.5 mg/kg/day PO for 2 years

Source: Wilbur JR, Sutow WW, Sullivan MP. The changing treatment of rhabdomyosarcoma in children, particularly in treatment for inoperable rhabdomyosarcoma of the nasopharynx and oropharynx. In: MD Anderson Hospital: Neoplasia of the Head and Neck. Chicago: Year Book Medical Publications; 1974:281.

The present method of management of these lesions involves resection of all disease, if possible, without creating a huge defect that aesthetically and functionally severely compromises the patient. The recent advances in head and neck reconstructive surgery, especially the use of musculocutaneous and free flaps, have permitted wider-field resections that will enable the surgeon to do more adequate cancer surgery without crippling the patient. If there is nodal involvement, a radical neck dissection is done.[41] Prophylactic neck dissections are not done because the incidence of cervical nodal involvement is only 7%.[42] It is apparent, however, that chemotherapy and irradiation are vital elements of the treatment plan. For large tumors with widespread local infiltration, a debulking procedure reduces the total tumor load for ablation by chemotherapy and irradiation. A carefully coordinated, well-planned, multidisciplinary approach has resulted in vastly improved survivorship. Although the delayed effects of the toxic medications and the high dose of irradiation are as yet undetermined and can only be speculated upon, the improved disease free survival rates certainly seem to justify such treatment.[33,38–40,42] Radiation doses are usually in 4500 cGy for microscopic residual disease and 5000 cGy when gross residual tumor is left behind. Parameningeal involvement is treated with 5000 cGy with an attempt to shield the eyes.

Current chemotherapy protocols include cycles of vincristine and dactinomycin for group I tumors with the addition of cyclophosphamide for groups II and III. Those tumors with embryonal histology respond better than those with an alveolar pattern.[36] The addition of doxorubicin and cisplatin improved survival rates in group III to 71%.[43] A more recent IRS-IV report on children with rhabdomyosarcoma at all sites in patients with nonmetastatic disease analyzed 883 previously untreated individuals with stages I to III. Three regimens were compared; the standard therapy vincristine, dactinomycin, and cyclophosphamide, the second; vincristine, dactinomycin, and ifosfamide; and the third vincristine, ifosfamide, and etoposide. The group III patients were further fractionated into standard radiotherapy and hyperfractionated radiotherapy. The radiation protocols had a 3-year tumor-free survival rate of 77% for conventional radiotherapy and 86% for hyperfractionation. The 3-year rates were little different between the three chemotherapeutic regimens, which varied between 75 and 77%. The 3-year survival for tumors of the eye or eyelid was 91%. Other sites in the head and neck were not fractionated out[44] in the analysis.

Paulino et al[45] looked at the long-term side effects of radiotherapy of the head and neck for rhabdomyosarcoma. In the time period between 1967 and 1994, 30 children were treated, 17 survived, and all were examined. Late side effects occurred in all patients. Retardation of facial growth was seen in 11 patients, neuroendocrine dysfunction in nine, visual and orbital problems in nine, dental abnormalities in seven, hearing loss in six, and hypothyroidism in three. One of the hearing loss complications may have occurred secondarily to the administration of cisplatin. In my own experience facial growth retardation is present in all cases.

◆ Fibrosarcoma

Fibrosarcoma is the third most common head and neck malignancy in children, with 25% of all pediatric fibrosarcomas occurring in this region.[27] Histologically there are two basic types, differentiated and undifferentiated. The well-differentiated tumors have a tendency to local recurrence but rarely metastasize. The poorly differentiated metastasize early and widely and therefore have an expectedly poor prognosis. The degree of differentiation, and even the distinction between fibrosarcoma and benign fibromatoses such as desmoid tumor, dermatofibrosarcoma, and nodular fasciitis, is a difficult problem. Moreover, the metastatic potential of a given lesion

is not always possible to predict for histological examination. In addition, the histological appearances of a variety of other soft tissue sarcomas mimic fibrosarcoma.

In both adults and children, fibrosarcomas have a predilection for males.[46] They can occur at any age and may even be present at birth.[47,48] **Figure 11.5** illustrates a well-differentiated fibrosarcoma in the alveolar ridge of the mandible in a 5-year-old boy. The tumor was excised with a marginal mandibulectomy, and he is now 3 years free of disease. Fortunately, the prognosis in children is better than that in adults.[49] This is exemplified by the 23 patients reviewed by Stout,[50] of whom nine had recurrences, two developed metastasis, but only three died of the disease. In Jaffe's series,[4] the 5-year disease-free survival rates were 79% for patients with well-differentiated lesions and 33% for those with the undifferentiated type. Fortunately, the cases of well-differentiated tumors outnumber those of poorly differentiated by a ratio of 3 or 4 to 1. The biological behavior of fibrosarcoma is unlike that of any other malignancy of the head and neck. The tumor presents as a painless mass that steadily and slowly enlarges.[51] However, one case reported by Chung and Enzinger[52] doubled in size in a period of 2.5 weeks. Late recurrences are not uncommon, with late appearances of recurrent disease appearing up to 15 years later.[53]

The most effective treatment is resection.[4] In Conley's series of 22 fibrosarcomas in children, only two were undifferentiated, and both patients died despite treatment.[1] The remainders of the tumors were well differentiated and were resected. Five years after surgery, 16 of the patients were alive and free of disease and four were alive with disease. Lymph node metastases are rare, so routine neck dissection is unwarranted. Because of the tendency for local recurrence, wide resection is the rule. Radiotherapy and chemotherapy do not result in cure.

◆ Neuroblastoma

Neuroblastoma, although the commonest solid tumor in the pediatric age group, is rare in the extracranial portion of the head and neck.[54] Ten percent of neuroblastomas are congenital, and half of all congenital tumors are neuroblastomas.[3] It usually arises in the cervical sympathetic chain. In the M.D Anderson series,[2] the head and neck region was the site of 7% of all neuroblastomas seen, whereas Bodian[55] reported 5% of 129 cases and Gross et al[56] 2% of 217 cases to be located in the head and neck. Although the tumor can arise di novo in cervical sympathetic ganglia, neuroblastomas in the head and neck often represent metastatic disease from distant sites.

This tumor demonstrates a rather curious biological behavior. Neuroblastomas are discovered in 0.5% of all autopsies done on infants under the age of 3 months.[57] Because the overall incidence of the tumor is 1/10,000, an active immune defense mechanism must exist for these neoplasms. Indeed, Hellstrom et al[58] have demonstrated antineuroblastoma activity in the lymphocytes and plasma of affected patients. Furthermore, Lauder and Aherne[59] have established that the duration of survival is positively related to the amount of round cell infiltration seen in reaction to the tumor.

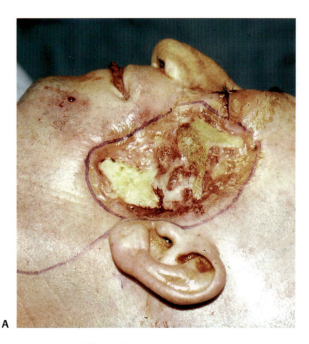

A

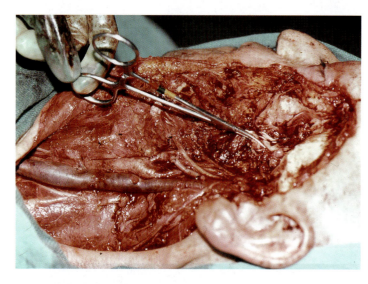

B

Fig. 12.2 Middle-aged man with extensive squamous cell carcinoma of facial skin with multiple prior Mohs excisions and full course radiation therapy. The local recurrence is extremely difficult to completely delineate. (**A**) Lesion prior to resection. (**B**) Large defect after wide-field resection of primary tumor and modified radical neck dissection for metastatic disease in the neck.

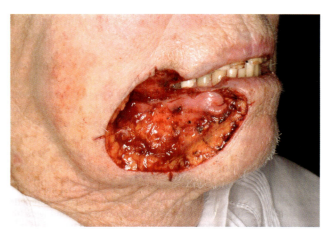

Fig. 12.3 Elderly woman with a through and through facial defect following Mohs resection of a large squamous cell carcinoma.

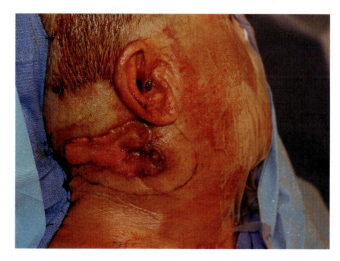

Fig. 12.4 Rodent ulcer.

storiform or pinwheel aggregate of tightly packed cells (**Fig. 12.7B**). Recurrent lesions tend to have a more mucoid appearance.

Wide excision is recommended because of its marked tendency for local recurrence, which is ~20%. Metastases are very uncommon.

Merkel Cell Carcinoma

Merkel cell carcinoma is a very uncommon malignancy. It appears as a dome-shaped nodule with or without ulcera-

tion and with a predilection for the periocular skin. It is often red to purplish in color with telangiectasia over the skin surface and is firm in consistency (**Fig. 12.8**).

It is poorly differentiated and consists of basaloid type, small cells in sheets, and anastomosing cords. It has been described as a neuroendocrine tumor of the skin. Its appearance has often been confused with nodular basal cell carcinoma or amelanotic malignant melanoma. Regional and distant metastasis is common. The tumor is made up of small, rather uniform undifferentiated cells confined mainly to the dermis. Tang and Toker[6] described the presence on electron

for ablation by chemotherapy and irradiation. A carefully coordinated, well-planned, multidisciplinary approach has resulted in vastly improved survivorship. Although the delayed effects of the toxic medications and the high dose of irradiation are as yet undetermined and can only be speculated upon, the improved disease free survival rates certainly seem to justify such treatment.[33,38–40,42] Radiation doses are usually in 4500 cGy for microscopic residual disease and 5000 cGy when gross residual tumor is left behind. Parameningeal involvement is treated with 5000 cGy with an attempt to shield the eyes.

Current chemotherapy protocols include cycles of vincristine and dactinomycin for group I tumors with the addition of cyclophosphamide for groups II and III. Those tumors with embryonal histology respond better than those with an alveolar pattern.[36] The addition of doxorubicin and cisplatin improved survival rates in group III to 71%.[43] A more recent IRS-IV report on children with rhabdomyosarcoma at all sites in patients with nonmetastatic disease analyzed 883 previously untreated individuals with stages I to III. Three regimens were compared; the standard therapy vincristine, dactinomycin, and cyclophosphamide, the second; vincristine, dactinomycin, and ifosfamide; and the third vincristine, ifosfamide, and etoposide. The group III patients were further fractionated into standard radiotherapy and hyperfractionated radiotherapy. The radiation protocols had a 3-year tumor-free survival rate of 77% for conventional radiotherapy and 86% for hyperfractionation. The 3-year rates were little different between the three chemotherapeutic regimens, which varied between 75 and 77%. The 3-year survival for tumors of the eye or eyelid was 91%. Other sites in the head and neck were not fractionated out[44] in the analysis.

Paulino et al[45] looked at the long-term side effects of radiotherapy of the head and neck for rhabdomyosarcoma. In the time period between 1967 and 1994, 30 children were treated, 17 survived, and all were examined. Late side effects occurred in all patients. Retardation of facial growth was seen in 11 patients, neuroendocrine dysfunction in nine, visual and orbital problems in nine, dental abnormalities in seven, hearing loss in six, and hypothyroidism in three. One of the hearing loss complications may have occurred secondarily to the administration of cisplatin. In my own experience facial growth retardation is present in all cases.

◆ Fibrosarcoma

Fibrosarcoma is the third most common head and neck malignancy in children, with 25% of all pediatric fibrosarcomas occurring in this region.[27] Histologically there are two basic types, differentiated and undifferentiated. The well-differentiated tumors have a tendency to local recurrence but rarely metastasize. The poorly differentiated metastasize early and widely and therefore have an expectedly poor prognosis. The degree of differentiation, and even the distinction between fibrosarcoma and benign fibromatoses such as desmoid tumor, dermatofibrosarcoma, and nodular fasciitis, is a difficult problem. Moreover, the metastatic potential of a given lesion

is not always possible to predict for histological examination. In addition, the histological appearances of a variety of other soft tissue sarcomas mimic fibrosarcoma.

In both adults and children, fibrosarcomas have a predilection for males.[46] They can occur at any age and may even be present at birth.[47,48] **Figure 11.5** illustrates a well-differentiated fibrosarcoma in the alveolar ridge of the mandible in a 5-year-old boy. The tumor was excised with a marginal mandibulectomy, and he is now 3 years free of disease. Fortunately, the prognosis in children is better than that in adults.[49] This is exemplified by the 23 patients reviewed by Stout,[50] of whom nine had recurrences, two developed metastasis, but only three died of the disease. In Jaffe's series,[4] the 5-year disease-free survival rates were 79% for patients with well-differentiated lesions and 33% for those with the undifferentiated type. Fortunately, the cases of well-differentiated tumors outnumber those of poorly differentiated by a ratio of 3 or 4 to 1. The biological behavior of fibrosarcoma is unlike that of any other malignancy of the head and neck. The tumor presents as a painless mass that steadily and slowly enlarges.[51] However, one case reported by Chung and Enzinger[52] doubled in size in a period of 2.5 weeks. Late recurrences are not uncommon, with late appearances of recurrent disease appearing up to 15 years later.[53]

The most effective treatment is resection.[4] In Conley's series of 22 fibrosarcomas in children, only two were undifferentiated, and both patients died despite treatment.[1] The remainders of the tumors were well differentiated and were resected. Five years after surgery, 16 of the patients were alive and free of disease and four were alive with disease. Lymph node metastases are rare, so routine neck dissection is unwarranted. Because of the tendency for local recurrence, wide resection is the rule. Radiotherapy and chemotherapy do not result in cure.

◆ Neuroblastoma

Neuroblastoma, although the commonest solid tumor in the pediatric age group, is rare in the extracranial portion of the head and neck.[54] Ten percent of neuroblastomas are congenital, and half of all congenital tumors are neuroblastomas.[3] It usually arises in the cervical sympathetic chain. In the M.D Anderson series,[2] the head and neck region was the site of 7% of all neuroblastomas seen, whereas Bodian[55] reported 5% of 129 cases and Gross et al[56] 2% of 217 cases to be located in the head and neck. Although the tumor can arise di novo in cervical sympathetic ganglia, neuroblastomas in the head and neck often represent metastatic disease from distant sites.

This tumor demonstrates a rather curious biological behavior. Neuroblastomas are discovered in 0.5% of all autopsies done on infants under the age of 3 months.[57] Because the overall incidence of the tumor is 1/10,000, an active immune defense mechanism must exist for these neoplasms. Indeed, Hellstrom et al[58] have demonstrated antineuroblastoma activity in the lymphocytes and plasma of affected patients. Furthermore, Lauder and Aherne[59] have established that the duration of survival is positively related to the amount of round cell infiltration seen in reaction to the tumor.

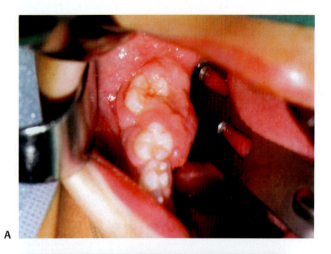

A

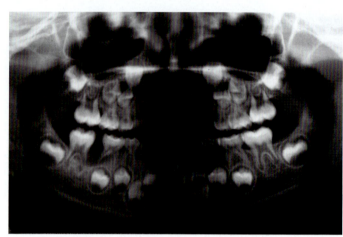

B

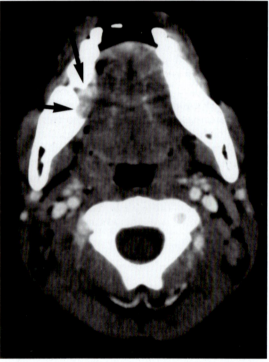

C

Fig. 11.5 Fibrosarcoma of the mandibular alveolus in a 5-year-old boy. (**A**) Fibrosarcoma of the distal alveolar ridge. (**B**) Panorex x-ray showing erosion of bone on the right distal mandibular alveolus over the unerupted third molar tooth. (**C**) Axial computed tomographic scans showing bone erosion on the lingual aspect of the mandible (see *arrows*).

The presence of a neuroblastoma causes the production of urinary catecholamines; specifically VMA (3 methoxy-4-acid) and cystathionine. Elevated levels of these metabolites not only indicate the presence of disease but are a reliable indicator of residual or recurrent disease as well.

The prognosis of the disease hinges on several factors. Patients under the age of 1 have a 60% chance of survival, but those over the age of 1 have only a 16% chance. The more differentiated the cells composing the tumor, the better the prognosis. Neuroblastomas of the head and neck have an overall better prognosis than those in any other site. In view of the aforementioned comments concerning the immunological reaction to these tumors, it is not surprising that they have a relatively high incidence of spontaneous regression. Another strange behavioral characteristic of these tumors is their tendency to differentiate into a mature ganglioneuroma.

When presenting in the head and neck, neuroblastomas usually appear as a rapidly growing cervical mass. Rarely, the primary tumor may originate in the nasopharynx, maxillary sinus, orbit, nose, scalp, or lip. The nasopharynx is the most common of these latter sites. The mass is initially painless and displaces or invades the surrounding structures. The supraclavicular fossa is a common cervical site, and invasion of the brachial plexus and even cervical vertebrae can occur, especially in the more undifferentiated varieties. Primaries occurring higher in the cervical sympathetic chain may invade the cranial nerves so that impairment of nerves X, XI, and XII may become apparent. Before initiating therapy, one must make a thorough search for metastatic disease, keeping in mind that the cervical disease may very likely represent a metastasis from a distant site. Olfactory neuroblastoma is very rare in the pediatric age group. Its biology is quite distinct in contrast to the cervical neuroblastoma that arises from the cervical sympathetics.

Localized disease is best managed by surgical resection. Severe compromise of function or drastic alterations in aesthetic appearance may be avoided by leaving some residual tumor and "mopping up" with postoperative irradiation of the bed. Although generally this principle is to be decried in the management of head and neck malignancy, it appears to be effective in curing neuroblastoma. Widespread metastatic disease can be eliminated, especially if the patient is less than 1 year of age.[4] The wide discrepancy of reported survival rates is indicated in **Table 11.10**.

Table 11.10 Survival Rates for Extraadrenal Neuroblastomas[*]

Authors	No. of Patients	Survival No.	Percent	Duration (years)
Bodian	51	19	37	1
Fortner et al	48	8	17	5
King et al	13	13	100	2
Koop	68	26	38	4
Phillips	20	7	35	3
Young et al	17	9	53	5

Source: Batsakis J. Neoplastic and non-neoplastic tumors of skeletal muscle. In: Tumors of the Head and Neck. Baltimore: Williams & Wilkins; 1974:206. Reprinted with permission.

The pathophysiological behavior of olfactory neuroblastoma (esthesioneuroblastoma) is related in part to its origin in the olfactory epithelium. Most of these tumors begin in the region of the cribriform plate. As such they tend to spread into the adjacent ethmoid sinuses and superiorly into the anterior cranial fossa. Excellent control is achieved by utilizing a craniofacial resection (see chapter 5). Postoperative radiotherapy adds little to the overall control of the disease, and the long-term complications in children do not warrant its use.

◆ Osteosarcoma

Osteogenic sarcomas, chondrosarcomas, and Ewing sarcoma are fortunately rare in children. The most usual site is the mandible or the skull. The zygoma and maxilla, especially the alveolar processes of the latter, may also be involved. The body of the mandible is most commonly affected.[60]

Most of the information on these tumors is derived from single-case reports. Ewing sarcoma is especially rare in the head and neck. Although the second commonest bony malignancy in children is Ewing sarcoma, the head and neck are the least common sites. In a review of the Massachusetts General Hospital experience over a 22-year period, 50 cases throughout the body were discovered.[61] Only two were located in the head and neck; one in the mandible of a 14-year-old child who died 30 months after resection, and another in the same site of a 29-year-old who was alive 2 years following irradiation therapy. A review of the litera-

ture by Rocca AM et al[62] that covered the period from 1949 to 1967 revealed 37 Ewing sarcomas of the jaw, with special note made of the frequency of mandibular involvement. Approximately 50 to 65% of these tumors occur in the first 2 decades of life, most commonly between the ages of 10 and 20.[63,64] Males are affected more than females by a ratio of 2:1. The tumor appears to originate in the mesenchymal cells of bone marrow and causes local swelling, pain, tenderness, and fever. A radiograph of a lytic lesion in the affected bone, showing increased density, expansion of the cortex, and increased periosteal thickening, coupled with the clinical picture, often creates confusion with an inflammatory lesion. Bloodborne and lymphatic metastases are common, with up to 25% of patients demonstrating metastases at the time of diagnosis.[65]

The most effective treatment is the judicious combination of surgery, radiation, and chemotherapy. Goeppert et al[64] demonstrated a 20% 5-year survival rate using this approach. Jaffe et al,[66] using mainly a combination of vincristine, actinomycin D, and cyclophosphamide coupled with irradiation therapy, treated 14 patients with Ewing sarcoma outside of the head and neck. Of the nine who had no metastases at the time of diagnosis, two died of pulmonary metastases, and the remaining seven are alive without disease at 4-month to 4-year follow-up. Those who had metastases at the time of diagnosis experienced decreased survival times. Tumor-free survival appears to be related to tumor volume at the time of treatment. According to Mendenhall et al,[67] tumor volume is an important prognostic factor. In their series those with a tumor volume greater than 100 mL had only a 17% chance of a 3-year tumor-free survival, whereas those with less than a 100 mL volume had a 78% survival. Some controversy exists over the efficacy of high-dose radiation versus wide-field resection.

Chondrosarcomas are exceptionally rare in the head and neck. Only 5 to 10% of all chondrosarcomas occur in the region of the head and neck.[68] The usual age of presentation of this tumor is at 30 to 45 years of age; however, one patient in Barnes et al's experience was only 16 months old.[68] Considerable difficulty is experienced in the histological differentiation between chondroma and chondrosarcoma. Moreover, the biological behavior is not always commensurate with the histological picture. To add further confusion, chondrosarcomatous foci may appear in an osteogenic sarcoma.[69] This latter fact prompted Conley[1] to group these lesions together as osteochondrosarcomas. Head and neck osteogenic sarcoma and chondrosarcoma are most commonly seen in the mandible and maxilla. The mandible[70] is the more frequent site for osteogenic sarcoma (a ratio of 2:1 over the maxilla), whereas the maxilla is a more common site of chondrosarcoma, accounting for ~60% of all cases involving bony structures of the head and neck.[60] Chondrosarcomas may arise in a preexisting benign chondroma. Individuals with Ollier disease (familial multiple exostoses and enchondromatosis) are highly predisposed to developing chondrosarcoma, with malignant degeneration tending to develop around the time of puberty.[70]

Bone that has been irradiated is predisposed to the development of osteogenic sarcoma. Kragh et al[71] report four cases of mandibular osteosarcoma that occurred following irradiation. Mandibular lesions tend to remain localized; they have a marked propensity for local recurrence but rarely cause regional or distant metastasis. Fibrous dysplasia is an additional predisposing factor, being a precursor in 12 cases of osteogenic sarcoma recorded by Yannopoulos et al.[72]

Both chondrosarcoma and osteogenic sarcoma are radioresistant, so that successful therapy depends upon the ability to adequately resect the lesion. The mandibular tumors have a fairly good prognosis. Kragh et al[71] reported a 33% 5-year survival rate in a study of 35 patients with osteosarcoma. Tumors of the maxillary alveolar ridge have a more favorable prognosis than those of the antrum in that the former can be adequately encompassed by a radical resection. Radical neck dissection is reserved for those individuals with manifest cervical metastases.

Mandibular reconstruction with an osseous free flap will successfully rehabilitate the child. Adjustment will have to be made and revisions will be required as growth proceeds.

◆ Malignant Hemangiopericytoma

This neoplasm arises from the pericytes of Zimmerman. Since its discovery in 1942 by Stout and Murray, 300 cases have been reported, of which approximately a third originated in the head and neck.[73] Kauffman and Stout[74] reported nine of 31 cases in children having developed in the head and neck. The sites of origin are the nose and paranasal sinuses, neck, oral cavity, scalp, skull, orbit, larynx, and nasopharynx.[4,73,74] Histological differentiation between benign and malignant forms is extremely difficult.

Management is by wide local excision because the tumor, despite its vascularity, is radioresistant. Regional metastases are far less common with head and neck lesions than with those located elsewhere. Because the major problem in management is the frequency of local recurrence, radical excision is essential. Radical neck dissection is reserved for lesions with manifest regional nodes. Malignant hemangiopericytomas have a marked tendency for late recurrence, with tumor reappearing 10 years and even longer after apparently successful excision.

◆ Chordoma

Chordoma is an unusual lesion that can affect any age and is seen in children in only 5% of cases, with the usual age of occurrence being in the third and fourth decades of life.[75] They arise from notochordal remnants in the spinal column and clivus, most commonly at each end of the spine. About 50% occur in the sacrococcygeal area and 35% at the base of the skull. Although the tumors are considered by some as benign because of their lack of metastasis, they often have a very malignant course invading bone and adjacent soft tissue. They usually remain extradural until they have been operated upon and the dura is violated. If recurrence supervenes then intradural and brain invasion is seen. Clival tumors and those with chondroid differentiation are more

commonly seen in the young. The tumor has a characteristically soft, fish-flesh appearance. Histologically it is characterized by the appearance of foamy, bubbly, vacuolated cells called physaliferous cells.

Clival chordomas usually present with visual disturbances, including diplopia, loss of visual fields, and headache. Nasal obstruction, purulent nasal drainage, and epistaxis are seen when the tumor obstructs the nasopharynx or invades the paranasal sinuses. The bulging in the posterior wall of the oropharynx or nasopharynx will be covered by normal-appearing pharyngeal mucosa. Lower cranial nerves become involved as the tumor spreads to the skull base. On physical examination a bulge is seen in the nasopharynx or high in the oropharynx if there are symptoms of nasal obstruction. Vocal cord paralysis, sternocleidomastoid and trapezius paralysis, as well as atrophy and deviation of the protruded tongue, are seen if the tenth, eleventh, and twelfth nerves are affected.

Computed tomographic (CT) scanning will show bone erosion and a soft tissue mass (**Fig. 11.6 and Fig. 11.7**). Magnetic resonance imaging (MRI) scans will show the extent of soft tissue involvement (**Fig. 11.6 and Fig. 11.7**).

Treatment is very complex and may require a multistage operation. Biopsy is obtained usually through the transoral/transoropharyngeal route. The initial phase of resection can be accomplished at this time, and in the cases of small tumors of limited extent, a complete removal can be accomplished. Extension of tumor up the foramen magnum can be resected using the far lateral approach, and an occipital-temporal or petroclival approach may be necessary for com-

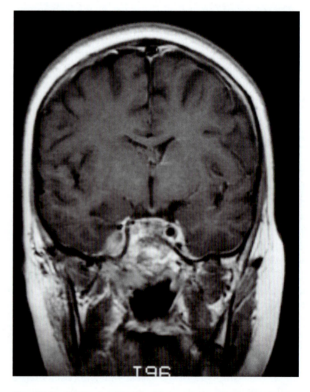

Fig. 11.6 A 14-year-old girl with a massive clivus chordoma.

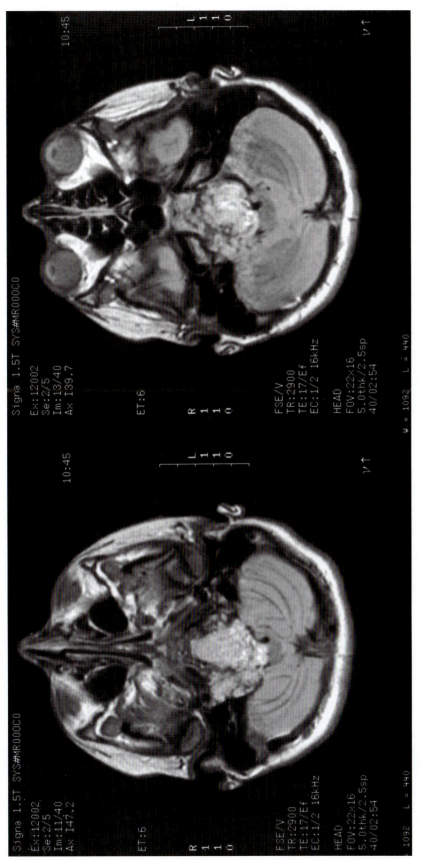

Fig. 11.7 A 15-year-old boy with a massive clivus chordoma extending into the posterior and middle cranial fossae.

plete tumor extirpation. The details of these resections have already been described in chapter 9. In advanced tumors, such as those illustrated in **Fig. 11.6** and **Fig. 11.7**, the tumor defies complete excision. Follow-up treatment with proton irradiation appears to hold some promise. The patients depicted in the figures died at 18 and 24 months, respectively, despite multiple aggressive skull base resections and proton beam irradiation.

◆ Rare Lesions

Angiosarcoma, liposarcoma, leiomyosarcoma, malignant schwannoma, and neuroepithelioma are very rarely seen in children. Guidance in therapy is usually based on individual case reports rather than series of cases containing significant numbers.

Angiosarcomas appear as purplish masses, usually in skin or mucous membrane, and are most commonly found in the scalp. As they spread in the dermal layer they impart a violaceous hue to the skin adjacent to the lesion. Conley[1] had only two angiosarcomas in his series of 88 pediatric tumors. Only one patient, who was treated by a radical maxillectomy, survived 5 years. Jaffe[4] also had two cases in his large series. Wide excision is the treatment of choice, with radiotherapy reserved for unresectable cases and chemotherapy for distant metastatic disease. These tumors are among the few types of sarcoma that metastasize to lymph nodes, with this occurring in 30 to 50% of cases.

Leiomyosarcoma is very rare but has a good prognosis. Treatment is wide excision. Liposarcoma is a curiosity in the head and neck, although a very common sarcoma elsewhere in the body. It usually occurs in persons over age 30. In our experience, a 10-year-old boy with this tumor in the buccal fat pad was treated by incomplete excision followed by radiation and chemotherapy. The patient succumbed to extensive local disease and widespread metastases 2 years later.

Malignant schwannoma usually occurs in patients suffering from von Recklinghausen disease. Multiple sites of origin may be found. Wide-field excision is essential because of the tumor's tendency to spread along the sheath of the involved nerve. Bloodborne metastases are common, and the prognosis is generally poor.[76]

Neuroepithelioma is also very rare in the pediatric age group and is amenable to radiotherapy.

◆ Group Description and Therapy

I. Localized disease, completely dissected, no lymphadenopathy
   A. Confined to muscle or organ of origin
   B. Contiguous infiltration of localized tissues
II. Total gross resection with evidence of regional spread
   A. Microscopic positive margins
   B. Regional disease with positive lymph nodes, negative margins
   C. Regional disease with positive lymph node in the most distal node and positive margins
III. Incomplete resections with gross residual disease
   A. Biopsy only
   B. More than 50% of the tumor left behind
IV. Presence of distant metastasis

References

1. Conley J. Concepts in Head and Neck Surgery. New York: Grune & Stratton; 1970:181–192
2. Sutow WW, Montague ED. Pediatric tumors. In: McComb WS, Fletcher GH, eds. Cancer of the Head and Neck. Baltimore: Williams & Wilkins; 1967:428–446
3. Cotton RT, Rothschild MA, Zwerdling T, Ballard ET, Meyer CM, Koch BL. Tumors of the head and neck in children. In: Thawley SE, Panje WE, Batsakis JG, Lindberg RD, eds. Comprehensive Management of Head and Neck Tumors. Vol 2. 2nd ed. Philadelphia: WB Saunders; 1999:1846–1902
4. Jaffe BF. Neck masses and malignant tumors of the head and neck. In: Ferguson CF, Kendig EL Jr, eds. Disorders of the Respiratory Tract in Children. Vol 2: Pediatric Otolaryngology. Philadelphia: WB Saunders; 1972:1135
5. Sutow WW, Sullivan MR, Ried HL, et al. Prognosis in childhood rhabdomyosarcoma. Cancer 1970;25:1384–1390
6. Kilman JW, Clatworthy HW, Newton WA, et al. Reasonable surgery for rhabdomyosarcoma: a study of 67 cases. Ann Surg 1973;178:346–351
7. Bailey RJ, Burget EO, Dahlin DC. Malignant lymphomas in children. Pediatrics 1961;28:985–992
8. Pierce MI. Lymphosarcoma and Hodgkin's disease in children. Fourth National Cancer Conference Proceedings, 1960. Philadelphia: JB Lippincott; 1961:559
9. Rosenberg SA, Diamond HD, Dargeon HW, et al. Lymphosarcoma in childhood. N Engl J Med 1958;259:505–512
10. Rappaport H. Tumors of the Hematopoietic System. Washington, DC: Armed Forces Institute of Pathology; 1966
11. Kinney MC, Swerdlow SH. Hematopoietic and lymphoid disorders. In: Barnes L, ed. Surgical Pathology of the Head and Neck. Vol 2. 2nd ed. New York: Marcel Dekker; 2001:1264
12. Lukes RJ, Collins RD. Tumors of the Hematopoietic System. Second Series, Fascicle 9. Washington, DC: Armed Forces Institute of Pathology; 1992
13. Kinney MC, Swerdlow SH. Hematopoietic and lymphoid disorders. In: Barnes L, ed. Surgical Pathology of the Head and Neck Vol 2. 2nd ed. New York: Marcel Dekker; 2001:1265
14. Kinney MC, Swerdlow SH. Hematopoietic and lymphoid disorders. In: Barnes L, ed. Surgical Pathology of the Head and Neck. Vol 2. 2nd ed. New York: Marcel Dekker; 2001:1267
15. Harris NL, Jaffe ES, Stein H, et al. A revised European-American classification of lymphoid neoplasms: a proposal from the International Lymphoma Study Group. Blood 1994;84:1361–1392
16. Ro G, Mierau GW, Favara BE. Tumors of the Head and Neck in Children. New York: Praeger; 1983:302
17. Weinstein HJ, Tarbell NJ. Leukemias and lymphomas of childhood. In: DeVita VT, Hellman S, Rosenberg SA, eds. Cancer Principles and Practice of Oncology. 5th ed. Lippincott Raven; 1997:chapter 44.2
18. Gobbi PG, Attardo-Parinello G, Lattanzio G, et al. Severe pruritus should be a B-symptom in Hodgkin's disease. Cancer 1983;51:1934–1936
19. Carbone PP, Kaplan HS, Mussoff K, et al. Report of the Committee on Hodgkin's Disease Staging Classification. Cancer Res 1971;31:1860–1861
20. Rosenberg SA, Diamond BD, Jaslowitz B, et al. Lymphosarcoma: a review of 1269 cases. Medicine 1961;40:31–84
21. Burkitt D. A sarcoma involving the jaws in African children. Br J Surg 1958;46:218–223
22. Burkitt D. Burkitt's lymphoma outside the known endemic area of Africa and New Guinea. Int J Cancer 1967;2:562–565
23. Wright DH. Burkitt's tumor: a postmortem study of 50 cases. Br J Surg 1964;51:245–251

24. Clift RA, Wright DH, Clifford P. Leukemia in Burkitt's lymphoma. Blood 1963;22:243–251

25. Williamson JJ. Blood dyscrasias. In: Gorlin RJ, Foldman HM, eds. Thoma's Oral Pathology. Vol 2. St. Louis: CV Mosby; 1970:948–951

26. Schnitzer B, Weaver DK. Lymphoreticular disorders. In: Batsakis JG, ed. Tumors of the Head and Neck. Baltimore: Williams & Wilkins; 1974:359–362

27. Healy GB. Malignant tumors of the head and neck in children: diagnosis and treatment. Otolaryngol Clin North Am 1980;13:483–488

28. Batsakis JG, ed. Neoplastic and non-neoplastic tumors of skeletal muscle. In: Tumors of the Head and Neck. Baltimore: Williams & Wilkins; 1974:206–210

29. Dito WR, Batsakis JG. Rhabdomyosarcoma of the head and neck: an appraisal of the biological behavior in 170 cases. Arch Surg 1962;84:112–118

30. Ro G, Mierau GW, Favara BE. Tumors of the Head and Neck in Children. New York: Praeger; 1983:363

31. Lawrence W Jr, Hays DM, Moon TE. Lymphatic metastasis with childhood rhabdomyosarcoma. Cancer 1977;39:556–559

32. Donaldson SS, Castro JR, Wilbur JR, et al. Rhabdomyosarcoma of the head and neck in children. Cancer 1973;31:26–35

33. Schuller DE, Lawrence TL, Newton WA. Childhood rhabdomyosarcoma of the head and neck. Arch Otolaryngol 1979;105:689–694

34. Sutow WW, Sullivan MR, Ried HL, et al. Prognosis in childhood rhabdomyosarcoma. Cancer 1970;25:1384–1390

35. Maurer HM, Moon T, Donaldsen M, et al. The Intergroup Rhabdomyosarcoma Study: a preliminary report. Cancer 1977;40:2015–2026

36. Malkin D. Cancers of childhood. In: DeVita VT, Hellman S, Rosenberg SA, eds. 5th ed. Lippincott Raven; 1997:2107–2113

37. Johnson DG. Trends in surgery for childhood rhabdomyosarcoma. Cancer 1975; 35(3, Suppl)916–920

38. Heyn RM, Holland R, Newton WA Jr, et al. The role of combined chemotherapy in the treatment of children with rhabdomyosarcoma. Cancer 1974;34:2128–214

39. Ghavimi F, Exelby PR, D'Angio GJ, et al. Multidisciplinary treatment of embryonal rhabdomyosarcoma in children. Cancer 1975;35:677–687

40. Wilbur JR, Sutow WW, Sullivan MP. The changing treatment of rhabdomyosarcoma in children, particularly in treatment for inoperable rhabdomyosarcoma of the nasopharynx and oropharynx. In: MD Anderson Hospital: Neoplasia of the Head and Neck. Chicago: Year Book Medical Publications; 1974:281–288

41. Lawrence W Jr, Hays DM, Moon TE. Lymphatic metastasis with childhood rhabdomyosarcoma. Cancer 1977;39:556–559

42. Healy GB, Jaffe N, Cassady JR. Rhabdomyosarcoma of the head and neck: diagnosis and management. Head Neck Surg 1979;1:334–339

43. Crist W, Gehan EA, Ragab AH, et al. The third intergroup rhabdomyosarcoma group study. J Clin Oncol 1995;13:610–630

44. Crist WM, Anderson JR, Meza JL, et al. Intergroup Rhabdomyosarcoma Study—IV: results for patients with non-metastatic disease. J Clin Oncol 2001;19:3091–3102

45. Paulino AC, Simon JH, Zhen W, Wen BC. Long-term effects in children treated with radiotherapy for head and neck rhabdomyosarcoma. Int J Radiat Oncol Biol Phys 2000;48:1489–1495

46. Stout AP, Lattes R, eds. Tumors of the Soft Tissues. Washington, DC: Armed Forces Institute of Pathology; 1966:101–106

47. Gross RE, Faber S, Martin LW. Neuroblastoma sympatheticum. Pediatrics 1959;23:1179–1191

48. Weingrad DN, Rosenberg SA. Early lymphatic spread of osteogenic and soft tissue sarcomas. Surgery 1978;84:231–240

49. Barnes L. Tumors and tumor-like lesions of the soft tissues. In: Surgical Pathology of the Head and Neck. New York: Marcel Dekker; 1985:968–969

50. Stout AP. Fibrosarcoma in infants and children. Cancer 1962;15:1028–104

51. Weiss SA, Goldblum JR. Fibrous tumors of infancy and childhood. In: Enzinger and Weiss's Soft Tissue Tumors. 4th ed. St. Louis: Mosby; 2001:377–382

52. Chung EB, Enzinger FM. Infantile fibrosarcoma. Cancer 1976;38:729–739

53. Horne CH, Slavin G, McDonald AM. Late recurrence of juvenile fibrosarcoma. Br J Surg 1968;55:102–103

54. DeLorimier AA, Bragg KU, Linden G. Neuroblastoma in childhood. Am J Dis Child 1969;118:441–450

55. Bodian M. Neuroblastoma. Pediatr Clin North Am 1959;6:449–472

56. Gross RE, Farber S, Martin LW. Neuroblastoma sympatheticum: a study and report of 217 cases. Pediatrics 1959;23:1179–1190

57. Beckwith JB, Perrin EV. In situ neuroblastomas: a contribution to the natural history of neural crest tumors. Am J Pathol 1963;43:1089–1104

58. Hellstrom I, Hellstrom KE, Sjogren NO, et al. Demonstration of cell-mediated immunity to human neoplasms of various types. Int J Cancer 1971;7:1–16

59. Lauder I, Aherne W. The significance of lymphatic infiltration in neuroblastoma. Br J Cancer 1972;26:321–330

60. Kragh LV. Bone tumors of the jaws. In: Gorlin RJ, Goldman HM, eds. Thoma's Oral Pathology. Vol 1. 6th ed. St. Louis: CV Mosby; 1970:560–576

61. Wang CC, Schultz MD. Ewing's sarcoma—a study of 50 cases treated at the Massachusetts General Hospital, 1930–1952 inclusive. N Engl J Med 1953;248:571–576

62. Roca AM, Smith JL, MacComb WS, et al. Ewing's sarcoma of maxilla and mandible. Oral Surg 1968;25:194–203

63. McCormack LJ, Dockerty MB, Ghormley RK. Ewing's sarcoma. Cancer 1952;5:85–89

64. Goeppert H, Rochlin DB, Smart CR. Palliative treatment of Ewing's sarcoma. Am J Surg 1967;113:246–250

65. Falk S, Alpert M. Clinical and roentgen aspects of Ewing's sarcoma. Am J Med Sci 1965;250:492–508

66. Jaffe N, Traggis I, Salian S, et al. Improved outlook for Ewing's sarcoma with combination therapy (vincristine, actinomycin D, cyclophosphamide) and radiation therapy. Cancer 1976;38:1925–1930

67. Mendenhall CM, Marcus RB Jr, Enneking WF, et al. The prognostic significance of soft tissue extension in Ewing's sarcoma. Cancer 1983;51:913–917

68. Barnes L, Verbin RS, Appel BN, Peel RL. Disease of the Bone and Joints. New York: Marcel Dekker; 1985:1142–1146

69. Spjut HJ, Darfman HD, Fechner RE, et al. Tumors of bone and cartilage. In: Atlas of Tumor Pathology, Fascicle 5. 2nd ed. Washington, DC: Armed Forces Institute of Pathology; 1971:104–110

70. Garrington GE, Scofield HH, Cornyn J, et al. Osteosarcoma of the jaws: analysis of 56 cases. Cancer 1967;20:377–391

71. Kragh LV, Dahlin DC, Erich JG. Osteogenic sarcoma of the jaws and facial bones. Am J Surg 1958;96:496–505

72. Yannopoulos K, Bom AF, Griffiths CO, et al. Osteosarcoma arising in fibrous dysplasia of the facial bones: case report and review of the literature. Am J Surg 1964;107:556–564

73. Walike JW, Bailey BJ. Head and neck pericytoma. Arch Otolaryngol 1971;93:345–353

74. Kauffman SL, Stout AP. Hemangiopericytoma in children. Cancer 1960;13:695–710

75. Barnes L, Verbin RS, Appel BN, Peel RL. Disease of the Bone and Joints. New York: Marcel Dekker: 1985:1151–1156

76. D'Agostino AN, Soule EN, Miller RH. Sarcomas of the peripheral nerves and somatic soft tissues associated with multiple neurofibromatosis (von Recklinghausen's disease). Cancer 1963;16:1015

12

Advanced Carcinoma of the Facial Skin

Paul J. Donald

Carcinoma of the facial and cervical skin is becoming a more common diagnosis, especially among those individuals who live in the so-called sun belt of the United States. The depletion of the ozone layer has rendered individuals, especially of fair complexion, more vulnerable to the damaging ultraviolet B rays of the sun. Malignant melanoma has been dealt with in chapter 10 and will not be covered in this chapter. Basal cell and squamous cell carcinomas make up the majority of cutaneous malignancies encountered in everyday practice. More unusual types such as Merkel cell carcinoma, eccrine carcinoma, and malignant fibrous histiocytoma protuberans each have a distinctive pathophysiology and will be covered in less detail. Attention will be more centered upon advanced basal cell and squamous cell carcinoma.

The head and neck surgeon faces the following problems in these difficult cases: (1) the management of the extensive tumor that requires wide-field resection and complex reconstruction (**Fig. 12.1**); (2) the management of the previously resected tumor, often with positive margins and postoperative radiation, that has recurred (**Fig. 12.2**); and (3) the reconstruction of large defects following Mohs resection (**Fig. 12.3**).

◆ Pathology

Basal Cell Carcinoma

In the United States basal cell carcinoma is seen in 19 out of 1000 of all males and 14 out of 1000 of all females.[1] The cell of origins are the cells of the basal layer of the epidermis. There is a strong association between fair complexion, sun exposure, and especially a history of sunburn, and basal cell cancer. Gailani et al[2] have shown a correlation of the loss of heterozygosity at chromosome 9q22 as the most frequent genetic mutation in tumors of patients with basal cell carcinoma. There is a limited relationship between this loss of heterozygosity and ultraviolet (UV) radiation possibly invoking other environmental factors in the etiology of basal cell carcinoma.

The commonest tumor is the nodular type. When it undergoes necrosis in the center, an ulceration forms that tends to undermine the edges producing the so-called rodent ulcer that characterizes it (**Fig. 12.4**). The most pernicious type is the morpheaform or sclerosing basal cell carcinoma. Its histological borders unlike the pushing pattern of the nodular variety (**Fig. 12.5A**) are often ill defined and difficult to establish on microscopic examination (**Fig. 12.5B,C**). This tumor also commonly spreads by perineural invasion.

Basal cell carcinomas appear to be the most invasive when they invade the lines of embryonic fusion, especially along the nasal facial groove and at the inner and outer canthi of the eyes. Lambert and Siegle[3] describe the so-called H zone as illustrated in **Fig. 12.6**, where the basal cell carcinomas are most likely to be most invasive. He describes three zones of relative invasiveness from highest to lowest with the most dangerous type being that within the H zone.

Basosquamous carcinoma is a troubling diagnosis, and the tumor usually behaves like a squamous carcinoma. It may represent a metaplasia or transitional form of squamous cell cancer and has the potential for regional and distant metastasis. Basal cell carcinomas almost never metastasize to regional lymph nodes and even more rarely to distant sites. In the author's experience only two patients ever had a distant metastasis from basal cell carcinoma, and they were to the lung.

Squamous Cell Carcinoma

The next most common malignancy of skin is squamous cell carcinoma, with an average incidence of ~60:100,00 Caucasians. In Northern Australia where sun exposure is extreme the incidence is 1300:100,00.[4] Most squamous cell cancers take origin in a previously existing actinic keratosis. Approximately 1:1000 actinic keratoses will develop into a squamous cell carcinoma each year.[5] Individuals with actinic keratosis have a 12 to 25% chance of developing a squamous cell carcinoma. Squamous cell carcinomas are a more

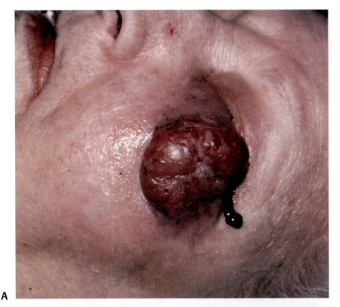

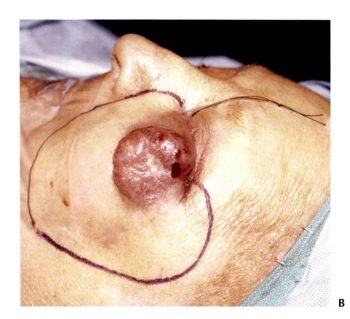

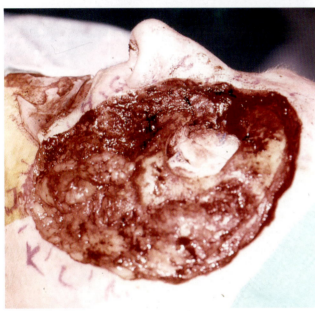

Fig. 12.1 (**A**) Elderly woman with Merkel cell carcinoma involving facial skin, orbit, and maxillary sinus. (**B**) Area of resection outlined. Note degree of subcutaneous resection extension requiring wide resection of skin. (**C**) Defect following resection.

serious problem than their basal cell counterparts because of their rapid growth potential and their ability to metastasize to regional lymph nodes. The marked irregularity of the borders so often encountered as the tumor advances locally renders it somewhat more difficult to encompass by Mohs type resection. Tumor also readily invades underlying muscle and bone. Perivascular and perineural spread are also not uncommon.

Metastasis to regional lymphatics from facial malignancies often goes to areas such as the parotid gland and the occipital regions of the upper neck, which are uncommonly involved in tumors primary to the upper aerodigestive tract. Distant metastases from squamous carcinoma of the facial skin are decidedly unusual.

Malignant Melanoma

This often highly and predictable tumor is discussed in chapter 10.

Dermatofibrosarcoma Protuberans

Dermatofibrosarcoma protuberans is a slowly growing but locally aggressive tumor of the skin that begins in the dermis. It can occur at any age but is more common in the elderly. Males are more commonly affected than females. It is an exophytic firm lesion of red or pink coloration with, in the larger tumors, numerous surface bosselations (**Fig. 12.7A**). Histologically they have a characteristic appearance of a

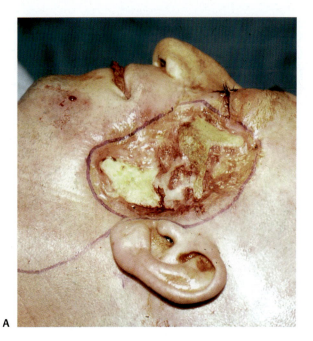
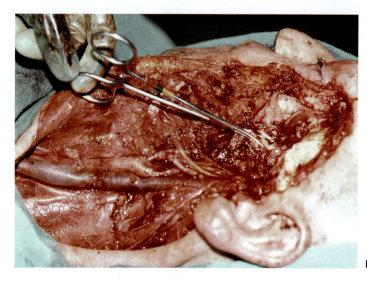

Fig. 12.2 Middle-aged man with extensive squamous cell carcinoma of facial skin with multiple prior Mohs excisions and full course radiation therapy. The local recurrence is extremely difficult to completely delineate. (**A**) Lesion prior to resection. (**B**) Large defect after wide-field resection of primary tumor and modified radical neck dissection for metastatic disease in the neck.

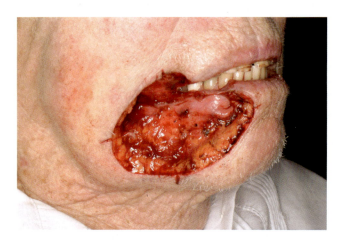

Fig. 12.3 Elderly woman with a through and through facial defect following Mohs resection of a large squamous cell carcinoma.

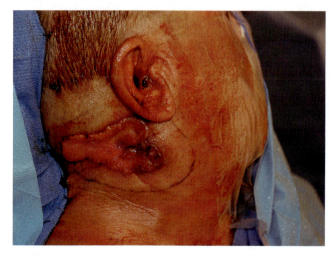

Fig. 12.4 Rodent ulcer.

storiform or pinwheel aggregate of tightly packed cells (**Fig. 12.7B**). Recurrent lesions tend to have a more mucoid appearance.

Wide excision is recommended because of its marked tendency for local recurrence, which is ~20%. Metastases are very uncommon.

Merkel Cell Carcinoma

Merkel cell carcinoma is a very uncommon malignancy. It appears as a dome-shaped nodule with or without ulcera-

tion and with a predilection for the periocular skin. It is often red to purplish in color with telangiectasia over the skin surface and is firm in consistency (**Fig. 12.8**).

It is poorly differentiated and consists of basaloid type, small cells in sheets, and anastomosing cords. It has been described as a neuroendocrine tumor of the skin. Its appearance has often been confused with nodular basal cell carcinoma or amelanotic malignant melanoma. Regional and distant metastasis is common. The tumor is made up of small, rather uniform undifferentiated cells confined mainly to the dermis. Tang and Toker[6] described the presence on electron

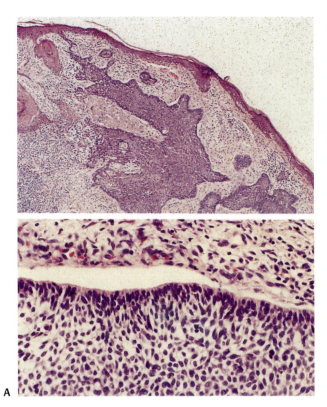

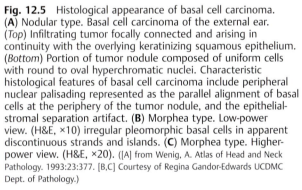

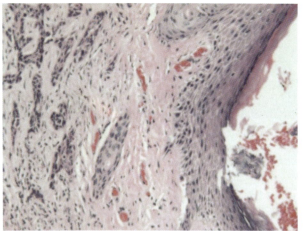

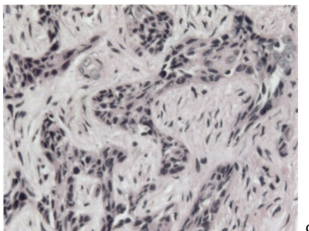

Fig. 12.5 Histological appearance of basal cell carcinoma. (**A**) Nodular type. Basal cell carcinoma of the external ear. (*Top*) Infiltrating tumor focally connected and arising in continuity with the overlying keratinizing squamous epithelium. (*Bottom*) Portion of tumor nodule composed of uniform cells with round to oval hyperchromatic nuclei. Characteristic histological features of basal cell carcinoma include peripheral nuclear palisading represented as the parallel alignment of basal cells at the periphery of the tumor nodule, and the epithelial-stromal separation artifact. (**B**) Morphea type. Low-power view. (H&E, ×10) irregular pleomorphic basal cells in apparent discontinuous strands and islands. (**C**) Morphea type. Higher-power view. (H&E, ×20). ([A] from Wenig, A. Atlas of Head and Neck Pathology. 1993:23:377. [B,C] Courtesy of Regina Gandor-Edwards UCDMC Dept. of Pathology.)

microscopy of dense-core granules in the cells of these tumors similar to those seen in the cells of the amine precursor uptake and decarboxylation (APUD) system. This has led to other names for Merkel cell tumor such as APUDoma, neuroendocrine carcinoma, and primary small cell carcinoma of the skin.

The tumor is usually fast growing and is infamous for frequent local and regional metastases and extensive subepithelial local spread. Wide excision is mandatory because of the indefinite border of the tumor and its high incidence of local recurrence.

◆ Pathophysiology

With the exception of melanoma and Merkel cell tumor, the majority of skin cancers usually tend to remain localized with infrequent metastases and spread by pushing margins. Basal cell carcinoma, which is by far the commonest, almost never metastasizes. In a greater than 30-year experience of handling problem cases of head and neck cancer I have seen only three patients who had metastatic basal carcinoma to the neck and one who had metastasis to the lung. Squamous cell cancer has a different biological behavior, but metastases are still not nearly as common as in upper aerodigestive tract tumors. Overall the metastatic rate for squamous cell cancer of the skin of the head and neck has been estimated to be 0.5[7] to 3.0%.[8,9] The low figure comes from an American study, whereas the other two studies are from Australia. However, I agree with Ruhoy et al[10] and Lund[11] that the study by Tavin and Persky[7] probably underestimates the actual number seen. Unfortunately regional and distant metastases carry a 35% mortality rate.

Determinates of metastatic disease are well outlined in the excellent article by Veness et al.[12] These factors include tu-

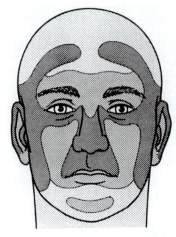
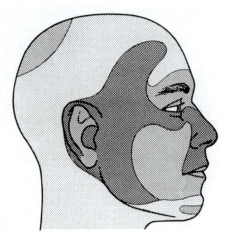

■ HIGHEST
□ INTERMEDIATE
□ LOWEST

Fig. 12.6 So-called H zone in which basal and squamous cell carcinomas appear to take on a more invasive character. (From Lambert DR, Siegle RJ. Skin cancer: a review with consideration of treatment options including Mohs micrographic surgery. Ohio Med 1980;86:745.)

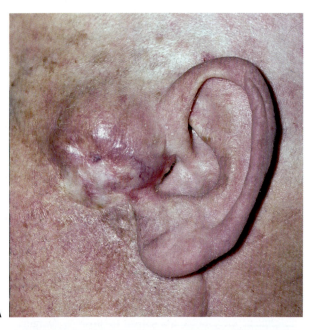

A

Fig. 12.7 (**A**) Dermatofibroma protuberans. (**B**) Histological appearance. Low-power (H&E, ×10) spindle cells in a streaming and whirling pattern with abundant fibrous tissue stroma. (**C**) Histological appearance. High power. (H&E, ×20) ([B,C] Courtesy of Regina Gandor-Edwards UCDMC Dept. of Pathology.)

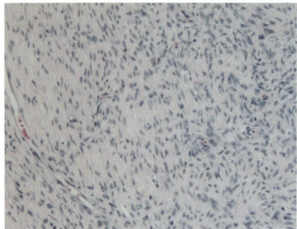

B

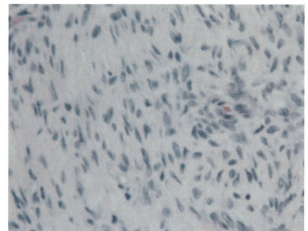

C

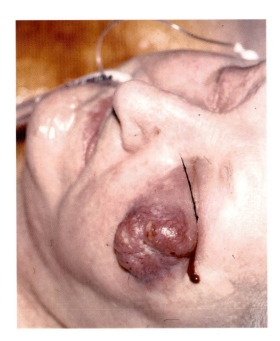

Fig. 12.8 Merkel cell carcinoma in an elderly woman.

mor size, depth of penetration, recurrence, and grade as well as histological evidence of perineural spread or lymphovascular invasion.

Location is an important determinant as well as the presence of immunosuppression in the patient. All cutaneous squamous cell carcinomas have the potential for metastatic spread through the lymphatics. In the literature the more dangerous tumors in this regard appear to be over 2 cm in diameter. We have, however, encountered very large tumors of the facial and neck skin, present for many years, that remained free of metastases (**Fig. 12.9**). Furthermore the presence of a small tumor is no guarantee against spread to lymph nodes. One review showed a metastatic rate of 30%

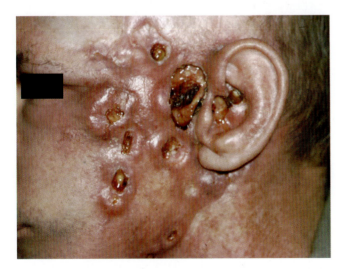

Fig. 12.9 Patient with multifocal squamous cell carcinomas of the face present for many years without metastasis.

for lesions larger than 2 cm in diameter and only a 9% rate for those less than 2 cm.[13]

Depth of penetration of tumor greater than 4 or 5 mm appears to have an important influence on regional metastatic rate. In a study by Kraus et al, of all the patients in their cohort with cutaneous head and neck squamous cell carcinomas who had metastatic lymphadenopathy, only 17% had lesions that were less than 4 mm in depth. The remaining 83% of metastatic skin tumors were thicker than 4 mm.[14] As in other sites in the head and neck, more poorly differentiated tumors have a higher incidence of neck metastatic disease than well differentiated ones. Two studies quoted by Veness et al[12] corroborate this conclusion. Breuninger et al[15] found in a series of 571 patients a 17% metastatic rate in the poorly differentiated tumors and a 4% rate in those that were well differentiated. Even more striking were the findings of Cherpelis et al,[16] who found a 44% incidence of neck metastasis in poorly differentiated tumors and a 5% rate of nodal secondaries in those with well-differentiated tumors. Desmoplasia is also accompanied by a higher metastatic rate. Recurrent tumors are more likely to metastasize than those treated for the first time. Both perineural spread and lymphovascular invasion are accompanied by a significantly increased metastatic rate of up to sixfold higher than those who show no evidence of this activity. Tumor location in the various head and neck sites is an indicator of metastatic rate. The anatomical sites of greatest propensity for metastatic spread are the upper lip, the nose, and the ear.[3] Tumors with a periauricular location have a higher incidence of lymphatic spread, usually to the parotid gland, and upper cervical lymph nodes.

◆ Treatment

Treatment Philosophy

It is a foregone conclusion that the majority of skin malignancies, at the present time, are managed by the dermatologist. The success of the Mohs technique for management of cutaneous cancers with complete excision, low recurrence rates usually resulting in minimal morbidity, and little cosmetic deformity have made this technique the treatment of choice. The original procedure as designed by Frederic Mohs[17–19] had the tumor fixed in situ, on the patient, with zinc chloride and then excised with close margins, the tumor carefully mapped with color-coded dyes, and all aspects of the tumor examined microscopically. The patient returned in a day or two, and any positive areas were again fixed with the chemical and resected the following day, similarly mapped, stained, and microscopically examined. Once the margins were all clear of tumor the wound was allowed to granulate in. The local recurrence rate in his original series of 2249 cases of squamous cell carcinoma of the skin operated upon between the years 1939 to 1968 was only 6%.[18] One of the major drawbacks to the original procedure was that the fixation process was very painful. The modern approach to this technique, thanks to the innovations of Tromovitch and Stegman,[20,21] eliminated the original painful zinc chloride fixation technique and replaced it with frozen sectioning of the fresh specimen and utilizing the "squeeze-down" technique

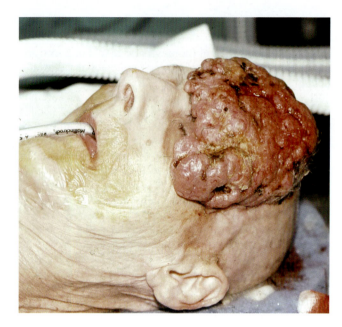

Fig. 12.10 Elderly woman with a massive basal cell carcinoma of the scalp present for many years who presented for treatment because the tumor prolapsed over her eye obscuring her vision.

of placing the resected tissue in the microtome cassette so once the specimen is frozen the blade passes through the entire resection margin as it produces the slices for examination. The modified Mohs technique is ideally designed for nodular basal cell and relatively small squamous cell carcinomas. The advantage in morpheaform basal cell tumors is that the small extensions and tendrils of tumor creeping under the epidermis can be tracked. One of the main limitations of the technique is that underlying bone and cartilage cannot be processed with frozen section, and most dermatologists have little to no experience with surgery involving hard tissues. The other problem is that of perineural spread of tumor, which in some neoplasms involves skip areas with narrow resection margins. As a result the resection may miss areas of persistent tumor in the perineural spaces.

Unfortunately the Mohs technique does not work all the time. Often failures are multifocal and may even be a reflection of new adjacent disease rather than a local recurrence. Tumor in bone and cartilage cannot be resected adequately with this technique. The Mohs surgeon may be lulled into a sense of false security based on past successes in soft tissue and may believe that tumor in periosteum or perichondrium, but with underlying grossly normal appearing cartilage or bone, requires no further surgery. Mohs technique on recurrent tumors is less successful than on previously treated patients with recurrent disease.

Although some patients will present with a large, fungating, previously untreated tumor (**Fig. 12.10**), most problem tumors seen by the head and neck oncological surgeon are going to be recurrences following prior Mohs excision or scalpel or hot knife excision (**Fig. 12.11**). The misconception by some surgeons that the presence of a positive margin following skin cancer excision is of no consequence is an utter fallacy. Irradiation of the tumor bed after incomplete excision is often

fraught with recurrence, and subsequent surgical salvage frequently presents one of the biggest challenges to the head and neck surgeon. The tumor depicted in **Fig. 12.12** is a recurrent squamous cell carcinoma of the scalp. This recurred despite the concerted efforts of an excellent Mohs surgeon and an experienced head and neck surgery team with postoperative radiation therapy. Margins on such recurrences have to be wide.

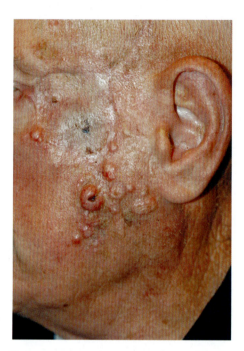

Fig. 12.11 Patient with an aggressive infiltrating basosquamous cell carcinoma of the lateral facial skin recurrent in the skin after multiple attempts at Mohs excision and conservative local resection and now with metastatic disease in the neck and parotid salivary gland.

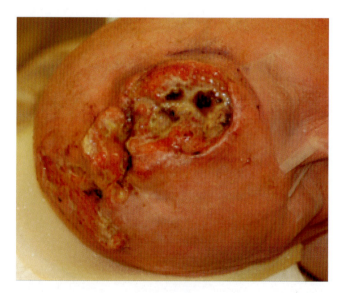

Fig. 12.12 Elderly man with recurrent squamous cell carcinoma in the scalp spreading to the calvarium and dura after repeated Mohs resections and postoperative irradiation.

Playing "catch-up" is a difficult problem. When in doubt take more tissue than you think. Cosmesis and the reconstructive effort are not a consideration until after the tumor exenteration is completed. Margins should not be hedged in these troublesome recurrent tumors.

An important principle of treatment of recurrent skin cancer is the necessity of being able to observe the operative site directly, unobscured by a reconstructive flap for at least 12 to 18 months after the definitive resection. The operative site should be covered with a split-thickness skin graft so that any early recurrence can be detected. Even when a partial or total rhinectomy has been done to completely excise the tumor, a skin graft and prosthesis should be used for coverage and cosmesis for a reasonable period of time until a reconstructive effort is initiated. Covering the resection site of a skin cancer, especially when there has been a failure of both repeated surgical excision and irradiation therapy, is a formula for disaster (**Fig. 12.13**).

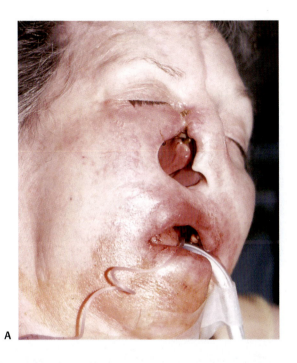

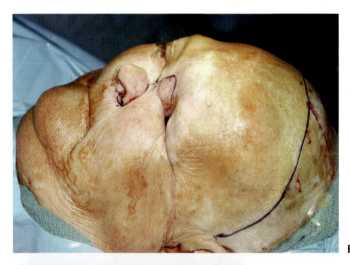

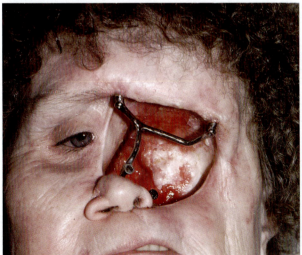

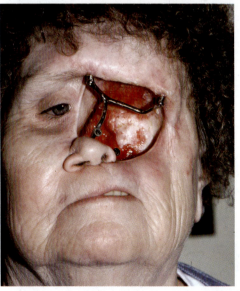

Fig. 12.13   (**A**) Patient with an aggressive basal cell carcinoma of the nose that had failed prior resection. A partial rhinectomy and immediate reconstruction was done using a midline forehead flap. Local recurrence evaded detection because of the obfuscation created by the flap. (**B**) Frontal view of patient just prior to attempt at salvage by anterior skull base approach. Blue marking outlines the cutaneous portion of tumor. (**C**) Calvarial bone flap and attached dura extensively invaded by tumor. (**D**) Patient after extensive craniofacial surgery including orbital exenteration. Metal frame in orbit is attached to implanted titanium fixtures for attachment of orbital-facial prosthesis.

In cancer of the facial skin an accompanying symptom of facial numbness is an ominous sign. **Figure 12.14** demonstrates magnetic resonance imaging (MRI) on a middle-aged man who had a squamous carcinoma of the cheek skin who within a year of excision complained of facial numbness. The symptom was passed over as "neuralgia" of some sort. The film displays marked enhancement of the infraorbital nerve by gadolinium suggesting perineural spread. A wide-field resection of facial skin, maxillectomy, and orbital exenteration were necessary to surgically encompass the tumor (**Fig. 12.15**). The perineural spread of cutaneous malignancy often extends far beyond the tumor's primary site. Unfortunately, current scanning methods can only predict gross tumor spread, and even then somewhat inconsistently.[22] However, a recent study of adenoid cystic perineural spread by Hanna et al[23] showed a high correlation with high-resolution computed tomographic (CT) scan and/or MRI and perineural spread as evidenced by nerve thickening or enhancement with gadolinium or foraminal erosion. Bone erosion of neural foramina is a late sign of perineural spread usually indicating spread far proximally from the nerve's exit from the skull (**Fig. 12.16**). **Figure 12.17** shows a man with the perineural spread of facial skin cancer that not only extended along the infraorbital nerve to the gasserian ganglion but also spread along the peripheral branches of V1+V3. He is now tumor free 7 years since his infratemporal fossa/middle fossa resection that included the anterior portion of the cavernous sinus and trigeminal ganglion.

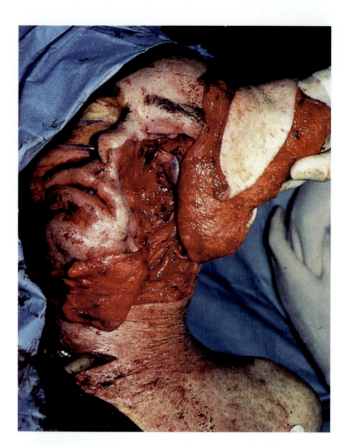

Fig. 12.15 Extensive surgery to eliminate tumor resulted in orbital exenteration and maxillectomy.

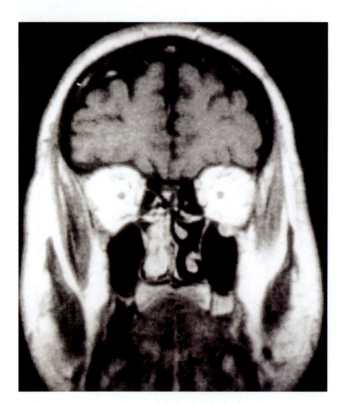

Fig. 12.14 Magnetic resonance imaging of a patient with a previously excised cutaneous squamous cell carcinoma who presented with facial numbness secondary to perineural spread along the infraorbital nerve.

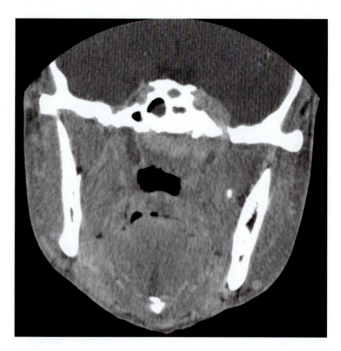

Fig. 12.16 Computed tomographic scan of patient with perineural spread of malignancy along the third division of the trigeminal nerve causing erosion of the foramen ovale. Tumor has spread from the dura of the Meckel cave to the cavernous sinus. ("Cavernous Sinus Malignancy" # 41).

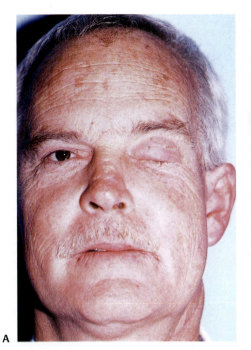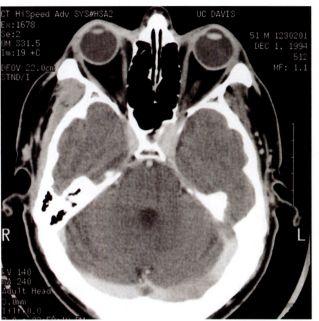

A

B

Fig. 12.17 (**A**) Patient with a history of carcinoma of the skin that invaded through the foramen rotundum to the gasserian ganglion and then antegrade to the cutaneous branches of V3. Patient is greater than 5 years post-partial resection of the cavernous sinus. (**B**) A computed tomographic scan showing cavernous sinus invasion.

◆ Treatment of Neck Metastases

As previously mentioned, neck metastasis from skin cancer is uncommon. From basal cell carcinoma it is a decided rarity, and it is very common in deeply invasive malignant melanoma and Merkel cell tumor, and only occasionally seen in squamous cell carcinoma. Neck metastasis follows on an only mildly predictive pattern. The use of sentinel node biopsy is still very much in the investigative stages as regards squamous carcinoma of the skin. As mentioned in chapter 8, the parotid nodes in the preauricular area are common sites for metastases from the temporal scalp, the auricle, and the lateral forehead region. Total parotidectomy coupled with a lateral temporal bone excision if the metastasis is close to the external auditory canal and a modified radical neck dissection including level 1 is the treatment of choice. Skin invasion requires a wide-field skin excision closed with either a facial rotation flap or a split-thickness skin graft.

Cancer of the lip, usually the lower lip, has less than a 10% incidence of lymph nodal metastasis.[24,25] Unfortunately the prognosis of these patients with this regional spread of disease is much worse than the more commonplace situation in which no metastasis occurs.[26] The spread is either to the submental or submandibular nodes (**Fig. 12.18**). A modified radical or radical neck dissection is done in these patients. Prophylactic neck dissection is not warranted in patients with no manifest neck nodes on palpation or CT scan. Scans are not usually done except in exceptionally large tumors in which bone erosion is suspected.

Squamous cell carcinoma of the scalp over the vertex or postauricular area may metastasize to the upper nodes in level 5. Dissection of the occipital nodes and those just under the trapezius muscle will also be usually necessary. Like the problem with melanoma, metastases from these parts of the scalp can be bilateral. Dissection of level 1 and 4 are usually not needed.

Reconstruction

For the simple straightforward case of skin cancer the options of reconstruction following resection are multiple and varied. They will only be touched upon because the purpose of the book is to discuss management of the difficult and complex case. The choices of closure of the wound vary from straight-line closure to the extreme of the transfer of free vascularized tissue. **Table 12.1** outlines the range of reconstructive options. In addition to wound closure by these methods another option that is commonly used in Mohs surgery of small wounds is closure by secondary intention, namely, letting the wound close over a period of time by the process of granulation and reepithelialization. This latter method is not applicable to the complex wounds under discussion in this chapter.

As previously stated, closure of defects created by extirpation of recurrent lesions following frequent surgical excision are best covered by a split-thickness skin graft. There are some instances when this is undesirable because of the need to protect vital structures or preserve function. This is particularly important when the eye is exposed or when dura or brain are open to a cavity such as a paranasal sinus or open to the environment as in calvarial resections for scalp carcinoma.

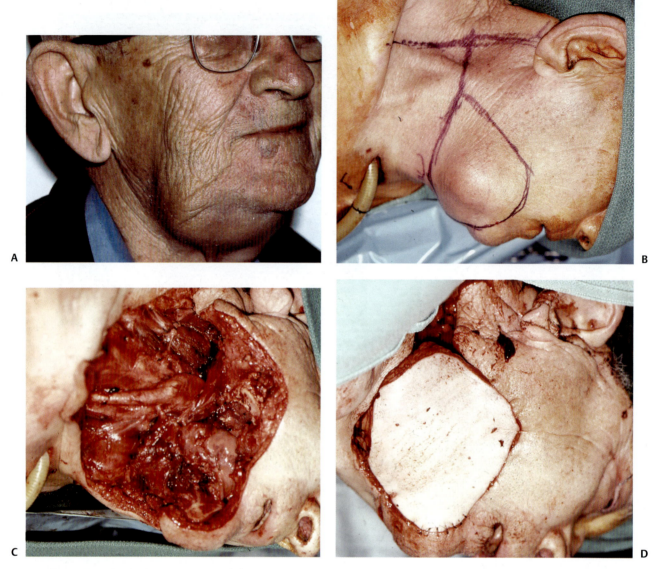

A

B

C

D

Fig. 12.18 (**A**) Elderly man with a metastasis from a carcinoma of the lip to the submandibular lymph node (the node of Star) that was stuck to the skin. (**B**) Despite a radical neck dissection, extensive skin excision, and (**C**) partial mandibulectomy, then (**D**) reconstruction with a pectoralis musculocutaneous flap, the patient died of pulmonary metastasis within the year.

Table 12.1 Reconstructive Choices in Closure of Cutaneous Wound

1. Primary closure	5. Musculocutaneous flaps
2. Skin grafts	a. Pectoralis
a. Split thickness	b. Trapezius
b. Full thickness	c. Sternomastoid
3. Local flaps	6. Free Flaps
a. Advancement	a. Radial forearm
b. Rotational	b. Thigh
c. Transposition	
4. Regional flaps	
a. Deltopectoral	
b. Forehead	
c. Nape of neck	

Case 1 (Figs. 12.19–12.26, pp. 423–425)

Mr. P.F. was a 60-year-old male with a history of multiple squamous cell carcinomas of the scalp that he had been troubled by for over 14 years. The site of the current problem was over the left temporal-parietal scalp where a cluster of tumors had persisted despite numerous attempts at local excision and skin grafting, then finally a full course of irradiation therapy. The last attempt to eradicate the tumor had been by Mohs resection but there had been positive margins on the calvarial periosteum. He presented to us for the first time with an open painless ulceration on the temporal-parietal scalp measuring 6 cm by 6 cm. A wide-field surgical excision of the previously placed skin graft and ulceration was done including a 10 cm by 10 cm resection of the outer table of the calvarium. The defect was then covered with a split-thickness graft.

He presented to us again 9 months later with a granulating defect following another series of Mohs excisions with persistent positive deep margins as depicted in **Fig. 12.19**.

A CT scan (**Fig. 12.20**) showed erosion of the bone under the cutaneous lesion. An attempt at conservative resection removing only the outer calvarial layer then grafting with split-thickness skin failed with a recurrence appearing ~9 months later.

A more aggressive resection was then attempted where a large section of scalp, skin graft, underlying calvarium, and dura were taken (**Fig. 12.21, Fig. 12.22**). All resection margins were negative. The dura was replaced with bovine pericardium (**Fig. 12.23**) and the resected calvarium with titanium mesh (**Fig. 12.24**). A 16 cm by 16 cm latissimus dorsi muscle microvascular free flap was placed to replace the missing scalp that was in turn covered by a split-thickness skin graft (**Fig. 12.25**). He has an excellent aesthetic and functional result and is now 2 years postoperative and free of disease (**Fig. 12.26**).

Discussion

This case is typical of the problem of the multifocal, pernicious scalp carcinoma that has recurred multiple times. Oftentimes the sun-damaged scalp skin resembles the scenario witnessed in the condemned mucosa of the upper aerodigestive tract seen in some smokers and drinkers who have had multiple primary mucosal carcinomas. Continuous surveillance is essential in such patients.

Repeated local application of topical 5-FU or other anticancer topical medications will rid the patient of most actinic keratosis and very superficially invasive cutaneous malignancies. Observation by the dermatologist or head and neck surgeon should be performed every 4 months, and monthly if the patient has had a neck dissection for cervical metastatic disease. When such tumors penetrate deeply into the galea and particularly when they invade the periosteum, the Mohs technique is much less successful than deep primary excision.

Case 2 (Figs. 12.27–12.32, pp. 426–427)

G.W. is a 59-year-old male who presented to his dermatologist with an 8-year history of a slowly growing nodular mass in the premastoid skin. The mass was slightly painful and had ulcerated and was periodically bleeding. On examination he had an ulcerated postauricular mass measuring ~4 cm in diameter. Biopsy revealed a basal cell carcinoma of the morphea type. An attempt at a radical Mohs excision was thwarted by persistent positive margins in the external auditory canal and in the tissues deep to the mastoid tip (**Fig. 12.27, Fig. 12.28**). A CT scan done before he presented to UCD revealed tumor in the external auditory canal skin but not extending to the tympanic membrane (**Fig. 12.29**).

A complete full-thickness excision of the prior scalp resection was carried down to bone (**Fig. 12.30**). Resection of the soft tissue in the infraauricular region extended to the facial nerve at which point negative margins were obtained. The parotid gland was not involved with tumor and was spared. A wide margin of scalp, neck skin, and underlying muscle was resected. A lateral temporal bone excision was executed with the osseous margin of resection ~3 mm lateral to the tympanic annulus (**Fig. 12.31**).

The wound was covered with a split-thickness skin graft. A free flap was not used because of the fear of covering any possible local recurrence. In ~18 to 24 months a free flap will be used to replace the skin graft if the patient desires. The patient is now 18 months postoperative and is disease free (**Fig. 12.32**).

Discussion

All tumor was encompassed by this aggressive procedure. The lateral temporal bone resection could spare the tympanic membrane because there was no evidence of mastoid extension of tumor and no invasion of the bone of the external auditory canal. Because the tumor was a basal cell carcinoma in contrast to a squamous cell cancer, the deep lobe of the parotid was spared. Because of the worry of the unavailability of early detection of a possible recurrence of disease if the defect were covered by flap, a split thickness skin graft was used. It is not uncommon for patients to decide against further reconstruction, as they are content with the appearance of the graft.

Case 3 (Figs. 12.33 and 12.34, p. 427)

T.C. was a 45-year-old man with a 10- to 12-year history of a slowly growing mass on the side of his face. At presentation he had a 12- to 14-cm lesion on the facial skin that was deeply invasive into the underlying soft tissue and zygoma (**Fig. 12.33**). Biopsy showed basal cell carcinoma. Surgical excision required removal of the skin of the side of the face up to the lateral canthus of the eye, over the forehead and parotid, down to the jaw line. Posteriorly, the preauricular and postauricular skin, as well as the pinna, was removed. A parotidectomy, resection of the temporalis and masseter muscles, as well as the zygoma, mandibular condyle, and a portion of the nose were required to clear the deep margins (**Fig. 12.34**). The wound was covered with a split-thickness skin graft to the external auditory canal, and the remainder of the wound was covered with a pectoralis major musculocutaneous flap. A revisional operation was required 2 months later because of two recurrences at the margin of the first resection. The patient is now over 6 years postoperative and free of disease.

Discussion

The latter two cases were examples of long-neglected tumors that despite their extensive nature were successfully resected. Case 3 had a local recurrence at ~2 months postoperatively as well as a second primary tumor in the scalp. These were resected and reconstructed with split-thickness skin grafts.

Two further resections for basal cell carcinomas and squamous cell carcinomas were done over the next 3 months. The appearance of multiple lymph nodal metastases 5 months from his initial procedure culminated in the performance of a radical neck dissection. He has done very well over the ensuing 4 years and has remained tumor free.

Case 4 (Figs. 12.35–12.38, pp. 427–428)

E.P. is an 82-year-old female who presented to her dermatologist with a "4-month history" of a mass on the right side of her face (**Fig. 12.35**). The mass was painless and had superficial erosion. She was fair skinned and had spent much of her life outdoors in California. Her state of systemic good health was exemplified by the fact that she had finally quit playing tennis just 2 years prior to presentation. On examination she had a deeply invasive squamous cell carcinoma of the skin of the lower face measuring 6 cm in diameter that extended almost to the periosteum of the mandible and was adherent to the buccal mucosa as well as penetrating the facial skin. The lower lip was invaded but the upper lip was spared.

Mohs surgery was preformed that resulted in a deep defect of the skin overlying the mandible just shy of the periosteum then through and through the facial skin and underlying buccal mucosa that included the lateral one third of the lower lip and commissure (**Fig. 12.36**).

Reconstruction consisted of primary approximation of the buccal mucosa then reestablishing the continuity of the oral sphincter by the use of a cross-lip Stein-Estlander flap (**Fig. 12.37**). The cheek defect was restored by the construction of a cervicofacial rotation flap that was swung into the defect (**Fig. 12.38**). The skin provided the necessary coverage and the subcutaneous fat and platysma muscle the missing bulk of buccal fat.

Discussion

The lack of recognition and/or denial of her facial carcinoma is seen not uncommonly in such patients as typified by the "4-month history" given by this otherwise alert, intelligent patient. Perhaps the lack of pain often experienced by such patients with these usually slowly growing lesions is responsible for this seeming self-neglect.

The lack of oral continuity experienced after Mohs surgery is a distressing symptom. Reestablishing the integrity of the oral sphincter is paramount even at the expense of microstomia, which fortunately was not a problem in this patient. The large rotation flap may on the surface appear to be excessive in extent, but when rotated into the large defect it ultimately provided excellent coverage. These flaps require a pedicle that is at least the diameter of the long axis of the defect, thus the large flap size. Such a tension-free closure allows excellent healing and a favorable aesthetic appearance.

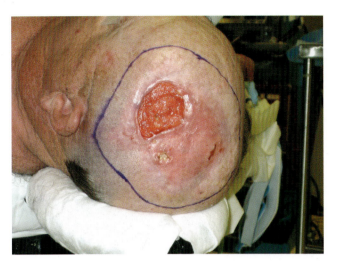

Fig. 12.19 *Case 1* Patient with Mohs excision for recurrent squamous cell carcinoma of the scalp with positive margins on the calvarium.

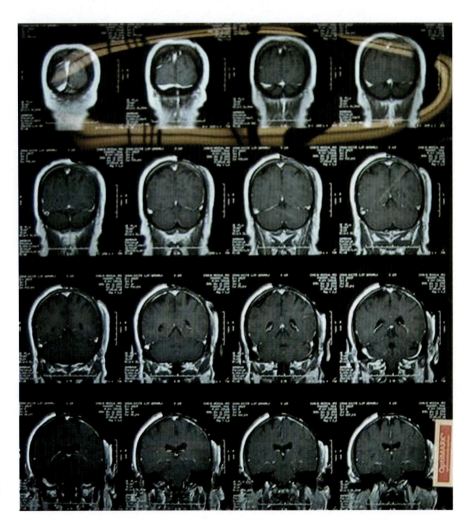

Fig. 12.20 *Case 1* Computed tomographic scan coronal view showing bone erosion of the calvarium.

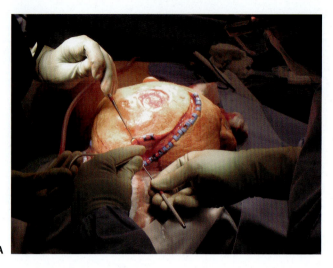

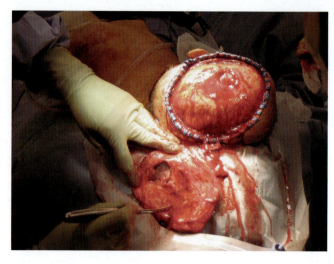

Fig. 12.21 *Case 1* (**A**) Resection of scalp, galea, and pericranium is begun. (**B**) Resection is completed. The central part of the tumor is still attached to calvarium and dura.

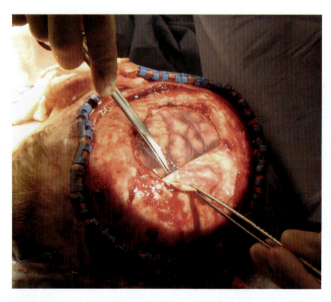

Fig. 12.22 *Case 1* Craniectomy completed and affected dura resected.

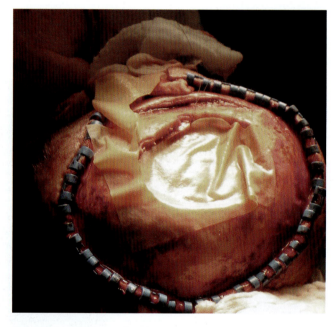

Fig. 12.23 *Case 1* Dural replacement with bovine pericardial graft.

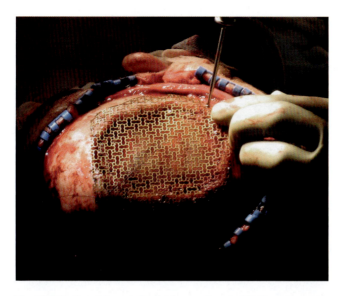

Fig. 12.24 *Case 1* Resected calvarium replaced with titanium mesh.

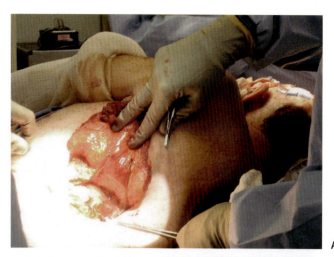

A

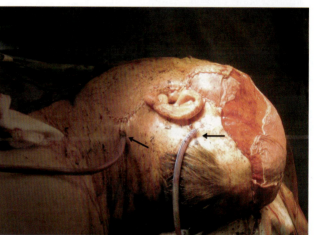

B

Fig. 12.25 *Case 1* (**A**) Reconstruction using latissimus dorsi muscle free flap covered with split-thickness skin. (**B**) Appearance after reconstruction completed. *Arrows* point to suction drains.

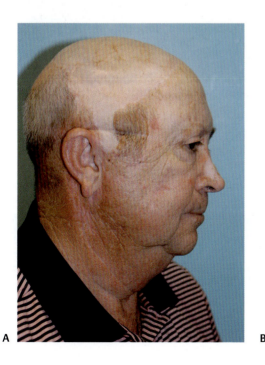

A

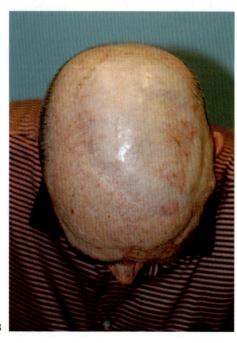

B

Fig. 12.26 *Case 1* Patient 2 years postoperatively with no evidence of local recurrence. (**A**) Lateral view. (**B**) Top view of skull.

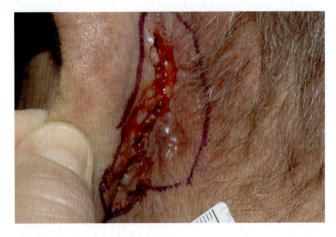

Fig. 12.27 *Case 2* Patient with large morphea type basal cell carcinoma of the postauricular skin previously treated by Mohs excision but with positive margins.

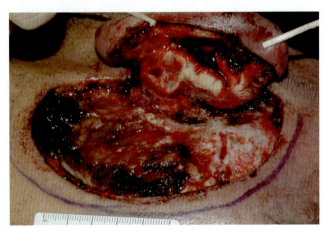

Fig. 12.28 *Case 2* Wound after aggressive Mohs resection but still with positive margins on the cartilage of the external auditory canal and mastoid periosteum.

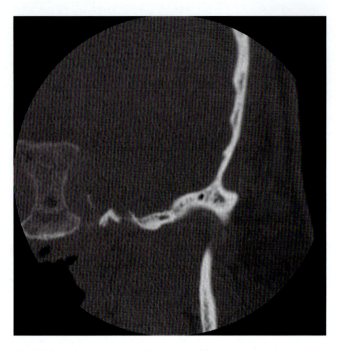

Fig. 12.29 *Case 2* Computed tomographic scan, coronal view illustrating tumor eroding through the auricular cartilage into the external auditory canal.

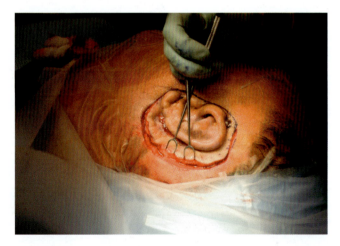

Fig. 12.30 *Case 2* Excision outlined to include auricle, scalp, and lateral temporal bone.

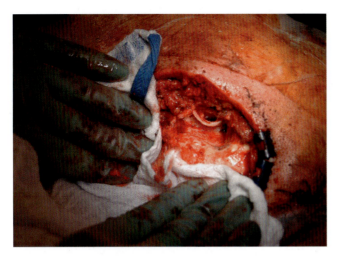

Fig. 12.31 *Case 2* Full-thickness scalp excision, auriculectomy including partial resection trapezius and upper aspect of sternocleidomastoid muscle. Mastoidectomy done with skeletonization of the external auditory canal ready for lateral temporal bone excision.

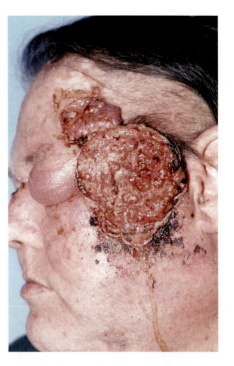

Fig. 12.33 *Case 3* Large neglected squamous cell carcinoma of the facial skin present for 10 to 12 years.

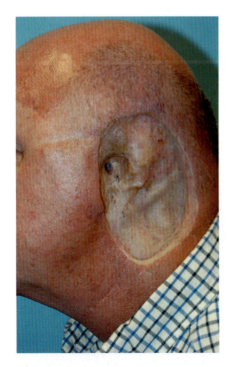

Fig. 12.32 *Case 2* Patient disease free 18 months later.

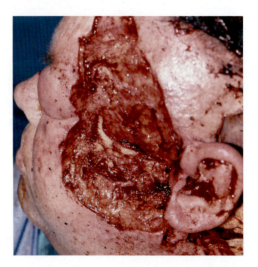

Fig. 12.34 *Case 3* Defect following wide-field resection. A revisional operation had to be done 6 weeks later because of a local recurrence.

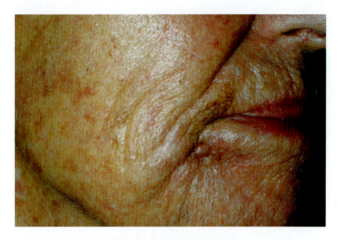

Fig. 12.35 *Case 4* Large deeply infiltrative basal cell carcinoma of the skin of the lower face adjacent to oral commissure.

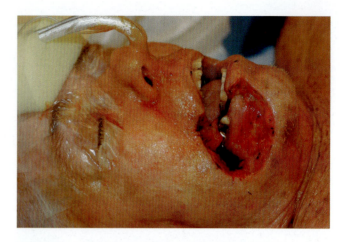

Fig. 12.36 *Case 4* Defect following Mohs resection.

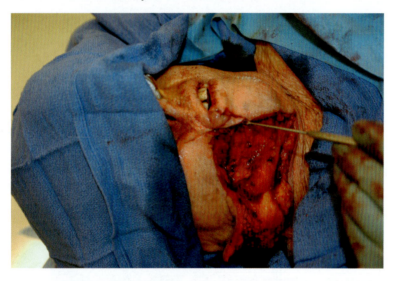

Fig. 12.37 *Case 4* Stein-Estlander flap used for lip reconstruction. Commissure-plasty to be done at a future time.

Fig. 12.38 *Case 4* Buccal mucosal closure done with local advancement flaps. Cutaneous closure achieved with a cervicofacial rotation flap. (**A**) Stein-Estlander flap and rotation flaps turned. (**B**) Reconstruction completed.

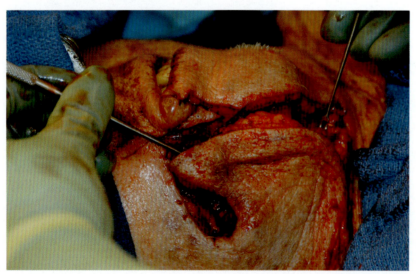

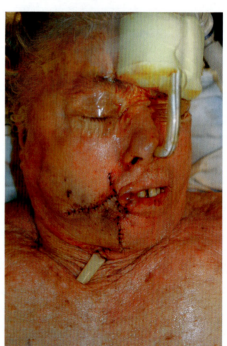

A

B

References

1. Gellin GA, Kopf GW, Garfinkle L. Basal cell epithelioma. Arch Dermatol 1965;91:38–45

2. Gailani MR, Leffel DJ, Ziegler A, et al. Relationship between sunlight exposure and a key genetic alteration in basal cell carcinoma. J Natl Cancer Inst 1996;88:349–354

3. Lambert DR, Siegle RJ. Skin cancer: a review with consideration of treatment options including Moh's micrographic surgery. Ohio Med 1990;86:745–747

4. Buettner PG, Raasch B. Incidence rates of skin cancer in Townsville, Australia. Int J Cancer 1998;78:587–593

5. Sober AJ, Burstein JM. Precursors to skin cancer. Cancer 1995; 75(2, Suppl)645–650

6. Tang CK, Toker C. Trabecular carcinoma of the skin: an ultrastructural study. Cancer 1978;42:2311–2321

7. Tavin E, Persky M. Metastatic squamous cell carcinoma of the head and neck region. Laryngoscope 1996;106(2, pt. 1):156–158

8. Joseph MG, Zulueta WP, Kennedy PJ. Squamous cell carcinoma of the skin: the incidence of metastases and their outcome. ANZ J Surg 1992;62:697–701

9. Czarnecki D, Staples M, Mar A, Giles G, Meehan C. Metastases from squamous cell carcinoma of the skin in Southern Australia. Dermatology 1994;189:52–54

10. Ruhoy SM, Flynn KJ, DeGuzman MJ, et al. Pathology of selected skin lesions of the head and neck. In: Barnes L, ed. Surgical Pathology of the Head and Neck. Vol 3. 2nd ed. New York: Marcel Dekker; 1985:1802–1809

11. Lund HZ. How often does squamous cell carcinoma of the skin metastasize? Arch Dermatol 1965;92:635–637

12. Veness MJ, Porceddu S, Palme CE, Morgan GJ. Cutaneous head and neck carcinoma metastatic to parotid and cervical lymph nodes. Head Neck 2007;29:621–631

13. Rowe DE, Carroll RJ, Day CD. Prognostic factors for local recurrence, metastasis, and survival rates in squamous cell carcinoma of the skin, ear and lip. J Am Acad Dermatol 1992;26:976–990

14. Kraus DH, Carew JF, Harrison LB. Regional lymph node metastasis from cutaneous squamous cell carcinoma of skin and vermillion surface. Arch Otolaryngol Head Neck Surg 1998;55:287–292

15. Breuninger H, Black R, Rassner G. Brief scientific statement: microstaging of squamous cell carcinomas of the skin. Am J Clin Pathol 1990;94:624–627

16. Cherpelis BS, Marcusen C, Lang PG. Prognostic factors for metastasis in squamous cell carcinoma of the skin. Dermatol Surg 2002;28:268–273

17. Mohs FE. Mohs micrographic surgery: a historical perspective. Dermatol Clin 1989;7:609–612

18. Mohs FE. Microscopically controlled surgery for skin cancer-past, present and future. J Dermatol Surg Oncol 1978;4:41–53

19. Mohs FE. Chemosurgery: Microscopically Controlled Surgery for Skin Cancer. Springfield, IL: Charles C Thomas; 1978

20. Tromovitch TA, Stegman SJ. Microscopically controlled excision of skin tumors: (Mohs) fresh technique. Arch Dermatol 1974;110:231–232

21. Tromovitch TA, Stegman SJ. Microscopically controlled excision of cutaneous tumors: fresh tissue technique. Cancer 1978;41:653–658

22. Nemzek WR, Hecht S, Gandour-Edwards R, Donald PJ, Mckennan K. The perineural spread of head and neck tumors: how accurate is MR imaging? AJNR Am J Neuroradiol 1998;19:701–706

23. Hanna E, Vural E, Prokopakis E, Carrau Rsnyderman C, Weissman J. The sensitivity and specificity of high-resolution imaging in evaluating perineural spread of adenoid cystic carcinoma to the skull base. Arch Otolaryngol Head Neck Surg 2007;133:541–545

24. Zitsch RP III. Carcinoma of the lip. Otolaryngol Clin North Am 1993; 26:265–267

25. Zitsch RP III, Park CW, Renner GJ, Rea JL. Outcome analysis for lip carcinoma. Otolaryngol Head Neck Surg 1995;113:589–596

26. Baker SR, Krause CJ. Carcinoma of the lip. Laryngoscope 1980;90:19–25

13

Advances in Radiotherapy for Head and Neck Cancer

Rachel H. Chou and Richard B. Wilder

Cancers of the head and neck region constitute 3% of all cancers, with ~40,000 new cases each year in the United States.[1] Smoking is the most common cause of head and neck cancer.[2] Alcohol abuse and poor oral hygiene also constitute common risk factors.[2] The role of genetic abnormalities are just now beginning to be elucidated. For example, p53 gene mutations are frequently observed in patients with head and neck cancer.[3,4] Epstein-Barr virus (EBV) or human papilloma virus type 6, 11, 16, and 18 infection may also play a role in the development of head and neck cancer.[2,5]

Treatment should involve a multidisciplinary team that provides prospective treatment recommendations and delivers dental care along with nutritional, psychological, and social support. The aims of a multidisciplinary approach are to maximize disease-free and overall survival while minimizing morbidity.

This chapter discusses general principles of radiation therapy and clinical applications. Many head and neck sites are discussed specifically, with an emphasis on technically challenging cases and recent advances.

◆ Radiation Physics and Biology and Radiotherapy

Radiotherapy has been used to treat cancer for over a century. Recently, important advances have been made in radiation physics and biology.

The most commonly used unit to describe the dose of radiation is the gray (1 Gy = 100 cGy = 100 rads), which refers to the energy deposited in tissue per unit mass (J/kg).

The most commonly used machines for external beam radiotherapy (EBRT) are linear accelerators. These machines produce photons (x-rays). A penetrating, high-energy (4 to 6 MV), x-ray beam is used to help reduce the dose of radiation that is delivered to the skin. In contrast, electrons or superficial x-rays have a more limited depth of penetration

in tissue and are only suitable for treating superficial lesions. Cobalt-60 machines are less popular because the beam edges are less sharp than those from linear accelerators. This makes it more difficult to safely match fields and spare critical adjacent normal structures such as the spinal cord. Radiation therapy can also be delivered using brachytherapy, which involves the implantation of radioisotopes such as iridium-192 (Ir-192) or cesium-137 (Cs-137) directly into unresectable cancers. With cobalt-60 or brachytherapy, gamma rays are emitted by the radioactive sources. Gamma rays have the same biological effect as x-rays.

At a small number of facilities around the world, charged particles such as protons or heavy ions are used. In contrast to photons or gamma rays, most of the energy is absorbed at the end of the particles' path through tissue (Bragg-peak phenomenon). The dose unit for charged particles is Gy equivalent (GyE). **Figure 13.1** compares the energy deposition patterns for 15 MV photons, 9 MeV electrons, 30 MeV neutrons, 160 MeV protons, and Ir-192. Charged particle therapy has not substantially gained in popularity, in part, because the equipment costs tens of millions of dollars to purchase and maintain. Also, the number of indications where charged particle therapy is advantageous over traditional radiotherapeutic techniques is limited: unresectable skull base and cervical spine tumors and choroidal melanomas. Results with charged particle therapy are presented in the Base of Skull section.

Histopathologically, vacuolation, swelling, nuclear pyknosis, and karyolysis eventually leading to cell death occur in response to radiotherapy.[6] Loss of function and mitotic ability are the major radiation effects at the cellular level.[7] Loss of function can be due to radiation-induced mutations or interphase cell death. Interphase cell death is also referred to as apoptosis or "programmed cell death."

Repair, repopulation, reoxygenation, and reassortment play important roles in the response of cancers to radiotherapy.[7] One can take advantage of the ability of normal tissue to repair itself more quickly than a cancer by delivering mul-

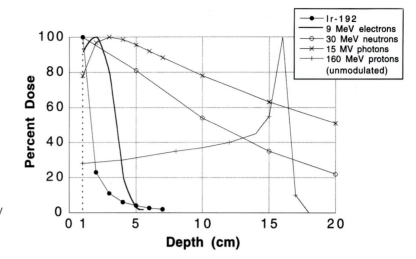

Fig. 13.1 Energy deposition patterns of 15 MV photons, 9 MeV electrons, 30 MeV neutrons, 160 MeV protons and Ir-192. (Courtesy of Mike Mulan, Ph.D., in the Department of Radiation Oncology at the Duke University Medical Center in Durham, NC.)

tiple, small doses of radiation over several weeks as opposed to a single, large dose of radiation in 1 day. Because cancer cells may start to repopulate more rapidly toward the end of a course of radiotherapy, two radiotherapy treatments rather than one may be delivered each day over the last 2 to 2.5 weeks of radiotherapy to increase cell killing. Hypoxic cancer cells are more resistant to radiotherapy. Reoxygenation of a poorly vascularized cancer due to changes in its blood supply can make it more radiosensitive. When radiotherapy is delivered over 1 day as opposed to several weeks, there may not be enough time for tumor reoxygenation to occur, reducing the effectiveness of the treatment. Normal tissues contain relatively few hypoxic cells. Oxygen increases the number of radiation-induced free radicals, which in turn damage cancer cells' DNA. *Reassortment* refers to the redistribution of cells into various phases of the cell cycle in response to radiation injury. The G_2 and M phases of the cell cycle are the most radiosensitive. By delivering radiotherapy over several weeks, cancer cells may be more likely to reassort themselves into the radiosensitive phases of the cell cycle during treatment.

Based on clinical experience, fractionation (i.e., the delivery of multiple, small rather than a single, large dose of radiation) has constituted a cornerstone of radiotherapy since the 1920s. Recently, there has been interest in altered fractionation schedules that differ from the traditional, once-a-day approach. The rationale for and results with altered fractionation are summarized in the Therapeutic Doses of Radiation: Microscopic versus Gross Disease section below.

◆ Clinical Applications of Radiotherapy

When early-stage disease has been treated with radiotherapy, two to three fields have traditionally been used. For more advanced disease, a three-field technique has traditionally been used, which includes coverage of the primary site as well as regional lymph nodes. The three fields typically include two opposed, lateral fields matched with an anterior, low anterior neck field.

Based on recent technical advances, newer techniques that differ from the traditional two- to three-field approach have been used to increase the likelihood of cure. One of the newer techniques is three-dimensional conformal radiotherapy (3D-CRT), wherein sophisticated computer programming is used to determine the optimal beam shape and field arrangement. A recent beam-collimating device known as a multileaf collimator allows for collimation of the x-ray beam during treatment. Using computer guidance, "dynamic" multileaf collimators can change shape during treatment, giving rise to intensity-modulated radiation therapy (IMRT). With IMRT, radiation therapy can be delivered more conformally than with 3D-CRT, allowing for the delivery of higher doses to the cancer. Both 3D-CRT and, more recently, IMRT are being used by leading radiation oncology centers throughout the world to treat head and neck cancer. Intraoperative radiation therapy (IORT) involves the delivery of a single, large dose of radiation to a target defined by the otolaryngologist in the operating room. IORT has been used at some centers in the treatment of advanced or recurrent head and neck cancers. As previously noted, brachytherapy and particle beam therapy have also been used to deliver conformal radiotherapy to head and neck cancers. Radiation oncology training programs in Europe and Canada tend to emphasize brachytherapy more than those in the United States, where fractionated EBRT remains popular.

Tissue Tolerance to Radiotherapy

Inherent to the safe delivery of radiotherapy is an understanding of the tolerance of critical normal structures. Tolerance depends upon many factors, including the volume of tissue irradiated, the dose per fraction, the total radiation dose, the delivery of chemotherapy, and coexisting medical conditions such as diabetes mellitus. The main, dose-limiting structures are the spinal cord, brain, optic nerves, optic chiasm, and retinas. Rubin and Casarett have suggested that a 5% risk of severe complications 5 years postirradiation ($TD_{5/5}$) be used as a method of expressing normal tissue tolerance.[8]

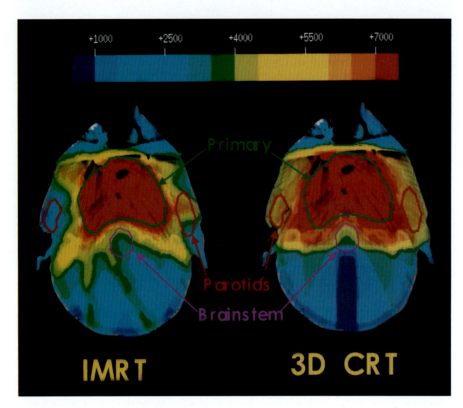

Fig. 13.2 Axial computed tomographic scan through the normal parotid glands in a patient with nasopharynx cancer. Colors are used to represent the dose (cGy) of radiation delivered with intensity modulated radiation therapy (left) versus three-dimensional conformal radiotherapy (3D-CRT) (right). Note that less normal tissue surrounding the primary tumor is treated to a high dose with intensity modulated radiation therapy than with 3D-CRT. (Courtesy of Kenneth Forster, Ph.D., in the Department of Physics at the University of Texas M. D. Anderson Cancer Center in Houston, Texas.)

Similarly, $TD_{50/5}$ is defined as a 50% risk of severe complications 5 years postirradiation.

In general, an attempt is made to limit the dose of radiation delivered to the spinal cord to 45.0 to 50.0 Gy when either 1.8 or 2.0 Gy is administered daily.[9] When part of the brain is included in the radiation fields, the dose should not exceed 60 Gy to limit the risk of necrosis to 5% at 5 years.[10] At many institutions, tolerance of the optic chiasm and optic nerves is considered to be 54 Gy in 30 fractions over 6 weeks.[11] When retina is included in the radiation fields, the dose should be limited to 45 Gy because retinal damage with eventual visual loss has been reported with higher doses.[12]

Though the salivary glands are generally not considered to be the "dose-limiting structures," EBRT to both parotid glands to ~30.0 Gy at 1.8 to 2.0 Gy per fraction results in permanently decreased salivation.[13] Xerostomia can be chronically bothersome to patients and increases their risk of developing caries. Prevention of xerostomia is more helpful than treatment. With regard to prevention, the most recent technical advance in radiation treatment planning is IMRT,[13,14] which allows one to conform the high-dose region to the cancer while minimizing the dose of radiation that is delivered to normal structures such as the radiosensitive parotid glands (see **Fig. 13.2 and Fig. 13.3**).

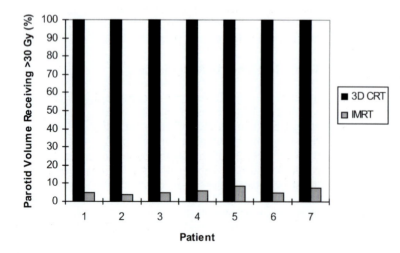

Fig. 13.3 Histogram illustrating that a much smaller volume of the parotid glands is treated to > 30 Gy with intensity-modulated radiation therapy than with three-dimensional conformal radiotherapy in seven consecutive patients with nasopharyngeal carcinoma. (Courtesy of Kenneth Forster, Ph.D., in the Department of Physics at the University of Texas MD Anderson Cancer Center in Houston, Texas.)

The dose delivered to a lacrimal gland should be limited to 30 Gy, if possible, to minimize the risk of a dry eye. The dose delivered to the mandible should be limited to 70 Gy to minimize the risk of osteoradionecrosis.[15] When the mandible is included in the radiotherapy fields, teeth extractions should be done prior to radiotherapy to reduce the risk of complications.

Therapeutic Doses of Radiation: Microscopic versus Gross Disease

In general, 44 to 50 Gy at 1.8 to 2.0 Gy per fraction is administered to regions with ≥ 15% risk of harboring microscopic disease.[16] Sixty-six to 70 Gy is usually prescribed for primary tumors measuring ≤ 2 cm that are associated with little or no lymphadenopathy.[17] For more advanced disease, doses ≥ 70 Gy are necessary to control the primary tumor and involved nodes when radiotherapy alone is delivered.[17] As a rule of thumb, the dose of radiation required for locoregional control increases as tumor size increases. For lymphadenopathy, EBRT alone can control over 90% of neck nodes ≤ 2 cm.[17] For lymph nodes measuring 3 cm, EBRT to doses ≥ 70 Gy controls only ~80% of nodes.[17] Lymph nodes that are larger than 3 to 4 cm are rarely controlled with EBRT alone and usually require a planned neck dissection. However, there are two exceptions: lymph node metastases due to nasopharyngeal or tonsillar carcinoma are more radiosensitive than metastases arising from primary tumors at other sites.

Locoregional control in advanced head and neck cancers is suboptimal when radiotherapy alone is administered using a once-a-day schedule. For radiobiological reasons, altered fractionation schedules, where two to three doses of radiation are delivered daily (≥ 6 hours apart to reduce toxicity), have been actively explored in the treatment of advanced head and neck cancer. "Hyperfractionation," which typically refers to twice-a-day fractionation (e.g., 1.2 Gy twice a day), throughout the course of radiotherapy, has been used as a way of decreasing the risk of late complications while achieving the same or better tumor control. "Accelerated fractionation" aims to decrease overall treatment time to reduce repopulation in rapidly proliferating cancers. One variant of this approach that was developed at the University of Texas M.D. Anderson Cancer Center, which is known as the "concomitant boost technique," consists of the delivery of twice-a-day treatments during the last 2 to 2.5 weeks of radiotherapy when tumor cells may begin to repopulate more rapidly. "Accelerated hyperfractionation" has also been studied as a way of increasing tumor cell killing without increasing the risk of late complications. Multiple trials have suggested that there is a benefit to altered fractionation (e.g., hyperfractionation or accelerated fractionation), compared with conventional, once-a-day fractionation.[18–24] The Radiation Therapy Oncology Group (RTOG) recently reported the 2-year results of a prospective, randomized trial (Protocol 9003) involving 1113 patients that compared once-a-day fractionation with hyperfractionation and two variants of accelerated fractionation.[24] In this study, stage III to IV cancers arising in the oral cavity, oropharynx, hypopharynx, or supraglottic larynx were examined (stage II base of tongue and hypopharynx cancers were also included). There was a trend toward improved locoregional control ($p = 0.07$) and disease-free survival ($p = 0.07$) with hyperfractiona-

tion compared with once-a-day fractionation. In addition, there was a significant advantage in terms of locoregional control ($p = 0.03$) and disease-free survival ($p = 0.04$) with the concomitant boost technique compared with once-a-day fractionation. As a result, the concomitant boost technique will constitute the control arm on future RTOG phase III trials for locally advanced head and neck cancers.

Preoperative versus Postoperative Radiotherapy

In general, early stages of head and neck cancer only require surgery or radiotherapy. For advanced lesions, however, both surgery and radiotherapy are necessary to maximize the likelihood of cure. Theoretical advantages of preoperative EBRT include the following: (1) the vascular supply remains intact, reducing the number of radioresistant, hypoxic cells in the cancer, thereby allowing a lower dose of radiation to be delivered; and (2) the sterilization of tumor cells that may be spilled at the time of surgery and give rise to metastases. There are several advantages of postoperative EBRT, including (1) pathological information from the surgery allows for the delivery of a higher dose of radiation to the area at greatest risk for recurrence; (2) fewer infections and wound complications develop; and (3) the treatment does not obscure the initial extent of disease and inappropriately lead to a more conservative resection. Postoperative radiotherapy should, in general, be initiated within 4 to 6 weeks of surgery.

Several studies have addressed the issue of preoperative versus postoperative radiotherapy. RTOG 73–03 randomized patients with advanced, operable squamous cell carcinoma of the supraglottic larynx or hypopharynx to receive either preoperative EBRT to 50 Gy or postoperative EBRT to 60 Gy. Patients with primary tumors in the oral cavity or oropharynx were randomized to preoperative EBRT, postoperative EBRT, or definitive radiation therapy to 65 to 70 Gy at 1.8 to 2.0 Gy per fraction.[25,26] Three-hundred and twenty patients were evaluable, with a medium follow-up of 60 months. Locoregional control was significantly better in the postoperative than in the preoperative group (65% vs 48%, $p = 0.04$).[25] When patterns of failure were analyzed, there were more local failures in the preoperative group than in the postoperative group during the first 2 years. However, after 2 years, distant metastases and second primary tumors predominated. Because of the shift in the pattern of failure and increase in intercurrent deaths with longer follow-up, no overall survival advantage was observed in the postoperative group.

Postoperative radiotherapy is generally indicated when patients have pathological evidence of extracapsular extension, a single positive node larger than 3 cm; multiple positive lymph nodes; close or positive margins; invasion of cartilage, bone, muscles, or blood vessels; or extensive subglottic extension, or when patients have undergone emergent tracheostomy with tumor cut-through.

Radiotherapy for Cancers of Specific Head and Neck Sites

Most of the cancers arising from the upper aerodigestive tract are squamous cell carcinomas or variants such as lymphoepithelioma or verrucous carcinoma. Mucoepidermoid carcinomas, malignant mixed tumors, adenoid cystic carcinomas, and adenocarcinomas are commonly found in the major and minor salivary glands. Overall, the management of an individual head and neck cancer patient depends upon many factors. Consequently, the following discussion should only be used as a general guideline for the management of such patients.

Nasopharynx

Cancers of the nasopharynx are primarily treated by chemoradiation because of their potential for spread to retropharyngeal nodes, making complete resection unlikely without undue morbidity. Also, nasopharyngeal cancer is more radiosensitive than cancers arising from other head and neck sites. It is relatively uncommon in North America compared with Southeast Asia. The etiology is multifactorial, including EBV infection and genetic factors. Unlike other head and neck cancers, it is not strongly associated with tobacco or alcohol abuse. Common presenting signs are unilateral hearing impairment, cervical adenopathy, otitis media, nasal obstruction, epistaxis, and/or cranial nerve palsies.

The nasopharynx has a rich lymphatic plexus, resulting in 50% bilateral neck involvement and 85 to 90% unilateral neck involvement at presentation.[27] Primary lymphatic drainage is to (1) parapharyngeal "junctional" nodes leading to the lateral, retropharyngeal "nodes of Rouvière"; (2) the jugular chain (especially the subdigastric nodes); and (3) spinal accessory nodes in the posterior neck. Patients with nasopharyngeal cancer have a relatively high incidence of distant metastases (e.g., to lungs or bones). As a result, they should be staged thoroughly prior to definitive chemoradiation.[28]

Most patients with cancers of the nasopharynx present with advanced disease. Therefore, a computed tomographic (CT) or magnetic resonance imaging (MRI) scan or both should be used to fully evaluate the extent of the disease, with special attention to the base of skull (the incidence of base of skull involvement at presentation is 25 to 33%). Nasopharyngeal carcinoma used to be treated with EBRT alone. Despite relatively good locoregional control with radiotherapy alone, the 5-year overall survival rates for stages III and IV were poor (36 to 58%) due to the high incidence of distant metastases.[29–34] Consequently, a randomized, intergroup study (number 0099) was conducted comparing radiotherapy alone versus radiation plus concurrent cisplatin chemotherapy for three cycles followed by 5-fluorouracil and cisplatin for three additional cycles.[35] The radiation doses in both arms were 70 Gy in 35 to 39 fractions, once-a-day, 5 days per week. At 3 years, the progression-free survival was significantly ($p < 0.001$) better in the combined modality group (69%) than in the radiotherapy alone group (24%). In addition, at 3 years, overall survival rate was better ($p < 0.001$) in the combined modality group (76%) than in the radiotherapy alone group (46%). Based on these results, the standard treatment for stage III and IV nasopharyngeal carcinoma is radiotherapy with concurrent cisplatin followed by 5-fluorouracil and cisplatin chemotherapy.

For stage I and II nasopharyngeal carcinoma, the role of chemotherapy is less well established. Five-year local control and overall survival rates for early-stage disease treated with radiotherapy alone are 82 to 100% and 48 to 76%, respectively.[30,31,36] Identification of a subset of early-stage patients who are at high risk for distant metastases may allow physicians to select which patients may benefit from chemotherapy.[37]

The recent development of IMRT has allowed radiation oncologists to escalate the dose of radiation delivered to tumors while minimizing the dose of radiation delivered to normal organs such as the parotid glands (see **Fig. 13.2 and Fig. 13.3**).[13,14,38]

If nasopharyngeal carcinoma recurs, retreatment with radiotherapy has been undertaken in patients who refused surgery and had recurrent disease confined to the nasopharynx or had only limited extension to the adjacent parapharyngeal space or base of skull. Five-year overall survival rates with this approach range from 21 to 55%.[39–42] However, severe complication rates are high, ranging from 4 to 34%.[40,41,43,44] Therefore, newer treatment techniques including IMRT with or without chemotherapy as a radiosensitizer are presently being investigated as treatment options for recurrent nasopharyngeal cancer in patients who elect not to undergo surgical salvage.[14,45]

Oral Cavity

Oral cavity structures include the lips, oral tongue, floor of mouth, hard palate, buccal mucosa, upper and lower gingiva, and retromolar trigone. Each of these sites is discussed separately.

Lip

Carcinoma of the lip is usually localized, spreading by direct invasion into surrounding soft tissue. Primary lymphatic drainage is to the submental, upper cervical, and facial nodes. Small lesions can be successfully treated with either surgery or radiotherapy.[46,47] Advanced lesions with nerve, bone, or nodal involvement are best treated with surgery and postoperative radiotherapy, though radiotherapy alone represents a reasonable approach in the elderly. The most commonly used EBRT regimens range from 40 Gy in 10 fractions to 70 Gy in 35 fractions. More rapid fractionation (e.g., 30 Gy in five fractions or 20 Gy in a single fraction) may be used when the late cosmetic result is not important and travel may be difficult for the patient (e.g., in a debilitated, elderly patient).[48]

Oral Tongue

Primary lymphatic drainage for the oral tongue is to the subdigastric (jugulodigastric), submandibular (submaxillary), and submental lymph nodes. Approximately one third of patients have nodal involvement at presentation.[27] Carcinoma of the oral tongue usually spreads by direct invasion into adjacent structures such as floor of mouth, mandible, base of tongue, or anterior tonsillar pillar. Distant metastases are uncommon.

For unilateral lesions ≤ 1 cm, surgery is preferred. These lesions can easily be excised without functional impairment. For small, exophytic lesions in patients who refuse surgery or are medically inoperable, EBRT that includes use of an intraoral cone (IOC) has been used. Local control rates for T1 and T2 lesions treated with EBRT, including an IOC, were 94% and 80%, respectively.[49]

For T3-T4 lesions and multiple nodal metastases, surgery and postoperative radiotherapy are recommended for optimal locoregional control.

In patients with advanced disease who refuse surgery or are medically inoperable, radiotherapy should be offered. When combining EBRT with brachytherapy, the EBRT dose should be kept below 40 Gy so that a higher boost dose can be delivered with brachytherapy, resulting in a cumulative dose of ~75 Gy. Crook and Esche[50] reviewed local control with this approach in 437 patients. The local control rate was 89% when the EBRT dose was kept below 40 Gy versus only 63% when the EBRT dose was greater than 40 Gy.

With brachytherapy, the mandibular dose can easily exceed tolerance. Therefore, every attempt should be made to minimize the volume of mandible within the high-dose region. When the mandibular dose exceeds 75 Gy, a 19% incidence of osteonecrosis has been reported by Delclos et al.[51]

Floor of Mouth

Carcinoma of the floor of mouth typically invades locally by direct extension into the lower alveolar ridge, tongue, and mandible. Primary lymphatic drainage is to the submandibular and subdigastric nodes followed by the midjugular nodes.[27] Lindberg et al[27] reported that for T1, T2, and T3-T4 lesions, the incidence of nodal involvement is 11%, 29% and 44 to 54%, respectively. In patients who present with clinically negative necks, at least 20% will develop nodal metastases if the neck is not treated.[52] The overall incidence of distant metastases is 6% for stages I to III and 26% for stage IV (T4N0-N1) cancers.[53] The most common sites for hematogenous metastases are the lungs, liver, and bones.

T1-T2N0 lesions can be treated with either surgery or radiotherapy.[53] For T1 lesions, local control with radiotherapy is greater than 90%, regardless of whether EBRT, brachytherapy, IOC, or a combination of these techniques is used.[53,54] For T2 lesions, a combination of EBRT and either brachytherapy or IOC should be used because the local control rate with EBRT alone is suboptimal (80 to 95% vs 64 to 82%).[52–55]

Hicks et al[56] have reported 5-year, disease-specific survival rates in pathological stage I through IV patients treated largely with surgery alone of 95%, 86%, 82%, and 52%, respectively. Hence, for stage IV disease, surgery and postoperative EBRT constitute the preferred approach.[53,56] In patients who refuse surgery, radiotherapy consisting of EBRT and either interstitial implant or IOC should be offered. Following treatment of floor of mouth cancer, there is a 31% likelihood that the patient will develop a second head and neck malignancy within 5 years.[57] In general, the annual incidence of second primary cancers following treatment for head and neck cancer is 4 to 7%.

Hard Palate

The hard palate is the most common site in the oral cavity for minor salivary gland cancers. Squamous cell carcinomas of the hard palate are rare. Primary lymphatic drainage is to the submandibular, subdigastric, and upper jugular nodes, and ~13 to 24% of patients have nodal involvement at presentation.[27,58]

Surgery is usually the preferred treatment. Radiotherapy is an option for superficial lesions of the hard palate that do not invade underlying bone based on CT scan or for medically inoperable patients. Chung et al[59,60] reported comparable local control rates for early-stage lesions treated with surgery or radiotherapy. Evans and Shah[61] at the Memorial Sloan-Kettering Cancer Center have reported their 15-year experience with hard palate carcinomas. The overall survival rates for stage I, II, and III (including postoperative radiotherapy in some stage II and III) patients were 75%, 46%, and 40%, respectively. For advanced cancers, the preferred treatment consists of surgery and postoperative radiotherapy.

Upper and Lower Gingiva

Approximately 80% of gingival carcinomas arise from the lower gingiva, and of these, 60% are located posterior to the bicuspid. Primary lymphatic drainage is to the submental, sudmandibular, subdigastric, and jugular nodes. Patients usually present with a history of ill-fitting dentures, nonhealing ulceration, or bleeding. Trismus can develop with locally advanced disease. Lesions of the upper gingiva frequently spread by direct extension into the maxillary sinus or the upper gingivobuccal sulcus, and the incidence of lymph node involvement at diagnosis is ~25%.[58] Half of patients with cancers in the lower gingiva have mandibular invasion, and clinical neck nodal involvement is seen in 18 to 52% of patients.[27,58]

For very early, superficial lesions, radiotherapy can yield results that are comparable to surgery.[62] However, the results achieved with radiotherapy alone for more advanced lesions have been poor. For example, MacComb et al[62] reported local control rates for T2, T3, and T4 lesions treated with radiotherapy alone of 70%, 59%, and 29%, respectively. For upper gingival lesions invading the maxilla, the role of postoperative radiotherapy is controversial when negative margins are achieved.[31] For lower gingival lesions invading the mandible, surgery and post-operative radiotherapy are recommended.[62]

Buccal Mucosa

Patients with buccal mucosa cancer often have preexisting leukoplakia or a history of chewing tobacco or betel nuts.[2] Primary lymphatic drainage is to the submandibular, subdigastric, and superior deep jugular lymph nodes. Approximately 9 to 31% of patients present with nodal metastases.[58] Patients with carcinomas more than 1 cm thick that invade the skin of the cheek have a relatively poor prognosis.[63]

Superficial (T1) lesions involving the oral commissure may be treated with either surgery or radiotherapy. Although stage

I-II cancers may be treated with surgery alone, surgery and postoperative radiotherapy are recommended for stage III-IV disease.[64] Nair et al[65] reported locoregional control rates for buccal mucosa cancers treated with radiotherapy alone using various techniques (EBRT, EBRT and brachytherapy, or brachytherapy alone). The locoregional control rates for T1N0, T2N0, T3N0, and T4N0 were 100%, 63%, 69%, and 42%, respectively. Radiotherapy alone resulted in only 41% and 18% regional control rates in patients with N1 and N3 disease, respectively.

Retromolar Trigone

Primary lymphatic drainage is to the submandibular and subdigastric followed by the midjugular nodes. The incidence of nodal metastases at diagnosis is 30 to 40%.[27] Distant metastases are rare. Small lesions can be treated with either surgery or definitive radiotherapy with comparable results.[49] Radiation therapy is less likely to cause necrosis if an IOC is used for part of the treatment. Advanced lesions typically require surgery and postoperative radiotherapy for local control to be achieved.

Lo et al[66] reviewed the University of Texas M.D. Anderson Cancer Center experience with radiotherapy for retromolar trigone or anterior faucial pillar squamous cell carcinomas in 159 patients. Local control rates were 71% for T1, 70% for T2, 76% for T3, and 60% for T4 cancers. Most of the radiotherapy failures were successfully salvaged with surgery. As a result, the ultimate local control rates for T1, T2, T3, and T4 cancers were 100%, 94%, 92%, and 80%, respectively. The 5-year, determinate survival rate was 83%.

Oropharynx

The oropharynx is divided into four sites: soft palate, tonsillar fossae and pillars, base of tongue, and pharyngeal wall between the pharyngoepiglottic fold and the nasopharynx.

Soft Palate

Approximately 45% of patients have nodal involvement at presentation. Primary lymphatic drainage is to the subdigastric and midjugular nodes.[27] For T1-T2 lesions, excellent local control can be achieved with either surgery or radiotherapy.[49,67–69] For example, local control rates for T1-T2 lesions treated with radiotherapy alone range from 83 to 100%.[49,68,69] Surgical excision of carcinomas < 1 cm causes little or no functional loss. However, for lesions measuring 1 to 4 cm, speech and swallowing impairment may be more severe after surgery than radiotherapy. Consequently, radiotherapy represents a reasonable treatment option in such patients. For T3-T4 lesions, surgery and postoperative radiotherapy constitute the preferred approach because the results with radiotherapy alone have been suboptimal.[67,69,70]

Tonsillar Fossa and Pillars

The most common site of oropharyngeal cancers is the tonsillar fossa/pillars. The incidence of occult disease in lymph nodes at presentation is ~50%.[27] Because of the high incidence of nodal metastases, treatment of the neck is essential.

Early tonsillar lesions can be treated with either surgery or radiotherapy. Local control rates with radiotherapy alone are 80 to 100%.[18,71] The ultimate local control rates for T1-T2 lesions are 85 to 100% after surgical salvage.[18,71] With small, lateralized lesions, 3D-CRT or IMRT may be used to reduce the dose of radiation delivered to the contralateral parotid gland, thereby reducing the incidence and severity of xerostomia. In patients with advanced disease, radiotherapy alone using a concomitant boost technique or EBRT followed by brachytherapy should be offered to patients who elect not to undergo surgery and postoperative radiotherapy. The European Organization for Research and Treatment of Cancer (EORTC) conducted a prospective, randomized trial comparing twice-a-day radiotherapy to 80.5 Gy in 70 fractions versus once-a-day radiotherapy to 70 Gy in 35 to 40 fractions in stage II-III oropharyngeal carcinomas, excluding base of tongue.[21] Locoregional control was improved with twice-a-day treatment (5-year rates: 59% vs 40%, $p = 0.007$). There was also a trend toward improved overall survival with twice-a-day treatment (40% vs 30%, $p = 0.08$). No difference in late toxicity existed between the two arms. Similar locoregional control and overall survival rates have been observed in patients with slightly more advanced (stage III-IV) disease treated with radiotherapy using a concomitant boost technique.[24] However, surgery and postoperative radiotherapy produce better locoregional control in such patients than EBRT alone.[72,73]

Puthawala et al[74] have reported the results of EBRT and interstitial Ir-192 implants in 80 patients with tonsillar carcinomas. Eighty-one percent of the patients had stage III-IV carcinomas, and 49% had nodal disease. Primary tumors were treated with EBRT to 45 to 50 Gy using conventional fractionation followed by an Ir-192 implant that delivered 20 to 25 Gy over 50 to 60 hours for T1-T2 lesions, and 30 to 40 Gy over 60 to 100 hours for T3-T4 lesions. Neck nodes also received an Ir-192 implant that delivered 20 to 40 Gy over 50 to 80 hours. Local control rates were 95% for T1-T2 lesions and 79% for T3-T4 lesions.

Base of Tongue

In 75% of cases, patients with carcinoma of the base of tongue present with nodal metastases.[27] The subdigastric nodes are most commonly involved. Metastases to the submandibular, superior deep jugular, and midjugular nodes develop slightly less frequently. Approximately one third of patients have bilateral neck disease at diagnosis.[27]

Early-stage disease involving the base of tongue can be treated with surgery or radiotherapy.[18,73,75] Local control and survival rates for small lesions are comparable with either approach.[18,73,75]

Surgery and postoperative radiotherapy result in the greatest likelihood of locoregional control for advanced disease. In patients who elect not to undergo surgery as part of a combined modality approach, EBRT using a concomitant boost technique or EBRT followed by an implant should be offered. Multiple series have reported excellent locoregional control rates with EBRT and brachytherapy.[74,76–78] Local control rates with EBRT and implant for T1, T2, T3, and T4 cancers range from 100%, 80 to 100%, 75 to 80%, and 67 to 100%, respectively.[74,76–78] Regional control rates of neck for N1, N2, and N3 disease range from 81 to 100%, 78 to 100%, and 50 to 100%, respectively. For all stages, the 5-year overall survival rates with EBRT and an implant range from 35 to 85%.[74,76–78]

Larynx

Cancers of the larynx are the most common cancers of the upper aerodigestive tract.[1,79] The supraglottis has a rich, submucosal lymphatic plexus that drains primarily to the subdigastric and midjugular nodes. The incidence of nodal involvement at diagnosis is 55%, with bilateral nodes in 16% of cases.[27] The true vocal cords lack any significant lymphatics. Consequently, nodal metastases develop more frequently after the supraglottis or the subglottis is invaded. The incidence of nodal involvement for T1, T2, T3, and T4 glottic tumors is 0 to 2%, 3 to 7%, 15 to 20%, and 20 to 30%, respectively.[80,81] Subglottic cancers are rare, constituting < 1% of laryngeal cancers. Approximately 20 to 50% of carcinomas of the subglottis exhibit nodal metastases at presentation.[82,83] Primary lymphatic drainage is to the prelaryngeal (Delphian), lower jugular, pretracheal, paratracheal, and mediastinal nodes.[27] Distant metastases also develop more often for supraglottic and subglottic than glottic cancers.

Supraglottic Larynx

Early-stage cancers can usually be treated with a supraglottic laryngectomy or radiotherapy with comparable excellent local control rates and voice preservation.[84–87] For moderately advanced supraglottic cancers, supraglottic laryngectomy with or without neck dissection and postoperative EBRT offer the best locoregional control.[84,85] A randomized trial conducted by the Department of Veterans Affairs Laryngeal Cancer Study Group suggested that natural speech preservation is possible in 64% of stage III-IV patients using three cycles of neoadjuvant 5-fluorouracil and cisplatin chemotherapy followed by EBRT.[88] Patients were randomized between neoadjuvant chemotherapy and EBRT versus total laryngectomy, neck dissection, and postoperative EBRT. Based on a median follow-up of 33 months, there was improved locoregional control (*p* = 0.0005) and a trend (*p* = 0.11) toward improved disease-free survival with the surgical approach. However, there was no difference in overall survival between the two groups, in part due to surgical salvage of chemoradiation failures.

A follow-up intergroup phase III study randomized stage III or IV laryngeal carcinoma patients to radiation alone versus induction chemotherapy followed by radiation versus concurrent chemoradiation with cisplatin every 3 weeks.[89] With a median follow-up of 3.8 years, better laryngeal preservation rates were demonstrated with the concurrent regimen (88%, 75%, and 70% for concurrent, induction, and radiation alone arms, respectively). The locoregional control rate was superior in the concurrent arm over both the induction and radiation alone arms (78%, 61%, 56%, respectively). No difference in overall survival was observed between these three arms. Of note, the concomitant regimen had increased mucosal toxicity.

More recently, higher locoregional control rates have been observed with altered fractionation rather than once-a-day EBRT for supraglottic carcinomas.[19,86]

Locoregional control rates for supraglottic cancers treated with altered fractionation are 71 to 100% for T1, 50 to 81% for T2, 38 to 70% for T3, and 26 to 46% for T4 diseases. The ultimate locoregional control rates are 82 to 100% for T1, 50 to 88% for T2, 49 to 83% for T3, and 29 to 67% for T4 lesions, including surgical salvage.[86,90–92] The lower percentage in each T stage was reported by Wang using split-course, accelerated, hyperfractionated EBRT.[92] The higher local control rates reported for each stage were achieved using hyperfractionated EBRT. Five-year, cause-specific survival rates range from 39 to 45%.[19,86]

Glottis

Carcinoma in situ of the glottis can be treated successfully with laser therapy, endoscopic stripping, or radiotherapy.[93,94] Fein et al[93] have reported the results achieved with radiotherapy at the University of Florida for carcinoma in situ. The 5-year local control rate with natural speech preservation was 93% and the ultimate local control rate was 100%. Smitt and Goffinet[94] reported a 10-year local control rate with radiotherapy of 89% and an ultimate local control rate of 100% with surgical salvage.

T1-T2 lesions can be treated with a hemilaryngectomy, cordectomy, or radiotherapy. With EBRT, the quality of the voice is often good to excellent following treatment. For T1-T2 lesions, local control rates for radiotherapy are 83 to 93% and 67 to 88%, respectively.[92,95–97] Because most radiotherapy failures can be salvaged surgically, the ultimate local control rates for T1 and T2 lesions are 94 to 99% and 86 to 95%, respectively. The 5-year, determinant survival rates are 96 to 97% for T1 and 88 to 91% for T2 lesions, respectively.[95–97]

Some T3 lesions have been treated initially with twice-a-day radiotherapy, reserving surgery for salvage.[98–100] The ultimate local control rates with this approach are 37 to 81%, and the 5-year, determinant survival rates range from 57 to 74%.[98–100] Based on the intergroup phase III laryngeal cancer study discussed earlier, concomitant chemoradiation therapy is favored over radiation twice-a-day treatment alone for laryngeal preservation.[89] For T4 lesions, locoregional control is most likely to be achieved with surgery and postoperative radiotherapy.

Subglottis

Most patients present with advanced disease at diagnosis and are best managed with surgery and postoperative radiotherapy. Warde et al[101] reported a local control rate of 70% and 5-year actuarial and determinate survival rates of 26% and 61%, respectively, for radiotherapy.

Hypopharynx

The hypopharynx includes the pyriform sinus, posterior pharyngeal wall, and postcricoid region. It has a rich lymphatic network. Primary lymphatic drainage is to the subdigastric and midjugular followed by the lower jugular nodes.[27] The incidence of nodal metastases is 75% for pyriform sinus cancers and 50% for posterior pharyngeal wall cancers.[27] Forty to 60% of patients develop nodal metastases.[102,103] The primary tumor typically spreads by submucosal extension.[104] Most patients present with advanced disease, and 20 to 30% develop distant metastases within 2 years, which is the second highest rate of distant metastasis in head and neck cancers.[104,105]

Pyriform Sinus

Radiotherapy may be offered to the uncommon patient with a T1-T2 lesion.[19,106] Mendenhall et al[106] reported a 2-year local control rate of 79% for T1-T2 lesions and an ultimate local control rate of 88% with surgical salvage. After radiotherapy, symptoms of local recurrence include odynophagia and ear pain and signs of local recurrence include major edema. If N1 disease is treated with radiotherapy, a neck dissection should be performed if any residual disease does not completely regress 4 to 6 weeks following the completion of treatment.[106,107] For T3-T4 lesions, better locoregional control is achieved with surgery and postoperative radiotherapy than surgery alone.[108] Radiotherapy alone should be offered to patients with a poor performance status. Bataini et al[107] reported 249 patients with pyriform sinus cancers treated with radiotherapy at the Institute of Curie. The 2-year local control rate for all patients was 55%, and the 2-year disease-free survival rate was 47%.

Although surgery and postoperative radiotherapy provide excellent locoregional control for advanced hypopharyngeal carcinomas, chemotherapy and radiotherapy have been studied as a way of reducing the incidence of distant metastases. Preliminary results from a randomized EORTC trial comparing two to three cycles of induction 5-fluorouracil and cisplatin chemotherapy followed by radiotherapy versus surgery and postoperative radiotherapy have been reported.[105] The local and regional control rates were similar for the two arms: 83% and 77%, respectively, in the chemotherapy and radiotherapy arm versus 88% and 81%, respectively, in the surgery and postoperative radiotherapy arm. The incidence of distant metastases was less in the chemotherapy and radiotherapy arm than in the surgery and postoperative radiotherapy arm (25% vs 36%, $p = 0.04$). The median survival of 44 months in the chemotherapy and radiotherapy arm was superior to the surgery and postoperative radiotherapy arm of 25 months ($p = 0.006$). Overall survival rates remain relatively low secondary to intercurrent deaths and second primary cancers.[108–111]

Pharyngeal Walls

T1-T2 cancers can be treated with surgery or radiotherapy. However, more advanced disease should be treated with surgery and postoperative radiotherapy. Five-year survival remains relatively poor for advanced cancers (22 to 33%).[102,112–114]

Postcricoid Region

Cancers of the postcricoid region are relatively rare, and patients usually present with advanced disease. Surgery and postoperative radiotherapy have traditionally been regarded as the standard approach. However, 5-year survival rates remain poor, ranging from 16 to 31%.[115–118] Radiotherapy alone is reserved for patients who refuse surgery or are medically inoperable.

Nasal Cavity/Paranasal Sinuses

Cancers of the nasal cavity and paranasal sinuses are relatively rare malignancies. Unlike most other cancers arising from the upper aerodigestive tract, tobacco and alcohol abuse are not predisposing factors. Rather, nasal cavity and paranasal sinus cancers have been associated with work-related exposures in saw mills (wood dust), leather tanneries, or nickel refineries.[119]

The incidence of nodal metastases is low, ranging from 0 to 15%.[119] The incidence of distant metastases is low as well. Eighty to 85% of sinonasal cancers are squamous cell carcinomas or their variants. The remaining histological types arise from minor salivary glands (e.g., adenocarcinoma, adenoid cystic carcinoma, or mucoepidermoid carcinoma in descending order of frequency).

Although early-stage lesions can be treated with either surgery or radiotherapy, many patients present with advanced disease that requires surgery and postoperative radiotherapy for optimal locoregional control.

Parsons et al[120] have reported results in 48 patients with cancers of the nasal cavity, ethmoid sinus, or sphenoid sinus. Forty-two of the patients were treated with radiotherapy alone, and the remainder were treated with surgery and radiotherapy. With the exception of adenoid cystic carcinoma, the ultimate local control rates at 10 years for all histologies were 40 to 60%. The 5-, 10-, 15-, and 20-year actuarial survival rates were 52%, 30%, 22%, and 22%, respectively. When patients are treated with radiotherapy alone, the risk of optic neuropathy or retinopathy is relatively high. In Parson et al's study, 33% of patients developed unilateral blindness 17 to 90 months posttreatment. Therefore, careful treatment planning (e.g., with IMRT) is mandatory when using radiotherapy alone for cancers of the nasal cavity, ethmoid sinus, or sphenoid sinus in an effort to reduce the risk of blindness.

Esthesioneuroblastoma of the nasal cavity is rare. Early-stage patients can be treated with surgery or radiotherapy. A review of the literature by Elkon et al[121] found no significant survival differences in outcomes with surgery, radiotherapy, or a combined approach.[121] For more-advanced disease, surgery and postoperative radiotherapy are preferred.[121]

Maxillary sinus cancers are generally treated with surgery and postoperative radiotherapy because most patients present with advanced disease. Jiang et al[122] reported 73 cases of maxillary sinus carcinomas treated at the University of Texas M.D. Anderson Cancer Center with surgery and postoperative radiotherapy. There were three T1, 16 T2, 32 T3, and 22 T4 carcinomas. The overall local control rate was 78%, and 5-year relapse-free survival rate was 51%. The nodal recurrence rate without initial elective neck treatment was 38% for squamous cell and undifferentiated carcinomas. Based on the high incidence of neck recurrences without elective treatment, the authors recommended elective nodal irradiation routinely to patients with squamous cell or undifferentiated carcinomas, with the exception of T1 lesions. Ryu recommends elective nodal irradiation for cancers that are poorly differentiated, T4 (e.g., invade the nasopharynx), or recurrent.[123]

Salivary Glands

The salivary glands include the parotid, submandibular, and sublingual glands. The minor salivary glands are located throughout the entire upper aerodigestive tract and are predominantly found in the hard palate, paranasal sinuses, tongue, and nasal cavity. The selection of treatment options for salivary gland tumors depends on the histology and extent of disease.

In general, adenoid cystic carcinomas of the head and neck have a long natural history and may ultimately prove fatal.[79] Although adenoid cystic carcinomas are often histologically low grade because they contain < 30% solid areas, they should be treated as high-grade cancers.[79] An adenoid cystic carcinoma that was completely excised and treated with postoperative radiotherapy can recur locally or distantly many years later. Even after distant metastases develop, patients can live for years. The usual approach at presentation consists of wide surgical excision and postoperative radiotherapy to a generous volume including the perineural pathways and ipsilateral neck.

In contrast, most benign mixed tumors require surgery only. Indications for postoperative radiotherapy include three or more previous recurrences, involvement of the deep lobe of the parotid, > 5 cm in greatest dimension, positive surgical margins, or malignant transformation.[124] For malignant tumors, postoperative radiotherapy is recommended for high-grade lesions, gross residual disease, positive or close surgical margins, intraoperative tumor spillage, multiple positive nodes, perineural invasion, involvement of the deep lobe of the parotid gland, facial nerve involvement, or extraglandular extension into adjacent structures.[125] For patients who refuse surgery or are medically inoperable, radiotherapy alone sometimes produces cures as well.[126] Most salivary gland tumors do not require elective neck treatment, with the exception of large or high-grade cancers.[127] Spiro et al[128] reported actuarial 5- and 10-year local control rates of 95% and 84%, respectively, for 62 patients with parotid cancers treated with surgery and radiotherapy. The actuarial 5- and 10-year, disease-free survival rates were 77% and 65%, respectively. For patients with positive or close surgical margins, Fu et al[129] reported local recurrence rates of 54% in the surgery alone group versus 14% in the surgery and postoperative radiotherapy group. Weber et al[130] also showed a benefit to postoperative radiotherapy in patients with submandibular gland carcinoma. In their study, the locoregional recurrence rate was 52% in the surgery alone group versus 18% in the combined modality group. For advanced minor salivary gland cancers, local control rates with surgery and radiotherapy range from 71 to 83%.[129,131]

Fast neutron beam radiotherapy has also been explored in the treatment of incompletely resected or inoperable salivary gland cancers. The Radiation Therapy Oncology Group of North America and Medical Research Council of England conducted a randomized trial comparing fast neutron beam radiotherapy with conventional photon beam radiotherapy in patients with incompletely resected or inoperable salivary gland cancers.[132] The trial was stopped after only 32 patients had been accrued because the fast neutron radiotherapy group had significantly improved locoregional control. With 10-year follow-up, the improved local control remains significantly better ($p = 0.009$) in the neutron group (65%) than in the photon group (15%). However, there was no difference in overall survival (15% vs 25%, $p > 0.05$). Distant metastases accounted for the majority of failures in the neutron radiotherapy group, whereas locoregional recurrences accounted for most failures in the conventional radiotherapy group. There was a greater incidence of severe complications in the neutron radiotherapy group, which helps to explain why this treatment approach hasn't gained substantially in popularity. Because locoregional control is more likely to be achieved in patients with salivary gland cancers ≤ 4 cm, initial surgical resection is advocated, if possible.[133] The installation of modern neutron machines and use of three-dimensional treatment planning at selected institutions should help to reduce the 11% incidence of severe complications with neutron radiotherapy.[134]

Base of Skull

The cranial nerves, brain stem, brain, optic chiasm, optic nerves, and retinas limit the dose of radiotherapy that can be safely delivered. For benign tumors such as chemodectomas, a relatively low dose of radiation is required: 45 to 54 Gy in 25 to 30 fractions.[135] Therefore, normal tissue tolerance poses much less of a problem. Based on a review of the literature, Springate and Weichselbaum[136] concluded that either surgery or radiotherapy produces a local control rate of 93% and a low incidence of complications in patients with temporal bone chemodectomas. Similarly, Powell et al[137] reported a 10-year actuarial local control rate of 90% and a 25-year actuarial local control rate of 73% for skull base glomus jugulare and glomus tympanicum tumors treated with radiotherapy. Morbidity was minimal.

For cancers, radiation doses greater than 59.4 to 60.0 Gy in 30 to 33 fractions are often necessary to achieve local control. This has traditionally posed a problem because higher doses cannot be delivered safely to normal structures. In the case of skull base tumors, charged particle radiotherapy has an advantage over conventional photon radiotherapy because it allows for highly localized energy deposition within cancers while sparing adjacent critical normal structures. Physicians at the Massachusetts General Hospital (MGH) and Harvard Cyclotron Laboratories have reported their extensive experience in treating skull base tumors.[138–144] Munzenrider and Liebsch[141] recently updated the MGH experience with combined photon-proton radiotherapy for chordomas and low-grade chondrosarcomas of the skull base and cervical spine treated from 1975 to 1998. Six hundred and twenty-one patients were analyzed: 60% had chordomas and 40% had chondrosarcomas. Eighty-four percent of the patients had skull base tumors and 16% had cervical spine tumors. Fifty-two percent were male and 48% were female. Local control was defined as the absence of tumor enlargement on follow-up imaging studies with neurological stability or improvement. For skull base tumors, local recurrence-free survival was significantly improved in patients with chondrosarcomas rather than chordomas: 94% versus 54% at 10 years ($p < 0.0001$). Overall survival was also significantly better for patients with chondrosarcomas rather than chordomas (88% vs 54% at 10 years, $p < 0.0001$). Male chordoma patients tended to fare better than their female counterparts. In contrast, the outcome of chondrosarcoma patients did not differ by gender. The probabilities of brain stem and cervical spinal cord injury were 8% and 13% 5 and 10 years postirradiation, respectively. The probability of temporal lobe injury was 13% 5 years postirradiation. Optic neuropathy developed in 4.4% of patients. Fifteen of 33 patients prospectively evaluated developed a hearing deficit 2 to 5 years postirradiation. Almost two thirds of patients receiving ≥ 62.7 GyE to the inner ear or the auditory nerve experienced progressive, severe hearing loss. Therefore, the dose to the inner ear should be limited to ≤ 62 GyE. Endocrinopathies and cranial nerve injuries were also noted.

Castro et al[142,143] at the Lawrence Berkley Laboratory have reported their experience in treating skull base tumors in 223 patients using helium or neon as the charged particles. The 5-year local control rate was 63% and 5-year overall survival rate was 75%. Because the results with charged particle radiotherapy compare favorably with conventional radiotherapy for skull base or cervical spine tumors, interest in charged particle radiotherapy has steadily been increasing.[144]

Because there are only a limited number of facilities that offer charged particle radiotherapy, 3D-CRT has also been explored.[145–148] Latz and associates described the outcome of 13 patients with clival chordomas treated with 3D-CRT to a median dose of 70 Gy.[148] Based on a median follow-up of 32 months, 12/13 patients were still alive. The local control rate was 69%. Only one patient developed endocrine dysfunction requiring hormonal replacement. No complications involving the optic pathway, cranial nerves, or brain stem were observed. IMRT is also a promising approach that is more widely available than charged particle radiotherapy.

◆ New Advances in Radiation Oncology

Three-Dimensional Conformal Radiotherapy

As previously discussed, 3D-CRT has been investigated for multiple different head and neck sites, including skull base tumors. Liebel et al[148a] compared three-dimensional conformal radiotherapy treatment plans with two-dimensional, conventional radiotherapy plans in 10 patients with newly diagnosed and five patients with locally recurrent nasopharyngeal carcinomas. For both tumor control probabilities and normal tissue complication probabilities, the 3D-CRT plans were superior to the two-dimensional plans. The probability of tumor control was increased by 15% with 3D-CRT versus 2D-conventional radiotherapy. Emami et al[149] at Washington University also demonstrated that 3D-CRT treatment plans are superior to conventional radiotherapy plans for head and

neck cancer patients.[149] Perez et al[150] have reported that the acute toxicity of 3D-CRT for head and neck cancer patients is comparable to or lower than that observed with conventional radiotherapy. Multileaf collimators significantly decrease the daily treatment time for 3D-CRT, making this approach feasible for busy practices.[151] Gademann et al[152] have described promising results with 3D-CRT in 195 patients with tumors arising in the head, neck, or brain. With a median follow-up of 22 months, 95% of patients treated with 3D-CRT only were still alive versus 86% of patients who received 3D-CRT simply during the last part of the radiotherapy. As in other studies,[38,153] the morbidity of 3D-CRT was minimal.

Intensity-Modulated Radiation Therapy

With 3D-CRT, the tumor and regions at risk for microscopic extension are contoured on each axial CT slice. The tumor volume is then visualized in three dimensions. The physicist and dosimetrists work together to construct a beam arrangement that will deliver the desired therapeutic dose to the tumor volume while minimizing the dose of radiation that will be delivered to adjacent normal tissues. IMRT differs from 3D-CRT in that each beam is broken up into many beamlets, and the intensity of each beamlet is then adjusted individually. Inverse planning is a process whereby a computer program takes the desired dose distribution and works backward to tell the physicist and dosimetrists the intensity of every beamlet to achieve the desired therapeutic dose. In contrast, with 3D-CRT, a trial and error approach is used with treatment planning in an attempt to obtain the desired therapeutic dose. IMRT fields can be efficiently treated using computer-controlled multileaf collimators. IMRT allows one to better conform the high-dose region to the tumor, thereby allowing for dose escalation. Multiple studies have demonstrated the potential advantages and feasibility of IMRT in the treatment of head and neck cancer.[13,38,45,154] Preliminary clinical studies by various investigators have been promising.[14,155,156]

Figure 13.2 is a color wash display depicting dose distributions for 3D-CRT versus IMRT in a patient with nasopharyngeal carcinoma. Note that less normal tissue surrounding the primary tumor is treated to a high dose with IMRT than with 3D-CRT. **Figure 13.3** demonstrates that a much smaller volume of the parotid glands is treated to > 30 Gy with IMRT than with 3D-CRT in seven consecutive patients with nasopharyngeal carcinomas. After IMRT, these patients did not experience prolonged xerostomia, a typical side effect associated with 3D-CRT for this disease.

Stereotactic Radiosurgery and Fractionated Stereotactic Radiotherapy

Stereotactic radiosurgery involves the precise delivery of a single, large dose of radiation to a target that typically measures less than 3.5 cm. Stereotactic radiosurgery can be delivered using a linear accelerator, gamma knife, or cyclotron. By limiting the treatment to a small target, a steep dose fall-off can be achieved in adjacent normal tissue. Because one goal of radiosurgery is to minimize the dose of radiation that is delivered to normal tissue, a stereotactic frame is used to im-

mobilize the patient during treatment. Besides immobilizing the patient, the frame also serves as a reference, allowing for precise target localization in three-dimensional space. Radiosurgery has been used in the treatment of skull base tumors and nasopharyngeal carcinomas.[157,158]

There are radiobiological advantages to treating cancers with multiple, small rather than a single, large dose of radiation.[159,160] Recently, fractionated stereotactic radiotherapy has been developed. This technique involves the use of a relocatable head frame for patient positioning during multiple, daily treatments.[160] The relocatable head frame does not allow for quite the same accuracy of target localization as a fixed head frame. Consequently, ~2 mm of additional normal tissue (e.g., cranial nerves), is included in the high-dose region. However, by delivering multiple, small rather than a single, large dose of radiation, one can actually reduce the risk of cranial nerve palsies when irradiating skull base tumors such as acoustic neuromas or pituitary adenomas, particularly when treating larger (i.e., 3 to 5 cm) tumors.[161–164]

Intraoperative Radiation Therapy

With IORT, a single, large dose of radiotherapy is delivered in the operating suite after the tumor bed and adjacent normal organs have been defined. With IORT, electrons rather than photons are administered because, with the former technique, the dose of radiation falls off rapidly with depth. This allows one to spare normal underlying tissues. The typical dose delivered with IORT is 12 to 20 Gy in a single fraction. Because of the advantage of rapid dose fall-off with depth, IORT has been investigated in the treatment of head and neck cancer, especially locally advanced or recurrent disease.[165–167] **Figure 13.4** shows an electron treatment cone being "docked" into position in the operating suite for the delivery of IORT to the tumor bed in the neck.

Freeman and coworkers reported IORT results in 104 patients with head and neck cancer.[165] Forty patients were initially treated with surgery and IORT, and the remaining pa-

tients received IORT for recurrent disease. IORT doses ranged from 15 to 20 Gy. The 2-year local control rate was 54%. Patients with microscopic disease at the time of IORT experienced better local control than those with gross disease. The complication rate was 14%. All of the patients with complications had previously undergone radiotherapy. Rate et al[166] reported the outcome of 47 patients with recurrent head and neck cancer who underwent resection and IORT. The 2-year actuarial local control rate was 62% and the 2-year survival rate was 55%. Toita et al[167] reported the outcome of 25 patients with advanced or recurrent head and neck cancer treated with surgery and IORT. The 2-year control rate within the IORT port was 0% for gross disease and 55% for microscopic disease. The 2-year complication rate was 33%. There was an increased incidence of complications with IORT doses ≥ 20 Gy.

Chemotherapy

Early studies typically used chemotherapy alone for recurrent or metastatic disease, and the results were relatively disappointing.[168,169] Next, chemotherapy was administered prior to radiotherapy in patients with previously untreated, locally advanced disease in an effort to increase the likelihood of natural speech preservation without compromising overall survival. Two randomized trials have supported this approach.[88,105] A meta-analysis of prospective, randomized trials suggested that chemotherapy improves local control at the cost of increased morbidity.[170] Nevertheless, chemotherapy can lead to an improvement in overall survival when it is administered concurrently with as opposed to prior to radiotherapy.[170]

Relatively recently, chemotherapy delivered concomitantly with altered fractionation radiotherapy has been investigated in patients with advanced head and neck cancer.[171–173] Brizel et al[172] at Duke University reported the results of a randomized trial wherein the outcome with twice-a-day radiotherapy and concurrent 5-fluorouracil and cisplatin chemotherapy was superior to that with twice-a-day radiotherapy alone. One hundred and sixteen patients with advanced head and neck can-

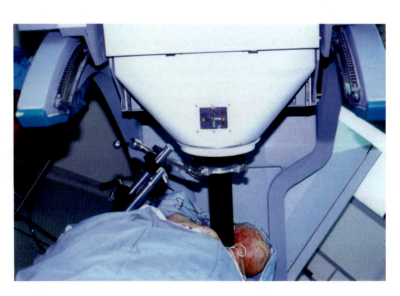

Fig. 13.4 An electron treatment cone is being "docked" into position in the operating suite for the delivery of intraoperative radiotherapy to the tumor bed. (Courtesy of Karen Fu, M.D., in the Department of Radiation Oncology at the University of California, San Francisco.)

cer were analyzed in this study, which had a median follow-up of 41 months. Locoregional control in the combined modality group was significantly better ($p = 0.01$) than in the radiotherapy alone group (3-year rates: 70% vs 44%, respectively). There was a trend toward improved relapse-free and overall survival in the combined modality group (3-year rates: 61% and 55%, respectively) relative to the radiotherapy alone group (3-year rates: 41% and 34%, respectively).

Image-Guided Radiation Therapy

With knowledge and data obtained from 3D imaging and IMRT studies, radiation oncologists have gained a better understanding of inherent uncertainties during the radiation treatment process. In an effort to minimize these uncertainties, including set-up variation (interfraction) and body or organ (intrafraction) motion, more technical and clinical advances have emerged to improve radiation delivery accuracy and precision, the so-called image-guided radiation therapy (IGRT).[173] IGRT allows one to manage external beam radiation interfraction and intrafraction motion in a real-time way much better than any other previous tools.

◆ Acute and Late Complications of Radiotherapy

Various site-specific complications may develop, depending on the treatment volume, fractionation, and prescribed dose. The most common acute side effects of radiotherapy include fatigue, mucositis, xerostomia, loss of taste, decreased appetite, esophagitis, and radiodermatitis. Most of these side effects spontaneously resolve within 4 to 6 weeks of the completion of radiotherapy. Patients are advised to take frequent sips of water throughout the day to help with their xerostomia. Weight loss during treatment is common and some patients may require supplemental tube feedings. Serous otitis externa and otitis media can also develop during or after the completion of treatment.[30,32,174] Most of these patients respond to hydrocortisone, neomycin, and polymyxin B otic solution and decongestants. These patients occasionally may also require myringotomy to relieve their discomfort and decreased hearing. Permanent hearing impairment can develop, especially when the dose to the inner ear exceeds 50 Gy.[174] In general, most acute reactions are more severe with altered fractionation and/or when chemotherapy is delivered concurrently with radiotherapy.[171–173] Sometimes a treatment break may become necessary due to the severity of the acute reactions (e.g., confluent, painful mucositis). In general, treatment breaks are kept as brief as possible to maximize the effectiveness of radiotherapy.

After the first few days of radiotherapy, patients will occasionally complain of swollen, tender parotid glands with/without a low-grade fever. Radiation-induced parotitis usually resolves within 1 to 2 weeks. Nonsteroidal, antiinflammatory medication provides symptomatic relief.

Xerostomia is the most common, chronic sequela of radiation therapy for head and neck cancer. Most patients experience a permanent dry mouth, with the severity depending upon the dose delivered to and volume of salivary glands included in the treatment fields. Permanent xerostomia can lead to multiple problems including dental caries. Therefore, good dental prophylaxis with topical fluoride and continuous dental care before, during, and after radiotherapy is crucial to reduce the incidence of dental problems. Loss of taste can also be permanent. However, most patients will regain at least some if not at all taste sensation over a period of months.

Osteonecrosis of the mandible may develop, especially after doses > 70.[14] Soft tissue necrosis may also occur.[175] However, they usually respond well to conservative management including good oral hygiene and antibiotics.[79] In severe cases, hyperbaric oxygen may be required.[79]

Fibrosis of masticatory muscles may lead to trismus in some patients.[175] Mandibular stretching exercises can help to reduce the incidence and severity of trismus. Neck fibrosis commonly develops after radiotherapy and can be exacerbated by a neck dissection.[175] Neck stretching exercises help to prevent the progression of fibrosis. Submental edema is a common side effect of radiotherapy that develops due to impairment of lymphatic drainage. It typically waxes and wanes and may last for a prolonged period of time.

Laryngeal edema occurs when the larynx is included in the radiotherapy fields.[176] The incidence of laryngeal edema increases with total dose, dose per fraction, and field size.[176] Most of the edema will resolve in response to voice rest, steroids, and occasionally antibiotics as necessary. If the edema persists longer than 3 months following the completion of radiotherapy, the patient has persistent disease until proven otherwise, and deep biopsies are indicated. Usually, a laryngectomy is required for severe laryngeal edema that does not respond to conservative management.

Transverse myelitis with resulting paralysis can also develop following the delivery of radiotherapy to the cervical spinal cord. Improved treatment planning and careful attention to the dose that is delivered to the spinal cord have made this complication a rare event.[175]

When base of skull or orbital structures are included in the radiotherapy fields, endocrine dysfunction, brain necrosis, cranial nerve dysfunction, optic neuropathy, retinopathy, and cataracts may develop. Therefore, careful attention to treatment planning is crucial if one is to minimize complications.[175] Technical advances such as proton beam therapy and IMRT make it easier for one to deliver a high dose of radiation to the cancer while sparing adjacent normal tissue.

◆ Conclusion

Advances in surgery have made it possible to resect cancers that had had previously been regarded as incurable. Similarly, advances in radiation oncology such as altered fractionation, IORT, proton beam therapy, IMRT, and fractionated stereotactic radiotherapy have helped to improve the outlook for patients with locally advanced or recurrent head and neck cancer. Preliminary results with radioprotectors such as amifostine[177] and glutamine[178] and chemopreventive agents such as 13-cis retinoic acid and interferon α[179,180] have also been encouraging, making this an exciting time for physicians involved in the multidisciplinary management of head and neck cancer.

Acknowledgments
The authors would like to thank Peggy Gravitte for her secretarial assistance.

References

1. Cancer Facts & Figures 2000. Atlanta: American Cancer Society; 2000

2. Johnson NW, Warnakulasuriy SW, Tavassoli M. Hereditary and environmental risk factors; clinical and laboratory risk markers for head and neck, especially oral, cancer and precancer. Eur J Cancer Prev 1996;5:5–17

3. Brennan JA, Boyle JO, Koch WM, et al. Association between cigarette smoking and mutation of the p53 gene in squamous cell carcinoma of the head and neck. N Engl J Med 1995;332:712–717

4. Paterson IC, Eveson JW, Prime SS. Molecular changes in oral cancer may reflect aetiology and ethnic origin. Eur J Cancer B Oral Oncol 1996;32B:150–153

5. Pearson GR, Weiland LH, Neel HB, et al. Application of Epstein-Barr virus (EBV) serology to the diagnosis of North American nasopharyngeal carcinoma. Cancer 1983;51:260–268

6. Warren S. Effects of radiation on normal tissue. Arch Pathol (Chic) 1942;34:749–787

7. Khan FM. The Physics of Radiation Therapy. 2nd ed. Baltimore: Williams & Wilkins; 1994

8. Rubin P, Casarett GW. Clinical Radiation Pathology. Vols 1,2. Philadelphia: WB Saunders; 1968

9. Phillips TL, Buschke F. Radiation tolerance of the thoracic spinal cord. Am J Roentgenol Radium Ther Nucl Med 1969;105:659–664

10. Kramer S, Southard ME, Mansfield CM. Radiation effects and tolerance of the central nervous system. Front Radiat Ther Oncol 1972;6:332–335

11. Parsons JT, Fitzgerald CR, Hood CI, et al. The effects of irradiation on the eye and optic nerve. Int J Radiat Oncol Biol Phys 1983;9:609–622

12. Parsons JT, Bova FJ, Firzgerald CR, et al. Radiation retinopathy after external-beam irradiation: analysis of time-dose factors. Int J Radiat Oncol Biol Phys 1994;30:765–773

13. Eisbruch A, Ten Haken RK, Kim HM, et al. Dose, volume, and function relationships in parotid salivary glands following conformal and intensity-modulated irradiation of head and neck cancer. Int J Radiat Oncol Biol Phys 1999;45:577–587

14. Kuppersmith RB, Greco SC, The BS, et al. Intensity-modulated radiotherapy: first results with this new technology on neoplasms of the head and neck. Ear Nose Throat J 1999;78:238–248

15. Beumer J, Harrison R, Sanders B, et al. Postradiation dental extractions: a review of the literature and a report of 72 episodes. Head Neck Surg 1983;6:581–586

16. Fletcher GH. Clinical dose-response curves of human malignant epithelial tumors. Br J Radiol 1973;46:1–12

17. Fletcher GH. Textbook of Radiotherapy. 3rd ed. Philadelphia: Lea & Febiger; 1980:180–219

18. Fein DA, Lee WR, Amos WR, et al. Oropharyngeal carcinoma treated with radiotherapy: a 30-year experience. Int J Radiat Oncol Biol Phys 1996;34:289–296

19. Garden AS, Morrison WH, Ang KK, et al. Hyperfractionated radiation in the treatment of squamous cell carcinoma of the head and neck: a comparison of two fractionation schedules. Int J Radiat Oncol Biol Phys 1995;31:493–502

20. Horiot JC, Bontemps P, van den Bogaert W, et al. Accelerated fractionation (AF) compared to conventional fractionation (CF) improves locoregional control in the radiotherapy of advanced head and neck cancers: results of the EORTC 22851 randomized trial. Radiother Oncol 1997;44:111–121

21. Horiot JC, Le Fur R, N'Guyen T, et al. Hyperfractionation versus conventional fractionation in oropharyngeal carcinoma: final analysis of a randomized trial of the EORTC cooperative group of radiotherapy. Radiother Oncol 1992;25:231–241

22. Peters LJ, Ang KK. The role of altered fractionation in head and neck cancers. Semin Radiat Oncol 1992;2:180–194

23. Parsons JT, Mendenhall WM, Stringer SP, et al. Twice-a-day radiotherapy for squamous cell carcinoma of the head and neck: the University of Florida experience. Head Neck 1993;15:87–96

24. Fu KK, Pajak TF, Trotti A, et al. A Radiation Therapy Oncology Group (RTOG) phase III randomized study to compare hyperfractionation and two variants of accelerated fractionation to standard fractionation radiotherapy for head and neck squamous cell carcinomas: preliminary results of RTOG 9003 (abstract). Proc 41st ASTRO Meeting. Int J Radiat Oncol Biol Phys 1999;41(3S):145

25. Kramer S, Gelber RD, Snow JB, et al. Combined radiation therapy and surgery in the management of advanced head and neck cancer: final report of study 73-03 of the Radiation Therapy Oncology Group. Head Neck Surg 1987;10:19–30

26. Tupchong L, Scott CB, Blitzer PH, et al. Randomized study of preoperative versus postoperative radiation therapy in advanced head and neck carcinoma: long-term follow-up of RTOG study 73-03. Int J Radiat Oncol Biol Phys 1991;20:21–28

27. Lindberg R. Distribution of cervical lymph node metastases from squamous cell carcinoma of the upper respiratory and digestive tracts. Cancer 1972;29:1446–1450

28. Ahmad A, Stefani S. Distant metastases of nasopharyngeal carcinoma: a study of 256 male patients. J Surg Oncol 1986;33:194–197

29. Chu AM, Flynn MB, Achino E, et al. Irradiation of nasopharyngeal carcinoma: Correlations with treatment factors and stage. Int J Radiat Oncol Biol Phys 1984;10:2241–2249

30. Hoppe RT, Goffinet DR, Bagshaw MA. Carcinoma of the nasopharynx: eighteen years' experience with megavoltage radiation therapy. Cancer 1976;37:2605–2612

31. Wang CC. Radiation Therapy for Head and Neck Neoplasms: Indications, Techniques, and Results. 2nd ed. Chicago: Year Book Medical Publishers; 1990

32. Mesic JB, Fletcher GH, Goepfert H. Megavoltage irradiation of epithelial tumors of the nasopharynx. Int J Radiat Oncol Biol Phys 1981;7:447–453

33. Bailet JW, Mark RJ, Abemayor E, et al. Nasopharyngeal carcinoma: results with primary radiation therapy. Laryngoscope 1992;102:965–972

34. Vikram B, Strong EW, Manolatos S, et al. Improved survival in carcinoma of the nasopharynx. Head Neck Surg 1984;7:123–128

35. Al-Sarraf M, LeBlanc M, Shanker PG, et al. Chemoradiotherapy versus radiotherapy in patients with advanced nasopharyngeal cancer: phase III randomized intergroup study 0099. J Clin Oncol 1998;16:1310–1317

36. Perez CA, Devineni VR, Marcial-Vega V, et al. Carcinoma of the nasopharynx: factors affecting prognosis. Int J Radiat Oncol Biol Phys 1992;23:271–280

37. Ho S, Leung WT, Yuen J, et al. Serum levels of CYFRA 21-1 in nasopharyngeal carcinoma and its possible role in monitoring of therapy. Eur J Cancer B Oral Oncol 1996;32B:377–380

38. Wu Q, Manning M, Schmidt-Ullrich R, et al. The potential for sparing of parotids and escalation of biologically effective dose with intensity-modulated radiation treatments of head and neck cancers: a treatment design study. Int J Radiat Oncol Biol Phys 2000;46:195–205

39. Wei WI, Ho CM, Lam KH, et al. Surgical resection for nasopharynx cancer. In: Johnson JT, Didolkar MS, eds. Head and Neck Cancer. Hong Kong: Elsevier Science; 1993;465

40. Pryzant RM, Wendt CD, Delclos L, et al. Re-treatment of nasopharyngeal carcinoma in 53 patients. Int J Radiat Oncol Biol Phys 1992;22:941–947

41. Fu KK, Newman H, Phillips TL. Treatment of locally recurrent carcinoma of the nasopharynx. Radiology 1975;117:425–431

42. Vikram V. Permanent iodine-125 implants for recurrent carcinoma of the nasopharynx: Early results. Endocrine Hypertherm Oncol. 1986;2:83–85

43. Yan JH, Hu YH, Gu XZ. Radiation therapy of recurrent nasopharyngeal carcinoma. Report on 219 patients. Acta Radiol Oncol 1983;22:23–28

44. Wang CC. Re-irradiation of recurrent nasopharyngeal carcinoma—Treatment techniques and results. Int J Radiat Oncol Biol Phys 1987;13:953–956

45. De Neve W, De Gersem W, Derycke S, et al. Clinical delivery of intensity modulated conformal radiotherapy for relapsed or second-primary head and neck cancer using a multileaf collimator with dynamic control. Radiother Oncol 1999;50:301–314

46. Wilder RB, Margolis LW. Skin cancer. In: Phillips TL, Leibel SA, eds. Textbook of Radiation Oncology. Philadelphia: WB Saunders; 1998:1165–1182

47. Ang KK, Morrison WH, Wilder RB, et al. Cutaneous carcinoma and melanoma. In: Cox JD, ed. Moss' Radiation Oncology: Rationale, Technique, Results. 8th ed. St. Louis: Mosby; in press

48. Traenkle HL, Mulay D. Further observations on late radiation necrosis following therapy of skin cancer. Arch Dermatol 1960;81:908–913

49. Wang CC, Biggs PJ. Technical and radiotherapeutic considerations of intra-oral cone electron beam radiation therapy for head and neck cancer. Semin Radiat Oncol 1992;2:171–179

50. Crook JM, Esche BA. The Role of interstitial radiation in oral cavity cancer. In Johnson JT, Didolkar MS, eds. Head and Neck Cancer. Hong Kong: Elsevier Science; 1993;3:697–705

51. Delclos L, Lindberg RD, Fletcher GH. Squamous cell carcinoma of the oral tongue and floor of mouth: evaluation of interstitial radium therapy. AJR Am J Roentgenol 1976;126:223–228

52. Fu KK, Lichter A. A carcinoma of the floor of mouth: an analysis of treatment results and sites and causes of failures. Int J Radiat Oncol Biol Phys 1976;1:829–837

53. Ildstad ST, Bigelow ME, Remensnyder JP. Intra-oral cancer at the Massachusetts General Hospital: squamous cell carcinoma of the floor of the mouth. Ann Surg 1983;197:34–41

54. Chu A, Fletcher GH. Incidence and causes of failures to control by irradiation of the primary lesions in squamous cell carcinomas of the anterior two-thirds of the tongue and floor of mouth. Am J Roentgenol Radium Ther Nucl Med 1973;117:502–507

55. Aygun C, Salazar O, Sewchand W, et al. Carcinoma of the floor of the mouth: a 20 year experience. Int J Radiat Oncol Biol Phys 1984;10:619–626

56. Hicks WL Jr, Loree TR, Garcia RI, et al. Squamous cell carcinoma of the floor of mouth: a 20-year review. Head Neck 1997;19:400–405

57. Zelefsky MJ, Harrison LB, Fass DE, et al. Postoperative radiotherapy for oral cavity cancers: impact of anatomic subsite on treatment outcome. Head Neck 1990;12:470–475

58. Mendenhall WM, Million RR, Cassisi NJ, et al. Elective neck irradiation in squamous cell carcinoma of the head and neck. Head Neck Surg 1980;3:15–20

59. Chung CK, Johns ME, Cantrell RW, et al. Radiotherapy in the management of primary malignancies of the hard palate. Laryngoscope 1980;90:576–584

60. Chung CK, Rahman SM, Lim ML, et al. Squamous cell carcinoma of the hard palate. Int J Radiat Oncol Biol Phys 1979;5:191–196

61. Evans JF, Shah JP. Epidermoid carcinoma of the palate. Am J Surg 1981;142:451–455

62. MacComb WS, Fletcher GH, Healey JE. Cancer of the Head and Neck. Baltimore: Williams & Wilkins; 1967:110

63. Fang FM, Leung SW, Huang CC, et al. Combined-modality therapy for squamous carcinoma of the buccal mucosa: treatment results and prognostic factors. Head Neck 1997;19:506–512

64. Mishra RC, Singh DN, Mishra TK. Post-operative radiotherapy in carcinoma of buccal mucosa, a prospective randomized trial. Eur J Surg Oncol 1996;22:502–504

65. Nair MK, Sankaranarayanan R, Padamanabhan TK. Evaluation of the role of radiotherapy in the management of carcinoma of the buccal mucosa. Cancer 1988;61:1326–1331

66. Lo K, Fletcher GH, Byers RM, et al. Results of irradiation in the squamous cell carcinoma of the anterior faucial pillar extramular trigone. Int J Radiat Oncol Biol Phys 1987;13:969–974

67. Weber RS, Peter LJ, Wolf P, et al. Squamous cell carcinoma of the soft palate, uvula, and anterior faucial pillar. Otolaryngol Head Neck Surg 1988;99:16–23

68. Lindberg RD, Fletcher GH. The role of irradiation in the management of head and neck cancer: analysis of results and causes of failure. Tumori 1978;64:313–325

69. Parsons JT, Mendenhall WM, Million RR, et al. The management of primary cancers of the oropharynx: combined treatment or irradiation alone? Semin Radiat Oncol 1992;2:142–148

70. Million RR. Squamous cell carcinoma of the head and neck: combined therapy: surgery and postoperative irradiation. Int J Radiat Oncol Biol Phys 1979;5:2161–2162

71. Wong CS, Ang KK, Fletcher GH, et al. Definitive radiotherapy for squamous cell carcinoma of the tonsillar fossa. Int J Radiat Oncol Biol Phys 1989;16:657–662

72. Zelefsky MJ, Harrison LB, Armstrong JG. Long-term treatment results of postoperative radiation therapy for advanced stage oropharyngeal carcinoma. Cancer 1992;70:2388–2395

73. Foote RL, Olsen KD, Davis DL, et al. Base of tongue carcinoma: patterns of failure and predictors of recurrence after surgery alone. Head Neck 1993;15:300–307

74. Puthawala AA, Syed AM, Eads DL, et al. Limited external beam interstitial iridium irradiation in the treatment of carcinoma of the base of tongue: a ten year experience. Int J Radiat Oncol Biol Phys 1988;14:839–848

75. Weber RS, Gidley P, Morrison WH, et al. Treatment selection for carcinoma of the base of tongue. Am J Surg 1990;160:415–419

76. Harrison LB, Zelefsky MJ, Sessions RB, et al. Base-of-tongue cancer treated with external beam irradiation plus brachytherapy: oncologic and functional outcome. Radiology 1992;184:267–270

77. Harrison LB, Kraus DH, Zelefsky MJ, et al. Long term results of primary radiation therapy for squamous cell cancer of the base of tongue (abstract). Proceedings of the 4th International Meeting on Head and Neck Cancer. 1996:71

78. Housset M, Bailet F, Dessard-Diana B, et al. A retrospective study of three treatment techniques for T1–T2 base of tongue lesions: implantation and external radiation alone. Int J Radiat Oncol Biol Phys 1987;13:511–516

79. Million RR, Cassissi NJ. Management of Head and Neck Cancer: A Multidisciplinary Approach. 2nd ed. Philadelphia: JB Lippincott; 1994

80. Kaplan MJ, Johns ME, Clark DA, et al. Glottic carcinomas: the roles of surgery and irradiation. Cancer 1984;53:2641–2648

81. Woodhouse RJ, Quivey JM, Fu KK, et al. Treatment of carcinoma of the vocal cords: a review of 20 years experience. Laryngoscope 1981;91:1155–1162

82. Lederman M. Cancer of the larynx, I: Natural history in relation to treatment. Br J Radiol 1971;44:569–578

83. McGavran MH, Bauer WC, Ogura JH. The incidence of cervical lymph node metastasis from epidermoid carcinoma of the larynx and their relationship to certain characteristics of the primary tumor: a study based on the clinical and pathological findings for 96 patients treated by primary en bloc laryngectomy and radical neck dissection. Cancer 1961;14:55–66

84. Bocca E. Surgical management of supraglottic cancer and its lymph node metastases in a conservation perspective. Ann Otol Rhinol Laryngol 1991;100:261–267

85. Robbins KT, Davidson W, Peters LJ, et al. Conservation surgery for T2 and T3 carcinomas of the supraglottix larynx. Arch Otolaryngol Head Neck Surg 1988;114:421–426

86. Mendenhall WM, Parsons JT, Stringer SP, et al. Carcinoma of the supraglottic larynx: a basis for comparing the results of radiotherapy and surgery. Head Neck 1990;12:204–209

87. Million RR. The larynx...so to speak: everything I wanted to know about laryngeal cancer I learned in the last 32 years. Int J Radiat Oncol Biol Phys 1992;23:691–704

88. Department of Veterans Affairs. Induction chemotherapy plus radiation compared with surgery plus radiation in patients with advanced laryngeal cancer. N Engl J Med 1991;324:1685–1690

89. Forastiere AA, Goepfert H, Maor M, et al. Concurrent chemotherapy and radiotherapy for organ preservation in advanced laryngeal cancer. N Engl J Med 2003;349:2091–2098

90. Harwood AR, Beale FA, Cummings BJ, et al. Supraglottic laryngeal carcinoma: an analysis of dose-volume factors in 410 patients. Int J Radiat Oncol Biol Phys 1983;9:311–319

91. Wall TJ, Peters LJ, Brown BW, et al. Relationship between lymph node status and primary tumor control probability in tumors of the supraglottic larynx. Int J Radiat Oncol Biol Phys 1985;11:1895–1902

92. Wang CC. Carcinoma of the larynx. In: Wang CC, ed. Indications, Techniques, and Results. Chicago: Year Book Medical Publishers; 1990:223

93. Fein DA, Mendenhall WM, Parsons JT, et al. Carcinoma in situ of the glottic larynx: the role of radiotherapy. Int J Radiat Oncol Biol Phys 1993;27:379–384

94. Smitt MC, Goffinet DR. Radiotherapy for carcinoma in situ of the glottic larynx. Int J Radiat Oncol Biol Phys 1994;28:251–255

95. Mendenhall WM, Parsons JT, Million RR. T1–T2 squamous cell carcinoma of the glottic larynx treated with radiation therapy: relationship of dose-fractionation factors to local control and complications. Int J Radiat Oncol Biol Phys 1988;15:1267–1273

96. Amornmarn R, Prempree T, Viravathana T, et al. A therapeutic approach to early vocal cord carcinoma. Acta Radiol Oncol 1985;24:321–325

97. Le QT, Fu KK, Kroll S, et al. Influence of fraction size, total dose, and overall time on local control of T1–T2 glottic carcinoma. Int J Radiat Oncol Biol Phys 1997;39:115–126

98. Mendenhall WM, Parsons JT, Stringer SP, et al. Stage T3 squamous cell carcinoma of the glottic larynx: a comparison of laryngectomy and irradiation. Int J Radiat Oncol Biol Phys 1992;23:725–732

99. van den Bogaert W, Aostyn F, van der Schueren E. The primary treatment of advanced vocal cord cancer: laryngectomy or radiotherapy? Int J Radiat Oncol Biol Phys 1983;9:329–334

100. Stewart JG, Jackson AW. The steepness of the dose response curve both for tumor cure and normal tissue injury. Laryngoscope 1975;85:1107–1111

101. Warde P, Harwood A, Keane T. Carcinoma of the subglottis: results of initial radical radiation. Arch Otolaryngol Head Neck Surg 1987;113:1228–1229

102. Cunningham MP, Caitlin D. Cancer of the pharyngeal wall. Cancer 1967;20:1859–1866

103. Shah JP, Shaha AR, Spiro RH, et al. Carcinoma of the hypopharynx. Am J Surg 1976;132:439–443

104. Harrison DF. Pathology of hypopharyngeal cancer in relation to surgical management. J Laryngol Otol 1970;84:349–367

105. Lefebvre JL, Chevalier D, Luboinski B, et al. Larynx preservation in pyriform sinus cancer: preliminary results of a European Organization for Research and Treatment of Cancer phase III trial. J Natl Cancer Inst 1996;88:890–899

106. Mendenhall WM, Parsons JT, Stringer SP, et al. Radiotherapy alone or combined with neck dissection for T1–T2 carcinoma of the pyriform sinus: an alternative to conservation surgery. Int J Radiat Oncol Biol Phys 1993;27:1017–1027

107. Bataini P, Brugere J, Bernie J, et al. Results of radical radiotherapeutic treatment of carcinoma of the pyriform sinus: experience of the Institut Curie. Int J Radiat Oncol Biol Phys 1982;8:1277–1286

108. El Badawi SA, Goepfert H, Fletcher GH, et al. Squamous cell carcinoma of the pyriform sinus. Laryngoscope 1982;92:357–364

109. Vandenbrouck C, Eschwege F, De la Rochefordiere A, et al. Squamous cell carcinoma of the pyriform sinus: retrospective study of 351 cases treated at the Institut Gustave-Roussy. Head Neck Surg 1987;10:4–13

110. Dubois JB, Guerrier B, Di Ruggiero JM, et al. Cancer of the pyriform sinus: treatment by radiation therapy alone and with surgery. Radiology 1986;160:831–836

111. Ho CM, Lam KH, Wei WI, et al. Squamous cell carcinoma of the hypopharynx: analysis of treatment results. Head Neck 1993;15:405–412

112. Spiro RH, Kelly J, Vega AL, et al. Squamous carcinoma of the posterior pharyngeal wall. Am J Surg 1990;160:420–423

113. Talton BM, Elkon D, Kim J, et al. Cancer of the posterior hypopharyngeal wall. Int J Radiat Oncol Biol Phys 1981;7:597–599

114. Fein DA, Mendenhall WM, Parsons JT, et al. Pharyngeal wall carcinoma treated with radiotherapy: impact of treatment technique and fractionation. Int J Radiat Oncol Biol Phys 1993;26:751–757

115. Inoue T, Shigematsu Y, Sato T. Treatment of carcinoma of the hypopharynx. Cancer 1973;31:649–655

116. Stell PM, Carden EA, Hibbert J, et al. Post-cricoid carcinoma. Clin Oncol 1978;4:215–226

117. Hennessy TPJ, O'Connell R. Carcinoma of the hypopharynx, esophagus, and cardia. Surg Gynecol Obstet 1986;162:243–247

118. Kajanti M, Mantyla M. Carcinoma of the hypopharynx: a retrospective analysis of the treatment results over a 25 year period. Acta Oncol 1990;29:903–907

119. Carrau RL, Myers EN, Johnson JT. Paranasal sinus carcinoma-diagnosis, treatment, and prognosis. Oncology 1992;6:43–50

120. Parsons JT, Mendenhall WM, Mancusco AA, et al. Malignant tumors of the nasal cavity and ethmoid and sphenoid sinuses. Int J Radiat Oncol Biol Phys 1988;14:11–22

121. Elkon D, Hightower SI, Lim ML, et al. Esthesioneuroblastoma: surgical treatment without radiation. Cancer 1979;44:1087–1094

122. Jiang GL, Ang KK, Peters LJ, et al. Maxillary sinus carcinomas: natural history and results of postoperative radiotherapy. Radiother Oncol 1991;21:193–200

123. Ryu JK. Nasal cavity and paranasal sinuses. In: Phillips TL, Leibel SA, eds. Textbook of Radiation Oncology. Philadelphia: WB Saunders; 1998:527–548

124. Liu FF, Rotstein L, Davison AJ, et al. Benign parotid adenoma: a review of the Princess Margaret Hospital experience. Head Neck 1995;17:177–183

125. Matsuba HM, Thawley SE, Devineni VR, et al. The parotid gland: effective use of planned combined surgery and irradiation. Laryngoscope 1985;95:1059–1063

126. Shidnia H, Hornbach NB, Hamaker R, et al. Carcinoma of major salivary glands. Cancer 1980;45:693–697

127. Armstrong JG, Harrison LB, Thaler HT, et al. The indications for elective treatment of the neck in cancer of the major salivary glands. Cancer 1992;69:615–620

128. Spiro IJ, Wang CC, Montgomery WW. Carcinoma of the parotid gland. Cancer 1993;71:2699–2705

129. Fu KK, Leibel S, Levine M, et al. Carcinoma of the major and minor salivary glands: analysis of treatment results and sites and causes of failures. Cancer 1977;40:2882–2890

130. Weber RS, Byers RM, Petit B, Wolf P, Ang K, Luna M. Submandibular gland tumors. Adverse histologic factors and therapeutic implications. Arch Otolaryngol Head Neck Surg 1990;116:1055–1060

131. Tran L, Sidrys J, Sadeghi A, et al. Salivary gland tumors of the oral cavity. Int J Radiat Oncol Biol Phys 1990;18:413–417

132. Laramore GE, Krall JM, Griffin TW, et al. Neutron versus photon irradiation for unresectable salivary gland tumors: final report of an RTOG-MRC randomized clinical trial. Radiation Therapy Oncology Group. Medical Research Council. Int J Radiat Oncol Biol Phys 1993;27:235–240

133. Douglas JG, Lee S, Laramore GE, et al. Neutron radiotherapy for the treatment of locally advanced major salivary gland tumors. Head Neck 1999;21:255–263

134. Krull A, Schwarz R, Brackrock S, et al. Neutron therapy in malignant salivary gland tumors: results at European centers. Recent Results Cancer Res 1998;150:88–99

135. Munzenrider JE, Adams J, Liebsch NJ. Skull base tumors: treatment with three-dimensional planning and fractionated x-ray and proton radiotherapy. In: Leibel SA, Phillips TI, eds. Textbook of Radiation Oncology. Philadelphia: WB Saunders; 1998

136. Springate SC, Weichselbaum RR. Radiation or surgery for chemodectoma of the temporal bone: a review of local control and complications. Head Neck 1990;12:303–307

137. Powell S, Peters N, Harmer C. Chemodectoma of the head and neck: results of treatment in 84 patients. Int J Radiat Oncol Biol Phys 1992;22:919–924

138. Austin-Seymour M, Urie M, Munzenrider J, et al. Consideration in fractionated proton radiation therapy: clinical potential and results. Radiother Oncol 1990;17:29–35

139. Benk V, Liebsch NJ, Munzenrider JE, et al. Base of skull and cervical spine chordomas in children treated by high-dose irradiation. Int J Radiat Oncol Biol Phys 1995;31:577–581

140. Terahara A, Niemierko A, Goitein M, et al. Analysis of the relationship between tumor dose inhomogeneity and local control in patients with skull base chordoma. Int J Radiat Oncol Biol Phys 1999;45:351–358

141. Munzenrider JE, Liebsch NJ. Proton therapy for tumors of the skull base. Strahlenther Onkol 1999;175:57–63

142. Castro JR, Linstadt DE, Bahary BP, et al. Experience in charged particle irradiation of tumors of the skull base. Int J Radiat Oncol Biol Phys 1994;29:647–655

143. Berson AM, Castro JR, Petti P, et al. Charged particle irradiation of chordoma and chondrosarcoma of the base of skull and cervical spine: the Lawrence Berkeley Laboratory experience. Int J Radiat Oncol Biol Phys 1988;15:559–565

144. Krengli M, Liebsch NJ, Hug EB, et al. Review of current protocols for protontherapy in USA. Tumori 1998;84:209–216

145. Mizerny BR, Kost KM. Chordoma of the cranial base: the McGill experience. J Otolaryngol 1995;24:14–19

146. Payne DG. Radiation therapy of tumors involving the skull base. Can J Neurol Sci 1985;12:363–365

147. Catton C, O'Sullivan B, Bell R, et al. Chordoma: long-term follow-up after radical photon irradiation. Radiother Oncol 1996;41:67–72

148. Latz D, Gademann G, Hawighorst H, et al. The initial results in the fractionated 3-dimensional stereotactic irradiation of clavus chordomas. Strahlenther Onkol 1995;171:348–355

148a. Leibel SA, Kutcher GJ, Harrison LB, et al. Improved dose distributions for 3D conformal boost treatments in carcinoma of the nasopharynx. Int J Radiat Oncol Biol Phys 1991;20:823–833

149. Emami B, Purdy JA, Simpson JR, et al. 3-D conformal radiotherapy in head and neck cancer: the Washington University experience. Front Radiat Ther Oncol 1996;29:207–220

150. Perez CA, Purdy JA, Harms W, et al. Three-dimensional treatment planning and conformal radiation therapy: preliminary evaluation. Radiother Oncol 1995;36:32–43

151. De Meerleer GO, Vakaet LAML, Bate M-T, et al. The single-isocentre treatment of head and neck cancer: time gain using MLC and automatic set-up. Cancer Radiother 1999;3:235–241

152. Gademann G, Schlegel W, Debus J, et al. Fractionated stereotactically guided radiotherapy of head and neck tumors: a report on clinical use of a new system in 195 cases. Radiother Oncol 1993;29:205–213

153. Ship JA, Eisbruch A, D'Hondt E, et al. Parotid sparing study in head and neck cancer patients receiving bilateral radiation therapy: one-year results. J Dent Res 1997;76:807–813

154. Claus F, Vakaet L, De Gershem W, et al. Postoperative radiotherapy of paranasal sinus tumors: a challenge for intensity modulated radiotherapy. Acta Otorhinolaryngol Belg 1999;53:263–269

155. Grant W III, Woo SY. Clinical and financial issues for intensity-modulated radiation therapy delivery. Semin Radiat Oncol 1999;9:99–107

156. Fraass BA, Kessler ML, McShan DL, et al. Optimization and clinical use of multisegment intensity-modulated radiation therapy for high-dose conformal therapy. Semin Radiat Oncol 1999;9:60–77

157. Kondziolka D, Levy EI, Niranjan A, et al. Long-term outcomes after meningioma radiosurgery: physician and patient perspectives. J Neurosurg 1999;91:44–50

158. Tate DJ, Adler JR Jr, Chang SD, et al. Stereotactic radiosurgical boost following radiotherapy in primary nasopharyngeal carcinoma: impact on local control. Int J Radiat Oncol Biol Phys 1999;45:915–921

159. Hall EJ, Brenner DJ. The radiobiology of radiosurgery: rationale for different treatment regimens for AVMs and malignancies. Int J Radiat Oncol Biol Phys 1993;25:381–385

160. Solberg TD, Selch MT, Smathers JB, et al. Fractionated stereotactic radiotherapy: rationale and methods. Med Dosim 1998;23:209–219

161. Lederman G, Lowry J, Wertheim S, et al. Acoustic neuroma: potential benefits of fractionated stereotactic radiotherapy. Stereotact Funct Neurosurg 1997;69(1–4 Pt 2):175–182

162. Mitsumori M, Shrieve DC, Alexander E III, et al. Initial clinical results of LINAC-based stereotactic radiosurgery and stereotactic radiotherapy for pituitary adenomas. Int J Radiat Oncol Biol Phys 1998;42:573–580

163. Tokuuye K, Akine Y, Sumi M, et al. Reirradiation of brain and skull base tumors with fractionated stereotactic radiotherapy. Int J Radiat Oncol Biol Phys 1998;40:1151–1155

164. Kalapurakal JA, Silverman CL, Akhtar N, et al. Improved trigeminal and facial nerve tolerance following fractionated stereotactic radiotherapy for large acoustic neuromas. Br J Radiol 1999;72:1202–1207

165. Freeman SB, Hamaker RC, Singer MI. Intraoperative radiotherapy of head and neck cancer. Arch Otolaryngol Head Neck Surg 1990;116:165–168

166. Rate WR, Garrett P, Hamaker R, et al. Intraoperative radiation therapy for recurrent head and neck cancer. Cancer 1991;67:2738–2740

167. Toita T, Nakano M, Takizawa Y, et al. Intraoperative radiation therapy (IORT) for head and neck cancer. Int J Radiat Oncol Biol Phys 1994;30:1219–1224

168. Endicott JN, Jensen R, Lyman G, et al. Adjuvant chemotherapy for advanced head and neck squamous carcinoma. Final Report of the Head and Neck Contracts Program. Cancer 1987;60:301–311

169. Jaulerry C, Rodriguez J, Brunin F, et al. Induction chemotherapy in advanced head and neck tumors: results of two randomized trials. Int J Radiat Oncol Biol Phys 1992;23:483–489

170. El-Sayed S, Nelson N. Adjuvant and adjunctive chemotherapy in the management of squamous cell carcinoma of the head and neck region: a meta-analysis of prospective and randomized trials. J Clin Oncol 1996;14:838–847

171. Glicksman AS, Wanebo HJ, Slotman G, et al. Concurrent platinum-based chemotherapy and hyperfractionated radiotherapy with late intensification in advanced head and neck cancer. Int J Radiat Oncol Biol Phys 1997;39:721–729

172. Brizel DM, Alders ME, Samuel RF, et al. Hyperfractionated irradiation with or without concurrent chemotherapy for locally advanced head and neck cancer. N Engl J Med 1998;338:1798–1804

173. Groh BA, Siewerdsen JH, Drake DG, et al. A performance comparison of flat-panel imager-based MV and kV cone-beam CT. Med Phys 2002;29:967–975

174. Grau C, Moller K, Overgaard M, et al. Sensori-neural hearing loss in patients treated with irradiation for nasopharyngeal carcinoma. Int J Radiat Oncol Biol Phys 1991;21:723–728

175. Lee AW, Law SC, Ng SH, et al. Retrospective analysis of nasopharyngeal carcinoma treated during 1976–1985: late complications following megavoltage irradiation. Br J Radiol 1992;65:918–928

176. Fu KK, Woodhouse RJ, Quivey JM, et al. The significance of laryngeal edema following radiotherapy of carcinoma of the vocal cord. Cancer 1982;49:655–658

177. Schonekas KG, Wagner W, Prott FJ. Amifostine—a radioprotector in locally advanced head and neck tumors. Strahlenther Onkol 1999;175(Suppl 4):27–29

178. Huang E-Y, Leung SW, Wang C-J, et al. Oral glutamine to alleviate radiation-induced oral mucositis: a pilot randomized trial. Int J Radiat Oncol Biol Phys 2000;46:535–539

179. Buntzel J, Kuttner K. Chemoprevention with interferon alfa and 13-cis retinoic acid in the adjunctive treatment of head and neck cancer. Auris Nasus Larynx 1998;25:413–418

180. Lingen MW, Polverini PJ, Bouck NP. Retinoic acid and interferon alpha act synergistically as antiangiogenic and antitumor agents against human head and neck squamous cell carcinoma. Cancer Res 1998;58:5551–5558

14

Restoration of Oral and Facial Defects Secondary to Tumor Ablation: A Multidisciplinary Approach

John Beumer III, Eleni D. Roumanas, and Bhavani Venkatachalam

Resection of tumors involving the oral-facial region may require removal of portions of the tongue-mandible, the hard and soft palate, and facial structures such as the orbital contents, the ear, the nose, and the cheek. These surgical resections can cause facial disfigurement and severe functional disabilities. These defects are best restored with a multidisciplinary approach, and this chapter describes how this is best accomplished.

◆ The Multidisciplinary Approach to Rehabilitation: Today's Standard of Care

Today, it is possible to restore almost all patients to near normal form and function enabling them to continue to have useful and productive lives. In the 1980s, technical advances were made, for example, the development of osseointegrated dental implants and free vascularized flaps—but in recent times the most significant improvements have been the result *of improved collaborations between medical and dental researchers and clinicians*. In the leading cancer centers of the world, rehabilitation specialists see and examine the patient prior to their cancer treatment and work with their colleagues in surgical oncology, reconstructive surgery, radiation oncology, and medical oncology to minimize posttreatment morbidities and to develop plans to rehabilitate the patient. Our colleagues in surgery and radiation therapy have begun to realize that minor alterations in their surgical procedures or subtle changes in the radiation treatment volume can have a significant impact on the eventual posttreatment function and appearance of the patient. Presently, with a proper multidisciplinary approach to patient care, *almost all patients* with oral or facial cancer can be effectively rehabilitated, retaining their ability to speak, swallow, chew, and control their saliva, enabling them to interact socially with family, friends, and professional colleagues.

In the not too distant past, the morbidities secondary to surgical resection were so severe that the phrase "the cure was worse than the disease itself" was often used to describe patients after treatment of their oral or facial cancer. Upon completion of treatment many patients had little prospect of partaking of the simple pleasures of life—for instance, enjoying a meal in a restaurant with family, sipping coffee with friends at a neighborhood café, or participating in a lively discussion with friends and colleagues. Equally important was that many if not most were prevented from carrying on with their profession—they were denied the ability to work and maintain a productive life. These patients felt stigmatized and ostracized by their friends and family, and along with these anxieties came the fear of abandonment. Concurrently the caregivers—surgeons, radiation oncologists, and maxillofacial prosthodontists—had to cope with their own feelings of inadequacy and helplessness.[1,2]

However, in recent years, with advances in surgical reconstruction and prosthetic restoration and with a multidisciplinary approach to rehabilitation, significant improvements have been made. One very good example is in patients with tongue–jaw tumors. The functional disabilities associated with resection of a portion of the tongue and the adjacent lower jaw are primarily dependent upon the amount of the tongue resected and how the tongue is reconstructed and the wound closed. In the not too distant past, following resection of cancers in this region the surgical wound was almost always closed primarily or with tongue flaps—for example, by suturing the tongue to the cheek. Following resection and closure, the bulk of the tongue was dramatically reduced and that which remained was immobilized. Such patients were unable to speak intelligibly, control their saliva, and control the bolus of food when attempting to chew, and they also found it difficult to swallow effectively. Today these functional deficits are preventable. Missing portions of the tongue, floor of mouth, and mandible can be replaced at the time of tumor ablation with free tissue transfers. The soft tissues of these flaps can be contoured and shaped so that the bulk and contour of the tongue can be restored to near normal (**Fig. 14.1**), and the bony elements of these flaps can be used to replace the missing portion of the mandible while preserving the complex jaw relationships that are necessary in providing the patient with a functional occlusion. After healing, osseointegrated dental implants can be placed to help restore the missing dentition (**Fig. 14.2**). Patients restored in this manner have the prospect of achieving near normal appearance and oral function. A major breakthrough has been the recognition of the importance of *making restoration of tongue function the first priority* as opposed to restoration of mandibular continuity. For decades now surgeons have had the ability to restore missing segments of the lower jaw that were lost secondary to the resection of oral cancers. However, restoration of the continuity of the mandible had little impact on restoring oral function, if significant portions of the tongue had also been removed during the resection of the tumor.

Another area where collaborative efforts in clinical care and research have had a great impact is in the restoration of

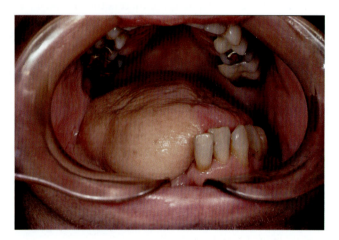

Fig. 14.1 Hemiglossectomy—hemimandibulectomy defect reconstructed with a scapula flap. Speech and swallowing were near normal.

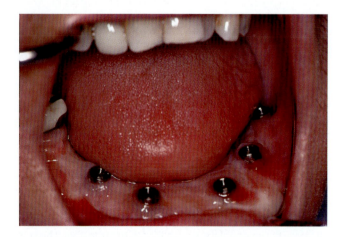

Fig. 14.2 Mandible restored with fibula free flap. Five implants have been placed.

individuals with facial defects secondary to surgical resection of facial parts because of skin cancers. The materials and technology exist today that enable us to restore such patients to near normal appearance. Silicone elastomers have been developed that are flexible, color stable, easily detailed, and colored to match the skin adjacent to the prostheses. They are light in weight and flexible, making the prosthesis comfortable to wear. In addition, variations of the designs used for osseointegrated dental implants have been developed for use in patients with craniofacial defects, and these implants provide excellent anchorage for the silicone facial prostheses. However, the quality of the aesthetic result is still primarily determined by the nature of the surgical resection of the tumor. If the surgical oncologist resects a nose or an ear infiltrated with cancer, ignores the factors that enable fabrication of an aesthetic facial prosthesis, and creates a surgical defect where adjacent facial contours and structures are distorted, it is difficult to achieve an acceptable aesthetic result with the facial prosthesis, in spite of these new materials and technologies. However, if the surgeon solicits a presurgical consultation from the prosthodontist, the surgical defect created will most likely be tailored to meet the demands of the facial prosthesis, superior aesthetic results will be consistently achieved, and the patient's disfigurement will be effectively hidden from the public, friends, and family.

Unfortunately, the pace of change given the technical advances made in reconstructive surgery, maxillofacial prosthodontics, and radiation oncology during the past 30 years has been far too slow. For example, the means of preventing postradiation dental caries secondary to radiation-induced xerostomia had been discovered in the mid-1970s,[3] yet radiation caries are still prevalent. Likewise it has been known for more than 20 years that by selectively removing teeth with moderate to advanced gum disease within the radiation field prior to radiation treatment, that the risk of the patient developing osteoradionecrosis of the mandible after radiation could be almost eliminated.[4–6] Yet today such infections still occur all too frequently. At the present time, free tissue transfers are being used by surgeons throughout the world to restore bony defects of the lower jaw, but still *far too many surgeons fail to understand that it is much more important to restore the bulk and contour of the tongue than to restore the continuity of the mandible if the patient is to have the ability to speak, chew, and swallow after cancer resection.*

◆ Restoration of Tongue-Mandible Defects

Surgical Modifications to Enhance Rehabilitation

Lateral Tongue–Mandible Resections

Minor alterations in the surgical resection of these tumors may improve the prospects of rehabilitation. In edentulous patients, if reconstruction of the mandible is not anticipated, the condyle and ascending ramus should be removed. If a condylar–coronoid fragment remains it is often retracted medially and anteriorly and approximates the maxillary

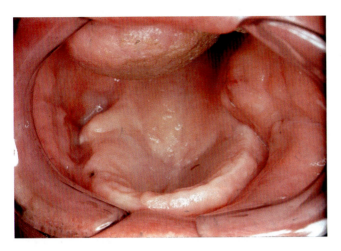

Fig. 14.3 Condyle and ramus segment were retained but not maintained in position. Result: buccal pouch area obliterated.

tuberosity (**Fig. 14.3**). In edentulous patients this prevents proper extension of the maxillary complete denture into the buccal pouch area and compromises its retention and stability. If mandibular reconstruction is planned at a later date it is vital to maintain the presurgical position of each mandibular fragment. These fragments are prone to displacement by scar contracture or contraction of the muscles of mastication. In a resection of the lateral portion of the mandible, the posterior resection line should be made vertically from the sigmoid notch to angle rather than horizontally across the ramus.[7] When the mandible is resected horizontally, the unopposed contraction of the temporalis muscle displaces the ramus fragment superomedially beneath the zygomatic arch, making it very difficult to retrieve later during reconstruction. When the mandible is resected vertically the fragment remains in a relatively normal anatomical position.

If there is a soft tissue deficit at the resected site some form of fixation is useful to stabilize the residual mandibular fragments. Internal fixation devices today primarily consist of titanium reconstruction plates of various designs. These should be considered as temporary means of fixation be-

cause they can fracture or loosen if left over an extended period of time. External pin fixation is an effective means of stabilizing mandibular fragments, particularly in those patients undergoing mandibular resection secondary to osteoradionecrosis.

Bony cuts through the dentulous portion of the mandible should be intraseptal rather than interproximal. This practice will result in higher levels of bone for the tooth adjacent to the surgical defect, making this tooth more suitable if necessary as a partial denture abutment. In addition, bony resections through the body of the mandible should be made as far posteriorly as possible. The more mandible remaining the better the prosthetic prognosis, particularly in edentulous patients. The presence and the condition of teeth profoundly influence the rehabilitation of mandibular resection patients. For example, mandibular guidance procedures are ineffective in the absence of teeth. Prior to surgery key teeth to be salvaged should be identified. Retention of the mandibular cuspids is especially beneficial.

Flaps—Their Use from a Prosthodontic Perspective

The functional disabilities associated with tongue–mandible resections are primarily dependent upon the amount of tongue resected and the method of closure. If the surgical wound is closed primarily (primary closure) by suturing the edges of the wound together (e.g., connecting the residual tongue to the buccal mucosa) the functional disabilities are compounded (**Fig. 14.4A**). Such practice leaves many patients incapacitated, lacking the ability to control their saliva, speak, or swallow. In addition, with primary closure, a concave facial defect is created by resection of the mandible and tongue because of the large bony and soft tissue deficit. The degree of facial disfigurement varies with the extent of surgery, the facial form exhibited by the patient, and the method of closure. In the 1960s the search for other means of wound closure led to development of the thoracoacromial (deltopectoral) flaps[8] and forehead flaps. The use of these flaps permitted the oncology surgeon to be more aggressive resulting in improved survival rates. However, they had only marginal impact on the postsurgical oral function. In addi-

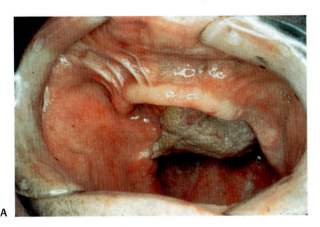
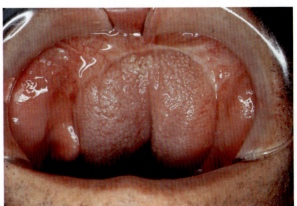

A   B

Fig. 14.4 (**A**) Tongue sutured to buccal mucosa following hemiglossectomy. (**B**) Tongue sutured to lip. In both patients all oral functions are compromised.

tion, these two methods each possessed distinct disadvantages. The thoracoacromial flaps needed to be staged, and the forehead flap left the patient profoundly disfigured.

The introduction of the myocutaneous flap in the late 1970s ameliorated some of the disabilities and deformities; thus this flap became a popular means of wound closure following tongue–mandible resections.[9] From a prosthodontic perspective these flaps were preferred over the methods previously available because they could replace resected soft tissues such as the missing portion of the tongue. The mobility of the residual tongue was somewhat improved and it was centered more normally beneath palatal structures. The result was improved speech, swallowing, and saliva control and less mandibular deviation. Skin paddles of appropriate size could be left attached to the muscle pedicle and be used to reline extensive areas of the oral cavity.

Free vascularized flaps were introduced in the mid-1980s and have had a dramatic impact on postsurgical rehabilitation of these patients. Like the musculocutaneous flaps, the technique enabled replacement of the resected soft tissues due to the resection of the tumor. A significant advantage of these flaps over the others was its improved blood supply, not only for the tissue being transferred but also to the tissues of the recipient site. The improved blood supply improves wound healing, ensures the survival of the flap even in irradiated tissues, and restores the defect with flexible soft tissues.

Postsurgical tongue function is less affected if the resected portion is restored with a free flap. Although the myocutaneous flap restores (referred to above) lost bulk and prevents severe mandibular deviation seen in patients closed primarily, these flaps became scarred and immobile, limiting the mobility of the residual tongue. In contrast, patients whose tongue is reconstructed with free flaps have the potential of achieving near normal speech. Free flaps restore lost bulk, as does the myocutaneous flap, but they do not become heavily scarred and immobile (**Fig. 14.1**). Thus the mobility of the residual and reconstructed tongue is improved dramatically and the quality of speech articulation and bolus control approaches normal limits in many patients.[10]

When implants are placed into the reconstructed mandible and a dental prosthesis is fabricated mastication efficiency approaches the tumor ablation levels.[11,12]

Anterior Floor of Mouth—Mandible Resections

When removal of these lesions requires resection of the mandible anteriorly, the disabilities are quite severe unless mandibular continuity is maintained or restored. If mandibular continuity is not restored the two remaining posterior fragments are pulled medially by the residual mylohyoid muscles and superiorly by the muscles of mastication. With loss of the anterior mandible, the patient appears to have lost the entire lower third of the face. The displacement of the mandibular remnants prevents intercuspation of teeth in dentulous patients and precludes construction and use of dentures in edentulous patients. In addition, with loss of its anterior attachment the tongue tends to retrude posteriorly and may occlude the airway. Primary closure of intraoral

wounds leads to impaired mobility of the tongue and loss of vestibules in the anterior region. Mastication is impossible, speech is unintelligible, and the patient drools constantly (**Fig. 14.4B**).

Given the predictability of free tissue transfers it is highly preferable to reconstruct anterior mandible discontinuity defects primarily. The fibula[10] is the preferred donor site unless the soft tissue deficit is unusually large. The osteotomized fibula provides sufficient length and bulk of bone. At a later date osseointegrated implants can be placed to retain and support a dental prosthesis (**Fig. 14.2**). If bony reconstruction is to be delayed, two objectives must be achieved to prepare the area for reconstruction: (1) stabilization of the mandibular fragments by placement of a fixation device and (2) adequate soft tissue restoration. These objectives can be achieved with the use of a titanium reconstruction plate in combination with a myocutaneous or a free flap.

Tonsillar Resections

In the past, defects secondary to resection of tonsillar tumors were closed either with a tongue flap, or occasionally with a forehead flap. These methods of closure predisposed the patient to both functional disabilities and significant cosmetic deformity. The use of tongue flaps was particularly disabling. Following such closures a large portion of the tongue was no longer available for function, and that which remained was relatively immobile and not properly centered beneath the palate so that speech, swallowing, and salivary control were severely compromised.

Since the early 1980s myocutaneous flaps have been used to close and reconstruct these defects (**Fig. 14.5A**). The most common musculocutaneous flap was based on the pectoralis major muscle. This flap is well suited for the reconstruction of the tonsillar region because the resected tissues are relatively immobile. Mandibular deviation is prevented and, if the tongue was not involved in the resection, its entire bulk remains available for speech and swallowing postsurgically. If a lateral segment of the mandible is removed during the resection, it need not be reconstructed. The musculocutaneous flap provides sufficient bulk to maintain a reasonably symmetrical lateral facial contour, and it also prevents deviation of the mandible. If the patient is dentulous, functional occlusal relationships can be maintained or reestablished quite easily. If the patient is edentulous, osseointegrated implants can be placed to retain and support removable overlay dentures. Residual velopharyngeal defects are best restored with an obturator prosthesis. The functional and cosmetic results are acceptable, and most patients are capable of normal speech, swallowing, and near normal mastication efficiency.

Similarly good results can be obtained with free flaps, the radial forearm flap being most commonly employed (**Fig. 14.5B**). If more than half of the lateral portion of the soft palate is removed, however, the surgeon must avoid tying the flap to the remaining two thirds of the soft palate. Such practice will prevent the reconstructed soft palate from elevating sufficiently to obtain velopharyngeal closure. Palatal lift prostheses have been ineffective in elevating these flaps, and proper obturator placement is difficult because of lack

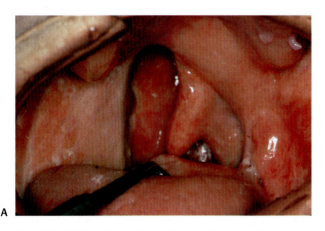 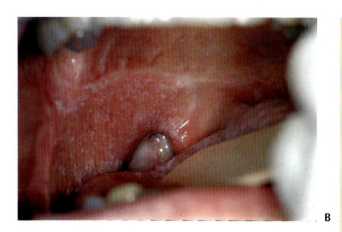

Fig. 14.5 **(A)** Tonsillar defect restored with Pectoralis myocutaneous flap. **(B)** Tonsillar defect restored with radial forearm flap.

of access. Obturation is simple, however, if the defect is left open and speech is restored to normal with this device.

Strategies and Methods Used in Rehabilitation

Palatal Speech and Swallowing Aids

If the reconstructed tongue does not possess the ability to elevate sufficiently to interact with the palatal structures, speech and swallowing can be improved with a maxillary re-shaping device[13,14] (**Fig. 14.6**). The contours of the prosthesis are developed with modeling plastic or tissue–conditioning material and eventually processed into acrylic resin. These aids are enjoying a resurgence of interest because of the effectiveness of tongue reconstruction with free flaps.

Mandibular Guidance Therapy

When mandibular continuity is not restored, methods used to correct mandibular deviation include intermaxillary fixation and mandibularly based or palatally based guidance restorations. The method of choice should be combined with a well-organized mandibular exercise program. Mandibular guidance therapy begins when the initial postsurgical pain and edema have subsided, usually in 2 to 3 weeks. Upon maximum opening, the mandible is displaced by hand as forcefully as possible toward the nonsurgical side. These movements tend to lessen scar contracture, reduce trismus, and improve maxillomandibular relationships.

If the mandible can be manipulated into an acceptable maxillomandibular relationship but the patient lacks the neuromuscular control to bring the mandible into occlusion, a cast mandibular resection prosthesis is appropriate.[15] This prosthesis consists of a removable partial denture framework with a metal flange extending 7 to 10 mm laterally and superiorly on the buccal aspect of the bicuspids and molars on the unresected side. This flange engages the maxillary teeth during mandibular closure, thereby directing the mandible into an appropriate intercuspal position. The partial denture framework must be stable and retentive to counteract the lateral forces generated on the flange during closure. The guidance flange is constructed of cast chrome-cobalt metal. Modifications can be made with acrylic resin.

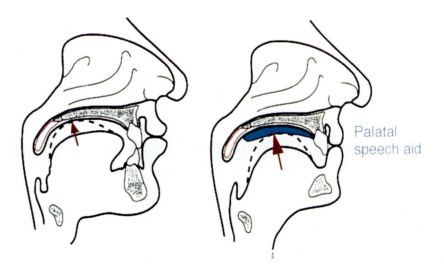

Palatal speech aid

Fig. 14.6 Palatal speech aid enables the dorsum of the reconstructed tongue to the valve against prosthetic palate.

A second design confines the guidance ramp and index to a maxillary prosthesis.[15] This form of guidance prosthesis is indicated when severe deviation prevents manipulation of the mandible into acceptable occlusal contact. Maxillary guidance ramps are more adjustable than mandibular guidance ramps. They are constructed of acrylic resin with wrought wire retainers because they usually serve only temporarily until an acceptable occlusion can be established (**Fig. 14.7**).

The success of mandibular guidance therapy depends on the nature of the surgical defect, its early initiation, and the full cooperation of the patient. Patients with extensive posterior base of tongue lesions that are closed primarily combined with a radical neck dissection and radiation therapy are often unable to achieve functional intercuspal relationships. Mandibular guidance therapy is most successful when the resection involves minimal soft tissue removal or when the soft tissue defects are restored with myocutaneous or free flaps. Following mandibular guidance therapy, occlusal equilibration or selective crown placement may be required to achieve optimal occlusal relationships.

Removable Partial Dentures

The functional outcome for patients fitted with removable partial dentures following resections of the tongue and mandible depends upon the function of the residual or reconstructed tongue. In patients with poor tongue function, only appearance and oral competence can be improved, whereas for patients with good tongue function, mastication is a reasonable objective. The usual principles of partial denture design and fabrication should be followed. Major connectors should be rigid; occlusal rests should direct occlusal forces along the long axis of teeth; guiding planes should be employed to provide stability and bracing; retention must be within the limits of physiological tolerance of the periodontal ligament of the abutment teeth; and maximum support should be gained from the adjacent soft tissues. Retainers, minor connectors, and proximal plates should be designed so that they do not subject the remaining teeth to excessive lateral forces during function.

In patients with lateral discontinuity defects, it may not always be possible to design a framework with retainers that disengage during function because of the altered patterns of force applied to the prosthesis. Viewed from the frontal plane, the arc of closure of the mandible is angular rather than vertical, with forces of occlusion confined to the nonresected side. Rotation of the mandible in the frontal plane causes the resected side to drop down out of occlusion as the force of contracture on the unresected side is increased, and, therefore, the location of the fulcrum line of a partial denture is not easily determined. A typical lateral mandibulectomy defect with a suggested prosthetic design is shown in **Fig. 14.8**. The forces of occlusion are unilateral, so the axis of rotation of the partial denture deviates from the norm. By placing the occlusal rest on the mesial of the premolar, it is possible to place a retainer on this tooth that disengages during application of occlusal forces in the distal extension area. However, a retainer cannot be positioned in a retentive area on the opposite cuspid that disengages during occlusal function. Consequently, this retainer must either be placed on the height of contour, or if placed in a retentive area it must be flexible so that an occlusal force will not subject the cuspid to undue stress. All partial denture frameworks should be physiologically adjusted.[15]

After the partial denture casting has been fabricated, verified, and adjusted, an altered cast impression is obtained of the edentulous areas. Particular attention should be paid to the lingual extension on the unresected side, especially the polished surfaces, which provide additional retention and stability. Maximum extension of the denture base is always attempted. Coverage of the buccal shelf and retromolar pad on the unresected side is essential to maximize support for the prosthesis. Centric relation records are made and occlusal schemes developed that are consistent with the unilateral mandibular movement patterns of mandibulectomy patients (**Fig. 14.9**).

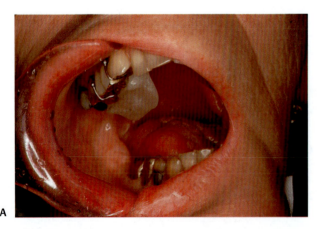

A

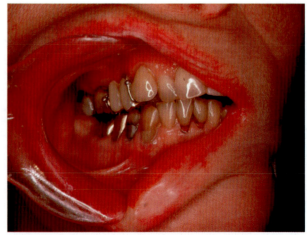

B

Fig. 14.7 (**A**) Resection guidance ramp. (**B**) After several weeks of physical therapy occlusion is restored. Prosthesis is discarded and occlusion idealized by equilibrated and/or restoration.

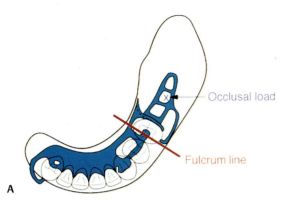

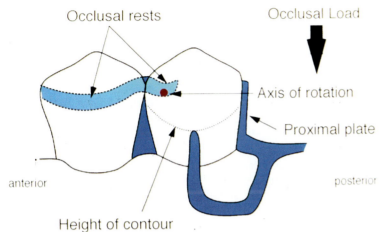

BUCCAL VIEW

Fig. 14.8 Suggested partial denture design for mandibular resection defect. (**A**) Occlusal view. (**B**) Buccal view of nonresected side. "I" bar retainer disengages when occlusal force is applied in extension area.

Complete Dentures

Dentures for edentulous patients with discontinuity defects of the mandible may provide aesthetic improvement by replacing teeth and improving lip and cheek contours, but unless the patient has extraordinary tongue mobility and control, mastication is generally not possible. Several factors affect the patient's ability to function with resection den-

tures: (1) the stability, support, and retention of the mandibular denture may be compromised by the resection; (2) the salivary flow may be reduced; (3) the angular pathway of mandibular closure tends to dislodge dentures; (4) the abnormal maxillomandibular relationships may prevent ideal placement of the denture teeth over their supporting structures; (5) the impairment of motor or sensory control of the tongue, lip, and cheek limits the patient's ability to control

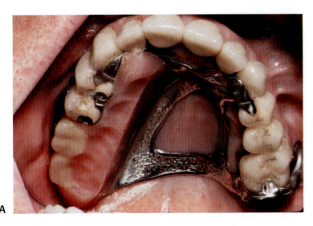

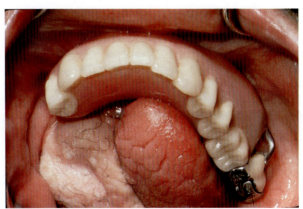

Fig. 14.9 Patient with lateral tongue mandibulectomy defect. (**A**) Maxillary prostheses in position. Note occlusal platform allowing patient to close in altered centric position. (**B**) Mandibular prosthesis in position.

dentures during function. In patients with good tongue bulk and control, implant-assisted resection dentures can overcome many of these difficulties, particularly those associated with compromised retention, stability, or support. Secondary to the resection, the status of the remaining tongue is obviously the most important prognostic factor. If tongue bulk is restored, motor or sensory control is retained on one side, and the tongue can be moved in several directions, resection denture stabilization simultaneous with control of the food bolus during function becomes possible.[15]

Edentulous patients with mandibular resections extending to the midline have a poor prosthetic prognosis. If the resection is limited to the ramus-molar or premolar regions anteriorly, the prosthetic prognosis is more favorable. In resections limited to the ramus, remnants of the masseter or medial pterygoid muscle may remain attached to the mandible, enabling the development of bilaterally balanced occlusion. These patients demonstrate more normal envelopes of mandibular motion, and near-normal ridge relationships, allowing for more favorable distribution of forces during mastication and swallowing.

During fabrication of resection dentures the occlusal plane should be lowered and the vertical dimension should be reduced in most patients. Following impressions, centric and lateral registrations and occlusal schemes should take into consideration the altered pattern of mandibular movements. At denture delivery, denture extensions can be verified with a disclosing wax, and excessive tissue displacement eliminated with the aid of pressure–indicating paste.[13]

◆ **Implant-Assisted and Supported Overlay Dentures** Patients with reasonable tongue bulk and mobility and with motor and sensory innervation intact on at least one side gain the most from implant-retained overlay prostheses. In such patients the tongue is no longer required to control the denture, so it functions mainly to manipulate the food bolus during mastication and swallowing. If the patient's speech is intelligible, the prognosis for effective bolus manipulation with implant-retained overlay prosthesis is very good.[15] In mandibular resection patients, if implants are to be placed into the mandible to retain and support an overlay prosthesis, consideration should be given to placing implants in the opposing maxilla. The unilateral occlusal forces and increased lateral forces generated during the chewing cycle tend to dislodge the maxillary denture. In addition, xerostomia secondary to a course of radiation therapy may compromise the peripheral seal of the maxillary denture. Therefore, implants should be considered if the retention and stability of a conventional maxillary denture are marginal (**Fig. 14.10**). In most patients, the only implant sites available in the edentulous resected mandible are located in the symphyseal region. A minimum of two implants should be placed (**Fig. 14.10**). However, if space allows, more are desirable and serve to improve the stability of the overlay prosthesis.

Implant success rates in free bone grafts used to restore mandibular continuity defects have been encouraging.[16] The data reflecting the use of implants in fibula free flaps have likewise been quite positive.[17]

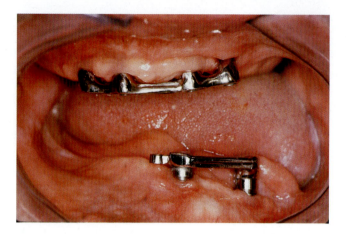

Fig. 14.10 Patient with an unrestored lateral mandible defect. Implants have been added to the maxilla to counteract the unilateral forces of occlusion caused by mandibular resection.

◆ Restoration of the Maxilla and Soft Palate Defects

Unrestored defects of the hard or soft palate produce a variety of problems. Hypernasality makes speech unintelligible; mastication is difficult, particularly for the edentulous patient, because dental structures or denture-bearing tissue surfaces are lost; swallowing is awkward because food and liquids may be forced up into the nasal cavity and out of the nose; the nasal mucous membranes become desiccated by abnormal exposure to the oral environment; nasal and sinus secretions collect in the defect area and may be difficult to control; and facial disfigurement can result from lack of midface bony support or resection of a branch of the facial nerve. In some cases, tumor invasion requires exenteration of the orbital contents or partial removal of the cheek.

Customarily, a temporary prosthesis, known as an immediate surgical obturator, is placed at the time of surgery. During the healing period, this prosthesis is relined periodically with temporary denture reliners to compensate for tissue changes secondary to organization and contracture of the wound. When the defect becomes well healed and dimensionally stable (usually 3 to 4 months after surgery), the definitive prosthesis is made.

Compromised retention, stability, and support for the obturator prosthesis are the main problems encountered when the patient attempts to use such a device. The remaining teeth or dental implants therefore become extremely valuable in providing support, retention, and stability for these restorations. The purpose of the obturator prosthesis is to restore palatal contours, to replace missing teeth, and to restore the physical separation between the oral and nasal cavities, thereby restoring speech, swallowing, and mastication and providing support for the lip and cheek.

Surgical Modifications to Enhance Rehabilitation

It is essential that the prosthodontist examine and consult with the patient before surgery. The sequence of treatment should be explained to the patient, and diagnostic casts and appropriate radiographs should be obtained. With this information, the prosthodontist is ready to consult with the surgeon about the design and fabrication of the surgical obturator. Modifications in the surgical plan that may improve the prosthetic prognosis without adversely affecting tumor removal should be discussed at this time. The surgeon can improve the prosthetic prognosis by considering the following modifications.[18,19]

Hard Palate

Significant portions of the hard palate, particularly the premaxillary segment, can often be identified as being free of disease. Retention of the premaxillary segment significantly improves the support, stability, and retention of the future prosthesis under function (**Fig. 14.11**). Retention of this segment is particularly helpful for the edentulous patient because the remaining palatal surface area provides more support for the obturator prosthesis, and the enhanced support leads to improved chewing efficiency. In addition, in edentulous patients the premaxilla is the most advantageous site for placing osseointegrated implants, and the more of this segment retained, the greater the number of implants can be placed.

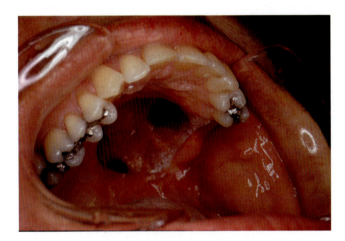

Fig. 14.11 Retention of premaxilla improves support and stability of future obturator prosthesis.

Transalveolar Resections

In dentulous patients, transalveolar bony cuts should be made as distant as possible from the tooth that will be adjacent to the palatal defect. The tooth adjacent to the defect is subject to significant occlusal forces (**Fig. 14.12**) and must be well anchored in bone. It is strongly suggested that bony cuts *not* be made interproximally (between adjacent teeth) because this results in the loss of bone on the defect side of the tooth, thereby compromising the tooth's periodontal support and predisposing it to premature loss. When possible, the next adjacent tooth should be extracted and the transalveolar cut made through the defect side of the extraction socket.

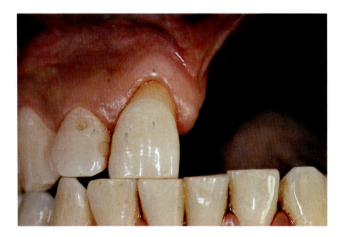

Fig. 14.12 Teeth adjacent to defect are exposed to significant occlusal forces. Note this incisor has healthy layer of bone and gingiva on defect side making it suitable for partial denture abutment.

This approach will result in a sufficient amount of bone on the defect side of the remaining tooth and thus make it a more suitable abutment for the support, stability, and retention of the obturator prosthesis. Retention of the cuspid is quite valuable because of its longer root and superior bony support as compared with its immediate neighbors.

Palatal Mucosa

In many instances, the surgeon can save some of the palatal mucosa normally included in the resection and use this keratinized mucosa to cover the margins of the cut palatal bone. If the exposed bony surface is allowed to granulate and epithelialize spontaneously, it may become lined with respiratory mucosa or poorly keratinized squamous epithelium and provides a decidedly inferior denture-bearing surface. The palatal margin of the defect, particularly in the edentulous patient, serves as the fulcrum around which the prosthesis rotates during function. A keratinized surface in this region will enhance patient comfort and improve the stability of the obturator prosthesis by providing resistance to lateral displacement during mastication and swallowing.

Soft Palate

In a maxillectomy or palatectomy that involves a significant portion of the soft palate or in resection of tumors primarily confined to the soft palate, the remaining portion of the velopharyngeal mechanism must be accessible to the prosthesis if proper velopharyngeal closure is to be achieved during speech and swallowing with an obturator prosthesis. If the resection includes the anterior and middle third of the soft palate, a posterior narrow nonfunctional band of intact soft palate may remain postsurgically (**Fig. 14.13**). These posterior third remnants lack musculature and/or neural innervation and therefore the capacity for elevation. These posterior bands become scarred and contract superiorly, preventing proper positioning of an obturator prosthesis designed to interface with the residual velopharyngeal musculature. Re-

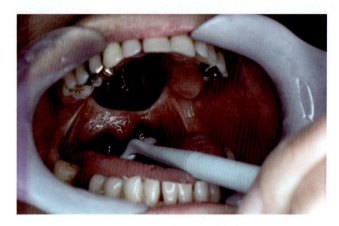

Fig. 14.13 Remaining soft palate was nonfunctional and contracted superiorly, blocking the residence muscles of velopharyngeal closure compromising the function of soft palate obturator.

sultant speech will be hypernasal, and leakage of fluids into the nose will occur during swallowing. Therefore, following a maxillectomy, if one third or less of the posterior aspect of the soft palate remains postsurgically on the resected side, the entire soft palate on that side should be removed. An exception should be made for an edentulous patient undergoing a radical maxillectomy. Retention of the obturator prosthesis is always difficult in such situations, and a distal extension of the obturator prosthesis placed onto the nasal side of the soft palate is an advantage that outweighs the possible speech and leakage problems previously mentioned. In such patients, osseointegrated implants can also be placed in the residual premaxillary segment, thereby providing retention for the anterior portion of the obturator prosthesis (**Fig. 14.14**).

Skin Grafts

The surgeon can dramatically improve the tolerance and retention of the obturator prosthesis if the reflected cheek flap and other adjacent raw tissue surfaces are lined with a split-

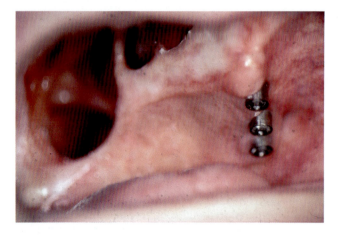

Fig. 14.14 Osseointegrated implants have been placed to retain obturator in this edentulous patient.

thickness skin graft (**Fig. 14.15**). Keratinized stratified squamous epithelium is more resistant to the abrasion caused by the obturator prosthesis than is respiratory epithelium

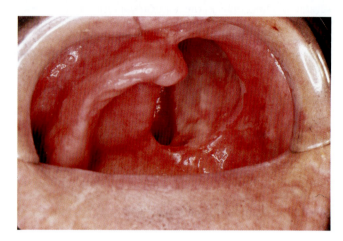

Fig. 14.15 Skin grafts should be used to line maxillectomy and palatectomy defects because they facilitate retention, stability, and support of the obturator prosthesis. Skin graft in this edentulous patient dramatically enhances retention and stability of the obturator.

or nonkeratinized stratified squamous epithelium. The latter types of epithelium will line the defect if it is allowed to granulate and epithelialize spontaneously. Placement of the skin graft also limits scar contracture and increases the flexibility of the cheek. This flexibility enables the prosthodontist to more effectively restore midfacial contours with the labial and buccal surfaces of the obturator prosthesis. In addition, a longitudinal scar band is formed at the junction of the skin graft and the oral mucosa, which creates a retentive pocket above and a support area below the band. Engaging the scar band superiorly and inferiorly with the obturator prosthesis enhances its stability, support, and retention. At surgery the amount of the skin graft survival and defect coverage is improved by the use of an immediate surgical obturator. This device supports a bolus placed into the defect, usually surgical gauze packing, and keeps the graft in place and properly adapted to the raw tissue surface of the cheek until healing. Thermoplastic material like gutta percha attached to the obturator and molded to the limits of the defect can also be used for this purpose.

Access to the Defect

The surgeon should provide access to the superior and lateral aspects of the defect for the prosthodontist. Extending the obturator up the lateral walls of the defect provides retention and stability for the prosthesis and alleviates stresses and strains on abutment teeth or implants. Engaging the lateral nasal side of the orbital floor provides vertical support for the obturator prosthesis. Such structures as the turbinates and bands of oral mucosa may prevent the prosthesis from engaging key areas of the defect, dramatically compromising its function (**Fig. 14.16**). If the postsurgical defect is large,

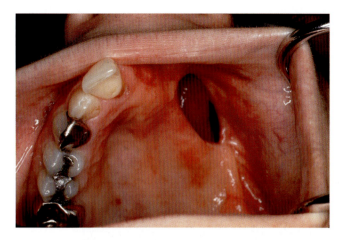

Fig. 14.16 There is inadequate access to this defect. The partial denture used to replace missing teeth and obdurate the defect will subject abutment teeth to excessive torquing forces. An ideal defect with proper extension of the prosthesis up the lateral wall would eliminate these torquing forces thereby better preserving the dentition.

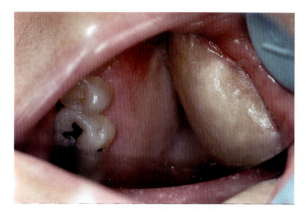

Fig. 14.17 Maxillary defect restored with a free flap. Flap distorts palatal contours impairing tongue space compromising speech articulation and preventing proper positioning of teeth and denture flanges compromising the cosmetic result. In addition, a removable partial denture used to replace missing dentition will torque abutment teeth and lead to premature loss of dentition.

these structures provide little benefit to the patient if oral integrity is not maintained, and severely limit the ability of the prosthodontist to seal the defect and provide proper obturation. Furthermore, the turbinates can enlarge secondary to irritation. The edematous turbinates may extend below the normal palatal plane, distorting the contour of the palatal portion of the prosthesis, impairing tongue space, and disrupting speech and swallowing. Consequently, these structures should be considered for inclusion in the resection. This suggestion may not apply to small midline defects of the hard–soft palate junction.

Osseointegrated Implants

In edentulous patients or when the prognosis for remaining dentition is poor, placement of osseointegrated implants at the time of tumor resection should be considered. These implants can be placed immediately upon tumor removal and require little additional operating time. The most suitable sites for implant placement are the remaining premaxillary segment and the maxillary tuberosity. In some edentulous patients, there may be sufficient bone remaining in the alveolar process below the maxillary sinus (**Fig. 14.14**). The use of bone sites within the defect should be discouraged except in extraordinary circumstances. Compromised oral hygiene access makes it difficult to maintain healthy peri-implant soft tissues around implants positioned in the surgical defect. The prospect of postoperative radiation may preclude the use of osseointegrated implants at these sites if the radiation dose is above 5000 cGy.[20]

Surgical Reconstruction of Palatal Defects

Attempts should not be made to close large defects of the hard palate by surgical means (**Fig. 14.17**). Such surgical closures disrupt normal contours and eliminate tongue space, resulting in difficulty in speech articulation and swallow-

ing. These flaps also make it difficult, if not impossible, for the patient to wear a prosthesis replacing the missing teeth, compromising aesthetics, and may also delay detection of recurrent tumor. An exception would be of defects of 2 cm or less of the palate or, at the other extreme, total palatectomy defects. In the latter, the fibula is the flap of choice because if successful the fibula provides ideal boney sites for placement of osseointegrated implants.

Likewise, most soft palate defects should not be reconstructed by surgical means. Surgical reconstruction of these defects may result in nonfunctional denervated tissues, which are incapable of functioning in a coordinated fashion with the residual velopharyngeal musculature. If the remaining velopharyngeal structures retain the capacity for some movement, properly contoured speech prosthesis will restore normal speech and eliminate almost all nasal leakage of food and liquids. The obturator prosthesis consists of a platform of acrylic resin positioned in the nasopharynx around which the surrounding velopharyngeal musculature functions in a coordinated manner (**Fig. 14.18**). If the peripheral musculature retains capacity for contraction, the patient is able to control the magnitude of nasal airflow, allowing for normal speech and swallowing. Therefore surgical closures that impair the function of the residual velopharyngeal musculature should be discouraged. For example, tethering the residual soft palate to a flap may limit palatal elevation and make difficult the proper positioning of an obturator prosthesis, leading to hypernasal speech and nasal leakage of liquids and bolus.

Immediate Surgical Obturators

Immediate obturators of a palatal defect with an obturator prosthesis will greatly facilitate the patient's postoperative course.[19] The obturator provides a matrix on which the surgical packing can be placed, minimizes contamination of the wound in the immediate postoperative period, and enables the patient to speak and swallow effectively immediately

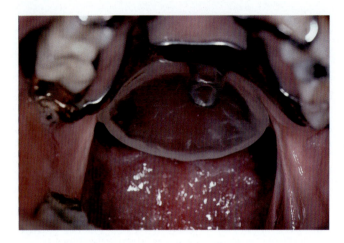

Fig. 14.18 Soft palate obturator in position. Note the space around the obturator. This space permits normal nasal breathing and production of nasal speech phonemes. When residual musculature of velopharyngeal mechanism (levator palatini and superior constrictor) contract, closure is complete and the patient can swallow without fear of nasal leakage and produce normal oral phonemes.

after surgery. The immediate surgical obturator is useful in both dentulous and edentulous patients.

Making the prosthesis is simple. An impression is obtained of the maxillary arch and the anterior portion of the soft palate, and a cast is made. The obturator's size is determined by the surgical boundaries of the resection, as indicated by the surgeon. In the dentulous patient, teeth in the path of the surgical resection are removed from the cast (**Fig. 14.19**). Care should be taken to extend the surgical obturator posteriorly past the proposed posterior soft palatal resection line to effectively seal the defect. These prostheses are processed in autopolymerizing methylmethacrylate. They can be altered at surgery by trimming or by adding a temporary denture reliner. The prosthesis is wired to remaining teeth,

alveolar ridge, or other available structures (e.g., zygomatic arch, anterior nasal spine) (**Fig. 14.20**).

After the surgical packing is removed (6 to 10 days after surgery), the prosthesis is relined with a temporary denture reliner. As healing progresses, the obturator is periodically relined and extended further into the defect, and adaptation is improved. Three to 5 months after surgery, and after initial wound contracture is complete, the definitive prosthesis is begun. Edentulous patients with maxillary defects often require a longer period of healing because the defect must be engaged more aggressively so as to maximize stability, support, and retention of the prosthesis.

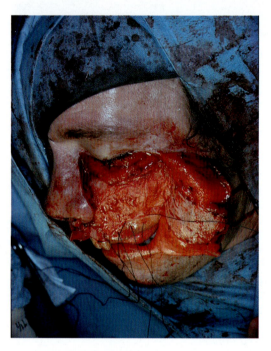

Fig. 14.20 The immediate surgical obturator wired in position with surgical parking placed on top to hold the skin graft in intimate contact with the cheek flap.

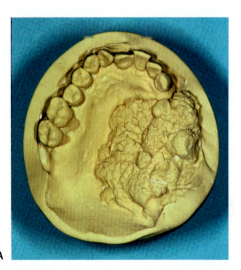

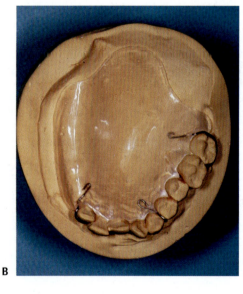

Fig. 14.19 (**A**) Cast of maxilla made. (**B**) Tumor and teeth in path of resection are removed from cast and an immediate surgical obturator prosthesis is fabricated.

A

B

Definitive Obturator Prostheses

Defects of the hard palate are restored effectively with a prosthesis. If teeth are present, they greatly improve the retention and stability of the obturator prosthesis. Speech, swallowing, mastication, and facial contours can be restored with proper extensions and obturation. The obturator should extend maximally up the lateral wall of the defect (**Fig. 14.21**). This high lateral extension improves retention and lateral stability and provides support for the lip and cheek. The movement of the medial surface of the ramus into the distolateral area of the defect must be accounted for during

border molding and final impression procedures. The extension superiorly along the medial margin of the defect should not exceed the level of the repositioned palatal mucosa. If it does, little mechanical benefit results, nasal breathing on the defect side is impaired, and painful ulceration of the respiratory mucosa lining the nasal septum may result. In some edentulous patients, extension onto the nasal surface of the soft palate or into the nasal aperture anteriorly may be necessary to facilitate obturator retention. When the completed prosthesis is inserted, speech and swallowing are restored to normal, and appearance is greatly improved.

Fabrication of an obturator prosthesis for an edentulous patient will challenge the ability of the most skilled clinician. In the presence of a sizable palatal defect, air leakage, compromised stability, and reduced bearing surface will compromise adhesion, cohesion, and peripheral seal of the prosthesis. However, the use of osseointegrated implants can resolve these difficulties[20,21] (**Fig. 14.22**). The obturator must still be extended up into the defect, particularly up the defect's lateral wall to minimize the torquing forces applied to the implants. On the defect side, engaging the skin-lined lateral wall and extending onto the nasal side of the soft palate will facilitate retention. Support for the prosthesis on the defect side can be obtained by extending the prosthesis superiorly to contact the lateral portion of the orbital floor. On the unresected side, the

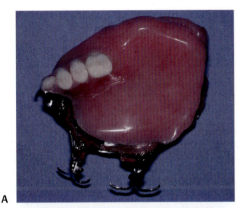

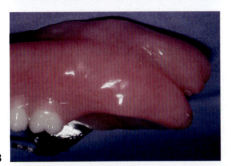

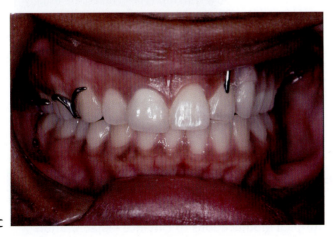

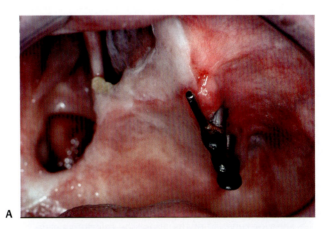

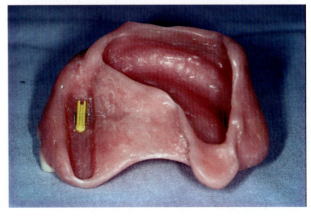

Fig. 14.21 (**A**) Occlusal view of obturator. (**B**) The obturator extends up of lateral into defect and (**C**) restores the partition between the oral nasal cavities. Palatal contours are restored to normal and teeth are properly positioned, enabling restortation of swallowing, speech, and aesthetics.

Fig. 14.22 (**A**) Tissue bar in maxillectomy defect. (**B**) This implant retained complete denture with obturator restored speech, mastication, and swallowing to their presurgical levels.

restoration obtains its retention from the retentive mechanism attached to the implants. Support is provided by engaging the residual palatal structures in the usual manner. The implant-secured overdenture retention mechanism must take into account the multiple axis of rotation of the prosthesis when occlusal forces are applied. In most patients it is advisable to first fabricate a trial denture followed by a dental index, thereby establishing the proper positioning of the denture teeth before the retentive mechanism is fabricated. In some patients the retentive apparatus can be a useful aid in making altered cast impressions or centric relation records. These records are then transferred to an articulator in the usual fashion. For most edentulous patients nonanatomical posterior teeth are preferred. Processing the prosthesis must take into account the special needs related to the retentive attachments. The resulting prosthesis can be gratifying to the patient as well as the clinician. In large defects dramatic improvements in function can be effected as a result of the improved retention and increased support and stability provided for the prosthesis by osseointegrated implants.

Definitive Soft Palate Prostheses

Velopharyngeal closure normally occurs when the soft palate elevates and contacts the contracting lateral and posterior pharyngeal walls of the nasopharynx. When a portion of the soft palate is excised or when the soft palate is perforated, scarred, or neurologically impaired, complete velopharyngeal closure cannot occur. Speech becomes hypernasal, and normal swallowing is not possible. With a pharyngeal obturator the patient will be able to reestablish velopharyngeal closure if the residual portion of the velopharyngeal mechanism still exhibits reasonable movement (see **Fig. 14.18**). Properly designed and fabricated, the obturator will not interfere with breathing, impinge on soft tissues during postural movements, or hamper the tongue during swallowing and speech. The soft palate obturator remains in a fixed position in the nasopharynx and does not attempt to duplicate normal movements of the soft palate. The inferior surface of the obturator remains level with the hard palate contour, which in most patients is approximately the level of the anterior tubercle of the atlas. The inferior margin of the posterior surface of the obturator contacts the Passavant pad, if present, and extends ~10 mm superiorly into the nasopharynx. During breathing and the production of nasal speech sounds, the space around the obturator reflects the potential for muscular contraction. During swallowing and the production of oral speech sounds, this sphincteric muscular network moves into contact with the stationary acrylic resin obturator, establishing velopharyngeal closure. A correctly positioned and constructed obturator *will result in the return of normal speech and swallowing for patients with acquired soft palate defects.*

◆ Restoration of Facial Defects

Restoration of facial defects is a difficult challenge for both the surgeon and the prosthodontist. Surgical reconstruction and prosthodontic restoration both have distinct limitations. The surgeon is limited by the availability of tissue, the damage to the local vascular bed in tumor patients, the need for periodic visual inspection of an oncological defect, and the physical condition of the patient. The prosthodontist is limited by movable tissue beds and the difficulty in retaining large prostheses, although this problem has largely been overcome by the use of osseointegrated implants. Whatever the mode of rehabilitation, the patient should be informed about these choices and should participate in the decision-making process. Prior to surgery, patients should be well-informed with realistic expectations about their rehabilitation.

Surgical Reconstruction versus Prosthetic Restoration

The choice between surgical reconstruction and prosthetic restoration of large facial defects is difficult and complex and depends on the size and etiology of the defect as well as the wishes of the patient. Surgical reconstruction of small facial defects is possible and in most cases is preferable. Many patients prefer masking a small defect with their own tissue rather than with a prosthetic restoration, even though it is difficult, if not impossible, for the surgeon to fabricate a facial part that is as effective in appearance as a well-made prosthesis. However, not everyone will accept an artificial part, and many would rather have a permanent, even if less aesthetic, partial nose or ear. The application of osseointegrated implants in facial defects has, in part, changed patient perceptions about facial prostheses because of the effectiveness of retention achieved.[22]

The following circumstances may dictate prosthetic restoration of facial defects:

1. When a large resection is necessary and reccurrence of tumor is likely, it is advantageous to be able to monitor the surgical site closely. Prosthesis permits such observation, whereas primary surgical reconstruction may make it more difficult.
2. Surgical restoration of large defects is technically difficult and requires multiple procedures and hospitalizations. Patients confronted with this type of defect are usually older and less able or willing to tolerate the multiple procedures required for surgical reconstruction.
3. Many of these types of tumors are treated with radiation therapy. Reduced vascularity, increased fibrosis, and scarring of the tissues bordering the defect increase the risk of complications associated with reconstruction. In many patients, full-course radiation therapy precludes successful surgical reconstruction.

Even when surgical reconstruction is deemed possible, significant delay may be necessary to ensure control of the tumor. Most surgeons prefer to wait at least 1 year after a large resection before beginning surgical reconstruction of a facial defect resulting from removal of a malignant or a benign tumor.

Surgical Modifications to Enhance Rehabilitation

Nasal Defects

When a total rhinectomy is contemplated, the nasal bones should be removed, even though these structures may not be infiltrated with tumor (**Fig. 14.23A**). If the nasal bones remain, the prosthesis must either terminate just above the superior surgical margin, compromising concealment of the prosthetic margin, or extend superiorly over the nasal bridge. Extension of the prosthesis over the nasal bones enables concealment of prosthesis margins but creates a thin, overcontoured prosthesis in these areas that is subject to tearing. Additionally, retained nasal bones will dictate the position and prosthetic contours of the nasal tip. The resultant nasal prosthesis may then appear larger than normal, leading to an unaesthetic result (**Fig. 14.23B**).

Whenever possible, care should be taken to avoid surgical displacement or distortion of the upper lip during resection and closure. If the lip is retracted posteriorly or displaced vertically to accomplish closure, it is not possible to fabricate a nasal prosthesis that can faithfully reproduce presurgical facial contours, particularly from the lateral perspectives. A retracted upper lip immediately draws attention to the patient's midfacial defect and compromises the concealment of the prosthetic margins (**Fig. 14.23B**).

During surgical resection of the tumor, care should also be taken to avoid undue distortion of the cheeks and nasolabial folds. Obliteration or displacement of the nasolabial folds adversely affects the contour and position of the nostril and columella portion of the prosthesis. During surgical resection, the nasal bones, alae, columella, and anterior portion of the nasal septum should be removed without distortion of adjacent facial contours. The osseous and soft tissue margins of the surgical defect should be smoothed and covered with skin grafts (**Fig. 14.24**). Primary closure of such defects

should be avoided because of the possibility of distorting midfacial contours. In selected patients, osseointegrated implants can be placed immediately following tumor resection. The preferred site is the floor of the nose. In dentulous patients care must be taken to avoid the roots of teeth during implant placement.

Orbital Defects

Resections confined to removal of the orbital contents are prosthetically easier to restore than those extending beyond the orbit. As surgical margins extend beyond the orbital confines, the prosthesis becomes less aesthetic because of the inability to camouflage lines of juncture between the skin and the prosthesis. Additionally, as the prosthesis extends beyond the orbit, mobile tissues are encountered. This results in further exposure of the lines of juncture and compromises retention of the prosthesis.

As with rhinectomy, the surgeon should avoid procedures that lead to distortion of adjacent facial structures. In particular, slight discrepancies in the position of the globe or eyebrow are noticed by even the most casual observer. Orbital defects should be lined with split-thickness skin grafts (**Fig. 14.25**). Flaps intended to fill the orbital cavity are discouraged because access to the defect and sufficient depth of defect are essential to fabricate an aesthetic orbital prosthesis (**Fig. 14.26**). When the orbital contents are resected, the eyelids should also be removed because retaining them only hinders access to the defect and often prevents the clinician from placing the globe in proper position.

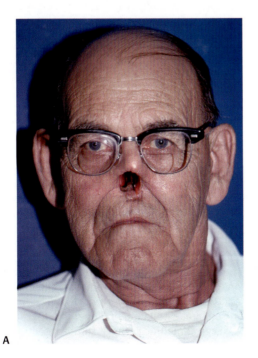
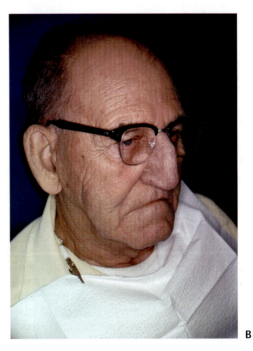

A   B

Fig. 14.23 (**A**) In this patient nasal bones were retained and the lip elevated and closed with the nasal mucosa. (**B**) The combination of retention of nasal bones and a shortened and retracted lip results in a *poor aesthetic result*.

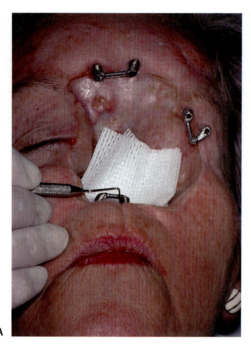
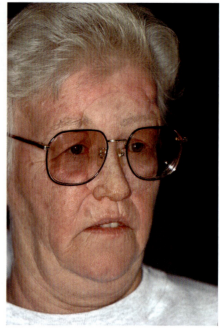

Fig. 14.28 (**A**) Patient with tissue bars in position. (**B**) Facial prosthesis secured in position.

Auricular Defects

If surgical reconstruction of the auricle is not contemplated, the entire ear should be removed, leaving a flat bed of tissue. This tissue bed can be lined with split-thickness skin grafts, full-thickness skin grafts, or pedicle flaps. Hair-bearing flaps should be avoided. The presence of hair precludes the placement of implants, and skin adhesives designed for retention of the prosthesis are difficult to use. The tragus should be retained because this structure helps hide the anterior lines of juncture between the prosthesis and the skin (**Fig. 14.29**). Residual tissue tags have no retentive value and may com-

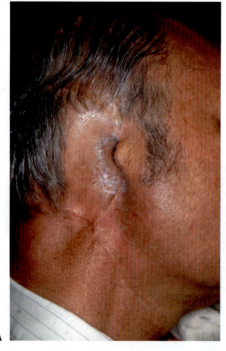
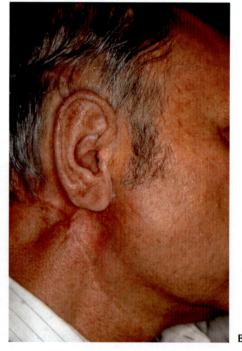

Fig. 14.29 (**A**) Only the tragus remains following resection. The resected area was lined with split-thickness skin graft. (**B**) Prosthesis in place. Note how the tragus helps to camouflage the anterior margin of the prosthesis.

be infiltrated with tumor (**Fig. 14.23A**). If the nasal bones remain, the prosthesis must either terminate just above the superior surgical margin, compromising concealment of the prosthetic margin, or extend superiorly over the nasal bridge. Extension of the prosthesis over the nasal bones enables concealment of prosthesis margins but creates a thin, overcontoured prosthesis in these areas that is subject to tearing. Additionally, retained nasal bones will dictate the position and prosthetic contours of the nasal tip. The resultant nasal prosthesis may then appear larger than normal, leading to an unaesthetic result (**Fig. 14.23B**).

Whenever possible, care should be taken to avoid surgical displacement or distortion of the upper lip during resection and closure. If the lip is retracted posteriorly or displaced vertically to accomplish closure, it is not possible to fabricate a nasal prosthesis that can faithfully reproduce presurgical facial contours, particularly from the lateral perspectives. A retracted upper lip immediately draws attention to the patient's midfacial defect and compromises the concealment of the prosthetic margins (**Fig. 14.23B**).

During surgical resection of the tumor, care should also be taken to avoid undue distortion of the cheeks and nasolabial folds. Obliteration or displacement of the nasolabial folds adversely affects the contour and position of the nostril and columella portion of the prosthesis. During surgical resection, the nasal bones, alae, columella, and anterior portion of the nasal septum should be removed without distortion of adjacent facial contours. The osseous and soft tissue margins of the surgical defect should be smoothed and covered with skin grafts (**Fig. 14.24**). Primary closure of such defects

should be avoided because of the possibility of distorting midfacial contours. In selected patients, osseointegrated implants can be placed immediately following tumor resection. The preferred site is the floor of the nose. In dentulous patients care must be taken to avoid the roots of teeth during implant placement.

Orbital Defects

Resections confined to removal of the orbital contents are prosthetically easier to restore than those extending beyond the orbit. As surgical margins extend beyond the orbital confines, the prosthesis becomes less aesthetic because of the inability to camouflage lines of juncture between the skin and the prosthesis. Additionally, as the prosthesis extends beyond the orbit, mobile tissues are encountered. This results in further exposure of the lines of juncture and compromises retention of the prosthesis.

As with rhinectomy, the surgeon should avoid procedures that lead to distortion of adjacent facial structures. In particular, slight discrepancies in the position of the globe or eyebrow are noticed by even the most casual observer. Orbital defects should be lined with split-thickness skin grafts (**Fig. 14.25**). Flaps intended to fill the orbital cavity are discouraged because access to the defect and sufficient depth of defect are essential to fabricate an aesthetic orbital prosthesis (**Fig. 14.26**). When the orbital contents are resected, the eyelids should also be removed because retaining them only hinders access to the defect and often prevents the clinician from placing the globe in proper position.

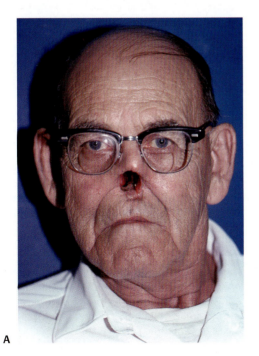
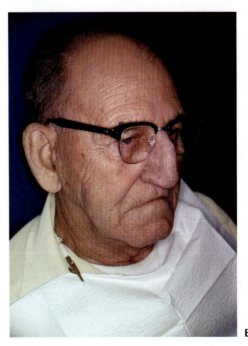

A B

Fig. 14.23 (**A**) In this patient nasal bones were retained and the lip elevated and closed with the nasal mucosa. (**B**) The combination of retention of nasal bones and a shortened and retracted lip results in a *poor aesthetic result*.

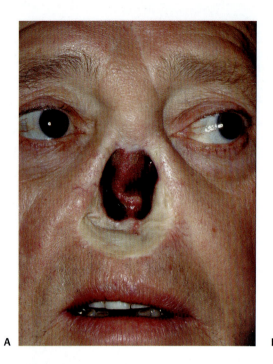

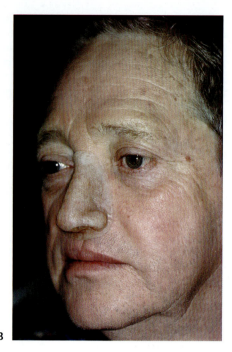

Fig. 14.24 **(A)** In this patient nasal bones were resected and skin graft interposed between the lip margin and mucosal margin of resection. **(B)** The lip is in a normal position and has relatively normal posture, leading to a superior aesthetic result.

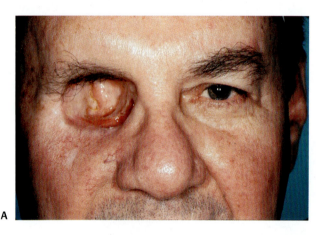

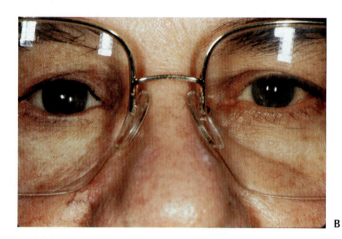

Fig. 14.25 **(A)** Orbital defect lined with a split-thickness skin graft. **(B)** Proper positioning of the globe and development of proper lid contours.

Midfacial Defects

These defects usually result from resection of advanced nasal or nasal cavity tumors and may lead to resection of the nose, upper lip, and orbital contents with extension into the oral cavity. The prosthetic prognosis is primarily dependent on the condition of the remaining teeth, the amount and contour of the residual hard palate, the functional status of the lower lip, and the motivation and adaptability of the patient. The presence of small amounts of upper lip is usually of little value, and in most defects it is not advisable to reconstruct the upper lip surgically. The reconstructed upper lip is often improperly positioned and inflexible, and access to the oral cavity is compromised as a result. In addition, the reconstructed lip can prevent normal lip valving during speech.

Furthermore, the poor aesthetics of the reconstructed upper lip often focuses more attention on the defect and the midfacial prosthesis. Usually, the reconstructed upper lip must be overlaid and covered with the prosthesis to restore speech and aesthetics. The small oral opening and impaired flexibility of the reconstructed oral stoma make it difficult for the prosthodontist to fabricate any necessary oral prostheses and make their insertion/removal difficult for the patient. In addition, oral hygiene procedures will invariably be compromised by the impaired oral opening (**Fig. 14.27**).

Surgical modifications at tumor resection that may be indicated include retention of key teeth to support and retain the combined facial and intraoral prosthesis, and preparation of the defect with the intent of creating skin-lined retentive pouches that can later be used to retain and stabilize

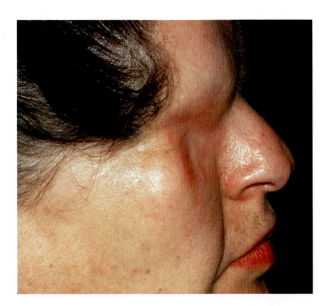

Fig. 14.26 The orbital defect was filled in with free flap. Fabrication of the orbital prosthesis was not possible.

the prosthetic restorations. Soft tissue undercuts created surgically should be lined with split-thickness skin grafts. A failure to do this will result in excessive contracture, and in some cases, loss of the created undercut. Additionally, these undercut areas if not lined with skin usually become epithelialized with nonkeratinized squamous epithelium or respiratory mucosa, thereby limiting their usefulness as a prosthesis-bearing surface. Keratinized tissue at the anterior palatal margin will also improve patient comfort. Skin grafting the nasal floor of the residual hard palate is particularly useful because this surface may be used to retain both the oral and the facial prostheses.

Placement of osseointegrated implants has had a dramatic impact on the function of these large and heretofore difficult to retain midfacial prostheses. Possible sites include the orbital rim, the floor of the nose, the residual malar or zygoma segments, and the glabela. With implants in position, these large facial prostheses can be retained effectively (**Fig. 14.28**). When possible, the implants should be placed at the time of the tumor resection.

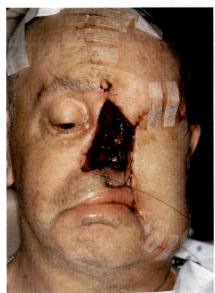

A

Fig. 14.27 (**A**) The upper lip has been reconstructed. (**B**) However, following healing it retracted and became inflexible, making insertion of the oral prosthesis difficult. (**C**) The lip had to be overlaid by facial prosthesis to enable proper lip valving for speech and to achieve a reasonable aesthetic result.

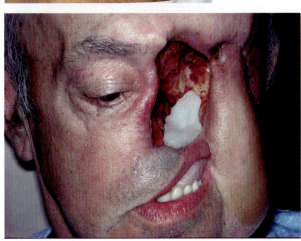

B

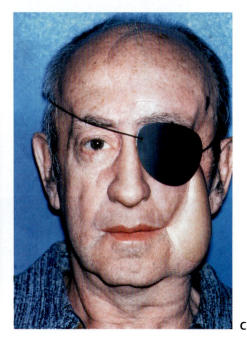

C

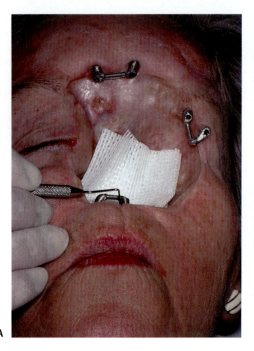
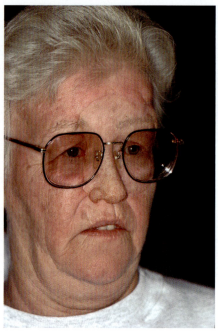

Fig. 14.28 (**A**) Patient with tissue bars in position. (**B**) Facial prosthesis secured in position.

Auricular Defects

If surgical reconstruction of the auricle is not contemplated, the entire ear should be removed, leaving a flat bed of tissue. This tissue bed can be lined with split-thickness skin grafts, full-thickness skin grafts, or pedicle flaps. Hair-bearing flaps should be avoided. The presence of hair precludes the placement of implants, and skin adhesives designed for retention of the prosthesis are difficult to use. The tragus should be retained because this structure helps hide the anterior lines of juncture between the prosthesis and the skin (**Fig. 14.29**). Residual tissue tags have no retentive value and may com-

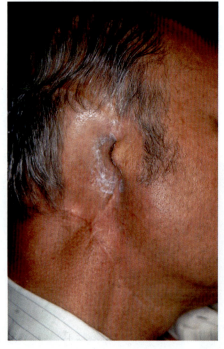
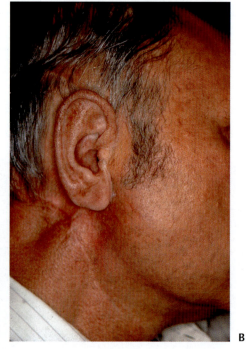

Fig. 14.29 (**A**) Only the tragus remains following resection. The resected area was lined with split-thickness skin graft. (**B**) Prosthesis in place. Note how the tragus helps to camouflage the anterior margin of the prosthesis.

plicate sculpture and positioning of a prosthetic ear that is symmetrical with the remaining auricle. In selected patients, implants can be placed during the same surgical session as tumor ablation.

Prosthetic Restorations

The challenge to the prosthodontist is to fabricate an aesthetically pleasing restoration. A conspicuous prosthesis may produce more anxiety and permit less social readjustment than a simple facial bandage or an eye patch. Because successful use of the restoration may depend on the patient's psychological acceptance of it, it is beneficial to have the patient seen by a social worker during the rehabilitation period. The most critical period is the first 2 to 3 days after delivery. The conflicting emotional responses of the patient should be anticipated and discussed before delivery. In some cases, a patient will not wear a facial prosthesis because of unrealistic expectations. Because all facial restorations are detectable under close scrutiny, the patient must understand that the prosthesis has two different roles: for family, close friends or business associates, it can only cosmetically replace the tissues excised; for the public at large, it generally provides enough concealment to render the reconstructed defect inconspicuous.

Materials Used for Facial Prostheses

Several materials have been used. These include wax, metals, and, recently, polymers. Current materials exhibit some excellent properties but some deficiencies. The materials most often used today are the silicone elastomers. The newest silicone elastomers have been shown to be the most clinically acceptable material. They are color stable and have achieved wide acceptance.

Osseointegrated Implants and Retention

A major development in recent years has been the use of osseointegrated implants for retention.[23] In eligible patients with sufficient bone at the desired sites, the result is an extremely well-retained prosthesis, allowing for vigorous physical activities. The tissue-adhesive systems used during the past 40 years are rapidly being discarded in favor of these new implant systems.

The use of osseointegrated implants is having a dramatic impact on restoration of facial defects. The retention and support derived from these implants eliminate some of the primary limitations of adhesive-retained facial restorations. Benefits derived from implant-retained prostheses include (1) improved retention and stability of the prosthesis, (2) elimination of the occasional skin reaction to the adhesives, (3) ease and enhanced accuracy of prosthesis placement (particularly important in orbital prostheses), (4) improved skin hygiene and patient comfort, (5) decreased daily maintenance associated with removal and reapplication of skin adhesives, (5) increased life span of the facial restoration, and (6) enhanced lines of juncture between the prosthesis and skin. When skin adhesives are used for retention, they must be removed and reapplied each day, leading to loss of colorants at the margin of the prosthesis, eventually rendering the prosthesis aesthetically less acceptable. When an implant prosthesis is fabricated, its margins can be made thinner, and positive pressure can be developed with the prosthesis. These two factors can be especially useful when a facial prosthesis extends into movable tissue beds.

When implants are to be placed, the clinician is best advised to develop a wax sculpting of the facial part to be replaced prior to implant placement. From this sculpting a surgical template can be fabricated and used at surgery to identify appropriate implant positions. In rhinectomy defects, two implants placed into the floor of the nose positioned so as not to distort the contours of the future nasal prosthesis are sufficient for retention and support. More implants are needed for orbital defects, not for retention but because of the higher rate of implant loss at this site. Two implants placed posterior and superior to the ear canal are suitable for retention of most auricular prostheses.

Surgical Placement of Facial Implants

The craniofacial implants are fabricated of commercially pure titanium. They are available in lengths of either 3 or 4 mm and have a 5 mm diameter flange (**Fig. 14.30A**). The short lengths are designed to allow placement in limited bone beds. The flange facilitates initial immobilization of the implant and prevents undue penetration into interior compartments.

A two-stage surgical procedure, the same as is used in the intraoral application, is employed.[23,24] Surgical placement can be conducted with local anesthesia but sterile conditions must be observed. A full-thickness flap is reflected and potential implant sites evaluated with the help of a surgical template. The implant sites are prepared and tapped in the usual manner (**Fig. 14.30B**). A titanium cover screw is placed into the implant to prevent ingrowth of bone and soft tissue during the 4- to 6-month healing period.

In the orbital area the supraorbital rim is usually the preferred site for the fixtures because the bone thickness is adequate in this area. A skin incision just below the eyebrow is made, a skin periosteal flap is reflected inferiorly, and, if the bone thickness allows, 4 mm or longer fixtures are used. Two to three fixtures are sufficient to retain an orbital prosthesis. In the nasal area, there are three possible sites for the installation of implant fixtures. If the patient is edentulous in the anterior maxillary area, two fixtures can be placed in the anterior nasal floor. When roots of teeth are present, the lateral wall of the piriform aperture can be used as implant fixture sites bilaterally. Sufficient bone volume does not always exist in this area, however, and if not, the glabela is another option. At this site one 4 to 7 mm fixture can be placed in what remains of the nasal bones or into the anterior wall of the frontal sinus. The nasolabial fold area should be avoided. Mobility of the tissues in this area from lip movement results in frictional irritation of the soft tissues around the implants, leading to inflammation and proliferation of granulation tissue. In the auricular region the surgical procedures are the same as described earlier. Usually two fixtures are sufficient. They should be placed posterior and superior to the ear canal.

At the second stage a transcutaneous abutment cylinder is attached. Special care must be directed toward thinning

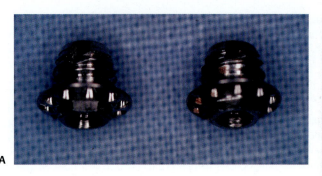

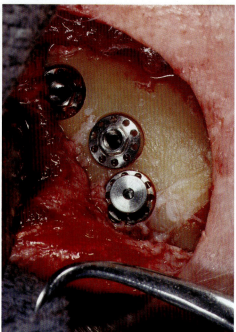

Fig. 14.30 (**A**) Titanium implants are designed for use in craniofacial defects. (**B**) Sites are prepared and tapped and implants inserted in the usual manner.

the tissue flap over the implant sites prior to placement of the abutments. This procedure will lead to the formation of their epithelial cuffs around the abutments and facilitate the maintenance of healthy peri-implant soft tissues. The surgical exposure of implants and the placement of the transepithelial abutments are generally performed 2 to 4 months after the initial placement. For the orbital area, the second stage procedure is similar to the technique described for the oral cavity. An incision is developed inferior to the eyebrow, and the flap reflected supraperiosteally. The cover screws are located and the periosteum over the implants is removed with a punch blade knife. The overlying soft tissue flap is thinned by removing subcutaneous tissue. This flap is then repositioned and the skin is perforated over the fixtures. The cover screws are removed and the abutments are connected on top of the fixtures. Healing caps are placed and polysporin-impregnated gauze is wrapped around the abutment sleeves to compress the soft tissue flap. Use of free skin grafts has not been necessary for the orbital rim region.

For the nasal area, the second-stage procedure is similar. However, due to the anatomical limitations and close approximation to the oral cavity, extreme care is necessary to avoid a through and through communication from the dermis layer into the oral cavity. A major goal during the second surgical stage is to reduce the thickness of the tissue flap to provide a nonmobile tissue bed around the implants and to use as short an abutment sleeve as possible. At second-stage surgery, great care should be taken to thin the subcutaneous tissues around the fixtures. In the auricular area if hair follicles are present in the skin covering the implants, the flap should be removed and replaced with a free, split-thickness skin graft.

Prosthesis Design Considerations

Although the details concerning fabrication of facial prostheses are beyond the scope of this chapter, a few basic principles should be mentioned. Impressions of the defect are usually obtained with elastic impression materials, taking care not to displace the tissues being recorded. The contours of the prostheses are sculpted in wax, both on the cast and on the patient. Surface characteristics, appropriate contour, coloration, and margin placement are equally important factors to be considered. Processing the materials used in facial restorations is complicated and requires special instrumentation. Special large flasks are necessary for processing large prostheses.

When using osseointegrated implants, the retentive mechanism must be contoured and positioned so as to avoid creating distortions of the facial prosthesis (**Fig. 14.31**). The silicone elastomers continue to be the most popular materials used for facial restorations. This material is easy to process, accepts extrinsic coloration, and exhibits acceptable color stability when exposed to the ultraviolet rays of the sun. However, its poor edge strength requires that templates of acrylic resin be fabricated to house the retentive network. These templates are fashioned to fit within the confines of silicone facial prostheses.

Prosthesis Coloration

Coloration of the prosthesis varies with the materials used and the preference of the clinician. Basic skin tones should be developed into a shade guide for each material. The base shade selected for a patient should be slightly lighter than

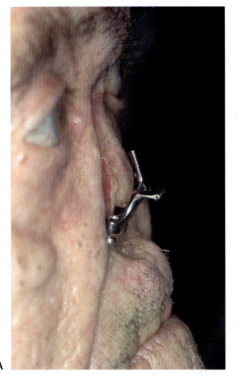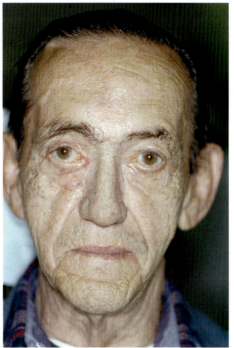

Fig. 14.31 (**A**) The retention bar is screwed to implants. (**B**) Prosthesis in position.

the lightest skin tones of the patient, because as color is added extrinsically the prosthesis will darken. Color may be applied either intrinsically or extrinsically. Intrinsic coloration is longer lasting and is therefore preferred, but it is more difficult to accomplish than extrinsic coloration.

Prosthesis Maintenance

Implant hygiene is achieved by sulcus style toothbrushes, proxy brushes, and other oral hygiene aids. If daily hygiene is not maintained, keratin and debris begin to accumulate on the abutment cylinders, resulting in inflammatory reactions and tissue hypertrophy. Three-month follow-up is recommended.

Results

The success rates of osseointegrated implants used to restore craniofacial defects have been quite good.[25] Success rates for auricular sites have exceeded 95% in most studies,[26] and few complications have been encountered. Success rates for the floor of nose sites are between 85% and 90%, almost as good as the auricular sites and about the same as oral implants placed in the premaxillary segment.[27] However, the success rates of implants placed in the frontal bone and the supraorbital rim have been disappointing. Failure rates seem to be three- to fourfold greater for these sites as compared with the auricular and floor of the nose sites.[27]

◆ Implants in Irradiated Tissues

Predictability of Success

Irradiation of head and neck tumors predisposes to changes in bone, skin, and mucosa that affect the predictability of osseointegrated implants. Successful long-term function of these implants is dependent on viable bone capable of modeling and remodeling as the implant is subjected to functional loading. However, the viability of irradiated bone may not be sufficient to ensure a predictable result at doses to bone above 5500 cGy.

Preliminary reports indicate that the success/failure rates in irradiated bone are dependent upon the anatomical site, total dose delivered to the site, and the use of hyperbaric oxygen. Animal experiments have shown the bone oppositional index is reduced.[28,29] Studies have also indicated that the quality of the bone in the implant–bone appositional zone is compromised, particularly in doses above 5500 cGy.[30]

Recent clinical reports appear to substantiate the concerns raised in the animal studies. Implants in irradiated sites have significantly lower success rating than implants at nonirradiated sites. The University of California–Los Angeles experience is particularly interesting. From 1987 to 1989 92 implants of the craniofacial type were placed in 30 patients to retain facial prostheses. About two thirds were placed in nonirradiated sites and one third were placed in irradiated sites. All irradiated sites received at least 5000 cGy. After

1-year follow-up the success rates were about the same for both groups. By the end of 3 years, 68% of the implants in irradiated sites remained in place as opposed to 84% of the implants placed in nonirradiated sites. At 10 years almost all of the implants in irradiated sites had failed (including 100% of those placed in the irradiated frontal bone), whereas all of the nonirradiated implants that had survived 3-year follow-up continued to be functional at 10-year follow-up.[27]

Similar results are seen for implants placed in the irradiated maxilla used to retain and stabilize maxillary obturator prostheses. At 5-year follow-up, success rates in nonirradiated sites exceed 80%, whereas the success rates of those placed in sites irradiated with doses of 5000 cGy or higher are ~60%.[18] Longer-term data are not available in the irradiated maxilla, but because of the compromised remodeling apparatus we expect the survival rates to continue to decrease over time. Because of these results some clinicians have attempted to improve the viability of irradiated bone with hyperbaric oxygen treatments prior to implant placement.[31] Results have been favorable. However, time and cost preclude this option for many patients.

Risk of Osteoradionecrosis

The risk of osteoradionecrosis secondary to implant placement is primarily confined to the mandible. There is little data available but an analysis of the bone necrosis rate reported in patients undergoing postradiation extraction of teeth in irradiated bone is a useful indicator of the risk. Based on these data, it should be relatively safe to place implants in irradiated mandible sites if the dose is below the equivalent of 5500 cGy. In the one report the risk of osteoradionecrosis secondary to implants placed in the irradiated mandible was 3.4%.[32] All the patients in this retrospective analysis received 6000 cGy to the implant sites. The risk would appear to be high for doses above 6500 cGy, and in these patients a course of hyperbaric oxygen would be prudent. In patients with doses to bone between 5500 and 6500 cGy, individual patient factors, such as dose per fraction, altered fractionation schedules, a previous radical neck dissection, and so forth may be important cofactors to consider when assessing the risk. In the maxilla, the risk of bone necrosis is probably negligible. The use of hyperbaric oxygen can only be justified at the prospect of possibly improving success rates.

Irradiation of Existing Implants

Irradiation of titanium implants already in place results in backscatter, and the bone and mucosa on the radiation source side receive a higher dose. The dose is increased ~15 to 20% at 1 mm from the implant surface. Backscatter associated with noble alloys approaches 50%. Based on these findings and clinical reports, we recommend that all abutments and superstructures made from noble alloys be removed prior to radiation and that healing abutments be secured to the implant fixtures prior to radiation. In the mandible following completion of radiation therapy, if the dose to the implant sites is above 6000 we recommend that the healing abutments remain in place. In the maxilla and the craniofacial sites the original abutments, superstructures, and so forth, can be replaced.

References

1. Ordway D. The crisis of cancer—challenge to change. J Prosthet Dent 1977;37:184–189
2. Ross B. The clinician and the head and cancer patient: psycho-dynamic interactions in maxillofacial rehabilitation. In: Beumer J, Curtis T, Marunick M, eds. Prosthodontic and Surgical Consideration. St. Louis: Ishiyaku Euro-America; 1996:15–24
3. Dreizen S, Daley T, Drane J. Prevention of xerostomia-related dental caries in irradiated cancer patients. J Dent Res 1977;56:99–104
4. Daley T, Drane J. Management of Dental Problems in Irradiated Patients. Houston: University of Texas, MD Anderson Cancer Center; 1972
5. Hayward JR, Kerr DA, Jesse RH, Castigliano SG, Lampe I, Ingle JI. The management of teeth related to treatment of oral cancer. CA Cancer J Clin 1969;19:98–106
6. Beumer J, Harrison R, Sanders B, Kurrasch M. Preradiation dental extractions and the incidence of bone necrosis. Head Neck Surg 1983;5:514–521
7. Schwartz H. Mandibular reconstruction of the head and neck cancer patient. In: Kagan R, Miles J, eds. Head and Neck Oncology. New York: Pergamon; 1989:167–206
8. Bakamjian VY. A two stage method for pharyngoesophageal reconstruction with a primary pectoral skin flap. Plast Reconstr Surg 1965;36:173–184
9. Ariyan S. The pectoralis major myocutaneous flap. Plast Reconstr Surg 1979;63:73–81
10. Markowitz B, Calcaterra T. Reconstruction of tongue mandible defects with free flaps in maxillofacial rehabilitation. In: Beumer J, Curtis T, Marunick M, eds. Prosthodontic and Surgical Considerations. St. Louis: Ishyaku; 1996:161–168
11. Garrett N, Roumanas E, Blackwell K, et al. Efficacy of conventional and implant supported mandibular resecrtion prostheses: study overview and treatment outcomes. J Prosthet Dent 2006;96:13–24
12. Roumanas ED, Garrett N, Blackwell K, et al. Masticatory and swallowing threshold performances with conventional and implant supported prostheses post mandibular fibula free flap reconstruction. J Prosthet Dent 2006;96:289–297
13. Cantor R, Curtis T, Shipp L, Beumer J, Vogel B. Maxillary speech prostheses for mandibular surgical defects. J Prosthet Dent 1969;22:253–260
14. Wheeler RL, Logemann J, Rosen M. Maxillary reshaping prosthesis; effectiveness in improving speech and swallowing of postsurgical oral cancer patients. J Prosthet Dent 1980;43:313–319
15. Beumer J, Marunick M, Curtis T, Roumanas E. Acquired defects of the mandible: etiology, treatment and rehabilitation in maxillofacial rehabilitation. In: Beumer J Curtis T, Marunick M, eds. Prosthodontic and Surgical Considerations. St. Louis: Ishyaku; 1996:114–231
16. Keller EE. Mandibular discontinuity reconstruction with composite grafts: free autogenous iliac bone, titanium mesh trays and titanium endosseous implants. Oral Maxillofac Surg Clin North Am 1991;3:877
17. Roumanas ED, Markowitz B, Lorant J, Calcaterra T, Jones N, Beumer J. Reconstructed mandibular defects: fibula free flaps and osseointegrated implants. Plast Reconstr Surg 1997;99:356–365
18. Beumer J, Nishimura R, Roumanas E. Maxillary defects: alterations at surgery to enhance the prosthetic prognosis. In: Zlotolow I, Esposito S, and Beumer J, eds. Proceedings of the First International Congress on Maxillofacial Prosthetics. 1996:22–26
19. Curtis T, Beumer J. Restoration of hard palate defects. In: Beumer J, Curtis T, Marunick M, eds. Maxillofacial Rehabilitation Prosthodontic and Surgical Considerations. St. Louis: Ishyaku; 1996:225–284
20. Roumanas ED, Nishimura R, Davis B, Beumer J. Clinical evaluation of implants retaining edentulous maxillary obturator prostheses. J Prosthet Dent 1997;77:184–190
21. Curtis T, Beumer J. Restoration of hard palate defects. In: Beumer J, Curtis T, Marunich M, eds. Maxillofacial Rehabilitation-Prosthodontic and Surgical Considerations. St. Louis: Ishyaku; 1996:240–247
22. Chang TL, Garrett N, Roumanas E, Beumer J. Treatment satisfaction with facial prostheses. J Prosthet Dent 2005;94:275–280

23. Tjellström A, Linstrom J, Hallen O, Albrektsson T, Branemark PI. Osseointegrated titanium implants in the temporal bone. Am J Otol 1981;2:304–310

24. Lundgren S, Moy P, Beumer J, Lewis S. Surgical considerations for endosseous implants in the craniofacial region: a 3 year report. Int J Oral Maxillofac Surg 1993;22:272–277

25. Tjellström A, Jansson K, Branemark PI. Craniofacial defects. In: Worthington P, Branemark PI, eds. Advanced Osseointegration Surgery. Chicago: Quintessence Publishing; 1992

26. Sugar A, Beumer J III. Reconstruction prosthetic methods for facial defects. Oral Maxillofac Surg Clin North Am 1994;6:755–764

27. Roumanas ED, Freymiller E, Chang T, Aghaloo T, Beumer J. Implant retained prostheses for facial defects: an up to 14 year followup report on the survival rates of implants at UCLA. Int J Prosthodont 2002;15:325–332

28. Hum S, Larson. The effect of radiation at the titanium bone interface in tissue integration in oral, orthopaedic and maxillofacial reconstruction. Lang W, Tolmer D, eds. Chicago: Quintessence Publishing; 1990:234

29. Weinlaender M, Beumer J, Kenney E, et al. Histomorphometric and fluorescence microscopic evaluation interfacial bone healing around 3 different implants before and after radiation therapy. Int J Oral Maxillofac Implants 2006;21:212–224

30. Nishimura R. Implants in irradiated bone. In: Zlotolow I, Esposito S, Beumer J, eds. Proceedings of the First International Congress on Maxillofacial Prosthetics. 1996:199–203

31. Granstrom G. Osseointegration in irradiated cancer patients: an analysis with respect to implant failures. J Oral Maxillofac Surg 2005;63:579–585

32. Esser E, Wagner W. Dental implants following radical oral cancer surgery and adjuvant radiotherapy. Int J Oral Maxillofac Implants 1997;12:552–557

15

Nursing Care of the Complex Head and Neck Cancer Patient

Ann E. F. Sievers

This chapter reviews the nursing care demanded by complicated head and neck cancer patients. These patients require very specially trained nurses who understand normal anatomy and physiology, surgical anatomy and physiology, postoperative care, and rehabilitation. Head and neck cancer patients have special care needs because of the tremendous insults of the tumor, surgical resections, and adjunct therapy.

It is important for nurses to understand that head and neck tumors can be locally and systemically very aggressive, leading to grave disability and death. Attempts to cure these tumors must also be very aggressive to sustain life. But in therapy to sustain life, disability and disfigurement occur. Head and neck cancer patients have alterations in facial appearance, verbal communication, changes in their methods of eating and breathing. Hearing and sight may often be impaired. Normal human facial expressions are altered, and disfigurement may occur. These impairments will definitely manifest if no cancer treatment is instituted.

Nowhere else in the body are scars, defects, and asymmetry as evident to others as in the face and head and neck area. The face is a focal point for communication, both verbal and facial expression. Identity and beauty are very important in societal norms. Tumors and wounds of the head and neck area not only cause disfigurement but also involve organs that function to meet the basic human needs of air, fluid, and food intake. These organs also serve to assess and interact with the environment via the special senses of vision, auditory processing, taste, deglutition, olfaction, and oral and expressive communication. Radical surgery for the treatment of head and neck cancer involves these tissues. It also may require the removal of, or changes in, the organs used for speech, swallowing, sight, breathing, and hearing. Any interference with facial appearance, the ability to obtain basic human needs, or the ability to communicate can be a devastating experience for the patient and family.[1]

Head and neck cancer patients require the care of a multidisciplinary team of experts. Staff nurses, clinical nurse specialists, physical therapists, social workers, dieticians, discharge planners, and speech pathologists are the core members. This cohort of professionals intimately interfaces with the physician team to complete the matrix that is required for care of these complicated patients.

Coordination of the team to facilitate communication is imperative, with the goal being accurate and consistent information and education from all involved. In a busy head and neck cancer center, team meetings can occur as often as twice weekly. Our own team meets once on Tuesdays to evaluate the current status of in-patients and then again following tumor board on Fridays to review new patients and triage any existing problems. The overall goal is ongoing consistent communication to solve problems and plan ahead for patient care. Ongoing informal communication links flow throughout the week. Nurses (especially female nurses) who care for patients following head and neck surgery need to be aware of their perceptions of patients with facial disfigurement and how their perceptions can influence the nursing care they provide.[2]

The most challenging aspect of care is to provide the emotional, psychological, and physical support needed to help patients return to as normal a life as possible, as well as to help patients attain the optimum level of functioning that they are capable of. The patients and families must be involved and must understand that this is a cooperative planning and decision-making effort. *The secret of the care of the patient is in caring for the patient.*[3]

Head and neck cancer patients usually present with multifactorial illnesses. This complex of illnesses often includes, in addition to the cancer, respiratory and cardiovascular diseases related to smoking, alcoholism, and malnutrition. Often, age-related diseases are manifest at this time because head and neck cancer usually occurs in the later decades of life. This multifactorial presentation makes nursing care difficult to integrate within a surgical setting. It makes the patient's needs more complex and requires more innovative health care resources.

◆ Preoperative Care

Many profound influences are directed at the patient and family at the initial diagnosis. These are stress, the crisis of a new diagnosis of cancer, and the decisions of therapy and the possibility of the finality of the disease. Timely intervention with education and support is critical to patient and family in the early days of diagnosis and planning of therapy. Many patients relate that they really don't understand or remember what is said to them between diagnosis and surgery. Therefore, there is a great need for information, instruction, and psychological support. Pain control is equally as important in this early stage as it is in the postoperative period.

Patients should be encouraged to stop smoking and drinking prior to their anesthesia. But, in reality, this is their pattern of life and defense, and it may not be possible to attain these goals prior to cancer surgery. According to Lillington and Sachs,[4] it has been shown that the elevated incidence of postoperative pulmonary complications (POPC) in current or previous smokers can be reduced significantly by persuading the patient to stop smoking prior to surgery, although there is no consensus on the minimal or optimal duration of preoperative abstinence. The risk for oral cancers (of the lip, mouth, tongue, and throat), according to Burns 1998[5] in the 1998 NCI monograph on cigar smoking, among daily cigar smokers who do not inhale is seven times greater than for nonsmokers. Even the risk of lung cancer among noninhalers who are daily cigar smokers is double that of the risk for nonsmokers.

Often because of the etiology of head and neck cancer, smoking and drinking to excess, the syndrome of Korsokoff affects the patients ability to process new information. Patients with Korsokoff syndrome often demonstrate antegrade and retrograde amnesia at times of stress, which makes the informed consent process and patient education much more challenging. The research of Jacobson and colleagues[6] suggests that, in addition to their amnesia, many patients with Korsokoff syndrome have sustained widespread cognitive deficits, affecting particularly visuoperceptual and abstracting function.[7]

Written information provided at the initial visit solidifies the explanations of diagnosis and proposed therapy. A patient and family information book can also help the patient and family scribe notes and reminders. These books serve as pathways for the patient throughout the health care process. Head and neck cancer information books are often taken home and not read until the day before surgery, if at all, again focusing on the crisis mode of learning. Adults learn best when they want to learn and when they perceive a need to learn.[8] The medical language is a language that most people do not choose to learn, especially in a time of crisis. Interpretation of medical language to a normal conversational language is a very effective role of the expert nurse. This is also more important with the plethora of information available on the Internet. Face-to-face human discussion cannot be replaced. Repeated attempts may be needed to inform the patient and family of the odyssey they are to undergo. The establishment of trust between the patient and treating team is a distinct and important goal.

It may be very beneficial to introduce the patient and family to another patient who has undergone similar therapy for a similar diagnosis. Many patients refuse this offer before surgery and delay this meeting until after recovery. The American Cancer Society and the International Association of Laryngectomees have support and counseling programs for patients to meet people who have undergone similar therapies. This can be a very beneficial adjunct to the process of education. Even when recommended, reality may become too overwhelming, and the patient often refuses to see a Cancer Society visitor.

Despite our best efforts at preoperative counseling, many patients with head and neck cancer still show evidence of inadequate counseling, particularly during the perioperative period. Learning in crisis is difficult, and this may account for the many misconceptions and misunderstandings. Patients have misunderstandings about their disease and its treatment, the physical sequel of laryngectomy, self-care, and the various steps involved in total rehabilitation. When the patient and close relatives are not informed about these matters, postoperative adjustment tends to become increasingly difficult and prolonged. The impact of this lack of presurgical counseling and learning was well documented by Keith et al in 1978[9] and again by Lambie in 1997.[10]

Preoperative pain management is best addressed immediately. The ideal goal of cancer pain management is the combination of comfort and function.[11] Pain is what the patient describes. The pain of untreated head and neck cancer can be as functionally debilitating as the disease itself. Opioid and nonopioid analgesics are employed as needed to treat the pain. Opioids are the drugs of choice in treating cancer pain. As pain has become the fifth vital sign, nurses have become more and more attuned to safe, adequate, and aggressive pain management, World Health Organization (WHO) standards.[12] Adequate pain control succeeds in making the patient more comfortable and establishing trust in the treating team. It also allows the treating team to evaluate the patient's ability to tolerate different types and combinations of pain medications. Agency for Health Care Policy and Research (AHCPR) clinical practice guidelines for acute pain management[13] (operative or medical) and for cancer pain management are invaluable in guiding the process of pain management, (AHCPR Clinical Practice Guidelines on Management of Cancer Pain).[14]

A major role of nursing is to, in consultation with the physician team, establish a plan of care and set guidelines for pain management in the preoperative period. Adequate dosing and evaluation of the effect of pain medication is imperative. Pain scales such as the 1 to 10 normative scale or OUCHER scale (for children) must be part of the armamentarium of the head and neck cancer nurse. The family and patient should have clear instructions on dosing and grading the response to the medication. As most of these patients are not in the hospital, a plan for reporting back should be in place to assess if the medication is managing the pain.

The pain medication delivery system is important to assess because of the impact of head and neck cancer on swallowing. If the patient is able to take oral medication, MS Contin (Purdue Pharma L.P., Stamford, CT), sustained release morphine, is an excellent choice. This drug provides excellent extended dosing over a long period of time. If oral routes are not feasible, small intraoral doses of concentrated drugs such as Roxanol (Boehringer Ingelheim Roxane, Inc., Columbus, Ohio) can still be effectively used. Duragesic (fentanyl patches) (Ortho-McNeil-Janssen Pharmaceuticals, Inc., Raritan, NJ) are excellent nonoral alternatives. The concomitant use of neuro desensitizing agents like anticonvulsants and even certain antidepressants can address the neuropathic pain often associated with peripheral and cranial nerve involvement. Stool softeners should be prescribed as part of the routine use of narcotics. Consideration of antiemetics is addressed because nausea is not an unexpected early side effect of narcotic administration. Often misdiagnosed as an adverse or allergic reaction to narcotics, the nausea usually abates with tolerance to the medication.

◆ The Tumor Board

The tumor board functions as a second and third objective opinion for patients. Staffed by a multidisciplinary team of surgeons, medical oncologist, radiation oncologist, nurses, dentists, speech pathologists, social workers, nutritionists, and support staff, the patient is offered the corporate combined knowledge. The tumor board also acts as a peer review process for the team. It is a series of checks and balances to ultimately afford the patient the best recommendations.

The role of the nurse expert in the tumor board is many faceted. Explaining the process to the patient and family eases the anxiety of presentation and decisions. The tumor board evaluates the entire patient and family as a system and develops a plan of care that encompasses the entire hospitalization, discharge, and return to clinic. The expert nurse has the opportunity to gain insight and provide knowledge into the treatment planning process and final plan of care.

Input regarding the patient's preferences is important during this time. Many patients and families will tell different stories and histories to different people and representatives of different disciplines. A nurse is often less threatening than a physician, and many patients will thus confide more information in the nurse. Time spent on accurate histories makes for much safer and improved patient care.

Tumor board recommendations are only a recommendation for therapy. It is entirely up to patients to understand and decide what therapy they feel is best. It is up to the physician and staff to explain the ramifications of the decision. Few patients when faced with head and neck cancer therapy choose no therapy. This, however, is an option and must be offered, and the consequences must be explained.

The tumor board is an excellent means for assessing both the patient and the family. This includes health habits, tobacco, alcohol, drugs, exercise, diet, alternative medicines, and herbal therapies. You should include directed questions regarding socioeconomic, respiratory, and nutritional status, as well as support structure, communication and literacy, handedness, coordination, and ability to ambulate. These factors play an important role in postoperative recovery, adjustment, and treatment. The goal of preoperative teaching

is to decrease anxiety and enlist the cooperation of the patient and family in the treatment process and to assess the patient's understanding of the physician's explanation of the diagnosis and proposed surgical procedure. Asking patients what concerns them the most about their surgery allows nurses to answer the most pressing questions first.

Preoperative teaching should review where each incision will be made and what facial and airway differences/ alterations are going to occur. The types of tube to be used, postoperative pain management, and early ambulation are explained. To give the patient and family some control, the patient is given specific types of tasks to perform in the immediate postoperative period: coughing and deep breathing and leg and foot exercises. Patients are instructed to do these exercises every hour or every time they look at the clock. They should practice these tasks preoperatively and have the family remind them postoperatively.

During the entire process of diagnosis, treatment, and follow-up, the patient may often feel a loss of control as well as a loss of privacy. The constraints, especially time limits that are often imposed upon the patient, can be overwhelming. Staff sometimes underestimate the patient's emotional need for control and self-determination. Patients who have extensive surgical procedures do require constant observation and intervention. But a balance is important. Allowing the patient and family time to themselves to think, talk, and conduct their own business often provides a welcome respite from medically related activities. This allowance of private time is often reciprocated by a patient who is more willing to endure frequent dressing changes and numerous required tests. The process of building a nursing care plan together with the patient allows the patients to actively participate in their own care. When the plan is developed and followed by both staff and patient, it is usually more successful in directing energies toward the patient's recovery.

Family and friends should not be ignored. They should be informed about where to wait during the surgery and be given updates every 4 hours. Information is important on how long the visiting hours are in the intensive care unit (ICU) and how long the patient will stay in ICU before being moved to the regular hospital floor. Factual information throughout the hospitalization can make the difference between an extremely anxious and untrusting family and one that feels enabled to participate in and understand the care of the patient.[3]

◆ Postoperative Care

Protocols

Head and neck cancer patients who have extensive surgical procedures and present with multifactorial illnesses require close monitoring following surgical resections. A combination of long anesthesia, an extensive smoking history, and significant reconstruction efforts dictates that postoperative care be exacting. Many institutions require complex head and neck cancer patients to be monitored in ICUs following their procedures. Standard postoperative ICU orders are time efficient and often improve the overall accuracy of patient care. Hupcey[16] found that ICU patients have an overwhelming need to feel safe. The perception of feeling safe was influenced by family and friends, ICU staff, religious beliefs, and feelings of knowing, regaining control, hoping, and trusting. Nurses in the ICU can intervene in numerous areas to foster the feeling of safety in critically ill patients.

Developed in conjunction with the attending surgeons, residents, ICU staff, and expert ear, nose, and throat (ENT) nurses, standard orders serve to provide consistency and accuracy of care. Allowances are made in standard orders for development of individual patient variations in care requirements. Standard orders should be reviewed annually and linked to quality of care programs. Standard orders are not cookbook medicine but they help refine the overall process of complex care needs.

Similarly, nursing care plans are suitable for standardization, again ensuring consistency and accuracy of care. Hospitals commonly use collaborative pathways or education pathways or both. The combination of these may serve a better purpose of educating nurses to better educate their patients (see **appendices 15.1** and **15.2**).

In the immediate postoperative period (the first 12 hours), close monitoring of vital signs, respiratory status, and fluid status is done until the patient is stable. This may mean every 15 minutes for 1 hour, every 30 minutes for 2 hours, and then every hour until stable. Then observations are advanced to every 2 to 4 hours as protocol and especially patient requirements dictate. The airway of head and neck cancer patients is the single most important issue that nursing must address. Nurses must integrate the effects of medication interactions, surgical stress, anesthesia, venous congestion, central airway disease, long smoking history, and edema. Early ambulation, coughing and deep breathing, and turning cannot be emphasized enough. These standard nursing care protocols that have been utilized for years are beneficial to counteract the effects of immobility. All the parameters of advanced nursing practice come to bear in taking care of otorhinolaryngology (ORL) patients.

Postoperative Care of the Wound

Suture lines are cleaned of crusts and debris with half-strength hydrogen peroxide and normal saline, using 4 × 4 fluffs. A very light application of an antibiotic ointment is applied to the suture line to act as a seal and antibiotic coverage. All suture lines should be inspected for purulent drainage, dehiscence, and skin color and temperature changes, which may indicate infection or necrosis. Overuse of antibiotic ointment on the suture line may result in skin maceration; some patients develop pustules from the base vehicle ointment, which may then lead to incision infections or breakdown. Intraoral flaps should be regularly inspected with a flashlight for the same changes noted as any external flap. Special care should be used to avoid trauma to the inside of the mouth. Oral suction should be minimized and directed to the side opposite the flap or suture line. The patient is almost always NPO, and nutrition is maintained by enteral feeding. Dietary consults are mandatory to begin early and aggressive nutrition for wound healing.

Patients may experience pain from venous congestion, edema, or muscle spasm, as well as incision pain, as a result of the positioning of the head during the surgical procedure. If there is extensive manipulation of the mandible, the facial pain may be more pronounced. Many patients complain of headache rather than incision pain. Headache may be from venous congestion, nicotine withdrawal, or caffeine withdrawal. Assess duration, location, and intensity of pain and treat appropriately. The use of nicotine patches, Cafergot (Novartis Pharmaceuticals, East Hanover, NJ), or even cool coffee through the nasogastric tube may be beneficial.

Following neck dissection, if a single jugular vein is resected, facial edema may result from the loss of venous egress from the head. Facial edema will decrease with time as the collateral circulation improves. With bilateral radical neck dissections and therefore bilateral jugular vein resections, cerebral and facial edema is significant and can temporarily impair cognitive function. Limitation of free fluid both during and following surgery assists in controlling this problem. Korsokoff syndrome and alcohol withdrawal may also contribute to the patient's confusion and agitation. Agitation protocols are extremely helpful in streamlining care. The careful use of benzodiazepines and pain medication titrated to control symptoms is very effective.

Postoperative Care of the Patient after Carotid Resection

Although not often necessary, carotid resection is required if the tumor is intimately involved with the arterial vascular structures of the neck. If the carotid artery is resected there is a potential for intracranial complications, specifically stroke. Most patients who have a planned carotid resection will have undergone a single photon emission computed tomographic (SPECT) scan and balloon test occlusion (BTO). These tests are done to assess the patient's ability to withstand carotid resection. BTO is done using angiography that first defines the anatomy competency of the cerebral arterial system and the ability of the patient to withstand 20 minutes of internal carotid occlusion, under observation. The patient is lightly sedated but conscious so as to be able to respond to neurological assessment questions, perform handwriting tasks, and enable assessment of foot and hand strength.

Following carotid resection the patient's neurological status should be assessed and documented at least every hour during the first 48 hours. Glasgow coma scale, pupil size, heart rate, blood pressure, extremity movement, and response to verbal commands must be monitored. Maintenance of an adequate blood pressure to sustain flow through the opposite carotid artery, vascular reconstruction, and supplemental cerebral arterial supply is probably one of the most important nursing parameters to monitor, and changes require immediate response.

The patient's written and verbal communication must be assessed for accuracy. Both written and verbal receptive and expressive aphasias are often sequelae of stroke following carotid resection. Changes in these parameters, as well as subjective complaints of headache, nausea, and vomiting should be immediately assessed. The difficulty in assessment results from the alteration in communication with artificial airways. This is an area where the ingenuity of expert nursing assessment comes into play.

Postoperative Care of the Patient after Reconstruction

A flap is any tissue that is transferred from a donor site to a recipient site while maintaining its own native blood supply. A free flap is tissue completely removed from a donor site. Types of flaps are cutaneous flaps, myocutaneous, myofascial, or free flaps. The first three mentioned are supplied by their native arterial vessel and drained by their venous outflow system. The latter, free flap, is tissue that is taken entirely from a distant site, with native artery and vein intact and, via microvascular anastomosis, sutured into recipient arterial and venous outflow systems. The types of free flaps that are most commonly used are the radial forearm, fibular, rectus, and abdominis flaps (**Fig. 15.1**).

Viability of the reconstruction flap is maintained by preventing internal and external pressure directly on the flap tissue or on the supporting vessels of the flap pedicle, which will compromise adequate blood flow through the artery and vein of the pedicle. Because of impaired lymph drainage and surgical trauma to tissues, edema can cause pressure on the vascular base of the flap and result in decreased circulation and venous congestion. Venous drainage is promoted by positioning the patient with the head of the bed elevated 30 to 40 degrees. Patients are instructed not to twist or turn their head into a position that will impede blood flow to the flap, and to keep their head in a specifically ordered range of positions. Head rolls or sandbags may be used to help maintain the correct position. Avoid lying the patient on the operative side; this promotes venous and lymphatic congestion.

Positioning the patient, with the head of the bed elevated 30 to 45 degrees will prevent hyperextension of the neck, re-duce edema, and help prevent tension on the reconstruction flaps or grafts. It will also improve pulmonary ventilation.

Observation of the flap's color, temperature, and capillary refill should be done every hour for the first 48 hours. The color may not exactly match the recipient site but should be close to the color of the donor site. The flap should feel warm to the touch. Good capillary refill is demonstrated when the flap returns to its previous color within 1 to 2 seconds when pressed gently with the finger. Reddish, slightly cyanotic skin, white color changes, temperature changes, bulging of the flap, all are indications of impaired blood supply or egress, and immediate response by the physician is indicated.

When a large flap such as the latissimus dorsi is used for reconstruction, observation of the neck skin under the flap for redness or irritation is essential. A dry sponge placed between the flap and neck will keep the area dry. Be aware that a patient who has been irradiated, or who is in poor nutritional status, is at an increased risk of infection and wound breakdown: therefore frequent observations of the flap and surrounding tissue should be made and interventions initiated.

Postoperative Care for the Patient with Free Flap Reconstruction

Free flaps are called "free" because they are taken entirely from their native location and placed in an alternate location to reconstruct the defect from the tumor resection. Postoperative care for free flaps is more complicated because a microvascular anastomosis is used to connect the vessels of the free flap to new recipient site vessels. Microvascular anastomosis requires the postoperative use of heparin and dextran. The vascular pedicle must be monitored by Doppler ultrasound technique. If the Dopplered pulse is lost or the flap becomes ischemic or displays venous congestion, the vascular

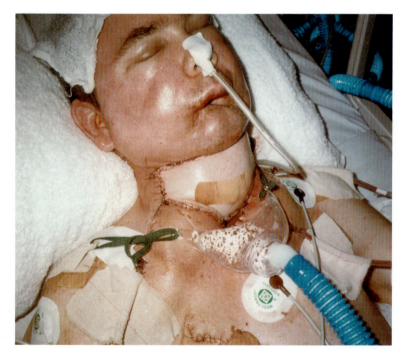

Fig. 15.1 Free rectus reconstruction flap to the anterior neck following resection of a locally invasive laryngeal tumor eroding through the skin of the anterior neck. The patient required total laryngectomy, bilateral neck dissections, pectoralis major myocutaneous flap, and rectus flap reconstruction.

anastomosis must be explored and repaired immediately. If the repair is done quickly, the flap can be salvaged. If the flap is lost, it is a catastrophic event given that the patient losses reconstructive tissue and must then undergo subsequent attempts at reconstruction.

With a fibular free flap, the donor site is the fibula, the non–weight bearing bone of the lower leg. Skin, bone, and fascia are harvested. The leg donor site requires elevation, a splint, and a period of non–weight bearing. The vascular pedicle must be Dopplered to monitor blood flow. The foot and toes must be monitored for neurovascular supply to the lower extremity.

A radial forearm free flap donor site is the volar, radial surface of the forearm. Usually skin and fascia, sometimes only muscle and fascia, are harvested. This flap is frequently used for intraoral or pharyngeal reconstruction. The donor site is skin grafted, wrapped, splinted, and elevated. The fingers and hand must be monitored for neurovascular adequacy. Occupational and physical therapy is indicated once the initial healing has occurred.

Postoperative Care of Surgical Drains

Surgical drains are placed into the wound beds at the completion of the resection. Drains prevent the accumulation of blood, fluids, and air underneath the reconstructed skin flaps. A Jackson-Pratt closed drain system (Allegiance Health Care Corp., IL) is often used. *Never* disconnect the drain for the purpose of hastening suction or to assess movement of fluid through the drains. Proper suctioning is checked by inspecting drainage tubes for fluid movement as they leave the body.

The Varidyne suction drains are numbered individually. Drains are securely fixed to the chest skin (**Fig. 15.2**). Tincture of benzoin (or any protective dressing) is first applied to the skin. Stomahesive sheets (ConvaTec, Greensboro, NC) are then applied to the skin, and Elastikon (Johnson&Johnson, Langhorne, PA) is tented over the drain to provide security. Each drain is attached to a single drainage canister. This is to very accurately measure the output of each drain. The drains are placed in specific anatomical locations to monitor output from that surgical bed. This also ensures immediate recognition of mechanical breakdown of the drain or bleeding from a specific geographic site. Drains are stripped every 1 to 2 hours to prevent clots from forming and occluding the drain. Drains are never to be open to the air or discontinued from their suction.

When stripping the drain, a test for proper suctioning is done by pinching the tube together close to the skin exit site and with the other finger and thumb stripping the flexible part of the drain tube. The pinched tube closest to the exit site is then released. If the tube remains compressed or without fluid, there is proper suction underneath the flaps. If the drainage tubes return to their usual roundness without the presence of fluid, or a sound is heard that stops when the tubing closest to the patient is pinched, there is an air leak or a problem with the suction machine. If this occurs, the surgeon should be notified immediately.

In rare instances, the drainage tubes will be taken off suction and placed on passive drainage. This is done to try to prevent an enteral-cutaneous fistula and infection. To determine malfunction of the equipment itself, pinch the tubing closest to the suction itself, and if the sound continues, the Varidyne suction is faulty and should be replaced. The amount and color of drainage should be measured and recorded every shift. Any sudden increase in bloody drainage may indicate bleeding in that geographic drainage area. When drainage has decreased to less than 30 mL in 24 hours, the Varidyne drain is removed. A pressure dressing is applied to the insertion site to prevent any fluid accumulation under the flap. This pressure dressing may be removed in 24 hours.

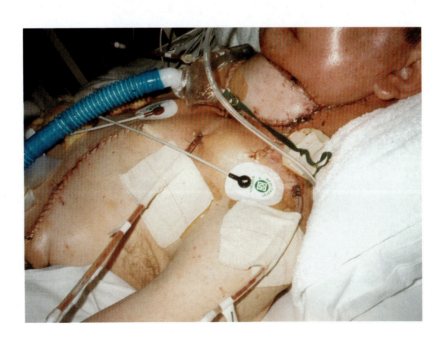

Fig. 15.2 Secured drains with skin preparation, Stomahesive (ConvaTec, Greensboro, NC), and elastic tape. Each drain is numbered individually and separately connected to collection/suction chambers for accurate recording of drainage.

Postoperative Care of the Donor Site

If primary closure of the operative site cannot be accomplished and therefore requires extra tissue for reconstruction, such as musculocutaneous flaps to close the wound, a split thickness skin graft (STSG) from the anterior thigh may also be used. Neck dissection, with the removal of the sternocleidomastoid muscle (SCM), lymph nodes and jugular vein, and spinal accessory nerve (CN XI), leaves the carotid artery bare. Many surgeons prefer to use dermis grafts placed over the carotid artery following the neck dissection and tumor resection. Others choose a double-layer closure that is protective of the carotid artery if the reconstruction flap were to fail or if there was fistula formation. The use of musculocutaneous flaps and therefore the need for STSG or full thickness skin graft (FTSG) leaves a large donor-site defect on the anterior thigh. The exposed nerve endings at the graft donor site are very sensitive to touch, pressure, and moving air. To protect this site and heal the wound, a hydrocolloid dressing such as Hydrogel dressing (Kendall Brand, Covidien, MA) is placed at the time of surgery (**Fig. 15.3**). The length of time for healing of the graft donor site will depend on the thickness of the graft and the patient's nutritional condition. The Hydrogel dressing can be changed every 1 to

2 days or PRN. The use of an island dressing, a piece of Hydrogel that has its own adhesive around the perimeter of the dressing, makes the dressing more secure. The dressing is changed every time fluid or blood accumulates under it. The Hydrogel is not covered with any type of occlusive dressing. Only the edges are secured if needed, until another dressing is obtained for placement.

Patients describe a significant decrease in pain with the use of this type of dressing. By the time of discharge, 7 to 10 days, the leg donor site should be completely healed enough so as not to use any dressing. Patients are instructed to massage the area with cream twice daily for at least 2 to 3 months to minimize scaring and promote maturation of skin healing.

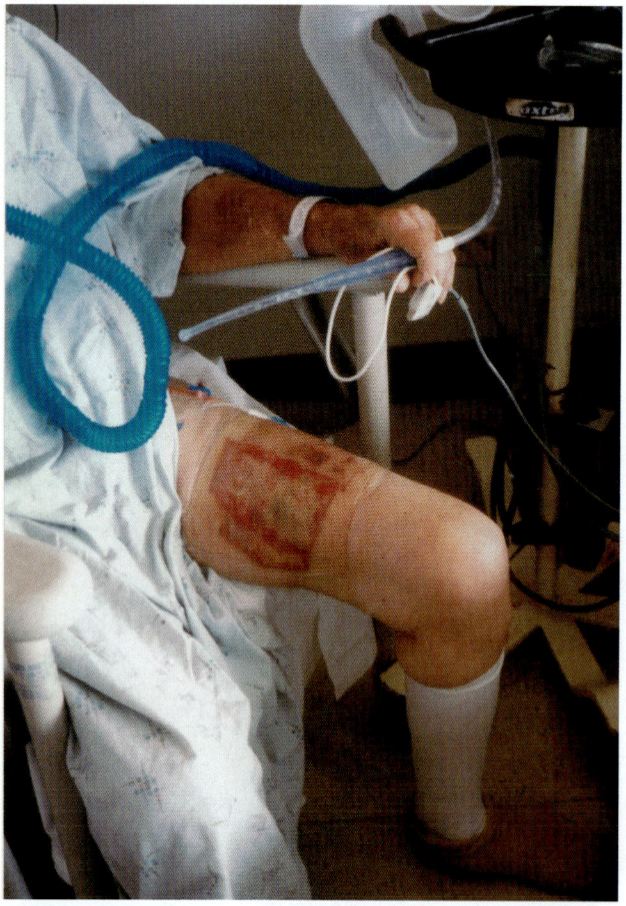

Oral Care

Postoperative infection of the surgically reconstructed oral mucosa may be minimized with meticulous oral hygiene. A Water Pik Dental Water Jet (Water Pik, Inc., Fort Collins, CO) on very low power may be used. If an intraoral flap is present or a suture line is present then very gentle oral care is done using a syringe catheter and normal saline. The catheter is placed in the mouth on the side *opposite* the suture line or reconstruction flap and gentle rinses are used. After healing, a very soft toothbrush as well as the Water Jet is encouraged.

A solution of weak H_2O_2 is useful in removing crusts and thick secretions. Once the oral mucosa is clean nothing more than normal saline is necessary for cleansing. The saline is used at room temperature or slightly warm. Commercial mouthwashes should be avoided because of their drying and irritating effects to the oral mucosa. Many of these preparations contain alcohol, which is destructive to the oral mucosa. A host of new nonalcohol-based products for intraoral care have been developed and should be strongly considered. These new products can also be used during and after radiation therapy. The goal is to keep the mouth clean, provide comfort to the patient, and do no harm to the surgical site and the mucosa.

Pain Management

The management of pain is an art, based in science. Nurses are trained to be experts at managing patients in pain. Early, aggressive pain management for the head and neck cancer patient is the goal in the postoperative period. Intermittent dosing and patient controlled analgesia (PCA) have been used successfully. The major focus in the early postoperative period is adequate dosing to control pain. Clinically, if pain is well controlled in the early postoperative period, less overall pain medication is used in the later postoperative period. Opioids are, as previously stated, the drugs of choice in controlling postoperative pain. Intravenous morphine or Dilaudid (Abbott Laboratories, Abbott Park, IL) are initially used for pain control, then the patient is progressed to codeine with acetaminophen by tube or orally. It is important to consider the amount of pain medication the patient was taking prior to surgery. Addressing a patient's prior history as to whether he or she is narcotic naive or has required significant medica-

Fig. 15.3 Management of the split-thickness donor site on the anterior thigh with hydrocolloid dressings.

tion helps in managing the postoperative pain. Knowledge of previous use may prevent narcotic withdrawal and allows for more appropriate dosing of pain medication in the postoperative period. Consultation with an established pain service is recommended.

Many head and neck cancer patients complain of pain not necessarily from the surgical site but from the reconstruction graft sites and donor sites. In the tumor resection many of the sensory nerves are cut during the dissection of tumor, thus not leaving the patient completely compromised with pain. However, the reconstruction sites are often quite painful and sensitive.

Joint stiffness in the early postoperative period is a frequent complaint. It is believed that this comes from the immobility during the long (6 to 18 hours) surgical procedures. Ambulation, turning side to side, and movement of legs and arms will alleviate this stiffness. If counseled preoperatively, most patients are more than willing to do leg exercises and shoulder shrugs to alleviate this postop stiffness. Judicious use of nonsteroidal antiinflammatory drugs (NSAIDs) may also be of benefit.

The pain from the STSG site on the anterior thigh can be the most distressing. Sensitive nerve endings are exposed, and the slightest pressure or puff of air can cause excruciating pain. The use of Hydrogel, a hydrocolloid dressing, almost alleviates this pain. The previous method of using petroleum-impregnated dressing and allowing it to dry is extremely painful and takes a very long time to heal. This new approach to wound care is excellent for pain management and for wound healing.

We have generally found that if postoperative pain is addressed early on with aggressive proactive management, patients overall are more comfortable and generally require less medication during their entire hospitalization.

Nutrition

Nutrition is a critical element in the care of complex head and neck cancer patients. Many head and neck cancer patients are malnourished for a variety of reasons: tumor invasion, alcohol abuse, inability to swallow because of tumor bulk, poor finances to purchase adequate foods, as well as the profound cachexia of cancer. Chapter 16 is devoted to nutritional aspects. Skilled dieticians on the treating team evaluate patients from a different perspective and offer a rich depth of knowledge in metabolic function.

Early intervention, prevention of weight loss, and long-term planning for nutrition cannot be overemphasized. Weight loss can be prevented during therapy, and there is little excuse for not intervening early. It is clinically well documented that patients who are better nourished and better hydrated have fewer side effects during radiation therapy. This is whether the radiation is the isolated form of therapy or in combination with sensitizing chemotherapy or standard radiation following surgical resection.

A nasogastric tube inserted at the time of surgery is placed to suction for the first 24 hours to decompress the stomach and prevent nausea and vomiting and ileus. The tube should be silastic, soft, and of sufficient internal diameter to ensure a good flow pattern of feeding. Once gastrointestinal motility has returned, feedings can be initiated. Feedings usually begin on postoperative day 2, with constant flow, and are then slowly advanced to bolus feedings as tolerance improves. Bolus feeding of breakfast, lunch, dinner, and snack simulates the normal pattern of eating. Secure the nasogastric tube properly with tincture of benzoin on the skin, a thin strip of Duoderm (ConvaTec, Greensboro, NC) and silk tape (**Fig. 15.4**). This method provides comfort and additional safety to keep the tube in correct position. Nares erosion can be prevented by this method of securing the tube. The dressing should be changed to keep the nose clean and free of debris.

If for some reason the tube accidentally comes out, especially in the early postoperative period, under *no* circumstances replace the tube without a specific physician order. Inadvertent placement through an internal oral, pharyngeal, or laryngeal suture line is possible. Always confer with the physician before tube replacement. Appropriate securing of the tube will prevent most of these unfortunate occurrences.

Many patients have gastrostomy tubes placed at the time of surgical resection. This is a matter of surgical team preference. Interruption of the belly makes the patient less likely to be able to cough well postoperatively. In view of significant smoking histories, chronic obstructive pulmonary disease (COPD), chronic bronchitis, and pulmonary secretion clearance are very important in smokers who develop head and neck cancer. Most patients have a component of COPD. With the alternative of percutaneous feeding tubes, placement can occur at any time surrounding the time of diagnosis. In our experience there are four reports of seeding the oral tumor to the gastrostomy site. Endoscopic placement of a gastrostomy tube should not be done in a patient with a large oropharyngeal or any hypopharyngeal tumor.

Swallowing

Although swallowing is well addressed in chapter 17 of this book, the nursing care of head and neck cancer patients who have undergone resection must included swallowing evaluation and rehabilitation. Both surgery and radiation have profound effects on swallowing.[16]

Bedside clinical evaluation, although giving excellent clinical information, cannot accurately define the site of problems, nor can it accurately quantify timing of the swallow. Silent aspiration often goes undetected if only the clinical exam is done. A thorough cranial nerve exam, taking into consideration surgical anatomical changes, is imperative in assessing the swallow. Auscultation of the larynx during swallowing and evaluating the laminar airflow or its disruption may give additional information that just observation is unable to give.

Dynamic swallow testing by cine-esophagram is the standard of care to assess not only the patient's ability to attain oral nutrition but to assess and plan rehabilitation and safe oral nutrition. Enteral feeding should be continued until it is proven that the patient can fully support oral nutrition without aspiration.

Speech therapy, by skilled speech–language pathologists in otolaryngology, is critical for swallow therapy and speech following head and neck cancer resection.[17]

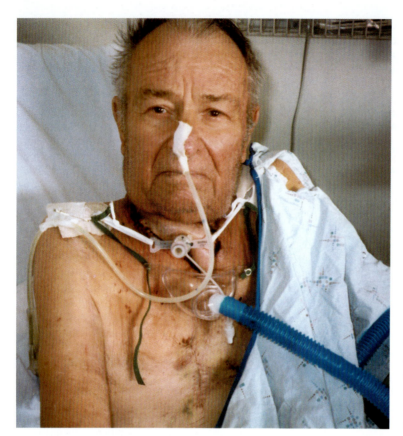

Fig. 15.4 Securing of the artificial airway to the shoulders to prevent pressure on the reconstructive flap. The nasogastric tube is secured with a skin protector to the nose and tape that is changed as needed. Also demonstrating use of the Bivona TTS tracheostomy tube (Smith's Industries, London, England) to prevent the reconstructed flap from prolapsing into the laryngectomy stoma.

Activity/Physical Therapy

Throughout the postoperative period, patients are encouraged to regain to the best of their ability their previous level of functioning. As early as postoperative day 1, if stable, patients can be ambulated, out of bed to chair, or out of bed in a cardiac chair. If patients are taught this preoperatively they are usually more than ready to ambulate. They and the family understand the plan and the consequences. Considerations must be made for cardiac or pulmonary instability and pain management regimen. Regular and early ambulation is mandatory to increase circulation, prevent complications, and increase self-esteem. The use of physical therapy and exercises is beneficial in performing range of motion exercises and increasing muscle strength. It has long been thought that chest physical therapy for pulmonary hygiene is efficacious in preventing and treating postoperative atelectasis.[18] Physical therapists must operate under a standard protocol for head and neck cancer patients. This should be developed with the ENT team. Physical therapists trained in the care of ORL patients are a huge asset to a multidisciplinary team. Physical therapy protocols guide practice for the rehabilitation of patients who undergo head and neck cancer resections. Special attention should be directed to range of motion of the shoulder following a neck dissection sacrificing the spinal accessory nerve CN XI. Range exercises may prevent frozen shoulder. Jaw range of motion is important for speech as well as oral nutrition.

Postoperative Care of the Patient with an Infected Wound

Although prophylactic antibiotics are used following resection of head and neck tumors, the patient is at risk for infection because of the contamination of the wound with the microbes of the upper aerodigestive tract. This could lead to flap necrosis, wound breakdown, fistula formation, and carotid artery exposure. Malnutrition and hypoalbuminemia are critical in the complex equation of wound healing. Close observation of the patient's wounds for increased redness and inflammation around the suture line, donor site, or recipient area is necessary. Wound dehiscence is frequently heralded by purulent, foul-smelling drainage from one small area. Once the wound is opened by incision and drainage, standard protocol is to profusely irrigate and pack the wound. Wound packing is usually done initially every 2 to 4 hours. This will remove necrotic tissue from within the wound and promote granulation. The goal is for the wound to heal from the base outward.

Different types of solutions may be used at the discretion of the physician. Normal saline is the most frequently used solution; it is bactericidal and aids in the removal of necrotic tissue. Hydrogen peroxide 2% strength, with normal saline oxidizes the wound and lowers surface tension to loosen necrotic tissue more effectively. Betadine (Purdue Pharma L.P., Stamford, CT), Dakins (Century Pharmaceuticals, Indianapolis, IN) solution, and ¼% acetic acid are other solutions of choice.

Large wounds are packed with a 4 × 4 or fluff opened up fully, soaked in solution, wrung dry, and packed gently into the wound. Do not use pressure because that may increase the wound size. Gently packing allows the wet dressing to touch all areas of the wound and debride the surface, removing necrotic debris. Strip packing with medications is used for smaller wounds and comes in ¼-, ½-, 1-, and 2-inch sizes. Choose the appropriate size to fit the wound and pack gently into the depths of the wound using a Q-tip, bayonet forceps, or similar instrument to pack the wound until fully healed.

Prevention of Flap Failure

Many factors contribute to circulatory embarrassment of the flap used in reconstruction. When evaluating a flap, distinction must be made as to the type of flap used and its arterial supply and venous egress. It is through understanding the surgical anatomy that clarification of the problem becomes easier to understand. Thorough discussions with the surgeons add to the armamentarium of the nurse in understanding both the surgical resection and the reconstruction.

Venous congestion is one of the initial vascular complications that can compromise flap survival. Improper positioning can result in tension, twisting, and kinking of the flap pedicle. Postoperative edema of the head and neck area due to the sacrifice of normal lymphatic channels, and removal of the jugular veins, as well as hematoma formation are culprits in compromise. A line of demarcation, the formation of vesicles, and cyanotic color are all signs of impending flap necrosis and possible loss.

Frequent assessment of the flap for any evidence of vascular impairment is a critical aspect of nursing observation. When gentle pressure is applied, the tissue should have a capillary refill of 1 to 2 seconds. Color can be divided into three basic parameters, knowing that no patient follows any guideline perfectly. Blue color with a quick refill signifies venous congestion; white—no arterial supply but with open venous egress; and red—vigorous arterial supply and partial venous congestion.

Often the impairment of vascular flow to or from the flap is a technical rather than physiological problem. The vascular pedicle may be kinked, twisted, or closed under tension. This may be the result of lying on the flap, use of a pressure bandage or ties around the pedicle of the flap, tight suturing, edema, or a compartmentalized hematoma. Release of sutures or evacuation of a hematoma may improve the blood flow to or from the flap. Careful attention should be given to the amount and rate of intravenous fluid because increased edema may also result in venous congestion. The use of intravascular expanders such as albumin or Hespan (HESpan B, Braun, Germany) rather than intravenous (IV) fluid may help in the management of edema.

Postoperative Care of the Patient with a Fistula

Cancer, previous radiation therapy, and malnutrition put the patient at increased risk for wound breakdown and fistula. The first indicator of poor healing is often seen in the early postoperative period, as evidenced by an elevated temperature, unusual odor, skin color changes, skin sloughing, and increased tenderness. A subsequent increases in drainage form the Varidyne or unusual drainage from the suture line may also indicate the formation of a fistula. A fistula is a communication between two body cavities or a cavity and the skin. Orocutaneous fistulae are between the surgical wound and the oral cavity and a pharyngocutaneous fistula, between the pharynx and the skin. The fistula is usually identified by a salivary stream in the bed of the wound.

In the early postoperative period any dehiscence in the suture line may indicate an impending fistula. Any obvious drainage should be suspect. The treatment is appropriate antibiotic therapy, incision, and drainage and packing of the fistula. A fistula may take weeks or months to heal. Once critical structures are covered, the infection treated, and the family taught to dress the wound the patient may leave the hospital. They should be followed very closely in the outpatient clinic, but if stable they do not require hospitalization.

When fully healed, reconstruction can be considered. Any patient undergoing surgical resection following radiation therapy must be carefully watched for fistula formation. Again, malnutrition and radiation therapy are leading causes of poor wound healing.

A chyle fistula results from a leak in the lymphatic duct system. This type of fistula occurs during a neck dissection and sometimes during a mediastinal dissection. The lymph vessels drain into the lymphatic duct (on the right) and the thoracic duct (on the left). The thoracic duct is a higher risk because it may loop as far as 4 to 6 cm into the neck before returning to the chest and entering the subclavian vein. The left (thoracic) duct contains chyle, the product of intestinal digestion, and the drainage from it is the fat content, which is opaque or milky. The amount of drainage through the wound or through the drains can be as much as 1500 mL in 24 hours. It can result, if not recognized and treated, in fluid and electrolyte imbalances. The volume of drainage and its characteristic color distinguish chyle from blood, serum, or saliva. The finding of free fat droplets in a sample of the drainage usually confirms the presence of a chyle leak. The management of chyle fistula may require surgery to oversew the duct, depending on the severity of the leak. In most cases, the existing surgical drain is cut off from suction and becomes a wick. A pressure dressing is placed over the site near the supraclavicular fossa. Feeding with a no fat or elemental diet will decrease the flow of chyle and seal the leak without surgical intervention.

Carotid Artery Precautions and Rupture

For nurses to recognize the patient at risk for carotid artery rupture they must be aware of the factors that influence tissue breakdown and healing. Identifying the patient at risk allows an anticipation of the nursing care needs. A comprehensive plan of care includes continuous assessment of the wound, preventive action to avoid further deterioration and infection, and guidelines for action in the event of a carotid artery rupture.

The common carotid arteries supply blood to the head and neck. The arteries ascend the lateral aspects of the neck, deep to the SCM. At approximately the level of the thyroid cartilage, the common carotid arteries bifurcate into the internal and external carotid arteries. The internal courses upward through the skull base to supply the brain. The carotid artery is made of three layers, the intima, the adventitia, and the media. The adventitial layer carries 80% of the blood supply to the remaining walls of the artery. It is very susceptible to drying, infection, and effects of radiation therapy.

During surgical resection it may be necessary to strip the tumor from the adventitial layer, thereby compromising the blood supply to the vessel. Those patients who have tumor recurrence, prior radiation therapy, or malnutrition have delayed or impaired wound healing. If the carotid artery is exposed to air, as in the case of carotid exposure following wound dehiscence or flap failure, the drying process destroys the tenuous blood supply to the vessel wall. Poor healing, tumor growth and invasion, exposure of the artery during the surgery, previous treatment with radiation and/or chemotherapy, and infection are all mechanisms that contribute to arterial wall necrosis. The artery may be exposed in the neck or in the pharynx. A carotid bleed from the pharynx is much harder to control because of the difficulty in adequate exposure to access and control the bleeding.

If the carotid artery is exposed, carotid protocol nursing care is instituted. The patient is moved close to the nursing station. Wound care is done every 2 hours with wet to soaked wet saline fluffs or gauze. The wound dressing is kept wet to avoid any chance of drying of the artery. In between dressing changes, if there is any suspicion of drying, saline pillows can be squirted on the dressing. Sterility is of utmost importance. Even though the wound may be draining saliva and in contact with the oral cavity, the nurse and physician should maintain the highest grade of sterility possible so as not to introduce further bacterial growth.

If the artery begins to show signs of a dark area or bleb, signaling death of tissue, the decisions must be made to resect the artery or allow nature to take its course with inevitable hemorrhage and death. If the patient has chosen not to be treated, then nursing should prepare the patient and family for the possibility of bleed and ensuing death. Whether in the hospital or at home, dark towels, available at the bedside, may lessen the impact of the enormous quantity of blood following a carotid bleed. There always is the chance that excellent nursing care will prevent the bleed and lead to healing, so wound care should proceed as ordered.

Sleep deprivation is an important element in the patient's ability to cooperate with frequent dressing changes. As the wound heals, is less infected, and becomes more stable, carotid dressing care can extend to every 4 hours during the night, usually from midnight to 6 am. The dressing is saturated with sterile saline every 2 hours in between changes, but this can be done without waking the patient.

Recognition of events preceding a carotid bleed may save the patient's life. A herald bleed, a small sentinel bleed, may be noted in the wound 24 to 48 hours preceding a full carotid bleed. However, this may not occur, so diligent observation is essential. Patients may also complain of epigastric pain or discomfort. This may be due to the separation of the layers of the artery and sympathetic nerve responses up and down

the vagus. The sensation of heartburn or of discomfort is a warning sign.

The most critical factor in the management of a carotid artery rupture is establishing a controlled situation in which life-threatening hemorrhage and stroke are avoided. A large-bore IV catheter should be in place at all times, preferable a peripherally inserted central catheter (PICC), as well as a peripheral IV, again as large as possible. Supplies that may be needed are placed at the bedside. This includes four boxes of fluffs or similar bandages, IV solution and tubing, and Hespan. Because of the shortage of blood products Hespan is an excellent substitute in emergency situations.

Hemorrhage may occur externally from the neck, or internally from within the oropharynx, or both, if a fistula is present. *Direct digital pressure* should be immediately applied to the site of bleeding. If hemorrhage occurs externally, the patient should be positioned supine with the head turned to facilitate drainage and prevent aspiration. Nursing goals include maintaining an airway and preventing aspiration of blood. The tracheotomy cuff should be inflated and blood suctioned immediately from the airway and the oral cavity. If no artificial airway is in place the patient may be intubated to control the airway. If hemorrhage occurs internally, in the oral cavity, pressure should be applied intraorally near the tonsillar fossa with one hand, and with the other hand apply counterpressure to the neck to control bleeding from both sides. Digital pressure on the common carotid artery below the level of the bleed may aid in control of the bleeding.

Under no circumstances should the direct digital pressure be released at any time, until a surgeon capable of handling the situation is present and ready to take control of the patient. Colleagues can assist in beginning IV therapy, medication administration, and alerting the operating room. Morphine sulfate may be administered for pain and anxiety. It may also decrease the systemic blood pressure, aiding in flow control.

Carotid rupture can be difficult for both the patient and family. It can be equally difficult for the nursing staff. Patients, when at all possible, must be informed that their carotid artery is in jeopardy and of the possibility of carotid rupture. Patients must understand the implications of bleeding, carotid ligation, and possibility of stroke in both instances. Sensitivity and compassion, when accompanied by technical competence, can be reassuring and life saving. Following carotid rupture the nursing staff should be debriefed, the situation discussed, and follow-up regarding their practice and the patient's outcome be made.

Airway Maintenance

Maintenance of an adequate airway is the utmost priority in the nursing care of head and neck cancer patients. A nursing goal is to maintain a moist patent airway with both tracheotomies and laryngectomy and to ensure adequate air exchange. A nurse skilled in care of the patient with an artificial airway responds to the physiological and psychological needs of the patient.

A cuffed tracheostomy tube is used to attempt to seal the airway for positive pressure ventilation and an attempt at prevention of aspiration of oral secretions or reflux. Tracheostomy or laryngectomy care should be done at least every 4 hours and PRN. Crust and dried secretions around the sutures and stoma should be cleaned with half-strength peroxide and normal saline. The inner cannula of the tracheostomy tube should be inspected and changed if needed at least once a shift. A drain sponge, a piece of Duoderm, or both should be placed under the faceplate of the tube to prevent excoriation of the skin. These dressings must be changed frequently to prevent infection from accumulated secretions. If the skin is clean and dry no dressing is required.

Tracheostomy ties are never circumferential (around the neck) to prevent any pressure on flaps and reconstructed tissue. Ties are secured to the shoulders (**Fig. 15.4**) in a similar way as drains are secured. Use tincture of benzoin on the skin, Stomahesive (ConvoTec), and Elastikon (Johnson & Johnson) to secure the ties; then secure the ties to the faceplate of the tracheostomy tube itself. With unilateral neck dissections, the ties on the unoperated side may be placed at the peak of the shoulder, or even slightly further back, whereas the ties on the operated side must be place laterally. Under no circumstance should ties or tubing be placed over a neck dissection incision or reconstructed flap. The tube itself may or may not be sutured in place. The sutures are removed on postoperative day 5 when the first tube change is done.

Pressure of the cuff on the tracheal wall creates a potential for necrosis, scarring, and stenosis. Standard orders are to leave the cuff *deflated* if the patient does not require positive pressure ventilation. If the patient requires positive pressure ventilation, measure cuff pressure each shift and maintain 20 to 25 mm Hg.[19] A spare tracheotomy tube should always be at the patient's bedside, and this should be the same size or one size smaller than the tube the patient has in place. Keep all parts of tubes together and check for similar sizes.

Saline is instilled to clear secretions.[20] Suction only PRN. Patients should cough and deep breath (as taught preoperatively) frequently every 1 to 2 hours for the first 24 hours or until ambulating and able to clear their own secretions. If patients require mechanical ventilation, suctioning, bagging, as well as the treatments of saline instillation, coughing, and turning are instituted. Saline should be instilled *very slowly* so as not to impair deep breathing or scare the patient. The use of saline spray bottles is much better tolerated. Particle deposition of the normal saline is a smaller droplet size. The patient is better able to cough to clear the secretions.[21] Deep suctioning may not be necessary.

Laryngectomy stoma care is important for the nurse to begin teaching as soon as the patient is able to listen. Teaching should begin early, as the nurse administers routine care. Initially the patient uses a mirror to see how to clean stomal suture lines and instill normal saline. One of the ways that people adapt to self-image changes is by their ability to control their environment via self-care initiatives. Care of their stoma is usually one of the major image changes.

SCT Single Cannula Tracheostomy (Shiley Mallinckrodt, Covidien, MA) tubes are very valuable tools in the nurse's armamentarium. Slightly longer than the standard tubes for the relative inner diameter these tubes are used for patients with thick necks, plunging trachea, or bulky flaps that require a longer reach to the trachea. The standard tube is cuffed but can be ordered as noncuffed for routine in hospital and home care.

Bivona (Smiths Industries, London, England) stoma buttons are excellent choices for total laryngectomy patients who require support for their stoma. Often, scar tissue forms at the suture line where skin and trachea are joined. This tissue may stenose the stoma, creating microstomia and a smaller-diameter airway. Bivona buttons provide gentle pressure on the scar tissue to keep the stoma open. The ultimate goal is for the patient not to wear any appliance.

Supportive Services

Because of the enormity of the impact of the disease and its treatment many disciplines are involved in the care of the patient. Discharge planning, social service, physical therapy, and dietary are integral in the team effort. In multidisciplinary rounds, staff education, communication, and experience enable the team to develop appropriate plans for each patient.

Speech Therapy

Support from speech pathology trained in otolaryngology and surgical procedures is invaluable in the preoperative counseling and postoperative care of head and neck cancer patients. The ability to communicate is extremely important in our society, and maintenance of a functioning language system can make a great deal of difference during the hospitalization and rehabilitation. All patients undergoing total laryngectomy optimally receive before surgery, *Looking Forward: A Guide Book for the Laryngectomee* by Robert Keith Mayo Foundation. Postoperatively they also receive *Self-Help for the Laryngectomee* by Edmund Lauder.

Speech therapists trained in swallowing evaluation and therapy are an invaluable aid to the patient and nursing staff.

◆ Psychological Aspects of Rehabilitation

The disfigurement and functional impairment that follow an ablative head and neck cancer surgery can be emotionally traumatic to the patient, family, and associates. Patients will react in their own way, and a rehabilitation plan must be individually tailored. Head and neck cancer is frequently described as the most emotionally traumatic of all cancers. The process of physical recovery encompasses the biophysiological adjustment of the patient under the conditions of disease, treatment, and perceived stress associated with the illness.[22]

It is best to establish self-care as a goal early in the diagnostic and treatment-planning phase and to reinforce it with each contact. Anxiety, depression, and problems of self-image are the most likely stresses seen in a patient following head and neck surgery. When these occur, our role encompasses not only providing information but also providing emotional support to both the family and the patient. Coping mechanisms should not be tampered with unless they can be carefully replaced with something better, such as patients' gradual understanding of their condition while maintaining a reasonable degree of emotional comfort.

Acknowledgment that patients' feelings are appropriate enhances their sense of being understood, and the recognition of their assets and strength by others will instill a greater sense of security, trust, and optimism. Dropkin[23] states that functional recovery may be intricately linked to social support. Recovery is predicated on a very complex system of physiological and psychological parameters. Coping, identity, and body image integration is integral in patients' recovery.[24] If we are able to acknowledge the pain, fear, loneliness, and isolation that these patients experience during their acute illness we must also acknowledge the challenges of recovery.

◆ Conclusion

Caring for the patient with head and neck cancer is one of the most challenging career choices that nurses can make. The continuous presence of a nurse at the bedside provides meaningful comfort and security to critically ill patients, and a nurse's watchful attentiveness, when accompanied by technical skill, is perceived by patients as evidence of caring.[25] Coupling technical skills and advanced knowledge with empathy and caring, the otolaryngology head and neck cancer nurse is a multifaceted professional. Use of ORL Nursing Practice Guidelines and the Society of Otorhinolaryngology Head and Neck Nurses (SOHN) Core Curriculum provides the nurse with a standard of practice that can only be expanded with experience in the field of otolaryngology head and neck cancer. The care of otolaryngology head and neck cancer patients makes personal and professional demands upon the staff delivering care. It also enriches the practice of nursing.

◆ Appendix 15.1

Patient Teaching Tools

Laryngeal Cancer Resection with or without Neck Dissection

◆ **Total or Partial Laryngectomy** *Source:* Adapted from University of California Davis Health System (UCDHS) Multidisciplinary Patient Education Protocol.

All patients and families will receive health care information throughout the hospitalization. The information will be accurate and relevant to their self-care. The goal is participative health care management throughout the process.

1. *State the type of cancer and the plan of care.*

Laryngeal cancer is usually caused by the combination of smoking and alcohol. The tumor arises from the violated mucosa of the larynx or from the growth of tumor from other affected areas of the aerodigestive tract. Explain the type and cause of cancer and the proposed/ongoing plan of care including the therapies of surgery, radiation therapy, combined surgery and radiation, or other modalities of

therapy. Each patient will receive the book, *Head and Neck Cancer, a Patient Information Book*, in the preoperative clinic setting. Each patient undergoing total laryngectomy will receive the book, *Looking Forward: A Guidebook for the Laryngectomy*.

2. *Define the type/extent of proposed resection.*

Each patient should be able to state the type of proposed surgery. Surgical resection includes the tumor site and at least a 2 mm margin around the tumor. The resection may also include adjacent tissue to ensure tumor-free margins. Total laryngectomy patients must know that they will have a permanent stoma. Partial laryngectomy patients must know that they may have a temporary tracheotomy. Both patients may have nasogastric feedings while in the hospital.

The exact extent of resection is decided by the physical location of the tumor. The tumor is staged by the tumor, nodes, metastasis (TNM) classification system according to size and location. The size and location of the tumor will define the extent of deficit following surgical resection. The type of reconstruction also depends on the size and location of the tumor.

This type of surgery may or may not include neck dissection, depending on nodal involvement. A neck dissection removes tumor in the neck, the neck lymph nodes, the SCM, Jugular vein, and spinal accessory nerve CN XI. The major deficit after neck dissection is limited to reduced movement of the shoulder and arm from the resection of CN XI. A more limited neck dissection may be performed at the discretion of the physician.

3. *State the purpose of panendoscopy, biopsy, and tumor mapping.*

Panendoscopy includes bronchoscopy, esophagoscopy, nasopharyngoscopy, inspection of the oral cavity, laryngoscope, tumor mapping, and tissue biopsy. This procedure defines the extent of the tumor and provides a tissue sample of the tumor for analysis.

4. *Discuss feelings of anxiety, fear, loss of control, coping and change in body image.*

Loss of voice, alteration in body image, control over self, coping, and inadequate preparation for surgical intervention when faced with the diagnosis of cancer are very traumatic for the patient. Give the patient the opportunity to discuss feelings, offer support, and answer questions concretely.

5. *State how to communicate after total laryngectomy or partial (voice conservation) laryngectomy.*

It is important to explain in detail, before surgery, the measures that will be used to help the patient communicate. Writing is the major mode of communication in association with universally understood hand and facial gestures. Assess the patient's ability to communicate by writing and reading English or his or her native language. Demonstrate the use of communication/writing boards. Explain call lights and the immediate callback system for the patient with permanent stomas and artificial airways.

All total laryngectomy patients will be seen by an ENT department speech pathologist. If possible, patients will also be seen by a laryngectomy visitor from the American Cancer Society, Lost Cord Club, preferably preoperatively. They will be informed of the methods for alaryngeal speech.

All partial laryngectomy patients (voice conservation) patients will also be referred to ENT speech pathology for voice rehabilitation and swallowing therapy. Voice changes will be discussed.

6. *Demonstrate the care of the permanent stoma (total laryngectomy patients) or the care of a temporary artificial airway (partial laryngectomy patients).*

Patient and family will be taught saline instillation, wound care, self-suctioning, coughing and deep breathing, changing laryngectomy/tracheotomy tube ties (if present), changing the stoma button or artificial airway, and emergency care of the patient with an artificial airway. Total laryngectomy patients should receive written information on care of their laryngectomy stoma.

Partial (voice conservation) laryngectomy patients should receive written information on home care with a temporary tracheotomy if they are to go home with one.

Each patient should be discharged with a suction machine and a laryngectomy discharge kit or tracheotomy discharge kit. Each patient should also be referred to a home health agency for in-home follow-up.

7. *State and demonstrate the importance of maintaining optimal pulmonary hygiene deep breathing, coughing, suctioning, self-suctioning, and saline instillation.*

The maintenance of adequate pulmonary hygiene is essential in the care of head and neck cancer patients. Preoperative teaching and deep breathing, early ambulation, saline instillation, and goals of airway care help the patient regain early mobility and independence. Preoperative teaching and preparation are imperative to prepare the patient for participative care during the postoperative period.

8. *State the importance of nutrition and demonstrate adequate oral intake, nasogastric feedings, or gastrostomy feedings.*

Patients with head and neck cancer often present with malnutrition from the inability to eat due to tumor effects and alcoholism. Adequate nutrition is important for wound healing following surgical resection. Adequate nutrition and hydration during radiation therapy can decrease side effects of the radiation therapy.

Head and neck cancer patients cannot eat orally following resection because of the need to bypass internal suture line, oropharyngeal swelling, potential for aspiration in the partial laryngectomy patient, and the large amount of tissue resected. Enteral feedings are always delivered until a dynamic swallow study is performed to determine the patient's ability to orally sustain nutrition. For the total laryngectomy patient, a routine barium swallow ascertains the integrity of the internal suture line. If no suture line dehiscence is observed on the study, the patient can begin oral nutrition.

The patient will know how to give enteral feedings by gastrostomy, nasogastric tube, or jejunal feedings. Feedings may be given by bolus, continuous, or combination, depending on individual needs of the patients. Dietary recommendations are important to follow. Twice weekly weights are standard to monitor loss or gain, and intake is calculated for both enteral feedings and free water. Insensible water loss is a very important component of the evaluation of the head and neck cancer patient. Because of both oral and airway suctioning, patients often require higher amounts of free water replacements.

9. *Begin safe oral nutrition. dynamic swallow study or barium swallow is completed and evaluated.*

Dynamic swallow study is primarily geared for patients with an intact larynx, but following laryngectomy it serves a dual purpose of (1) evaluating the integrity of the internal suture line and (2) evaluating the patient's ability to begin esophageal voice training.

10. *Demonstrate oral hygiene after laryngeal cancer resection.*

Oral care is important to decrease the level of oropharyngeal microbial growth, particularly the incidence of thrush and mucositis, and protect from superinfections during radiation therapy.

11. *Communicate pain and need for pain medication.*

Pain medication is tantamount to the comfort and recovery of all patients. Head and neck cancer patients should be aggressively treated for pain in the postoperative period. As they progress in their hospitalization, advancing to nasogastric and, as allowed, oral medications. Communication of need for medication should be established preoperatively. Nursing assessments must always include pain levels, response to medications, and appropriate medication administration.

12. *Demonstrate wound care for home.*

Standard stoma care of saline administration and cleaning should begin as early as the first postop day. Incorporation of stoma care as a normal activity of daily living will lead patients to become self-sufficient in their own stoma care.

Patients whose wounds require packing or extensive dressing changes should be knowledgeable in their care. Teaching of their families and significant others should begin as early as possible.

Home nursing for laryngectomy patients is always arranged by the discharge planner. Discharge supplies and suction machines are part of the teaching preparation for home care.

13. *State follow-up appointments and plan of care after discharge.*

Patients and their families should be able to state the follow-up plan of care and importance of return appointments in the ENT clinic. All cancer patients should be seen in clinic within a week after discharge.

14. *State emergency procedure in the outpatient/home setting.*

Patients and their families should be aware of the 911 system, emergency breathing via stoma, and methods of cleaning the stoma to prevent airway obstruction by secretions. MedicAlert bracelets are important to wear as well as enrolling in a CPR class. Families must be instructed in mouth-to-stoma breathing techniques.

15. *State how each member of the multidisciplinary team is involved in the care plan.*

All patients should be able to state the care they will/have received from the ENT multidisciplinary team, both as inpatients and as outpatients

16. *List one source of support available in the community.*

American Cancer Society, American Lung Association, International Association of Laryngectomees, MedicAlert program.

◆ Appendix 15.2

Patient Teaching Tools

Oropharyngeal Cancer Resection with or without Neck Dissection

Source: Adapted from UCDHS Multidisciplinary Patient Education Protocol

All patients with oropharyngeal cancer undergoing oropharyngeal (composite) resections will receive this teaching. The multidisciplinary team is involved in the ongoing process of care planning.

1. *State the type of cancer and proposed ongoing plan of care.*

Oropharyngeal cancer is usually caused by the combination of smoking, alcohol, cigar smoking, and tobacco chewing. The tumor arises from the violated mucus membrane of the oropharynx/upper aerodigestive tract. Explain the type of cancer and the proposed/ongoing plan of care including the therapies of surgery, radiation therapy, combined surgery and radiation, or other modalities of therapy. Each patient will receive the book, *Head and Neck Cancer, a Patient Information Book* in the preoperative clinic setting.

2. *Define the type/extent of proposed resection.*

Surgical resection includes the tumor site and at least a 2 mm margin around the tumor. It also may include a partial glossectomy, partial pharyngectomy, partial mandibulectomy, and neck dissection if there is nodal involvement.

The exact extent of resection is decided by the physical location of the tumor. The tumor is staged by the TNM classification system according to size and location. Tumor size and location will define the extent of deficit following surgical resection. The type of reconstruction also depends on the size and location of the tumor. A neck dissection removes tumor in the neck, the neck lymph nodes, the SCM, jugular vein, and spinal accessory nerve CN XI.

3. *State the purpose of panendoscopy, tumor mapping, and biopsy.*

Panendoscopy includes bronchoscopy, esophagoscopy, nasopharyngoscopy, inspection of the oral cavity, tumor mapping, and tissue biopsy. This procedure defines the extent of the tumor and provides a tissue sample of the tumor for analysis.

4. *Discuss feelings of anxiety, fear, loss of control, and change in body image.*

Loss of control and inadequate preparation for surgical intervention when faced with the diagnosis of cancer is very traumatic for the patient. Allow the patient the opportunity to discuss feelings, offer support, and answer questions concretely.

5. *State how to communicate postop with an artificial airway in place.*

Explain in detail, before surgery, the measures that will be used to help the patient communicate. Writing is the major mode of communication in association with universally understood hand and facial gestures. Assess patients' ability to communicate by writing and reading English or their native language. Demonstrate the use of communication/writing boards. Explain call lights and the immediate callback system for patients with artificial airways. As the patient progresses, most patients with oropharyngeal cancer resections can learn to speak with a tracheostomy tube in place. After healing has occurred, teach patients how to cover the tube with their fingers and to speak on exhalation. Speech therapy consult via the ENT speech department is appropriate.

6. *Demonstrate care of the temporary artificial airway by discharge.*

Patients and significant others will be taught saline instillation, wound care, self-suctioning, coughing and deep breathing, changing tracheostomies, changing the tracheostomy tube, and emergency care of the artificial airway. Each patient should be taught using written information about tracheostomy care. Patients should go home with an artificial airway *only* after they have demonstrated ability to care for themselves. The majority of patients should be able to change their own tracheostomy tubes before discharge. All patients are discharged with a suction machine and a tracheostomy discharge kit. Each patient must be referred to a home health agency.

7. *State and demonstrate the importance of maintaining optimal pulmonary hygiene: deep breathing, coughing, suctioning, self-suctioning, and saline instillation.*

The maintenance of adequate pulmonary hygiene is essential in care of head and neck cancer patients. Most patients have long smoking histories and either chronic bronchitis or COPD. Preop teaching of coughing and deep breathing, early ambulation, saline instillation, and goals of tracheostomy care help the patient attain early mobility and independence. Preoperative teaching and preparation are imperative to prepare the patient for participative care during the postoperative period.

8. *State importance of nutrition and demonstrate nasogastric or gastrostomy feedings by discharge.*

Patients with head and neck cancer often present with malnutrition from the inability to eat due to tumor effects and alcoholism. Adequate nutrition is important for wound healing following surgical resection. Adequate nutrition and hydration during follow-up radiation therapy can decrease side effects of the radiation therapy. Head and neck cancer patients cannot eat orally immediately following resection because of the need to bypass the internal suture line, oropharyngeal swelling, potential for aspiration, and the large amount of tissue resected. Enteral feedings are always delivered until a dynamic swallow study is performed to determine the patient's ability to orally sustain nutrition. The patient will know how to give enteral feedings by gastrostomy, nasogastric tube, or jejunal feedings. Feedings may be given by bolus, continuous, or combination, depending on individual needs of the patients.

Dietary recommendations are to be followed. Twice weekly weights are standard to monitor loss/gain, and intake is calculated for enteral feedings and free water. Caloric and protein requirements are calculated based on height, weight, metabolic requirements, and current protein status. A general figure for calculating caloric requirements is 33 to 35 kcal per kg/ideal body weight (IBW). Following surgery, protein requirements are generally 1.3 to 1.5 g per kg/IBW. Water replacements are ~22 to 23 mL/kg of body weight. Accurate intake and output, accurate weights, weekly chem 7 or 20 are essential in calculating the effect of enteral nutrition in the postop period.

9. *Begin safe oral nutrition after dynamic swallow study is completed and evaluated.*

Because of extensive resections, potential for aspiration, and importance of nutrition during the postop period, all head and neck cancer patients will have dynamic swallow studies before beginning oral nutrition. This study will evaluate the patient's ability to swallow after resection and reconstruction and will protect the airway. Studies are videotaped and replayed to the patient for teaching purposes. Speech evaluation is done at the same time under fluoroscopic visualization.

10. *Demonstrate oral care after oropharyngeal cancer resection.*

Oral care is important after upper aerodigestive tract cancer resections. Immediately after surgery, oral care consists of gently suctioning and rinsing with saline and hydrogen peroxide solution. As the internal sutures heal, more aggressive cleaning can be initiated. Do not clean or suction directly over the internal suture line, oral skin grafts, or myocutaneous/myofacial reconstruction flaps. Oral swishing and suctioning on the unoperative side are indicated.

11. *Communicate pain and need for pain medication.*

Immediately postop, patients can be placed on a PCA protocol with basal and PCA dosing. By the time of transfer from ICU, most patients should be transitioned to enteral or oral pain medication. PCA will be reinstituted if necessary. Home transition will again be to oral or enteral pain medications. During postoperative radiation therapy, the patient may require a higher level of pain control therapy and, following radiation therapy, will be transitioned to oral or enteral medications.

For postoperative anxiety small adjuvant doses of benzodiazepines given in alternating doses with the pain medications are indicated.

12. *Demonstrate wound care for home.*

Even if intraoral or external neck wounds have not healed completely, the patient may be able to be discharged to home, with assistance. Standard wound care includes cleaning the suture line with hydrogen peroxide and saline combination. Antibacterial ointment may or may not be used. Wound care at discharge is usually three to four times a day and as needed. Clean technique is used at home. Large open wounds usually associated with orocutaneous fistula are treated as clean wounds and packed with fluffs or Nu-Gauze. Patients and families can be taught to change dressings in the home with home health support.

13. *State follow-up appointments and plan of care after discharge.*

State follow-up plan of care and importance of returning to clinic for follow-up. All newly discharged cancer patients are seen in clinic within the first week.

14. *State emergency procedure in the outpatient/home setting.*

Patients and families should be well versed in how to assess for emergency needs. Patients should understand how to access 911, hospital operators, and their ENT physician on call. Transport in the event of a real emergency should be to the nearest emergency room.

15. *State how each member of the multidisciplinary team is involved in the care plan.*

All patients should be able to state the plan of care they will receive form the ENT multidisciplinary team as inpatients and outpatients.

16. *List one source of support available in the community.*

American Cancer Society. American Lung Association, MedicAlert Foundation.

References

1. Keith CF. Wound management following head and neck surgery: the challenge of complex nursing intervention. Nurs Clin North Am 1979;14:761–778
2. Lockhart JS. Nurses' perceptions of head and neck oncology patients after surgery: severity of facial disfigurement and patient gender. ORL Head Neck Nurs 1999;17:12–25
3. Sievers A. Nursing aspects. In: Donald PJ, ed. Care of the Complicated Case. Philadelphia: WB Saunders 1984
4. Lillington GA, Sachs DPL. Preoperative smoking reduction, all or nothing at all. Chest 1998;113:856–857
5. Burns DM. Cigar smoking: overview and current state of the science. Smoking and tobacco control. Monograph No. 9. U.S. Department of Health and Human Services. National Institutes of Health NIH Publication; 1998
6. Jacobson RR, Acker CF, Lishman WA. Patterns of neuropsychological deficit in alcoholic Korsakoff's syndrome. Psychol Med 1990;20:321–334
7. Spies CD, Rommelspacher H. Alcohol withdrawal in the surgical patient: prevention and treatment. Anesth Analg 1999;88:946–954
8. Knowles MS. The Modern Practice of Adult Education, Andragogy versus Pedagogy. New York: Association Press; 1976

9. Keith RL, Lingebaaugh D, Cox B. Presurgical counseling needs of laryngectomee: a survey of 78 patients. Laryngoscope 1978;88:1660–1665

10. Lambie D. A Phenomenological Study, Quality of Life in Head and Neck Cancer Patients. Unpublished master's thesis, California, State University, Sacramento, 1997

11. Levy MH. Pharmacologic management of cancer pain. Semin Oncol 1994;21:718–739

12. World Health Organization. Standards on Pain. Geneva: World Health Organization; 1990

13. Acute Pain Management Panel. Operative or Medical Procedures and Trauma. Clinical Practice Guideline. AHCPR Publication No 92–0032. Rockville, MD: Agency for Health Care Policy and Research, US Department of Health and Human Services; 1992

14. Cancer Pain Management Panel. Management of Cancer Pain. Clinical Practice Guideline No 9. AHCPR Publication No 94–0592. Rockville, MD: Agency for Health Care Policy and Research, Public Health Service, US Department of Health and Human Services; 1994

15. Kendall KA, McKenzie S, Leonard R, Jones C. Structural mobility in deglutition after single modality treatment of head and neck carcinomas with radiotherapy. Head Neck 1998;20:720–725

16. Hupcey JE. Feeling safe: the psychosocial needs of ICU patients. J Nurs Scholarsh 2000;32:361–367

17. Kendall K, Leonard B, eds. Assessment and Treatment of Dysphagia. San Diego: Plural Publishing 2007

18. Kigin CM. Chest physical therapy for the postoperative or traumatic injury patient. Phys Ther 1981;61:1724–1736

19. Carroll RG. Evaluation of tracheal tube cuff design. Crit Care Med 1973;1:45–46

20. Hudak M, Bond-Domb A. Postoperative head and neck cancer patients with artificial airways: the effects of saline lavage on tracheal mucus evacuation and oxygen saturation. ORL Head Neck Nurs 1996;14:17–21

21. Sievers AE, Donald PJ. The use of bolus normal saline instillations in artificial airways: is it useful or necessary? Heart Lung 1987;16:342–343

22. Dropkin MJ. Head and neck cancer: a recovery perspective. Developments in Supportive Care, 3(20:49–52)1999

23. Dropkin MJ. Coping with disfigurement and dysfunction after head and neck cancer surgery: a conceptual framework. Semin Oncol Nurs 1989;5:213–219

24. Scott-Dorsett D. Quality of living. In: Corless IB, Germino BB, Pittman M, eds. Dying, Death, and Bereavement: Theoretical Perspectives and Other Ways of Knowing. Boston: Jones & Bartlett; 1994:189–219

25. Stein-Parbury J, McKinley S. Patients' experiences of being in an intensive care unit: a select literature review. Am J Crit Care 2000;9:20–27

◆ Suggested Reading

American Joint Committee on Cancer. AJCC Cancer Staging Manual. 5th ed. Philadelphia: Lippincott-Raven; 1997:29–30

Grealy L. Autobiography of a Face. Boston: Houghton Mifflin; 1994

Harris L, Huntoon M. Core Curriculum for Otolaryngology and Head and Neck Nursing. New Smyrna Beach, FL: Society of Otorhinolaryngology and Head and Neck Nurses; 1998

Keith R. Looking Forward . . . A Guide Book for the Laryngectomy Mayo Foundation. New York: Thieme; 1995

Netter F. Atlas of Human Anatomy. 2nd ed. Novartis (IOCN Learning Systems, Yardley, PA); 1989

Sigler BA, Schuring LT. Ear, Nose, and Throat Disorders. St. Louis: Mosby; 1993

Society of Otorhinolaryngology and Head and Neck Nurses Inc. Nursing Practice Guidelines. New Smyrna Beach, FL: SOHN; 1990

The nurse oncologist. Semin Oncol 1980;7(1):1–87

◆ Web References

http://www.cancer.org: American Cancer Society

http://www.lungusa.org: American Lung Association

http://www.larynxlink.com: International Association of Laryngectomees (IAL)

http://www.medicalert.org: MedicAlert Foundation

http://rex.nci.nih.gov: National Cancer Institute/National Institutes of Health

http://www.who.int/home: World Health Organization

www.drkoop.org: Dr. Koop medical web site

http://www.mallinckrodt.com: Shiley Airway products

http://portex.com: Portex airway products

http://www.bosmed.com: Boston Medical airway products

http://bivona.com: Bivona airway products

http://hoodlabs.com: Hood Laboratories

http://sohnnurse.com: Society of Otorhinolaryngology Head-Neck Nurses Inc.

http://altmed.od.nih.gov: Office of Alternative Medicine Cancer Research Center

http://nccam.nih.gov: National Center for Complementary and Alternative Medicine, NIH

http://support-group.com: Patient and family support group

http://acor.org: Association of cancer online resources

http://oncolink.upenn.edu: Oncolink support groups

http://www.oncochat.org: Chat rooms for oncology

http://www.rivendell.org: Grief net

http://www.aao-hns.org: American Academy of Otolaryngology—Head and Neck Surgery (AAO-HNS)

http://www.ons.org: Oncology Nursing Society (ONS)

http://www.cdc.gov: Centers for Disease Control

16

Nutrition in Head and Neck Cancer Patients

Ann E. F. Sievers and Beverly Lorens

The incidence of malnutrition in hospitalized patients was described in an article by Butterworth in 1974 that brought to the forefront the state of nutritional support in hospitals.[1] That article, "The Skeleton in the Closet," began a serious investigation into the state of nutrition of hospitalized patients. Protein-calorie malnutrition and involuntary weight loss continue to be prevalent among hospitalized and long-term care patients, particularly the elderly. Malnutrition occurs in as many as 30 to 40% of acute-care facility patients, in 50% of long-term care facility patients, and in up to 85% of nursing home residents.[2]

Malnutrition is reported frequently in cancer patients. Patients with head and neck malignancies are at particular risk of developing nutritional deficiencies.[3] This malnutrition is a source of morbidity, mortality, and significant quality of life issues. One of the objective definitions of malnutrition is weight < 80% ideal body weight (IBW) and/or an unintended weight loss of > 10% usual body weight (UBW) in the past 6 months. Van Bokhorst-de Van der Schuer et al identified a preoperative weight loss of > 10% to be the salient predictive parameter for the occurrence of major postoperative complications.[4] The predictive value of a low serum albumin for postoperative complications was also directly associated with weight loss.

The patient who presents with oncological malnutrition may have multiple causative factors, including cancer cachexia, pain, chemotherapy/radiation therapies, substance abuse, smoking, and comorbidity illness states. Often just the physical obstruction of the aerodigestive tract by a tumor can impede oral nutrition and result in weight loss. It is also known from the literature that the immune system is frequently affected in head and neck cancer patients.[5] Two important factors characterize head and neck cancer patients: immunosuppression and malnutrition. The former, which is very frequent and strong, is due to the immunosuppressive capacity of the tumor. The stress of surgery is an additional causative factor.[6] Of importance, immunosuppression is thought to be more frequent and severe in head and neck cancer patients than in those with malignancies involving other sites.[7] This lack of nutritionally induced immune response is seen in cell-mediated immunity and is demonstrated by a decreased lymphocyte production. The lowered immunity is also characterized by a decreased cytokine release and a lower antibody response to vaccines.

Head and neck cancer patients have an urgent requirement for professional attention to nutrition. The inclusion of a dietitian in the overall care of the patient is mandatory and may prevent complications, save extended hospitalizations, and improve quality of life.

◆ Causes of Malnutrition

Nutrition is a balance of caloric intake and caloric expenditure.[8] Caloric needs of all individuals vary with age, activity, and health. An individual's normal pattern of energy intake and expenditure is severely altered during the diagnosis, treatment, and recovery from cancer. Patients present with protein calorie malnutrition, but nutrient and mineral depletion is of equal concern. The ultimate undesired consequence of a compromised nutritional status for the cancer patient is the occurrence of cachexia, a profound wasting syndrome characterized by weight loss, anorexia, and asthenia[9] (**Fig. 16.1**).

Head and neck cancer patients present with unique problems associated with the development of nutritional difficulties. Some studies have found that > 60% of head and neck cancer patients present with mild to moderate malnutrition.[4] The anatomical location of the tumor by itself can cause physical obstruction to food. Pain affects the ability and willingness to eat. When pain emanates from the aerodigestive tract the problems of oral nutrition are magnified. If the pain is managed correctly, the patient may be better able to orally consume nutrients. The type and character or consistency of food ingested may drastically change form, from solid to soft to liquid. Usually the protein and calorie content of the food decreases along with this change.

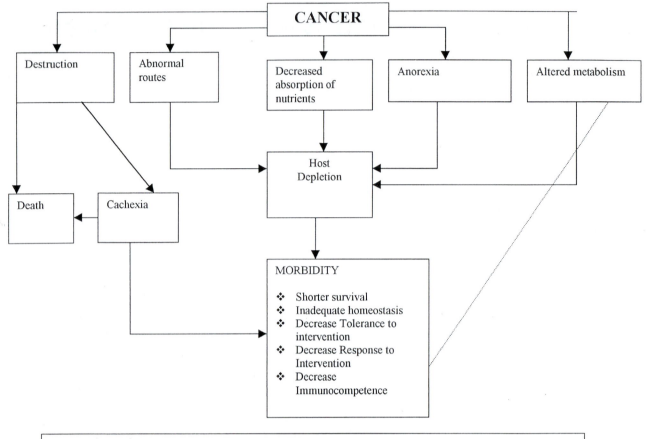

Daly JM, Thom AK:Neoplastic Diseases. IN Nutrition and Metabolism in Patient Care, Kinney JM et al (eds),
WB Saunders, Philadelphia, 1988. P.568.

Fig. 16.1 Cancer cachexia is a leading cause of morbidity and mortality in many neoplastic diseases. Nutritional support throughout the patient's trajectory is of critical importance.

Head and neck cancer is often a disease of the older population because of the length of time of exposure to the environmental carcinogens of smoking and alcohol. The elderly often have insufficient energy intake. Their energy requirements increase when they have cancer. Elderly patients at high risk for preexisting malnutrition are those who weigh < 80% of IBW, or are greater than 20% above their IBW or have a weight loss of > 10% UBW in the prior 6 months. Also at risk are those who take multiple drugs, have malabsorption syndromes, or have comorbid states such as diabetes, pulmonary disease, arthritis, and cardiac and renal disease. Dental issues are very frequently a major problem due to loss of teeth from lack of dental care and hygiene. The most significant factors that influence nutritional intake, however (in

nursing homes), are inadequate staffing, lack of knowledge about how to feed residents, and inadequate supervision by professional nurses.[10]

The abuse of alcohol in the elderly is an often silent, hidden, but not infrequent component. Excess alcohol intake plays a major part in nutritional deficiency. Alcohol is a significant factor in the development of head and neck cancer. As early as the 1850s an awareness of the dangers of drinking began to emerge.[11] Alcohol abuse continues to contribute to the risk factors of head and neck cancer. Alcohol calories may displace calories from other foods that are nutrient dense. It disrupts absorption of nutrients and damages the pancreas and liver. The toxic effects of alcohol are detectable once intake exceeds 15% of calories and may be severe at or above

30% of calories. Alcoholics often demonstrate deficiency in folic acid, pyridoxine, thiamin, and iron. They may have deficiencies of zinc, magnesium, and vitamins D, K, and A. This is predominantly due to inadequate or unbalance nutritional intake.

Psychosocial and socioeconomic difficulties are often a recurrent underlying theme in elderly individuals providing for themselves. About 35 to 85% of nursing home residents are malnourished.[12] We have often heard patients state that they don't have enough money to buy food or tube feedings. The true answer is that they are concerned about providing for their families, their medications, or their pets. Many insurance companies also do not provide for enteral feeding or supplementation as outpatients. Federal Medicare will not pay for enteral feeding if it is to be utilized for less than 3 months.

Obese patients are equally considered malnourished and present yet another complex set of nutritional and medical concerns. Those patients with a body mass index (BMI) of > 27 are considered at nutritional risk. Obesity is the most common chronic disease in the world and is associated with an increased risk for mortality.[13] Another concern is that excess adipose tissue can mask the otherwise visible altered muscle mass induced from a decrease protein and energy intake.

The impact of medical treatment on nutritional status confounds the clinical picture. Surgery, radiation, and chemotherapy interrupt the patient's ability to secure consistent nutrition. Perioperatively the patient may spend hours and even days NPO waiting for tests or surgical procedures. Radiation and chemotherapy induce a further set of problems, with mucositis, fatigue, anemia, nausea, and pain as hallmarks. Oral complications from radiotherapy originate from radiation injury to the salivary glands and oral mucosa. Clinical sequelae of such injury (depending on the intensity, duration, and port of therapy) include dryness of the mouth, "mouth blindness" (loss of taste discretion), dental caries, mucositis, osteoradionecrosis, oral infections, and trismus.[14] Nayel et al found in 1992 that by nutritionally supplementing patients before and during radiotherapy they were able to maintain or increase body weight.[15] An astonishing 58% of the patients that were *not* supplemented lost weight during the course of therapy. Mucosal reaction was of a lesser degree and shorter duration in the supplemented group. None of the patients in the supplemented group had a delay in treatment caused by side effects of radiotherapy. This is a very important study that clearly demonstrated the effectiveness of successful nutritional intervention and one that these authors support.

Anorexia, nausea, and vomiting constitute a spectrum of symptoms and signs that result in a reduction of food intake.[16] There are several causes of anorexia in advanced cancer. Identified as early as the 1960s these include abnormalities of taste and smell, disorders of the hunger-satiety mechanism, and possibly, production by the tumor of intermediate metabolites that can affect central and peripheral mediators of hunger and satiety, the so-called anorexiogenic metabolite hypotheses.[17]

Appetite may also be significantly affected by the metabolic changes that occur with tumor growth. Taste distortions are frequently encountered that are as yet not well understood. Some postulate that taste bud cells decrease in size with the presence of tumor, thus decreasing taste. Others feel that the metabolic abnormalities that occur affect the threshold of taste. The altered thresholds then affect perceptions of taste. The most striking effect of cancer in many patients is malignant cachexia, clinically manifested by anorexia, marked asthenia, significant loss of body fat and muscle, anemia, water and electrolyte abnormalities, and increased basal metabolic rate. The clinical spectrum of cachexia ranges from the patient in the early stages with an undiagnosed neoplasm and minimal weight loss to someone with end-stage disease who has marked weakness and muscle wasting. Wasting of the temporalis major, masseter, and hypothenar muscles is a primary indicator of this process.[18]

◆ Nutritional Evaluation

Nutritional screening at the patient's initial presentation at tumor board has been extremely beneficial in elucidating nutritional status and estimating nutritional requirements (**Fig. 16.2**). The Joint Commission on the Accreditation of Healthcare Organizations (JCAHO) mandates all patients must be nutritionally screened soon after admission to the hospital.[19] Screening and intervention make a significant impact in at-risk patients. Mears screened 177 hospitalized patients and found 22 patients were at severe risk, and appropriate nutritional intervention was initiated.[20] Those patients who were supplemented had a 12-day shorter average length of stay when compared with an unsupplemented group with the same degree of nutritional risk.

Both screening and comprehensive nutritional evaluations require consideration of a patient's anthropometric characteristics, dietary intake, relevant clinical and physical findings, and socioeconomic considerations. Himes states that measures of body weight, BMI, and midarm muscle circumference can provide estimates of somatic protein stores.[2] Laboratory measures of albumin, prealbumin, transferrin, hemoglobin, and total lymphocyte count indicate visceral protein levels. As part of the patient assessment, it is important to distinguish between causes due to nutritional deficiencies, which are potentially reversible with nutritional support, and disease-related causes (e.g., cancer, renal disease, and sepsis), which may not respond to nutritional intervention.[2] Significant changes in weight trends and hydration or unintentional weight loss in a patient, signal the need for a comprehensive nutritional evaluation.

Comprehensive assessment will thoroughly investigate each of these areas; for example, dietary intake will be assessed in terms of calories, protein, vitamins, minerals, and fluid, and evaluated for adequacy based on the patient's individual needs.[21] An optimal scheme of nutritional assessment enables the clinician to quickly detect the presence of malnutrition and provides guidelines for nutritional therapy.[22]

BMI is calculated.[23] Generally the criteria for a more thorough investigation predicates from a BMI < 22 or > 27. The calculation of weight loss based on recalled weight has been shown to be more accurate than that based on ideal weight

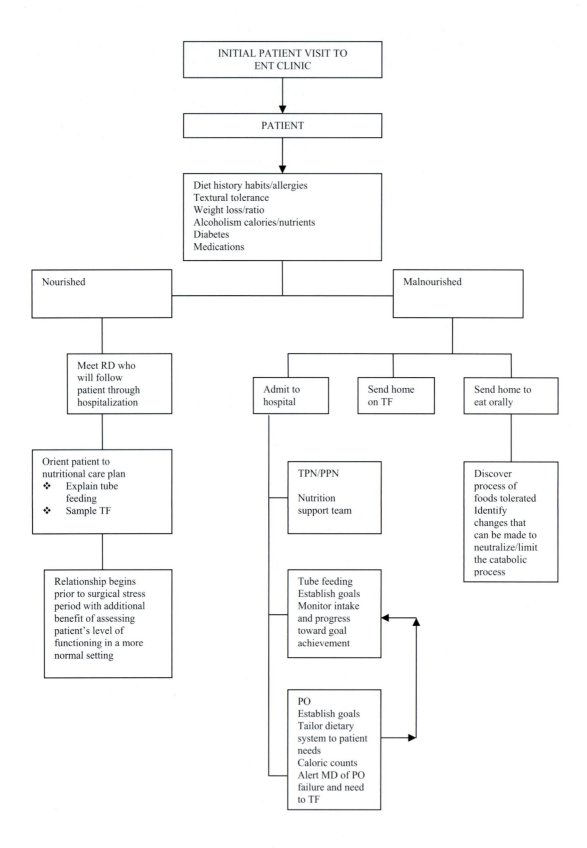

Fig. 16.2 Algorithm for patient nutritional care at initial tumor board presentation.

Calculation of Percentage of Weight Loss

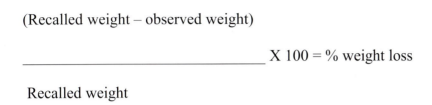

$$\frac{(\text{Recalled weight} - \text{observed weight})}{\text{Recalled weight}} \times 100 = \% \text{ weight loss}$$

Fig. 16.3 Equation for percent weight loss. Copland 1979

derived from standard tables.[24] The percent of weight loss can be calculated by the equation in **Fig. 16.3**.[25]

Weight change over time is a clear indicator of nutritional inadequacy, particularly if the weight loss is unintended. Blackburn et al describes in **Table 16.1** the difference in adjusting for weight change over time from significant to severe weight loss.[23,25] Patients presenting with a significant or severe loss must have nutritional intervention if therapy for the cancer is indicated. Rombeau et al (**Table 16.2**) describes the evaluation on nutritional status based on a percentage of weight.[26] This is another method of calculating the status of the patient with weight loss. Both methods give important patient information in evaluating their possible nutritional status and risk.

Perhaps the most important aspect of the initial nutritional assessment is the diet interview. A consistent method of documentation of the interview is an important tool for the dietitian (see appendix 16.1). It is important to consider more than laboratory data and calculated weight or BMI. A history including social and psychological factors will give very valuable information. Food allergies, intolerance, and food preferences, and the patient's own descriptions of the problem are very important in making an accurate assessment. *It is most important to take time to listen to the patient and family.* Family members and friends may reveal even further and sometimes more accurately the patient's nutritional intake. Family members may disclose a more thorough picture of the patient's difficulties. This interview often reveals more information than all the laboratory data available.[27]

During the interview, it is important to address the use of alcohol, drugs, and alternative therapies. Caffeine intake (coffee and cola products) is evaluated. Withdrawal symptoms from alcohol and drugs must be addressed before surgical procedures are undertaken because the withdrawal symptoms can be life threatening. Caffeine withdrawal can cause significant frontal headaches that are generally refractory to conventional opioids; acetaminophen with codeine is the treatment of choice.

Alternative medicine and herbal therapies may be considered as nutritional supplements by individuals. Because of the interactions with medications and anesthesia it is critically important that each type of homeopathic therapy be documented. Patients and family may not be aware of the significant interactions of herbs and administered medications and therapies. Use of supplemental vitamins in excessive quantities or "immune potentiators" are a potential for risk factor with the mix of medications and anesthesia.

Cultural and religious factors are of great importance. Those patients who are vegetarian sometimes find it difficult to increase their protein and caloric intake. Inability to eat "usual" foods let alone "usual cultural" foods can lead to depression and isolation. Food disturbance during holiday times also contributes to isolation and withdrawal.

Allergies to both foods and drugs should be investigated for their interaction with medications and nutrition. Food

Table 16.1 Evaluation of Weight Change[23]

Time	Significant Weight Loss (% of Change)	Severe Weight Loss (% of Change)
1 week	1–2	> 2
1 month	5	> 5
3 months	7.5	> 7.5
6 months	10	> 10

Table 16.2 Evaluation of Nutritional Status Based on a Percentage of Weight[26]

Malnutrition	% of Ideal Body Weight	% of Usual Body Weight
Mild	80–90	85–95
Moderate	70–79	75–84
Severe	0–69	0–74

preferences should be documented and incorporated into the treatment plan.

Thiamin deficiency and malnutrition are present in a patient who abuses alcohol. Protein-energy malnutrition with a resultant loss of body fat and lean body mass occurs when excess alcohol is substituted for nutrient-dense and protein-rich foods. Micronutrient deficiencies, particularly thiamin deficiency, are also common in people who are alcoholic and can occur when consumption of alcohol is excessive and the variety of foods in the diet is limited. Thiamin deficiency, if untreated, can result in Wernicke encephalopathy and eventually Korsakoff syndrome.[28] Alcohol-related neurological disease affects a person's memory and ability to process thoughts. This makes informed consent and patient education much more difficult. It is well documented that memory does lapse with these conditions, especially in stressful situations.

Standard laboratory data for evaluation includes a complete metabolic panel (CMP), phosphorus and magnesium levels, and a complete blood count (CBC). If diabetes mellitus presents as a history of high blood sugars, hemoglobin A1C is useful to establish the prior level of glucose control. The inclusion of a lipid panel, though not necessary, adds to the clinical picture. If available, a prealbumin provides a refined review of the visceral protein state. Of particular nutrition relevance are abnormal values in potassium, blood urea nitrogen (BUN), albumin, phosphorus, magnesium, hemoglobin, mean corpuscle volume (MCV), and cholesterol. Diminished nutrition status will be reflected in abnormally low values of the preceding parameters, with the exception of an elevated MCV, in folic acid or vitamin B12 deficiency.[29]

Physical examination includes thenar and hypothenar wasting, skin turgor, color, abdominal girth, presence of ascites, nonhealing wounds, edema, bruising, tongue furrows, or lip commissure sores. Presence of any one of these findings can be an indicator of protein, calorie, vitamin, or mineral deficiencies.

◆ Interventions to Meet Nutritional Needs

If shortcomings in nutritional intake are identified, recommendations are made to the patient and the patient's support system for changes in diet that will arrest further decline and improve nutrition.

Nutritional intervention must be provided early enough to prevent a catabolically induced decline in lean muscle mass, which can impair wound healing. The mechanisms of digestion are reduced in times of physiological stress, and cancer and cancer therapy constitute a stress state. Consumption, conversion, and expenditure of energy are essential for the performance of mechanical, chemical, and electrical work and for the growth of tissue. This is true in healthy as well as disease states.[13] More aggressive nutritional management and a greater understanding of the role of nutrition and weight gain in wound healing can result in more effective patient care.[2] Because patients can quickly lose energy and weight on basic intravenous solutions; supplementary methods of nutrition must be invoked to minimize or prevent the effects of the catabolic process. *Tissue nutrition is a high-energy metabolic activity.*

Educating the patient is the first step in improving nutrition. Counseling regarding improved eating habits is of great importance. Oral supplementation is the next step and is simply the addition of greater nutrition to the patient's basic diet. Written recommendations are valuable to an already overwhelmed patient population (see appendix 16.2).

Methods of Intervention

Dense calorie support is an interesting, effective, but not intrusive way to increase caloric intake. One approach for patients who cannot tolerate larger volumes, which are greater than 8 ounces at a time, may be to use a 2 cal/mL drink. The patient who is given 30 mL of a 2 calorie supplement receives 60 calories contained in a very small quantity. Therefore, 30 mL six times a day = 360 additional calories. This additional calorie and protein supplement may be the only intervention required to improve a catabolic patient.[9,10]. Head and neck cancer patients should be taught early on that food is a medication, equal to any other medication and possibly more potent in their recovery. Strict attention to nutrition is important in the perioperative treatment period. High calorie, high protein, oral supplementation may be indicated in the form of additional food or specially prepared shakes in addition to meals. Because of the physical alteration of the normal aerodigestive tract, the increased metabolic needs, and the pain involved in swallowing, patients and their families must be given instruction and support to alter their current noneffective method of eating.

Oral feeding is preferred because of the normalcy and psychological aspects of eating. Increased caloric intake can be achieved if patients are willing and able to address their needs. Normal deglutition requires the mobility of oral and pharyngeal structures to prepare the bolus, propel the bolus into the pharynx, open the upper esophageal sphincter, and protect the airway. Preoperative nutrition may be difficult for oropharyngeal and laryngeal cancer patients. The cancer may be the cause of aspiration. Following head and neck surgery, oral nutrition may also be extremely difficult due to the loss of the normal tissues of deglutition from surgical resection. Tissue fibrosis secondary to radiotherapy may decrease the mobility of these vital structures and therefore alter the ability to swallow.[30] Both pre- and postoperatively aspiration is a dreaded occurrence. The incidence of aspiration pneumonia is very high in patients with tumor in the oropharyngeal laryngeal complex and also in those who are undergoing radiation or radiotherapy combined with chemotherapy for their cancer therapy. Oral nutrition becomes more difficult with tumor growth, radiation therapy, and surgical resection. In evaluating the extent of dysphagia, the clinician must be observant for signs of altered swallow, coughing, and struggle with eating and noise of aspiration. In concert with the physical and the cranial nerve examinations, auscultation of the larynx may elicit very valuable information (**Fig. 16.4**). Laminar airflow through the larynx with quiet breathing is normal. Disruption of this laminar airflow during deglutition is abnormal. Accompanied with struggle and other associ-

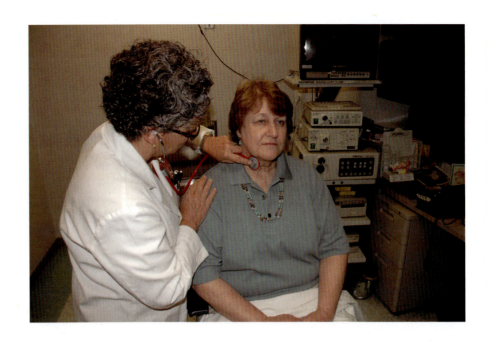

Fig. 16.4 Laryngeal auscultation.

ated signs this indicates aspiration. Radiographic definitive proof is obtained by a dynamic swallow study.[31]

Syringe feeding is a very adequate method of temporary alternative nutritional assistance. Usually used only for support until the patient can learn oral adequacy, this is a technique predominantly attempted postoperatively (**Fig. 16.5**). To make the syringe feeder, use a 20 or 30 mL syringe and a 14 gauge suction catheter, cut off the thumb control and the multieye tip to control direction, and attach to the syringe. Placement in the mouth is critical to success. Place the tube far enough into the mouth to prevent oral incontinence, and yet far enough back to ensure proper placement. Do not stimulate the gag reflex. Keep the tube away from the internal suture lines (if present), and position the patient in an upright sitting position. It is imperative that the patient be safe using this method for prevention of aspiration. A dy-

namic swallow study is beneficial to determine accurate oral catheter placement for the prevention of aspiration and to determine a safe swallow.[32]

Intervention is necessary if adequate oral nutritional consumption is impossible, and moderate to severe malnutrition is diagnosed. If patients are unable to sustain their nutrition by oral methods then enteral feeding must be seriously considered. The head and neck cancer patient, although unable to sustain oral nutrition, usually has the ability to utilize the gastrointestinal tract for enteral nutrition. Therefore, total parenteral nutrition (TPN) is rarely necessary in this population. The choice of intervention and the type of feeding are based on the patient's estimated need for energy, protein, fluid, vitamins, and minerals. Enteral intervention is indicated if the patient (1) is malnourished and unable to eat for > 5 to 7 days, (2) is normally nourished but unable to

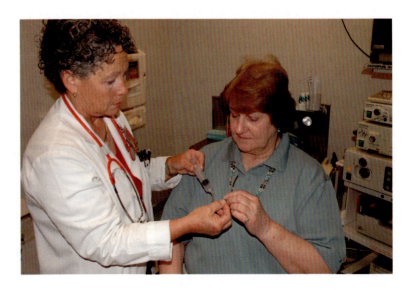

Fig. 16.5 Syringe for safe oral feeding.

eat for > 7 to 9 days, (3) has short bowel syndrome, (4) has undergone severe trauma or burns, or (5) experiences failure of oral intake.[13]

Early enteral feeding maintains gut integrity and immune competence, prevents gut atrophy, maintains gut function, diminishes bacterial translocation, improves gut healing (in gastrointestinal surgery), and stimulates hepatic cells. Early enteral feeding decreases sepsis and wound infections and prevents continuing weight loss. Close ongoing evaluation with a dietitian is critical to change an ever-increasing weight loss pattern.

There is interplay of medical, nutritional, institutional, and regulatory considerations that must be appreciated in choosing a formula. The product is chosen based on the indication for use and formulary availability. If the patient is the appropriate weight-for-height and in good nutritional status a choice would be a fiber formula that is near iso-osmolar, greater than or equal to 16% calories as protein, meeting the Recommended Dietary Intake (RDI) for vitamins and minerals at a 1200 to 1500 calorie level. If the patient is obese or has diabetes, with no renal insufficiency, select a higher protein formula greater than or equal to 23% calories as protein, near iso-osmolar with fiber. This meets the RDI for vitamins and minerals at about the 1200 calorie level. If the patient is underweight, with or without indications of protein malnutrition, select a fiber formula, near iso-osmolar at greater than or equal to 16% calories as protein. This meets the RDI for vitamins and minerals at 1200 to 1500 calories level. In this patient the calorie end point will be higher than for the weight-appropriate patient so the actual protein provision will be higher, approaching 1.5 to 1.8 g of protein per kilogram actual weight. In all patients, monitoring for initial bowel movements is critical for continued tolerance of tube feeding. Patients are prone to constipation from the effects of anesthesia, narcotic pain medication, bed rest, and fiber or nonfiber formula with possible insufficient intraluminal fluid due to water restriction or third spacing of fluid.

Nutritional Components of Intervention

Energy is stored as carbohydrates, fat, and protein. Carbohydrates are stored in the liver and muscle as glycogen. Fat is stored as triglycerides in the fat cells. Protein may also be considered to be an energy store, although all body protein is believed to be functional, and thus mobilization of protein to meet energy demands is detrimental. Extraction of energy from protein requires protein hydrolysis to individual amino acids.[33]

◆ **Energy** Carbohydrates and fats are required for wound healing and tissue remodeling; they supply cellular energy, and they spare protein. The preferred oxidative fuel of the body is glucose. Fat is the most calorically dense form of stored energy available and in particular manufactures cell membranes. A deficiency results in visceral and muscle protein use for energy. The information in **Table 16.3** gives target goals for weight gain or loss. These targets must be correlated with the current and anticipated energy expenditure of the patient.

Table 16.3 Average Daily Caloric Requirements for Healthy Adults[13]

Weight maintenance	25–30 Cal/Kg
Weight gain	35–40 Cal/kg
Weight loss	20 Cal/kg

Source: Data from Gottschlich M (2001) p. 34–35.

◆ **Protein** Protein is used in wound healing and repair of tissues. Deficiency in protein leads to poor tissue perfusion and resulting edema and is also integral in clotting factors and white blood cell (WBC) production. **Table 16.4** details the protein requirement for most individuals. Again specific individuals' requirements must be calculated to fit their personal needs.

Table 16.4 Average Protein Requirements for Adults[13]

Healthy adults	0.8 g/kg body weight
Elderly	1.0–1.25 g/kg
Disease state	1.5–2.5 g/kg

Source: Data from Gottschlich M (2001) p. 34.

◆ **Fluids** Water is important in the digestion, absorption, transport, and utilization of nutrients and the elimination of toxins and waste products. Water provides structure to cells and is a vital component of thermoregulation. It is the most abundant substance in the human body and composes ~60% of body weight in adult males and 50% of body weight in adult females. Fluid regulation varies with environment and metabolic activity, usually 1 mL/Kcal of energy expenditure.[13] Ear, nose, and throat (ENT) patients have a very high insensible water loss. Normal water loss per day is ~400 mL. In an ENT patient with an artificial airway, water loss is ~500 to 600 mL insensible volume with an additional 600 to 700 mL per day with suctioning. Replacement requirements must be carefully calculated to ensure proper hydration.

◆ **Vitamins and Minerals** Replacement utilizing an adult multivitamin with minerals is usually sufficient if taking oral nutrition. If enterally fed, most commercial formulas are sufficiently fortified with nutrients so that a standard multivitamin–mineral or intravenous multivitamin is not needed. Exceptions to this are conditions requiring repletion of thiamin, folic acid, potassium, magnesium, phosphorus, and possibly zinc.[34] These may include deficiencies induced from excessive alcohol ingestion, extreme overall nutritional depletion, or the increased needs of the body as metabolism upregulates with resumption of substrates availability.

◆ Assessment and Monitoring of Enteral Feeding

Standard postoperative orders for feeding and monitoring make the system efficient in instituting feeding protocols.

Standard orders include postoperative nutritional consultation. Because most of the patients have been seen preoperatively this is a continuation of their nutritional intervention. There is no substitute for careful evaluation and monitoring of tolerance of feeding. Safe and successful tube feeding depends on choosing the right patient, formula, route, and technique, as well as on expert vigilance and care.[35]

In the 1999 review article on wound healing, Himes defines normal wound healing.[2] It involves three overlapping phases: an inflammatory phase (1–3d after injury), a proliferative phase (3–10d after injury), and a remodeling or maturation phase (2 to 3 weeks to 1 to 2 years). During the inflammatory phase, platelets aggregate at the wound site, stimulating the release of growth factors and recruiting WBCs and local immune defenses to the wound site. This early phase is associated with a catabolic state. Increases in inflammatory mediators, oxidant activity, and catabolic hormones in conjunction with a decrease in the activity of endogenous anabolic hormones results in a net increase in protein degradation and significant tissue protein losses. In the proliferative phase, fibroblasts synthesize collagen and proteoglycans to form the scaffolding for wound and lean muscle repair. In the final remodeling stage, collagen is deposited into the wound as new tissue is formed. The strength and integrity of the new tissue during normal repair depend on collagen crosslinking and deposition. Wound healing is an anabolic, energy-requiring process, necessitating an increased protein and calorie intake to rebuild tissue. Slow-to-heal or nonhealing wounds result from a derangement of the normal wound healing process.[2]

Following surgical resection of head and neck cancers, the patient requires an ongoing nutritional evaluation, which includes a comprehensive plan of care (**Table 16.5**).

◆ Complications and Failure of Enteral Feeding

One of the most frequent complications of tube feeding is tube obstruction with the resultant inability to deliver feeding. The majority of time this complication can be prevented by flushing the tube with water before and after feeding and medication administration.[36] Keeping medications from coagulating or mechanically obstructing the tube is accomplished with water flushes. When available, use elixir or liquid forms of medication, with strict attention to the timing of medication and feeding.[37] In tubes that are placed with a stylette never attempt reinsertion of the stylette to unclog a tube. This could result in tube or digestive tract perforation.[38] Although relatively safe, there are complications with enteral feeding. Most complications are related to the position of the enteral tube and the patient's ability to tolerate the chosen enteral formula. Mechanical, gastrointestinal, and metabolic complications of enteral feeding are outlined in **Tables 16.6, 16.7,** and **16.8**.

Diarrhea is often indicted as a complication of tube feeding, but in reality diarrhea can be traced to a multiplicity of causes. The rate of tube feeding, especially in the beginning of enteral feeding, is often the cause of intolerance diarrhea. "Too fast" equals intolerance in many cases. Insufficient wa-

Table 16.5 Nutrition Monitoring Postsurgical Resection

Data	Acute Frequency	Stable Frequency
Body weight	Three times/week	Weekly to monitor stability or achievement of goals
Laboratories: Basic metabolic panel Phosphorus Calcium Magnesium	Daily times 3–5 days or until stable at nutritional goal, then twice weekly	PRN after stability is achieved
Laboratory: Albumin	Preoperative workup Preoperative surgery Postoperative weekly	Weekly until normalizes
Laboratory: Prealbumin C-reactive protein	Twice weekly while establishing efficacy of protein provision	Repeat prealbumin only when C-reactive levels normalize
Calorie counts Oral diet	Daily times 3–5 days or until stable at nutritional goal	Then weekly if intake remains at target goals
Intake of tube feeding	Daily while in hospital	1 to 2 times/week when weight and metabolic stable
Stool Pattern	Daily until tolerance of nutrition is established	Weekly if no interval changes
Texture	Frequency, volume and consistency	

ter or high osmolality can also cause untoward complications. Medications in elixir form are very high in sorbital and may be the culprit.[37,38] Changing to a fiber formula may be all that is required. When diarrhea occurs with enteral feeding, it is essential to understand that the causes other than the feeding are responsible the majority of the time. One must blame the feeding only after excluding these and after observing resolution of the diarrhea when the feeding is interrupted.[39,40] Administration of common antidiarrheal medication should be in the armamentarium.

Reflux or gastroesophageal reflux (GER) is a very common problem in orally fed as well as enterally fed patients. With the advancement of medications that alter the pH on the stomach and improve gastric emptying this serious problem is coming under better understanding and control. Reflux is thought to be one of the main risk factors leading to pneumonia in the critically ill patient with enteral feeding.[41,42] Ibáñez et al found that there is a high incidence of GER in critically ill patients and that semirecumbency does not prevent GER, but there is less incidence of GER when patients are in the supine position.[43] Coben et al found that both gastric distention and rapid transgastric bolus feeding contribute to the relaxation of the lower esophageal sphincter (LES) with resultant reflux.[44] Heyland et al found that postpyloric feeding reduces gastroesophageal reflux and that by feeding in this method we may be able to prevent subsequent pulmonary infections in high-risk populations.[45]

Aspiration, according to Maloney and Metheny, is a risk in critically ill patients who are receiving enteral feeding; these patients are susceptible to the pulmonary aspiration of gas-

Table 16.6 Enteral Feeding: Mechanical Complications, Causes, Prevention, and Treatment

Problem	Cause	Prevention/Treatment
Aspiration pneumonia	Delayed gastric emptying Gastroparesis Reflux Dysphagia of all types Migration of tube into esophagus	Reduce infusion rate Fed beyond the pylorus Check gastric residuals Minimize compromise of the LES with small tubes Initially and regularly check tube placement Position upright for and after feeds
Pharyngeal irritation, otitis and sinusitis Nasolabial, esophageal and mucosal irritation and erosion	Prolonged use of nasal tubes Poor method of securing tube to nares Prolonged use of nasal tubes especially large-bore Use of rubber or plastic	Use small bore tubes Consider GT/JT Secure properly Protect the nose with skin barriers and then tape Use smaller caliber tubes Consider GT/JT
Irritation and leakage at ostomy site Tube lumen obstruction	Drainage of digestive juices form stoma site Thickened formula residue Formation of insoluble formula-medication complexes	Skin and stoma care Maintain proper tube placement Irrigate tube frequently with water, especially before and after medications and formula

Abbreviations: GT, gastrostomy tube; JT, jejunostomy tube; LES, lower esophageal sphincter.

Source: Adapted from Ross Laboratories. Enteral Nutrition Reference Manual for Case Managers. A Guide to medical nutrition therapy. 1993.

Table 16.7 Gastrointestinal Complications, Causes, Prevention, and Treatment

Problem	Cause	Prevention/Treatment
Diarrhea	Low residue formula Rapid formula administration Hyperosmolar formula Bolus feeding using syringe force Hypoalbuminemia Nutrient malabsorption Microbial contamination Disuse atrophy Rapid GI transit time Prolonged antibiotic treatment or other drug therapy	Select fiber formula Initiate feedings at low rate or temporarily decrease rate Reduce rate of administration Use isotonic formula or dilute concentration and gradually increase strength Reduce rate Review medication profile and method of administration Repopulate normal gut flora Consider medication alternatives Consider alternate formulas Use elemental formulas Consider PPN/TPN until regulated
Cramping, gas, abdominal distention	Nutrient malabsorption Rapid intermittent administration of refrigerated formula Intermittent feeding using syringe force	Use continuous feedings Room temperature Reduce rate Choose alternate formula
Nausea and vomiting	Rapid formula administration Gastric retention	Initiate feeding at low rate and gradually advance to desired rate Temp decrease rate Use isotonic or dilute formulas Reduce rate of administration Consider low fat formulas Consider post pyloric feeding
Constipation	Opioids Inadequate fluid intake Insufficient bulk Inactivity	Decrease use of narcotics Increase fluid intake Select fiber formulas Encourage ambulation

Abbreviations: GI, gastrointestinal; PPN, peripheral parenteral nutrition; TPN, total parenteral nutrition.

Source: Adapted from Ross Laboratories. Enteral Nutrition Reference Manual for Case Managers: A Guide to Medical Nutrition Therapy. 1993.

tric contents.[46–50] Measures to enhance the early detection of aspiration include the tinting of feedings with the food dye FD&C blue no. 1. During sepsis, gastrointestinal permeability increases because of enterocyte death and loss of barrier function at intercellular gaps. Thus substances that are otherwise nonabsorbable may be absorbed during sepsis. An inhibition of mitochondrial oxidative phosphorylation by blocking electron transport or by blocking the generation of adenosine triphosphate (ATP) is the presumed path of cellular absorption of the dye. The cellular permeability during

Table 16.8 Metabolic Complications, Causes, Prevention, and Treatment

Problem	Cause	Prevention/Treatment
Dehydration	Inadequate fluid intake or excessive losses	Supplement intake with appropriate fluids Monitor hydration status
Overhydration	Rapid refeeding Excessive fluid intake	Reduce rate of administration, especially in severe malnutrition or major organ failure Monitor hydration status
Hyperglycemia	Inadequate insulin production for the amount of formula being given Stress	Initiate feeding at low rate Monitor blood glucose Use oral agents or insulin PRN Use low CHO formulas
Hypernatremia	Inadequate fluid intake or excessive losses	Assess fluid and electrolyte status Supplement with appropriate fluid
Hyponatremia	Inadequate intake Fluid overload Inappropriate antidiuretic Hormone secretion syndrome Excessive GI fluid losses Chronic feeding with low sodium enteral formulas as the sole source of dietary sodium	Assess fluid and electrolyte status Supplement Na sodium (Na^+) Restrict fluids Use diuretics Replace with fluids of similar composition
Hypophosphatemia	Aggressive refeeding of malnourished patients Insulin therapy	Monitor serum levels Replenish phosphorus levels before refeeding
Hypercapnia	Excessive carbohydrate loads given patients with respiratory dysfunction and CO_2 retention	Select low CHO high fat formulas
Hypokalemia	Aggressive refeeding of malnourished patient	Provide potassium (K^+) Monitor serum levels
Hyperkalemia	Excessive K intake Decreased excretion	Reduce potassium (K^+) levels Monitor serum levels

Abbreviations: CHO, carbohydrate; CO_2, carbon dioxide; GI, gastrointestinal; K^+, potassium; Na^+, sodium.

Source: Adapted from Ross Laboratories. Enteral Nutrition Reference Manual for Case Managers: A Guide to Medical Nutrition Therapy. 1993.

acidosis is altered and the dye is then absorbed. Therefore *judicious* use of food dye to detect aspiration is indicated, particularly in critically ill patients.

There is a strong relationship between a multiplicity of various factors and aspiration: (1) decreased level of consciousness, (2) supine position, (3) nasogastric tubes, (4) malpositioned feeding tube, (5) tracheal intubation/mechanical ventilation, (6) vomiting, and (7) delivery methods.[50] Other factors include high-risk disease/injury conditions, neurological disorders, major abdominal and thoracic trauma/surgery, diabetes mellitus, poor oral health, inadequate registered nurse staffing levels, and advanced age. The two main concerns identified by Metheny are decreased level of consciousness and sustained supine position.

Bacterial contamination: Mixing or diluting feedings appears to represent an increased risk of bacterial contamination. The growth of gram-negative bacilli (GNB) may produce adverse effects. Undiluted, canned enteral feedings were significantly less contaminated than those requiring mixing of powder. Contaminated enteral feedings may have become reservoirs for contamination of other body sites. Long hanging times and frequent interruption of the enteral feeding system with medications and water may be the source of contamination.[51]

Refeeding syndrome is best thought of broadly as the occurrence of severe fluid and electrolyte shifts, especially but not exclusively phosphorus, and their associated complications in malnourished patients undergoing refeeding either orally, enterally, or parenterally. In treatment it is important

to monitor potassium, magnesium, and glucose metabolism, vitamin deficiency, and especially the fluid volume.[52] Daily body weight is necessary to address the issue of fluid overload. Many head and neck cancer patients receive large volumes of fluid during long surgical procedures. Those patients at risk for refeeding syndrome are listed in **Table 16.9**.

Solomon recommendations to avoid the refeeding syndrome are included in **Table 16.10**, with a caution that to be aware of the syndrome and a little nutrition support is good, but a lot can be lethal. *Hypophosphatemia* is one of the main complications seen in refeeding syndrome (**Table 16.11**). *Hypomagnesiumemia* can occur with critically ill patients who abuse alcohol. This is a total body deficit of magnesium. During alcohol withdrawal, serum concentrations decrease further due to intracellular shifts. The result is a decrease in muscle function and cardiac arrhythmias. The treatment

Table 16.9 Patients at Risk for Refeeding Syndrome[52]

1. Anorexia nervosa
2. Classic kwashiorkor
3. Classic marasmus
4. Chronic malnutrition-underfeeding
5. Chronic alcoholism
6. Morbid obesity with massive weight loss
7. Patient unfed in 7–10 days with evidence of stress and depletion
8. Prolonged fasting

Table 16.10 Recommendations to Avoid the Refeeding Syndrome[52]

1. Be aware of the syndrome
2. Recognize the "patient at risk"
3. Carefully test for and correct electrolyte abnormalities before initiating nutrition support
4. Judiciously restore circulatory volume, monitor pulse rate, and intake and output
5. Increase caloric delivery *slowly* taking 2–4 days to achieve goals
6. Administer vitamins and minerals routinely
7. Carefully monitor the electrolytes over the first week, including phosphorus, potassium, magnesium, glucose, urinary electrolytes
8. *"A little nutrition support is good, too much is lethal"*

is slow, careful intravenous (IV) replacement in addition to enteral feedings.

Dumping syndrome occurs when the patient cannot tolerate the osmolar concentration of the formula, and free water leaves the systemic circulation and enters the gastrointestinal tract. This manifests as a form of shock and intravascular volume depletion. The symptoms are flushing, sweating, and diarrhea, and usually occur following enteral feeding. The migration of an enteral feeding tube into the small intestine and the continuation of large bolus feedings into the small intestine can cause dumping.[53]

Chyle leak occurs during neck dissection. Chyle is a fat-containing fluid that is formed in the lacteals of the intestine during digestion. It is transported via lymphatics and enters the venous circulation via the thoracic duct (near the subclavian veins). Approximately 70% of ingested dietary fat passes through this system.[54] Chyle is identified as milky white fluid (**Table 16.12**). During neck dissection the thoracic duct or

Table 16.11 Severe Sequelae of Hypophosphatemia[52]

Cardiac	Altered myocardial function, arrhythmia, congestive heart failure, sudden death
Hematological	Altered RBC, morphology, hemolytic anemia, WBC dysfunction, thrombocytopenia, depressed platelet function, hemorrhage
Hepatic	Liver dysfunction (especially in cirrhotics)
Neuromuscular	Acute areflexic paralysis, confusion, coma, cranial nerve palsies, diffuse sensory loss, Guillain-Barre-like syndrome, lethargy paresthesia, rhabdomyolysis, seizures, weakness
Respiratory	Acute ventilatory failure
Skeletal	Osteomalacia

Table 16.12 Chyle Properties[54]

Total lipid content	0.4 to 4.0 g/dL
Triglycerides	150–1100 mg/dL
Cholesterol	< 200 mg/dL
Lymphocytes	400–7000 cells × 10⁸ dL
Total protein	> 3 g/dL
pH	Alkaline > 7

jugular ducts may be interrupted and chyle spills into the wound. Upon postoperative feeding, chyle is produced in the gut, drains into the lymph channels, and then can be identified coursing through the surgical drains. This situation if untreated can lead to hypovolemia, electrolyte imbalances, alteration in protein and fat metabolism, and hemodynamic instability.[55] The treatment is a diet very low in long chain triglycerides (LCTs) and with increased protein for wound healing. Surgical repair is usually unnecessary if aggressive nutritional intervention is begun early and continued until drainage stops for 3 to 5 days. TPN can be used as a trial to halt the fat metabolism in the gut.

Hyponatremia may be caused by too much fluid resuscitation during or after the surgical procedure or the use of diuretics. The patient should be evaluated for whole body depletion of sodium to establish a dilution effect. Salt may be added to the tube feeding to increase the sodium intake or by ordering tube-feeding flushes with normal saline. Normal saline is 154 mEq sodium per liter of fluid. In the hospital, unless otherwise specified, the nurse adds the salt to the tube feeding flush. The salt may be provided by diet in the form of packets containing sodium chloride. Preferably obtain NaCl from pharmacy as 1 g NaCl tablets (43 mEq sodium). The nurse needs to crush the tablets.

Upon discharge the orders need to be translated from specific mEq of sodium into household measures such as ½ teaspoon. As an example the patient may add ~¼ tsp salt per day to every two cans of formula. Refer to **Table 16.13** for NaCl equivalents.

Table 16.13 Sodium Equivalents

¼ tsp table salt = 25 mEq sodium = 575 mg sodium = 1.25 g NaCl			
½ tsp table salt = 50 mEq sodium = 1150 mg sodium = 2.5 g NaCl			
1 tsp table salt = 100 mEq sodium = 2300 mg sodium = 6 g NaCl			

Recurrent cancer is a possibility if all methods of nutrition fail, or there are multiple ongoing complications that are not easily resolved. In our experience, this has occurred infrequently but it is a very real possibility when dealing with these very complex and fragile patients.

◆ Care of the Patient

The nursing care of head and neck cancer patients is covered in chapter 15, but interrelated is the role of nursing in nutrition. Nursing care and nutritional support are often the two main reasons the patient remains in the hospital. Accurate documentation of intake and output cannot be overemphasized. Feeding interruption for testing, ambulation, and presurgical fasting wreaks havoc on a consistent program of nutrition. A clearly documented nutritional history tells a story over time, and the accuracy of the history enables the clinicians to have a clearer picture of the patient's progress.

◆ Choice of Methods of Enteral Feeding

The choice of site and type of tube for enteral feeding is dependent on the estimated length of enteral feeding program, physiology of the patient's gastrointestinal tract, and the patient's and physician's choice of therapy (**Table 16.14**). Head and neck cancer patients have many choices available dependent upon the integrity of each patient's gastrointestinal tract. The choices of routes of administration are nasogastric, nasoduodenal or nasojejunal, gastrostomy (open or percutaneous), transgastric jejunostomy, and jejunostomy. There are advantages and disadvantages to all routes and these must be discussed in detail with the patient so an informed choice can be made. If a gastrostomy feeding tube is pulled or pushed through an area in the pharynx that has cancer, the tube may be contaminated with the tumor. Thus, in patients

Table 16.14 Selection of Feeding Tube Site

Access Site	Advantages	Disadvantages
Nasogastric	• Minimally invasive, easy placement • Suitable for short-term use • Transitional to bolus feeding • Radiographic confirmation not necessarily required	• Cosmetic—feeding tube visible unless patient self-inserts feeding tube at each feeding • Risk of sinusitis • Lack of intact gag reflex may (not necessarily) indicate increased aspiration risk • Stomach must be uninvolved with primary disease
Nasoduodenal	• Minimally invasive • Suitable for short-term use • Reduced risk of pulmonary aspiration • Useful in conditions of gastroparesis or impaired stomach emptying • Useful if esophageal reflux present • Allows for feeding when bowel sounds are diminished or absent	• Requires radiographic confirmation of placement • Cosmetic—feeding tube is visible • Requires 43-inch length feeding tube • May not remain placed in duodenum due to tube migration • Typically, smaller diameter tube than NG, more prone to plugging if not properly maintained • Bolus feeding contraindicated • Risk of sinusitis
Nasojejunal	• Same advantages as nasoduodenal • Placement of tip further down GI tract minimizes dislocation to stomach • 60-inch length tubes available offering even greater placement security	• Similar disadvantages as nasoduodenal except placement of tip more secure
Cervical esophagostomy	• Improved cosmetic appeal as insertions site of tube more easily concealed • Ease of feeding over gastrostomy as do not need to undress • More suitable for long-term feeding	• Although more suitable for long-term feeding, the lower esophageal sphincter is stented open and same concerns for gastric and esophageal reflux with possible pulmonary aspiration are present as with the NG feeding tube
Gastrostomy	• Suitable for long-term feeding • Cosmetically more appealing than a nasally place tube • Minimizes risk of tube migration and aspiration due to voluntary or accidental dislocation of nasoenteric tube by patient • Percutaneous placement available (PEG) • Some GT have large bore tubes, which minimizes occlusion from medications and high viscosity formulas • Most suitable of all tubes for use of homemade formula provided tip is placed in stomach and it is a large bore tube • Bolus feeding option available if tip of tube in stomach	• Potential risk of pulmonary aspiration • Lack of intact gag reflex and/or presence of esophageal reflux may indicate increase risk of aspiration • Insertion site care needed • Potential skin excoriation at stoma site from leakage of gastric secretions • Potential fistula at insertion site after GT removal • If GT feeding tip port is place in duodenum, usually a smaller bore tube is used and it is subject to higher occlusion risk
Jejunostomy	• Suitable for long-term feeding • Minimizes risk of aspiration • Positive gag reflex need not be present • Useful if esophageal reflux is present • Does not depend on functioning stomach • Percutaneous placement (PEJ)	• Typically smaller bore tube than a GT and risk of occlusion from medication or viscous formula • Stoma care needed • Potential skin excoriation at stoma site from leakage of gastric secretions • Bolus feeding not an option • Potential fistula at stoma site after JT removal
Tracheal esophageal puncture (TEP) for speech prosthesis	• Feeding tube primary function is to act as a stent for the tracheal esophageal fistula, however, if tube reaches the stomach, it can be used for feeding with same advantages as cervical esphagostomy	• Same as cervical esphagostomy

Abbreviations: GI, gastrointestinal; GT, gastrostomy; NG, nasogastric; PEG, percutaneous endoscopic gastrostomy; PEJ, percutaneous endoscopic jejunostomy.

Source: Data from Gottschlich M; Matarese L,; Shronts E, eds. *Nutrition Support Dietetics Core Curriculum 1993,* 2nd ed., American Society for Parenteral and Enteral Nutrition; 1993.

with head and neck cancer, pull or push procedures have a potential for direct implantation of tumor cells at the enterostomy site and thus may be less desirable because of this risk than other methods of tube insertion.[56]

The appropriate choice of a nasogastric tube includes the type of feeding, comfort, position/placement, and longevity of use. In the immediate postoperative period a Silastic (Dow Corning Corp., Midland, MI) sump tube is indicated because of the flexibility of the tube and sump properties. In the event of a postoperative ileus the sump can function to decompress the stomach. The Silastic properties are beneficial for comfort and decreased tissue damage along the tract of the tube. If traditional nasogastric tubes are in place for over 10 days they become very hard because of the interaction of the tube with the acid in the stomach. For routine enteral feeding the choice of a simple, soft tube size 12 to 14 French is indicated for gastric feeding. If jejunal feeding is indicated then the same criteria stand of simple, soft, and flexible with a length sufficient for true jejunal feeds. Types of feeding tubes are shown in **Figs. 16.6, 16.7, 16.8, 16.9, and 16.10**.

The proper method of nasogastric tube placement is based on the understanding of normal and surgical head and neck anatomy. This basic anatomical understanding holds true for most of surgical nursing care practice. The patient is, if possible, placed in a sitting position, head and chin forward, often called the sniffing position. The use of neosynephrine is very helpful in shrinking the mucus membranes to allow for passage of the tube through the narrow part of the nares. The patient is then locally anesthetized with a viscous topical anesthesia or an anesthetic spray, allowing sufficient time for the anesthesia to take effect. Cotton swabs with anesthesia gel are placed in the nasal vestibule and advanced posteriorly

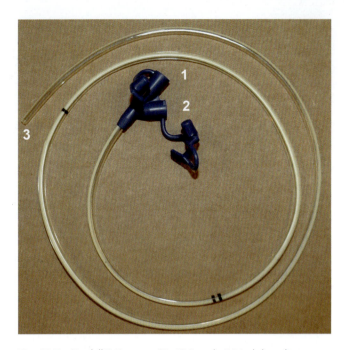

Fig. 16.7 Kendall™ Kangaroo™, 12 French, 36-inch length, unweighted (Tyco/Healthcare). Y-connector with (1) feeding port, (2) irrigation/medication port, (3) open end tip with exit ports in tubing.

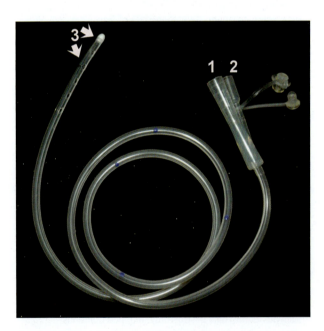

Fig. 16.6 Kendall™ Argyle™ Silicone Salem Sump™ tube, 16 French, 48-inch length (Tyco/Healthcare). Dual lumen, Y-connector with (1) suction drainage lumen/feeding port, (2) suction vent lumen, (3) closed-end tip with multiple exit ports.

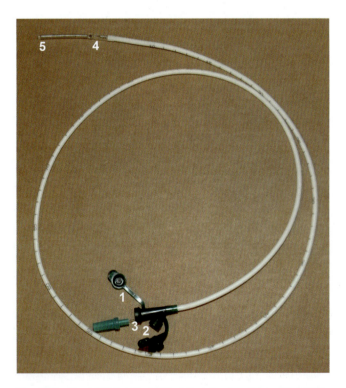

Fig. 16.8 Kendall™ Entriflex™ Dual Port Feeding Tube with FLOW THROUGH™ Stylet, 12 French, 43-inch length (Tyco/Healthcare). Y-connector with (1) feeding port, (2) irrigation/medication port, (3) stylet, (4) exit ports, (5) weighted tip.

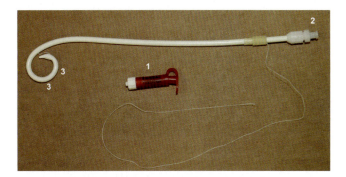

Fig. 16.9 Deutsch Gastrostomy Catheter (Cook Medical, Inc., Bloomington, IN) with AQ Hydrophilic Coating, 16 French, 25 cm long with Cook-Cope-type locking loop. (1) Enteral feeding adapter with male fitting, (2) leur lock tube opening, (3) exit ports.

through the most patent nares. Each swab is left in place and local anesthesia is reapplied as needed to create adequate anesthesia. The nasogastric tube is slowly advanced into the nares along the floor of the nose and then in a downward direction into the nasopharynx and pharynx. An understanding of the anatomy of the nose and upper aerodigestive tract is implicit in appreciating the downward direction the tube must take. Ask the patient to swallow his or her own saliva to advance the tube. Many clinicians advise the use of water to swallow, but in head and neck cancer patients (and many stroke or traumatic brain injury (TBI) patients) this is *not* advisable because of the possibility of aspiration.

Once the level of the epiglottis is reached, the patient may cough because of the stimulation of the supraglottic tissues. Usually after a cough the patient will swallow and the tube is then advanced further into the esophagus. A *slow* and *steady* advancement is advised. If the coughing continues, the tube may be in the supraglottis or larynx. Slowly remove the tube ~2 inches to allow the patient to relax and attempt placement again. Repositioning of the patient in the sniffing position is often necessary before attempting to reinsert the tube.

Measure the length of the tube and estimate the amount to insert leaving a measurable length outside the patient. Both of these lengths should be documented for reference in the event of tube migration. Auscultation of the stomach with insufflation of air into the tube verifies placement of its distal end in the stomach. Double checking placement by aspirating gastric secretions is a secondary and important measure. Usually with larger-bore tubes, auscultation and aspiration provide adequate confirmation. If there is any doubt about placement, radiographic verification is appropriate.[50] Secure the enteral feeding tube to prevent migration by taping the tube to the dorsum of the nose, protecting the skin with a piece of thin skin protector, and paying particular attention to the intranasal position so as not to place torque on the nares. There is no excuse for nasal tip erosion.

If the nurse is patient and proceeds *slowly* with the procedure there will be minimal trauma and the patient is well able to tolerate an uncomfortable procedure.

In early postoperative head and neck cancer patients, if the nasogastric tube inadvertently is removed, it is advised not to replace it without intimate knowledge of the internal surgical suture lines. Perforation of these suture lines with the tip of the tube can lead to fistula formation. This may be one of only a few indications for TPN. Until the fistula can heal an alternate feeding route must be secured.

Gastrostomy is indicated if the patient is unable or unwilling to tolerate the nasogastric tube for a long period of time. This route may be chosen if the patient has recurrent sinusitis because of the obstruction of normal sinus drainage. A feeding gastrostomy can be surgically, endoscopically, or laparoscopically placed. Percutaneous endoscopic gastrostomy (PEG) tubes can also be placed under local anesthesia by interventional radiologists.

◆ Methods of Enteral Feeding

The method of feeding (continuous, bolus, or combination) is dependent on the specific location of the tube in the gastrointestinal tract. The location often determines the rate of feeding that the patient can tolerate.

Bolus feeds can be delivered by gravity drip or by pump into the stomach. Continuous feedings can also be delivered by gravity or pump, but pump is preferred because of the required slow rates of feeding. Continuous feeding is usually into the jejunum but may be done into the stomach until transition to bolus is achieved.

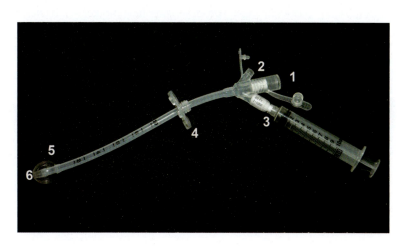

Fig. 16.10 Kimberly-Clark™ MIC™ gastrostomy feeding tube, 20 French, 7 to 10 mL balloon (Kimberly-Clark/Ballard Medical Products, Roswell, GA). (1) Feeding port, (2) irrigation/medication port, (3) balloon valve port, (4) external retention disc, (5) balloon, (6) open-tip exit port.

The interaction of drugs and tube feedings is an ongoing discussion by the nutrition experts. An example of this is the requirement to stop enteral feedings for 1 hour before and 1 hour after the administration of phenytoin (Dilantin).[57]

Feeding sources must be identified and queried as to their coverage of enteral feeds. Some insurance will not pay for feeding because food is a common need to all, not just patients. Therefore home enteral nutrition must be secured before discharge. Medicare will only pay for enteral nutrition if it is ongoing for greater than 90 days and so documented.

Local products or generic brands of enteral feeding can be used as well as Instant Breakfast–type drinks (Carnation Instant Breakfast Essentials; Nestlé S.A., Switzerland). A dietitian should be involved in making decisions regarding tube feeding product type; protein, carbohydrate, and calorie levels; and tube feeding regimens.

Often home regimens can mimic breakfast, lunch, and dinner. So, as an example a feeding regimen could be two cans of feeding by slow bolus three times a day with one can in the evening. This simulates normal feeding patterns and allows the patient free time from feeding. Patients, because of issues related to reflux, may require jejunal tube feeding. This almost always mandates a continuous feeding regimen, and portable backpack pumps offer much needed mobility. Maintenance of a feeding schedule is essential to the patient attaining nutritional goals. Once patients have mastered the process of tube feeding and nutritional maintenance is tolerated, the strict reg-

imens can often be liberalized to life patterns. Patients can be instructed to take the prescribed number of cans at their own rate and volume. A slow bolus is often the secret to tolerance.

The discharge from the hospital of a patient with head and neck cancer is a complex multidisciplinary task. The discharge process should begin early on, preferably before surgery, in the outpatient clinic.

At discharge, a kit for enteral feeding should be given to the patient and family to ensure adequate supplies and feeds until home health and support companies can begin intervention in the home. Continued nutritional evaluation in the home setting is just as important as in the hospital.

◆ Conclusion

When disease affects the aerodigestive tract, impairment of the nutritional state must be considered. The involvement of a multidisciplinary team allows the patient to benefit from the expertise of each member. Nutrition is a very specialized field. Food is not only a mixture of chemicals, it is a symbol of cultural identity, love, connectedness, and holidays. Recognition of food's involvement in providing the substrates for life, for maintenance, and for healing of the organism requires a balance. With the recognition of the science of nutrition and the balance of care for the patient we are better able to attend to the needs of the individual.

◆ Appendix 16.1

NAME: UNIVERSITY OF CALIFORNIA MEDICAL CENTER

MR#:   SACRAMENTO

DOB: **OPD PROGRESS RECORDS**

OTOLARYNGOLOGY CLINIC – Clinical Dietetics   DATE: _____

□ Tumor Board Visit: _____

□ Clinic Visit. Reason for referral: _____

Age: _____   Ht: _____   UBW: _____   IBW: _____   Wt Change (+) (–): _____

Wt: _____   %UBW: _____   %IBW: _____   % Δ: _____   Over Length of Time? _____

DIET: □ Oral _____ □ Tube Feeding   □ NG   □ GT Formula: _____

□ Dysphagia   □ Odynophagia   Do either alter food intake? (YES) (NO)

(YES) (NO) Has physician been informed of pain affecting nutrition intake? Action: _____

Supplements: (Home): Vitamin / Minerals? (YES) (NO) _____ Vitamin E?   (YES) (NO) _____

Herbal / Alternative Supplements? (YES) (NO) _____

Tolerance to Milk? (YES) (NO)

Barriers to Learning:

     □ None   □ Anxiety / Stress   □ Unable to Write

     □ Language   □ Culture / Religion   □ Unable to Read

     □ Vision Loss   □ Pain / Fatigue / Weakness   □ Other _____

     □ Hearing Loss   □ Unable to Speak

Comprehension:

    ☐ Verbalizes / Indicates understanding

    ☐ Identifies appropriate foods to choose / avoid

    ☐ Unable to comprehend

    ☐ Person with patient indicates understanding

Written Information Given:

    ☐ High Calorie Eating   ☐ Tube Feeding Guide

    ☐ Food Pyramid   ☐ Your Guide to Home Tube Feeding

Nutrition Goals if pertinent: _____Calories/d; _____ grams Protein/d; _____ cc/day for Maintenance Fluid

Assessment / Plan:

_____

RD Signature

◆ Appendix 16.2 Ideas for Increasing Food Intake

What Can You Do?

1. If you have *pain* when eating, be sure to *tell your doctor*. There may be medications to help with the pain. If you are in less pain, you will likely eat more.

2. If solids are hard to chew or swallow, make liquids *nutritionally complete. How?* If you tolerate milk, add Instant Breakfast to milk, two or three times a day. Further increase calories in your Instant Breakfast beverage by adding ice cream to make a milkshake. In about the same volume you have in 1 glass of milk, you now have ¼ of your vitamins and minerals for the day and double or triple the calories. Commercial liquid supplements (Ensure Plus [Abbott Nutrition, Columbus, OH], Boost Plus [Nestlé S.A.]) are useful if you do not tolerate milk, but check out the generic brands for cost savings. Think about using Lactaid milk (McNeil Nutritionals LLC, Ft. Washington, PA) with Instant Breakfast if you do not tolerate milk.

Foods you used to eat can easily be put in a food processor or blender—let the machine do your chewing! Add broth, gravy, or other liquids that complement the food to add moisture while blending or processing.

3. Soups are a favorite. Choose higher calorie soups such as split pea, lentil, or cream of tomato made with milk. Add powdered milk to further increase protein. Start by adding 2 to 3 tablespoons and increase according to taste. Broth-based soups can fill you up by their volume but are not nutritional powerhouses.

4. Foods traditionally eaten at breakfast can be eaten at other times of the day. Eggs can be prepared in different ways to give variety. Eggs are easy to chew and an excellent choice for protein. Now may not be the time to be watching your cholesterol intake.

5. Eat more frequently. Food is a medicine. You should eat even if your appetite has changed.

6. Take a multivitamin with minerals pill. Check the label for one that has zinc. If it is hard for you to swallow a pill, try a children's *chewable* vitamin. They taste *better* than adult vitamin pills. If it is hard for you to chew, the chewable vitamins can be crushed and put in applesauce or pudding. If you choose a liquid vitamin, be sure it includes minerals.

◆ High Calorie, High Protein Recipes

Milkshakes can be an easy way to increase your calorie and/or your protein intake. Many recipes can become a meal replacement or a meal addition if you are limited with the solid foods you can eat. If you want to gain weight, add shakes to what you are currently eating. Create your own shakes or try some of these recipes to help increase your calorie intake.

General Shake Recipe

Ingredients:

Base: ½ to 1 cup of any of the following: whole milk, 2% milk, fortified milk*, extra-rich milk, half-and-half, evaporated milk, condensed milk, non-dairy creamer, lactose-reduced milk, or fortified soy milk

Additions: ½ to 1 cup of any of the following: ice cream, sherbet, fruit, fruit juice
¼ cup Instant Breakfast or Slim-Fast powder (Unilever USA Inc., Englewood, NJ)
¼ cup nonfat dry milk
¼ cup egg substitute
1–2 tablespoons of fruit juice concentrate

Flavorings: To taste: vanilla or other essence, honey, sugar, cinnamon, nutmeg, powdered soft drink mix, chocolate or strawberry syrup, instant pudding mix, powdered milk, cocoa mix, peanut butter, instant coffee granules, or rum food flavoring

Garnish: As desired: maraschino cherry, sprig of mint, whipping cream, or nutmeg

Place all ingredients in blender and blend well. Pour into glass. Use your favorite garnish. Experiment with your favorite ingredients and keep a record of the recipes you enjoy!

*Fortified Milk
(Makes ~4 cups)
(220 calories, 15 g protein <u>per cup</u>)
4 cups whole milk
1 cup nonfat dry milk powder

Beverages Using Instant Breakfast

Hawaiian Float
(400 calories, 16 g protein)
2 tablespoons orange-pineapple juice concentrate (undiluted)
1 package or ¼ cup vanilla Instant Breakfast
or Slim-Fast powder
½ cup ice
½ cup evaporated whole milk
¼ cup lime sherbet

Milkshakes

Milk is used for the base of these recipes.

Any type of milk can be used, but try to use whole milk, evaporated milk, or extra-rich milk for extra calories.

2% milk can be used if you need to increase your protein.

Nonfat dry milk can be also be added to increase the protein as in fortified milk.

Orange Vanilla Drink
(325 calories, 15 g protein)
½ cup orange juice
½ cup whole or 2% milk
½ cup vanilla ice cream
¼ cup liquid egg substitute
1 teaspoon vanilla extract

Peanut Butter Drink
(625 calories, 19 g protein)
½ cup whole or 2% milk
3 tablespoons smooth peanut butter
3 tablespoons chocolate syrup
½ cup vanilla ice cream

Orange Cooler
(465 calories, 22 g protein)
⅓ cup orange juice concentrate
¾ cup nonfat powdered milk
1 cup ice water
½ cup vanilla ice cream

Pineapple Soda
(315 calories, 7 g protein)
¼ cup crushed pineapple
½ cup whole or 2% milk
½ cup vanilla ice cream
½ cup pear nectar

Instant Breakfast Nog
(425 to 565 calories, 25 g protein)
1 cup half-and-half or whole or 2% milk
½ cup ice cream (any flavor)
1 package or ¼ cup Instant Breakfast or Slim-Fast powder
¼ cup liquid egg substitute

Peach Shake
(205 calories, 10 g protein)
1 canned peach half
3 tablespoons dry milk powder
⅓ cup ice water
1 package or ¼ cup vanilla Instant Breakfast or Slim-Fast powder
¼ cup vanilla ice cream

Place all ingredients in blender and mix well.

Eggnog
(315 calories, 15 g protein)
½ cup half-and-half
½ cup whole or 2% milk
¼ cup liquid egg substitute
Sugar, vanilla and nutmeg to taste

Place all ingredients in blender and blend well. Pour into glass.
Use your favorite garnish: maraschino cherry, sprig of mint, whipping cream or lemon, lime, or orange wedges.

*Fortified Milk
(Makes ~4 cups)
(220 calories, 15 g protein per cup)
4 cups whole milk
1 cup nonfat dry milk powder

Yogurt Smoothies

Banana Berry Shake
(325 calories, 11 g protein)
½ cup boysenberry or blueberry yogurt
½ cup raspberry sherbet
⅓ cup cranberry juice
¼ cup liquid egg substitute

Lemony Pear Shake
(415 calories, 11 g protein)
½ cup pear nectar
½ cup lemon yogurt
½ cup lemon sherbet
½ cup chopped pear
¼ cup liquid egg substitute

Fruit and Tofu Smoothie
(380 calories, 18 g protein)
½ cup soft tofu, drained
1 cup flavored yogurt
½ cup canned fruit
1–2 ice cubes

Banana Yogurt Shake
(240 calories, 11 g protein)
½ cup whole or 2% milk
½ cup plain yogurt
1 ripe banana

Peachy Orange Shake
(330 calories, 12 g protein)
½ cup peach nectar
½ cup peach yogurt
½ cup orange sherbet
½ cup peach or apricot, sliced
¼ cup liquid egg substitute

Pineapple Smoothie
(215 calories, 12 g protein)
¼ cup crushed pineapple w/ juice
½ cup vanilla yogurt
½ cup whole or 2% milk
1 teaspoon lemon juice

Raspberry/Rice Smoothie
(550–700 calories, 10 g protein)
½ cup cooked brown rice
1 ripe banana
1 cup frozen raspberries (in syrup)
1 cup plain or flavored yogurt
1–2 teaspoons honey

Place all ingredients in blender and blend well. Pour into glass.
Use your favorite garnish: maraschino cherry, sprig of mint, whipping cream or lemon, lime, or orange wedges.

Sherbet Shakes

These shakes use sherbet as the base. They are high in calories, but low in protein.
To increase the protein content, add ¼ cup nonfat dry milk to these recipes.

Apricot Raspberry Shake
(225 calories, 2 g protein)
½ cup apricot nectar
4 apricot halves, chopped
½ cup raspberry sherbet

Orange Shake
(285 calories, 4 g protein)
½ cup orange juice
½ cup mandarin orange sections, drained
½ cup orange sherbet

Banana Grape Shake
(275 calories, 4 g protein)
⅓ cup grape juice
⅓ cup whole or 2% milk
½ banana
½ cup lemon sherbet

Pineapple Berry Freeze
(315 calories, 5 g protein)
1/3 cup whole or 2% milk
½ cup fresh or canned (drained) pineapple
¾ cup raspberry sherbet

Banana Orange Shake
(230 calories, 2 g protein)
½ cup orange juice
½ cup orange sherbet
½ banana

Pineapple Lemon Shake
(240 calories, 2 g protein)
½ cup pineapple juice
½ cup lemon sherbet
2 pineapple slices, chopped, drained

Berry Freeze
(295 calories, 5 g protein)
⅓ cup whole or 2% milk
¾ cup raspberry sherbet
6 to 8 fresh or frozen strawberries
¾ cup lemon sherbet

Banana Raspberry Shake
(255 calories, 2 g protein)
½ cup cranberry juice
½ cup raspberry sherbet
½ banana

**Cranberry Lemon Shake
(200 calories, 2 g protein)**
½ cup cranberry juice
½ cup lemon sherbet
½ banana

**Strawberry Banana Shake
(365 calories, 7 g protein)**
½ cup whole or 2% milk
½ banana
6 fresh or frozen strawberries

**Citrus Sipper
(265 calories, 2 g protein)**
¼ cup grapefruit juice
¼ cup pineapple juice
½ cup orange juice
½ tablespoon sugar
½ cup lime sherbet

Place all ingredients in blender and blend well. Pour into glass.
Use your favorite garnish: maraschino cherry, sprig of mint, whipping cream or lemon, lime or orange wedges.

References

1. Butterworth CE. The skeleton in the hospital closet. Nutr Today 1974; 9:4–8

2. Himes D. Protein-calorie malnutrition and involuntary weight loss: the role of aggressive nutritional intervention in wound healing. Ostomy Wound Manage 1999;45:46–55

3. van Bokhorst-de Van der Schuer MA, Langendoen SI, Vondeling H, Kuik DJ, Quak JJ, Van Leeuwen PA. Perioperative enteral nutrition and quality of life of severely malnourished head and neck cancer patients: a randomized clinical trial. Clin Nutr 2000;19:437–444

4. van Bokhorst-de Van der Schuer MA, van Leeuwen PA, Sauerwein HP, Kuik DJ, Snow GB, Quak JJ. Assessment of malnutrition parameters in head and neck cancer and their relation to postoperative complications. Head Neck 1997;19:419–425

5. Riso S, Aluffi P, Brugnani M, Farinette F, Pia F, D'Andrea F. Postoperative enteral immunonutrition in head and neck cancer patients. Clin Nutr 2000;19:407–412

6. Kerrebijn JD, Simons PJ, Tas M, et al. The effects of thymostimulin on immunological function in patients with head and neck cancer. Clin Otolaryngol Allied Sci 1996;21:455–462

7. Lichtenstein A, Zighelboim J, Dorey F, Brossman S, Fahey JL. Comparison of immune derangement's in patients with different malignancies. Cancer 1980;45:2090–2095

8. Krause M, Mahan K. Food, Nutrition and Diet Therapy. 10th ed. Philadelphia: WB Saunders; 2000:353

9. Olin AO, Osterberg P, Hadell K, Armyr I, Jerstrom S, Lungqvist O. Energy-enriched hospital food to improve energy intake in elderly patients. JPEN J Parenter Enteral Nutr 1996;20:93–97

10. Carnevali P. Nursing management for the elderly. In: Karkeck J, Worthington-Roberts B, eds. Nutrition. Philadelphia: JB Lippincott; 1993: 3–21

11. Musto DF. Alcohol in American history. Sci Am 1996;274:78–83

12. Kayser-Jones J. Starved for attention. Reflect Nurs Leadersh 2001;27:10–14

13. Saltzman E, Shah A, Shikora SA. Obesity. In: Gottschlich MM, Furhman MP, Hammond KA, Holcomb BJ, Saidner DL, eds. The Science and Practice of Nutrition Support: A Case-Based Core Curriculum. Dubuque, IA: Kendall/Hunt; 2001:677–682.

14. Dreizen S, Daly TE, Drane JB, et al. Oral complications of cancer radiotherapy. Postgrad Med 1977;61:85–92

15. Nayel H, El-Ghoneimy F, El-Haddad S. Impact of nutritional supplementation on treatment delay and morbidity in patients with head and neck tumors treated with irradiation. Nutrition 1992;8:13–18

16. Harris JG. Nausea, vomiting and cancer treatment. CA Cancer J Clin 1978;28:194–201

17. Holroyde CP, Reichard GA Jr. General metabolic abnormalities in cancer patients: anorexia and cachexia. Surg Clin North Am 1986;66:947–956

18. Gilmore SA, Robinson G, Posthaure ME, Raymond J. Clinical indicators associated with unintentional weight loss and pressure ulcers in elderly residents of nursing homes. J Am Diet Assoc 1995;95:984–992

19. Joint Commission on Accreditation of Health Care Organizations. Accreditation Manual for Hospitals, Standards Vol 1. Oakbrook Terrace, IL: Joint Commission on Accreditation of Health Care Organizations; 1995

20. Mears E. Prealbumin and nutrition. In: Dietetic Currents. Columbus, OH: Ross Products Division, Abbott Laboratories; 1994:1–4

21. Krause M, Mahan K. Food, Nutrition and Diet Therapy. 10th ed. Philadelphia: WB Saunders; 2000:353,867–876

22. Lorens B. Nutritional concerns and assessment. In: Leonard R, Kendall K, eds. Dysphagia Assessment and Treatment Planning, A Team Approach. San Diego: Plural Publishing Group; 2008

23. Blackburn GL, Bistrian BR, Maini BS, et al. Nutritional and metabolic assessment of the hospitalized patient. JPEN J Parenter Enteral Nutr 1977;1:11–22

24. Shopbell JM, Hopkins B, Shronts EP. Nutritional screening and assessment. In: Gottschlich MM, Furhman MP, Hammond KA, Holcomb BJ, Seidner DL, eds. The Science and Practice of Nutrition Support: A Case-Based Core Curriculum. Dubuque, IA: Kendall/Hunt; 2001:118–119

25. Morgan DB, Hill GL, Burkinshaw L. The assessment of weight loss from a single measurement of body weight: the problems and limitations. Am J Clin Nutr 1980;33:2101–2105

26. Rombeau JL, Caldwell MD, Forlaw L, Guenter PA, eds. Atlas of Nutritional Support Techniques. Boston: Little, Brown; 1989

27. Sievers A. Nursing evaluation and care of the dysphagic patient. In: Leonard R, Kendall K, eds. Dysphagia Assessment and Treatment Planning, A Team Approach. San Diego: Plural Publishing Group; 2008

28. Bridges KJ, Trujillo E, Jacobs D. Alcohol related thiamine deficiency and malnutrition. Crit Care Nurse 1999;19:80–85

29. Measurement of visceral protein status in assessing protein and energy malnutrition: standard of care, Prealbumin in Nutritional Care Consensus Group. Nutrition 1995;11:169–171

30. Kendall KA, McKenzie S, Leonard RJ. Structural mobility in deglutition after single modality treatment of head and neck carcinomas with radiotherapy. Head Neck 1998;20:720–725

31. Hamlet S, Genney D, Formolo J. Stethoscope acoustics and cervical auscultation of swallowing. Dysphagia 1994;9:63–68

32. Sievers A, Leonard R, McKenzie S. The safe use of an adaptive early feeding device for impaired patients. ORL Head Neck Nurs 1992;10:3–17

33. Theologides A. Anorexia producing intermediary metabolites. Am J Clin Nutr 1976;29:552–558

34. Doerr TD, Marks SC, Shamsa FH, Mathog RH, Prasad AS. Effects of zinc and nutritional status on clinical outcomes in head and neck cancer. Nutrition 1998;14:489–495

35. Dudrick SJ, Ruberg RL. Principles and practice of parenteral nutrition. Gastroenterology 1971;61:901–910

36. Bockus S. Troubleshooting your tube feedings. Am J Nurs 1991;91:24–28

37. Cutie AJ, Altman E, Lenkel L. Compatibility enteral products with commonly employed drug additives. JPEN J Parenter Enteral Nutr 1983; 7:186–191

38. Kohn-Keeth C. How to keep feeding tubes flowing freely. Nursing 2000; 30:58–59

39. Edes TE, Walk BE, Austin J. Diarrhea in tube-fed patients: feeding formula not necessarily the cause. Am J Med 1990;88:91–93

40. Heimburger DC. Diarrhea with enteral feeding: will the real cause please stand up? Am J Med 1990;88:89–90

41. Belafsky PC, Postma GN, Amin MR, Koufman JA. Symptoms and findings of laryngopharyngeal reflux. Ear Nose Throat J 2002;89:10–13

42. Coben RM, Weintraub A, DiMarino AJ Jr, Cohen S. Gastroesophageal reflux during gastrostomy feeding. Gastroenterology 1994;106:13–14

43. Ibáñez J, Peñafiel A, Raurich JM, Marse P, Jordá R, Mata F. Gastroesophageal reflux in intubated patients receiving enteral nutrition: effect of supine and semi-recumbent positions. JPEN J Parenter Enteral Nutr 1992;16:419–422

44. Coben RM, Weintraub A, DiMarion AJ, Cohen SJ. Gastroesophageal reflux during gastrostomy feeding. Gastroenterology 1994;106:13–14

45. Heyland DK, Drover JW, MacDonald S, Novak F, Lam M. Postpyloric feeding reduces gastroesophageal regurgitation in critically ill patients. Crit Care Med 2001;29:1495–1501

46. Maloney JP, Halbower AC, Fouty BF, et al. Systemic absorption of food dye in patients with sepsis. N Engl J Med 2000;343:1047–1048

47. Metheny NA, Clouse RE. Bedside method of detecting aspiration in tube-fed patients. Chest 1997;111:724–731

48. Metheny NA, St John RE, Clause RE. Measurement of glucose in tracheobronchial secretions to detect aspiration of enteral feedings. Heart Lung 1998;27:285–292

49. Metheny NA, Aud MA, Wenderlich RJ. A survey of bedside methods used to detect pulmonary aspiration of enteral formulas in intubated tube-fed patients. Am J Crit Care 1999;8:160–167

50. Metheny NA. Risk factors for aspiration. JPEN J Parenter Enteral Nutr 2002;26:S26–S33

51. Freedland CP, Roller RD, Wolfe BM, Flynn NM. Microbial contamination of continuous drip feedings. JPEN J Parenter Enteral Nutr 1989;13:18–22

52. Solomon SM, Kirby D. The refeeding syndrome: a review. JPEN J Parenter Enteral Nutr 1990;14:90–97

53. Pagana KD. Preventing complications in jejunostomy tube feedings. Dimens Crit Care Nurs 1987;6:28–38

54. Spain DA, McClave SA. Chylothorax and chylous ascites. In: Gottschlich MM, Furhman MP, Hammond KA, Holcomb BJ, Seidner DL, eds. The Science and Practice of Nutrition Support: A Case-Based Core Curriculum. Dubuque, IA: Kendall/Hunt; 2001:479–490

55. McCray S, Parrish CR. When chyle leaks: nutrition management options. Pract Gastroenterol 2004;17:60–74

56. Sinclair JJ, Scolapio JS, Star ME, Hinder RA. Metastasis of head and neck carcinoma to the site of percutaneous endoscopic gastrostomy: case report and literature review. JPEN J Parenter Enteral Nutr 2001;25:282–285

57. Copeland EM III, Daly JM, Dudrick SJ. Nutritional concepts in the treatment of head and neck malignancies. Head Neck Surg 1979;1:350–365

17

Ablative Procedures of the Head and Neck: Implications for Speech, Voice, and Swallowing

Rebecca J. Leonard

Ablative procedures of the head and neck can affect speech and swallowing in profound ways. Alterations of oral or oropharyngeal structures may impair a speaker's ability to shape the vocal tract in the complex ways required for the articulation of speech sounds, or to manipulate airflows and air pressures in accordance with normal speech requirements. The ability to manipulate foods and liquids in a manner that leads to effective swallowing may also be impaired. Lesions that require laryngeal ablation alter phonation, which is a feature of all speech sounds that require vibration of the vocal folds [i.e., vowels and voiced consonants (b, m, w, v, th, z, zh, j, n, d, g]. If the entire larynx is removed, alternative voicing sources must be considered. But even less extensive resections that affect the true vocal folds are likely to produce deleterious changes in the quality of the voice, as well the speaker's ability to manipulate its pitch and loudness characteristics. If laryngeal structures are unable to protect the airway, or if the usual sensory signals that alert us to foods or liquids in the airway are missing or absent, swallowing may become unsafe.

In short, any one, or all, of these problems represent significant liabilities to a patient who has survived disease and hopes to resume the most normal lifestyle possible. Alterations in such basic functions as eating, breathing, and speaking, as well as changes in cosmesis, may present an emotional challenge that rivals the seriousness of the patient's physical well-being. This chapter reviews our current understanding of the liabilities to speech and swallowing posed by ablative procedures of the head and neck, considers differential effects on speech and swallowing of treatment modalities and reconstruction strategies, and summarizes current speech and swallowing therapeutic approaches to the rehabilitation of patients who have these functional deficits.

◆ Classification of Head and Neck Cancer

For epidemiological purposes, head and neck cancer may be described by general location, as of the lip, tongue, mouth, pharynx, or larynx. Further specification in the medical/surgical literature may localize cancers to the tonsil, soft palate, floor of mouth, various parts of the tongue (base, tip, lateral), mandible, maxilla, pharynx, and other structures. Cancers may also be classified according to a staging system proposed by the American Academy of Otolaryngology–Head and Neck Surgery[1] and based on both the site and the extent of a lesion. In this schema, for example, an oral cavity lesion no greater than 2 cm in diameter is designated T1; a T4 classification would denote a tumor larger than 4 cm in diameter with deep invasion of other structures. In the oropharynx, a T1 classification would again describe a lesion less than 2 cm in diameter, whereas a T4 lesion would be larger than 4 cm, with possible invasion of bone, soft tissues of the neck, or deep muscles of the tongue root.

Tumor staging is a part of the physician's pretreatment diagnostic evaluation of a patient. A more definitive classification may emerge as treatment is actually undertaken. Regardless of the descriptive scheme utilized, it is important to recognize that treatment of a cancer described as originating in the tongue, floor of mouth, tonsil, larynx, or any single structure may actually involve ablation of parts of surrounding tissues. A careful review of treatment records, comprehensive clinical examination, and consultation with physicians involved in the patient's care may all be required to understand the extent of a patient's deficit, the specific type and intent of reconstructive procedure utilized, and the functional status of remaining tissues.

◆ Effects of Head and Neck Resection

Implications of Oral/Oropharyngeal Resection for Speech

All structures making up the oral cavity, oropharynx, and hypopharynx, collectively, the upper airway, contribute to speech. However, the relative importance of these structures to speech is not equivalent. Ablative procedures that involve the tongue are most likely to have serious implications for speech, and the consequences of glossectomy are emphasized in this section. Of the remaining structures, the lips, mandible, and palate should be noted. During speech, the lips may assume a particular shape, for example, rounded or spread as in the words *who'd* or *heed*, respectively. In other cases, the lips contribute to generating or articulating the speech sound, as in /p, b, m, f, v/. If the integrity of the lips is sufficiently interrupted, words requiring labialization may be distorted or difficult to understand.

Mandibular movements during speech typically encompass less than a centimeter.[2] Thus mandibular excisions that permit some motion of the mandible at normal velocities may not interfere significantly with speech intelligibility. A more serious consequence for speech is presented by disruption of the structural continuity of the mandible, particularly if the disruption is complete and involves the middle portion of the mandibular body or extends across the midline symphysis.[3,4]

Surgical excision of the palate presents perhaps the greatest ablative deterrent to normal speech in the immediate posttreatment period. Effective separation of oral and nasal cavities during speech is critical to the production of all sounds except the nasals /m, n/ and /ng/. If this separation is not maintained, as when some portion of the soft palate is resected, the vocal tract becomes larger, and its natural resonances change. Speech sounds are affected differentially, with those requiring the greatest amounts of intraoral pressure and flow (fricatives, e.g., /s, sh/; plosives, e.g., /p, t, k/; and affricates, e.g., /ch, j/) being most vulnerable to the effects of nasalization. With larger lesions, extending from the palate into other portions of the maxilla and perhaps involving sinuses, the speaker may labor to effect appropriate airflows and pressures for speech. Changes in articulation, timing, and phrasing characteristics are likely sequelae. Fortunately, current capabilities for restoration of palatal function via surgical or prosthetic approaches significantly reduce the residual impairment.[5–8]

As noted, resections that affect the tongue are likely to have the most profound effects on speech. Early studies of the consequences of glossectomy for speech described unusual placements for lingual consonants, altered grooving patterns for lingual fricatives, alterations in burst characteristics of stop consonants, difficulties in effecting vowel transitions, and aberrant vowel formants.[9–19]

Other investigators have attempted to relate extent of glossal resection to degree of speech impairment. Heller et al reported that patients with tongue lesions less than 3 cm in size experienced mild distortions of speech initially but were typically perceived as having normal speech within 6 months of surgery.[20] Similarly, Pruszewicz and Kruk-Zagajewsky reported good intelligibility postoperatively in patients undergoing resection of T1 (less than 2 cm) and T2 (2 cm to 4 cm) tumors.[21] Recently, Colangelo et al described significant differences in speech understandability depending on clinical T stage for patients with oral or oropharyngeal resections, respectively.[22] Differences at 3 months posthealing were noted between stages T1-T2 and T3 (> 4 cm) and T4 (invades other structures), respectively, for patients with oral resections. In all cases, a larger T-staging was associated with greater impairment. Severe problems associated with lesions greater then 3 to 4 cm have been substantiated by other authors, as well.[23–25]

Our own studies indicate that degree of impairment is not a simple function of extent of resection.[26] For example, impairment in subtotal glossectomy speakers was found to be greater than that in total glossectomees, possibly because the subtotal resections included structures in addition to the tongue (i.e., palate, pharynx, mandible). Patients with total glossectomy had more than two thirds of the tongue removed, but other structures remained essentially intact. We also found that anterior resections produced highly variable impairment depending on whether ventral or dorsal tongue was involved, and on whether an accompanying mandibulectomy crossed the midline symphysis. Other authors have speculated regarding the relative effects of *extent* versus *mobility* of residual tongue tissue as predictors of speech, with mobility generally regarded as the more critical variable.[27–32]

The relationship between speech impairment and type of reconstruction has been increasingly considered as surgical reconstructive techniques have broadened. These now include primary closure, secondary granulation, tongue flaps, local or regional flaps, pedicle flaps, myocutaneous flaps, and free flaps. McConnel et al reported that patients with T2 and T3 lesions (greater than 2 cm in size, no deep tissue invasion) reconstructed with split-thickness skin grafts had better oral function than patients with myocutaneous or hemitongue flaps, respectively.[33] In a subsequent study of patients with small anterior or base of tongue resections, McConnel et al reported that primary closures of defects produced equal or better speech function than flap reconstructions.[34]

Pauloski et al used correlational analyses to determine relationships between speech outcome measures and 14 treatment variables in patients with varying types of glossectomy.[35] Percent of oral tongue resected was more predictive of speech outcome in patients who underwent reconstruction with pedicled or free flaps, which are typically used for larger defects. Patients with primary closures or split-thickness skin graft reconstructions were less affected by percent of oral tongue resected. These findings received support from the McConnel et al study in which patients with primary closures for glossal defects were found to have better conversational intelligibility than patients who underwent reconstruction with distal flaps.[34] No differences in speech were found for reconstructions with distal myocutaneous flaps versus microvascular free flaps. Though these studies provide insights into the differential effects of reconstruction, the issue is likely to remain unclear until factors of lesion site and extent of resection are controlled for in research designs, for example, by using different reconstructive options in patients with very similar resections and treatment histories.

Effects of Radiation

The effects of radiation therapy on oral/oropharyngeal structures have not been extensively described. Mirza and Dikshit reported short-term effects of radiation on oral tissues as including mucositis and mucosal soreness, and lost or diminished sensations of taste or smell.[36] Among the long-term effects noted by these authors were dryness of the mouth due to destruction of salivary glands, reduced blood supply to tissues, and increased connective tissue fibrosis. Certainly, our clinical impression has been that radiation exacerbates impairment already produced by surgical resection. However, Pauloski et al reported on nine patient pairs matched for extent and location of oral/oropharyngeal resection, half who underwent postsurgical radiation and half who underwent surgery only.[37] No differences in speech were found between the two groups at posttreatment intervals up to 12 months. Hamlet et al described similar results in a group of five patients who were assessed postsurgically, and again following radiation.[38]

Speech Rehabilitation

Perspective on the dilemma of the glossectomized speaker can be gained from Stevens's description of the "quantal" nature of speech.[39] According to Stevens, there are areas of the vocal tract where even very small articulatory changes, that is, small movements of structures, produce significant acoustic (and thus perceptual) changes. Conversely, there are other regions of the tract in which even large articulatory alterations are of little acoustic consequence. In terms of the speaker with glossectomy, at least three possibilities for "dequantization" exist. The first is that residual tongue movements are relatively discrete and wide ranging, but do not take place in acoustically sensitive areas of the tract. For example, tongue movements that extend over a considerable range but cannot come within at least a centimeter of a critical location, such as anterior or posterior sites along the palate, may be ineffective in producing acoustic differentiations appropriate for some vowels or consonants.[40] Residual tongue that is mobile but relatively small might be representative of this type of deficit.

A second possibility is that residual tongue is present in acoustically sensitive areas but is not capable of making small, very precise adjustments within an area to produce a broad range of acoustic outcomes—as, for example, the small differences between "heat" and "hit," or "suit" and "soot." In the worst case, there is not sufficient tongue, or tongue function, in any area, to allow for shape changes of the vocal tract. Interestingly, each of these conditions would seem to represent different problems for rehabilitation. Approaches to therapy, whether behavioral, prosthetic, or reconstructive, might usefully consider the likely sequelae of an individual resection from this "quantal" perspective, and direct therapy objectives accordingly.

Assessment

Patients recovering from ablative procedures undergo changes in tissues and functional status for many weeks following initial resection, so that assessment is perhaps best viewed as a process that takes place continually throughout healing and rehabilitation. With medical/surgical therapies completed, more comprehensive assessments of phonological integrity directed toward speech rehabilitation can be considered. Meaningful assessment of these capabilities may require special considerations and unconventional approaches.

One of the particular challenges of assessment stems from the possibility that the redundancy, or multiplicity, of perceptual cues typically present in conversational speech may be missing, ambiguous, or confusing in the speaker with glossectomy who demonstrates multiple articulation errors. That is, when large numbers of phonetic segments are affected by ablation, it becomes difficult to determine to what extent perception of an individual sound as inaccurate is related to inappropriate features of the sound itself or to its embedding in a context of other sounds that are inaccurately produced. This characteristic of impairment is perhaps more prevalent in this patient population than in other groups of disordered speakers, and, as noted, must be given serious consideration when selecting assessment and treatment strategies.

Conventional *articulation tests* that sample speech in words or sentences may be useful in identifying sounds in error. If impairment is severe, however, it may be necessary to sample sound productions in highly structured, uniform contexts, that is, in environments which minimize the possibility that a particular sound will be judged as in error because it is surrounded by other sounds that are defective. Further, because both vowel and consonant errors are a likely consequence of ablation, both must be carefully sampled. Sets of single-word utterances that vary by only one phonetic segment, vowel or consonant (i.e., *heed, hid, head, had, hod, hood, who'd*) may be particularly useful for the error identification task.

Other measures that should be considered are the speaker's overall level of *intelligibility,* and/or the *severity* of the disorder. Such measures provide an indication of degree of impairment, or disability, as it relates to speech. Standardized tests that require listeners to make judgments about a speaker's productions of single word utterances can be used for intelligibility testing. Rating scales, as from 1 to 7 in which 1 represents normal and 7, most impaired or abnormal, are frequently used for severity estimates. Patients' own appraisal of their *communicative effectiveness*, in different situations, in noise, with various types of listeners, and with and without repetition, may also be useful. In whatever combinations, intelligibility and/or severity measures are particularly valuable in allowing the clinician, other professionals involved in the patient's care, and the speaker-patient to stay apprised of speech function and communicative effectiveness across treatment and posttreatment stages.

When oral/oropharyngeal structures are altered by ablative procedures, the three-dimensional shape of the upper airway, or "vocal tract," is altered, as are the capabilities of structures within the tract to effect constrictions and occlusions appropriate for speech production. Selected *acoustic analyses* of speech, for example, of vowel "formants," which reflect the resonance characteristics of the vocal tract, provide excellent insights into these alterations. Resonances are properties of all air-filled tubes, including the vocal tract. They are frequency locations at which most energy will be concentrated if the air within the tube is excited, as by a sound, or pressure, disturbance. Resonance locations are determined by the tube's three-dimensional shape or configuration. When the shape of the vocal tract changes, as it does in unique ways for each vowel sound, the resulting resonances are also unique and provide the major cue to a listener regarding which vowel was heard. Formants reflect the tract's resonance characteristics in output spectra and can be observed and measured in spectrographic displays of spoken vowels (**Fig. 17.1**). Because a major effect of ablative procedures is a reduced capability to change the vocal tract's shape, the degree of compression of a speaker's formant frequency range can provide an objective index of what might be considered the "acoustic effects" of ablation.

Our experience suggests strongly that the single most important factor in speech outcomes for glossectomy patients is mobility of residual structures. In fact, our feeling is that, after eradication of disease, and regardless of site/extent of resection or type of reconstruction, the surgeon's primary objective should be maximizing mobility. Thus, in addition to phonological assessment, evaluations that provide information about the range and variability of movement of oral and pharyngeal structures need to be considered. In our own clinical setting, patients with glossectomy who are undergoing dynamic videofluoroscopic x-ray studies as a part of swallowing evaluations are also routinely asked to produce speech stimuli. From the videotaped recordings, it is possible to determine the tongue's range of motion for vowel sounds (**Fig. 17.2A–D**), and to ascertain how closely the tongue approximates the palate for /t/ and /k/ sounds. Examination of the radiographic study can also reveal locations in the oral cavity and pharynx (i.e., anterior, mid, and posterior) where tongue movements may be more or less extensive. Similarly, insights into the independence of tongue and jaw movements, as well as the movement capabilities of velar, pharyngeal, and other structures, may be forthcoming. Such information can be useful in planning subsequent therapy objectives and is particularly valuable if a prosthetic appliance to improve speech is being considered.

Prosthetic Appliances in Speech Rehabilitation

The use of prosthetic appliances to improve speech (and swallowing) in speakers with glossectomy has been reported by numerous authors.[41-58] Although providing strong evidence for the value of glossal prostheses in individual patients,

these studies have generally not attempted to systematize approaches to prosthesis design for speech that could be generalized to any treatment candidate. Nor have they considered, experimentally, speech and speaker variables that may influence the success of prosthetic reconstruction.[27] If the value of prostheses is to be maximized in this patient population, such approaches must be forthcoming.

There are two major types of appliances, including palatal reshaping prostheses,[51] which have a wide application, and mandibular, or "glossal" prostheses,[48] which have been described for patients with total glossectomy. A palatal reshaping prosthesis may enable residual tongue to approximate constrictions and occlusions in selected areas of the vocal tract that are critical to speech articulation. In total glossectomy, when most or all of the tongue has been excised, an optimally shaped prosthesis that rides passively on the mandible may allow the speaker to achieve constrictions in anterior and posterior locations of the oral cavity that otherwise could not be achieved.

Speech Therapy

As we have come to understand the differential effects of resection on speech, we have attempted to tailor our own speech therapy efforts in a similarly differential fashion. Initial emphasis was on *oral motor exercises* designed to maximize mobility and strength in residual tissues. We reasoned that, if patients strive to improve or retain as much oral skill as possible after surgery and during radiation, their prognosis for speech posttreatment is improved. More recently, these exercises have been associated with speech because it is the resumption of motor activity specific to speech targets that is desired.

The objective of *speech therapy* with resected patients has been to reestablish acoustically "sensitive" areas of the vocal tract, that is, areas where constrictions frequently occur in the production of speech sounds, and to then maximize acoustic differentiations that can be effected in these areas. If exact articulatory targets cannot be restored, emphasis is on improving the speaker's ability to produce acoustically differentiated speech sounds, that is, sounds that may not be normal, but that are close enough to normal, and sufficiently different from other sounds, that a listener may perceive

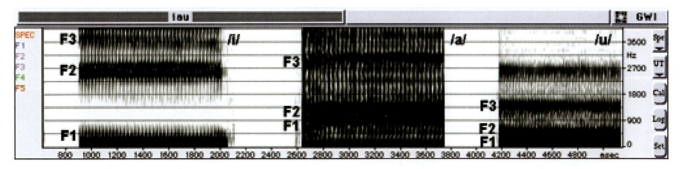

Fig. 17.1 "Formants," which reflect the natural resonance characteristics of the vocal tract for a particular size and shape, are revealed in a spectrographic analysis. Dark, horizontal bands labeled F1, F2, and F3 reflect concentrations of sound energy at particular time and frequency locations. These differ for every vowel sound, and cue the listener to what vowel sound was heard.

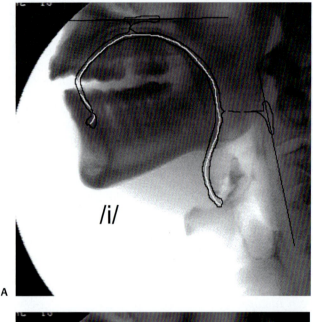

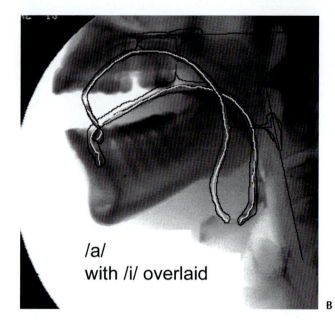

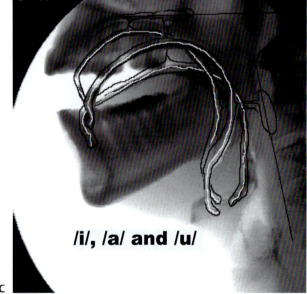

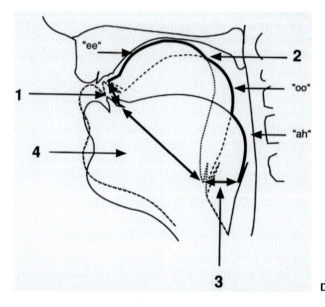

Fig. 17.2 From videofluoroscopic studies, lateral views of the vocal tract during the production of the vowels /i/, as in *heed*, /a/, as in *hod*, and /u/, as in *who'd* are obtained. From these, the range of tongue + jaw motion, representing the extremes of tongue positions for American English vowels, can be determined. **(A)** Vowel shape for /i/ (from a normal speaker) is traced and attached to reference lines superiorly and posteriorly. **(B)** Vowel shape for /i/ is overlaid on /a/ and referent lines are aligned. **(C)** Vowel /u/ is overlaid and aligned. **(D)** Outer boundary for all vowels is traced. Inferior border is indicated by straight line from valleculae to referent on anterior jaw. Numbers indicate dark lines representing boundaries, that is, (1) anterior, (2) superior, (3) posterior, and (4) inferior. Total range of tongue + jaw motion for the three vowels (in cm^2) is calculated. In addition, total range can be divided into "independent" area, that is, area utilized by one vowel only, and "shared" area, that is, area utilized by more than one vowel. Radiopaque disk of known diameter is in the field of filming so that quantitative measures can be made.

them as the speaker intended.[59] This therapy emphasizes heavily the speaker's ability to successfully effect *minimal differences*—units of speech that differ by only one sound— first with monosyllables, then in short phrases, and finally, in sentences. In patients with posterior tongue resections, this work has been directed primarily to vowel productions because these represent the category of speech sound most affected. In patients with anterior resections, consonants are targeted. In a retrospective review of 26 patients, therapy based on these principles appeared to produce significant improvements in speech.[60]

In contrast to a growing literature describing the profound and often debilitating effects on speech of glossal resection, there is no prospective, experimental evidence regarding the effects of speech therapy in any population of speakers with glossectomy. Pauloski et al found no recovery in speech or swallow function at 1, 3, and 12 months posttreatment in a group of glossectomy patients reconstructed with distal flaps.[61] Dysfunction in this group was severe as well as persistent, and the authors questioned whether the uniform lack of speech therapy (less than 3 hours) received by the patients may have been a factor. Historically, this situation has been in part related to the often poor prognoses associated with many oral or oropharyngeal cancers, and perhaps to the significant challenge the speech sequelae of this disease and its treatment pose to the speech pathologist. Although medical and surgical advances appear to have enhanced the rehabilitative potential for many of these patients, positive outcomes with respect to speech have not been demonstrated.

Implications of Oral/Oropharyngeal Resection for Swallowing

Glossal function is perhaps the major determinant of the success of the oral stage of swallowing, implicated not only in the formation, control, and direction (from anterior to posterior) of a bolus in the oral cavity but also in the propulsion of the bolus into the pharynx in prelude to the pharyngeal stage of swallow.[62–65] Less obvious, but equally important, is the role of the tongue in airway protection, that is, in the anterior elevation of the hyoid–larynx complex, and in the displacement of the epiglottis.[66] Both of these events, but particularly the former, are critical to "safe" swallowing, that is, swallowing without aspiration. Similarly, although the cause–effect nature of coordinated interactions between tongue and pharynx is unclear, it does appear that the tongue is involved in initiating the swallow reflex and in pharyngeal peristalsis. Since the timely, patterned sequencing of all of these events is responsible for the relaxation of the upper esophageal sphincter, and thus the initiation of the esophageal stage of swallow,[63] it is not unreasonable to view the tongue as contributing critically to all stages of swallow.

There have been numerous reports of swallowing difficulty associated with glossal resection.[25,49,63,67–71] At least one group has stated that impairment correlates more highly with extent of resection than with residual tongue mobility.[69] Conversely, several authors have reported that the maintenance or restoration of tongue mobility is the most important functional consideration in glossectomy.[21,72,73]

If it is clear that swallowing can be affected by ablative procedures of the oral cavity and/or pharynx, it is less obvious how such impairment is related to treatment variables associated with oral/oropharyngeal cancer. Method of reconstruction is of particular importance because there may be more than one reconstructive option available to the surgeon. Evidence that a specific technique offered certain advantages to individual patients could facilitate the surgeon's decision-making process at this stage of treatment.

McConnel and Mendelsohn noted that swallowing impairment is greater when residual tongue is used in closing a defect than when other types of reconstructive flaps are used for this purpose.[74] McConnel and O'Connor suggested the use of myocutaneous flaps when large volumes of tongue (i.e., T4

lesions) are resected, and free flaps when primary closure or skin grafts cannot be used.[75] These authors added that primary closure is likely to provide the best functional results for swallowing if tongue mobility can be maintained, even in some large resections, such as the removal of one half of the anterior two thirds of the tongue and floor of mouth tissue. However, according to McConnel and Mendelsohn, use of a primary closure technique when more than half of the tongue base has been resected tethers the tongue and significantly reduces its mobility.[75] These authors further described lateral tongue/pharyngeal wall resections (composite resection) as much less debilitating, functionally, when the mandible is preserved to the maximum extent possible. In fact, according to McConnel and O'Connor, emphasis is increasingly on preservation of the mandible with flaps or grafts, and away from composite resections.[75]

Total glossectomy with preservation of the larynx presents a unique challenge for swallowing rehabilitation because the primary means of bolus control in the oral cavity and pharynx are missing. If resection also involves the anterior mandible, elevation of the larynx, and opening of the upper esophageal sphincter (UES) are compromised. In such cases, McConnel and O'Connor recommended elevating the hyoid bone, which also serves to shorten the oral cavity.[75] Improved airway protection, and a more direct path to the pharynx, are the desired results. As previously described, both mandibular and palatal prosthetic appliances may facilitate swallowing and speech in these patients.[48]

Investigations that focus on specific alterations in swallowing and/or causes of dysphagia in resected patients, and not just the presence or absence of aspiration, are relatively few. Logemann and Bytell reported that patients with anterior floor of mouth resections had difficulty with preparation for swallow, and with oral transit, whereas patients with base of tongue resections demonstrated reduced times for both oral and pharyngeal stages of swallow.[73] Research in our own laboratory demonstrated a high correlation between base of tongue resection and poor pharyngeal constriction. More surprising was evidence that some patients with anterior tongue/floor of mouth resections also had difficulty effecting appropriate pharyngeal constriction and clearing. Further scrutiny revealed that this was true when tongue was used to close the floor of mouth defect. Patients who had primary closures or skin graft reconstructions were less affected. Hamlet et al reported that patients with active, unresected cancers of the pharynx or tongue base demonstrated alterations in the sequencing of swallow events, as compared with normals.[76] In these patients, pharyngeal stripping was found to precede velar closure, whereas in normals, the two events occurred simultaneously.

Additional observations regarding characteristics of swallowing associated with oral/oropharyngeal resection and reconstruction are in a preliminary state, or raise questions that remain unresolved. For example, though there has been an increased effort among surgeons to reestablish sensation in reconstructive flaps, for example, the potential functional benefits of these attempts have yet to be demonstrated. Similarly, changes in swallow function over time are not well understood. Pauloski et al used videofluoroscopy to assess swallowing in patients with anterior tongue/floor of mouth resections and distal flap reconstructions at 1 and 3 months posttreatment.[61] The authors found no recovery in their subjects over this time period, and persistent, severe dysfunction characterized by significant delays in oral transit times and oral residue. Somewhat similarly, 15 of 35 study patients in our own study demonstrated penetration and/or aspiration on liquid swallows. In general, these were patients who had undergone large unilateral resections or extensive base of tongue resections. All patients in the study were 1 year posttreatment and eating orally. Nevertheless, risks associated with chronic aspiration (i.e., pneumonia, weight loss, inadequate nutrition) were considered significant.

Swallowing Rehabilitation

One way to view the upper airway for swallowing is as a series of valves and chambers. "Chambers" describes the cavities, or spaces of the airway, such as the nose, oral cavity, pharynx, and esophagus. For swallow, it is imperative that most of these chambers be able to expand to accommodate bolus material, and to then constrict and shorten. Compression resulting from the latter is critical to effecting pressure differences necessary for bolus flow through the aerodigestive tract. "Valves" include those structures that open and close, thereby regulating the transfer of bolus material from one chamber to the next. For example, valving between the tongue and soft palate helps retain material in the oral cavity prior to swallow initiation. When this valve relaxes or opens, the material can be propelled into the oropharynx. Closure of the laryngeal valves, including the aryepiglottic folds and the false and true vocal folds, prevents bolus material from entering the airway and, of course, opening of the UES valve permits entry of bolus material into the esophagus.

Though simplistic, this model can be useful in considering swallowing difficulties in patients with oral/oropharyngeal resection. An analysis of the capabilities of individual valves and chambers provides insights into specific causes of dysphagia, as well as into specific objectives for intervention. If chambers, for example, the oropharynx or hypopharynx, cannot constrict appropriately, then we would expect to see problems with clearing of bolus material, and intervention would be focused on ways of effecting clearing. Depending on the nature of valving dysfunction, bolus material may enter chambers early or inappropriately or be prevented from entering a chamber. Subsequent intervention would be directed to strategies that might improve bolus flow. The assessment and treatment alternatives described next have a common focus on the capabilities of valves and chambers critical to swallow function.

Assessment

Three types of assessment have become standard inclusions in the speech-language pathologist's management of patients with dysphagia resulting from oral/oropharyngeal ablation. A *bedside swallow study* can be performed within days of the patient's surgery. Objectives of the exam are to evaluate oral anatomy and function, and to observe the patient during swallowing of selected materials. Insights into the patient's ability to manage different amounts and types of foods in the oral cavity, as well as clues regarding the integrity of airway protection, may be forthcoming. In addition, the swallowing therapist assesses the patient's readiness to undergo more extensive evaluations that will provide significant details of the patient's swallowing function, as well as specific deficits that can be addressed therapeutically.

One of these exams is a videofluoroscopic x-ray study, referred to as a *modified barium swallow*[63] or, in our clinic, a *dynamic swallow study*. For this exam, the patient is filmed in lateral and anterior-posterior views during swallowing of graded boluses. The study is initiated with a small amount of radiopaque liquid (1 mL). As the material is swallowed, its progress through the upper aerodigestive tract, from oral cavity to upper esophagus, is observed. If the patient is able to manage this without aspiration, the study advances to larger liquid boluses, and then to different consistencies of bolus material (i.e., pudding, paste, solids).

Evidence of aspiration before, during, or after the swallow; penetration, pooling, or residue of the bolus at various anatomical sites; inappropriate opening of the upper esophageal sphincter; or other abnormalities are noted (**Fig. 17.3**). In addition, physiological deficits that are producing these symptoms, such as poor control of oropharyngeal structures that leads to early loss of the bolus, poor pharyngeal constriction, reduced laryngeal elevation, or limited opening of the UES, can be observed and quantified for comparison to normal. The therapist conducting the study will note whether certain bolus consistencies or sizes can be handled more safely or efficiently than others and may also have the patient attempt various strategies or facilitative maneuvers (breath-holding, repeat swallow, effortful swallow) or postural changes (chin

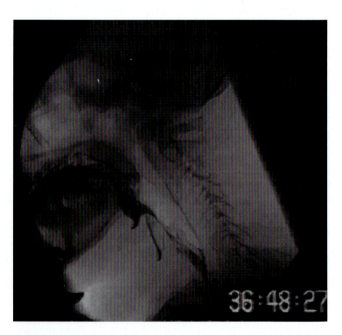

Fig. 17.3 Patient with base of tongue resection fails to constrict the pharynx during swallow. Residue is significant and patient is at risk for aspiration.

tuck, side-lying) that may improve swallowing efficiency or safety (**Fig. 17.4A,B**). Information from the study will be used to determine if, and with what restrictions, patients can return to oral feeding. Typically, this information will also form the basis of swallowing therapy for an individual patient.

A third exam that is useful is flexible endoscopic evaluation of swallowing (FEES).[77] This study follows the same progression as the videofluoroscopic x-ray exam but is performed with a flexible nasopharyngoscope attached to a small video camera. With the scope positioned in the oropharynx (and nose, if nasal reflux is suspected), different amounts and consistencies of bolus materials are introduced and the patient's attempts to manage them are observed on a video monitor. FEES does not provide all the same information as the modified barium swallow does, but it can provide information about alterations in anatomy that may not be apparent on fluoroscopy, for example, a vocal fold paresis or paralysis, or asymmetries in pharyngeal constriction from right to left.

In addition, the noninvasiveness of FEES allows it to be used when it is of interest to follow a patient over the course of a meal, or repeated swallows, as when there is a question of a patient fatiguing over time. FEES may also be indicated when a patient is unable to undergo videofluoroscopy, or when the aspiration risk is sufficiently high that it is desirable to observe only dry swallows. Not surprisingly, FEES is an excellent tool for teaching strategies, such as breath-holding, or observing the effects of various strategies, because both therapist and patient can observe the real-time study on a video monitor. *Scintigraphy*[78] and combined videofluoroscopy with *manometry*[79] have also been used in swallowing assessments with this patient population.

Swallowing Therapy

Swallowing therapy can be initiated within days after surgery and is typically predicated on the identification of specific deficits that need to be addressed, and on compensatory behavioral strategies that enable the patient to move away from nonoral to oral feeding as quickly and completely as possible. Demonstration of the effectiveness of such strategies, via videofluoroscopic or endoscopic viewing, provide the basis for their use. Swallow function that permits adequate nutrition, doesn't require excessive time, and represents minimal risk to pulmonary health, is a primary objective of swallowing therapy.

In cases where there is clear evidence of limited motion, endurance, or agility of gestures involved in swallowing, *exercise* of involved structures can be implemented. If sensory deficits are identified, alternative or improved sources of feedback may need to be introduced (as described with FEES) to maximize the benefits of exercise. Specific exercises are typically directed to improving capabilities of residual, impaired swallowing gestures, or to those gestures that have the greatest compensatory potential, and may involve the lips, mandible, tongue, pharynx, or larynx.

Other strategies for improving swallowing can take several forms. For example, *bolus manipulation* according to size, viscosity, placement (a particular site on the tongue or in the oropharynx), and sensory properties (e.g., temperature or taste) may be considered. Liquids are easily deformed and move readily in response to gravity and compression, requiring more skill in agility and coordination and less in strength of constriction, whereas thicker substances move

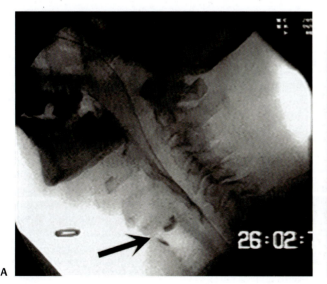
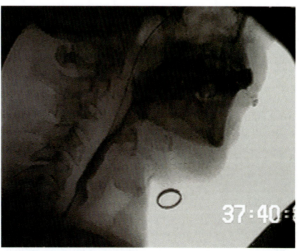

Fig. 17.4 (**A**) Glossectomy patient in lateral view demonstrates aspiration (bolus material is apparent in airway). (**B**) Glossectomy patient reclined to the left, tightly holding breath, and head turned to right. Upper esophageal sphincter opens and no aspiration occurs.

more slowly but require greater constriction and mucosal/salivary compensation. In addition, bolus material that is more deformable may pass through narrow sites in transit but may also be aspirated. Less deformable boluses, on the other hand, may obstruct the airway. Consideration of an individual patient's particular strengths and deficits, as well as the highly structured and cautious treatment probing of a variety of bolus manipulations, done with x-ray or FEES, helps determine what is most appropriate.

Postural compensations, such as tilting the upper body or head, can be attempted to redirect bolus material in a manner that improves efficiency or safety of swallowing. Such maneuvers not only change the direction of bolus flow by influencing gravity but may also impact size/shape of the pharyngeal chamber or opening of the UES. If the upper body is tilted laterally or posteriorly, for example, bolus material will flow on the downward side, away from the airway. Capital flexion, or "chin-tuck," enlarges the oropharynx but also reduces the size of the hypopharynx, which is also helpful to airway protection. Again, careful treatment probing based on feedback from videofluoroscopic or endoscopic evidence is useful in identifying compensations that may be of value.

Facilitative maneuvers are gestures that have similarly been found to facilitate safe and/or effective swallow. These strategies must be learned by the patient and require greater sensorimotor integrity and ability to understand and implement than strategies that can be to some extent imposed on a swallower by a feeder. Increased effort on swallow, repeat swallows, breath-holding, supraglottic swallow, super supraglottic swallow, and prolongation of maximum hyoid elevation (Mendelsohn maneuver) are examples of such maneuvers.[80] Desirable effects of these gestures include improved pharyngeal clearing with less residue; early, prolonged, or increased airway protection; and early, prolonged, or increased degree of UES opening. *Facilitative devices,* ranging from specialized instruments for eating to a palatal reshaping prosthesis, mandibular prosthesis, or palatal lift, may also be considered.[81]

◆ **Effectiveness/Efficacy of Swallowing Therapy** The reasonableness of these treatment objectives notwithstanding, there is, as noted, scant experimental evidence that they are effective. Similarly, those factors that predispose patients to greater or lesser degrees of dysphagia, according to resection category or other treatment variables, have generally not been elaborated for any group of oropharyngeal cancer patients. On the other hand, the effectiveness of therapeutic interventions is demonstrated frequently in individual patients who undergo radiographic or other investigations specifically for this purpose. That is, if a patient aspirates or fails to clear the pharynx during a typical swallow but avoids both when implementing a facilitative maneuver or postural compensation, and this is clearly apparent on x-ray, then the success of the strategy is demonstrated. If the patient successfully learns how to apply the strategies, avoids pulmonary complications or weight loss over a period of time, and demonstrates on repeat studies that swallowing is completed without aspiration or poor pharyngeal clear-

ing, this too must be considered as positive evidence of the value of intervention. It is hoped that experimental inquiries addressing the effectiveness of behavioral interventions in groups of patients will be forthcoming.

Implications of Laryngeal Resection for Voice and Speech

As surgical and medical management of laryngeal cancer has improved, conservation treatments that restore or preserve laryngeal structures have been introduced. Though the emphasis rightfully continues to be on eradication of disease, these new approaches have expanded the possibilities for voice restoration in many laryngeal cancer patients. At the same time, it has become clear that preservation of laryngeal tissue does not always translate into improvements in all laryngeal functions. This is in part a reflection of the diverse roles of the larynx in airway protection and maintenance, and phonation. That is, what may suffice as a voicing source may not work equally well as an airway protector.

Ablative procedures of the larynx can be generally divided into partial and total laryngectomies. Total laryngectomy involves removal of the entire larynx and is typically indicated in large lesions. Carcinoma in situ and microinvasive disease involve only the vocal fold cover and are sometimes managed by endoscopic excision. Partial or total cordectomy, in which only one true vocal fold is involved, is indicated for T1–T2 lesions and is typically treated with either radiotherapy or surgery. Other partial laryngectomy procedures include vertical, which may be either a standard or an extended hemilaryngectomy, and horizontal, also referred to as a supraglottic laryngectomy, standard or extended. A subtotal laryngectomy implies greater extent of resection and typically a neoglottic reconstruction. In the next section, the specific effects on voice and speech associated with each type of resection, as well as rehabilitation strategies unique to each, will be discussed.

Total Laryngectomy and Speech Rehabilitation

◆ **Implications for Speech** If the larynx is completely resected, voice produced by the true vocal folds is lost, and the patient is unable to produce vowel sounds and all voiced consonant sounds. Even with the airway diverted to the neck, however, most individuals can quickly learn to use residual air in the oral and pharyngeal cavities to produce voiceless speech sounds (/p, wh, f, t, s, sh, ch, k/). One exception to this is the sound /h/, which is articulated by the vocal folds. Articulation of other speech sounds, and the speaker's ability to effect resonance changes in the vocal tract, typically remain intact.

Alternatives for the alaryngeal speaker are numerous. In the earlier edition of this text, a historical review of the developments of many of these was presented in detail. In the intervening time, however, alternatives for these patients have been directed primarily to three options, including electronic devices (i.e., artificial larynges), esophageal speech, and tracheoesophageal speech. In keeping with both the contemporary popularity and the prevalence of these rehabitation strategies, our discussion here will address only these alternatives.

◆ **Artificial Larynx** The electrolarynx, or "artificial larynx," is one of the most enduring voice options for speakers with total laryngectomy. These battery-powered instruments produce sound electronically and then transmit this sound into the upper airway. If sound energy sufficient to excite this column of air is delivered, the speaker should be able to articulate voiced speech sounds. There are two major types of these instruments, a neck type and an intraoral type. The neck or throat device is placed on tissues of the neck (or perhaps cheek) and sound is transmitted through transcervical tissues of the body into the airway (**Fig. 17.5**). An intraoral device transmits sound directly from the electronic source into the oral cavity through a plastic tube that the speaker holds in the corner of the mouth (**Fig. 17.6**). These instruments may be indicated in patients with thick or fibrotic neck tissues that preclude use of a neck-type electrolarynx. Other devices may be encased in a dental prosthesis and attached inside the oral cavity.

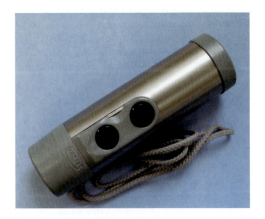

Fig. 17.5 Throat type electrolarynx (Servox Electrolarynx, Asyst, Indian Creek, IL). The diaphragm is positioned on the tissues of the neck and sound is transmitted into the upper airway.

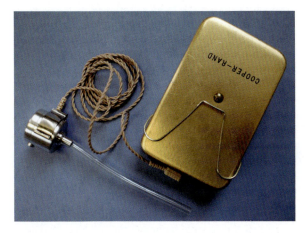

Fig. 17.6 Intraoral type electrolarynx (Cooper-Rand Voice Prosthesis, Lauder, San Antonio, TX). Plastic tube is held just inside the oral cavity and sound is introduced into the vocal tract.

The advantages of electrolarynges include their applicability, availability, and ease of use. That is, most alaryngeal speakers are candidates for these instruments, have access to them, and can quickly learn to use them shortly after surgery. They do require the use of one hand, and generally preclude talking and engaging in complex manual activities at the same time. In addition, the sound produced by most instruments does not closely approximate human vocal quality, pitch, or loudness variability. A related problem is that, unlike natural speech, which includes both voiced and unvoiced sounds, all speech sounds produced with the electrolarynx are voiced. Newer developments in electrolarynx technology have focused on greater intensity generation and pitch variability, but devices that permit speech that sounds more natural, or that is unique to the speaker, are generally not available at this time.

◆ **Esophageal Speech** Esophageal speech refers to the use of the UES, also referred to as the pharyngoesophageal segment (PES), as a vibratory sound source to support speech. To speak in this fashion, speakers must learn to inject or inhale air into the esophagus and to then direct this back over the PES. Even in the best esophageal speakers, voice production is typically lower in frequency than normal, with fewer syllables produced per air expulsion. But, produced by the speaker's own tissues, it does have the advantage of being unique to the speaker (and distinct from other speakers), requires no batteries or free hands, and represents a viable alternative for those individuals who are able to learn it.

There are several characteristics of the structure of the PES that can influence its ability to produce sound. For example, hypertonicity or spasm of the PES, as well as excessive flaccidity, can interfere with sound quality. PES dilation, pharyngeal neurectomy, myotomy, and botulinum toxin have all been used in the treatment of hypertonicity.[82] The application of compression to the neck in the area of the PES, either by hand or with a neck band, can sometimes be effective in patients with a flaccid segment. Izdebski et al reported that patients who developed esophageal (or electrolaryngeal or tracheoesophageal speech) following laryngectomy but prior to radiotherapy experienced deleterious changes in voice and speech during radiotherapy.[82] The authors attributed this to changes in the impaired mobility and vibratory capability of the esophageal wall and mucosa, to fibrosis of the submandibular region, and to trismus. Speech and voice function was generally restored to preradiotherapy levels within weeks of the end of radiation, however.

◆ **Tracheoesophageal Speech** The third alternative for alaryngeal speakers is tracheoesophageal speech, popularly referred to as TE speech or TEP speech. This method is based on a series of historical attempts to surgically establish a route for air from the trachea to the cervical esophagus. In 1979, Singer and Blom described a surgically created fistula from the posterior wall of the trachea into the cervical esophagus through which a one-way silicon valve (i.e., tracheoesophageal prosthesis), could be placed.[83] To produce voice, the speaker occluded the stoma and exhaled, allowing air to be diverted into a small inferior port in the tracheal portion of the prosthesis and then through the valve into the esophagus. When air pressure under the PES was adequate, esophageal sound could be produced and used to support speech (**Fig. 17.7**). A major advantage of this method, as compared with traditional esophageal speech, is in the number of syllables that can be produced on one exhalation. This is due to the fact that the esophagus can deliver only a small amount of air (80 to 100 mL) to power the PES, as compared with the much greater amount of pulmonary air typically available. Other advantages of TE speech over esophageal speech include a higher, and closer to normal, fundamental frequency.[84] Factors that may adversely affect a patient's ability to use a tracheoesophageal prosthesis include stoma size, manual skills, and the integrity of the PES as a sound generator.

Since its introduction, TE speech has become widely accepted and utilized. The procedure was first described as a secondary procedure to laryngectomy but can also be performed at the time of laryngectomy. At least two studies have reported no difference in speech quality whether the TE surgery is done as a primary or secondary procedure. Nor does prior radiation therapy appear to affect the complication rate of the TE surgical procedure or speech outcome.[85–89] Another advantage of TE speech is that it may be used effectively in patients who have undergone pharyngectomy and laryngectomy and have then been reconstructed with radial forearm or jejunum flaps.[90,91] However, quality of speech is likely to be significantly poorer in these patients than in patients with total laryngectomy, only.[92]

In the 20-plus years since their introduction, tracheoesophageal prostheses have undergone several modifications. These include increases in the diameter of the valve and modifications of the esophageal port to achieve lower

resistances (and greater ease in sound generation), variations in design of the esophageal portion of the prosthesis to prevent flow of material from the esophagus into the airway, and alterations designed to minimize fungal colonization[93,94] and improve airway humidification. In addition, a prosthetic valve that automatically occludes in response to certain levels of tracheal air pressure, eliminating the need for digital occlusion, and "in-dwelling" prostheses designed to eliminate the need for frequent removal and cleaning of the device, have been introduced (**Fig. 17.7**).[95–97] Several devices are available (e.g., Blom-Singer, Provox, Groningen, Voice Master, Nijdam), and a few investigations have compared speech characteristics between or among prostheses.[98–101]

In our own experience, patients have generally not preferred devices with automatic valves, in particular, if they are capable of a wide range of exercise levels that have differing respiratory requirements. We have also noted a direct relationship between increased diameters of valves and degree of leaking around the prosthesis, and have attempted to strive for the least resistance possible without also incurring excessive leakage. Our own philosophy has been to ensure that patients are proficient at both maintaining (i.e., removing, cleaning, inserting) and using TEPs prior to dismissal from therapy, in part because many of our patients live far away from our center and have few resources for expedient help should they experience difficulty. The first indwelling devices required physician insertion and replacement and minimal patient involvement. Newer materials and insertion techniques have made some of these more "user friendly" for patients, however, and they have become increasingly popular.

Few studies are available to suggest which of these three major alternatives for alaryngeal speakers is predominant in this country. Those data that are available are widely disparate. For example, artificial larynx use among alaryngeal speakers has been reported at rates ranging from 5 to 66%.[102] The prevalence of traditional esophageal speech is similarly in doubt but may be less now than prior to the emergence of the TE prosthesis. A prospective study by Gates et al in 1982 revealed that 26% of patients acquired functional esophageal speech.[103] Interestingly, a retrospective study by these same authors revealed a much greater success rate of 62%. The authors interpreted the large differences as evidence of selection bias associated with the retrospective study paradigm. In another prospective study, St Guily et al reported that only 5% of patients acquired esophageal speech.[104] Use of TEP speech has been reported to range from 30 to 93%.[102]

A few studies have attempted to compare the relative prevalence of the three alaryngeal speech methods. Two surveys among head and neck surgeons reported the acquisition rate of TEP speech as between 30 and 38%, the rate of esophageal speech acquisition between 38 and 49%, and artificial larynx use between 21 and 48%.[103] In a survey of 151 experienced speech–language pathologists, TEP speech was reported to be their "preferred" rehabilitation alternative, and the electrolarynx, their least preferred method. However, the electrolarynx was reportedly the most frequently used method. Fifty percent of the speech–language pathologists surveyed reported that fewer than six therapy sessions were required for patients to become competent with TEPs; 20% reported

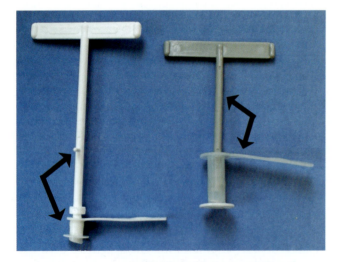

Fig. 17.7 On the left is a Blom-Singer tracheoesophageal prosthesis (InHealth Technologies, Carpinteria, CA). *Arrow* at top indicates inserter; arrow at bottom indicates prosthesis. On the right, a Blom-Singer indwelling prosthesis is shown. Again, *arrow* at top indicates inserter and *arrow* at bottom indicates actual prosthesis.

the need for 10 or more therapy sessions.[105] In the most extensive study to date, Hillman et al described functional outcomes, including voice and speech, in patients who received either surgery and radiation, or radiation and induction chemotherapy, for treatment of T3 and T4 laryngeal squamous cell carcinoma.[102] Of 166 patients who underwent total laryngectomy followed by radiation therapy, 6% developed esophageal speech or remained nonvocal (8%), 55% used an electrolarynx, and 31% successfully used TE prostheses.

Nontotal Laryngectomy and Voice

◆ **Carcinoma In Situ/Microinvasion** Lesions that are minimally invasive and amenable to either surgical or radiation therapy may nonetheless have consequences for voice. The epithelial layer of the vocal fold affected is the outer layer of the fold's vibratory margin, and voice quality following treatment is likely to be influenced by how much mucosa is excised, as well as the straightness of the edge of the fold. Several authors have noted the potential for harm in "stripping" the vocal fold for this type of lesion due to the increased amount of mucosa removed with this procedure, and the increased likelihood for vocal ligament damage. Several authors have reported good results for postoperative voice using the CO_2 laser. Other authors believe best results are achieved with careful microdissection using "cold" phonomicrosurgical techniques.[92]

◆ **Cordectomy** For lesions (typically T1 or T2) that involve one vocal fold, partial cordectomy is achieved with surgical or radiation therapy. Voice posttreatment is likely to be affected by the amount of tissue loss, the degree of contact between both true vocal folds on voicing, and the condition of the mucosa. If treated with laser excision, scar tissue eventually replaces the missing tissue and is covered by mucosa. However, the underlying stiffness of the fold at this site may be revealed by the lack of a mucosal wave on stroboscopic imaging and may contribute to poorer voice quality. Well-known effects of radiation include necrosis, mucositis, edema, xerostomia, and fibrosis, all of which may affect the vibratory source and resulting voice quality posttreatment.[106]

Several authors have described improvements in voice and phonatory function from 8 weeks to 2 years postradiation treatment.[107-109] Tsunoda et al reported follow-up stroboscopic findings in 10 patients who had undergone radiotherapy for T1N0M0 lesions.[110] At 6 months posttreatment, the presence of a mucosal wave was first identified, and by 1 year posttreatment, all patients demonstrated a mucosal wave. However, Lehman et al noted continued alterations from normal in radiated patients as long as 20 years following treatment.[111] These included increased perturbation factors in voice (possibly perceived as instability or roughness in the voice), decreased maximum phonation durations, increased subglottal pressures required for voicing, diminished mucosal wave activity, and an increase in supraglottic hyperperfusion. Other authors have reported similar, continued differences from normal voice at varying times postradiation.[112-114] Benninger et al reported postradiation voices to be worse when patients continued smoking, had bilateral involvement, and had undergone stripping rather than biopsy on initial diagnosis.[115]

McGuirt et al described similar phonatory function findings in patients who were 6 months post–laser resections for their disease.[116] Subjective judgments of patients' voice quality by speech–language pathologists were also included in this study. On a scale of 1 to 5, with 1 representing "normal quality," the mean rating was 2.68, as judged from the reading of a standardized passage. The range extended from near normal to mildly abnormal. Casiano et al described continued alterations from normal voice in six patients at 6 months following treatment.[117] These authors also noted the presence of anterior webs and granuloma in some patients at this posttreatment interval.

In a comparison of postradiation voice to postlaser voice, Hirano et al noted that both were different from normal, and very similar to each other, although the laser-treated patients in this study were perceived as slightly more hoarse than patients who had undergone radiation.[118] A comparison by Ott et al found no significant differences in voice quality or harmonic:noise ratios in patients who had undergone either radiation or laser treatment, respectively.[119] In both patient groups, vibratory characteristics of the true folds were different from normal.

McGuirt et al investigated voicing characteristics in patients with T1 lesions. Thirteen were treated with radiation, and 11 were treated with the CO_2 laser.[120] All subjects were male, and all were at least 6 months posttreatment. In this study, patients in the laser group tended to do more poorly than patients treated with radiation in terms of glottal resistance, maximum phonation duration, and subjective ratings of voice quality. On other measures, findings were similar between the groups. Other studies that have compared posttreatment voice in laser and radiated patients have generally found either no differences, or slightly better results in patients undergoing radiation therapy (6400 to 6600 cGy).[121-123] However, a recent study by Delsupehe et al considered perceptual ratings of voice before surgery and at various treatment intervals up to 2 years posttreatment.[124] Twelve patients with early glottic carcinoma were treated with radiotherapy and 30 with a narrow-margin CO_2 laser cordectomy. Although voice results were worse in the immediate posttreatment period for the laser group, no significant differences between groups were noted at 6 and 24 months posttreatment.

Rosier et al retrospectively compared results of radiation therapy, laser microsurgery, and partial laryngectomy for the treatment of T1N0M0 glottic carcinomas.[125] The authors reported a trend toward decreased patient satisfaction, increased hoarseness, and increased breathiness in patients who underwent partial laryngectomy, as compared with the other groups. Ott et al investigated signal-to-noise ratios in 39 patients treated with either primary radiation, cordectomy or frontolateral partial resections for T1 and T2 glottic cancers.[126] These authors reported no differences in patients treated with radiotherapy or cordectomy, and significantly poorer results in patients who underwent partial resections.

In total cordectomy, the entire vocal fold, from the vocal process of the arytenoid to the anterior commissure, is involved. Approaches to treatment include endoscopic or through a laryngofissure. To our knowledge, there are few comparisons of voice resulting from these procedures. Olsen et al performed a chart review on 95 patients who had undergone one or the other of these procedures.[127] The authors noted poor voice in 17% of patients, apparently not specifically related to one or the other of these procedures. Bockler et al recently described voice quality posttreatment in patients treated with transoral endolaryngeal laser surgery versus patients treated with an anterolateral partial laryngectomy.[128] Several voice and phonatory function measures were considered, and results indicated no significant differences between the groups. However, a tracheotomy was avoided in patients undergoing laser surgery.

Collective review of these studies appear to demonstrate clearly only that poorer voice is associated with partial laryngectomy than with radiotherapy or laser microsection, and that voice may not return to normal regardless of treatment modality. Although the weight of the available evidence may suggest more benign effects of radiotherapy than laser microsurgery, there is at least some evidence that voice results may not differ significantly between these two modalities. It should also be noted that procedural problems with much of the available research make findings problematic in some cases, and comparisons among studies difficult. A lack of pretreatment comparisons across patients, insufficient control over lesion type and extent, some patients' receipt of multiple treatment modalities, variability in time of evaluation posttreatment, and variability in voicing measures obtained are a few of the factors contributing to this dilemma.

◆ **Hemilaryngectomy** In a standard hemilaryngectomy (vertical laryngectomy), the true vocal fold, false vocal fold, ventricle, and anterior thyroid cartilage are removed. The epiglottis remains intact. In an extended hemilaryngectomy, the ipsilateral arytenoid cartilage and part of the contralateral true fold are involved as well. Voice is affected at least moderately by such procedures, and numerous strategies for reconstructing the excised side have been described, including strap muscle flaps, epiglottic laryngoplasty, corniculate-cuneiform flaps, and several types of local flaps (as from pyriform sinus, platysma, false fold, or aryepiglottic fold). Mandell et al recently examined 42 patients who had undergone vertical partial laryngectomy with various types of reconstruction.[129] These authors found that the contralateral false vocal fold was the most common site of vibration, followed by contralateral arytenoid mucosa and then contralateral true vocal fold. No differences were found in quality of voice with respect to site of vibration, and voice quality was judged similar for pyriform mucosa flap reconstructions and other types of reconstruction. Salam et al described excellent voice quality in 21/30 patients who were reconstructed with pyriform sinus mucosa following vertical partial laryngectomy.[130]

Of further interest is Hirano et al's report of 54 patients who underwent reconstruction with a sternohyoid muscle flap.[118]

Although Hirano performed all procedures, voice outcomes were markedly variable. In all patients, maximum phonation duration was decreased (mean of 13 seconds, normal = 15 to 25 seconds); airflow was increased (275 cc/s, normal = 100 to 150 cc/s); fundamental frequency range was decreased (mean of 18 semitones, normal = 24 to 30 semitones); and intensity range was limited (mean of 21 dB, normal = 30 to 35 dB). Voice produced by patients was characterized as rough, breathy, and strained, and evidence of hyperfunction was noted. Similar findings were reported by Blaugrund et al.[131] These authors found that glottic closure was incomplete in 80% of hemilaryngectomy patients, and hyperfunction of supraglottic structures on voicing was present in most patients. These authors also noted severely restricted fundamental frequency and intensity variability in their hemilaryngectomy patients.

A study by Leeper et al of unreconstructed hemilaryngectomy patients provides an interesting comparison to Hirano's reconstructed group.[132] Leeper found a mean maximum phonation duration of 10 seconds, mean airflow of 201 cc/s, fundamental frequency range of 13 semitones, intensity range of 25 dB, and a mean severity rating of 5 on a 1 to 7 scale with 1 indicating normal voice. Procedural differences between the two studies make direct comparisons difficult. However, the data suggest the value of reconstruction, even though resulting voice and phonatory function clearly do not approximate normal. Questions regarding the best alternative for reconstruction in these patients, however, are complicated by wide variability in both treatment modalities and reconstruction options, and the generally small numbers of subjects within each group available for study. To our knowledge, differential effects of surgery versus radiation on voice in this patient group have not been reported.

◆ **Supraglottic Laryngectomy** This procedure involves excision of the epiglottis and preepiglottic space, aryepiglottic folds, false vocal folds, upper third of the thyroid cartilage, a radical neck dissection, and possibly the hyoid bone. The true vocal folds are left intact, and voice is typically good to excellent following treatment. If poor, factors to consider are edema, radiation fibrosis, aspiration effects, and impaired mobility of residual structures.

◆ **Other Nontotal Laryngectomy Types** Other partial laryngectomy surgical procedures have been attempted, although few systematic investigations of voice outcomes associated with these procedures have been reported. One exception is a study by Laccourreye et al, who compared voice in 28 patients with supracricoid partial laryngectomies with voice in 14 normal adults.[133] Results demonstrated excessive air escape in the patient group due to incomplete neoglottic closure, and a significantly decreased maximum phonation duration. Voices of patients also contained excessive noise, and fundamental frequencies were higher than normal. Pearson et al described "near total laryngectomy," in which the larynx is entirely removed except for retained portions of the subglottis and segments of true vocal fold and arytenoid cartilage.[134] These remnants are surgically formed into a tissue shunt that allows air to enter it with the stoma occluded. The interaction of air and tissue produces sound that, in some patients, supports speech. Hoasjoe et al and Hoyt et al described great variability in voice production across patients, a finding that appeared related to small tissue differences resulting from either or both resection and reconstruction.[135,136] High fundamental frequencies and significant noise in the voicing signal, as well as hyperfunctional behaviors, were also characteristic of speakers investigated.

In cancers that affect both true vocal folds anteriorly (i.e., transglottic carcinoma), other types of near total laryngectomy procedures have been described. For example, Lu and Dong reported results for 32 patients reconstructed with platysmal myocutaneous flaps.[137] Laurian and Zohar described the use of a composite nasal mucoseptal graft to bridge the laryngeal defect.[138] Zanaret et al described neoglottic reconstruction with the epiglottis following total laryngectomy,[139] and several authors have reported results of cricohyoepiglottopexy or cricohyoidopexy.[140–143] Only a few of these studies offer objective data regarding voice outcomes, but most describe resulting voice as at least "functional."

Nontotal Laryngectomy and Voice Rehabilitation

◆ **Assessment**   As previously noted, patients who have undergone major ablative procedures will experience changes in tissues and functional status for days or weeks following initial resection. Assessment is thus best viewed as a continuing process that considers an individual's particular needs at each stage of recovery. Initially, a patient's ability to write legibly or to use a communication board may be priorities. With additional healing, more definitive treatment options can be considered. These will be determined to a large extent by the nature of the patient's resection and the integrity of residual structures. But it is equally important to assess those aspects of the individual that are likely to influence treatment progress, for example, the ability to learn new skills. In every case, a patient's specific needs, desires, and capabilities must be determined and then matched to the most optimal treatment alternative available.

Also important to assessment are those measures selected to evaluate voice at each treatment stage. Care providers' subjective impressions of voice are not sufficient for this purpose. And, though listeners' perceptions of voice, obtained in an objective manner, are a primary determinant of success, they provide limited insights into the details of phonatory function that explain why the voice is perceived as it is. However, there are problems with the use of more objective measures, as well. For example, though there are myriad acoustic measures that can quantify differences between normal and abnormal voice, they are usually made from sustained vowel sounds or very limited speech samples. Although these may be quite useful for intrasubject pre- and posttreatment comparisons, they may not be highly correlated with perceptual judgments of voice in conversation. In addition, they require careful attention in collection and interpretation. Measures of laryngeal function, such as airflow, glottal resistance, and subglottal pressure provide excellent insights into voice, and the effort required to produce voice. But these measures also require care and time in collection and may not be readily available in many clinical settings.

Perhaps the best approach to assessing voice and speech in these patients is one that incorporates multiple purposes. For example, one purpose is how *functional* the voice is, that is, how well it serves the speaker in daily life. For this purpose, measures directed to how durable, or resistant to fatigue, the voice is, and how easily understood speech is to listeners, in quiet or noise, or how often messages must be repeated, are valuable. Some routine voice evaluation measures, such as maximum phonation duration (length of a vowel sound produced on one breath), or fundamental frequency and intensity variability in voice, provide insights into functionality, as well.

Related to functionality are measures that provide insights into *ease of production*. One example is the number of syllables the speaker can produce on one exhalation. This measure tells us something about the speaker's rate of production, and of how often there must be inspiratory breaks to replenish the air supply. Laryngeal function measures, as noted, are also useful to this purpose. Another purpose might be an appraisal of *satisfaction*; that is, how pleasant to listen to or easy to understand is voice/speech to both speaker and listener? Other measures may provide insights into *treatment directions*, whether behavioral or surgical.

In our opinion, the best protocol for assessing voice in this patient population is one that does include measures designed to serve multiple purposes. Ideally, these purposes would include at least some that are useful to medical professionals, speech–language pathologists, the patient and his or her constellation of family and other caregivers, and those third parties that provide funding for treatment. Beyond this, the protocol should include only those measures that can be collected and interpreted accurately, compared with normative data and, given the exigencies of most clinical settings, be obtained in an expedient manner.

◆ **Voice Therapy**   Specific objectives for voice therapy in nontotal laryngectomy patients will be determined by the ablative treatment(s) undergone. Unfortunately, there are scant available data describing particular treatment protocols for any group of these patients, or describing effectiveness or efficacy of treatment. With limited resections, perhaps affecting only one vocal fold, the primary problem is likely to be voice quality related to alterations in the composition of the vibratory source. Stretching exercises (i.e., going from high to low in fundamental frequency in sweep or stair-step fashion) or vocal trills may be useful in increasing compliance and elasticity of residual tissue. Our usual practice is to recommend that patients perform such exercises several times a day, but for only a few minutes each session. We also encourage vocal hygiene measures, such as keeping well hydrated, practicing at least conservative reflux precautions, and avoiding vocal hyperfunction.

In more extensive resections, such as cordectomy, vertical partial laryngectomy, or subtotal procedures, voice therapy may be focused on involving residual or reconstructed tissues in sound generation. We have found the use of the flexible nasopharyngoscope quite useful to this purpose, both for the clinician attempting to maximize voicing potential, and as a feedback tool for patients who are learning to use a neoglottis. Vocal hygiene measures and the avoidance of vocal hyperfunction are also considered. Typically, supraglottic laryngectomy is associated with good voice, and the voice clinician's primary role here may be to troubleshoot possible factors that are preventing this outcome. In our experience, neoglottic reconstructions for near total laryngectomy have been quite variable. A viable sound source appears to be largely dependent on the success of surgery. If adequate sound is possible, then attempts to increase duration and perhaps achieve some variability in pitch or loudness may be explored. Prevention of hyperfunctional behaviors is also a realistic objective.

Implications of Laryngeal Resection for Swallowing

Total Laryngectomy and Swallowing

In total laryngectomy, the diversion of the airway precludes aspiration. Nevertheless, this patient population is not without dysphagia. Alterations in the UES caused by surgery or radiation may produce incomplete opening that prevents expedient entrance of material into the esophagus. Other authors have implicated the loss of laryngeal elevation as a factor in poor UES opening in these patients.[144] McConnel et al pointed out that increased resistance in the pharynx following laryngectomy could alter bolus flow and produce both longer transit times and increased activity by the tongue during bolus propulsion.[145] Strictures are other sources of dysphagia in this patient group, as illustrated in **Fig. 17.8A,B** and **Fig. 17.9**. Sometimes noted on videofluoroscopic studies (**Fig. 17.10**) is a pseudoepiglottis or scar band that acts to retain food and liquid.[146,147] In the example illustrated in

Fig. 17.9, the pocket was so large that material collected was eventually refluxed into the nose. Alterations in smell and taste are likely to influence food management independent of patients' ability to swallow.

Few data regarding the prevalence of dysphagia in patients with total laryngectomy are available, and there is broad variability across reported estimates.[148–150] In addition, swallowing difficulty among laryngectomy patients may be obscured by patients' successful attempts to accommodate their difficulty, as by modifying their diets or adapting facilitative techniques. Hillman et al reported few differences in swallowing difficulty at 2 years posttreatment in two treatment groups, one treated with laryngectomy and radiation; the second treated with radiation and induction chemotherapy.[102] In both groups, ~30% of patients continued to report swallowing difficulty.

More patients in the surgery plus radiation group (24%) reported diet modifications at 2 years than were noted for the chemotherapy plus radiation group (13%). Diet modifications, in order of frequency of occurrence, included soft mechanical texture, soft pureed, liquid, and tube feeding. Sixty-four percent of patients in the surgery plus radiation group continued to have taste abnormalities at 24 months; fewer than 45% of patients in the chemotherapy plus radiation group had similar complaints. Interestingly, in a subgroup of patients who had undergone chemotherapy and radiation with the larynx preserved, over 30% experienced alterations in taste 24 months posttreatment. Also reported by Hillman et al were data indicating that weight loss in the immediate posttreatment period was significantly less frequent in patients undergoing radiation than in patients undergoing surgery plus radiation.[104] By 24 months posttreatment, however, weight loss was reported in only 9% of patients in the surgery plus radiation group, and in less than 15% of patients in the chemotherapy plus radiation group.

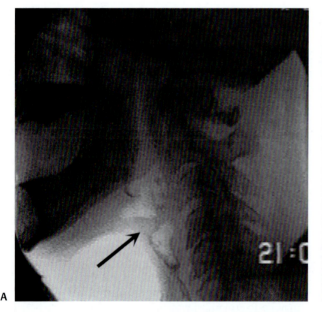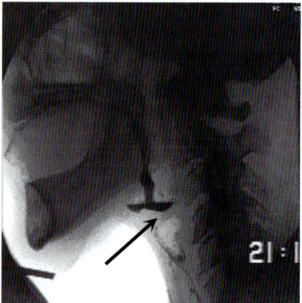

Fig. 17.8 (A) Stricture in laryngectomy patient. (B) Some bolus material trickles into lower pharynx.

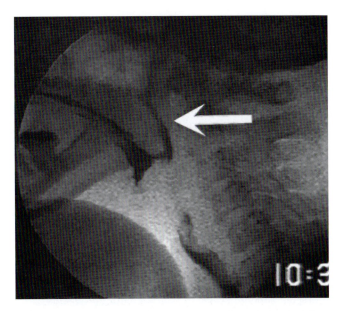

Fig. 17.9 Scar band is so large in this patient that bolus material is refluxed into the nose.

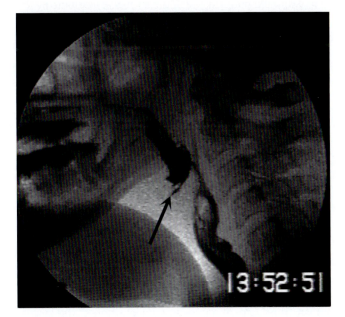

Fig. 17.10 Pseudoepiglottis in laryngectomy patient retains food and liquid.

Nontotal Laryngectomy and Swallowing

In nontotal laryngectomy, swallowing problems range from minimal to severe. With partial laryngectomy procedures, the airway remains intact. Airway protection and aspiration thus become potentially serious risks to patients. If resection involves only the intrinsic muscles of the larynx, then airway protection is likely to be the primary problem. As extent of resection increases to involve extrinsic muscles and structures, however, problems extend beyond airway protection

to other difficulties, including appropriate and adequate bolus propulsion and UES opening.

◆ **Glottic Carcinoma** Schneider et al reported on a group of 56 patients with T1-T2 glottic lesions, 40 of whom were treated by CO_2 laser surgery and 16 by primary radiotherapy.[151] According to these authors, patients in the surgery group scored significantly better than irradiated patients on survey questions related to swallowing solid foods and xerostomia. A 5-year follow-up study of 55 patients undergoing cricohyoepiglottopexy for T1 and T2 glottic carcinomas reported normal swallow function in 75% of cases, and occasional aspiration of liquids in 25% of cases.[139] Similar results for 98 patients who underwent cricohyoidopexy and 51 who underwent cricohyoidoepiglottopexy have been reported by de Vincentiis et al.[140] Partial laryngectomy involving reconstruction of a neoglottis using the epiglottis was described by Zanaret et al.[139] The procedure was performed on 57 patients with T1 or T2 glottic carcinoma. Although voice recovery, which was the main objective of the reconstruction, was unpredictable, all patients were reportedly swallowing between 5 and 22 days after surgery.

◆ **Hemilaryngectomy** This form of partial laryngectomy typically requires separating the infrahyoid musculature from the hyoid (and tongue base), the inferior constrictor muscle from the thyroid lamina, and cutting of the anterior cricothyroid muscle.[151] As a consequence, the residual laryngeal complex is likely to assume a lowered position in the neck. This situation can make elevation of the larynx to a protective position under the tongue base problematic. In an investigation of 11 hemilaryngectomy patients, Schoenrock et al found asymmetric laryngeal elevation and good tongue–larynx approximation only on the unoperated side.[152] In addition, the unilateral absence of a true vocal fold, false vocal fold, and aryepiglottic fold pose further problems for adequate protection of the airway during swallowing. If a pyriform sinus is closed, perhaps as a consequence of using its mucosa to reconstruct the involved side, bolus material can be funneled directly to the glottis to pose a serious challenge to residual airway protection mechanisms. Loss of sensation that may result if the superior laryngeal nerve is involved in resection may jeopardize awareness of impending or present bolus material in the airway.

Rademaker et al compared postoperative swallowing in patients undergoing different types of partial laryngectomy surgeries.[153] A measure of swallow "efficiency," defined as the percent of bolus material actually swallowed into the esophagus divided by oropharyngeal transit time, was obtained from a videofluoroscopic study. In addition, times to achievement of oral intake, removal of feeding tube, preoperative diet, and normal swallow were considered. Nine out of 12 patients with hemilaryngectomy (two patients had preoperative radiotherapy and one had postoperative radiotherapy) achieved all outcomes. The median time to achievement of normal swallow was 25 days in patients with the vocal process removed, and 50 days in patients with some portion of the anterior commissure involved in resection. The swallow efficiency measure calculated for liquids at 2 weeks postsurgery was found to be predictive of time to achieve oral intake, feeding tube removal, and return to preoperative diet. For example, for every 10-point increase in swallowing efficiency, there was about a 20% increase in the probability that preoperative diet would be achieved.

Another factor likely to influence swallowing outcome in hemilaryngectomy is type of reconstruction. To our knowledge, however, there have been no investigations comparing effects of reconstruction type on swallowing. In other cases, little or no objective information is provided regarding swallowing function in patients reconstructed with a particular technique. Calcaterra described the use of a superiorly based sternohyoid myofascial flap to reconstruct the larynx in 31 patients and noted that swallowing was achieved in all patients without significant aspiration.[154] In addition, all patients were eventually extubated. Chantrain et al described the use of a radial forearm free flap, including the tendon of the palmaris longus and a sensory branch of the radial nerve, in reconstructing patients with a vertical hemilaryngectomy and pharyngectomy.[155] According to these authors, swallowing was functional even in these patients with extended resections. Other materials used have included nasal septal cartilage and auricular cartilage. Sekercioglu et al report findings for 12 patients with this type of reconstruction and noted an average of 19 days to decannulation. Little detail is provided regarding swallowing function, however, except to say it was satisfactory.[156] McConnel and O'Connor have noted that arytenoid fixation as a consequence of radiation, or resection of the arytenoid, can produce dysphagia in hemilaryngectomy due to glottic incompetence, loss of arytenoid–tongue contact, and impaired ZUES opening.[75] They stress mucosal coverage of all exposed cartilage in cases where the laryngectomy follows radiation failure, and reconstruction of the vocal fold with a muscle flap or cartilage graft if the arytenoid is resected.

◆ **Supraglottic Laryngectomy** Although the true vocal folds typically remain intact in supraglottic laryngectomy, loss of the false vocal folds, epiglottis, and aryepiglottic folds poses a serious challenge to airway protection. In addition, the loss of the valleculae and the shallowness of the pyriform sinuses eliminate two potential "holding areas" available when bolus material is not transported through the oro- or hypopharynx in an appropriate or timely manner. Not surprisingly, it is this group of laryngectomy patients who are generally considered to have the greatest swallowing deficits posttreatment. Weaver et al noted that 16/23 (70%) patients with supraglottic laryngectomy were still experiencing chronic mild to severe aspiration 6 months postoperatively, although only 1/23 (4%) was not eating orally.[157]

Strijbos et al described 37/56 (66%) patients eating normally at 1 year, but continued occasional aspiration in 32 of the 56 (57%) patients at 3 years postsurgery.[158] These results are similar to those reported by Maceri et al for 33 supraglottic laryngectomy patients.[159] These authors noted that, by 3 years postsurgery, 20/33 (61%) patients were not demonstrating aspiration, 9/33 (27%) demonstrated some aspiration, and 4/33 (12%) were still nonoral.

In an investigation of swallowing in patients with various types of partial laryngectomy, Rademaker et al found that supraglottic laryngectomy patients required a median time to "normal" swallow of 106 days.[160] In supraglottic patients whose surgeries were extended (i.e., involved the pyriform sinus, arytenoid cartilage, or tongue base), this time was greatly increased, requiring 6 months to a year. In fact, a return to normal swallow had not been achieved at 1 year in a significant percentage of these patients.

McConnel and Mendelsohn found three factors that appeared to predispose supraglottic laryngectomy patients to aspiration.[74] These included, first, a lowered resting position of the larynx in the neck that prevented its elevation during swallow to a protected position under the tongue base. Second, incomplete contact between the tongue and larynx prevented residue that may have fallen on glottic structures from being swept posteriorly into the esophagus. Third, some patients who did demonstrate laryngeal elevation did so in delayed fashion, thus rendering the airway insufficiently protected and vulnerable to aspiration during swallow.

Logemann et al described similar results for a group of nine supraglottic laryngectomy patients.[160] As compared with control subjects, the laryngectomy patients 2 weeks postsurgery exhibited poor closure of the laryngeal vestibule by the arytenoid cartilage and base of tongue, poor movement of the tongue base to the posterior pharyngeal wall, reduced laryngeal elevation, increased width of cricopharyngeal opening, and later onset of airway closure and tongue base movement. By 3 months postsurgery, those patients who were able to eat orally demonstrated significantly longer duration of tongue base contact to the pharyngeal wall, longer duration of airway closure, and greater movement of the arytenoid cartilage. Based on these findings, the authors suggested that swallowing therapy in supraglottic laryngectomy patients should be directed to improved posterior tongue base movement and anterior tilting of the arytenoid to facilitate closure of the laryngeal vestibule.

Schweinfurth and Silver performed a retrospective review of videofluoroscopic studies and other records on nine supraglottic laryngectomy patients.[161] According to the authors, factors that predisposed these patients to a higher risk of aspiration included a lowered larynx position and delayed oropharyngeal transit times. Conversely, those patients who did relatively better demonstrated shorter oropharyngeal transit times and an anterosuperior position of the larynx. Five of nine patients resumed a regular diet, including thin liquids, within 1 year of surgery. In some contrast to these findings, Hirano et al investigated records of 38 supraglottic laryngectomy patients and noted that the standard supraglottic procedure, including surgical approximation of the larynx to the base of the tongue and cricopharyngeal myotomy, did not produce serious deglutition problems.[162] However, when removal of an arytenoid cartilage or asymmetrical removal of the false vocal folds occurred, problems were exacerbated. Only three of the 38 patients in this study continued to eat nonorally after 60 days postsurgery. Hirano's results were mirrored by Flores et al in 46 patients with supraglottic laryngectomy.[163] These authors considered effects on deglutition of preservation of the hyoid bone, arytenoid resection, base of tongue resection, vagus paralysis, and cricopharyngeal myotomy. Arytenoid resection was the only variable found to be significantly related to poorer swallow function.

Steiniger et al compared morbidity in two groups of supraglottic carcinoma patients, 12 patients who underwent surgery only, and 17 patients who underwent surgery and postoperative radiotherapy.[164] According to the authors, there were nonsignificant trends toward greater tracheotomy dependence (24% vs 0%), aspiration pneumonia (35% vs 9%), and delayed swallowing (34.8 weeks vs 7.8 weeks) in patients who received the combined therapy. Another factor reported to influence swallowing outcomes in supraglottic laryngectomy patients is pulmonary function. Beckhardt et al noted that a ratio of forced expiratory volume in 1 second to forced vital capacity ($FEV_1 : FVC$) of less than 50% signified a greater risk for severe aspiration and deglutition complications, whereas extensions of the standard procedure did not correlate significantly with increased problems in the group of patients they studied.[165]

◆ **Subtotal Laryngectomy** Although numerous subtotal laryngectomy procedures have been reported, few details of their effects on swallowing have been noted. As previously noted, Pearson et al described a subtotal laryngectomy procedure that preserved a myomucosal segment of intrinsic glottic musculature attached to the recurrent laryngeal nerve and formed into a mucosa-lined tube that could act as a neoglottis for voicing, and constrict to close during swallowing.[134] Initial results for seven patients revealed no significant aspiration.

Effects of Radiation

As previously noted, radiation effects on head and neck tissues are likely to affect both speech and swallowing. In the case of laryngeal cancer, the UES is within the field for external beam radiotherapy of the adjacent larynx, and in fact apparently receives the full radiation dose. Gaze et al investigated the effects of laryngeal irradiation, 13 to 71 months posttreatment, on pharyngoesophageal motility in 19 patients with T1 to T3 glottic carcinomas.[166] Results were compared with findings in 23 healthy controls. Using manometric techniques, the authors measured lower esophageal sphincter pressure, distal peristaltic contraction, tonic UES pressure, and several pharyngoesophageal dynamics during bread and water swallows. Findings included evidence of decrements in peristaltic wave velocity and increases in wave duration that were inversely related to posttreatment interval. No effects were noted on upper or lower sphincter tone. Delayed effects of radiation, as these relate to swallowing (or voice), have not been widely reported.

Swallowing Rehabilitation in Laryngectomy

◆ **Assessment** The same techniques described for swallowing assessment in patients with oral/oropharyngeal cancer, including a bedside or clinical swallow evaluation, videofluoroscopic study, and FEES are equally appropriate for laryngectomy patients and won't be reviewed again here. However, the clinician's focus for each of these assessment tools is likely to differ with laryngectomy patients. For example, if a total laryngectomy patient is experiencing dysphagia, factors that interfere with successful transport of bolus material into the esophagus, such as strictures or obstructions, are often suspected. And, unless the tongue base or pharynx has been involved in the resection, oral and perhaps oropharyngeal components of swallow are likely to remain intact, whereas hypopharyngeal and laryngeal components may be missing or greatly altered. As previously described, radiographic studies performed within 2 weeks of surgery may be useful not only in identifying specific causes of dysphagia but also in predicting eventual outcomes related to return to oral feeding or normal swallow.[62]

Other assessment tools provide valuable insights into the impact of swallowing disability on a patient's quality of life. These have been demonstrated to be particularly useful when completed by patients, as opposed to caregivers, and when administered at various times over the course of treatment. Though quality of life measures do not provide specific information regarding causes of dysphagia, they do direct attention to related issues, such as xerostomia and excessive mucus, which may be as much of a burden to patients as an inability or altered ability to manage food and liquids. The inclusion of this type of information in clinical trials research designed to evaluate treatment outcomes has become increasingly apparent. Several currently available quality of life instruments address swallowing, as well as voice and speech. These include the Performance Status Scale for Head and Neck Cancer Patients, which includes diet, speech, and eating in public subscales[167]; the European Organization for Research and Treatment of Cancer Quality of Life Questionnaire (EORTC)[168]; and the FACT-HN (Functional Assessment of Cancer Therapy-Head and Neck), a multidimensional quality of life measure.[169]

◆ **Swallowing Therapy** From the perspective of the "valves" and "chambers" model described before, at least two causes of dysphagia are likely to be predominant in this patient population. If resection is confined to the true vocal folds, then it is closure of the laryngeal valve that will need to be addressed. If resection has involved the vocal folds and other laryngeal valves, and has also disassociated the larynx from its usual suspensory association with pharyngeal and oral cavity structures, problems will be more extensive. Airway protection, adequate opening of the UES, and poor clearing of the hypopharynx, in particular, may all need to be considered.

Swallowing therapy can be initiated within days after surgery and is designed to move patients from nonoral to safe and effective oral feeding as quickly as possible. The specific behavioral strategies noted previously, including *exercise, bolus manipulation, postural compensations,* and *facilitative maneuvers,* constitute the basis of behavioral swallowing therapy and can be applied when radiographic and other evidence suggests their appropriateness and advisability.

In our experience, airway protection is typically a preliminary and primary therapeutic target for this group of patients. For example, Mozolewski et al noted that breath holding during normal swallow typically requires 1.3 seconds; for patients with supraglottic laryngectomy, this may be increased to 9 or 10 seconds.[170] A single objective, such as learning to maximize length and extent of vocal fold closure, or improving arytenoid to tongue base approximation, may be sufficient to ensure safe swallowing. In other cases, or when problems extend beyond vocal fold valving, combined strategies may be required, that is, maximizing extent and duration of laryngeal closure, performing a chin tuck, and swallowing a nonliquid bolus that is directed to the most intact side by assuming a side-lying position. Visual feedback from a FEES study can be an effective tool for teaching patients particular strategies and for demonstrating their effects. In other instances, evidence from radiographic or FEES studies is crucial to identifying problems for which other types of intervention are appropriate. Strictures, spasms, or pouches that are observed on a dynamic swallow study, for example, may require dilation or surgery.

Data pertinent to the benefits of swallowing therapy for patients with laryngeal cancer are generally unavailable. Denk et al considered several variables, including swallowing therapy, that influenced swallow recovery in 35 patients with various types of head and neck cancer.[171] The authors found a positive correlation between early onset of behavioral therapy and eventual recovery of oral swallow, and suggested early intervention based on videoendoscopic and fluoroscopic findings. Logemann et al similarly urged the use of videofluoroscopy and swallowing therapy in the first 3 months following treatment for various types of head and neck cancer.[172] These authors also reported preliminary findings supporting the use of range of motion exercises for improving swallowing (and speech) in head and neck cancer patients.

Changes in Residual/Reconstructed Tissues

In addition to a *loss* of tissue, ablative procedures of the head and neck produce alterations in residual tissue. Both speech and swallowing are influenced or regulated by sensory capabilities of receptors in the skin, muscles, and joints of pertinent structures. Certainly, touch-pressure and kinesthetic and proprioceptive sensory receptors in head and neck structures might be expected to undergo temporary or permanent alteration as a consequence of ablative and reconstructive surgical procedures. Exactly what these changes might be, however, and how they might contribute to degree of impairment, is not known.

Other structures involved in resection, residual innervation, pre- or postoperative radiation, and repeated surgeries (each with attendant scarring), represent other variables for which effects are still not well understood. The possible influence on speech and swallowing of these factors—loss of sensation, diminished hydration, decreased blood supply, and fibrosis of at least some tissue components in the oral cavity, pharynx, and larynx—is at this time primarily a matter of speculation. Determination of the precise relationship between any one of these variables and speech or swallow-

ing is further clouded by an individual's ability to compensate, or to reorganize, in the face of alterations to structure and function. However rudimentary our understanding, an elaboration of speech and swallowing characteristics related to ablative procedures must consider the consequences not only of loss of tissue, but also, of alterations in residual and reconstructed tissues.

◆ Summary

As stated at the outset, ablative procedures of the head and neck can have profound, deleterious consequences for voice, speech, and swallowing. Recovery from disease may not mean a return to normal good health. The course of rehabilitation may be marked by serious functional deficits that affect a patient's physical and emotional health in equal parts. The challenges to patients and their families are sometimes enormous. It is also true that the challenge to care providers charged with improving speech and swallowing can be formidable. For certain of the head and neck populations, in fact, there is little evidence from groups of patients that our interventions are even recommended or attempted. And until we provide the experimental evidence that they should be, the situation is not likely to change.

The need for experimental inquiry into our own specific treatment strategies, applied to specific populations, in a manner that permits valid and reliable outcome data, is critical. Beyond this, we have a unique opportunity to collaborate with surgeons and other care providers in designing investigations that answer questions regarding, for example, optimal reconstructive strategies as these relate to speech and swallowing, or to specific effects of various treatment modalities on speech and swallowing. As issues regarding survival from head and cancer permit, physicians are able to focus to a greater extent on functional outcomes, including speech, voice, and swallowing. Our combined efforts to consider these is likely, ultimately, to provide significant insights into what constitutes optimal management, and to produce the best results for patients.

References

1. Robbins KT, ed. Pocket Guide to Neck Dissection. Classification and TNM Staging of Head and Neck Cancer. Alexandria, VA: American Academy of Otolaryngology–Head and Neck Surgery and Oncology Foundation; 1991

2. Sussman HM, MacNeilage PF, Hanson R. Labial and mandibular dynamics during the production of bilabial consonants: preliminary observations. J Speech Hear Res 1973;16:397–420

3. Bloomer H, Hawk H. Speech considerations: speech disorders associated with ablative surgery of the face, mouth and pharynx—ablative approaches to learning. ASHA Reports 1972;8:42–61

4. Cantor R, Curtis T. Prosthetic management of edentulous mandibulectomy patients, I: Anatomic, physiologic and psychologic considerations. J Prosthet Dent 1971;25:446–457

5. Majid AA, Weinberg B, Chalian B. Speech intelligibility following prosthetic obturation of surgically acquired maxillary defects. J Prosthet Dent 1974;32:87–96

6. Masuda M, Kida Y, Ohtani T. Oral rehabilitation by prosthetic restoration after maxillectomy for malignant tumors. Int J Oral Surg 1979;8:356–362

7. Fletcher SG, Soodi I, Frost SD. Quantitative and graphic analysis of prosthetic treatment for "nasalance" in speech. J Prosthet Dent 1974;32:284–291

8. Plank DM, Weinberg B, Chalian V. Evaluation of speech following prosthetic obturation of surgically acquired maxillary defects. J Prosthet Dent 1981;45:626–638

9. Fletcher SG. Speech production following partial glossectomy. J Speech Hear Disord 1988;53:232–238

10. Allison GR, Rappaport I, Salibian A. Adaptive mechanisms of speech and swallowing after combined jaw and tongue reconstruction. Am J Surg 1987;154:419–422

11. Barry WJ, Timmerman G. Mispronunciations and compensatory movements of tongue-operated patients. Br J Disord Commun 1985;20:81–90

12. Morrish L. Compensatory vowel articulation of the glossectomee. Br J Disord Commun 1984;19:125–134

13. Leonard R, Gillis R. Effects of a prosthetic tongue on vowel intelligibility and food management in a patient with total glossectomy. J Speech Hear Disord 1982;47:25–30

14. Georgian DA, Logemann J, Fisher H. Compensatory articulation patterns of a treated oral cancer patient. J Speech Hear Disord 1982; 47:154–159

15. Bradley PJ, Hoover L, Stell P. Assessment of articulation after surgery in the tongue. Folia Phoniatr (Basel) 1980;32:334–341

16. LaRiviere C, Seilo M, Dimmick K. Report on the speech intelligibility of a glossectomee: perceptual and acoustic observations. Folia Phoniatr (Basel) 1975;27:201–214

17. Amerman JD, Laminack K. Evaluation and rehabilitation of glossectomy speech behavior. J Commun Disord 1974;7:365–374

18. Skelly M, Spector D, Donaldson R, et al. Compensatory physiologic phonetics for the glossectomee. J Speech Hear Disord 1971;36:101–114

19. Massengill R Jr, Maxwell S, Pickrell K. An analysis of articulation following partial and total glossectomy. J Speech Hear Disord 1970;35:170–173

20. Heller KS, Levy J, Sciubba JJ. Speech patterns following partial glossectomy for small tumors of the tongue. Head Neck 1991;13:340–343

21. Pruszewicz A, Kruk-Zagajewska A. Phoniatric disturbances in patients after partial tongue resection for malignant neoplasms. Folia Phoniatr (Basel) 1984;36:84–92

22. Colangelo LA, Logemann JA, Pauloski BR, Pelzer JR, Rademaker AW. T stage and functional outcome in oral and oropharyngeal cancer patients. Head Neck 1996;18:259–268

23. Weber RS, Ohlms L, Bowman J, Jacob R, Goepfert H. Functional results after total or near total glossectomy with laryngeal preservation. Arch Otolaryngol Head Neck Surg 1991;117:512–515

24. Salibian AH, Allison GR, Rappaport I, Krugman ME, McMicken BL, Etchepare TL. Total and subtotal glossectomy: function after microvascular reconstruction. Plast Reconstr Surg 1990;85:513–524

25. Mitrani M, Krespi YP. Functional restoration after subtotal glossectomy and laryngectomy. Otolaryngol Head Neck Surg 1988;98:5–9

26. Leonard R, Goodrich S, McMenamin P, Donald P. Differentiation of speakers with glossectomies by acoustic and perceptual measures. Am J Speech Lang Pathol 1992;1:56–63

27. Leonard RJ. Computerized design of speech prostheses. J Prosthet Dent 1991;66(3):224–230

28. Salibian AH, Allison GR, Krugman ME, et al. Reconstruction of the base of the tongue with the microvascular ulnar forearm flap: a functional assessment. Plast Reconstr Surg 1995;96:1081–1091

29. Michi K, Imai S, Yamashita Y, Suzuki N. Improvement of speech intelligibility by a secondary operation to mobilize the tongue after glossectomy. J Craniomaxillofac Surg 1989;17:162–166

30. Bradley PJ, Hoover L, Stell P. Assessment of articulation after surgery in the tongue. Folia Phoniatr (Basel) 1980;32:334–341

31. Rentschler GJ, Mann M. The effects of glossectomy on intelligibility of speech and oral perceptual discrimination. J Oral Surg 1980;38:348–350

32. Skelly M, Spector D, Donaldson R, et al. Compensatory physiologic phonetics for the glossectomee. J Speech Hear Disord 1971;36:101–114

33. McConnel FM, Teichgraeber J, Adler R. A comparison of three methods of oral reconstruction. Arch Otolaryngol Head Neck Surg 1987;113:496–500

34. McConnel FM, Pauloski BR, Logemann JA, et al. Functional results of primary closure vs. flaps in oropharyngeal reconstruction: a prospective study of speech and swallowing. Arch Otolaryngol Head Neck Surg 1998;124:625–630

35. Pauloski BR, Rademaker AW, Logemann JA, et al. Surgical variables affecting speech in treated patients with oral and oropharyngeal cancer. Laryngoscope 1998;108:908–916

36. Mirza FD, Dikshit JV. Use of implant prostheses following radiation therapy. J Prosthet Dent 1978;40:663–667

37. Pauloski BR, Logemann JA, Colangelo LA, Rademaker AW. Speech and swallowing in irradiated and nonirradiated postsurgical oral cancer patients. Otolaryngol Head Neck Surg 1998;118:616–624

38. Hamlet SL, Mathog RH, Patterson RL, Fleming SM. Tongue mobility in speech after partial glossectomy. Head Neck 1990;12:210–217

39. Stevens K. The quantal nature of speech: evidence from articulatory-acoustic data. In: Penes P and David E, eds. Human Communication: A Unified View. New York: McGraw-Hill; 1972:51–65

40. Stevens KN, House A. An acoustical theory of vowel production and some of its implications. J Speech Hear Res 1961;4:303–320

41. Leonard RJ, Gillis R. Differential effects of prostheses in glossectomized patients. J Prosthet Dent 1990;64:701–708

42. Logemann JA, Kahrilas PJ, Hurst P, Davis J, Krugler C. Effects of intraoral prosthetics on swallowing in patients with oral cancer. Dysphagia 1989;4:118–120

43. Davis JW, Lazarus C, Logemann J, Hurst P. Effect of a maxillary glossectomy prosthesis on articulation and swallowing. J Prosthet Dent 1987;57:715–719

44. Izdebski K, Ross J, Roberts W, deBoie R. An interim prosthesis for the glossectomy patient. J Prosthet Dent 1987;57:608–611

45. Robbins KT, Bowman J, Jacob R. Postglossectomy deglutitory and articulatory rehabilitation with palatal augmentation prostheses. Arch Otolaryngol Head Neck Surg 1987;113:1214–1218

46. Knowles JC, Chalian V, Shanks J. A functional speech impression used to fabricate a maxillary speech prosthesis for a partial glossectomy patient. J Prosthet Dent 1984;51:232–237

47. Leonard RJ, Gillis RE. Effects of a prosthetic tongue on vowel formants and isovowel lines in a patient with total glossectomy. J Speech Hear Disord 1983;48:423–426

48. Gillis RE, Leonard RJ. Prosthetic treatment for speech and swallowing in a patient with total glossectomy. J Prosthet Dent 1983;50:808–814

49. Leonard R, Gillis R. Effects of a prosthetic tongue on vowel intelligibility and food management in a patient with total glossectomy. J Speech Hear Disord 1982;47:25–30

50. Lauciello FR, Vergo T, Schaaf N, Zimmerman R. Prosthodontic and speech rehabilitation after partial and complete glossectomy. J Prosthet Dent 1980;43:204–211

51. Wheeler RL, Logemann J, Rosen J. A maxillary reshaping prosthesis: its effectiveness in improving the speech and swallowing of postsurgical oral cancer patients. J Prosthet Dent 1980;43:491–495

52. Rentschler GJ, Mann M. The effects of glossectomy on intelligibility of speech and oral perceptual discrimination. J Oral Surg 1980;38:348–354

53. Hufnagle J, Pullon P, Hufnagle K. Speech considerations in oral surgery, II: Speech characteristics of patients following surgery for oral malignancies. Oral Surg Oral Med Oral Pathol 1978;46:354–361

54. LaRiviere C, Seilo M, Dimmik K. Report on the speech intelligibility of a glossectomee: perceptual and acoustic observations. Folia Phoniatr (Basel) 1975;27:201–214

55. Moore DJ. Glossectomy rehabilitation by mandibular tongue prosthesis. J Prosthet Dent 1972;28:429–433

56. Lehman WL, Hulicka IM, Mehringer E. Prosthetic treatment following complete glossectomy. J Prosthet Dent 1966;16:344–350

57. Duguay MJ. Speech after glossectomy. N Y State J Med 1964;64:1836–1838

58. Logemann JA, Kahrilas PJ, Hurst P, Davis J, Krugler C. Effects of intraoral prosthetics on swallowing in patients with oral cancer. Dysphagia 1989;4:118–120

59. Leonard R. Speech characteristics in speakers with glossectomy and other oral/oropharyngeal ablation. In: Bernthal J, ed. Child Phonology: Characteristics, Assessments, and Intervention with Special Populations. New York: Thieme; 1995

60. Leonard R, Goncalves M. Speech rehabilitation post-glossectomy. In: Robbins T, Murry T, eds. Head and Neck Cancer: Organ Preservation, Function and Rehabilitation. San Diego: Singular; 1998

61. Pauloski BR, Logemann JA, Rademaker AW, et al. Speech and swallowing function after oral and oropharyngeal resections: one-year follow-up. Head Neck 1994;16:313–322

62. Dodds WJ, Man KM, Cook IJ, Kahrilas PJ, Stewart ET, Kern MK. Influence of bolus volume on swallow-induced hyoid movement in normal subjects. AJR Am J Roentgenol 1988;150:1307–1309

63. Logemann JA. Evaluation and Treatment of Swallowing Disorders. San Diego: College Hill; 1983

64. Hrycyshyn AW, Basmajian J. Electromyography of the oral stage of swallowing in man. Am J Anat 1972;133:333–340

65. Bosma JF. Deglutition: pharyngeal stage. Physiol Rev 1957;37:275–300

66. Fink B. The Human Larynx: A Functional Study. New York: Raven; 1975

67. Donald P. Head and Neck Cancer: Management of the Difficult Case. Philadelphia: WB Saunders; 1984

68. Wheeler RL, Logemann J, Rosen J. A maxillary reshaping prosthesis: its effectiveness in improving the speech and swallowing of postsurgical oral cancer patients. J Prosthet Dent 1980;43:313–319

69. Doberneck RC, Antoine A. Deglutition after resection of oral, laryngeal and pharyngeal cancers. Surgery 1974;75:87–90

70. Conley JJ. Swallowing dysfunction associated with radical surgery of the head and neck. Arch Surg 1960;80:602–612

71. Shedd D, Scatliff J, Kirchner J. The buccopharyngeal propulsive mechanism in human deglutition. Surgery 1960;48:846–853

72. McConnel FM, Tiechgraeber J, Alder R. A comparison of three methods of oral reconstruction. Arch Otolaryngol Head Neck Surg 1987;113:496–500

73. Logemann JA, Bytell DE. Swallowing disorders in three types of head and neck surgical patients. Cancer 1979;44:1095–1105

74. McConnell FM, Mendelsohn M. The effects of surgery on pharyngeal deglutition. Dysphagia 1987;1:145–151

75. McConnel FM, O'Connor A. Dysphagia secondary to head and neck cancer surgery. Acta Otorhinolaryngol Belg 1994;48:165–170

76. Hamlet S, Jones L, Mathog R, Bolton M, Patterson R. Bolus propulsive activity of the tongue in dysphagic cancer patients. Dysphagia 1988;3:18–233

77. Langmore SE, Schatz K, Olsen N. Fiberoptic endoscopic examination of swallowing safety: a new procedure. Dysphagia 1988;2:216–219

78. Hamlet SL, Muz J, Patterson R, Jones L. Pharyngeal transit time: assessment with videofluoroscopic and scintigraphic techniques. Dysphagia 1989;4:4–7

79. McConnel FM, Cerenko D, Mendelsohn MS. Manofluorographic analysis of swallowing. Otolaryngol Clin North Am 1988;21:625–635

80. Leonard R, Kendall K. Dysphagia Assessment and Treatment Planning: A Team Approach. San Diego: Singular; 1997

81. Zormeier MM, Meleca RJ, Simpson ML, et al. Botulinum toxin to improve tracheoesophageal speech after total laryngectomy. Otolaryngol Head Neck Surg 1999;120:314–319

82. Izdebski K, Fontanesi J, Ross JC, Hetzler D. The effects of irradiation on alaryngeal voice of totally laryngectomized patients. Int J Radiat Oncol Biol Phys 1988;14:1281–1286

83. Blom ED, Singer MI. Tracheoesophageal puncture: a surgical prosthetic method for post laryngectomy speech restoration. Proceedings of the 3rd International Symposium on Plastic and Reconstructive Surgery of the Head and Neck, 1979

84. Izdebski K, Reed CG, Ross JC, Hilsinger RL Jr. Problems with tracheoesophageal fistula voice restoration in totally laryngectomized patients. a review of 95 cases. Arch Otolaryngol Head Neck Surg 1994;120:840–845

85. Wenig BL, Mullooly V, Levy J, Abramson AL. Voice restoration following laryngectomy: the role of primary versus secondary tracheoesophageal puncture. Ann Otol Rhinol Laryngol 1989;98(1 Pt 1):70–73

86. Kao WW, Mohr RM, Kimmel CA, Getch C, Silverman C. The outcome and techniques of primary and secondary tracheoesophageal puncture. Arch Otolaryngol Head Neck Surg 1994;120:301–307

87. Trudeau MD, Schuller DE, Hall DA. The effects of radiation on tracheoesophageal puncture: a retrospective study. Arch Otolaryngol Head Neck Surg 1989;115:1116–1117

88. Artazkoz del Toro JJ, Lopez Martinez R. Surgical voice rehabilitation: influence of postoperative radiotherapy on tracheoesophageal fistulas: long-term follow-up study. Acta Otorrinolaringol Esp 1997;48:299–304

89. LaBruna A, Klatsky I, Huo J, Weiss MH. Tracheoesophageal puncture in irradiated patients. Ann Otol Rhinol Laryngol 1995;104(4 Pt 1):279–281

90. McAuliffe MJ, Ward EC, Bassett L, Perkins K. Functional speech outcomes after laryngectomy and pharyngolaryngectomy. Arch Otolaryngol Head Neck Surg 2000;126:705–709

91. Deschler DG, Doherty ET, Reed CG, Anthony JP, Singer MI. Tracheoesophageal voice following tubed free radial forearm flap reconstruction of the neopharynx. Ann Otol Rhinol Laryngol 1994;103:929–936

92. Simpson CB, Postma GN, Stone RE Jr, Ossoff RH. Speech outcomes after laryngeal cancer management. Otolaryngol Clin North Am 1997;30:189–204

93. Izdebski K, Ross JC, Lee S. Fungal colonization of tracheoesophageal voice prosthesis. Laryngoscope 1987;97:594–597

94. Eerenstein SE, Grolman W, Schouwenburg PF. Microbial colonization of silicone voice prostheses used in laryngectomized patients. Clin Otolaryngol 1999;24:398–403

95. Graville D, Gross N, Andersen P, Everts E, Cohen J. The long-term indwelling tracheoesophageal prosthesis for alaryngeal voice rehabilitation. Arch Otolaryngol Head Neck Surg 1999;125:288–292

96. Leder SB, Erskine MC. Voice restoration after laryngectomy: experience with the Blom-Singer extended-wear indwelling tracheoesophageal voice prosthesis. Head Neck 1997;19:487–493

97. Cavalot AL, Magnano M, Nazionale G, Rosso S, Ferrero V, Cortesina G. The use of indwelling phonatory valve in the rehabilitation of laryngectomized patients: preliminary results in 30 patients. Acta Otorhinolaryngol Ital 1997;17:109–114

98. Delsupehe K, Zink I, Lejaegere M, Delaere P. Prospective randomized comparative study of tracheoesophageal voice prosthesis: Blom-Singer versus Provox. Laryngoscope 1998;108:1561–1565

99. van den Hoogen FJ, Van den Berg RJ, Oudes MJ, Manni JJ. A prospective study of speech and voice rehabilitation after total laryngectomy with the low-resistance Groningen, Nijdam and Provox voice prostheses. Clin Otolaryngol 1998;23:425–431

100. Chung RP, Patel P, Ter Keurs M, Van Lith Bijl JT, Mahieu HF. In vitro and in vivo comparison of the low-resistance Groningen and the Provox tracheoesophageal voice prostheses. Rev Laryngol Otol Rhinol (Bord) 1998;119:301–306

101. Henley-Cohn JL, Hausfeld JN, Jakubeczak G. Artificial larynx prosthesis: comparative clinical evaluation. Laryngoscope 1984;94:43–45

102. Hillman RE, Walsh MJ, Wolf GT, Fisher SG, Hong WK. Functional outcomes following treatment for advanced laryngeal cancer. Ann Otol Rhinol Laryngol Suppl 1998;172:1–27

103. Gates GA, Ryan W, Cooper J, et al. Current status of laryngectomee rehabilitation, I: Results of therapy. Am J Otolaryngol 1982;3:1–7

104. St Guily JL, Angelard B, El-Bez M, et al. Postlaryngectomy voice restoration; a prospective study of 83 patients. Arch Otolaryngol Head Neck Surg 1992;118:252–255

105. Culton GL, Gerwin JM. Current trends in laryngectomy rehabilitation: a survey of speech-language pathologists. Otolaryngol Head Neck Surg 1998;118:458–463

106. Hoyt DJ, Lettinga J, Leopold K. The effect of head and neck radiation therapy on voice quality. Laryngoscope 1992;102:477–480

107. Murry T, Bone RC, Von Essen C. Changes in voice production during radiotherapy for laryngeal cancer. J Speech Hear Disord 1974;39:194–201

108. Stoicheff ML. Voice following radiotherapy. Laryngoscope 1975;805:608–618

109. Colton RH, Sagerman RH, Chung C, Yu Y, Reed G. Voice change after radiotherapy: some preliminary results. Radiology 1978;127:821–824

110. Tsunoda K, Soda Y, Tojima H, et al. Stroboscopic observation of the larynx after radiation in patients with T1 glottic carcinoma. Acta Otolaryngol Suppl 1997;527:165–166

111. Lehman JJ, Bless D, Brandenburg J. An objective assessment of voice production after radiation therapy for stage I squamous cell carcinoma of the glottis. Otolaryngol Head Neck Surg 1988;98:121–129

112. Rovirosa A, Martinez-Celdran E, Ortega A, et al. Acoustic analysis after radiotherapy in T1 vocal cord carcinoma: a new approach to the analysis of voice quality. Int J Radiat Oncol Biol Phys 2000;47:73–79

113. Dagli AS, Mahieu HF, Festen JM. Quantitative analysis of voice quality in early glottic pharyngeal carcinomas treated with radiotherapy. Eur Arch Otorhinolaryngol 1997;254:78–80

114. Aref A, Dworkin J, Devi S, Denton L, Fontanesi J. Objective evaluation of the quality of voice following radiation therapy for T1 glottic cancer. Radiother Oncol 1997;45:149–153

115. Benninger MS, Gillen J, Thieme P, Jacobson B, Dragovich J. Factors associated with recurrence and voice quality following radiation therapy for T1 and T2 glottic carcinomas. Laryngoscope 1994;104:294–298

116. McGuirt WF, Blalock D, Koufman J, Feehs R. Voice analysis of patients with endoscopically treated early glottic carcinoma. Ann Otol Rhinol Laryngol 1992;101:142–146

117. Casiano RR, Cooper J, Lundy D, Chandler J. Laser cordectomy for T1 glottic carcinoma: a 10-year experience and videostroboscopic findings. Otolaryngol Head Neck Surg 1991;104:831–837

118. Hirano M, Kurita S, Matsuoka H. Vocal function following hemilaryngectomy. Ann Otol Rhinol Laryngol 1987;96:586–589

119. Ott S, Klingholz F, Willich N, Kastenbauer E. Assessing the quality of the speaking voice after therapy of T1 and T2 vocal cord cancers. Laryngorhinootologie 1992;71:236–241

120. McGuirt WF, Blaylock D, Koufman J, et al. Comparative voice results after laser resection or irradiation of T1 vocal cord carcinoma. Arch Otolaryngol 1994;120:951–958

121. Cragle SP, Brandenburg JH. Laser cordectomy or radiotherapy: cure rates communication and cost. Otolaryngol Head Neck Surg 1993; 108:648–654

122. Epstein BE, Lee DJ, Kashima H, et al. Stage T1 glottic carcinoma: results of radiation therapy or laser excision. Radiology 1990;175:567–570

123. Rydell R, Schalen L, Fex S, et al. Voice evaluation before and after laser excision vs. radiotherapy of T1A glottic carcinoma. Acta Otolaryngol 1995;115:560–565

124. Delsupehe KG, Zink I, Lejaegere M, Bastian RW. Voice quality after narrow-margin laser cordectomy compared with laryngeal irradiation. Otolaryngol Head Neck Surg 1999;121:528–533

125. Rosier JF, Gregoire V, et al. Comparison of external radiotherapy, laser microsurgery and partial laryngectomy for the treatment of T1N0M0 glottic carcinomas: a retrospective evaluation. Radiother Oncol 1998; 48:175–183

126. Ott S, Klingholz F, Willich N, Kastenbauer E. Assessing the quality of the speaking voice after therapy of T1 and T2 vocal cord cancers. Laryngorhinootologie 1992;71:236–241

127. Olsen KD, Thomas JV, DeSanto LW, et al. Indications and results of cordectomy for early glottic carcinoma. Otolaryngol Head Neck Surg 1993;108:277–282

128. Bockler R, Bonkowsky V, Seidler T, Hacki T. Comparative voice quality evaluation after laser surgical versus fronto-lateral partial laryngectomy in T1b and T2 vocal cord carcinoma. Laryngorhinootologie 1999;78:512–515

129. Mandell DL, Woo P, Behin DS, et al. Videolaryngostroboscopy following vertical partial laryngectomy. Ann Otol Rhinol Laryngol 1999;108(11 Pt. 1):1061–1067

130. Salam MA, el-Kahky M, el-Mehiry H. The use of pyriform sinus mucosa for reconstruction after vertical partial laryngectomy. J Laryngol Otol 1992;106:900–902

131. Blaugrund SM, Gould WJ, Haji T, et al. Voice analysis of the partially ablated larynx: a preliminary report. Ann Otol Rhinol Laryngol 1984;93:311–317

132. Leeper HA, Heeneman H, Reynolds C. Vocal function following vertical hemilaryngectomy: a preliminary investigation. J Otolaryngol 1990;19:62–67

133. Laccourreye O, Hans S, Borzog-Grayeli A, Maulard-Durdux C, Brasnu D, Housset M. Complications of postoperative radiation therapy after partial laryngectomy in supraglottic cancer: a long-term evaluation. Otolaryngol Head Neck Surg 2000;122:752–757

134. Pearson BW, Woods RD, Hartman DE. Extended hemilaryngectomy for T3 glottic carcinoma with preservation of speech and swallowing. Laryngoscope 1980;90:1950–1961

135. Hoasjoe DK, Martin GF, Doyle PC, et al. A comparative acoustic analysis of voice production by near-total laryngectomy and normal laryngeal speakers. J Otolaryngol 1992;21:39–43

136. Hoyt DJ, Lettinga JW, Leopold KA, et al. The effect of head and neck radiation therapy on voice quality. Laryngoscope 1992;102:477–480

137. Lu X, Dong P. The use of platysmal cryocutaneous flaps in laryngeal reconstruction. Lin Chuang Er Bi Yan Hou Ke Za Zhi 1997;11:56–58

138. Laurian N, Zohar Y. Laryngeal reconstruction by composite nasal mucoseptal graft after partial laryngectomy: three years follow-up. Laryngoscope 1981;91:609–616

139. Zanaret M, Giovanni A, Gras R, et al. Near total laryngectomy with epiglottic reconstruction: long-term results in 57 patients. Am J Otolaryngol 1993;14:419–425

140. de Vincentiis M, Minni A, Gallo A, DiNardo A. Supracricoid partial laryngectomies: oncologic and functional results. Head Neck 1998;20:504–509

141. Lallement JG, Bonnin P, el-Sioufi I, Bousquet J. Cricohyoepiglottopexy: long-term results in 55 patients. J Laryngol Otol 1999;113:532–537

142. Naudo P, Laccourreye O, Weinstein G, Hans S, Laccourreye H, Brasnu D. Functional outcome and prognosis factors after supracricoid partial laryngectomy with cricohyoidopexy. Ann Otol Rhinol Laryngol 1997;106:291–296

143. Laccourreye O, Crevier-Buchman L, Weinstein G, Biacabe B, Laccourreye H, Brasnu D. Duration and frequency characteristics of speech and voice following supracricoid partial laryngectomy. Ann Otol Rhinol Laryngol 1995;104:516–521

144. Hamlet SL, Patterson R, Fleming S, Jones L. Sounds of swallowing following total laryngectomy. Dysphagia 1992;7:160–165

145. McConnel FM, Mendelsohn M, Logemann J. Examination of swallowing after total laryngectomy using manofluorography. Head Neck Surg 1986;9:3–12

146. Davis RK, Vincent ME, Shapshay SM, Strong MS. The anatomy and complications of "T" versus vertical closure of the hypopharynx after laryngectomy. Laryngoscope 1982;92:16–22

147. Kirchner JA, Scatliff J, Dey F, Shedd D. The pharynx after laryngectomy. Laryngoscope 1963;73:18–33

148. Gates GA, Ryan W, Cooper JC, et al. Current status of laryngectomy rehabilitation: results of therapy. Am J Otolaryngol 1982;3:1–7

149. Ackerstaff AH, Hilgers FJM, Aaronson NK, Balm AJM. Communication, functional disorders and lifestyle changes after total laryngectomy. Clin Otolaryngol 1994;19:295–300

150. Balfe DM, Koehler R, Setzen M, Weyman P, Baron R, Ogura J. Barium examination of the esophagus after total laryngectomy. Radiology 1982;143:501–508

151. Schneider A, Guidicelli M, Stockli SJ. Quality of life after treatment of laryngeal carcinoma: surgery versus radiotherapy. Schweiz Med Wochenschr Suppl 2000;116:31S–34S

152. Schoenrock LD, King AY, Everts EC, Schneider HJ, Shumrick DA. Hemilaryngectomy: deglutition evaluation and rehabilitation. Trans Am Acad Ophthalmol Otolaryngol 1972;76:752–757

153. Rademaker AW, Pauloski BR, Logemann JA, Shanahan TK. Oropharyngeal swallow efficiency as a representative measure of swallowing function. J Speech Hear Res 1994;37:314–325

154. Calcaterra TC. Sternohyoid myofascial flap reconstruction of the larynx for vertical partial laryngectomy. Laryngoscope 1983;93:422–424

155. Chantrain G, Deraemaecker R, Andry G, Thill MP, Greant P. Vertical hemipharyngolaryngectomy: reconstruction with the radial forearm free flap. Eur J Surg Oncol 1989;15:564–567

156. Sekercioglu N, Cansiz H, Gunes M. Reconstruction with composite nasal septal cartilage and auricular cartilage in extended partial laryngectomy. J Laryngol Otol 1996;110:739–741

157. Weaver AW, Fleming S. Partial laryngectomy: analysis of associated swallowing disorders. Am J Surg 1978;136:486–489

158. Strijbos M, van den Broek P, Manni JJ, Huygen PL. Supraglottic laryngectomy: short- and long-term functional results. Clin Otolaryngol Allied Sci 1987;12:265–270

159. Maceri DR, Lampe HB, Makielski KH, Passamani PP, Krause CJ. Conservation laryngeal surgery: a critical analysis. Arch Otolaryngol 1985;111:361–365

160. Logemann JA, Gibbons P, Rademaker AW, et al. Recovery of postoperative swallowing in patients undergoing partial laryngectomy. Head Neck 1993;15:325–334

161. Schweinfurth JM, Silver SM. Patterns of swallowing after supraglottic laryngectomy. Laryngoscope 2000;110:1266–1270

162. Hirano M, Kurita S, Tateishi M, Matsuoka H. Deglutition following supraglottic horizontal laryngectomy. Ann Otol Rhinol Laryngol 1987;96(6 Pt 1):7–11

163. Flores TC, Wood BG, Levine HL, Koegel L Jr, Tucker HM. Factors in successful deglutition following supraglottic laryngeal surgery. Ann Otol Rhinol Laryngol 1982;91(6 Pt 1):579–583

164. Steiniger JR, Parnes SM, Gardner GM. Morbidity of combined therapy for the treatment of supraglottic carcinoma: supraglottic laryngectomy and radiotherapy. Ann Otol Rhinol Laryngol 1997;106:151–158

165. Beckhardt RN, Murray JG, Ford CN, Grossman JE, Brandenburg JH. Factors influencing functional outcome in supraglottic laryngectomy. Head Neck 1994;16:232–239

166. Gaze MN, Wilson JA, Gilmour HM, MacDougall RH, Maran AG. The effect of laryngeal irradiation on pharyngeoesophageal motility. Int J Radiat Oncol Biol Phys 1991;21:1315–1320

167. List MA, Ritter-Sterr C, Lansky SB. A performance status scale for head and neck cancer patients. Cancer 1990;66:564–569

168. Bjordal K, Hammerlid E, Ahlner-Elmquist M, et al. Quality of life in head and neck cancer patients: validation of the European Organization for Research and Treatment of Cancer Quality of Life Questionnaire-H&N35. J Clin Oncol 1999;17:1008–1019

169. Cella DF, Tulsky DS, Gray G, et al. The Functional Assessment of Cancer Therapy scale: development and validation of the general measure. J Clin Oncol 1993;11:570–579

170. Mozolewski E, Sulikowski M, Wysocki R. Mechanism of swallowing following horizontal laryngectomy: a radiological study. Ann Acad Med Stetin Supl. 1978;15:71–84

171. Denk DM, Swoboda H, Schima W, Eibenberger K. Prognostic factors for swallowing rehabilitation following head and neck cancer surgery. Acta Otolaryngol 1997;117:769–774

172. Logemann JA, Pauloski BR, Rademaker AW, Colangelo LA. Speech and swallowing rehabilitation for head and neck cancer patients. Oncology 1997;11:651–664

Index

Note: Page numbers followed by *f* and *t* indicate figures and tables, respectively.

Cushing disease, medullary thyroid carcinoma and, 266
Cystadenocarcinoma
  ovarian, laryngeal metastases, 117
  of salivary glands, 315
Cytomegalovirus (CMV) laryngitis, in immunocompromised host, 117

D

3D-CRT. *See* Radiation therapy, three-dimensional conformal
Deep cervical vein, 374, 376*f*
Deglutition. *See* Swallowing
Dehydration, enteral feeding and, 495*t*
Delphian node(s), 123–124, 124*f*
  involvement in laryngeal cancer, 189
Deltopectoral flap, 447–448
  for oropharyngeal reconstruction after glossectomy, 52*f*, 53
  for pharyngoesophageal reconstruction, 85–86, 85*f*, 86*f*, 89*f*
  with gastric pull-up, 91, 91*f*, 92*f*
Dental care, radiation therapy and, 440
Dental implants, 446, 446*f*
  osseointegrated, for maxilla and soft palate defects, 455
Dental rehabilitation, after anterior resection of oral cavity, 27
Dentition
  and malnutrition, 486
  restoration, 446, 446*f*
Dentures
  complete, 451–452
  implant-assisted, 452, 452*f*
  and oral cancer, 1, 4*f*
  removable partial, 450, 451*f*
  supported overlay, 452
Denture sore, 1, 4*f*
Dermatofibrosarcoma protuberans, of facial skin, 409–410, 412*f*
Desmoid tumor, of head and neck, 352
Diagnosis, patient education/information about, 469
Diarrhea, enteral feeding and, 493, 494*t*
Diet interview, 489, 500–501
Dilaudid, for postoperative pain control, 474
Dingman mouth gag, 56, 56*f*
Doppler ultrasound, postoperative monitoring of free flap, 472–473
Drain(s), surgical, postoperative care for, 473, 473*f*
Dry mouth. *See* Xerostomia
Dumping syndrome, 496
Duragesic, for preoperative pain control, 470
Dynamic swallow study, 512–513, 512*f*, 513*f*
Dysphagia, 76, 77
  after laryngectomy, 523–524
  after oral/oropharyngeal resection, 511–512

E

Ear(s)
  adenocarcinoma, 287, 287*t*
    distribution, 286*f*
  adenoid cystic carcinoma, distribution, 286*f*
  basal cell carcinoma, 284–285, 285*t*, 286*f*
    distribution, 285, 286*f*
    Mohs chemosurgery for, 289, 290, 290*f*–292*f*
    spread, 285, 286*f*
  cancer, 284–309
    distribution, 284–285, 286*f*
    pathology, 284–289
    spread, 285, 286*f*
    surgical management, 289–308
  glandular neoplasms, 285–287, 287*t*
EBRT. *See* External beam radiation therapy (EBRT)
Edema
  facial, postoperative, 471
  laryngeal, radiation-related, 440
  postoperative
    management, 477
    prevention, 477
  submental, radiation-related, 440

eIF4E proto-oncogene, and head and neck cancer, 136
Elderly
  alcohol abuse in, 486
  average daily protein requirements, 492, 492*t*
  malnutrition in, 486–487
Endocrinomas, laryngeal, 113
Endoscopic stripping, for carcinoma in situ of glottis, 435
Endoscopy
  contact, of larynx, 136
  of laryngeal cancer, 134–136
    anesthesia for, 134–135
    techniques for, 135–136
Energy
  average daily requirements, for healthy adults, 492, 492*t*
  intake, increasing, recipes for, 501–504
Enteral feeding
  assessment, 492–493
  bacterial contamination in, 495
  bolus feeds, 499
  complications, 493–496
    gastrointestinal, 494*t*
    mechanical, 494*t*
    metabolic, 495*t*
  continuous feeds, 499
  and drug administration, 500
  early, benefits, 492
  failure, 493–496
  formula selection, 492
  formulas for, 500
  home regimens, 500
  indications for, 491–492
  insurance coverage for, 500
  methods, 499–500
  monitoring, 492–493
  postoperative, 471
  principles, 491–492
  tubes for
    selection, 497–499, 497*t*
    sites, 497–499, 497*t*
    types, 497–499, 497*t*, 498*f*, 499*f*
Enteral nutrition. *See* Enteral feeding
Epiglottectomy, laser, 138
Epiglottis, 118, 119, 119*f*, 125
  management, with tongue-base surgery, 55, 55*f*
Epiglottoplasty, pull-down, 104
Epithelium, olfactory, 236*f*
Epstein-Barr virus (EBV)
  and head and neck cancer, 428
  and nasopharyngeal carcinoma, 354
Erythroplakia, malignant potential, 2
Esophageal carcinoma. *See also* Cervical esophagus, cancer
  apple core appearance, 78, 79*f*
  metastases, 76, 76*f*
    submucosal, 74
  pathophysiology, 76
Esophageal speech, 515
Esophagectomy, total, 90
Esophagoscopy, 78
Esophagostoma, in laryngopharyngectomy, 84–85, 85*f*
Esophagus
  cervical. *See* Cervical esophagus
  invasion by regional thyroid cancer, 117
  lamina propria, lymphatics, 76, 76*f*
  submucosal layer
    histology, 76, 77*f*
    lymphatics, 76, 76*f*
Esthesioneuroblastoma
  in children, 403
  invasion of ethmoid sinus, 235
  of nasal cavity, 217–218, 218*f*, 219*f*
    treatment, 436
  spread, 236
Ethmoid bone
  chondrosarcoma, presenting as nasal or paranasal sinus cancer, 235
  chordoma, presenting as nasal or paranasal sinus cancer, 235

Ethmoid sinus(es)
  anatomy, 212, 213*f*
  cancer
    advanced, craniofacial resection for, 232–235, 232*f*, 233*f*
    bone erosion, 234*f*, 235
    clinical presentation, 219*f*, 220*f*
    epidemiology, 216, 216*t*
    imaging, 221*f*
    treatment, 436
  lymphatics, 215
Eustachian tube
  oropharyngeal carcinoma extending into
    case report, 65–66, 69*f*
    resection, 56, 62, 62*f*
  pharyngeal end, resection, 56
  resection, 363
Ewing sarcoma
  in children, 394*t*, 403–404
  of ear and temporal bone, 288*t*
External auditory canal
  adenoid cystic carcinoma, 287, 287*t*
  glandular neoplasms, 285–287, 287*t*
  tumors, 284–285, 286*f*
External beam radiation therapy (EBRT)
  for cancer of floor of mouth, 433
  for cancer of oral tongue, 433
  for cancer of tongue base, 434–435
  for cancer of tonsillar fossa/pillars, 434
  doses, in microscopic versus gross disease, 431
  equipment for, 428
  for lip carcinoma, 432
  postoperative
    advantages, 431
    indications for, 431
  preoperative, advantages, 431
  for supraglottic laryngeal cancer, 435
External carotid artery. *See* Carotid artery(ies)
Eye(s), loss of, with nasal/paranasal sinus cancer, 231*f*, 239

F

Facial defects, restoration, 458–465
  prosthetic, 463–465
    indications for, 458
  surgical modifications that enhance, 458–463
  surgical versus prosthetic, 458
Facial edema, postoperative, 471
Facial lesions, anterior, treatment, 225–232, 229*f*–232*f*
Facial nerve
  anatomy, 310, 313*f*
  paralysis, 321, 321*f*
Facial prostheses, 446
  materials for, 463
Facial skin
  advanced carcinoma
    case reports, 419–420, 421*f*–426*f*
    depth of penetration, and metastatic rate, 413
    large previously untreated, 414, 414*f*
    location, and metastatic rate, 413
    management, 408, 409*f*
    metastases, 411–413
    neck metastases, treatment, 417, 418*f*
    pathology, 408–411
    pathophysiology, 411–413, 413*f*
    perineural spread, 231, 414, 416, 416*f*, 417*f*
      imaging, 416, 416*f*, 417*f*
    previously operated, 414–415, 414*f*, 415*f*
      management, 408, 410*f*
    reconstruction
      after Mohs resection, 408, 410*f*
      after resection, 417, 418*f*, 418*t*
    recurrence, 414–415, 414*f*, 415*f*
      management, 408, 410*f*
    size, and metastatic rate, 413
    treatment, 413–416
  basal cell carcinoma, 408, 410*f*–412*f*
    metastases, 411
    pathophysiology, 411

538

Index

539